ANNALS OF
THE NEW YORK ACADEMY
OF SCIENCES

Volume 877

EDITORIAL STAFF

Managing Editor
JUSTINE CULLINAN

Associate Editor
STEVEN E. BOHALL

The New York Academy of Sciences
2 East 63rd Street
New York, New York 10021

THE NEW YORK ACADEMY OF SCIENCES
(Founded in 1817)

BOARD OF GOVERNORS, October 1998 – September 1999

ELEANOR BAUM, *Chairman of the Board*
BILL GREEN, *Vice Chairman of the Board*
RODNEY W. NICHOLS, *President and CEO* [ex officio]

Honorary Life Governors
WILLIAM T. GOLDEN   JOSHUA LEDERBERG

JOHN T. MORGAN, *Treasurer*

Governors

D. ALLAN BROMLEY	LAWRENCE B. BUTTENWIESER	PRAVEEN CHAUDHARI
JOHN H. GIBBONS	RONALD L. GRAHAM	HENRY M. GREENBERG
ROBERT G. LAHITA	MARTIN L. LEIBOWITZ	JACQUELINE LEO
WILLIAM J. McDONOUGH	KATHLEEN P. MULLINIX	SANDRA PANEM
CHARLES RAMOND	SARA LEE SCHUPF	JAMES H. SIMONS
	TORSTEN WIESEL	

RICHARD A. RIFKIND, *Past Chairman of the Board*
HELENE L. KAPLAN, *Counsel* [ex officio]   PETER KOHN, *Secretary* [ex officio]

ADVANCING FROM THE VENTRAL STRIATUM TO THE EXTENDED AMYGDALA

IMPLICATIONS FOR NEUROPSYCHIATRY AND DRUG ABUSE

IN HONOR OF LENNART HEIMER

ANNALS OF THE NEW YORK ACADEMY OF SCIENCES
Volume 877

ADVANCING FROM THE VENTRAL STRIATUM TO THE EXTENDED AMYGDALA

IMPLICATIONS FOR NEUROPSYCHIATRY AND DRUG ABUSE

IN HONOR OF LENNART HEIMER

Edited by Jacqueline F. McGinty

The New York Academy of Sciences
New York, New York
1999

Copyright © 1999 by the New York Academy of Sciences. All rights reserved. Under the provisions of the United States Copyright Act of 1976, individual readers of the Annals are permitted to make fair use of the material in them for teaching or research. Permission is granted to quote from the Annals provided that the customary acknowledgment is made of the source. Material in the Annals may be republished only by permission of the Academy. Address inquiries to the Executive Editor at the New York Academy of Sciences.

Copying fees: *For each copy of an article made beyond the free copying permitted under Section 107 or 108 of the 1976 Copyright Act, a fee should be paid through the Copyright Clearance Center, Inc., 222 Rosewood Drive, Danvers, MA 01923. The fee for copying an article is $3.00 for nonacademic use; for use in the classroom, it is $0.07 per page.*

⊖*The paper used in this publication meets the minimum requirements of the American National Standard for Information Sciences—Permanence of Paper for Printed Library Materials, ANSI Z39.48-1984.*

Cover: *Schematic drawings showing the human basal forebrain at the level of the accumbens (upper figure) and the amygdala (lower figure). Striatum is colored blue, pallidum salmon, and basal nucleus of Meynert red. Olfactory cortex is shown in magenta, extended amygdala in yellow and green, and small-celled interface islands in light blue and black. (Art by Medical and Scientific Illustration, Crozet, Virginia.)*

Library of Congress Cataloging-in-Publication Data

Advancing from the ventral striatum to the extended amygdala : implications for neuropsychiatry and drug abuse : in honor of Lennart Heimer / edited by Jacqueline F. McGinty
   p. cm. — (Annals of the New York Academy of Sciences, 0077-8923 ; v. 877)
   Includes bibliographical references and index.
   ISBN 1-57331-178-2 (cloth : alk. paper)
   ISBN 1-57331-179-0 (pbk. : alk. paper)
   I. McGinty, Jacqueline F. II. Series.

99-34750
CIP

GYAT / PCP
Printed in the United States of America
ISBN 1-57331-178-2 (cloth)
ISBN 1-57331-179-0 (paper)
ISSN 0077-8923

ANNALS OF THE NEW YORK ACADEMY OF SCIENCES
Volume 877
June 29, 1999

ADVANCING FROM THE VENTRAL STRIATUM TO THE EXTENDED AMYGDALA[a]

IMPLICATIONS FOR NEUROPSYCHIATRY AND DRUG ABUSE

IN HONOR OF LENNART HEIMER

Editor and Conference Organizer
JACQUELINE F. MCGINTY

Conference Committee
GEORGE ALHEID, HENDRIK J. GROENEWEGEN, SUZANNE N. HABER,
PETER W. KALIVAS, LASZLO ZABORSZKY, AND DANIEL S. ZAHM

CONTENTS

Introduction. *By* JACQUELINE F. MCGINTY	xiii
The Concepts of the Ventral Striatopallidal System and Extended Amygdala. *By* JOSE S. DE OLMOS AND LENNART HEIMER	1

Part I. Functional Organization of the Ventral Striatopallidal System

The Concept of the Ventral Striatum in Nonhuman Primates. *By* SUZANNE N. HABER AND NIKOLAUS R. MCFARLAND	33
Convergence and Segregation of Ventral Striatal Inputs and Outputs. *By* HENK J. GROENEWEGEN, CHRISTOPHER I. WRIGHT, ARNO V.J. BEIJER, AND PIETER VOORN	49
Involvement of the Pallidal-thalamocortical Circuit in Adaptive Behavior. *By* PETER W. KALIVAS, LYNN CHURCHILL, AND ANASTASIA ROMANIDES	64
Functional Specificity of Ventral Striatal Compartments in Appetitive Behaviors. *By* ANN E. KELLEY	71
Mesolimbic Neuronal Activity across Behavioral States. *By* DONALD J. WOODWARD, JING-YU CHANG, PATRICIA JANAK, ALEXEY AZAROV, AND KRISTIN ANSTROM	91

[a]This volume is the result of a conference, entitled **Advancing from the Ventral Striatum to the Extended Amygdala: Implications for Neuropsychiatry and Drug Abuse—In Honor of Lennart Heimer**, held in Charlottesville, Virginia on October 18–21, 1998, by the New York Academy of Sciences and the National Institute of Mental Health.

Part II. Modulation of Ventral Striatopallidal Compartments

Functional-anatomical Implications of the Nucleus Accumbens Core and Shell Subterritories. *By* DANIEL S. ZAHM 113

Regulation of Neurotransmitter Interactions in the Ventral Striatum. *By* JACQUELINE F. MCGINTY 129

The Synaptic Framework for Chemical Signaling in Nucleus Accumbens. *By* G.E. MEREDITH 140

Modulation of Cell Firing in the Nucleus Accumbens. *By* PATRICIO O'DONNELL, JENNIFER GREENE, NINA PABELLO, BARBARA L. LEWIS, AND ANTHONY A. GRACE 157

Opioid Modulation of Ventral Pallidal Inputs. *By* T. CELESTE NAPIER AND IGOR MITROVIC 176

Cross-species Studies of Sensorimotor Gating of the Startle Reflex. *By* NEAL R. SWERDLOW, DAVID L. BRAFF, AND MARK A. GEYER 202

Part III. Organization and Functions of the Extended Amygdala

The Intrinsic Organization of the Central Extended Amygdala. *By* MARTIN D. CASSELL, LORIN J. FREEDMAN, AND CHANGJUN SHI 217

The Medial Extended Amygdala in Male Reproductive Behavior: A Node in the Mammalian Social Behavior Network. *By* SARAH WINANS NEWMAN 242

The Extended Amygdala and Salt Appetite. *By* ALAN KIM JOHNSON, JOSE DE OLMOS, CINTHIA V. PASTUSKOVAS, ANDREA M. ZARDETTO-SMITH, AND LAURA VIVAS 258

The Extended Amygdala: Are the Central Nucleus of the Amygdala and the Bed Nucleus of the Stria Terminalis Differentially Involved in Fear versus Anxiety? *By* MICHAEL DAVIS AND CHANGJUN SHI 281

Brain and Sexual Behavior. *By* KNUT LARSSON AND SVEN AHLENIUS 292

Part IV. Interactions of the Extended Amygdala with Other Brain Regions

Cortical Afferents to the Extended Amygdala. *By* ALEXANDER J. MCDONALD, SARA J. SHAMMAH-LAGNADO, CHANGJUN SHI, AND MICHAEL DAVIS 309

The Basal Forebrain Corticopetal System Revisited. *By* L. ZABORSZKY, K. PANG, J. SOMOGYI, Z. NADASDY, AND I. KALLO 339

Basal Forebrain Afferent Projections Modulating Cortical Acetylcholine, Attention, and Implications for Neuropsychiatric Disorders. *By* MARTIN SARTER, JOHN P. BRUNO, AND JANITA TURCHI 368

Prefrontal Cortical Networks Related to Visceral Function and Mood. *By* JOSEPH L. PRICE 383

Functions of the Amygdala and Related Forebrain Areas in Attention and Cognition. *By* MICHELA GALLAGHER AND GEOFFREY SCHOENBAUM .. 397

Associative Processes in Addiction and Reward: The Role of Amygdala-Ventral Striatal Subsystems. *By* BARRY J. EVERITT, JOHN A. PARKINSON, MARY C. OLMSTEAD, MERCEDES ARROYO, PATRICIA ROBLEDO, AND TREVOR W. ROBBINS 412

Functional and Anatomical Relationships among the Amygdala, Basal Forebrain, Ventral Striatum, and Cortex: An Integrative Discussion. *By* THACKERY S. GRAY 439

Part V. Implications for Drug Abuse

The Role of the Striatopallidal and Extended Amygdala Systems in Drug Addiction. *By* GEORGE F. KOOB 445

Drug Addiction as a Disorder of Associative Learning: Role of Nucleus Accumbens Shell/Extended Amygdala Dopamine. *By* G. DI CHIARA, G. TANDA, V. BASSAREO, F. PONTIERI, E. ACQUAS, S. FENU, C. CADONI, AND E. CARBONI 461

The Bed Nucleus of the Stria Terminalis: A Target Site for Noradrenergic Actions in Opiate Withdrawal. *By* GARY ASTON-JONES, JILL M. DELFS, JONATHAN DRUHAN, AND YAN ZHU 486

The Role of Dopamine, Dynorphin, and CART Systems in the Ventral Striatum and Amygdala in Cocaine Abuse. *By* YASMIN L. HURD, PERNILLA SVENSSON, AND MARJAN PONTÉN 499

D_3 Dopamine and Kappa Opioid Receptor Alterations in Human Brain of Cocaine-overdose Victims. *By* DEBORAH C. MASH AND JULIE K. STALEY 507

Functional Magnetic Resonance Imaging of Brain Reward Circuitry in the Human. *By* HANS C. BREITER AND BRUCE R. ROSEN 523

Part VI. Implications for Neuropsychiatry

Epilepsy, Schizophrenia, and the Extended Amygdala. *By* JANICE R. STEVENS 548

Mesolimbic Activity Associated with Psychosis in Schizophrenia: Symptom-specific PET Studies. *By* JANE EPSTEIN, EMILY STERN, AND DAVID SILBERSWEIG 562

Ventromedial Temporal Lobe Pathology in Dementia, Brain Trauma, and Schizophrenia. *By* GARY W. VAN HOESEN, JEAN C. AUGUSTINACK, AND SARAH J. REDMAN 575

D_3 Receptors and the Actions of Neuroleptics in the Ventral Striatopallidal System of Schizophrenics. *By* JEFFREY N. JOYCE AND EUGENIA V. GUREVICH 595

Prefrontal Cortical-Amygdalar Metabolism in Major Depression. *By* WAYNE C. DREVETS 614

On Some Clinical Implications of the Ventral Striatum and the Extended Amygdala: Investigations of Aggression. *By* MICHAEL R. TRIMBLE AND LUDGER TEBARTZ VAN ELST 638

Part VII. Poster Papers

Anatomy, Chemistry, and Physiology of the Ventral Striatopallidal and Extended Amygdaloid Systems

The Interstitial Nucleus of the Posterior Limb of the Anterior Commissure: A Novel Layer of the Central Division of Extended Amygdala. *By* GEORGE F. ALHEID, SARA J. SHAMMAH-LAGNADO, AND CARLOS A. BELTRAMINO 645

Projections of the Amygdalopiriform Transition Area (APir): A PHA-L Study in the Rat. *By* SARA J. SHAMMAH-LAGNADO AND ADRIANA C. SANTIAGO 655

The Ventral Striatum of the Syrian Hamster. *By* LUKE R. JOHNSON AND RUTH I. WOOD 661

Afferent Connections to the Ventral Striatum from the Medial Prefrontal Cortex (Area 25) and the Thalamic Nuclei in the Macaque Monkey. *By* K. NAKANO, T. KAYAHARA, AND T. CHIBA 667

Expression of Enkephalin in Pallido-Striatal Neurons. *By* PIETER VOORN, SERGE VAN DE WITTE, GUNO TJON, AND ALLERT JAN JONKER 671

Terminals from the Rat Prefrontal Cortex Synapse on Mesoaccumbens VTA Neurons. *By* DAVID B. CARR AND SUSAN R. SESACK 676

Dopamine D_4 Receptors Are Strategically Localized for Primary Involvement in the Presynaptic Effects of Dopamine in the Rat Nucleus Accumbens Shell. *By* ADENA L. SVINGOS, SUNDARI PERIASAMY, AND VIRGINIA M. PICKEL 679

Glutamatergic Modulation of Subcortical Motor and Limbic Circuits. *By* DANIEL J. HEALY AND JAMES H. MEADOR-WOODRUFF 684

Modulation of Ventral Tegmental Area Dopamine Cell Activity by the Ventral Subiculum and Entorhinal Cortex. *By* CHRISTOPHER L. TODD AND ANTHONY A. GRACE 688

Electrophysiological Properties of Anatomically Identified Ventral Pallidal Neurons in Rat Brain Slices. *By* C. PETER BENGTSON AND PEREGRINE B. OSBORNE 691

Neurons of the Bed Nucleus of the Stria Terminalis (BNST): Electrophysiological Properties and Their Response to Serotonin. *By* DONALD G. RAINNIE 695

Distribution of [^{3}H]Citalopram Binding Sites in the Nonhuman Primate Brain. *By* HILARY R. SMITH, JAMES B. DAUNAIS, MICHAEL A. NADER, AND LINDA J. PORRINO 700

Antidepressants and Atypical Neuroleptics Induce Fos-like Immunoreactivity in the Central Extended Amygdala. *By* M. MORELLI AND A. PINNA 703

Stimulation of Dopamine Release in the Bed Nucleus of Stria Terminalis: A Trait of Atypical Antipsychotics? *By* EZIO CARBONI, ALESSANDRA SILVAGNI, MARIA T.P. ROLANDO, AND GAETANO DI CHIARA 707

Functions and Dysfunctions of the Ventral Striatopallidal and Extended Amygdaloid Systems

Involvement of the Ventral Pallidum in Working Memory Tasks With or Without a Delay. *By* STAN B. FLORESCO, DEANNA N. BRAAKSMA, AND ANTHONY G. PHILLIPS 711

NMDA Glutamatergic Blockade of Nucleus Accumbens Disrupts Acquisition but Not Consolidation in a Passive Avoidance Task. *By* P.A. GARGIULO, G. MARTÍNEZ, C. ROPERO, A. FUNES, AND A.I. LANDA 717

Disrupted and Undisruptable Latent Inhibition following Shell and Core Lesions. *By* I. WEINER, G. GAL, AND J. FELDON 723

Freezing Behavior in BNST-lesioned Wistar Rats. *By* DANIELA SCHULZ AND
RESIT CANBEYLI 728

A Functional Role for Dopamine Transmission in the Amygdala during
Condtioned Fear. *By* FAY A. GUARRACI, RUSSELL J. FROHARDT,
STACEY L. YOUNG, AND BRUCE S. KAPP 732

Effect of Amygdala Kindling on Emotional Behavior and Benzodiazepine
Receptor Binding in Rats. *By* LISA E. KALYNCHUK, DEBRA M.
PEARSON, JOHN P.J. PINEL, AND MICHAEL J. MEANEY 737

Does Chronic Activity-Stress Produce Hippocampal Atrophy and Basal
Forebrain Lesions? A Preliminary Analysis. *By* KELLY G. LAMBERT,
PRINCY QUADROS, CATHERINE AURENTZ, CATHERINE LOWRY, AND
CRAIG H. KINSLEY 742

Role of the Basolateral Amygdala in Panic Disorder. *By* A. SHEKHAR,
T.S. SAJDYK, S.R. KEIM, K.K. YODER, AND S.K. SANDERS 747

Changes in Nociceptive and Anxiolytic Responses following Herpes Virus-
mediated Preproenkephalin Overexpression in Rat Amygdala Are
Naloxone-reversible and Transient. *By* WEN KANG, STEVEN P. WILSON,
AND MARLENE A. WILSON 751

Enduring Neurochemical Effects of Early Maternal Separation on Limbic
Structures. *By* S.L. ANDERSEN, P.J. LYSS, N.L. DUMONT, AND
M.H. TEICHER 756

Prenatal Stress-induced Modifications of Neuronal Nitric Oxide Synthase in
Amygdala and Medial Preoptic Area. *By* STEPHEN D. MILLER, ERIC
MUELLER, GORDON W. GIFFORD, AND CRAIG HOWARD KINSLEY 760

Amygdaloid and Hippocampal β-Adrenoceptors in the Olfactory Bulbectomy
Syndrome: Effects of Desipramine. J. STEVEN RICHARDSON AND
ALEC H. K. TIONG 764

Cholinergic, M_1 Receptors in the Nucleus Accumbens Mediate Behavioral
Depression: A Possible Downsteam Target for Fluoxetine. *By*
DAVID CHAU, PEDRO V. RADA, REBECCA A. KOSLOFF, AND
BARTLEY G. HOEBEL 769

Pattern of Disturbance of Different Ventral Frontal Functions in Organic
Depression. *By* FRIEDEL M. REISCHIES 775

The Relationship of the Ventral Striatopallidal and Extended Amygdaloid Systems to Drug Abuse

Phasic Accumbal Firing May Contribute to the Regulation of Drug Taking
during Intravenous Cocaine Self-administration Sessions. *By*
LAURA L. PEOPLES, ANTHONY J. UZWIAK, FRED GEE, ANTHONY T.
FABBRICATORE, KATHRYN J. MUCCINO, BINAIFER D. MOHTA, AND
M.O. WEST 781

Cocaine Is Self-administered into the Shell Region of the Nucleus Accumbens
in Wistar Rats. *By* D.L. MCKINZIE, Z.A. RODD-HENRICKS, C.T.
DAGON, J.M. MURPHY, AND W.J. MCBRIDE 788

Involvement of Acetylcholine in the Nucleus Accumbens in Cocaine
Reinforcement. *By* GREGORY P. MARK, ANTHONY E. KINNEY,
MICHELE C. GRUBB, AND ALAN S. KEYS 792

Cocaine-seeking Behavior and Fos Expression in the Amygdala Produced by Cocaine or a Cocaine Self-administration Environment. *By* DAVID A. BAKER, RITA A. FUCHS, LY T.L. TRAN-NGUYEN, ART J. PALMER, JOHN F. MARSHALL, RON J. MCPHERSON, AND JANET L. NEISEWANDER 796

Differences in Receptor System Participation between Nicotine- and Cocaine-induced Dopamine Overflow in Nucleus Accumbens. *By* ISTVAN SZIRAKI, HENRY SERSHEN, MYRON BENUCK, AUDREY HASHIM, AND ABEL LAJTHA 800

Modulation of Cocaine-induced Sensitization by κ-Opioid Receptor Agonists: Role of the Nucleus Accumbens and Medial Prefrontal Cortex. *By* VLADIMIR CHEFER, ALEXIS C. THOMPSON, AND TONI S. SHIPPENBERG 803

SPECT following Intravenous Procaine in Cocaine Addiction. *By* BRYON ADINOFF, MICHAEL D. DEVOUS, SUSAN BEST, MARK S. GEORGE, DEANNA ALEXANDER, AND KELLY PAYNE 807

A Multicomponent Learning Model of Drug Abuse: Drug Taking and Craving May Involve Separate Brain Circuits Underlying Instrumental and Classical Conditioning, Respectively. *By* JOHN L. HARACZ, DEBORAH C. MASH, AND RATNA SIRCAR 811

Mesoaccumbens Dopamine and the Self-administration of Amphetamine. *By* DANIEL S. LORRAIN, GRETCHEN M. ARNOLD, AND PAUL VEZINA 820

Amphetamine Microinfusion in the Dorso-Ventral Axis of the Prefrontal Cortex Differentially Modulates Dopamine Neurotransmission in the Shell-Core Subterritories of the Nucleus Accumbens. *By* GAËL HEDOU, JUDITH HOMBERG, JORAM FELDON, AND CHRISTIAN A. HEIDBREDER ... 823

Amphetamine Injections into the Nucleus Accumbens Enhance the Reward of Stimulation of the Subiculum. *By* K.L. SWEET AND D.B. NEILL 828

Asymmetrical Effects of Ethanol in Basal Ganglia Aldehyde Dehydrogenase Activity. *By* V.I. SATANOVSKAYA AND L.R. BARDINA 831

Index of Contributors 833

Financial assistance was received from:
Supporters:
- OFFICE OF RESEARCH AND GRADUATE STUDIES, AND SCHOOL OF MEDICINE, EAST CAROLINA UNIVERSITY
- UNIVERSITY OF VIRGINIA HEALTH SCIENCES CENTER

Contributors:
- HOECHST MARION ROUSSEL, INC.
- MERCK RESEARCH LABORATORIES
- PFIZER INC.
- PHARMACIA AND UPJOHN
- RESEARCH BIOCHEMICALS INC.
- UNIVERSITY OF WISCONSIN HEALTH EMOTIONS RESEARCH INSTITUTE

The New York Academy of Sciences believes it has a responsibility to provide an open forum for discussion of scientific questions. The positions taken by the participants in the reported conferences are their own and not necessarily those of the Academy. The Academy has no intent to influence legislation by providing such forums.

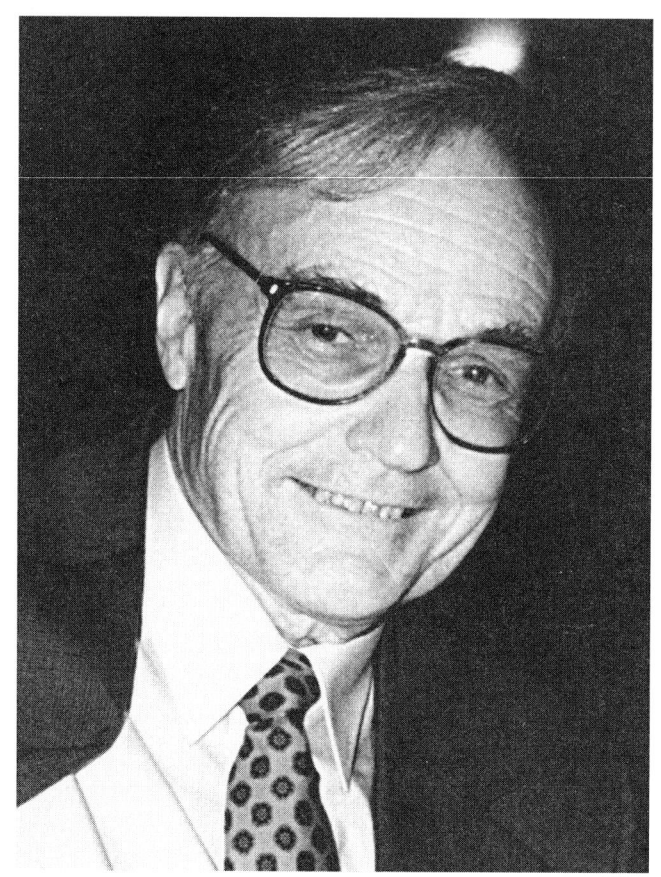

Lennart Heimer, M.D.

Introduction

JACQUELINE F. MCGINTY

Department of Anatomy and Cell Biology, East Carolina University, School of Medicine, Greenville, North Carolina 27858, USA

The conference held by the New York Academy of Sciences on the ventral striatum and the extended amygdala was a three-day symposium held in Charlottesville, Virginia on October 18–21, 1998. The meeting brought together basic and clinical investigators to explore the relationships among the anatomy, neurochemistry, and function of the basal forebrain systems implicated in neuropsychiatric and addictive disorders.

The energy of the conference participants was palpable at the first reception and remained audible throughout the meeting. The major reason for this enthusiastic response was that everyone came to honor one of the most distinguished leaders of the field, Dr. Lennart Heimer. Heimer and colleagues pioneered the now-vintage concept of the ventral striatum as well as the nascent concept of the extended amygdala. Together these systems mediate goal-directed behavior triggered by reward-related incentives. Although not everyone accepts the organization of the extended amygdala that Heimer and colleagues have posited, everyone at the meeting seemed to have an opinion about it! In fact, because the extended amygdala is a controversial subject, it provided a tangible framework for spirited debate.

The presentations on day one concerned the functional organization of the ventral striatum. In her plenary lecture, Suzanne Haber highlighted many studies that suggest sophisticated interactions between the dorsal and ventral striatal systems in species from rodent to human. She introduced images of ever-expanding "spirals" that integrate the entire striatum from medial to lateral and dorsal to ventral. Thereafter, spirals became the buzzword of the meeting. Several speakers discussed the characteristics and connections of the medium spiny projection neurons at the origin of these spirals in the ventral striatum, specifically in the nucleus accumbens. These neurons are organized into functional ensembles with different input–output relationships (Groenewegen), and they have one of the highest convergence ratios in the brain (Meredith), indicating a profound degree of integration. The neuronal ensembles are found in the core and shell subcompartments of the nucleus accumbens that have specific connections to motor-related basal ganglia structures or reward-related structures, respectively (Zahm). These circuits are activated by psychostimulants that release dopamine and glutamate and trigger intracellular cascades in medium spiny neurons that result in long-term changes in gene expression (McGinty). Convergent glutamatergic inputs from the subiculum, amygdala, and prefrontal cortex selectively gate the pattern of activity of these neurons in ventral striatal compartments (O'Donnell). Similarly, patterns of neuronal activity in mesolimbic regions linked to the ventral striatum shift dynamically during reward-related tasks when the target reward changes (Woodward). The ventral pallidum is one of the nodal points of this network. It is an equal partner with the ventral striatum in processing dynamic reward-related information (Napier). The selective relationships among subcompartments in these interconnected structures form the basis of the functional specificity within the ventral striatopallidal system. Examples include the mesoaccumbens-pallidal-prefrontal subcircuits that mediate drug-reinforced behavioral responding, as well as the learning of spatial-discriminative and response-reinforcement tasks (Kalivas, Kelley) and the mescoaccumbens–lateral hypothalamic–brain stem circuitry that mediates feeding behavior (Kelley). Toward the end of the day, implications were drawn that disruptions at different levels in this complex circuitry may underlie many neuropsychiatric disorders, including schizophrenia (Swerdlow). Finally, a lively and crowded poster session before dinner provided many outstanding short papers for presentation in this volume.

The second day was devoted to the extended amygdala. The highlight of the meeting was the plenary lecture presented by Drs. de Olmos and Heimer on why their concept of the extended amygdala is a logical strategy for understanding basal forebrain organization. The focal point of their concept is that the ventral striatopallidal system and the centromedial amygdala extend structurally, neurochemically, and functionally into the bed nucleus of the stria terminalis, forming a continuum throughout the basal forebrain. Immediately following their elegant presentation, Dr. Cassell seemed to take the opposite point of view: that the concept of the amygdala itself needs to be reorganized. Dr. Cassell made a case for the central nucleus of the amygdala as a striatopallidal-like structure on the basis of the organization of its GABAergic output neurons, its GABA-GABA connections, and other histochemical and hodological patterns. Considering that the basolateral amygdala has been considered cortical-like for many years, and that the medial amygdala is closely aligned with the hypothalamus, by the end of the day, the amygdala as a unitary entity was severely endangered! For the rest of the meeting, people could be found in small groups discussing "Just what is the amygdala?" As far apart as the Heimer and Cassell camps appear to be, however, they are part of a common groundswell that aims to clarify the relationships of the heterogeneous amygdaloid subcompartments with their structurally and functionally related neighbors.

The disappearance of the structure formerly known as the amygdala did not daunt the remaining speakers of the day who convincingly attributed specific functions, such as reproductive behavior (Newman), blood volume and cardiovascular homestasis (Johnson), fear and anxiety (Davis), attention and cognition (Gallagher), and conditioned reinforcement (Everitt) to conventionally defined amygdalar subdivisions, the connections of which were laid out in detail (McDonald, Price). Not to be outdone by the amygdalophiles, Drs. Zaborszky and Sarter described the relationships of the noncholinergic and cholinergic neurons of the basal forebrain to their heterogeneous neighbors. The day culminated with a banquet and a program packed with colleagues and former students of Lennart Heimer, who presented a stream of entertaining anecdotes about the Olympic-quality skier and scientist who inspired them to seek excellence in their own careers and lives.

Day three was marked by exciting presentations on drug abuse in the morning and neuropsychiatry in the afternoon. The tone for the day was set by Dr. Koob who discussed similar effects of the major substances of abuse, including alcohol and nicotine, on common neuromodulatory systems underlying reinforcement and withdrawal. He emphasized that decreased responsiveness of brain reinforcement systems, coupled with increased recruitment of brain-stress systems in the extended amygdala, moves the hedonic set point in a direction that favors compulsive drug seeking. The remaning morning speakers chronicled changes in specific neurotransmitters in the ventral striatum and extended amygdala, such as dopamine (Di Chiara), norepinephrine (Aston-Jones), serotonin and dynorphin (Hurd), and D_3 and kappa opioid receptors (Mash) that mark different phases of drug reinforcement, withdrawal, and delirium in rodents and humans. Functional magnetic resonance images of cocaine-induced euphoria and craving in these basal forebrain regions reinforced the significance of the preclinical research to the human condition (Breiter).

In the final afternoon, clinical studies predominated that related the forebrain structures and organizational concepts discussed throughout the meeting with case studies of epilepsy (Stevens, Trimble), dementia (Van Hoesen), trauma (Van Hoesen, Trimble), schizophrenia (Silbersweig, Joyce), and depression (Drevets). Of these, the most striking were the images of increased dopamine D_3 receptors in the ventral striatum of schizophrenics (Joyce) and the dynamic metabolic dysregulation in cortico-amygdalar circuits in patients with depression (Drevets).

To hear such outstanding presentations and passionate discussion intermingled with overwhelming camaraderie and admiration for Lennart Heimer was a rare and unique opportunity. The theme of each presentation underscored the enormous role Lennart has played in our thinking about, and our exploration of, the basal forebrain. This volume represents the attempt of the organizers to share this experience with the rest of Lennart Heimer's extended family.

ACKNOWLEDGMENTS

I would like to thank the organizing committee for their consistent kindling of this Festschrift from a small flame at a reception in Charlottesville in November 1996 to a veritable bonfire in the same location two years later. Together we would like to thank Rashid Shaikh (Director of Science and Technology Meetings), Sue Davies (Development Manager), Ken McDonald (Public Information Officer), and Steven Bohall (associate editor for this volume) at the New York Academy of Sciences for their professionalism, encouragement, and support. Most of all we are indebted to Renée Wilkerson at the Academy, who coordinated all phases of this conference with exquisite attention to detail, always using her secret weapon, unfailing good humor. We also would like to thank the outstanding speakers, poster presenters, and participants for making the content of this conference a resounding success. Finally, we are deeply grateful to our cosponsor, the National Institute of Mental Health, for providing us with such generous financial and intellectual support.

The Concepts of the Ventral Striatopallidal System and Extended Amygdala

JOSE S. DE OLMOS AND LENNART HEIMER[a]

Instituto de Investigación Médica, Córdoba, Argentina and Departments of Otolaryngology–Head and Neck Surgery, and Neurological Surgery, University of Virginia, Charlottesville, Virginia 22908, USA

ABSTRACT: The concepts of the ventral striatopallidal system and extended amygdala have significantly improved our understanding of basal forebrain organization. As a result of these and other advances during the last twenty years, many of the most prominent basal forebrain structures, including the nucleus accumbens, olfactory tubercle, and amygdaloid body, have all but lost their relevance as independent functional anatomical units. In order to appreciate the distinct differences that exist between the ventral striatopallidal system and the extended amygdala, and as a way of explaining the choice of the terms *ventral striatopallidal system* and *extended amygdala*, we will review the discovery and subsequent elaboration of these two systems. On the background of these discussions, we will then proceed to dispel some recently published misgivings regarding the usefulness of the extended amygdaloid concept.

INTRODUCTION

The application of newly developed silver impregnation techniques in the late sixties led to the discoveries that provided the foundation for both the ventral striatopallidal system and the extended amygdala. This in itself is hardly surprising. No less an expert than Ramon y Cajal liked to remark that "discoveries are a function of the methods used." It is interesting to realize, however, that the two methods, the Fink and Heimer modification of the Nauta-Gygax method[27] and the cupric-silver method of de Olmos,[19] which facilitated the discoveries of the ventral striatopallidal system and the extended amygdala, respectively, represent two rather different silver impregnation procedures. With the introduction and subsequent elaboration of the ventral striatopallidal system and the extended amygdala, it has become evident that the term "substantia innominata" has become superfluous, because its various parts have been clearly identified as belonging to either the magnocellular basal forebrain complex (including the basal nucleus of Meynert), the ventral parts of the basal ganglia (that is, the ventral striatopallidal system), or to extensions of the centromedial amygdala that link it via subpallidal cell columns with the bed nucleus of the stria terminalis, that is, the extended amygdala. The magnocellular basal forebrain system has been analyzed and discussed at length in many scientific reports and book chap-

---

[a]To whom correspondence should be addressed: Lennart Heimer, MD, Department of Otolaryngology, Box 430, University of Virginia Health Sciences Center, Charlottesville, VA 22908. Voice: 804-924-5889; fax: 804-982-4535; lh2c@virginia.edu

ters, in large part because of its apparent relationship to Alzheimer's disease. We will devote this chapter to the ventral striatopallidal system and extended amygdala.

THE VENTRAL STRIATOPALLIDAL SYSTEM

The terms *ventral striatum* and *ventral pallidum* were first used in the rat, where experimental neuroanatomical studies provided convincing evidence that cortico-striato-pallidal projections are as characteristic for allocortex (hippocampus and olfactory cortex) as they are for neocortex.[46] In other words, the main idea advanced by the concept of the ventral striatopallidal system is that the whole cortical mantle, including both neocortex and allocortex, is related to the basal ganglia. The ventral parts of the basal ganglia, that is, the ventral striatum and ventral pallidum, which receive input from allocortical regions (hippocampus and olfactory or prepiriform cortex), were identified by using a combination of different techniques, including cytoarchitectural, histochemical, and tract-tracing techniques. Although the concept of the ventral striatopallidal system was first presented at the Golgi Centennial Symposium in Italy in 1973, several observations with direct bearing on the concept were included in earlier publications[37,38] as part of studies on higher-order olfactory connections.

The Subcortical Projections of the Prepiriform Cortex

The rat has a prominent olfactory (prepiriform) cortex, which can be easily approached for the specific manipulations needed for the experimental study of higher-

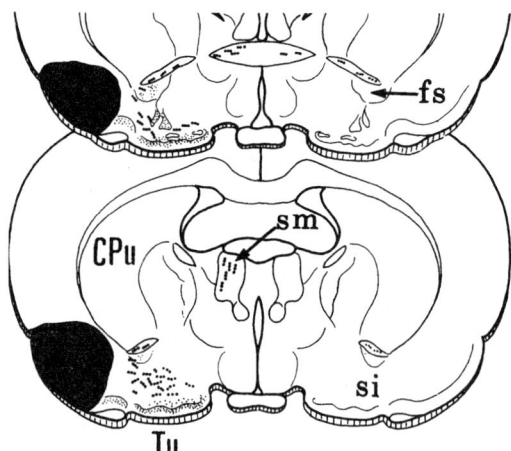

FIGURE 1. Pattern of degeneration (small dots, terminal degeneration; large dots, degenerating fibers) in the basal forebrain following a lesion (black area) in the prepiriform cortex. The terminal degeneration is located in the fundus striati (fs) and olfactory tubercle (Tu), as well as in columns of cells that bridge the gap between the tubercle and the fundus striati. sm, stria medullaris; si, substantia innominata; Tu, tubercle; CPu, caudate-putamen. (Heimer.[38] With permission from Karger, Basel.)

order olfactory pathways. The discoveries of allocortical projections to ventral extensions of the basal ganglia were facilitated by the development of more sensitive silver methods, which made it possible to outline more precisely the areas of terminations of axonal projections than was the case with earlier procedures. To make a long story short, aided by the newly developed silver impregnation procedures,[27] complemented by electron microscopic identification of degenerating terminals, it became apparent that the major targets for prepiriform projections in the mediobasal forebrain are extrahypothalamic rather than within the hypothalamus.[38] This contradicted earlier experimental tracing studies that had promoted the widely held opinion, based on normal anatomical studies, that the olfactory cortex projects massively into the region of the preoptic-anterior hypothalamic continuum. Instead, it turned out that the major areas of termination were located in the olfactory tubercle, accumbens, and the subcommissural "striatal pocket," sometimes referred to as the "fundus striati,"[70] underneath the temporal limb of the anterior commissure. Terminal degeneration was also present in striatal cell columns that bridge the gap between the me-

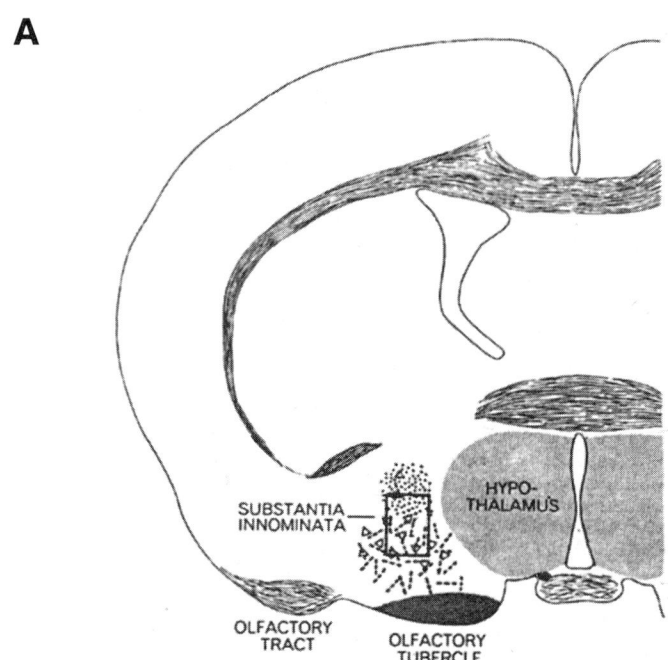

FIGURE 2. A superficial heat lesion in the olfactory tubercle (**A**) results in a characteristic pattern of degeneration in the region that used to be called the substantia innominata. Note that the area of terminal degeneration, which caps an area with degenerating fibers, is well confined and located in the dorsal part of the substantia innominata. The high-power microphotograph in **B** (corresponding to the rectangle in **A**) demonstrates a clear distinction between the area with degenerating fibers of passage (lower half of figure) and the dorsally located area of terminal degeneration (degenerating boutons and terminal axonal branches). The target area for the fibers from the olfactory tubercle was later identified as a ventral extension of the pallidal complex. (**A** only, Heimer.[37] With permission from *Scientific American*, New York.)

dium-sized cell assemblies of the olfactory tubercle, on one hand, and the accumbens and ventral parts of the caudate-putamen, on the other (FIG. 1).

The Subcortical Projections of the Olfactory Tubercle

A distinctly different picture of "higher order olfactory connections" was obtained in another set of experiments in which laminar heat lesions were made in the olfactory tubercle,[37] which at the time was generally considered to be part of the olfactory cortex. The olfactory tubercle was reached via a subtemporal approach,

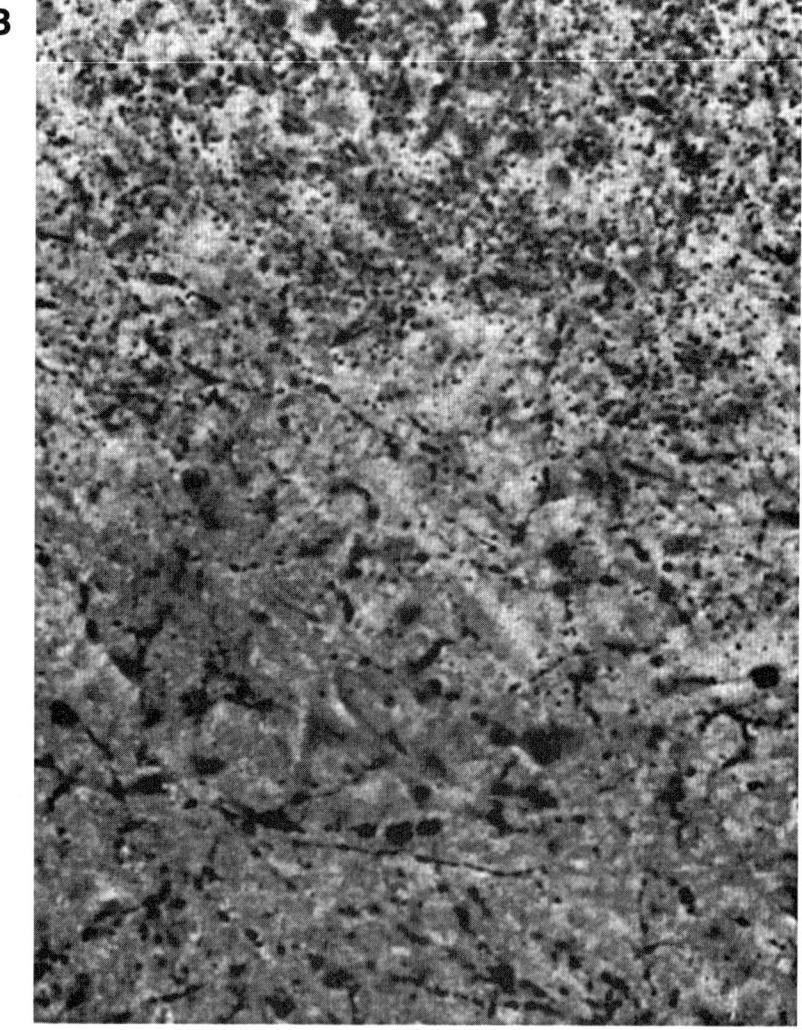

FIGURE 2B.

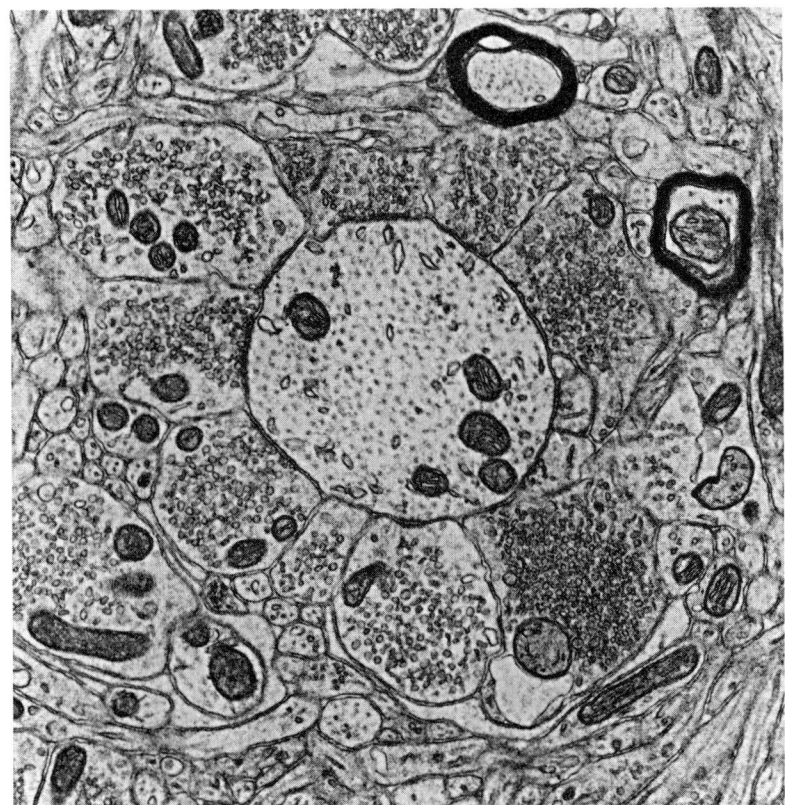

FIGURE 3. Dendrite in the dorsal part of the substantia innominata, which corresponds to the area with terminal degeneration in FIG. 2. The dendrite is completely surrounded by boutons, which establish primarily symmetrical contacts, reminiscent of the situation in the globus pallidus (Heimer.[37] With permission from *Scientific American*, New York.)

which made it possible to make a laminar heat lesion by placing a heated (70 degrees Celsius) silver plate on the surface of the tubercle for a few seconds without interfering with structures deep to the tubercle. As a result of such lesions, a characteristic pattern of axonal and terminal degeneration appeared in the region, which was then known either as the lateral preoptic area or as the substantia innominata (FIG. 2A). In particular, there was a striking topographic distinction between a confined area of terminal degeneration (capping the region of the diagonal band) and the diagonal band, which in turn contained primarily degenerating fibers of passage (FIG. 2B). The neuropil corresponding to the area of dense terminal degeneration was characterized by long dendritic profiles encased by a continuous sheath of boutons, establishing primarily symmetric synaptic contacts (FIG. 3), reminiscent of that in the globus pallidus. In the experimental material it was confirmed that several of the boutons were degenerating as a result of the lesion in the tubercle.[37]

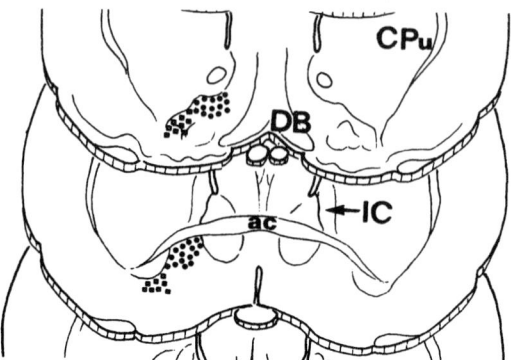

FIGURE 4. A schematic illustration of striatal projections to the ventral pallidum. The dots represent terminal degeneration resulting from a lesion in the accumbens, whereas the squares represent terminal degeneration from a lesion in the olfactory tubercle. The terminal areas for the projections from these two striatal structures form a continuum, which in turn is continuous with the globus pallidus behind the anterior commissure (ac). CPu, caudate-putamen; DB, diagonal band of Broca; IC, internal capsule. (Heimer & Wilson.[46] With permission from Raven Press, New York.)

When these studies of higher order olfactory connections were analyzed and compared with observations obtained in regular Nissl preparations and in recently developed histochemical preparations stained for acetylcholinesterase, both of which showed a distinct difference between the prepiriform cortex and the olfactory tubercle as well as striking similarities between the tubercle and the dorsally adjacent caudate-putamen, the idea that the olfactory tubercle represents a striatal structure rather than a cortical olfactory structure could hardly be dismissed. Subsequent studies only served to solidify this viewpoint.[45] This was consistent with the fact that the projection from the tubercle to the substantia innominata had the signatures of a striatopallidal projection, as described above. The projection from the prepiriform cortex to the olfactory tubercle would thus represent a cortico-striatal projection rather than a cortico-cortical association pathway, as generally believed at the time. This conclusion was further supported by the fact that the projection from the prepiriform cortex to the olfactory tubercle is not reciprocated, as is generally the case with cortical association pathways.

When the results from the above-mentioned studies of higher order olfactory connections were compared with experiments on the accumbens projections (R.D. Wilson; The neural associations of the nucleus accumbens septi. Masters thesis, M.I.T., Cambridge, MA), which were also aided by the Fink-Heimer silver impregnation methods, the continuity of the pallidal-like components related to the olfactory tubercle and accumbens was easily appreciated (FIG. 4). It was also evident that these pallidal components were directly continuous with the main part of the pallidal complex, that is, the globus pallidus. The striatal character of the accumbens was also firmly established by Swanson and Cowan,[89] who based their assessment both on developmental and connectional data. As indicated earlier, the terms ventral striatum and ventral pallidum were introduced to account for these apparent ventral extensions of the basal ganglia. The ventral striatum, which in the rat consists of the accumbens, ventral parts of the caudate-putamen, and extensive parts of the olfactory tubercle, is directly continuous with the dorsal parts of the striatal complex. The ventral pallidum occupies most of what was previously referred to as the anterior or subcommissural substantia innominata, and, as in the case of the striatum, there is no distinct border between the ventral and dorsal parts of the pallidal complex.

Cortico-subcortical Reentrant Circuits Through the Ventral Parts of the Basal Ganglia

Consistent with the situation in the dorsal parts of the basal ganglia, where the cortico-subcortical reentrant circuits through the basal ganglia proceed via the ventral anterior-ventral lateral thalamic nuclei back to the frontal cortex, we suggested a similar type of reentrant circuit for the ventral striatopallidal system. However, a specific thalamic relay for the circuits through the ventral parts of the basal ganglia had not been identified. A few years later the available evidence pointed to the mediodorsal nucleus as the thalamic relay for the cortico-subcortical reentrant circuits related to the ventral striatopallidal system[39] (see also FIG. 5). This was confirmed

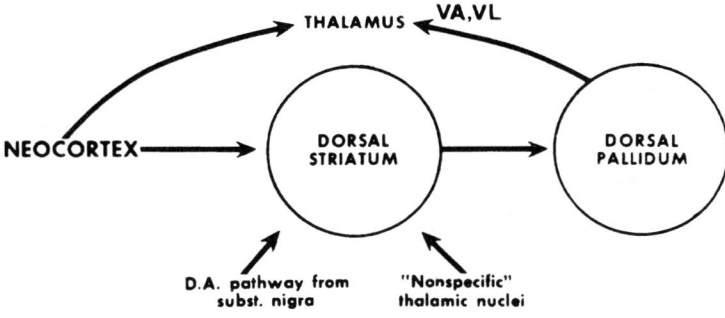

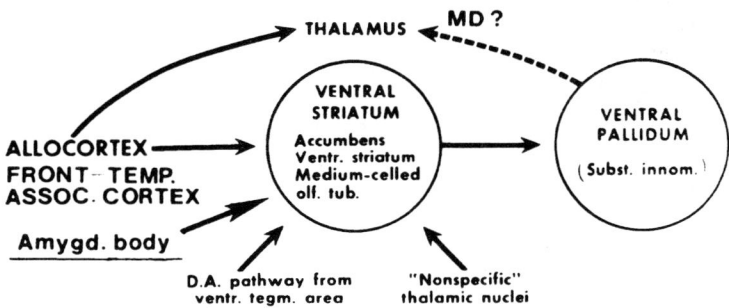

FIGURE 5. Schematic figure illustrating the striking similarities in cortico–subcortical relations between the neocortex and the allocortex. See FIG. 6 for abbreviations. (Heimer.[39] With permission from Plenum Press, New York.)

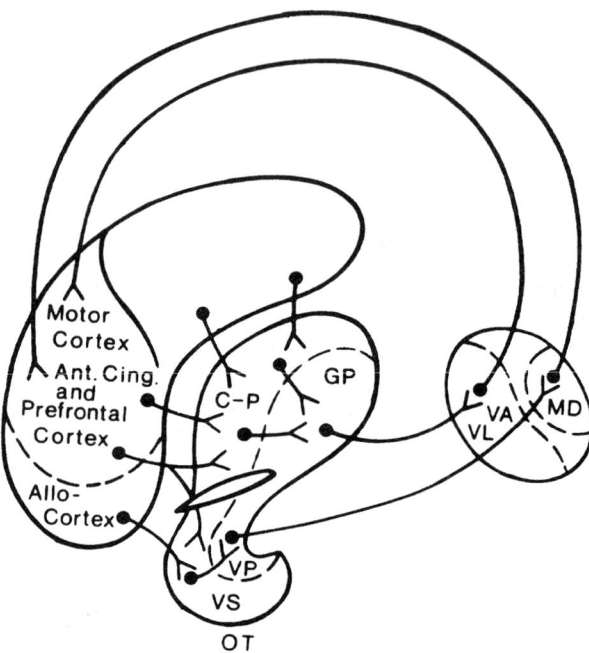

FIGURE 6. The cortico-subcortical reentrant circuit through the ventral striatopallidal system (VS, ventral striatum; VP, ventral pallidum) and mediodorsal thalamic nucleus (MD) back to prefrontal cortex is parallel to the well-known dorsal reentrant circuit through the dorsal parts of the basal ganglia (C-P, caudate-putamen, GP, globus pallidus) and ventrolateral thalamus (VA, ventral anterior nucleus; VL, ventral lateral nucleus) back to the motor–premotor cortex. OT, olfactory tubercle. (Heimer, L., R.D. Switzer & G.W. Van Hoesen. 1982. Trends Neurosci. **5(3):** 83-87, with permission.)

in subsequent studies aided by modern immunohistochemical and tract-tracing methods.[31,95,100] The discovery of an allocortical projection to the ventral parts of the basal ganglia and from there to the prefrontal cortex via the mediodorsal thalamus defined a cortico-subcortical reentrant circuit that is parallel to the well-known neocortical reentrant circuit through the dorsal parts of the basal ganglia and the VA/VL thalamic nuclei (FIG. 6). This was the beginning of the idea of parallel cortical-basal ganglia-thalamocortical reentrant circuits, which has become a productive and functionally relevant concept especially through the work of Alexander and coworkers.[1,2] To date, at least six different circuits have been identified, of which some are related to the ventral striatopallidal system.[33,98] To what extent these reentrant circuits represent separate processing channels is still being debated, as reviewed elsewhere;[48] the situation is especially complicated with regard to the ventral parts of the basal ganglia, where it appears that some of the circuits are organized in a feed-forward manner from olfactory cortex and other allocortical areas towards the premotor and supplementary motor areas.[98]

Even before the studies of cortico-subcortical reentrant circuits through the ventral striatum were completed, the striatal nature of the tubercle was firmly estab-

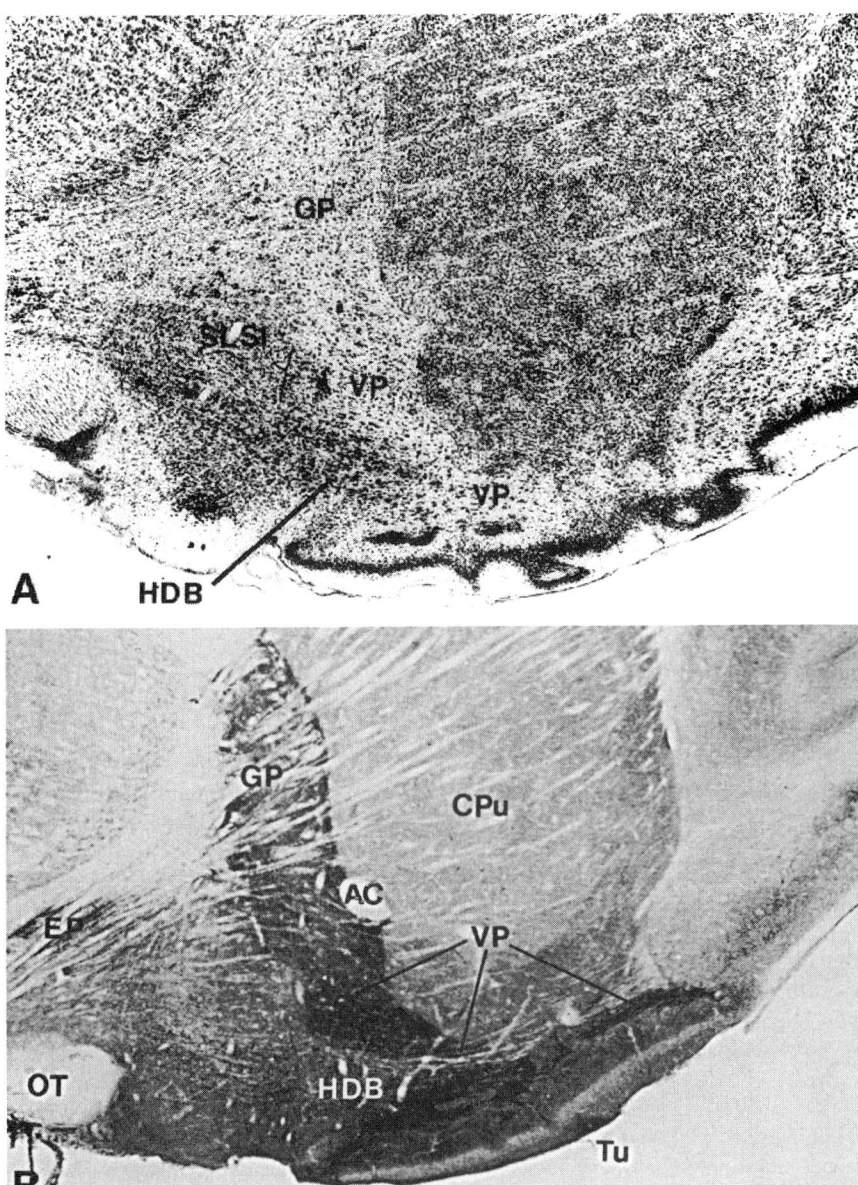

FIGURE 7. Adjacent parasagittal sections through the basal forebrain of the rat stained with the Nissl method (**A**) and with Perl's method for iron (**B**), which was used as a pallidal marker. The rostral part of the brain is to the right. Both pictures show a clear distinction between the sublenticular part of the substantia innominata (SLSI) and the subcommissural substantia innominata, which is occupied by the ventral pallidum (VP). The sublenticular substantia innominata is now recognized as the sublenticular part of the extended amygdala. Note how the ventral pallidum extends into the multiform layer of the olfactory tubercle (Tu). AC, anterior commissure; EP, entopeduncular nucleus; OT, optic tract. (Heimer *et al.*[47] With permission from Alan R. Liss, Inc.)

lished on the basis of cytoarchitectural, connectional, and histochemical studies.[25,39,64,68,69,95,99,100] It also became apparent that several finger-like extensions of the ventral pallidum were reaching well into the deep multiform layer of the olfactory tubercle.[36,47,64,92,99,100] The fact that the pallidal complex reaches ventrally into the deep part of the tubercle is best displayed in paramedian sagittal sections stained for a "pallidal" marker, such as iron or epidermal growth factor (FIG. 7B), but can also be appreciated in regular Nissl-stained preparations at certain levels (FIG. 7A).

The Two Divisions of the Substantia Innominata

The two sections in FIGURE 7 demonstrate another important fact, that is, that the region dorsal to the large collection of magnocellular neurons (representing the nucleus of the horizontal limb of the diagonal band, HDB) contains two cytoarchitectonically different regions (FIG. 7A). The anterior part, which is often referred to as the subcommissural part of the substantia innominata, and which is populated with rather loosely organized, large neurons, represents a ventral extension of the pallidal complex, that is, the ventral pallidum (VP). This can be easily demonstrated by the aid of a "pallidal" marker (FIG. 7B). The posterior, or sublenticular part of the substantia innominata (SLSI), which can be differentiated from the ventral pallidum already in a regular Nissl preparation because of smaller and more densely distributed neurons (FIG. 7A), represents the sublenticular corridor of the extended amygdala. This two-part division of the substantia innominata is one of the cornerstones in our conceptualization of the basal forebrain. We will return to this basic subdivision of the substantia innominata in the next section where we discuss in more detail the distinct differences that exist between the ventral striatopallidal system and the extended amygdala.

As a result of the studies mentioned above, the concept of the basal ganglia has been widened considerably to include several regions below the temporal limb of the anterior commissure, part of which previously belonged to the enigmatic forebrain region known as the substantia innominata or to the olfactory cortex (such as the olfactory tubercle). The fact that cortico-striatopallidal-thalamocortical reentrant circuits are as characteristic for allocortex as they are for neocortex represented, at the time, a distinct departure from the prevailing view, according to which neocortex and allocortex (including the hippocampus and prepiriform cortex) were characterized by differences rather than similarities in their subcortical projections. In other words, whereas neocortex was known to project to the basal ganglia, the allocortex, as part of the "limbic system," was assumed to be related to the hypothalamus rather than to the basal ganglia.

The early history of the development of the ventral striatopallidal system clearly reflects the role played by histotechnical advances. It also demonstrates the incremental nature of scientific inquiry. Both of these elements are prominently displayed also in subsequent studies, as various aspects of the ventral striatopallidal system have been analyzed by people in many laboratories during the last twenty years. Inasmuch as many of the recent advances related to the ventral striatopallidal system will be discussed in other chapters of this volume, we would like to refer only to some of the studies that have addressed the question of subterritories in the accum-

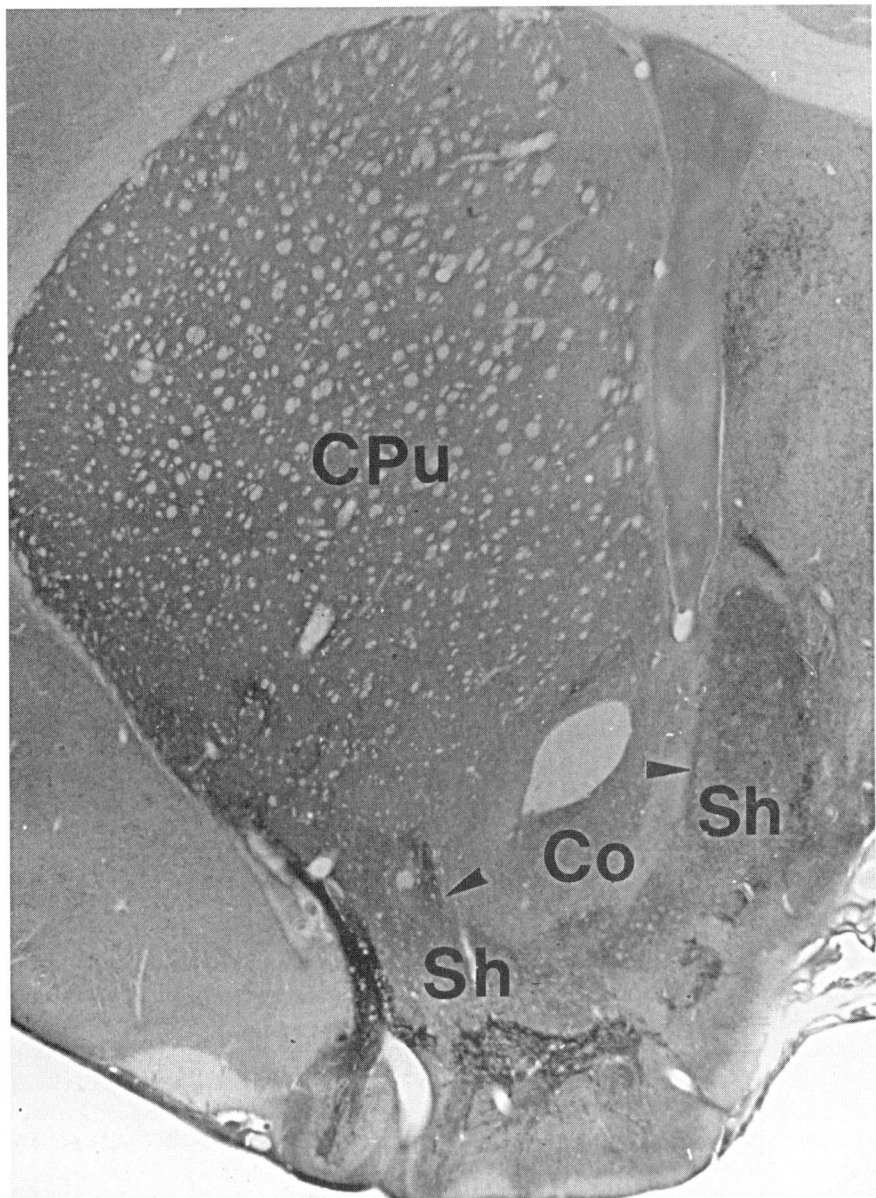

FIGURE 8. Coronal section through the forebrain of the rat showing substance P immunoreactivity. Note that a border beween the core (Co) and the dorsally adjacent main part of the striatal complex, caudate-putamen (Cpu), cannot be clearly identified, whereas the border between the core (Co) and the shell (Sh) is distinct (arrowheads). (Courtesy of Dr. Daniel S. Zahm).

bens, especially because that subject provides a natural transition to the next section on the extended amygdala.

The Core–Shell Dichotomy of the Accumbens

The accumbens can be subdivided into a central core, which is surrounded on its medial and ventral sides by a shell.[96] The core is in most respects similar to the rest of the caudate-putamen, and it is all but impossible to identify a distinct dorsal border of the core towards the rest of the striatal complex (FIG. 8). The border between the core and the shell, on the other hand, is distinct in most histochemical stains. Furthermore, in addition to its striatal characteristics, the shell has a number of features that are atypical for a striatal structure, but that are reminiscent of the extended amygdala with which it is directly continuous.[3,6,63] Nonetheless, it seems important to emphasize that the shell, like the core and the rest of the striatal complex, is characterized by being part of the so-called cortico-subcortical reentrant circuits, which eventually reach the frontal cortex via relays in the mediodorsal thalamus.[33,97] In this respect, the shell is different from the extended amygdala and should not be included as an integral part of the extended amygdala, notwithstanding the fact that it is directly continuous with one of its major components, that is, the central division of the extended amygdala (see below).

Because the caudomedial shell, in particular, does have a number of features in common with the central division of the extended amygdala, it is difficult to define a border between the caudomedial shell and the central division of the extended amygdala. The lack of a distinct border between the caudomedial shell and the extended amygdala is, furthermore, accentuated by the presence of apparent associative connections between the caudomedial shell and other parts of the central division of the extended amygdala.[40,49] However, it is only fair to admit that the associative connections between the caudomedial shell and the extended amygdala are considerably weaker than the long association fibers that characterize the extended amygdala. Nonetheless, the absence of a clearly defined boundary between parts of the striatopallidal system and the extended amygdala has led to the concept of transition areas between the two systems.[5,40] On the other hand, Zahm has recently questioned the usefulness of referring to a transition area in the caudomedial region of the shell, primarily on the basis that the caudomedial shell and the central amygdaloid nucleus (the prototypical central extended amygdaloid structure) are characterized by substantially different output channels.[97] These differences of opinion, no doubt, emphasize the difficulty that presents itself at the border between the accumbens and the extended amygdala, and for that matter throughout most of the area where the striatopallidal system adjoins the extended amygdala. Other areas of transition between the two systems will be discussed in the next section on the extended amygdala (see *Interstitial Nucleus of the Posterior Limb of the Anterior Commissure*) and in the section entitled **CRITICISM OF THE EXTENDED AMYGDALA** (see *The Two-part Division of the Substantia Innominata*).

In recent years, an increasing number of physiologists and pharmacologists have explored the functional differences between the core and the shell. Several of the chapters in this volume pay special attention to the so-called core–shell dichotomy and to more recent discoveries of subterritorial organization within the accumbens.

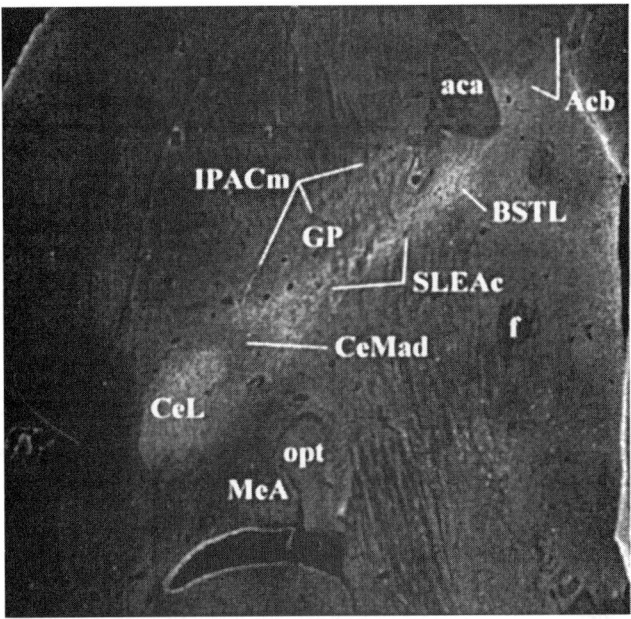

FIGURE 9. Dark-field image of cupric-silver stained horizontal section in a normal rat brain showing the granular argyrophilic neuropil in the central division of the extended amygdala. aca, anterior limb of the anterior commissure; Acb, accumbens; BSTL, lateral bed nucleus of the stria terminalis; CeL, lateral subdivision of the central amygdaloid nucleus; CeMad, anterodorsal part of the medial subdivision of the central amygdaloid nucleus; f, fornix; GP, globus pallidus; IPACm, medial part of the interstitial nucleus of the posterior limb of the anterior commissure; MeA, medial amygdaloid nucleus; SLEAc, central subdivision of the sublenticular extended amygdala; opt, optic tract. (Alheid et al.[5] With

THE EXTENDED AMYGDALA

A large amount of data has been gathered, particularly in the last ten years, to support the theory of a neuronal continuum, known as the extended amygdala within the basal forebrain.[5] The concept originated with the pioneering comparative and developmental studies by J.B. Johnston,[55] who suggested a close relationship between the bed nucleus of the stria terminalis and the centromedial amygdaloid nuclei. In particular, he noted in the human embryos and in lower vertebrates that these two territories form a continuum, and he maintained that this continuity is still evident in adult mammals through more or less continuous cell columns in the stria terminalis. Almost half a century later, de Olmos[19,20] revived the concept when he discovered that even in adult mammals the continuity between the centromedial amygdala and the bed nucleus of the stria terminalis includes columns of gray matter located in the subpallidal (sublenticular) substantia innominata (see below). The extended amygdala, in other words, appears as a large ring formation around the internal capsule. In fact, the extended amygdala can be divided into two parallel divisions or ring

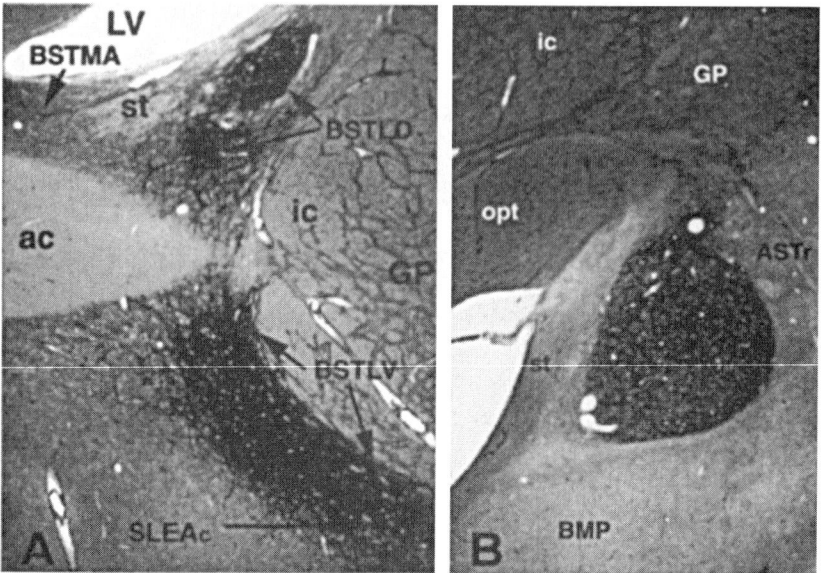

FIGURE 10. Low-power photomicrograph of cupric-silver stained coronal section through the normal rabbit brain. Note that these two photographs are from the right side of the brain, whereas all the other figures in this chapter represent the left side of the brain. The photograph in **A**, at the level of the crossing of the anterior commissure (ac), demonstrates the granular argyrophilic neuropil in the dorsal and ventral parts of the bed nucleus of the stria terminalis (BSTLD and BSTLV). The granular argyrophilia is continuous in a ventrolateral direction into the central subdivision of the sublenticular extended amygdala (SLEAc). The photograph in **B**, at a somewhat more caudal level, demonstrates the argyrophilic neuropil in the central amygdaloid nucleus. ASTr, amygdalostriatal transition area; BMP, posterior part of basomedial amygdaloid nucleus; GP, globus pallidus; ic, internal capsule; LV, lateral ventricle; opt, optic tract; st, stria terminalis.

formations. The central division includes the central amygdaloid nucleus and the lateral bed nucleus of stria terminalis, in addition to cell columns that bridge the gap between these two structures both within the stria terminalis and in the subpallidal region. The medial division of the extended amygdala, which is named after the medial amygdaloid nucleus and its rostral partner, the medial bed nucleus of stria terminalis, also includes cell columns within the stria terminalis and in the subpallidal area.

It is important to emphasize that the term *extended amygdala* denotes extensions of only the centromedial amygdala into the bed nucleus of the stria terminalis. In other words, the extended amygdala is a centromedial amygdala-bed nucleus of the stria terminalis continuum, which does not include the large cortical-laterobasal part of the amygdala. The cortical-laterobasal complex, however, provides important input to the extended amygdala, as it does to the ventral striatopallidal system.

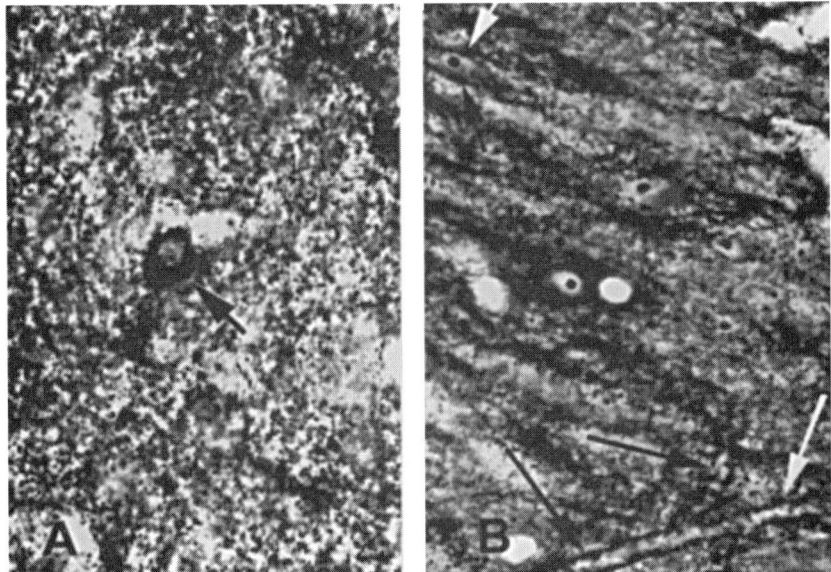

FIGURE 11. High-power microphotographs from cupric-silver stained coronal sections of a normal macaque monkey, demonstrating granular argyrophilic neuropil in the dorsal part of the lateral bed nucleus of stria terminalis (**A**) and in the central division of the sublenticular extended amygdala (**B**). Compare the typical peridendritic and perisomatic arrangement of the granular argyrophilia (arrows) in **B** with the more irregular pattern in **A**. The arrow in **A** points to an argyrophilic neuron.

The Central Division of the Extended Amygdala

The existence of a histochemically distinct neuronal continuum linking the central amygdaloid nucleus to the lateral bed nucleus of stria terminalis through the subpallidal area was first discovered by the aid of the cupric-silver technique. With this method, in which the oxidative action of the copper ions in the preimpregnation solution causes the suppression of normal axons and cell bodies, de Olmos demonstrated the presence of argyrophilic neurons and neuropil in the above-mentioned continuum in the basal forebrain of normal rats (FIG. 9). Similar results were obtained in brains of other mammals: armadillo, rabbit (FIG. 10), guinea pig, dog, and New and Old World monkeys (FIG. 11). The two high-power photomicrographs in FIGURE 11 demonstrate the appearance of granular argyrophilic neuropil (silver-stained axons and axon terminals) and argyrophilic neurons in the lateral bed nucleus of the stria terminalis (A) and the central division of the sublenticular extended amygdala (B) in a normal macaque monkey.

Major Extrinsic Connections of the Central Division of the Extended Amygdala

Once the central amygdaloid-lateral bed nucleus continuum was established, it became important to study its major extrinsic connections. One of the most striking

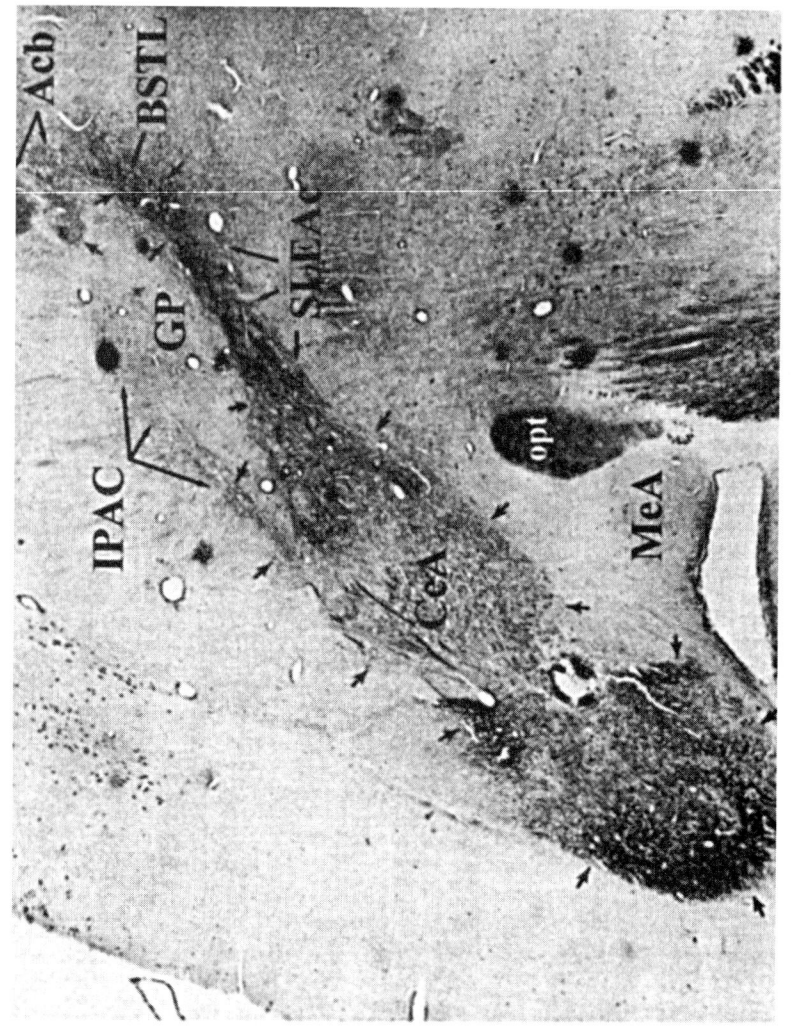

FIGURE 12. Cupric-silver stained horizontal section in the rat brain showing degenerating fibers and terminals throughout the extended amygdala following a lesion two days earlier in the laterobasal amygdaloid complex. Modified from de Olmos[20] to include current terminology. (See FIG. 9 for abbreviations).

findings from these studies[20] was that lesions in the laterobasal amygdaloid complex produced an uninterrupted terminal field along the whole length of the continuum, consisting of the central amygdaloid nucleus, the lateral bed nucleus of the stria terminalis, and cell columns in the sublenticular area (FIG. 12). Moreover, laminar heat lesions in the amygdalo-piriform area[20] also produced a unified field of degenerating terminals throughout the continuum, consisting of the central amygdaloid nucleus, the sublenticular substantia innominata, and the bed nucleus of the stria terminalis.

The importance of the centromedial amygdala-bed nucleus of the stria terminalis continuum was addressed only occasionally in the literature in the 1970s.[39] In 1982, however, Schwaber and his colleagues[80] demonstrated an unbroken continuum of retrogradely labeled cells extending from the central amygdaloid nucleus along the ventromedial border of the internal capsule into the lateral bed nucleus of the stria terminalis, following injections of the tracer in the vagal-solitary complex. A similar picture of labeled cells in a central amygdaloid-lateral bed nucleus of the stria terminalis continuum following injection of the retrograde tracer in the parabrachial nuclear complex was obtained by Jackson and Crossman.[53] These studies were later confirmed in many tract-tracing studies, including experiments with injections of retrograde tracers in brain stem autonomic centers. [34,50,66,81]

In subsequent studies, de Olmos and his colleagues injected retrograde fluorescent tracers in each of the three major components of the central continuum, that is,

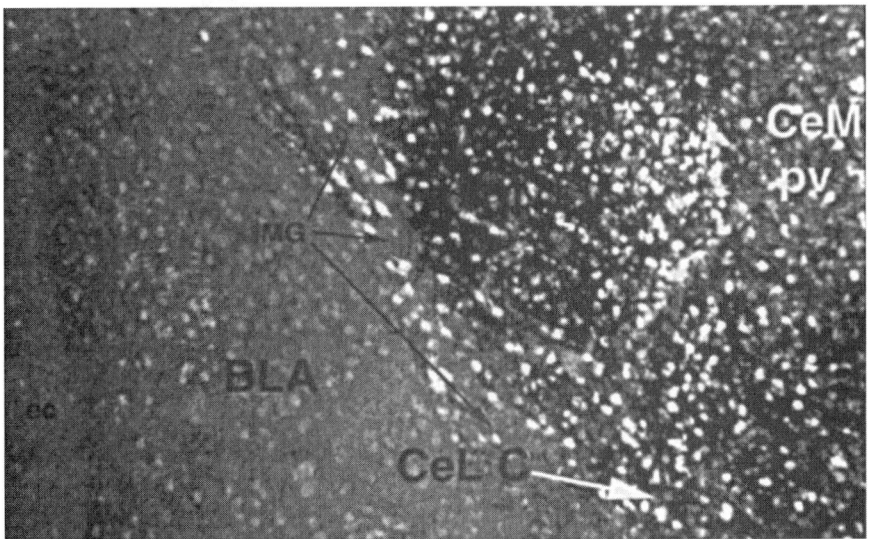

FIGURE 13. Cupric-silver stained coronal section showing part of the central amygdaloid nucleus in a rat brain in which the retrograde fluorescent tracer, Fluoro Gold, was injected into the sublenticular part of the central division of the extended amygdala. The retrogradely labeled cells appear as bright white dots surrounded by the black silver precipitate representing the granular argyrophilic neuropil. BLA, basolateral amygdaloid nucleus; CeLC, lateral subdivision of central amygdaloid nucleus, capsular part; CEM pv, medial subdivision of central amygdaloid nucleus, posteroventral part; ec, external capsule; IMG, intramedullary grisea.

the central amygdaloid nucleus, the sublenticular substantia innominata, and the lateral bed nucleus of stria terminalis. In all experiments of this kind, retrogradely labeled cells can be seen throughout the central division of the extended amygdala. For instance, following an injection of retrograde tracer in the central division of the sublenticular extended amygdala, labeled cells appear not only in the central amygdaloid nucleus (FIG. 13) and lateral bed nucleus of stria terminalis, but also in a more or less continuous column of neurons within the lateral part of the stria terminalis. This indicates that the different parts of the central extended amygdaloid continuum are interrelated by means of intrinsic associative connections.

In addition to a laterally located cell column within the stria terminalis, small clusters of neurons are also located in the medial part of the stria, and we have recently suggested that they belong to the medial division of the extended amygdala.[4] The cell columns within the stria terminalis itself are, like the sublenticular cell columns, continuous with the bed nucleus of stria terminalis in the rostromedial forebrain and with the centromedial amygdala in the temporal lobe. These columns of cells within the stria terminalis, that is, the supracapsular part of the bed nucleus of stria terminalis, provided important evidence for J.B. Johnston's original concept of a large neuronal forebrain continuum,[55] which we now recognize as the extended amygdala. The supracapsular part of the extended amygdala has been described in detail not only in the rat[4] but also in the human.[42,88]

Support for the concept of the extended amygdala comes from a number of different sources. The publication by Alheid et al.[5] is especially important in this context, because the authors have provided convincing evidence for a far-reaching symmetry between the centromedial amygdala and the bed nucleus of the stria terminalis. For almost every subdivision of the central and medial amygdaloid nuclei, corresponding subdivisions can be found in the lateral and medial bed nuclei of the stria terminalis. Although all of these prototypical subdivisions may not be present in the intervening cell columns, that is, at the level of the sublenticular substantia innominata and within the supracapsular stria terminalis, it is nevertheless important to emphasize that the cells within these two areas form two parallel, more or less continuous columns, that are in direct continuity with the central and medial amygdaloid nuclei, on one hand, and with the lateral and medial bed nuclei of the stria terminalis, on the other hand. Other compelling evidence for the concept of the extended amygdala comes from the distribution of neuropeptides and receptors as well as from various tract-tracing studies, as reviewed in several papers.[5,6,42,44] Nonetheless, the concept has become the focus of some sharp negative criticism during the last few years. This controversy will be discussed in some detail below.

Interstitial Nucleus of the Posterior Limb of the Anterior Commissure

The term *interstitial nucleus of the posterior limb of the anterior commissure* (IPAC) was introduced by de Olmos[20] to denote a narrow band of cells accompanying the posterior limb of the anterior commissure. Although its close association with the amygdala was noted at the time, it was only later that the region was included in the concept of the extended amygdala, or more precisely, as a rostral arm of the central division of the extended amygdala. In the process, the definition of IPAC was also expanded when it became apparent that a rather large territory surrounding the posterior limb of the anterior commissure has, contrary to the rest of the striatum,

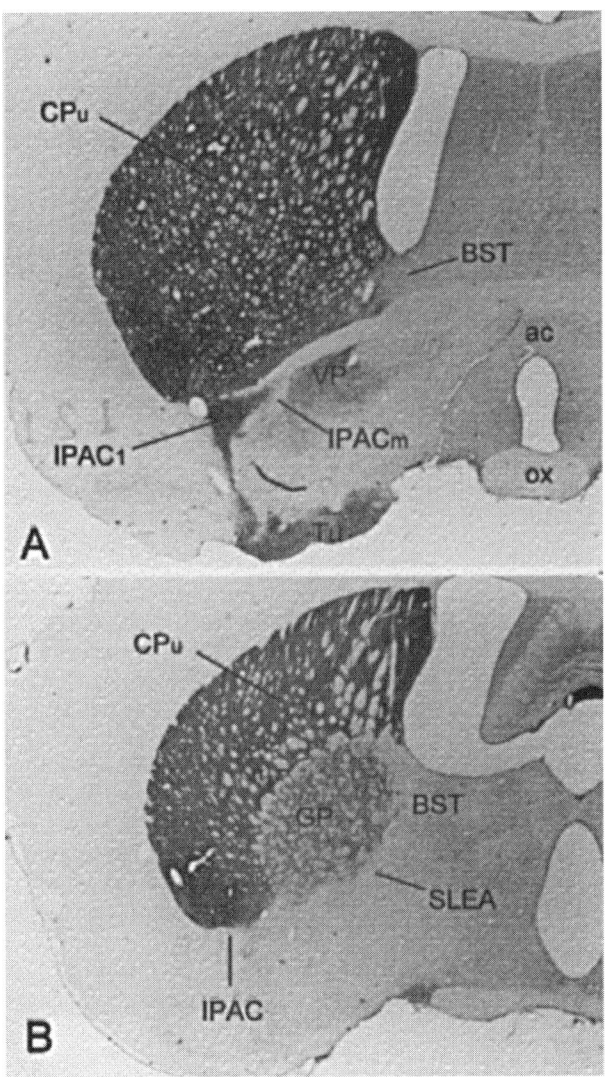

FIGURE 14. Distribution of A_{2A}-adenosine receptor-like immunoreactivity in coronal sections through the rat forebrain. Dense labeling of the neuropil can be seen in the striatal complex (CPu, caudate-putamen; $IPAC_l$, lateral part of the interstitial nucleus of the posterior limb of the anterior commissure; Tu, olfactory tubercle), including a striatal cell bridge (CB) between IPAC and the tubercle. Labeling in the pallidal complex (VP, ventral pallidum; GP, globus pallidus) is somewhat lighter. The extended amygdala, on the other hand, including the medial part of the interstitial nucleus of the posterior limb of the anterior comissure (IPACm), is not stained for adenosine receptors. ac, anterior commissure; ox, optic chiasm. (Modified from Rosin et al.[76] Courtesy of Dr. Diane Rosin.)

many of the same characteristics as the rest of the central division of the extended amygdala. Features typical for the central division of the extended amygdala include downstream projections to brain stem autonomic centers and the staining of a number of peptides and receptors, which are also characteristic for other parts of the central division of the extended amygdala.

A couple of recent papers[76,82] have contributed significantly to settling some of the uncertainties with regard to the IPAC. Rosin and her collaborators, who have studied the distribution of the striatal marker, adenosine A_{2A} receptors in the rat, have confirmed the many reports that tend to distinguish the extended amygdala (which is not stained for adenosine receptors) from the striatopallidal system, which is specifically stained for adenosine receptors. They have also shown that the anterolateral part of the IPAC, as outlined in a recent atlas of the rat brain,[71] does express adenosine receptors to approximately the same extent as the rest of the striatum (FIG. 14). This is somewhat reminiscent of the idea suggested originally by Alheid and his collaborator, that the medial part of the IPAC is an integral part of the central division of the extended amygdala, whereas the lateral part of IPAC is more difficult to specify. Based on the results obtained in a recent study of the afferent pathways of the IPAC, Shammah-Lagnado *et al.*[82] suggested that the anterolateral part of the IPAC be considered as a transitional area between the extended amygdala and the striatum.

The Medial Division of the Extended Amygdala

Evidence for the existence of a second ring-like gray continuum, that is, the medial extended amygdala, was first obtained in experiments in which the retrograde fluorescent tracer Fast Blue was injected in the accessory olfactory bulb in the rat.[22] Following such injections retrogradely labeled cells appeared in a continuous column extending from the rostrodorsal aspect of the medial amygdaloid nucleus through the posteroventral part of the sublenticular region (FIG. 15) to the caudal ventrolateral part of the large-celled subdivision of the posterior medial bed nucleus of stria terminalis. Similar results were obtained following injection of retrograde tracers in the medial preoptic area and ventromedial hypothalamus (de Olmos, unpublished results). In these experiments, labeled cells were seen, not only in the medial amygdaloid-medial bed nucleus continuum located in the sublenticular region, but also at different levels within the medial part of the supracapsular stria terminalis.

As in the case of the central division of the extended amygdala, the various subdivisions of the medial amygdaloid nucleus do, in general, have their counterparts in the medial bed nucleus of stria terminalis.[5] Similar to the situation in the central division, there is a rich system of local interconnections within the medial division of the extended amygdala.[11,15] This point is also illustrated in FIGURE 15, which demonstrates Nuclear Yellow labeled neurons in the medial division of the sublenticular extended amygdala following injection of the retrograde tracer in the medial amygdaloid nucleus. For detailed discussions of these and other histochemical features in support of the medial division of the extended amygdala in the rat and human, see chapters by de Olmos *et al.*,[22] Alheid *et al.*,[5] and Heimer *et al.*[42]

From a functional point of view, it is important to emphasize that the two divisions of the extended amygdala are, in large part, characterized by different efferent targets. Whereas the central division of the extended amygdala is characterized fore-

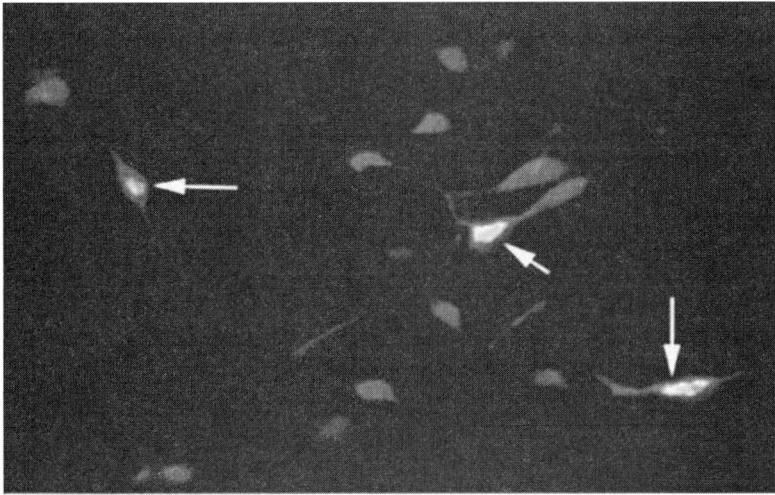

FIGURE 15. High-power microphotograph demonstrating retrogradely labeled cells in the medial division of the sublenticular extended amygdala in the rat following injection of Fluoro Gold in the accessory olfactory bulb and Nuclear Yellow in the medial amygdaloid nucleus. The Fluoro Gold labeled cells appear homogenuously gray, whereas the Nuclear Yellow–labeled neurons are characterized by bright white nuclei. Note that the three neurons (arrows), which project to the accessory olfactory bulb, are double labeled. In other words, they project both to the accessory bulb and the medial amygdaloid nucleus.

most by direct projections to the lateral hypothalamus and to somatomotor and autonomic brain stem centers, the medial extended amygdala is closely related to the medial hypothalamus (FIG. 16).

CRITICISM OF THE EXTENDED AMYGDALA

In a couple of recent articles, Swanson and his collaborators take issue with our proposal that the extended amygdala is a useful anatomical concept[11,90] (see also the chapter by Cassell, this volume). Instead, they propose that the centromedial amygdala is a striatal structure, and they consider the bed nucleus of stria terminalis, together with the substantia innominata, to be a related pallidal structure. In this section we will analyze their objections to the concept of the extended amygdala.

Cytoarchitectural and Histochemical Criteria Define the Extended Amygdala

Swanson and Petrovitch[90] suggest on page 326 that our concept of the extended amygdala is based on the fact that "... amygdala innervates the bed nuclei of the stria terminalis (BST) and intervening regions of the substantia innominata (ventral pallidum), and because the latter two regions share with the amygdala similar patterns of descending projections, the BST and caudodorsal regions of the substantia innom-

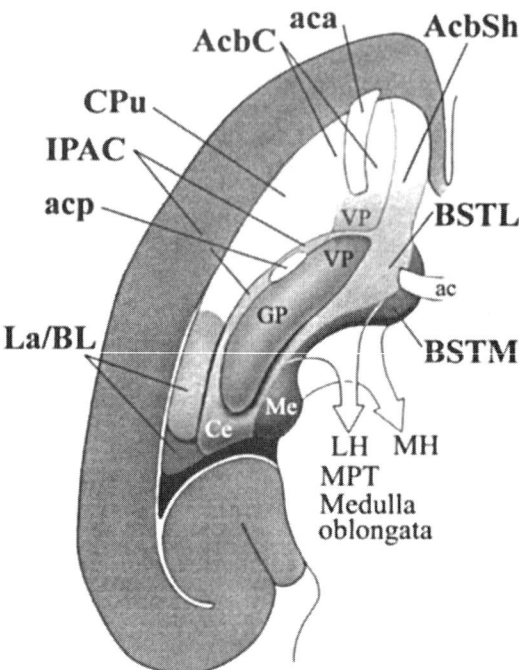

FIGURE 16. Schematic, partly three-dimensional drawing, of the basal forebrain of the rat in horizontal view. The two major subcortical forebrain structures, the basal ganglia and the extended amygdala, form large diagonally oriented "columns." The septum-diagonal band system and the hypothalamus are not included in the drawing. Striatum (in white) is represented by the caudate-putamen (CPu) and the core and shell of the accumbens. Note that the core of the accumbens can generally be distinguished from the shell. However, there is no clear border beween the core and the rest of the striatal complex, that is, the caudate-putamen. The pallidal complex (medium gray) is represented by the globus pallidus (GP) and the ventral pallidum (VP). The ventral pallidum disappears underneath the interstitial nucleus of the posterior limb of the anterior commissure (IPAC) and the ventral striatum (accumbens) in order to approach the ventral surface of the brain in the region of the olfactory tubercle. This rostroventral extension of the ventral pallidum underneath the core of the accumbens has only been implied by a gradually disappearing light gray color so as not to compromise the rendition of the core–shell dichotomy of the accumbens. The extended amygdala, finally, is indicated by two different shades of gray, that is, light gray for the central division and dark gray for the medial division.

The broad arrows illustrate how the two divisions of the extended amygdala are characterized by, in general, different descending projections. The central division of the extended amygdala projects to the lateral hypothalamus (LH) and to autonomic and somatomotor centers in the brain stem. The medial division is closely related to the medial hypothalamus (MH). aca, anterior limb of the anterior commissure; acp, posterior or temporal limb of the anterior commissure; BSTL, lateral bed nucleus of stria terminalis; BSTM, medial bed nucleus of stria terminalis; Ce, central amygdaloid nucleus; La/BL, lateral and basolateral amygdaloid nuclei (laterobasal amygdaloid complex); Me, medial amygdaloid nucleus. AcbC, accumbens' core; AcbSh, accumbens' shell; MPT, mesopontine tegmentum. (Modified from Heimer et al.[44] Original drawing by Medical and Science Illustrations, Crozet, VA, USA.)

inata belong to the (extended) amygdala as well ...." As indicated earlier, in relation to the central division of the extended amygdala, we are basing the concept of the extended amygdala on the fact that various parts of the continuum share similar cytoarchitectural and histochemical characteristics. In fact, in a recent paper by Alheid et al.,[5] the various subdivisions of the central nucleus has been matched, part by part, with corresponding subdivisions in the lateral bed nucleus with regard to both cytoarchitecture and histochemistry. Therefore, instead of basing our concept of the central extended amygdala on similarities in descending connections from its different parts, as suggested by Swanson and Petrovitch, we base the concept on the fact that the different parts of the central extended amygdala form a cytoarchitecturally and histochemically distinct continuum. On this basis we predict that the various parts of the continuum will show similarities in their descending projections, which in general appears to be the case (see above). Similarly, one would predict that all or most of the central extended amygdala would share similar inputs. References to that effect are included in several recent reviews.[7,21,22,43,97] Incidentally, a similar reasoning applies to the medial division of the extended amygdala, although the evidence for this second ring-like formation was first obtained in retrograde tract-tracing experiments (see above).

The Two Divisions of the Extended Amygdala

A similar misunderstanding is, in part, responsible for the rejection by Swanson and his collaborators of the idea that the extended amygdala contains two major components, a central and a medial division corresponding to the extensions of the central respective medial amygdaloid nucleus. The argument by Canteras, Simerly, and Swanson[11] that "... there are no clear differences between medial and central parts of the extended amygdala in the substantia innominata ..." (p. 241) is based on their studies of central and medial amygdaloid projections to the region of the substantia innominata (see below) and on a misinterpretation of the results obtained by Grove,[34] as reflected in FIGURE 6B in her article. The figure by Grove, however, on which Canteras and his collaborators base their argument depicts two divisions in the sublenticular part of the substantia innominata, as discussed in more detail by Heimer et al.[44] The divisions by Grove were labeled the dorsal division (corresponding to the sublenticular part of our central extended amygdala) respective to the ventral division (corresponding to the sublenticular part of our medial extended amygdala). It is remarkable to realize how well Grove's description of the sublenticular substantia innominata and its connections[34,35] fit with our conceptualizations of the extended amygdala, a fact that was duly recorded by Grove.

The presence of two distinct subdivisions of the extended amygdala is evident also in the supracapsular component of the extended amygdala,[4] which corresponds to what is generally called the supracapsular part of the bed nucleus of the stria terminalis. Swanson and his collaborators,[11,90] on the other hand, suggest that these neurons align along the sulcus terminalis and represent a dorsal extension of only the medial amygdaloid nucleus. It is difficult to see on what evidence they base this proposition, especially because the laterally located cell column within the stria terminalis, which is by far the largest of the two columns within the stria, is clearly continuous with the lateral bed nucleus and the central amygdaloid nucleus.[4] One explanation for this misconception may be the reliance of Swanson on the description by Geeraedts et al.[30] and Paxinos and Watson,[70] who seem to refer not to cells within the boundaries of the stria terminalis, but rather to a small cell group on the medial side of the stria that is "... rather densely crowded with preponderantly small and some medium-sized, oval-shaped and rather pale-staining neurons ...."[30] This description on page 518 in the paper by Canteras et al.[11] is not relevant to the medial part of the supracapsular bed nucleus, but is consistent rather with a small group of neurons in the thalamus on the medial side of the stria terminalis.[4] It is evident from our studies, that the main cell group within the supracapsular stria terminalis of the rat is located in its lateral part. It is also clear that this cell group is part of the central division of the extended amygdala, as evident by its continuity with the central amygdaloid nucleus as well as with the lateral bed nucleus of stria terminalis, as described in considerable detail by Alheid et al.[4]

It is sometimes difficult or even impossible, especially in the more anterior parts of the stria, to separate the lateral cell column of the supracapsular part of the extended amygdala from the neuronal population in the caudate-putamen. This situation, however, is no different from that in other regions of the forebrain, where part of the extended amygdala, for example, the central amygdaloid nucleus or IPAC (see above), is directly continuous with the striatal complex without easily recognizable borders.[3,5,82] It should be emphasized, however, that the situation with regard to the supracapsular part of the extended amygdala appears to be more clear-cut in the human than in the rat. In the human brain, a large parvicellular interface island, the paracaudate island,[79] is located at the interface between the caudate nucleus and the stria terminalis alongside the entire course of the stria terminalis, thereby effectively separating the supracapsular bed nucleus of stria terminalis from the caudate nucleus proper.[42]

The Two-part Division of the Substantia Innominata

Swanson and Petrovich[90] suggest that the "caudodorsal region of the substantia innominata," which corresponds to the sublenticular substantia innominata, is part of the ventral pallidum like the rest of the substantia innominata. It appears that they base this argument primarily on the fact that the centromedial amygdala (which in their opinion is part of the striatum) projects to the caudodorsal region of the substantia innominata. To suggest that all of the substantia innominata represents the ventral pallidum ignores the important fact that the posterior or sublenticular region is very different from the anterior, subcommissural part. In fact, the sublenticular region does not have any intrinsic cytoarchitectural or histochemical features reminiscent of a pallidal structure. The sublenticular or caudodorsal region of the substantia innominata is located behind the ventral pallidum, from which it can be distinguished already in Nissl preparations (FIG. 7A), and it is not stained with a "pallidal" marker such as epidermal growth factor (FIG. 7B). Instead, it appears, based on what we have presented earlier in this section, that the caudodorsal region of substantia innominata of Swanson and Petrovich shares cytoarchitectural, histochemical, and connectional characteristics with the centromedial amygdala and the bed nucleus of the stria terminalis. As indicated earlier, we consider the centromedial amygdaloid projections to the sublenticular region to be part of a widespread intrinsic association system within the extended amygdala.

The division of the substantia innominata into a primarily rostral, subcommissural "ventral pallidal" part and a posterior, subpallidal (sublenticular) "extended amygdaloid" part (FIG. 7) is an important distinction, which has guided much of our work in the basal forebrain. Unfortunately, however, the difference between these two parts is not always as obvious as shown in FIGURE 7, primarily, it seems, because elements of the extended amygdala to some extent invade the subcommissural ventral pallidum.[3,41] In other words, part of the territory referred to as the rostral, subcommissural substantia innominata does appear to represent a zone of transition between the extended amygdala and the ventral pallidum. However, this may not be a satisfying explanation for the assertion of Canteras *et al.*,[11] that efferents from both the central and medial amygdaloid nuclei reach not only the posterior, sublenticular part of the substantia innominata, but also to some extent its rostral parts. It is perhaps more important to acknowledge that the interstitial nucleus of the posterior limb of the anterior commissure, which, as an integral part of the central division of the extended amygdala is a recipient of association fibers within the extended amygdala, is located quite rostral in front of the ventral pallidum.

More detailed experimental connectional and histochemical studies on both the light- and electron-microscopic level are needed in order to elucidate the neuronal circuits related to the apparent transitional area between the extended amygdala and the striatopallidal system in this part of the brain, but the fact remains that intermingling of elements of the two systems in certain places are minor in comparison to the fundamental differences that exist between the two systems.

The proposal by Swanson and Petrovich[90] that the bed nucleus of stria terminalis is a pallidal structure is especially difficult to understand. Except for their suggestion that the bed nucleus is derived from the medial ganglionic eminence ("pallidal ridge"[b]), which is quite reasonable,[44,87] there is hardly any evidence, cytological, histochemical, or otherwise, that the bed nucleus of stria terminalis is a pallidal structure. An earlier observation that a restricted part of the ventral medial bed nucleus of stria terminalis is lightly stained for epidermal growth factor[26] suggests only a transition between the bed nucleus and adjacent ventral pallidum.

Summary of Pronounced Differences between the Striatopallidal System and the Extended Amygdala

Without going into further discussion of the conceptual framework proposed by Swanson and his colleagues, we do like to offer the following additional arguments for the wisdom of keeping a distinction between these two systems, regardless of how one might like to name them. First, as already indicated, the striatopallidal system is characterized by a set of "parallel" cortical-basal ganglia-thalamocortical reentrant circuits, which is not the case for the extended amygdala. The extended amygdala, on the other hand, is characterized by long associative pathways, which connect various parts of the extended amygdala with each other. Second, whereas the

---

[b]The renaming of the lateral and medial ganglionic eminence to "striatal" and "pallidal" ridges, respectively, is unfortunate, especially because there is still considerable uncertainty as to the origin of the pallidal complex. According to Song and Harlan, globus pallidus derives from the more caudal portion of the ventricular wall, where there are hardly any distinctions between a lateral and a medial eminence, and where it is customary to refer only to a lateral ganglionic eminence (Harlan, personal communication).

central extended amygdala, like the basal ganglia, has some efferent pathways to the somatomotor system, it projects, in contrast to the basal ganglia, to brain stem autonomic structures. The medial division of the extended amygdala, on the other hand, is characterized foremost by its projections to the endocrine-related medial hypothalamus (FIG. 13). In other words, the extended amygdala represents a strategically placed ring formation capable of coordinating the activities of multiple forebrain regions permitting coherent processing of information for the development of behavioral responses through the above-mentioned output channels. Third, whereas the dorsal striatum (caudate-putamen) and ventral striatum are characterized by large cholinergic interneurons and to a large extent, at least, by populations of parvalbumin interneurons,[13,16,17,57] such interneurons do not appear to be part of the intrinsic circuits of the extended amygdala. Fourth, whereas serotonin 2 receptors[67] and adenosine A_{2A} receptors[76] are prominent in the striatopallidal system, they are not present in the extended amygdala (see also *The Interstitial Nucleus of the Posterior Limb of the Anterior Commissure* in the previous section). Fifth, many receptors and other neuroactive substances are characteristic for one or both divisions of the extended amygdala and are not present to any significant degree in the striatopallidal system. Examples of such chemicals include Lyn protein,[14] regulated endocrine-specific protein-18,[18] pituitary adenylate cyclase activating polypeptide,[73] vasopressin and oxytocin receptors,[29,93,94] androgenic receptor (ref. 44, and Harlan, personal communications), and receptors for calcitonin and calcitonin gene-related peptides,[84,85] as well as many peptides, including cholecystokinin, angiotensin 11, somatostatin, and secretoneurin.[5,44] In fact, without reference to the extended amygdaloid concept, the distribution of many of these substances would be confusing indeed.

The examples mentioned above are only some of the most prominent in a rapidly increasing list of significant differences between the striatopallidal system and the extended amygdala. Not surprisingly, these anatomical differences appear to be matched by equally pronounced functional distinctions between the two systems, although reference is not always made to the extended amygdaloid concept in studies where the centromedial amygdala and the bed nucleus of stria terminalis have been the major foci of functional experiments. The prevailing view, at least in the past, has been one in which the bed nucleus of stria terminalis is conceived of as a relay in downstream projections from the centromedial amygdala.[12,24,28,51,59,83] This past appreciation is changed by the concept of the extended amygdala in which the centromedial amygdala and the bed nucleus of stria terminalis and associated subpallidal and supracapsular cell columns represent a cellular continuum. Published pictures, however, do give a clear indication that the authors are dealing instead with a forebrain continuum, that is, the extended amygdala,[52,54,77] rather than with two separate forebrain structures, that is, the centromedial amygdala and the bed nucleus of stria terminalis, serially connected in a descending pathway.

CONCLUDING REMARKS

The concepts of the ventral striatopallidal system and the extended amygdala were developed primarily on the basis of experimental studies in the rat. However, it appears, based on comparative anatomical studies in a number of different mammalian and nonmammalian species, that both systems are organized according to a general plan shared by all tetrapods.[10,60,61] From a clinical point of view, it is of special importance to realize that the ventral striatopallidal system and the extended amygdala are as prominent in the human brain as they are in the rat. In the human, as in the rat, they occupy a large territory, which for over a century has been referred to as the substantia innominata.[6,8,21,42] The third component of the human substantia innominata is the basal nucleus of Meynert. In fact, the cell groups formed by the magnocellular, mostly cholinergic neurons of the basal nucleus of Meynert in the human are so strikingly displayed in Nissl preparations that the term substantia innominata has sometimes been used as a synonym for the basal nucleus of Meynert. It is interesting to realize, however, that the basal nucleus, at least volumetrically, constitutes a relatively minor part of the substantia innominata in comparison with the other two systems.[42]

As reflected in several chapters in this book, the ventral striatopallidal system and extended amygdala have captured the imagination of clinical neuroscientists studying the neuronal mechanisms of neuropsychiatric disorders and drugs of abuse. Efforts to explain various symptoms in mood disorders, schizophrenia, Alzheimer's disease, and obsessive-compulsive disorders, as well as stress and anxiety-related disorders are increasingly relying on the neuronal circuits related to the ventral striatopallidal system and the extended amygdala.[23,32,56,62,65,78,91] It is also important to realize that prefrontal and medial temporal lobe structures, which are known to be involved in a number of neuropsychiatric disorders, do provide major inputs to both the ventral striatopallidal system and the extended amygdala. As reflected in several of the chapters in this volume, it is also the case that scientists advancing theories of drug abuse are increasingly focusing their interest on the large forebrain continuum, consisting of the shell of the accumbens and the extended amygdala.[58,72,74,75]

ACKNOWLEDGMENTS

We thank Dr. John Jane Sr. for his unwavering support for over a quarter of a century and Dr. George Alheid for long-lasting collaboration on various aspects of the systems reviewed in this chapter. We also thank Drs. Norman Knorr, Robert Cantrell, and Robert Carey for supporting our research effort by providing excellent facilities for Lennart Heimer at the University of Virginia School of Medicine. Drs. Scott Zahm and Richard Harlan made valuable suggestions, and Dr. Frank Schottler and Soledad de Olmos provided technical support. This work was supported by the National Council of Science (INIMEC-CONICET) of Argentina, PMT-PICT 0094 Prestamo BID 82/OC-AR and PMT-PICT 05-00000-00624 (J. de O.), and by US-PHS Grant NS-17743 (L.H.).

REFERENCES

1. ALEXANDER, G.E., M.D. CRUTCHER & M.R. DELONG. 1990. Basal ganglia-thalamo-cortical circuits: parallel substrates for motor, oculomotor, "prefrontal" and "limbic" functions. *In* The Prefrontal Cortex: Its Structure, Function and Pathology. H.B.M. Uylings, C.G. Van Eden, J.P.C. De Bruin, M.A. Corner & M.P.G. Feenstra, Eds.: 119–146. Elsevier. Amsterdam.

2. ALEXANDER, G.E., M.R. DELONG & P.L. STRICK. 1986. Parallel organization of functionally segregated circuits linking basal ganglia and cortex. Annu. Rev. Neurosci. **9:** 357–381.
3. ALHEID, G.F., C.A. BELTRAMINO, A. BRAUN, R.R. MISELIS, C. FRANÇOIS & J.S. DE OLMOS. 1994. Transition areas of the striatopallidal system with the extended amygdala in the rat and primate: observations from histochemistry and experiments with mono- and transsynaptic tracer. *In* The Basal Ganglia IV. New Ideas and Data on Structure and Function. G. Percheron, J.S. McKenzie & J. Feger, Eds.: **41:** 95–107. Plenum Press. New York.
4. ALHEID, G.F., C.A. BELTRAMINO, J.S. DE OLMOS, M.S. FORBES, D.J. SWANSON & L. HEIMER. 1998. The neuronal organization of the supracapsular part of the stria terminalis in the rat: the dorsal component of extended amygdala. Neuroscience **84:** 967–996.
5. ALHEID, G.F., J.S. DE OLMOS & C. A. BELTRAMINO. 1995. Amygdala and extended amygdala. *In* The Rat Nervous System, 2nd Ed. G. Paxinos, Ed.: 495–578. Academic Press, Inc. San Diego.
6. ALHEID, G.F. & L. HEIMER. 1988. New perspectives in basal forebrain organization of special relevance for neuropsychiatric disorders: the striatopallidal, amygdaloid, and corticopetal components of substantia innominata. Neuroscience **27:** 1–39.
7. ALHEID, G.F. & L. HEIMER. 1996. Theories of basal forebrain organization and the "emotional motor system." Prog. Brain Res. **107:** 461–484.
8. ALHEID, G.F., L. HEIMER & R. C. SWITZER. 1990. Basal ganglia. *In* The Human Nervous System. G. Paxinos, Ed.: 483–582. Academic Press, Inc. San Diego, CA.
9. ALVAREZ-BOLADO, G., M.G. ROSENFELD & L.W. SWANSON. 1995. Model of forebrain regionalization based on spatiotemporal patterns of POU-III homeobox gene expression, birthdates, and morphological features. J. Comp. Neurol. **355:** 237–295.
10. BRUCE, L.L. & T.J. NEARY. 1995. The limbic system of tetrapods: a comparative analysis of cortical and amygdalar populations. Brain Behav. Evol. **46:** 224–234.
11. CANTERAS, N.S., R.B. SIMERLY & L.W. SWANSON. 1995. Organization of projections from the medial nucleus of the amygdala: a PHAL study in the rat. J. Comp. Neurol. **360:** 213–245.
12. CARR, K.D., T.H. PARK, Y. ZHANG & E.A. STONE. 1998. Neuroanatomical patterns of fos-like immunoreactivity induced by naltrexone in food-restricted and ad libitum fed rats. Brain Res. **779:** 26–32.
13. CELIO, M.R. 1990. Calbindin D-28k and parvalbumin in the rat nervous system, Neuroscience **35:** 375–475.
14. CHEN, S., R. BING, N. ROSENBLUM & D. E. HILLMAN. 1996. Immunohistochemical localization of Lyn (p56) protein in the adult rat brain. Neuroscience **71:** 89–100.
15. COOLEN, L.M. & R.I. WOOD. 1998. Bidirectional connections of the medial amygdaloid nucleus in the syrian hamster brain: simultaneous anterograde and retrograde tract tracing. J. Comp. Neurol. **399:** 189–209.
16. COTE, P.-Y., A.F. SADIKOT & A. PARENT. 1991. Complementary distribution of calbindin D-28k and parvalbumin in the basal forebrain and midbrain of the squirrel monkey. Eur. J. Neurosci. **3:** 1316–1329.
17. COWAN, R.L., C.J. WILSON, P.C. EMSON & C.W. HEIZMANN. 1990. Parvalbumin-containing GABAergic interneurons in the rat neostriatum. J. Comp. Neurol. **302:** 197–205.
18. DARLINGTON, D.N., R.E. MAINS & B.A. EIPPER. 1996. Location of neurons that express regulated endocrine-specific protein-18 in the rat diencephalon. Neuroscience **71:** 477–488.
19. DE OLMOS, J.S. 1969. A cupric-silver method for impregnation of terminal axon degeneration and its further use in staining granular argyrophilic neurons. Brain Behav. Evol. **2:** 213–237.
20. DE OLMOS, J.S. 1972. The amygdaloid projection field in the rat as studied with the cupric silver method. *In* The Neurobiology of the Amygdala. B.E. Eleftheriou, Ed.: 145–204. Plenum Press. New York.
21. DE OLMOS, J.S. 1990. Amygdala. *In* The Human Nervous System. G. Paxinos, Ed.: 583–710. Academic Press. Inc., San Diego, CA.

22. DE OLMOS, J.S., G.F. ALHEID & C.A. BELTRAMINO. 1985. Amygdala. *In* The Rat Nervous System. G. Paxinos, Ed.: 223–334. Academic Press. Sydney.
23. DEUTCH, A.Y. 1993. Prefrontal cortical dopamine systems and the elaboration of functional corticostriatal circuits: implications for schizophrenia and Parkinson's disease. J. Neural. Transm. **91**: 197–221.
24. DEVRIES, G.J. & H.A. AL-SHAMMA. 1990. Sex differences in hormonal responses of vasopressin pathways in the rat brain. J. Neurobiol. **21**: 686–693.
25. FALLON, J.H. 1983. The islands of Calleja complex of rat basal forebrain. II. Connections of medium and large sized cells. Brain Res. Bull. **10**: 775–793.
26. FALLON, J.H., K.B. SEROOGY, S.E. LOUGHLIN, R.S. MORRISON, R.A. BRADSHAW, D.J. KNAUER & D.D. CUNNINGHAM. 1984. Epidermal growth factor immunoreactive material in the central nervous system: location and development. Science **224**: 1107–1109.
27. FINK, R.P. & L. HEIMER. 1967. Two methods for selective silver impregnation of degenerating axons and their synaptic endings in the central nervous system. Brain Res. **4**: 369–374.
28. FLANAGAN-CATO, L.M. & B.S. MCEWEN. 1995. Pattern of Fos and Jun expression in the female rat forebrain after sexual behavior. Brain Res. **673**: 53–60.
29. FREUND-MERCIER, M.J., M.M. DIETL, M.E. STOECKEL, J.M. PALACIOS & P. RICHARD. 1988. Quantitative autoradiographic mapping of neurohypophysial hormone binding sites in the rat forebrain and pituitary gland. II. Comparative study on the Long-Evans and Brattleboro strains. Neuroscience **26**: 273–281.
30. GEERAEDTS, L.M., R. NIEUWENHUYS & J.G. VEENING. 1990. Medial forebrain bundle of the rat. III. Cytoarchitecture of the rostral (telencephalic) part of the medial forebrain bundle bed nucleus. J. Comp. Neurol. **294**: 507–536.
31. GROENEWEGEN, H.J. 1988. Organization of the afferent connections of the mediodorsal thalamic nucleus in the rat, related to the mediodorsal-prefrontal topography, Neuroscience **24**: 379–431.
32. GROENEWEGEN, H.J. 1996. Cortical-subcortical relationships and the limbic forebrain. *In* Contemporary Behavioral Neurology. M.R. Trimble & J.L. Cummings, Eds.: 29–48. Blue Books of Practical Neurology, Vol. 16. C.D. Marsden & A.K. Ashbury, Series Eds. Butterworth-Heineman. Boston.
33. GROENEWEGEN, H.J. & H.W. BERENDSE. 1994. Anatomical relationships between the prefrontal cortex and the basal ganglia in the rat. *In* Motor and Cognitive Functions of the Prefrontal Cortex. A.M. Thierry, J. Glowinski, P.S. Goldman-Rakic & Y. Christen, Eds.: 31–77. Springer-Verlag. Berlin, Heidelberg.
34. GROVE, E.A. 1988. Efferent connections of the substantia innominata in the rat. J. Comp. Neurol. **277**: 347–364.
35. GROVE, E.A. 1988. Neural associations of the substantia innominata in the rat: afferent connections. J. Comp. Neurol. **277**: 315–346.
36. HABER, S.N. & W.J. NAUTA. 1983. Ramifications of the globus pallidus in the rat as indicated by patterns of immunohistochemistry. Neuroscience **9**: 245–260.
37. HEIMER, L. 1971. Pathways in the brain. Sci. Am. **225**: 48–60.
38. HEIMER, L. 1972. The olfactory connections of the diencephalon in the rat. An experimental light- and electron-microscopic study with special emphasis on the problem of terminal degeneration. Brain Behav. Evol. **6**: 484–523.
39. HEIMER, L. 1978. The olfactory cortex and the ventral striatum. *In* Limbic Mechanisms. K.E. Livingston & O. Hornykiewicz, Eds.: 95–187. Plenum Press. New York.
40. HEIMER, L., G.F. ALHEID, J.S. DEOLMOS, H.J. GROENEWEGEN, S.N. HABER, R.E. HARLAN & D.S. ZAHM. 1997. The accumbens beyond the core shell dichotomy. J. Neuropsychiatry Clin. Neurosci. **9**: 354–381.
41. HEIMER, L., G.F. ALHEID & D.S. ZAHM. 1993. Basal forebrain organization: an anatomical framework for motor aspects of drive and motivation. *In* Limbic Motor Circuits and Neuropsychiatry. P.W. Kalivas & C.D. Barnes, Eds.: 1–43. CRC Press. Boca Raton, Florida.
42. HEIMER, L., J. DE OLMOS, G.F. ALHEID, J. PEARSON, M. SAKAMOTO, J. MARKSTEINER & R.C. SWITZER III. 1999. The human basal forebrain, part 2. *In* Handbook of

Chemical Neuroanatomy, Vol. 15. The Primate Nervous System, Part III. F.E. Bloom, A. Björklund & T. Hökfelt, Eds. Elsevier. Amsterdam. In press.
43. HEIMER, L., J. DE OLMOS, G.F. ALHEID & L. ZABORSZKY. 1991. "Perestroika" in the basal forebrain: opening the border between neurology and psychiatry. [Review] Prog. Brain Res. **87:** 109–165.
44. HEIMER, L., R.E. HARLAN, G.F. ALHEID, M. GARCIA & J. DE OLMOS. 1997. Substantia innominata: a notion which impedes clinical-anatomical correlations in neuropsychiatric disorders. Neuroscience **76:** 957–1006.
45. HEIMER, L. & G.W. VAN HOESEN. 1979. Ventral striatum. In The Neostriatum. I. Divac & G.E. Oberg, Eds.: 147–158. Pergamon Press. New York.
46. HEIMER, L. & R.D. WILSON. 1975. The subcortical projections of allocortex: similarities in the neuronal associations of the hippocampus, the piriform cortex and the neocortex. In Golgi Centennial Symposium Proceedings. M. Santini, Ed.: 173–193. Raven Press. New York.
47. HEIMER, L., L. ZABORSZKY, D.S. ZAHM & G.F. ALHEID. 1987. The ventral striatopallidothalamic projection. I. The striatopallidal link originating in the striatal parts of the olfactory tubercle. J. Comp. Neurol. **255:** 571–591.
48. HEIMER, L., D.S. ZAHM & G.F. ALHEID. 1995. Basal ganglia. In The Rat Nervous System, 2nd edition. G. Paxinos, Ed.: 579–628. Academic Press. San Diego, CA.
49. HEIMER, L., D.S. ZAHM, L. CHURCHILL, P.W. KALIVAS & C. WOHLTMANN. 1991. Specificity in the projection patterns of accumbal core and shell in the rat. Neuroscience **41:** 89–125.
50. HOLSTEGE, G., L. MEINERS & K. TAN. 1985. Projections of the bed nucleus of the stria terminalis to the mesencephalon, pons, and medulla oblongata in the cat. Exp. Brain Res. **58:** 379–391.
51. HORN, C.C. & M.I. FRIEDMAN. 1998. Methyl palmoxirate increases eating behavior and brain fos-like immunoreactivity in rats. Brain Res. **781:** 8–14.
52. HUBSCHLE, T., M.J. MCKINLEY & B.J. OLDFIELD. 1998. Efferent connections of the lamina terminalis, the preoptic area and the insular cortex to submandibular and sublingual gland of the rat traced with pseudorabies virus. Brain Res. **806:** 219–231.
53. JACKSON, A. & A.R. CROSSMAN. 1981. Basal ganglia and other afferent projections to the peribrachial region in the rat: a study using retrograde and anterograde transport of horseradish peroxidase. Neuroscience **6:** 1537–1549.
54. JAKAB, R.L., T.L. HORVATH, C. LERANTH, N. HARADA & F. NAFTOLIN. 1993. Aromatase immunoreactivity in the rat brain: gonadectomy-sensitive hypothalamic neurons and an unresponsive "limbic ring" of the lateral septum-bed nucleus-amygdala complex. J. Steroid Biochem. Mol. Biol. **44:** 481–498.
55. JOHNSTON, J.B. 1923. Further contribution to the study of the evolution of the forebrain. J. Comp. Neurol. **35:** 337–481.
56. JOYCE, J.N. 1993. The dopamine hypothesis of schizophrenia: limbic interactions with serotonin and norepinephrine. Psychopharmacology **112:** S16–S34.
57. KITA, H., T. KOSAKA & C.W. HEIZMANN. 1990. Parvalbumin-immunoreactive neurons in the rat neostriatum: a light and electron microscopic study. Brain Res. **536:** 1–15.
58. KOOB, G.F. & M. LEMOAL. 1997. Drug abuse: hedonic homeostatic dysregulation., Science **278:** 52–58.
59. MAKINO, S., P.W. GOLD & J. SCHULKIN. 1994. Effects of corticosterone on CRH mRNA and content in the bed nucleus of the stria terminalis; comparison with the effects in the central nucleus of the amygdala and the paraventricular nucleus of the hypothalamus. Brain Res. **657:** 141–149.
60. MARIN, O., W.J. SMEETS & A. GONZALEZ. 1997. Basal ganglia organization in amphibians: development of striatal and nucleus accumbens connections with emphasis on the catecholaminergic inputs. J. Comp. Neurol. **383:** 349–369.
61. MEDINA, L., E. MARTI, C. ARTERO, A. FASOLO & L. PUELLES. 1992. Distribution of neuropeptide Y-like immunoreactivity in the brain of the lizard Gallotia galloti. J. Comp. Neurol. **319:** 387–405.

62. MEGA, M.S. & J.L. CUMMINGS. 1994. Frontal-subcortical circuits and neuropsychiatric disorders. J. Neuropsychiatry **6:** 358–370.
63. MEREDITH, G.E. & S. TOTTERDELL. 1999. Microcircuits in nucleus accumbens' shell and core involved in cognition and reward. Psychobiology. In press.
64. MILLHOUSE, O.E. & L. HEIMER. 1984. Cell configurations in the olfactory tubercle of the rat. J. Comp. Neurol. **228:** 571–597.
65. MODELL, J.G., J.M. MOUNTZ, G.C. CURTIS & J.F. GREDEN. 1989. Neurophysiologic dysfunction in basal ganglia/limbic striatal and thalamocortical circuits as a pathogenetic mechanism of obsessive-compulsive disorder. J. Neuropsychiatry Clin. Neurosci. **1:** 27–36.
66. MOGA, M.M., H. HERBERT, K.M. HURLEY, Y. YASUI, T.S. GRAY & C.B. SAPER. 1990. Organization of cortical, basal forebrain, and hypothalamic afferents to the parabrachial nucleus in the rat. J. Comp. Neurol. **295:** 624–661.
67. MORILAK, D.A., S.J. GARLOW & R.D. CIARANELLO. 1993. Immunocytochemical localization and description of neurons expressing serotonin2 receptors in the rat brain. Neuroscience **54:** 701–717.
68. MUGNAINI, E. & W.H. OERTEL. 1985. An atlas of the distribution of GABAergic neurons and terminals in the rat CNS as revealed by GAD immunohistochemistry. *In* Handbook of Chemical Neuroanatomy, Vol. 4. GABA and Neuropeptides in the CNS, Part 1. A. Björklund & T. Hökfelt, Eds.: 436–608. Elsevier. Amsterdam.
69. NEWMAN, R. & S.S. WINANS. 1980. An experimental study of the ventral striatum of the golden hamster. II. Neuronal connections of the olfactory tubercle. J. Comp. Neurol. **191:** 193–212.
70. PAXINOS, G. & C. WATSON. 1986. The Rat Brain in Stereotaxic Coordinates, 2nd Edition. Academic Press. Sydney.
71. PAXINOS, G. & C. WATSON. 1997. The rat brain. *In* Stereotaxic Coordinates, 3rd Edition. Academic Press. San Diego.
72. PIERCE, R.C. & P.W. KALIVAS. 1995. Amphetamine produces sensitized increases in locomotion and extracellular dopamine preferentially in the nucleus accumbens shell of rats administered repeated cocaine. J. Pharmacol. Exp. Ther. **275:** 1019–1029.
73. PIGGINS, H.D., J.A. STAMP, J. BURNS, B. RUSAK & K. SEMBA. 1996. Distribution of pituitary adenylate cyclase activating polypeptide (PACAP) immunoreactivity in the hypothalamus and extended amygdala of the rat. J. Comp. Neurol. **376:** 278–294.
74. PONTIERI, F.E., G. TANDA & G. DI CHIARA. 1995. Intravenous cocaine, morphine, and amphetamine preferentially increase extracellular dopamine in the "shell" as compared with the "core" of the rat nucleus accumbens. Proc. Natl. Acad. Sci. USA **92:** 12304–12308.
75. PONTIERI, F.E., G. TANDA, F. ORZI & G. DI CHIARA. 1996. Effects of nicotine on the nucleus accumbens and similarity to those of addictive drugs. Nature **382:** 255–257.
76. ROSIN, D.L., A. ROBEVA, R.L. WOODARD, P.G. GUYENET & J. LINDEN. 1998. Immunohistochemical localization of adenosine A_{2A} receptors in the rat central nervous system. J. Comp. Neurol. **401:** 163–186.
77. SAGAR, S.M., K.J. PRICE, N.W. KASTING & F.R. SHARP. 1995. Anatomic patterns of Fos immunostaining in rat brain following systemic endotoxin administration. Brain Res. Bull. **36:** 381–392.
78. SALLOWAY, S. & J. CUMMINGS. 1994. Subcortical disease and neuropsychiatric illness. J. Neuropsychiatry **6:** 93–99.
79. SANIDES, F. 1957. Die Insulae terminales des Erwachsenen Gehirns des Menschen. J. Hirnforsch. **3:** 243–273.
80. SCHWABER, J.S., B.S. KAPP, G.A. HIGGINS & P.R. RAPP. 1982. Amygdaloid and basal forebrain direct connections with the nucleus of the solitary tract and the dorsal motor nucleus. J. Neurosci. **2:** 424–1438.
81. SCHWANZEL-FUKUDA, M., J.I. MORRELL & D.W. PFAFF. 1984. Localization of forebrain neurons which project directly to the medulla and spinal cord of the rat by retrograde tracing with wheat germ agglutinin. J. Comp. Neurol. **226:** 1–20.

82. SHAMMAH-LAGNADO, S.J., G.F. ALHEID & L. HEIMER. 1999. Afferent connections of the interstitial nucleus of the posterior limb of the anterior commissure and adjacent amygdalostriatal transition area in the rat. Neuroscience. Submitted.
83. SIMERLY, R.B. & L.W. SWANSON. 1987. Castration reversibly alters levels of cholecystokinin immunoreactivity within cells of three interconnected sexually dimorphic forebrain nuclei in the rat. Proc. Natl. Acad. Sci. USA **84:** 2087–2091.
84. SKOFITSCH, G. & D.M. JACOBOWITZ. 1985. Calcitonin gene-related peptide: detailed immunohistochemical distribution in the central nervous system Peptides **6:** 721–745.
85. SKOFITSCH, G. & D.M JACOBOWITZ. 1992. Calcitonin- and calcitonin gene-related peptide: receptor binding sites in the central nervous system. *In* Handbook of Chemical Neuroanatomy, Vol. 11. Neuropeptide Receptors in the CNS. A. Björklund, T. Hökfelt & M.J. Kuhar, Eds.: 97–144. Elsevier. Amsterdam,
86. SONG, D.D. & R.E.HARLAN. 1993. Ontogeny of the proenkephalin system in the rat corpus striatum: its relationship to dopaminergic innervation and transient compartmental expression. Neuroscience **52:** 883–909.
87. SONG, D.D. & R.E. HARLAN. 1994. The development of enkephalin and substance P neurons in the basal ganglia: insights into neostriatal compartments and the extended amygdala. Dev. Brain Res. **83:** 247–261.
88. STRENGE, H., E. BRAAK & H. BRAAK. 1977. Über den Nucleus striae terminalis im Gehirn des erwachsenen Menschen. Z. Mikrosk. Anat. Forsch. Leipzig **91:**1.S. 105–118.
89. SWANSON, L.W. & W.M. COWAN. 1975. A note on the connections and development of the nucleus accumbens. Brain Res. **92:** 324–330.
90. SWANSON, L.W. & G.D. PETROVICH. 1998. What is the amygdala? Trends Neurosci. **21:** 323–331.
91. SWERDLOW, N.R. & G.F. KOOB. 1987. Dopamine, schizophrenia, mania and depression: toward a unified hypothesis of cortico-striato-pallido-thalamic function. Behav. Brain Sci. **10:** 197–245.
92. SWITZER, R.C., J. HILL & L. HEIMER. 1982. The globus pallidus and its rostroventral extension into the olfactory tubercle of the rat: a cyto- and chemoarchitectural study. Neuroscience **7:** 1891–1904.
93. TRIBOLLET, E. 1992. Vasopressin and oxytocin receptors in the rat brain. *In* Handbook of Chemical Neuroanatomy, Vol. 11. Neuropeptide Receptors in the CNS. A. Björklund, T. Hökfelt & M.J. Kuhar, Eds.: 289–320. Elsevier. Amsterdam.
94. VEINANTE, P. & M.J. FREUND-MERCIER. 1997. Distribution of oxytocin- and vasopressin-binding sites in the rat extended amygdala: a histoautoradiographic study. J. Comp. Neurol. **383:** 305–325.
95. YOUNG, W.S., G.F. ALHEID & L. HEIMER. 1984. The ventral pallidal projection to the mediodorsal thalamus: a study with fluorescent retrograde tracers and immunohistofluorescence. J. Neurosci. **4:** 1626–1638.
96. ZABORSZKY, L., G.F. ALHEID, M.C. BEINFELD, L.E. EIDEN, L. HEIMER & M. PALKOVITS. 1985. Cholecystokinin innervation of the ventral striatum: a morphological and radioimmunological study. Neuroscience **14:** 427–453.
97. ZAHM, D.S. 1998. Is the caudomedial shell of the nucleus accumbens part of the extended amygdala? A consideration of connections. Crit. Rev. Neurobiol. **12:** 245–265.
98. ZAHM, D.S. & J.S. BROG. 1992. On the significance of subterritories in the "accumbens" part of the rat ventral striatum. Neuroscience **50:** 751–767.
99. ZAHM, D.S. & L. HEIMER. 1987. The ventral striatopallidothalamic projection. III. Striatal cells of the olfactory tubercle establish direct synaptic contact with ventral pallidal cells projecting to mediodorsal thalamus. Brain Res. **404:** 327–331.
100. ZAHM, D.S., L. ZABORSZKY, G.F. ALHEID & L. HEIMER. 1987. The ventral striatopallidothalamic projection. II. The ventral pallidothalamic link. J. Comp. Neurol. **255:** 592–605.

The Concept of the Ventral Striatum in Nonhuman Primates

SUZANNE N. HABER[a] AND NIKOLAUS R. McFARLAND

Department of Neurobiology and Anatomy, University of Rochester School of Medicine, 601 Elmwood Avenue, Rochester, New York 14642, USA

ABSTRACT: The concept of the ventral striatum was first put forth by Heimer and Wilson to describe the extension of basal ganglia elements into the olfactory tubercle. The ventral striatum includes the conventional nucleus accumbens, which has been closely associated with reward and motivation. This paper uses the afferent connections to the ventral striatum to define this region in monkeys. Furthermore the shell and core subterritories are discussed with respect to their histochemistry and specific connections.

INTRODUCTION

This chapter addresses how the primate ventral striatum and the subterritories within it might be defined based on afferent connections from structures associated with reward and motivation. The nucleus accumbens is that part of the ventral striatum that has long been associated with the limbic system or with that group of structures thought to mediate motivational and emotional responses to environmental stimuli. This association is based on, among other things, its afferent connections from the amygdala and prefrontal cortical areas, considered to be involved in mechanisms of reward and positive reinforcement. The concept of the ventral striatum was originally developed in the classic paper by Heimer and Wilson in 1975 that describes the relationship between the nucleus accumbens and the olfactory tubercle in rats. The authors showed that striatal-like and pallidal-like elements of the olfactory tubercle constitute a ventral continuation of the striatum, and, therefore, together with the nucleus accumbens, these structures should be referred to as the ventral striatum.[1] Since then, the ventral striatum and its connections have been at the center of the reward circuit, and, as such, have been a research focus of the neurobiological mechanisms underlying drug addiction and mental disorders.[2-4] Thus, our concept of the striatal region implicated in reward has evolved to include more than the traditional boundary of the nucleus accumbens, and it extends into the ventral forebrain.

SUBTERRITORIES OF THE VENTRAL STRIATUM

Recently, a subterritory of the ventral striatum, the shell region, has been identified dividing the ventral striatum into two parts, a medial/ventral shell region, and a

---

[a]Voice: 716-275-4538; fax: 716-442-8766; suzanne_haber@urmc.rochester.edu

central core region.[5] Experiments aimed at delineating the functional significance of these two regions have been instrumental in understanding the circuitry underlying goal-directed behaviors, behavioral sensitization, and changes in affective states. Studies in rodents have been particularly important in demonstrating the organization of the shell and core and their relationship to distinct ventral striatal afferent and efferent projections. These studies provide critical information on how interactions between specific transmitter/receptor pathways mediate the transition between motivating stimuli and motor outcome.[6–11] Whereas several transmitter and receptor distribution patterns distinguish the shell/core subterritories, calbindin-28 is the most consistent marker for the shell across species.[12]

In primates, as in rodents, the ventral striatum is divided into two territories: the inner core, which is calbindin rich, and the outer crescent-shaped shell, which is calbindin poor. Although a calbindin poor region marks the subterritory of the shell, staining intensity of other histochemical markers varies both within the shell and in distinguishing it from the core. These markers include enkephalin; acetylcholinesterase; neurotensin; the μ opiate receptor; the growth-associated protein, GAP-43; the AMPA subunits, GluR1, GluR2/3, and GluR4; the dopamine transporter; and serotonin. In general, compared to the core, the shell is rich in GluR1, GAP-43, acetylcholinesterase, μ receptor binding, serotonin, and substance P[13–18] (FIG. 1). Substance P is distributed in patches throughout the striatum but is particularly dense in the shell. Acetylcholinesterase is very dense in the medial part of the shell. More laterally, however, the staining blends into the core and becomes indistinguishable from that observed in the remainder of the ventral striatum. Immunoreactivity for neurotensin is relatively low throughout the striatum; however, staining is dense in the medial rim of the shell. Enkephalin immunoreactivity is patchy throughout the striatum and does not show a remarkable differential pattern between the shell and core. Serotonin staining is dense in the shell, with the highest immunoreactivity in the medial dorsal portion. The dopamine transporter is relatively low throughout the ventral striatum, including the core. This pattern is consistent with the fact that the dorsal tier dopamine neurons express relatively low levels of mRNA for the dopamine transporter compared to the ventral tier.[19] Whereas GAP-43 immunoreactivity is found throughout the adult striatum, the shell region stands out with the strongest antisera reaction. The μ receptor distribution is dense but patchy in the ventral striatum. There are dense patches in the medial and ventral shell, with the remainder remarkably free of receptor. By contrast, the core shows numerous patches of immunoreactivity that extend into the medial wall of the ventral caudate. Most of the excitatory amino acid receptors do not distinguish the dorsal striatum and ventral striatum. However, the AMPA receptor subunits do. The GluR1 subunit shows particularly dense immunoreactivity in the shell, with patches of reactivity in the core. By contrast, the GluR4 subunit shows weaker immunoreactivity in the shell than in the rest of the striatum. Taken together, neurotransmitters and receptors help distinguish the ventral and medial borders of the ventral striatum and the shell/core subterritories within it. However, the dorsal and lateral boundaries are more problematic. Here, the ventral striatum merges imperceptibly with the dorsal striatum.

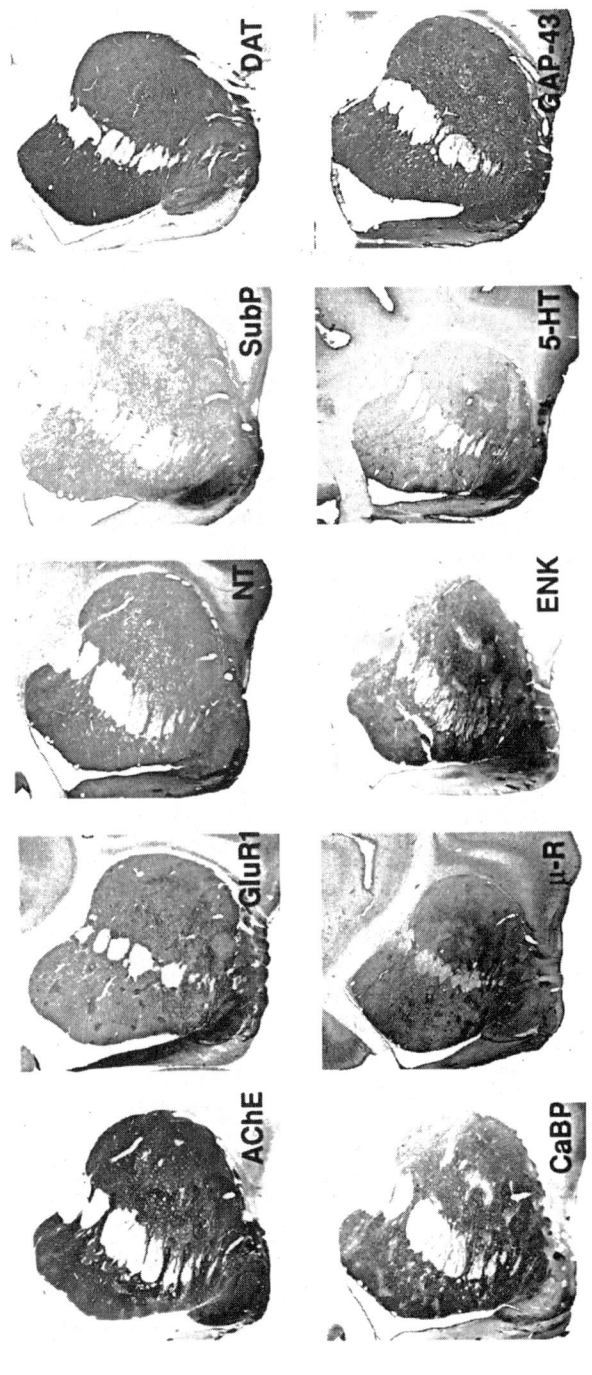

FIGURE 1. Photomicrographs of the striatum at the level of the shell and core, immunostained for various transmitter-related molecules. AChE, acetylcholinesterase; NT, neurotensin; SubP, substance P; DAT, dopamine transporter; CaBP, calbindin-28; μ-R, μ-opiate receptor; ENK, enkephalin; 5-HT, serotonin; GAP-43, growth-associated protein-43.

DISTINGUISHING THE VENTRAL FROM DORSAL STRIATAL TERRITORY

Several morphological characteristics are unique to the ventral striatum. It contains smaller and more densely packed neurons than the more homogenous dorsal striatum. Furthermore the organization of striosome (patch)-matrix compartments observed in the dorsal striatum is not characteristic of the ventral striatum. Instead, a complex relationship between transmitter systems exists that is not easily defined by a two-compartment system. Finally, unlike the dorsal striatum, the ventral striatum is invaded by many pallidal elements.[13,20,21] Although these are important distinguishing features, neither these cytoarchitectonic distinctions nor histochemical markers indicate a clear boundary between it and the dorsal striatum. Thus, the border between the core and the dorsal striatum is ambiguous. Given the central importance of this region for understanding the motivational neuronal networks and the fact that it is the target of studies that focus on the underlying mechanisms of response to emotional stimuli, we set out to gain a better definition of what to include in the ventral striatal territory in nonhuman primates and how to distinguish it from the dorsal striatum.

Because the ventral striatum is considered to be that part of the striatum associated with "reward," an operational anatomic definition of its boundaries should be based on afferent projections from brain regions important for mediating the development of reward-associated responses. The main afferent projection to the striatum is from the cortex. Frontal cortical inputs to the striatum are massive and represent the defining feature of separate functional circuits.[22–25] Information flow through the basal ganglia begins in functionally distinct regions of the frontal cortex as nodal points, with projections to anatomically distinct sectors of the striatum, the pallidum, the substantia nigra, and the thalamus. The thalamocortical pathway completes the circuit to frontal cortex. These pathways form functionally distinct loop systems that include the sensorimotor circuit (sensorimotor cortex); strategic planning and procedural memory circuit (dorsolateral prefrontal cortex); and the development of reward-associated responses, or the limbic circuit (medial and orbital prefrontal cortex, OMPFC). In addition to cortex, the other two main inputs to the striatum are from the thalamus and midbrain. All three afferent projecting systems are multifunctional, in that they contain distinct nuclear groups or regions, each involved specifically in sensorimotor, cognitive, or emotive processing. Our criteria for defining the ventral striatal region is that the afferent connections be derived from the OMPFC and thalamic and midbrain regions associated with reward, and exclude inputs from other cortical, thalamic, and midbrain regions. We used retrograde tracer techniques to characterize the afferent organization to the striatum from cortex, thalamus, and midbrain.[26–30]

Frontal Cortical Projections to the Striatum

The association of the frontal cortex with specific functions is well established. The orbital and medial prefrontal cortex (OMPFC) is involved in linking primary rewards with motivational and emotional features and plays a key role in the development of reward-guided behaviors. Lesions result in an inability to initiate and carry out goal-directed behaviors.[31-35] The recruitment of activity in the OMPFC with be-

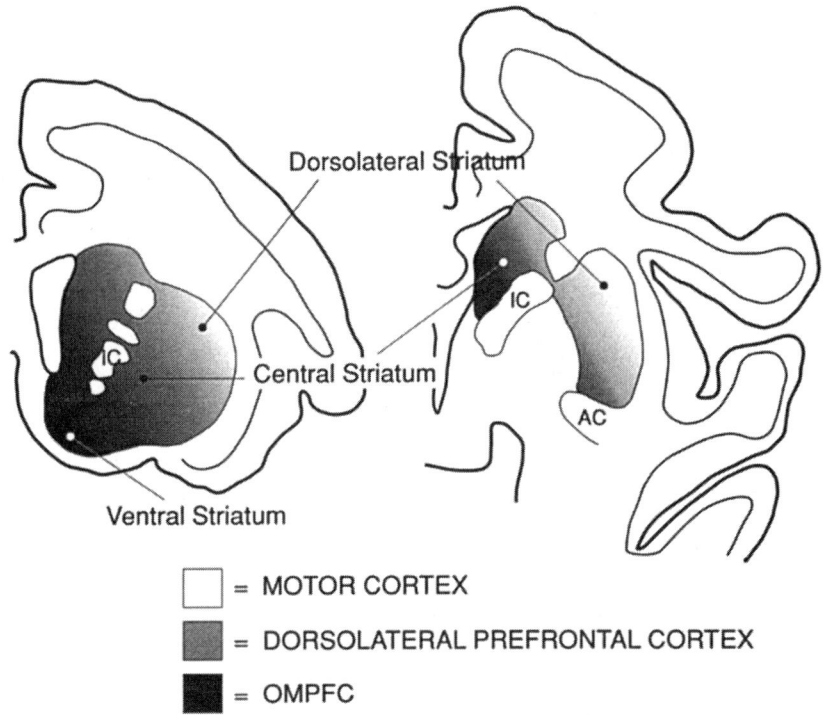

FIGURE 2. Schematic of corticostriatal topography.

haviors dependent on motivation and positive reinforcement is consistent with anatomical and physiological studies of the OMPFC. It receives input from, and can be stimulated by, olfactory, gustatory, and visceral sensations, all related to the assessment of palatable foods. These sensory afferent projections, coupled with visual input that associates food reward with an object, and inputs from the amygdala, attach emotional components to the primary reward.[36–43] By contrast, motor, premotor, and supplementary motor cortices (areas 4, 6, and 8) are involved in motor and sensorimotor function and integration, and the dorsolateral prefrontal cortex (areas 46, 45, and 9) is involved in procedural learning and strategic planning.[22, 25]

Projections from frontal regions form a functional gradient of inputs from the ventromedial sector through the dorsolateral striatum, with the OMPFC terminating in the ventromedial part, and the motor cortex terminating in the dorsolateral region (see FIG. 2). Within this gradient, our studies indicate that the cortical projections to the striatum are quite precise, and, depending on the location of relatively small injection sites, only specific cortical regions contain labeled cells (FIG. 3). In general, motor areas (areas 4, 6, and 8), but not from the OMPFC, project to the dorsolateral striatum. By contrast, the OMPFC (areas 24, 25, 32, 14, 13, and 12) projects to the ventral striatum, but not to the dorsolateral striatum. The dorsolateral prefrontal cortex (areas 9, 46, and 45) projects centrally, with little or no afferent projection to the calbindin-poor shell region or to the ventral rostral putamen, the ventral caudate nu-

Cortical Area	Ventromedial Cases								Central				Dorsolateral Cases								
	82	28	33	13	94W	38	35		89	94L	96		39	32	44	43	45	29	37	66L	102
4	-	-	-	-	-	-	-		-	-	-		+++	-	+++	++++	++	++	+++	++++	++++
6	-	-	-	-	-	-	-		++	-	-		+++	++	++++	++++	+++	++	++	+	+
24c	-	-	-	-	-	-	-		++	++	+++		-	-	+	+	+	++	++++	+++	++
8	-	-	-	-	-	-	-		-	++	++++		-	-	-	-	-	-	-	-	-
9	-	-	-	-	-	-	-		+++	+	+		-	-	-	-	-	-	-	-	-
45/46	-	-	-	-	-	-	+		++++	+++	++++		-	-	-	-	-	-	-	-	-
12	-	+	++	++	++	+++	++		+++	++	++		-	-	-	-	-	-	-	-	-
11	-	-	++	++	-	++++	+		+	+	+		-	-	-	-	-	-	-	-	-
13	-	-	+	-	++	+++	++		++	+	-		-	-	-	-	-	-	-	-	-
13a/b	-	++	++	++++	++	++	+		+	-	-		-	+	-	-	-	-	-	-	-
24a/b	-	++++	++++	++++	+	++	++++		+++	+	++		-	-	-	-	-	-	-	-	-
32	+	++	++	++	++	+	-		++	-	-		-	-	-	-	-	-	-	-	-
14	++	+++	++	++	++	++	-		+	-	-		-	-	-	-	-	-	-	-	-
Ia	++++	+++	++++	++++	+	++	-		-	-	-		-	-	-	-	-	-	-	-	-
25	++++	++++	++++	++++	++	++	++		+	-	-		-	-	-	-	-	-	-	-	-

FIGURE 3. Corticostriatal projections. Relative density of retrogradely labeled neurons in frontal cortical areas after injections of retrograde tracers into ventral, central, and dorsolateral striatal regions.

cleus, and the medial wall of the rostral caudate nucleus. Thus, the ventral striatum in primates can be viewed as that part of the striatum that receives prefrontal lobe input from the OMPFC but not from the dorsolateral prefrontal cortex or the sensorimotor cortex.

Thalamic Projections to the Striatum

Projections to the striatum from the thalamus are derived from the midline, the intralaminar nuclei, and the ventral tier nuclear group. The midline thalamic nuclei are most closely associated with the limbic system by virtue of their connections to the amygdala, hypothalamus, and cingulate cortex. The ventral tier nuclei and the centromedian nucleus of the intralaminar group are most closely aligned with the motor system via their connections to the motor and premotor cortex. Finally, the parafascicular nucleus of the intralaminar group and the dorsomedial nucleus are associated with the dorsolateral prefrontal area.[44,47] Although the boundaries within the intralaminar group are difficult to define, the more lateral portions of the intralaminar complex are connected to the motor cortex, whereas the medial regions are connected to the prefrontal areas. The midline nuclei and the medial parafascicular nucleus project to the ventral striatum, whereas the ventral tier and the centromedian nucleus project to the dorsolateral "sensorimotor" striatum. The midline thalamic nuclei and medial part of the parafascicular nucleus do not project to the

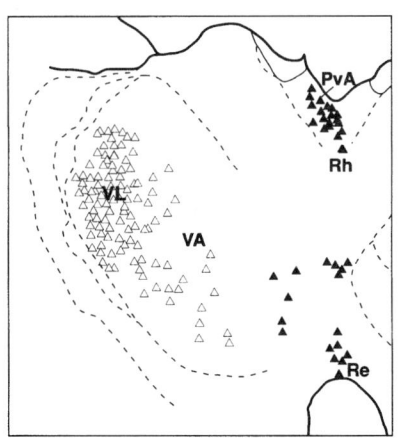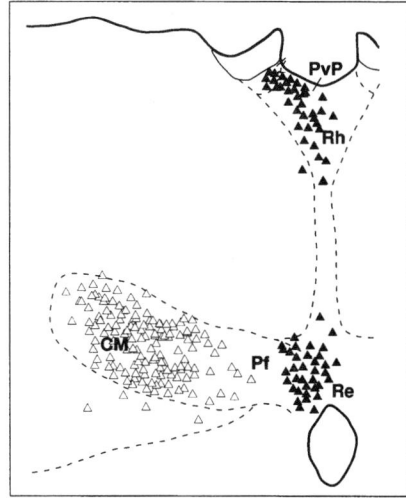

FIGURE 4. Thalamostriatal projections. Distribution of labeled cells in the thalamus after injections of retrograde tracers into the dorsolateral and ventral striatum. Filled triangles, distribution of cells labeled following ventral striatal injection sites; unfilled triangles, distribution of cells labeled following dorsolateral injection sites. CM, center median nucleus; Pf, parafascicular nucleus; PvA, anterior paraventricular nucleus; PvP posterior paraventricular nucleus; Rh, rhomboid nucleus; Re, nucleus reuniens; VA, ventral anterior nucleus; VL, ventral lateral nucleus.

dorsal striatum, and, conversely, the centromedian nucleus and the ventral tier nuclei do not project to the ventral striatum. In contrast to the ventral striatum, the dorsolateral striatum receives input from the lateral intralaminar nuclei (FIG. 4). These thalamostriatal projections support the notion that inputs to the striatum are organized along functional domains, with the ventral striatum receiving its thalamic input from the neurons located on or near the midline.

Midbrain Dopamine Projections to the Striatum

The midbrain dopamine neurons are divided into two groups: a dorsal tier and a ventral tier. The dorsal tier includes both the dorsal substantia nigra, pars compacta (SNc) and the contiguous ventral tegmental area (VTA). Cells in this region are oriented horizontally and are calbindini positive. The ventral tier cells are calbindin negative and include both the densocellular cell group and the cell columns that extend deep into the pars reticulata (FIG. 5a). Inputs to all striatal regions are from the entire rostrocaudal extent of the substantia nigra. The midbrain input to the sensorimotor-related striatum is from the ventral tier of dopaminergic neurons, both the densocellular region and the cell columns. The dorsal tier (the VTA and the dorsal SNc) do not project here.[30] Within the densocellular region, groups of cells that project to the sensorimotor striatum are found in the lateral two thirds; these cells do not extend to its medial border with the VTA. The projections to the ventral striatum originate primarily from the medial half of the midbrain neurons, but from both the dorsal and ventral tiers. However, it is only the densocellular region of the ventral tier that projects here: the cell columns do not.[30,48] The midbrain projections to the central region of the striatum are derived from a wide range of dopaminergic neurons in both the dorsal and ventral tiers. The majority come from the densocellular part of the ventral tier, but some come also from the dorsal SNc. Thus, three groups of neurons can be distinguished: the dorsal tier, which projects to the ventral striatum; the cell columns, which project to the dorsolateral striatum; and an intermediate area, the densocellular part of the ventral tier, which projects primarily to the central striatum (FIG. 5b). However, within the densocellular group, there is some intermingling of cells that project to different striatal territories. This results in a large area of the striatum that is modulated by inputs from the densocellular group.

Summary of Corticostriatal Topography

Based on the afferent projections from cortex, thalamus, and midbrain, we can define the ventral striatum as that part of the striatum that receives inputs from the OMPFC but not from motor, premotor, or supplementary motor regions of the frontal cortex and few, if any, from areas 9 and 46. In addition, the amygdala, the most widely recognized structure associated with emotional behavior projects extensively to the ventral striatum.[49–54] Our experiments demonstrate that, in contrast to the ventral striatum, there were no labeled cells in the amygdala following retrograde tracer injections into the dorsolateral (sensorimotor) striatum. It receives input from the midline thalamic nuclei and the medial-most part of the intralaminar nuclear group. The lateral part of the intralaminar nuclei and the ventral lateral nucleus do not project here. Finally, the dorsal tier of the midbrain dopamine neurons and the dorsal part of the densocellular group project to the ventral striatum. By contrast, the cell

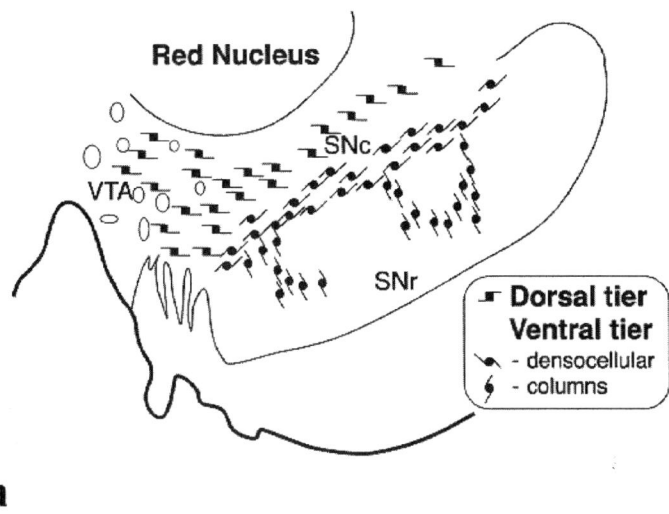

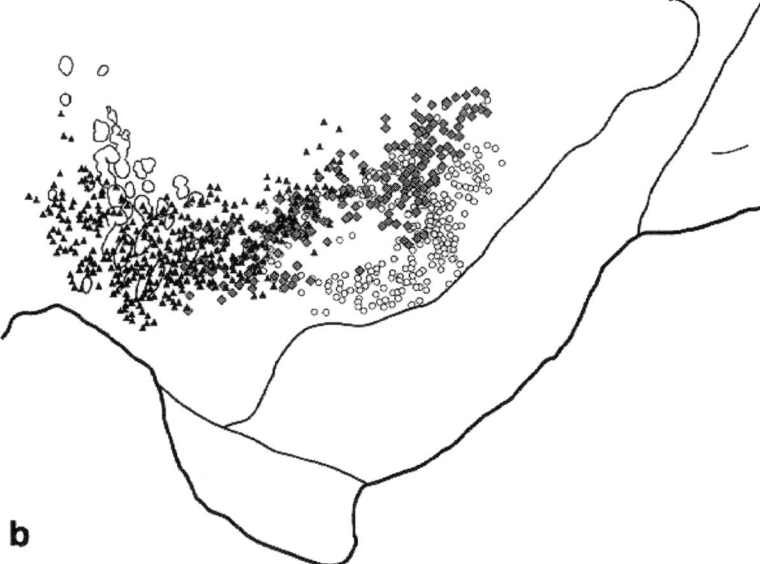

FIGURE 5. a: Schematic of the substantia nigra in the tiers of the midbrain dopamine neurons. VTA, ventral tegmental area; SNc, substantia nigra, pars compacta; SNr, substantia nigra, pars reticulata. **b:** Midbrain striatal projections. Distribution of labeled cells in the midbrain after injections of retrograde tracers into the dorsolateral and ventral striatum. Filled triangles, distribution of cells labeled following ventral striatal injection sites; filled diamonds, distribution of cells labeled following central injection sites; unfilled circles, distribution of cells labeled following dorsolateral injection sites.

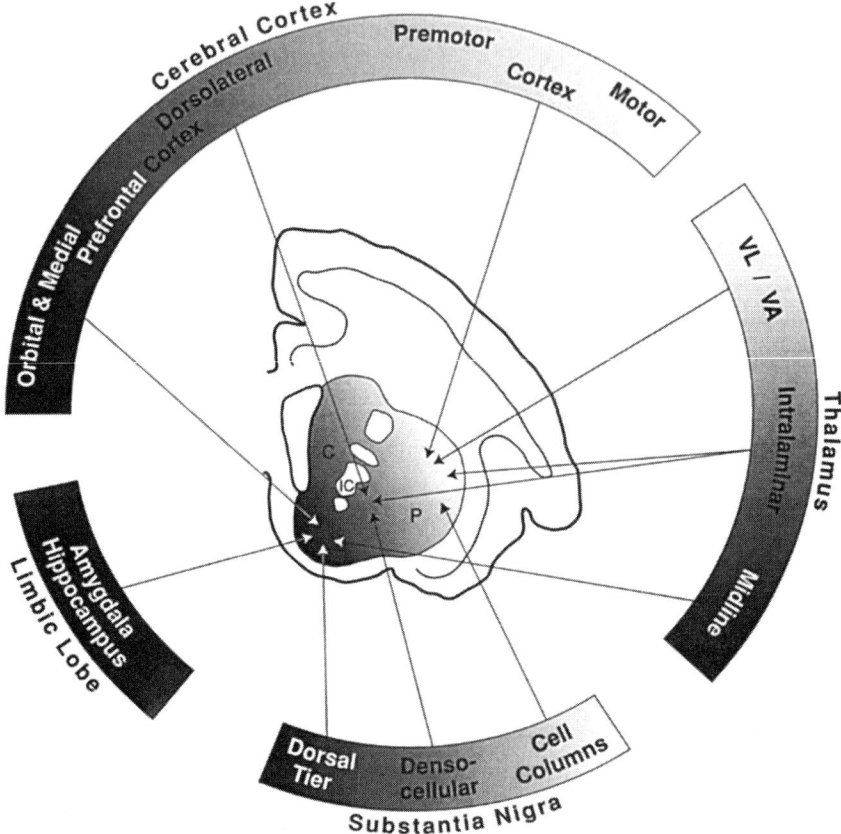

FIGURE 6. Summary diagram illustrating striatal territories based on inputs from specific cortical, thalamic, and midbrain regions.

columns do not. The ventral striatum receives little, if any, input from the dorsolateral prefrontal cortex. However, at the junction between the ventral striatum and the central striatum, projections from the OMPFC and dorsolateral prefrontal cortex do overlap. This transition region also receives mixed innervation from the intralaminar nuclei of the thalamus and the densocellular midbrain group (FIG. 6).

SPECIFICITY OF PROJECTIONS TO THE VENTRAL STRIATUM

OMPFC Projections

The OMPFC includes the anterior cingulate cortex, medial and lateral orbital cortex, and agranular insular cortex (Ia).[55] Based on clinical, behavioral, and connectional studies, the OMPFC can be divided into general areas: a medial prefrontal region (areas 25, 24a/b, and 32), a medial orbital region (areas 13a/b, 11, and 14), and a lateral region (areas 12, 13m, and 131). Areas 25 and Ia are most closely linked to connections with the amygdala. Areas 24 a/b, 14, and 13a/b are in a pivotal position. Like areas 25 and Ia, they receive input from the amygdala, albeit less. Area 13 receives the least input from the amygdala. Thus, these prefrontal cortical areas are arranged, such that areas 24 a/b and 13a/b provide a bridge between areas receiving a dense projection from the amygdala and those that do not.[38,39]

Our retrograde studies show that the shell receives the densest OMPFC innervation from medial areas 25.14 and 32, 24a/b, and Ia. The medial shell has the most limited inputs, which are from areas 25, 14, and Ia. In addition to afferent projections from these areas, the ventral shell receives input from areas 24 a/b and area 32. Medial areas 25, 14, 24, and 32 also project to the medial wall of the caudate nucleus. This area of the caudate nucleus also receives a dense innervation from areas 13a/b and from parts of the dysgranular insular cortex. By contrast, the central and more

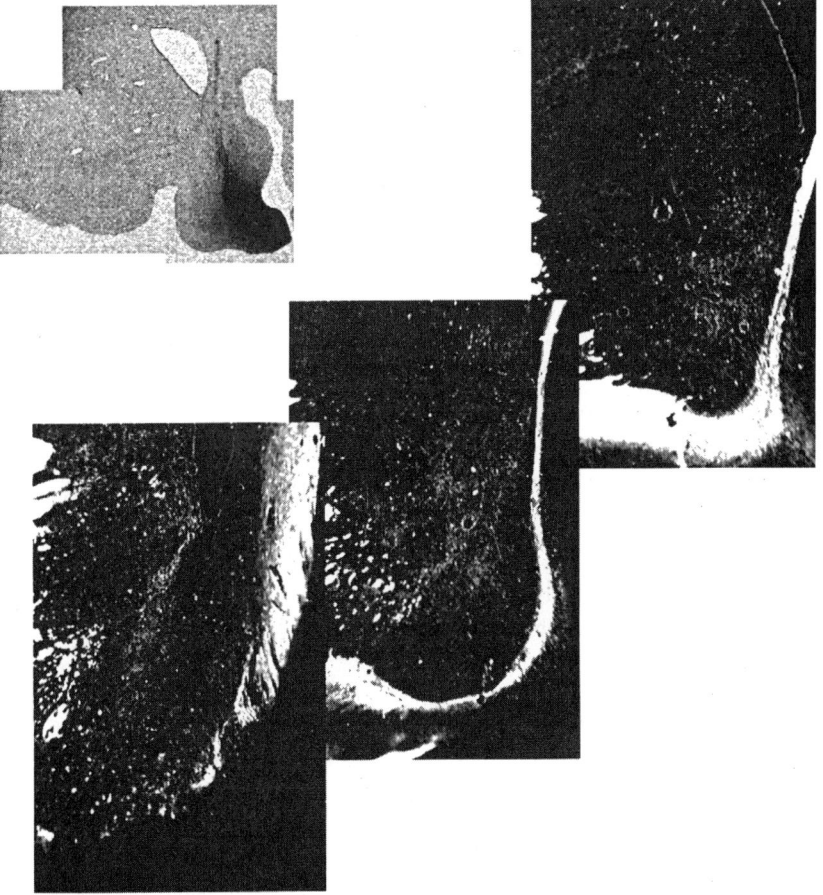

FIGURE 7. Fiber distribution in the rostral striatum following an anterograde tracer injection into the medial prefrontal cortex.

lateral core receives fewer inputs from areas 25 and Ia, and a denser projection from lateral OMPFC regions, areas 13 and 12, and the dysgranular insular cortex.[26-28] It is of interest to note that the part of the cingulate cortex, area 24c, that is closely connected to motor areas does not project to the ventral striatum.

Injections of anterograde tracers confined to areas 14 and 13a of the OMPFC confirmed the retrograde experiments. Clusters of fibers are distributed in the ventral striatum, just rostral to and at the level of the anterior commissure. There were no terminals in the dorsolateral striatum. Fibers are primarily located in the core, with a few patches in the shell. The densest projection field was along the medial wall of the ventral caudate nucleus. Fibers extend rostrally through the rostral caudate nucleus (FIG. 7). Here, they are no longer limited to the ventral part of the striatum, but they appear in the central regions as well. In summary, the CaBP-poor shell region receives the most limited OMPFC projection. This projection is derived primarily from medial areas 25, 32, 24a/b, and from Ia. The core receives more widespread OMPFC projections. Of particular interest is that the OMPFC projection extends dorsally and rostrally from the conventionally defined nucleus accumbens into the ventral caudate nucleus and throughout a large part of its rostral pole.

Thalamic Projections to the Striatum

All regions of the ventral striatum receive dense projections from the midline thalamic nuclei and from the medial parafascicular nucleus.[29] The midline nuclei include the anterior and posterior paraventricular, parataenial, rhomboid, and reuniens thalamic nuclei. The shell of the nucleus accumbens receives the most limited projection. The medial shell is innervated almost exclusively by the anterior and posterior paraventricular nuclei and the medial parafascicular nucleus. The ventral shell receives input from these nuclei as well as from the parataenial, rhomboid, and reuniens midline groups. The medial wall of the caudate nucleus receives projections, not only from the midline and the medial intralaminar nuclei, but also from the central superior lateral nucleus, and a limited input from the magnocellular subdivision of the ventral anterior nucleus. By contrast, the central core receives a limited projection from the midline thalamic nuclei, predominantly from the rhomboid nucleus. It also receives input from the parafascicular nucleus and the central superior lateral nucleus. In summary, midline nucleus thalamic input to the medial shell is mostly confined to a specific group of cells. The ventral shell receives a more widespread midline nucleus afferent projection. Additional thalamic nuclear groups project to the medial wall of the caudate nucleus. Finally, the central core receives the smallest midline thalamic projection.

Midbrain

The neurons innervating the shell of the nucleus accumbens originate from the dorsal tier of mesencephalic neurons, including the dorsal SNc and the VTA.[48] These cells project to all ventral striatal regions. The ventral tier (densocellular part) also projects throughout the ventral striatum, with the exception of the medial shell region. This projection is derived from the medial and dorsal part only (primarily the VTA), and it varies in intensity in different ventral striatal regions. The ventral shell receives a very limited projection from the densocelluilar group, from cells located in the most medial and dorsal region. The midbrain projections to the medial wall of the caudate nucleus is from a wider medial-lateral range of the densocellular group, but are located in its dorsal portion. The central and lateral core region derives the least amount of its afferent projection from the dorsal tier. More laterally and ventrally placed cells of the ventral tier project to the core, compared to the shell or medial wall of the caudate nucleus. Injections of retrograde tracers into the rostral striatum label the most dorsal group of densocellular neurons. Thus the topography of the midbrain-ventral striatal projection is such that input to the medial shell is derived only from the dorsal tier. Input to the ventral shell is primarily from the dorsal tier, with only a few cells that project there from the medial, dorsal densocellular group. Both the dorsal tier and the dorsal densocellular group project to the medial wall of the caudate and to the central and lateral core.

THE VENTRAL STRIATAL TERRITORY

Taken together, the ventral striatum in primates encompasses a large ventromedial region, the bulk of which extends from the anterior commissure to the rostral pole of the caudate nucleus. The shell receives the most limited input from the cortex, thalamus, and midbrain. This input is from areas 32, 25, 14, and Ia, the midline thalamic nuclei, and the dorsal tier of the midbrain dopamine neurons. Each of these areas is most closely aligned with other brain structures that mediate emotional responses, including the amygdala and hypothalamus. Within the shell there is a relative difference in afferent projections to the medial and ventral parts. The medial region, just beneath and medial to the ventricle, receives the most restricted input, which is derived almost entirely from areas 25 and Ia, the paraventricular midline thalamic nucleus, and the medial dorsal tier (the VTA) of the midbrain. In addition to these regions, the ventral shell receives input from areas 24a/b and 13a/b, the rhomboid and parataenial midline thalamic nuclei, and a limited input from the medial densocellular midbrain group. The medial wall of the caudate nucleus receives input from the same areas as the shell but also from additional cortical, midbrain, and thalamic areas that do not project extensively to the shell. These include other OMPFC areas, denser labeling in nonmidline thalamic regions, and wider spread input from the densocellular group of midbrain neurons.

These studies illustrate that although the inputs to the shell region in primates are more restricted than to other parts of the ventral striatum, they are not unique. Medial OMPFC areas innervate the shell and medial caudate nucleus. In addition, more lateral areas, 13 and 12, project throughout the core. The midline thalamic nuclei project most densely to the medial caudate nucleus and to the shell region. In addition, however, the medial caudate nucleus also receives a dense innervation from several thalamic nuclei (i.e., the ventral anterior nucleus) that do not project to the shell. Finally, the shell receives input from the dorsal tier of the midbrain dopaminergic neurons but not from the ventral tier. By contrast, both the dorsal and ventral tier neurons project to the rest of the ventral striatum. Thus in monkeys we can define a relatively small shell region that receives a specific and limited afferent projection most closely linked to the amygdala and hypothalamus. However, extending beyond the CaBP-negative borders is a more extensive area that also receives inputs from areas associated with reward. FIGURE 6 illustrates the more restricted inputs to the shell region that blend with additional inputs in the medial ventral striatum. The connectional similarities between the shell and the medial wall of the caudate nucleus suggest that although the medial wall is not CaBP negative, it may be a transitional zone between the shell and the core.

ACKNOWLEDGMENTS

This work was supported by NIH Grants NS22511 and MH45573 and a Grant from the Lucille P. Markey Charitable Trust to S.N.H. and MH 11661 to N.R.M.

REFERENCES

1. HEIMER, L. & R.D. WILSON. 1975. The subcortical projections of the allocortex: similarities in the neural associations of the hippocampus, the piriform cortex, and the neocortex. *In* Golgi Centennial Symposium: Perspectives in Neurobiology. M. Santini, Ed.: 177-193. Raven Press. New York.
2. KOOB, G.F. & E.J. NESTLER. 1997. The neurobiology of drug addiction. J. Neuropsychiatry Clin. Neurosci. **9**: 482-497.
3. KALIVAS, P.W., L. CHURCHILL & M.A. KLITENICK. 1993. The Circuitry mediating the translation of motivational stimuli into adaptive motor responses. *In* Limbic Motor Circuits and Neuropsychiatry. P.W. Kalivas & C. D. Barnes, Eds.: 237–275. CRC Press, Inc. Boca Raton.
4. MOGENSON, G.J., S.M. BRUDZYNSKI, M. WU, C.R. YANG & C.C.Y. YIM. 1993. From motivation to action: a review of dopaminergic regulation of limbic -> nucleus accumbens -> ventral pallidum -> pedunculopontine nucleus circuitries involved in limbic-motor integration. *In* Limbic Motor Circuits and Neuropsychiatry. P.W. Kalivas & C. D. Barnes, Eds.: 193 - 236. CRC Press, Inc. Boca Raton.
5. ZABORSZKY, L., G.F. ALHEID, M.C. BEINFELD, L.E. EIDEN, L. HEIMER & M. PALKOVITS. 1985. Cholecystokinin innervation of the ventral striatum: a morphological and radioimmunological study. Neuroscience **14** (No. 2): 427-453.
6. ZAHM, D.S. & J.S. BROG. 1992. On the significance of subterritories in the "accumbens" part of the rat ventral striatum. Neuroscience **50** (No. 4): 751-767.
7. BROG, J.S., A. SALYAPONGSE, A.Y. DEUTCH & D.S. ZAHM. 1993. The patterns of afferent innervation of the core and shell in the "accumbens" part of the rat ventral striatum: immunohistochemical detection of retrogradely transported fluoro-gold. J. Comp. Neurol. **338**: 255-278.
8. HEIMER, L., D.S. ZAHM, L. CHURCHILL, P.W. KALIVAS & C. WOHLTMANN. 1991. Specificity in the projection patterns of accumbal core and shell in the rat. Neuroscience **41** (No. 1): 89-125.
9. O'DONNELL, P. & A.A. GRACE. 1993. Dopaminergic modulation of dye coupling between neurons in the core and shell regions of the nucleus accumbens. J. Neurosci. **13**(8): 3456-3471.
10. GROENEWEGEN, H.J., C.I. WRIGHT & A.V.J. BEIJER. 1996. The nucleus accumbens: gateway for limbic structures to reach the motor system? *In* Progress in Brain Research. G. Holstege, R. Bandler & C. P. Saper, Eds.: 485-511. Elsevier Science.
11. PENNARTZ, C.M., H.J. GROENEWEGEN & F.H. LOPES DA SILVA. 1994. The nucleus accumbens as a complex of functionally distinct neuronal ensembles: an integration of behavioural, electrophysiological and anatomical data. Prog. Neurobiol. **42**(6): 719-761.
12. MEREDITH, G.E., A. PATTISELANNO, H.J. GROENEWEGEN & S.N. HABER. 1996. Shell and core in monkey and human nucleus accumbens identified with antibodies to calbindin-D28k. J. Comp. Neurol. **365**: 628-639.

13. ALHEID, G.F. & L. HEIMER. 1988. New perspectives in basal forebrain organization of special relevance for neuropsychiatric disorders: the striatopallidal, amygdaloid, and corticopetal components of substantia innominata. Neuroscience **27**: 1-39.
14. MARTIN, L.J., M.G. HADFIELD, T.L. DELLOVADE & D.L. PRICE. 1991. The striatal mosaic in primates: patterns of neuropeptide immunoreactivity differentiate the ventral striatum from the dorsal striatum. Neuroscience **43** (No. 2/3): 397-417.
15. IKEMOTO, K., K. SATOH, T. MAEDA & H.C. FIBIGER. 1995. Neurochemical heterogeneity of the primate nucleus accumbens. Exp. Brain Res. **104**: 177-190.
16. HURD, Y.L. & M. HERKENHAM. 1995. The human neostriatum shows compartmentalization of neuropeptide gene expression in dorsal and ventral regions: An in situ hybridization histochemical analysis. Neuroscience **64**: 571-586.
17. VOORN, P., L.S. BRADY, H.W. BERENDSE & E.K. RICHFIELD. 1996. Densitometrical analysis of opioid receptor ligand binding in the human striatum. I. Distribution of μ opioid receptor defines shell and core of the ventral striatum. Neuroscience **75**: 777-792.
18. MARTIN, L.J., C.D. BLACKSTONE, R.L. HUGANIR & D.L. PRICE. 1993. The striatal mosaic in primates: striosomes and matrix are differentially enriched in ionotropic glutamate receptor subunits. J. Neurosci. **13**: 782-792.
19. HABER, S.N., H. RYOO, C. COX & W. LU. 1995. Subsets of midbrain dopaminergic neurons in monkeys are distinguished by different levels of mRNA for the dopamine transporter: comparison with the mRNA for the D2 receptor, tyrosine hydroxylase and calbindin immunoreactivity. J. Comp. Neurol. **362**: 400-410.
20. HABER, S.N. & R. ELDE. 1982. The distribution of enkephalin immunoreactive fibers and terminals in the monkey central nervous system: an immunohistochemical study. Neuroscience **7**: 1049-1095.
21. HEIMER, L., G.F. ALHEID, J.S. DE OLMOS, H.J. GROENEWEGEN, S.N. HABER, R.E. HARLAN & D.S. ZAHM. 1997. The accumbens: beyond the core-shell dichotomy. J. Neuropsychiatry Clin. Neurosci. **9** (3): 354-381.
22. ALEXANDER, G.E. & M.D. CRUTCHER. 1990. Functional architecture of basal ganglia circuits: neural substrates of parallel processing. Trends Neurosci. **13**: 266-271.
23. HABER, S.N., E. LYND-BALTA & W.P.T.M. SPOOREN. 1994. Integrative aspects of basal ganglia circuitry. In The Basal Ganglia IV. G. Percheron, J.S. McKenzie & J. Féger, Eds.: 71-80. Plenum Press. New York.
24. PARTHASARATHY, H.B., J.D. SCHALL & A.M. GRAYBIEL. 1992. Distributed but convergent ordering of corticostriatal projections: analysis of the frontal eye field and the supplementary eye field in the macaque monkey. J. Neurosci. **12**(11): 4468-4488.
25. GOLDMAN-RAKIC, P.S. & L.D. SELEMON. 1986. Topography of corticostriatal projections in nonhuman primates and implications for functional parcellation of the neostriatum. In Cerebral Cortex Vol. 5. E.G. Jones & A. Peters, Eds.: 447-466. Plenum Publishing Corp. New York.
26. HABER, S.N., K. KUNISHIO, M. MIZOBUCHI & E. LYND-BALTA. 1995. The orbital and medial prefrontal circuit through the primate basal ganglia. J. Neurosci. **15**: 4851-4867.
27. CHIKAMA, M., N. MCFARLAND, D.G. AMARAL & S.N. HABER. 1997. Insular cortical projections to functional regions of the striatum correlate with cortical cytoarchitectonic organization in the primate. J. Neurosci. **17**(24): 9686-9705.
28. KUNISHIO, K. & S.N. HABER. 1994. Primate cingulostriatal projection: limbic striatal versus sensorimotor striatal input. J. Comp. Neurol. **350**: 337-356.
29. GIMÉNEZ-AMAYA, J.M., N.R. MCFARLAND, S. DE LAS HERAS & S.N. HABER. 1995. Organization of thalamic projections to the ventral striatum in the primate. J. Comp. Neurol. **354**: 127-149.
30. LYND-BALTA, E. & S.N. HABER. 1994. The organization of midbrain projections to the striatum in the primate: sensorimotor-related striatum versus ventral striatum. Neuroscience **59**: 625-640.
31. CUMMINGS, J.L. 1995. Anatomic and behavioral aspects of frontal-subcortical circuits. Ann. N. Y. Acad. Sci. **769**: 1-13.

32. FILLEY, C.M. 1995. Frontal lobe syndromes. *In* Neurobehavioral Anatomy. 149-162. University Press of Colorado. Niwot, CO.
33. FUSTER, J.M. 1989. Lesion Studies. *In* The Prefrontal Cortex Anatomy, Physiology, and Neuropsychology of the Frontal Lobe. 51-82. Raven Press. New York.
34. ROLLS, E.T., M.J. BURTON & F. MORA. 1980. Neurophysiological analysis of brain-stimulation reward in the monkey. Brain Res. **194:** 339-357.
35. BUTTER, C.M. 1969. Perseveration in extinction and in discrimination reversal tasks following selective frontal ablations in *Macaca mulatta*. Physiol. Behav. **4:** 163-171.
36. BENJAMIN, R.M. & H. BURTON. 1968. Projection of taste nerve afferents to anterior opercular-insular cortex in squirrel monkey. Brain Res. **7:** 221-231.
37. BAYLIS, L.L. & D. GAFFAN. 1991. Amygdalectomy and ventromedial prefrontal ablation produce similar deficits in food choice and in simple object discrimination learning for an unseen reward. Exp. Brain Res. **86:** 617-622.
38. AMARAL, D.G. & J L. PRICE. 1984. Amygdalo-cortical projections in the monkey *(Macaca fascicularis)*. J. Comp. Neurol. **230:** 465-496.
39. CARMICHAEL, S.T. & J. PRICE. 1996. Limbic connections of the orbital and medial prefrontal cortex in macaque monkeys. J. Comp. Neurol. **363:** 615-641.
40. BAYLIS, L.L., E.T. ROLLS & G.C. BAYLIS. 1995. Afferent connections of the caudolateral orbitofrontal cortex taste area of the primate. Neuroscience **64:** 801-812.
41. PORRINO, L.J., A.M. CRANE & P.S. GOLDMAN-RAKIC. 1981. Direct and indirect pathways from the amygdala to the frontal lobe in rhesus monkeys. J. Comp. Neurol. **198:** 121-136.
42. ROLLS, E.T. & L.L. BAYLIS. 1994. Gustatory, olfactory, and visual convergence within the primate orbitofrontal cortex. J. Neurosci. **14:** 5437-5452.
43. PASSINGHAM, R.E. 1995. The Frontal Lobes and Voluntary Action. Oxford University Press. Oxford.
44. JONES, E.G. 1985. The Thalamus. Plenum Press. New York.
45. AKERT, K. & K. HARTMANN-VON MONAKOW. 1980. Relationships of precentral, premotor and prefrontal cortex to the mediodorsal and intralaminar nuclei of the monkey thalamus. Acta Neurobiol. Exp. **40:** 7-25.
46. FRANCOIS, C., G. PERCHERON, A. PARENT, A.F. SADIKOT, G. FENELON & J. YELNIK. 1991. Topography of the projection from the central complex of the thalamus to the sensorimNew York.otor striatal territory in monkeys. J. Comp. Neurol. **305:** 17-34.
47. VOGT, B.A. 1993. Neurobiology of cingulate cortex and limbic thalamus. Birkhauser. Boston.
48. LYND-BALTA, E. & S.N. HABER. 1994. The organization of midbrain projections to the ventral striatum in the primate. Neuroscience **59:** 609-623.
49. RUSSCHEN, F.T., I. BAKST, D.G. AMARAL & J.L. PRICE. 1985. The amygdalostriatal projections in the monkey. An anterograde tracing study. Brain Res. **329:** 241-257.
50. POLETTI, C.E. & G. CRESSWELL. 1977. Fornix system efferent projections in the squirrel monkey: an experimental degeneration study. J. Comp. Neurol. **175:** 101-128.
51. KUNISHIO, K. & S.N. HABER. 1994. The primate striatal projections from the amygdala and hippocampus: a retrograde study. Soc. Neurosci. Abstr. **1:** 333-330.
52. KUNISHIO, K. & S.N. HABER. 1995. The topographic organization of the amygdaloid projections to specific regions of the ventral striatum in the primate. Neuroscience.
53. AGGLETON, J.P. 1993. The contribution of the amygdala to normal and abnormal emotional states. Trends Neurosci. **16:** 328-333.
54. LEDOUX, J.E., P. CICCHETTI, A. XAGORARIS & L.M. ROMANSKI. 1990. The lateral amygdaloid nucleus: sensory interface of the amygdala in fear conditioning. J. Neurosci. **10**(4): 1062-1069.
55. CARMICHAEL, S.T. & J.L. PRICE. 1994. Architectonic subdivision of the orbital and medial prefrontal cortex in the macaque monkey. J. Comp. Neurol. **346:** 366-402.

Convergence and Segregation of Ventral Striatal Inputs and Outputs

HENK J. GROENEWEGEN,[a] CHRISTOPHER I. WRIGHT,[b] ARNO V.J. BEIJER, AND PIETER VOORN

Graduate School Neurosciences Amsterdam, Research Institute Neurosciences Vrije Universiteit, Department of Anatomy, Vrije Universiteit, Amsterdam, The Netherlands

ABSTRACT: The ventral striatum, which prominently includes the nucleus accumbens (Acb), is a heterogeneous area. Within the Acb of rats, a peripherally located shell and a centrally situated core can be recognized that have different connectional, neurochemical, and functional identities. Although the Acb core resembles in many respects the dorsally adjacent caudate-putamen complex in its striatal character, the Acb shell has, in addition to striatal features, a more diverse array of neurochemical characteristics, and afferent and efferent connections. Inputs and outputs of the Acb, in particular of the shell, are inhomogeneously distributed, resulting in a mosaical arrangement of concentrations of afferent fibers and terminals and clusters of output neurons. To determine the precise relationships between the distributional patterns of various afferents (*e.g.*, from the prefrontal cortex, the basal amygdaloid complex, the hippocampal formation, and the midline/intralaminar thalamic nuclei) and efferents to the ventral pallidum and mesencephalon, neuroanatomical anterograde and retrograde tracing experiments were carried out. The results of the double anterograde, double retrograde, and anterograde/retrograde tracing experiments indicate that various parts of the shell (dorsomedial, ventromedial, ventral, and lateral) and the core (medial and lateral) have different input–output characteristics. Furthermore, within these Acb regions, various populations of neurons can be identified, arranged in a cluster-like fashion, onto which specific sets of afferents converge and that project to particular output stations, distinct from the input–output relationships of neighboring, cluster-like neuronal populations. These results support the idea that the nucleus accumbens may consist of a collection of neuronal ensembles with different input–output relationships and, presumably, different functional characteristics.

INTRODUCTION: VENTRAL STRIATUM AND NUCLEUS ACCUMBENS

The term *ventral striatum* denotes an area of the striatum that receives inputs from such limbic structures as the hippocampus, entorhinal cortex, and amygdala, as well as dopaminergic afferents from the ventral mesencephalon. These striatal afferents are largely confined to the ventral and medial parts of the striatum, although in

---

[a]Address for correspondence: H.J. Groenewegen, M.D. Ph.D., Department of Anatomy and Embryology, Faculty of Medicine, Vrije Universiteit, Van der Boechorststraat 7, 1081 BT Amsterdam, The Netherlands. Voice: 31-20-444-8040; fax: 31-20-444-8054; hj.groenewegen.anat@med.vu.nl

[b]Present address: Department of Neurology, Harvard Medical School, Brigham and Women's Hospital, Boston MA, USA.

particular, in rostral and caudal striatal areas, some of these "limbic" afferents might reach also more dorsal parts of the striatum. Outputs from the ventral striatum reach ventral pallidal areas, the hypothalamus, the ventral tegmental area (VTA), the substantia nigra pars compacta and pars reticulata, and more caudal mesencephalic areas as the retrorubral area and the caudal mesencephalic tegmentum (for reviews, see refs. 1 and 2). The nucleus accumbens (Acb) is a nuclear mass in the rostroventral part of the ventral striatum bordered medially by the septum and ventrally by the olfactory tubercle (FIG. 1). Following the initial suggestion by Stevens[3] that the Acb plays a role in the pathophysiology of schizophrenia, over the past decades, this nucleus has been the focus of an increasing number of neuroanatomical, electrophysiological, and pharmacobehavioral studies. Important in this respect have also been the seminal papers by Heimer and Wilson,[4] proposing that the Acb forms an integral part of the striatum, and Mogenson et al.,[5] suggesting that the Acb is the neural substrate for limbic-motor interactions. In more recent years, the Acb has played a prominent role in theories of reward and motivation, and disturbances at the level of this nucleus have been implicated in a number of other affective disorders, such as schizophrenia and drug abuse.[6,7] More caudal parts of the ventral striatum, which appear to share many inputs and outputs with the Acb, have also received attention in this context. These areas, which include among others the so-called interstitial nucleus of the posterior limb of the anterior commissure (IPAC), are thought to belong to the territory of the extended amygdala[1] and are dealt with in other chapters in this volume.

NUCLEUS ACCUMBENS: SHELL–CORE DICHOTOMY

Within the Acb, primarily on the basis of (immuno)histochemical characteristics, a distinction can be made between a shell and a core region.[8–10] It is generally accepted that the differential distribution of the calcium-binding protein, calbindin D_{28K} (CaB), provides the most reliable distinction between shell and core[10,11] (FIG. 2). The medial, ventral, and lateral parts of the Acb, which are lightly to moderately immunoreactive for CaB, are considered to consitute the shell, whereas the central and dorsal parts of the Acb, which are more strongly immunoreactive for CaB belong to the core.[c] In accepting the differential distribution of CaB-immunoreactivity as a marker for shell and core, the lightly staining rostral part of the Acb must be included in the shell;[11] (see, however, ref. 12). It must further be noted, however, that

---

[c]The Acb core imperceptibly merges with the dorsally adjacent caudate-putamen complex. Connections of the patch and matrix compartments of the Acb core, summarized below, in most cases include the same compartments of the adjacent caudate-putamen, even though not explicitely stated in the text.

FIGURE 1. Photomicrographs of two transverse sections through the rat Acb stained for Nissl substance (**A**, rostral; **B**, caudal). Note the inhomogeneous distribution of cells and the existence of clusters of neurons (arrowhead in **A**). In **B**, arrows mark the border between shell (AcbSh) and core (AcbC); compare with FIGURE 2. The large arrowhead in **B** indicates the major island of Calleja. ac, anterior commissure; CPu, caudate-putamen complex; OT, olfactory tubercle.

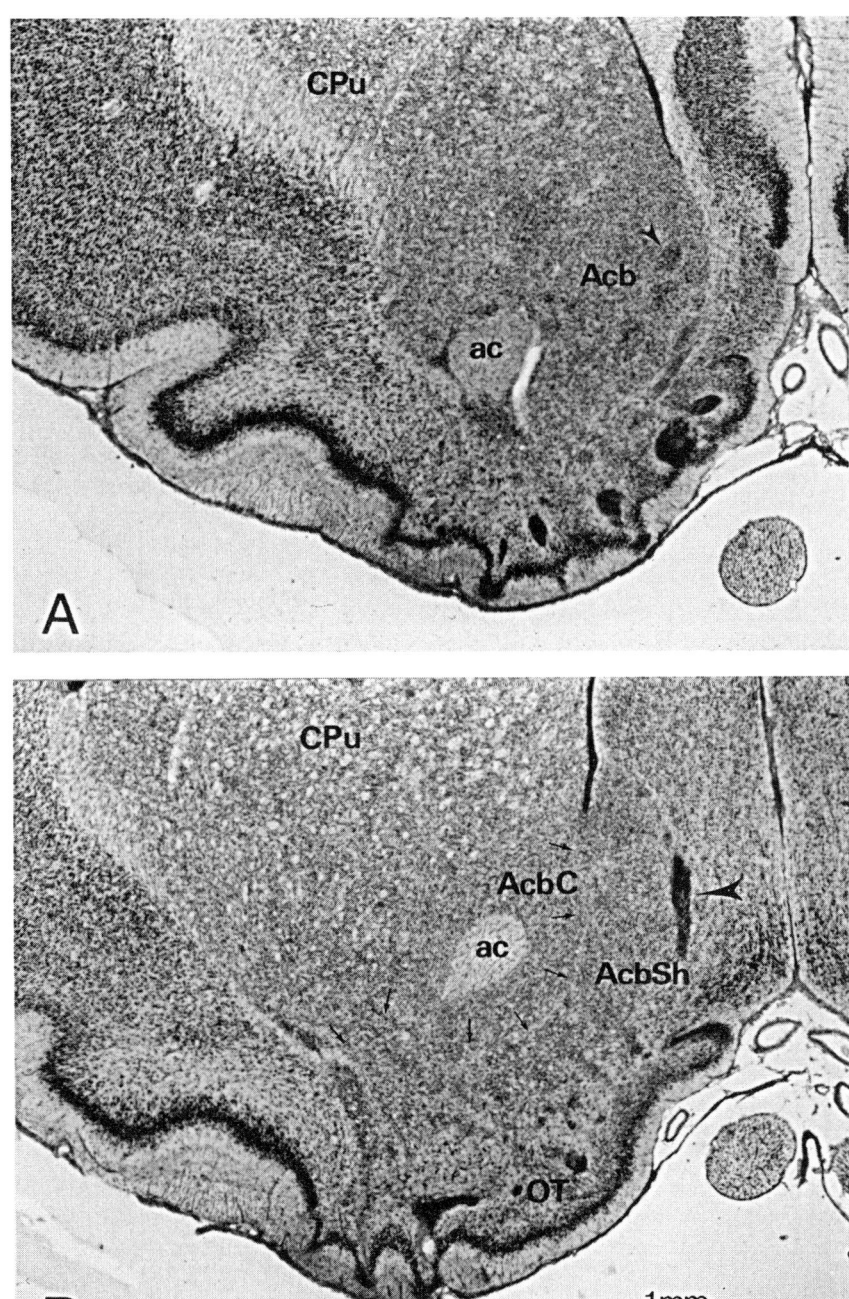

TABLE 1[a]

	CaB	ENK	NAL	DA	D_1	D_2	D_3	SP	NT
CORE	+++	++	+	++	++	++	+	++	++
patch	++	+++	+++	+				+++	+++
matrix	+++	++	+	++				++	+
"rostral zones"	+++	+++	+++	+				+	
SHELL	++	+++	+	+++	+++	+	++	+++	+++
cell clusters	+	+	+++	+				+	+
cone-shaped area	++	+++	++	+++				+++	+++

[a]The distribution of a limited number of neurochemical substances and neurotransmitter receptors in shell and core of the Acb (grey rows), and identifiable "compartments" therein,[9,10] is represented in a three-level scale: +++, dense; ++, moderate; +, weak. The distribution of the dopamine receptors D_1, D_2, and D_3 has not been described in such detail that a further subdivision within the shell and core is justified. For the various substances, the references contain the original data. CaB, calbindin D_{28K};[9–11,13] ENK, enkephalin;[9,14] NAL naloxon;[14] DA, dopamine;[9] D_1, dopamine D_1 receptor;[15] D_2, dopamine D_2 receptor;[15] D_3, dopamine D_3 receptor;[16] SP, substance P;[9,10] NT, neurotensin.[17,18]

both shell and core exhibit distinct inhomogeneities for cellular density (FIG. 1) and CaB-immunoreactivity (TABLE 1; FIG. 2). The lateral shell exhibits a moderate immunoreactivity for CaB, whereas medial, ventral, and rostral shell areas show much lower levels of CaB-immunoreactivity. Within the medial shell, cell cluster areas in Nissl-stained sections exhibit almost no CaB-immunoreactivity, whereas in its caudo-dorsal part, collections of CaB-immunoreactive neurons are present.[10] The core of the Acb, much like the ventromedial parts of the adjacent caudate-putamen complex, contains distinct areas of low CaB-immunoreactivity which coincide with the striatal patches expressing high concentrations of μ-opioid receptors.[19,20] TABLE 1 summarizes the differential distribution of a number of neurochemical substances and neurotransmitter receptors in the various parts of the Acb shell and core. At least five, but presumably more, different compartments can be recognized in the Acb. It must be noted that, for a variety of substances and receptors that are not represented in this table, also, inhomogeneous patterns of distribution have also been described, but that a complete picture of the precise mutual relationships between these patterns is still largely lacking.

FIGURE 2. Photomicrographs of three transverse sections through the Acb, immunostained for CaB. **A,** rostral; **C,** caudal. Arrows in **B** and **C** indicate the border between shell (AcbSh) and core (AcbC) of the Acb. Note that the shell shows much less CaB immunoreactivity than the core but that the shell is inhomogeneous in itself, exhibiting moderate immunoreactivity in the lateral shell and almost no immunoreactivity for CaB in its medial part (compare also FIG. 4A). The large arrowhead in **C** indicates the major island of Calleja. The core, exhibiting mostly high levels of CaB, contains, in addition, patches of light or moderate levels of immunoreactivity for CaB. The rostral part of the Acb (**A**), with the exception of a lateral region, is lightly immunoreactive for CaB and has been included in the shell on the basis of this characteristic by Jongen-Rêlo et al.[11] ac, anterior commissure.

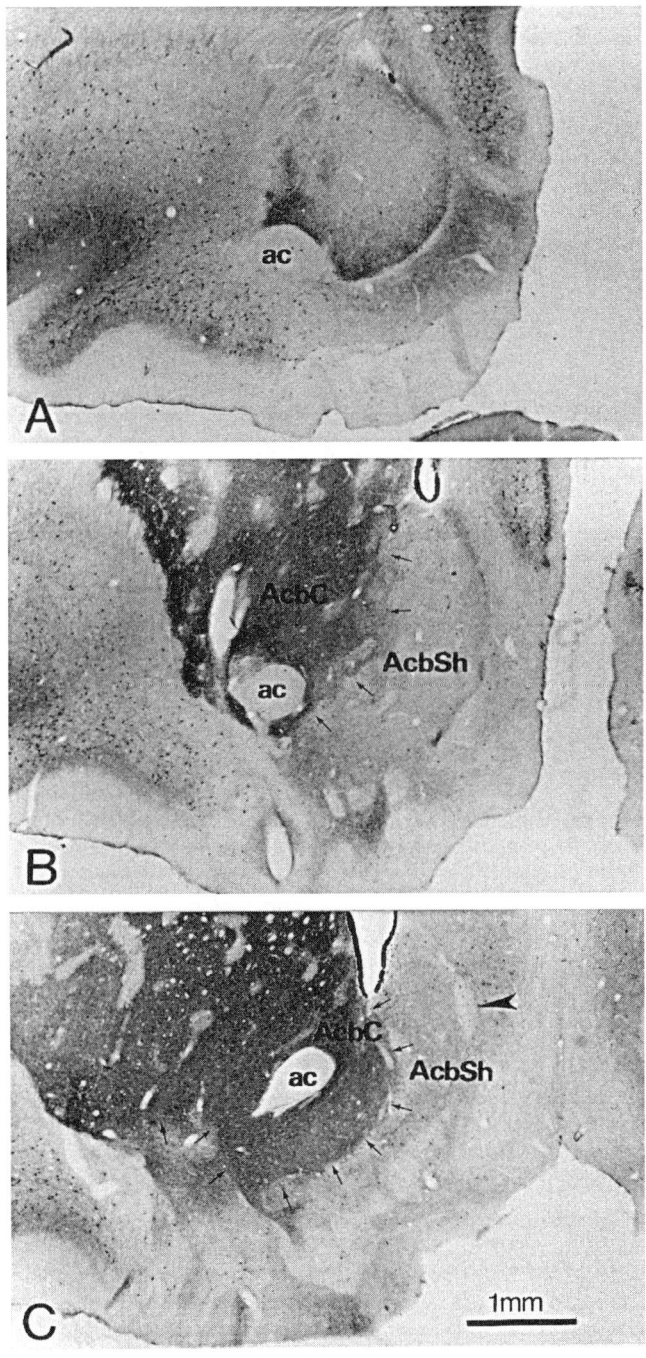

RELATIONSHIPS OF AFFERENTS AND EFFERENTS WITH SHELL AND CORE

The Acb receives inputs from the hippocampal region, basal amygdaloid complex, prefrontal cortex, midline and intralaminar thalamus, ventral pallidum, the dopaminergic ventral tegmental (A10) and retrorubral (A8) cell groups, the serotonergic median raphe nucleus, and the noradrenergic A2 cell group in the nucleus of the solitary tract.[1,21,22–24] The projections of none of these structures are restricted to the Acb, but they extend either into the ventrally adjacent striatal parts of the olfactory tubercle and/or into the dorsally adjacent caudate-putamen complex and more caudal ventral striatal areas. Within the Acb, the projections of most of these afferent structures are inhomogeneously distributed, and they show particular relationships with the shell and core, or subregions therein (FIG. 3). However, there are no afferent systems that are exclusively related to either Acb shell or core. Thus, whereas the projections from the hippocampal subicular and CA1 regions predominently target the medial, ventral, and rostral parts of the Acb shell, these hippocampal projections also extend into the medial part of the Acb core (refs. 21 and 22; and Beijer and Groenewegen, unpublished observations).

Likewise, the medial entorhinal area projects predominantly to the Acb shell, but these projections are by no means restricted to the shell, and they appear to also invade the Acb core. The lateral entorhinal area projects primarily to the Acb core but targets also the lateral part of the shell (ref. 25; and Beijer and Groenewegen, unpublished observations).

Afferents from different nuclei of the basal amygdaloid complex terminate in different parts of the Acb in a highly complex arrangement.[24] Whereas the caudal part of the parvicellular basal nucleus sends fibers predominently to the dorsomedial shell, it targets, in addition, the patches in the core. The rostral part of the magnocellular basal nucleus sends fibers to the lateral part of the Acb shell and, additionally, to the patches of the lateral Acb core. The midrostrocaudal part of the accessory basal nucleus issues fibers to the ventral part of the shell as well as to the matrix of the core. The caudal parts of the accessory basal and the magnocellular basal nuclei project to the ventromedial shell, whereas these nuclei have additional projections to the patches in the medial core of the Acb.[24]

The thalamic projections from the midline and intralaminar thalamic nuclei to the Acb likewise show specific arrangements in projecting to distinct parts of the Acb shell and either the patch or matrix compartments in the Acb core.[22,26] The anterior part of the thalamic paraventricular nucleus has a strong projection to the medial shell, as well as to the patches in the medial core of the Acb. More posterior parts of the paraventricular nucleus send fibers to more ventral and lateral parts of the shell. The intermediodorsal thalamic nucleus, a caudal representative of the midline thalamic nuclei, projects heavily to the Acb core, in particular targeting the matrix and avoiding its patches. The projections from the rostrally located parataenial nucleus include predominantly the ventral and rostral parts of the shell, avoiding its most medial and lateral parts. Additional projections reach the Acb core, but these are less dense and not strictly bound to either patch or matrix. The central medial thalamic nucleus and the medial part of the parafascicular nucleus send fibers to the rostral part of the Acb core and, in addition, extensively to the medial part of the caudate-putamen complex.[22,26]

The projections from different areas in the prefrontal cortex to the Acb are also topographically arranged. Moreover, the detailed arrangements with respect to specific compartments within the shell and core appear to depend upon the layer of origin of the prefrontal cortical projections.[13,23,27] The infralimbic cortex projects to a peripheral, band-like region in the medial and ventral parts of the shell, as well as to a region including the lateral part of the medial shell and the medial part of the core of the Acb. The lateral shell receives its cortical inputs predominantly from the ventral agranular insular area in the depth of the rostral part of the rhinal sulcus. The deep laminae (deep layer V) of the ventral prelimbic area send fibers to the dorsomedial part of the shell, as well as to the patches of the Acb core; its superficial laminae (superficial layer V and layer III) project to the matrix of the core. Similar arrangements exist for the deep versus superficial projections from the dorsal prelimbic area to, respectively, the patch and matrix compartments of the Acb core.[23,27] However, the projections from the dorsal prelimbic area extend further rostrally into the Acb and more dorsally into the medial caudate-putamen than those from the ventral prelimbic area. The dorsal agranular insular area in the lateral part of the prefrontal cortex primarily projects to the core of the Acb and extensive parts of the ventral caudate-putamen. Superficial layers project more heavily to the matrix, deep layers to the patches of the core.[23,28] The projections from the dorsal agranular insular and the dorsal prelimbic areas to the Acb core, in part, overlap in caudal parts of the Acb, but the dorsal prelimbic area tends to project more medially and rostrally in the Acb than the dorsal agranular insular area.

There is a clear, reciprocal point-to-point relationship between the Acb and the ventral pallidum: the medial shell and the core project to the ventromedial and the dorsal parts of the ventral pallidum, respectively.[29-31] In addition, the lateral shell projects to the ventrolateral part of the ventral pallidum (ref 31; and Groenewegen and Wright, unpublished observations). The return projections from the ventral pallidum to the Acb are organized in a comparable topographical fashion.[22,32]

The relationships of the Acb with the dopaminergic and nondopaminergic cell groups in the ventral mesencephalon are rather complex. Whereas the A10 cell group in the VTA projects predominantly to the medial and ventral parts of the shell, its fibers are by no means restricted to this area and terminate also in the medial core and adjacent regions of the caudate-putamen complex. Within the medial shell, an inhomogeneous distribution of dopaminergic fibers is apparent: whereas the cone-shaped area contains the highest density of dopaminergic fibers, the cell clusters that border this region receive virtually no such fibers (TABLE 1).[33] The retrorubral A8 cell group projects more laterally in the Acb, whereas the A9 projections in the Acb do not reach further ventrally than the core.[22,34,35] The accumbal projections to the ventral mesencephalon are arranged as follows. The medial shell sends fibers to the medial VTA; more lateral parts of the shell, that is, its ventromedial and ventral parts, innervate the lateral part of VTA, the dorsal tier of the substantia nigra pars compacta and the retrorubral area. A small number of fibers extend even further caudally to reach the midbrain tegmentum and lateral part of the central grey matter.[2,29,35,36] For the projections from the core, a distinction must be made between the patch and matrix compartments. The patches project to the substantia nigra pars compacta; the matrix sends fibers to a restricted dorsomedial part of the pars reticulata.[29,35,37-39]

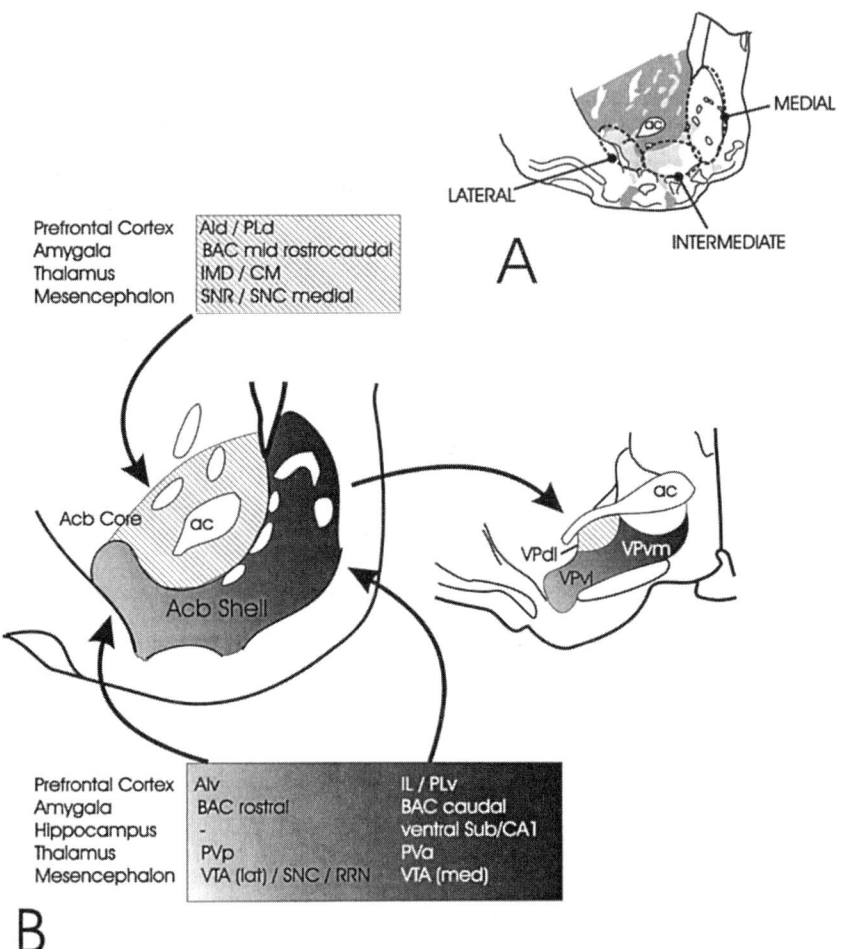

FIGURE 3. Tentative subdivision of the Acb shell and the topographical arrangements of inputs and outputs of the Acb. **A:** In a drawing of a transverse CaB-stained section through the Acb, the subdivision of the shell into medial, lateral, and intermediate parts is indicated. **B:** The broad topography of the main afferents and the ventral pallidal efferents of the core and the medial and lateral parts of the shell is represented in a transverse section through the Acb (left) and the ventral pallidum (right). ac, anterior commissure; Acb, nucleus accumbens; AId, dorsal agranular insular cortex; AIv, ventral agranular insular cortex; BAC, basal amygdaloid complex; CA1, cornu Ammonis field 1; CM, central medial nucleus; IL, infralimbic cortex; IMD, intermediodorsal nucleus; PLd, dorsal prelimbic cortex; PLv, ventral prelimbic cortex; PVa, anterior paraventricular nucleus; PVp, posterior paraventricular nucleus; SNC, substantia nigra pars compacta; SNR, substantia nigra pars reticulata; Sub, subiculum; VPdl, dorsolateral ventral pallidum; VPvl, ventrolateral ventral pallidum; VPvm, ventromedial ventral pallidum; VTA, ventral tegmental area.

An important distinction between the Acb core and shell is that the latter, at least its medial part, sends projections to the lateral preoptic and lateral hypothalamic areas.[29,31,40]

SUBDIVISIONS OF THE SHELL OF THE NUCLEUS ACCUMBENS

Taking together the immunohistochemical differentiation, for example, for CaB immunoreactivity, and the differential arrangements of afferents and efferents of the shell of the Acb, it may be suggested that this region consists of at least three subregions. Thus, a distinction can be made between a medial, a ventral, and a lateral shell (FIG. 3A). The medial shell, with its reciprocal relationships with the VTA and its strong input from the anterior paraventricular thalamic nucleus, the ventral subiculum, and the caudal basal amygdaloid nucleus, is clearly distinct from the lateral shell, which has more direct relationships with the substantia nigra pars compacta, the posterior paraventricular thalamic nucleus, and the rostral magnocellular basal amygdaloid nucleus (FIG. 3B). As discussed above, the ventral, intermedate part of the shell receives, at least to a large degree, inputs from yet another set of afferents, among which are the dorsal subiculum and midstrocaudal parts of the basal and accessory basal amygdaloid nuclei. The borders between the ventral part of the shell on the one hand and the medial and lateral parts of the shell on the other hand are not sharp, and, as yet, no immunohistochemical markers have been described that distinguish clearly between these areas in the shell. Yet, their specific input–output relationships suggest an involvement in different functional aspects of the Acb.

Within the medial shell further distinctions should probably be made, in view of the heterogeneities in the distribution of neurochemical substances, neurotransmitter receptors, and afferent and efferent connections (see refs. above and, e.g., 41 and 42). Purely for descriptive reasons, the terms ventromedial and dorsomedial shell have been introduced (e.g., refs. 13 and 42). Functional studies indicate that the ventromedial shell may indeed be a distinct r egion of the Acb.[43]

Both neuroanatomical[12,44,45] and functional studies[46,47] suggest that there exist also rostrocaudal differences within the Acb. Zahm and Heimer,[12] on the basis of an efferent connectivity pattern distinct from the "typical" projections patterns of both shell and core, designated the rostral part of the Acb as the so-called "rostral pole." Further studies are needed to substantiate the specific identity of the rostral part of the Acb, distinct from shell and core.

SHELL OF THE NUCLEUS ACCUMBENS: COLLECTION OF ENSEMBLES OF NEURONS?

The immunohistochemical and tract-tracing data reviewed above indicate that the shell and core of the Acb should not be considered as anatomical and functional units but rather that they can be further subdivided into different subregions. Thus, the medial, intermediate, and lateral parts of the shell of the Acb, as well as the medial and lateral parts of the core, receive different combinations of inputs from cortical and subcortical sources and project to different pallidal, hypothalamic, and mesencephalic targets. Moreover, within these subregions of the shell and core, the terminal fields of different sources of inputs and the neurons that give rise to different outputs are very heterogeneously distributed.[2,13,24,28,35,48,49] This leads to intricate relationships of various afferent systems in different parts of the Acb. For example, the results of double anterograde tracing experiments have shown that within the medial shell and core of the Acb the inhomogeneously distributed afferents from the anterior paraventricular thalamic nucleus, the caudal parvicellular basal amygdaloid nucleus, and the ventral prelimbic and infralimbic cortices form intricate patterns of convergence and segregation.[13] Similar arrangements of convergence and nonconvergence appear to exist in the lateral parts of the shell and core of the Acb with respect to afferents from the other parts of the midline thalamus, basal amygdaloid complex, and the (lateral) prefrontal cortex.[28] The results of retrograde tracing experiments, with small injections of retrograde tracers in one of the projection areas of the Acb, show that the Acb output neurons are organized in a clustered fashion.[2,35,49] An important question, that largely remains to be answered, is if and how the cluster-like organization of output neurons is related to the heterogeneous mosaic of convergent and segregated inputs of the Acb. In other words, to what extent does this organization reflect the existence of specific input–output channels through the Acb? Preliminary results of experiments, in which rats were injected with an anterograde tracer in one of the input structures of the Acb combined with a retrograde tracer in one of the Acb target areas, indicate that indeed particular clusters of output neurons may receive rather specific sets of inputs.[48,49]

In view of the wide range of behavorial aspects in which the Acb is presumed to play a role, Pennartz et al.,[50] in a recent review, argued that the nucleus consists of a collection of neuronal ensembles, or groups, with different functional and behavioral connotations. An ensemble is thought to be formed by a population of Acb neurons that is temporarily and (nearly) synchronously activated by a specific set of excitatory inputs. The coherent activity of these inputs could thus lead to the activation of a particular set of outputs of the Acb. Each distinct ensemble may be capable of generating a spatiotemporally coded output that is transferred to a set of target structures characteristic for this ensemble, and hence may induce behavioral effects that are specifically linked to this particular ensemble;[50] (see also O'Donnell et al., this volume). It is not a prerequisite for the idea of the existence of neuronal ensembles in the Acb that such ensembles of neurons are "bound" to a cluster of spatially closely related neurons. However, it is tempting to speculate that the experimentally shown clusters of output neurons in the above-mentioned retrograde tracing experiments, which receive different and specific combinations of converging inputs, form the anatomical substrates of such ensembles (FIG. 4A). Because only a strong exci-

---

FIGURE 4. Schematic representation of the input–output relationships of clusters of neurons in the shell of the nucleus accumbens. **A:** Different clusters of neurons (ensembles?) receive different combinations of converging inputs and project to distinct targets, including the ventral pallidum, the lateral hypothalamus, and the ventral mesencephalon. **B:** The various (limbic) cortical and subcortical structures that project to the Acb are strongly and, in a number of cases, reciprocally interconnected. Note that the Acb, via the ventral pallidum and the mediodorsal thalamic nucleus is involved in a closed thalamocortical–basal ganglia loop.[1,2] VTA, ventral tegmental area. Acb, nucleus accumbens; MD, mediodorsal thalamic nucleus; PV, paraventricular thalamic nucleus.

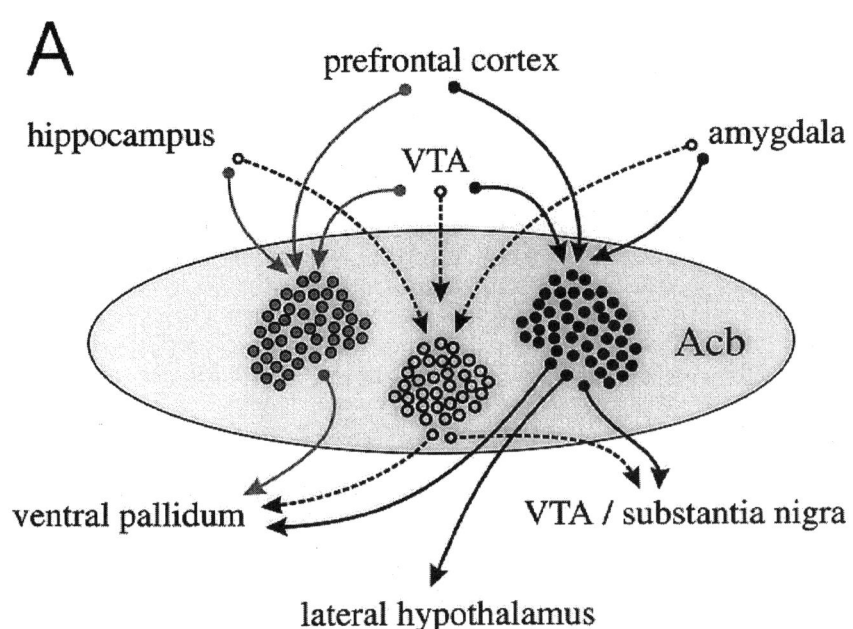

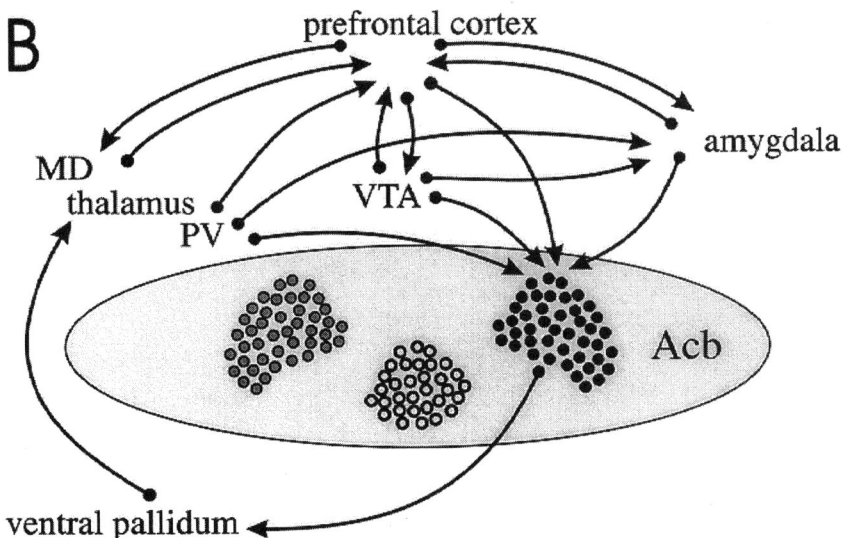

tatory input is thought to be able to electrophysiologically activate striatal output neurons (see below), it is important to realize that the major cortical, thalamic, and limbic inputs of the Acb have extensive, and in most cases, reciprocal interconnections (FIG. 4B). This extensive interconnectivity of the afferent structures of the Acb could be the anatomical basis for the temporarily coherent and synchronous activation of the populations of neurons that constitute the ensembles in the Acb (FIG. 4).

As indicated above, for an understanding of the way in which ensembles of Acb neurons may be activated, it is of great interest to consider the specific physiological properties of the Acb output cells, that is, the medium-sized spiny neurons. These spiny output neurons, both in the caudate-putamen complex [51] and the Acb, [52] have a bistable membrane potential, that is, they are mostly in a state with a hyperpolarized membrane potential of −85 to −90 mV ("down state"), but occasionally they reach a state with a relatively depolarized membrane potential of approximately −55 mV ("up state"). Only in neurons in the up state, of which the membrane potential is close to the spike threshold, can firing of action potentials be induced; neurons in the down state are physiologically "silent." It is thought that excitatory inputs from a particular source can bring striatal output neurons from the down state into the up state, but that excitatory inputs from yet another source are necessary to induce firing activity.[50–52] For example, hippocampal activation may bring Acb output neurons in their up state and, in this way, facilitate the throughout of prefrontal cortical activity via the Acb, as observed by O'Donnell and Grace,[52] in an intracellular electrophysiological study. Following lesions of the hippocampal afferents to the Acb, the Acb output neurons remain in their down state, and prefrontal cortical activity is not able to evoke Acb neuronal firing. Therefore, O'Donnell and Grace[52] have suggested that hippocampal inputs "gate" the prefrontal cortical throughput through the Acb. In an extracellular electrophysiological study, investigating the interactions between hippocampal and amygdaloid afferents in the Acb, Mulder *et al.*[53] found that amygdaloid activation facilitates hippocampal throughput through the nucleus but that, in contrast, hippocampal activation may close a gate for amygdaloid inputs. Although the observations of O'Donnell *et al.*[52] and Mulder *et al.*[53] cannot be completely reconciled with each other, they suggest that various afferents of the Acb interact with each other at the level of the output neurons, one of the possible consequences being that two or more afferents have to be active in temporal and spatial coherence to activate output neurons of the Acb. In that respect, it is of great importance to study in detail the input–output patterns at the level of the Acb, in order to understand the various possible interactions of inputs and, in this way, the activation or modulation of a multitude of outputs of the nucleus.

CONCLUDING REMARKS

The above reviewed data, with respect to the functional anatomical organization of the Acb, as part of the ventral striatum, indicate that this nucleus consists of various different subregions (e.g., medial and lateral shell and core, etc.) and that within these subregions functionally distinct ensembles of neurons exist, possibly organized in anatomical compartments and activated by specific sets of afferents that are primarily derived from (subregions of) limbic structures. It is thus important to note that the Acb neuronal ensembles must be viewed in close association with groups of neurons in prefrontal cortical, amygdaloid, and midline/intralaminar thalamic structures (as described above), which, in turn, have strong mutual interconnections (FIG. 4B). Such interconnections between structures that are afferent to the Acb may be crucial for the spatially and temporally coherent activation of the presumed ensembles in the Acb. How and under which functional circumstances the Acb neuronal ensembles are activated, and whether they can influence each other, are all important questions that need to be answered in order to further our understanding of the functional anatomy of the nucleus accumbens.

REFERENCES

1. HEIMER, L., D.S. ZAHM & G.F. ALHEID. 1995. Basal ganglia. In The Rat Nervous System, 2nd Edition. G. Paxinos & C. Watson, Eds.: 579–628. Academic Press. San Diego, CA.
2. GROENEWEGEN, H.J., C.I. WRIGHT & A.V.J. BEIJER. 1996. The nucleus accumbens: gateway for limbic structures to reach the motor system? In The Emotional Motor System, G. Holstege, R. Bandler & C.B. Saper, Eds. Prog. Brain Res. **107:** 485–511.
3. STEVENS, J.R. 1973. An anatomy of schizophrenia? Arch. Gen. Psychiatry. **29:** 177–189.
4. HEIMER, L. & R.D. WILSON. 1975. The subcortical projections of the allocortex: similarities in the neural associations of the hippocampus, the piriform cortex, and the neocortex. In Golgi Centennial Symposium: Perspectives in Neurobiology. M. Santini, Ed. :177–193. Raven Press. New York.
5. MOGENSON, G.J., D.L. JONES & C.Y. YIM. 1980. From motivation to action: functional interface between the limbic system and the motor system. Prog. Psychobiol. **14:** 60–97.
6. KOOB, G.F. 1992. Drugs of abuse: anatomy, pharmacology and function of reward pathways. Trends Pharmacol. Sci. **13:** 177–184.
7. ROBBINS, T.W. & B.J. EVERITT. 1996. Neurobehavioural mechanisms of reward and motivation. Curr. Opin. Neurobiol. **6:** 228–236.
8. ZÁBORSZKY, L., G.F. ADELHEID, M.C. BEINFELD, L.E. EIDEN, L. HEIMER & M. PALKOVITS. 1985. Cholecystokinin innervation of the vental striatum: a morphological and radioimmunological study. Neuroscience **14:** 427–453.
9. VOORN, P., C.R. GERFEN & H.J. GROENEWEGEN. 1989. The compartmental organization of the ventral striatum of the rat: immunohistochemical distribution of enkephalin, substance P, dopamine, and calcium binding protein. J. Comp. Neurol. **289:** 189–201.
10. ZAHM, D.S. & J.S. BROG. 1992. On the significance of subterritories in the "accumbens" part of the rat ventral striatium. Neuroscience **50:** 751 – 767.
11. JONGEN-RÊLO, A.L., P. VOORN & H.J. GROENEWEGEN. 1994. Immunohistochemical characterization of the shell and core territories of the nucleus accumbens in the rat. Eur. J. Neurosci. **6:** 1255–1264.
12. ZAHM, D.S. & L. HEIMER. 1993. Specificity in the efferent projections of the nucleus accumbens in the rat: comparison of the rostral pole projection patterns with those of the core and shell. J. Comp. Neurol. **327:** 220–232.
13. WRIGHT, C.I. & H.J. GROENEWEGEN. 1995. Patterns of convergence and segregation in the medial nucleus accumbens of the rat: relationships of prefrontal cortical, midline thalamic and basal amygdaloid afferents. J. Comp. Neurol. **361:** 383–403.
14. JONGEN–RÊLO, A.L., H.J. GROENEWEGEN & P. VOORN. 1993. Evidence for a multicompartmental histochemical organization of the nucleus accumbens in the rat. J. Comp. Neurol. **337:** 267–276.
15. JONGEN-RÊLO, A.L., G.J. DOCTER, A.J. JONKER & P. VOORN. 1995. Differential localization of mRNAs encoding dopamine D1 or D2 receptors in cholinergic neurons in the core and shell of the rat nucleus accumbens. Mol. Brain Res. **28:**169–174.

16. LE MOINE, C. & B. BLOCH. 1996. Expression of the D_3 dopamine receptor in peptidergic neurons of the nucleus accumbens: comparison with the D_1 and D_2 dopamine receptors. Neuroscience **73:** 131–143.
17. ZAHM, D.S. 1987. Neurotensin-immunoreactive neurons in the ventral striatum of the adult rat: ventromedial caudate-putamen, nucleus accumbens and olfactory tubercle. Neurosci. Lett. **81:** 41–47.
18. ZAHM, D.S. & L. HEIMER. 1988. Ventral striatopallidal parts of the basal ganglia in the rat: I. Neurochemical compartmentation as reflected by the distributions of neurotensin and substance P immunoreactivity. J. Comp. Neurol. **272:** 516–535.
19. HERKENHAM, M. & C.B. PERT. 1981. Mosaic distribution of opiate receptors, parafascicular projections and acetylcholinesterase in rat striatum. Nature **291:** 415–418.
20. MANSOUR, A., C.A. FOX, S. BURKE, H. AKIL & S.J. WATSON. 1995. Immunohistochemical localization of the cloned mu opioid receptor in the rat CNS. J. Chem. Neuroanat. **8:** 283–305.
21. GROENEWEGEN, H.J., E. VERMEULEN-VAN DER ZEE, A. TE KORTSCHOT & M.P. WITTER. 1987. Organization of the projections from the subiculum to the ventral striatum in the rat: a study using anterograde transport of *Phaseolus vulgaris*-leucoagglutinin. Neuroscience **23:** 103–120.
22. BROG, J.S., A. SALYAPONGSE, A.Y. DEUTCH & D.S. ZAHM. 1993. The patterns of afferent innervation of the core and shell in the "accumbens" part of the rat ventral striatum: immunohistochemical detection of retrogradely transported fluoro-gold. J. Comp. Neurol. **338:** 255–278.
23. BERENDSE, H.W., Y. GALIS-DE GRAAF & H.J. GROENEWEGEN. 1992. Topographical organization and relationship with ventral striatal compartments of prefrontal corticostriatal projections in the rat. J. Comp. Neurol. **316:** 314–347.
24. WRIGHT, C.I., A.V.J. BEIJER & H.J. GROENEWEGEN. 1996. Basal amygadaloid complex afferents to the rat nucleus accumbens are compartmentally organized. J. Neurosci. **16:** 1877–1893.
25. TOTTERDELL, S. & G.E. MEREDITH. 1997. Topographical organization of projections from the entorhinal cortex to the striatum of the rat. Neuroscience **78:** 715–729.
26. BERENDSE, H.W. & H.J. GROENEWEGEN. 1990. The organization of the thalamostriatal projections in the rat, with special emphasis on the ventral striatum. J. Comp. Neurol. **299:** 187–228.
27. GERFEN, C.R. 1989. The neostriatal mosaic: striatal patch-matrix organization is related to cortical lamination. Science **246:** 385–388.
28. WRIGHT, C.I. & H.J. GROENEWEGEN. 1996. Patterns of overlap and segregation between insular cortical, intermediodorsal thalamic and basal amygdaloid afferents in the nucleus accumbens of the rat. Neuroscience **73:** 359–373.
29. HEIMER, L., D.S. ZAHM, L. CHURCHILL, P.W. KALIVAS & C. WOHLTMANN. 1991. Specificity in the projection patterns of the accumbal core and shell in the rat. Neuroscience **41:** 89125.
30. ZAHM D.S. & L. HEIMER. 1990. Two transpallidal pathways originating in the rat nucleus accumbens. J. Comp. Neurol. **302:** 437–446.
31. USUDA, I., K. TANAKA & T. CHIBA. 1998. Efferent projections of the nucleus accumbens in the rat with special reference to subdivisions of the nucleus—biotinylated dextran amine study. Brain Res. **797:** 73–93.
32. GROENEWEGEN, H.J., H.W. BERENDSE & S.N. HABER. 1993. Organization of the output of the ventral striatopallidal system in the rat. Ventral pallidal efferents. Neuroscience **57:** 113–142.
33. VOORN, P., B. JORRITSMA-BYHAM, C. VAN DIJK & R.M. BUIJS. 1986. The dopaminergic innervation of the ventral striatum in the rat: a light- and electron-microscopical study with antibodies against dopamine. J. Comp. Neurol. **251:** 84–99.
34. BECKSTEAD, R.M., V.B. DOMESICK & W.J.H. NAUTA. 1979. Efferent connections of the substantia nigra and ventral tegmental area in the rat. Brain Res. **175:** 191–217.
35. BERENDSE, H.W., H.J. GROENEWEGEN & A.H.M. LOHMAN. 1992. Compartmental distribution of ventral striatal neurons projecting to the ventral mesencephalon in the rat. J.Neurosci. **12:** 2079–2103.

36. NAUTA, W.J.H., G.P. SMITH, R.L.M. FAULL & V.B. DOMESICK. 1978. Efferent connections and nigral afferents of the nucleus accumbens septi in the rat. Neuroscience **3:** 385–401.
37. GERFEN, C.R., M. HERKENHAM & J. THIBAULT. 1987. The neostriatal mosaic: II. Patch- and matrix-directed mesostriatal dopaminergic and non-dopaminergic systems. J.Neurosci. **7:** 3915–3934.
38. DENIAU, J.M., A. MENETREY & A.M. THIERRY. 1994. Indirect nucleus accumbens input to the prefrontal cortex via the substantia nigra pars reticulata: a combined anatomical and electrophysiological study in the rat. Neuroscience **61:** 533–545.
39. GROENEWEGEN, H.J., H.W. BERENDSE & F.G. WOUTERLOOD. 1994. Organization of the projections from the ventral striatopallidal system to ventral mesencephalic dopaminergic neurons. *In* The Basal Ganglia IV. G. Percheron & J.S. McKenzie, Eds.: 81–93. Plenum Press. New York.
40. GROENEWEGEN, H.J. & F.T. RUSSCHEN. 1984. Organization of the efferent projections of the nucleus accumbens to pallidal, hypothalamic, and mesencephalic structures: a tracing and immunohistochemical study in the cat. J. Comp. Neurol. **223:** 347–367.
41. CURRAN, E.J. & S.J. WATSON. 1995. Dopamine receptor mRNA expression patterns by opioid peptides in the nucleus accumbens of the rat: a double *in situ* hybridization study. J. Comp. Neurol. **361:** 57–76.
42. DIAZ, J., D. LÉVESQUE, C.H. LAMMERS, N. GRIFFON, M.P. MARTES, J.C. SCHWARTZ & P. SOKOLOFF. 1995. Phenotypical characterization of neurons expressing the dopamine D_3 receptor in the rat brain. Neuroscience **65:** 731–745.
43. MALDONADO-IRIZARRY, C.S., C.J. SWANSON & A.E. KELLEY. 1995. Glutamate receptors in the nucleus accumbens shell control feeding behavior via the lateral hypothalamus. J. Neurosci. **15:** 6779–6788.
44. VOORN, P. & G.J. DOCTER. 1992. A rostrocaudal gradient in the synthesis of enkephalin in nucleus accumbens. NeuroReport **3:** 161–164.
45. VOORN, P., G.J. DOCTER, A.L. JONGEN-RÊLO & A.J. JONKER. 1994. Rostrocaudal subregional differences in the response of enkephalin, dynorphin and substance P synthesis in rat nucleus accumbens to dopamine depletion. Eur. J. Neurosci. **6:** 486–496.
46. LADURELLE, N., G. KELLER, B.P. ROQUES & V. DAUGE. 1993. Effects of CCK8 and of the CCKB-selective agonist BC264 on extracellular dopamine content in the anterior and posterior nucleus accumbens: a microdialysis study in freely moving rats. Brain Res. **628:** 254–263.
47. HEIDBREDER, C. & J. FELDON. 1998. Amphetamine-induced neurochemical and locomotor responses are expressed differentially across the anteroposterior axis of the core and shell subterritories of the nucleus accumbens. Synapse (NY) **29:** 310–322.
48. BEIJER, A.V.J. & H.J. GROENEWEGEN. 1996. Specific anatomical relationships between hippocampal and basal amygdaloid afferents and different populations of projection neurons in the nucleus accumbens of rats. Soc. Neurosci. Abstr. **22:** 413.
49. HEIMER, L, G.F. ALHEID, J.S. DE OLMOS, H.J. GROENEWEGEN, S.N. HABER, R.E. HARLAN & D.S. ZAHM. 1997. The accumbens: beyond the core-shell dichotomy. J. Neuropsychiatry Clin. Neurosci. **9:** 354–381.
50. PENNARTZ, C.M.A., H.J. GROENEWEGEN & F.H. LOPES DA SILVA. 1994. The nucleus accumbens as a complex of functionally distinct neuronal ensembles: An integration of behavioural, electrophysiological and anatomical data. Prog. Neurobiol. **42:** 719–761.
51. WILSON, C.J. 1993. The geneartion of natural firing patterns in neostriatal neurons. Prog. Brain Res. **99:** 277–297.
52. O'DONNELL, P. & A.A. GRACE. 1995. Synaptic interactions among excitatory afferents to nucleus accumbens neurons: hippocampal gating of prefrontal cortical input. J.Neurosci. **15:** 3622–3639.
53. MULDER, A.B., M. GIJSBERTI HODENPIJL & F.H. LOPES DA SILVA. 1998. Electrophysiology of the hippocampal and amygdaloid projections to the nucleus accumbens of the rat: convergence, segregation, and interaction of inputs. J. Neurosci. **18:** 5095–5102.

Involvement of the Pallidal-thalamocortical Circuit in Adaptive Behavior

PETER W. KALIVAS,[a,c] LYNN CHURCHILL,[b] AND ANASTASIA ROMANIDES[a]

[a]*Department of Physiology and Neuroscience, Medical University of South Carolina, Charleston, South Carolina, USA*
[b]*Department of VCAPP, Washington State University, Pullman, Washington, USA*

ABSTRACT: Interconnections among the ventral mesencephalon, nucleus accumbens, and ventral pallidum are critical in the initiation of adaptive behavioral responses to environmental stimuli. Within this circuit are two highly topographically organized subcircuits that are differentially interconnected with limbic and motor circuitry in the brain. However, there is not a great deal of anatomical interconnection between the limbic and motor subcircuits. A polysynaptic connection between the two subcircuits involves projections from the limbic ventral pallidum to the mediodorsal thalamus to the prefrontal cortex back to the motor regions of the nucleus accumbens. In the present report we show that this connection is critical in the expression of motor behavior elicited by opioids and the capacity of a rat to perform in a task requiring spatial working memory.

INTRODUCTION

There is a well-developed literature describing the role of the projection from the nucleus accumbens to the ventral pallidum in mediating the initiation of adaptive behavioral responses.[1,2] This projection is embedded in the circuit shown in FIGURE 1A that has been termed the *motive circuit*.[3] The motive circuit mediates the translation of motivationally relevant stimuli into adaptive motor responses.[3–5] This translational function can be viewed in three stages: the receipt of motivationally relevant information via afferent innervation from limbic nuclei and the extended amygdala; the integration of this information within the motive circuit to determine the intensity of the adaptive motor response; and the initiation of the motor response via efferent projections to motor nuclei, such as the substantia nigra, subthalamic nucleus, and pedunculopontine motor region. These stages are reflected in the relatively discrete topography of projections within the motive circuit. FIGURE 1B illustrates that the afferent limb of the motive circuit involves interconnections among the ventral tegmental area (VTA), the shell of the nucleus accumbens, and the ventromedial ventral pallidum (VPm), whereas the efferent component of the motive circuit consists of interconnections among the substantia nigra, the core of the nucleus accumbens, and the dorsolateral ventral pallidum (VPl).[6,7] The relatively discrete topography of the limbic and motor subcircuits of the motive circuit provides anatomical substrates

---

[c]Send correspondence to Peter Kalivas, Ph.D., Department of Physiology and Neuroscience, Medical University of South Carolina, 167 Ashley Avenue, Suite 607, P.O. Box 25077, Charleston, South Carolina 29425. Voice: 843-792-4424; fax: 843-792-4423; kalivasp@musc.edu

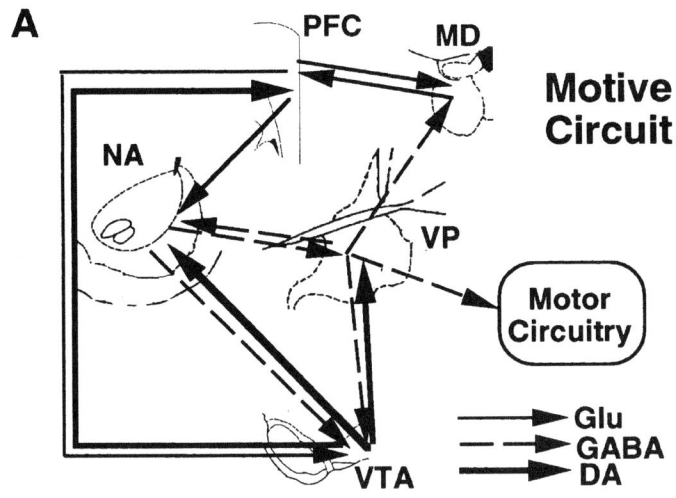

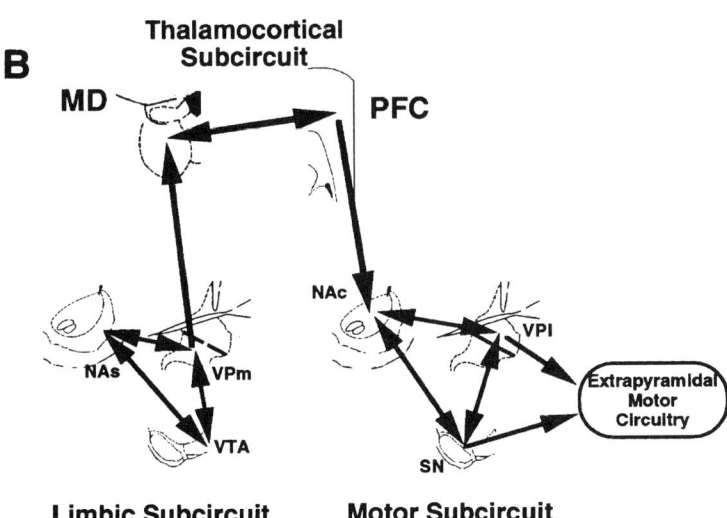

FIGURE 1. Illustration of the motive circuit and the topographically organized subcircuits constituting the motive circuit. MD, mediodorsal thalamus; NA, nucleus accumbens; NAc, core of the nucleus accumbens; NAs, shell of the nucleus accumbens; SN, substantia nigra; PFC, prefrontal cortex; VP, ventral pallidum; VPl, dorsolateral ventral pallidum; VPm, ventromedial ventral pallidum; VTA, ventral tegmental area.

for the first and third stages of the translational function of the motive circuit, namely the receipt of motivationally relevant information from limbic nuclei and the initiation of adaptive behavioral responses, respectively.

The second functional component of the motive circuit that mediates the integration of information requires communication between the afferent limbic and the efferent motor subcircuits. One anatomical substrate potentially responsible for communication between the subcircuits is the projection from the VPm to the mediodorsal thalamus (MD; see FIG. 1B). Neurons in the VPm project to the MD which has reciprocal connections with the dorsal prefrontal cortex (PFC).[8,9] This region of the PFC, including the prelimbic and anterior cingulate cortices, projects to the core and not to the shell of the nucleus accumbens.[10] Thus, the topography of this thalamocortical circuit provides a mechanism for transferring information from the limbic to the motor subcircuits.[6,7,11] Neither the projection from the VPm to the thalamus nor the projection from the PFC to the core of the nucleus accumbens is reciprocal. Thus, the flow of information is rectified and will move from the limbic to the motor subcircuit.

This article will review the relative functional importance of the thalamocortical connection between the limbic and motor subcircuits. Two behaviors involving the motive circuit were examined in order to assess the relative importance of the thalamocortical connection between the two subcircuits. The first behavior examined was the pharmacological induction of motor activity via microinjecting neurotransmitter agonists into the VP or MD. The second behavior was performance in a delayed spatial memory task following pharmacological manipulations in the VP, MD, and PFC.

THALAMOCORTICAL CIRCUIT AND MOTOR ACTIVITY

The stimulation of glutamate receptors with AMPA, dopamine receptors with dopamine, or mu opioid receptors with DAMGO in the VP elicits motor activation.[12,13] To determine involvement of the MD in the motor responses, the local anesthetic procaine was microinjected into the MD 5 min prior to injecting drug into the VP. Only the motor stimulant effect of DAMGO was blocked by procaine microinjection into the MD, whereas the behavioral activation by AMPA and dopamine was unaffected.[14]

To further examine the involvement of the thalamocortical circuit in motor stimulation, neurotransmitter analogues were microinjected directly into the MD.[15] Inhibiting MD cells with either the $GABA_B$ agonist baclofen or the mu agonist DAMGO produced motor stimulation. Moreover, the motor stimulant response was associated with alterations in dopamine transmission in the prefrontal cortex and core of the nucleus accumbens. This supports the involvement of the projection from the MD to the PFC and on to the nucleus accumbens.

THALAMOCORTICAL CIRCUIT AND WORKING MEMORY

A T-maze was used to assess the fidelity of spatial working memory in rats. The T-maze used has been described in detail elsewhere.[16] Slightly fasted (15 gm food/day) rats were trained (10 trials/day) to alternate entry into the arms of the T-maze in order to obtain a food reward. A 10 s delay was used between trials, and animals

TABLE 1. Effect of neurotransmitter analogue microinjection on working spatial memory as assessed by delayed alternation in a T-maze

Treatment	N	Dose (nmol)	% Correct
Prefrontal Cortex			
Control	12		91 ± 5
CNQX	5	0.5	86 ± 3*
CNQX	7	5	79 ± 4*
Control	6		87 ± 3
CPP	5	0.15	90 ± 4
CPP	6	1.5	65 ± 7*
Control	8		90 ± 6
MCPG	8	10.0	89 ± 4
Mediodorsal Thalamus			
Control	7		87 ± 2
Baclofen	7	0.03	83 ± 7
Baclofen	7	0.1	67 ± 9*
Baclofen	7	0.3	39 ± 10*
Ventral Pallidum			
Control	5		80 ± 3
DAMGO	7	0.01	74 ± 4
DAMGO	5	0.1	61 ± 5*

*$p < 0.05$, comparing drug treatment to controls within each brain area using a one-way ANOVA followed by a Dunnett's test. Control was saline for all drugs expect CNQX, which was 10% DMSO.

were trained to 80% correct prior to beginning experiments. To determine if glutamate transmission in the PFC was important in performing the delayed alternation task, the AMPA antagonist, CNQX, the NMDA blocker, CPP, or the metabotropic glutamate antagonist, MCPG, were microinjected into the PFC 5 min prior to beginning behavioral testing (TABLE 1). Both CNQX and CPP significantly reduced performance with minimum effective doses of 0.15 and 1.5 nmol, respectively. By contrast, a relatively high dose of MCPG (10 nmol) was ineffective. Having established a role for glutamate transmission in the PFC, it was determined if the glutamatergic projection from the MD to the PFC was important. The inhibition of neurons in the MD by microinjecting baclofen produced a dose-dependent reduction in performance in the T-maze. Because DAMGO microinjection into the VP was shown to produce a motor stimulant response that involved the MD (see above), the capacity of DAMGO microinjection into the VP to inhibit performance in the T-maze was examined. TABLE 1 shows that DAMGO in the VP significantly reduced the number of correct responses in the T-maze.

FUNCTIONAL RELEVANCE OF THE THALAMOCORTICAL CIRCUIT

The data described in this report support a functional role for the thalamocortical connection between the limbic and motor subcircuits of the motive circuit. In both behavioral tests pharmacological modulation of the thalamocortical circuit modified behavioral output. A role for the thalamocortical projection in regulating behavior has been implicated in other studies. Procaine microinjection into the MD inhibits hoarding behavior, and lesions of the MD disrupt a number of behaviors related to memory and learning, as well as the psychomotor stimulant–induced behavioral activity.[17–21]

Given the drugs employed in the studies described above and the transmitters present in the projection neurons of the motive circuit, the effects on both motor activity and working memory may arise from similar actions. Inhibition of the projection from the MD to the PFC with baclofen stimulated motor activity and inhibited performance in the T-maze. This is consistent with the fact that ionotropic glutamate antagonists microinjected into the PFC also inhibited T-maze performance. Inasmuch as the inhibition of the glutamatergic projection to the PFC is critical, it can be postulated that stimulation of the GABAergic neurons in the VP will also affect behavior by inhibiting neurons in the MD. In this regard it is perhaps surprising that the motor response arising via stimulation of the VP neurons with microinjected AMPA did not involve the thalamocortical circuit. It was also surprising that DAM-

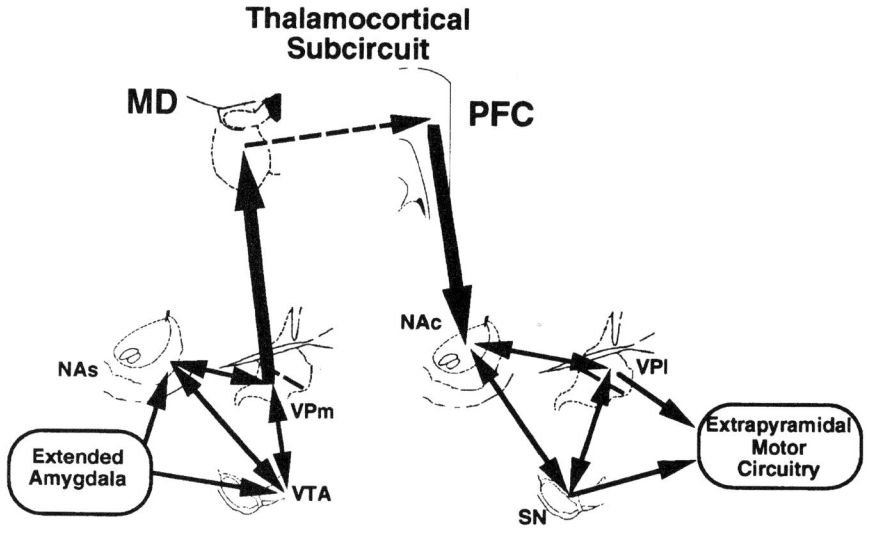

FIGURE 2. Illustration of changes in the thalamocortical subcircuit mediating increased locomotor activity and a disruption of spatial working memory. It is proposed that both behavioral alterations can be produced by increasing activity of the GABAergic projection from the VPm to the MD, decreasing glutamate transmission from the MD to the PFC, and increasing glutamate output from the PFC.

GO engaged the thalamocortical circuit, inasmuch as in most situations the stimulation of mu receptors is inhibitory to neuronal activity.[22] Therefore, one would predict that the motor response from DAMGO microinjection into the VP would include inhibition, not stimulation, of the GABAergic neurons projecting from the VP to the MD. This apparent contradiction can perhaps be explained by the fact that in addition to being on VP neurons, mu opioid receptors are located presynaptically on GABAergic afferents from the nucleus accumbens.[23] Moreover, GABA release is reduced by stimulating mu receptors in the VP (unpublished observations). Thus, the predominant effect from pharmacologically stimulating mu receptors in the VP may be to inhibit GABA release and thereby disinhibit the VP to MD projection.

FIGURE 2 illustrates the organization and shows the postulated changes produced in thalamocortical activity that affected locomotor activity and spatial working memory. These include an increase in GABAergic activity in the VP to MD projection, a decrease in glutamate transmission between the MD and PFC, and an increase in corticofugal glutamate transmission from the PFC to the core of the nucleus accumbens.

In summary, the motive circuit consists of topographically organized subcircuits. The limbic subcircuit is the afferent component receiving information coding motivationally relevant stimuli from limbic nuclei and the extended amygdala. By way of reciprocal interconnections within the limbic subcircuit, this information is integrated and passed through the PFC for evaluation via the thalamocortical circuit. Combined with cortical input this information is passed to the motor subcircuit, which ultimately communicates directly with extrapyramidal motor systems to initiate the appropriate behavioral response.

REFERENCES

1. MOGENSON, G.J., D.J. JONES & C.Y. YIM. 1980. From motivation to action: functional interface between the limbic system and the motor system. Prog. Neurobiol. **14:** 69–97.
2. LEMOAL, M. & H. SIMON. 1991. Mesocorticolimbic dopaminergic network: functional and regulatory roles. Physiol. Rev. **71:** 155–234.
3. KALIVAS, P.W., L. CHURCHILL & M.A. KLITENICK. 1993. The circuitry mediating the translation of motivational stimuli into adaptive motor responses. In Limbic Motor Circuits and Neuropsychiatry. P. W. Kalivas & C. D. Barnes, Eds.: 237–287. CRC Press. Boca Raton.
4. MOGENSON, G.J., S.M. BRUDZYNSKI, M. WU, C.R. YANG & C.C.Y. YIM. 1993. From motivation to action: a review of dopaminergic regulation of limbic- nucleus accumbens- pedunculopontine nucleus circuitries involved in limbic-motor integration. In Limbic Motor Circuits and Neuropsychiatry. P. W. Kalivas & C. D. Barnes, Eds.: 193–236. CRC Press. Boca Raton.
5. SWERDLOW, N.R. & G.F. KOOB. 1987. Dopamine, schizophrenia, mania and depression: toward a unified hypothesis of cortico-striato-pallido-thalamic function. Behav. Brain. Sci. **10:** 197–245.
6. HEIMER, L., D.S. ZAHM, L. CHURCHILL, P.W. KALIVAS & C. WOHLTMANN. 1991. Specificity in the projection patterns of accumbal core and shell in the rat. Neuroscience **41:** 89–125.
7. ZAHM, D.S. & J.S. BROG. 1992. On the significance of subterritories in the "accumbens" part of the rat ventral striatum. Neuroscience **50:** 751–767.
8. CHURCHILL, L., D.S. ZAHM & P.W. KALIVAS. 1996. The mediodorsal nucleus of the thalamus. I. Forebrain GABAergic innervation. Neuroscience **70:** 93–102.

9. PIROT, S., T.M. JAY, J. GLOWINSKI & A. THIERRY. 1994. Anatomical and electrophysiological evidence of an excitatory amino acid from the thalamic mediodorsal nucleus to the prefrontal cortex in the rat. Eur. J. Neurosci. **6:** 1225–1234.
10. DEUTCH, A.Y., A.J. BOURDELAIS & D.S. ZAHM. 1993. The nucleus accumbens core and shell: accumbal compartments and their functional attributes. *In* Limbic Motor Circuits and Neuropsychiatry. P. W. Kalivas & C. D. Barnes, Eds.: 45–88. CRC Press. Boca Raton.
11. GROENEWEGEN, H.J. 1988. Organization of afferent connections of the mediodorsal thalamic nucleus in the rat, related to mediodorsal-prefrontal topography. Neuroscience **24:** 379–431.
12. NAPIER, T.C. 1993. Transmitter actions and interactions on pallidal neuronal function. *In* Limbic Motor Circuits and Neuropsychiatry. P. W. Kalivas & C. D. Barnes, Eds.: 125–154. CRC Press. Boca Raton.
13. JOHNSON, K., L. CHURCHILL, M.A. KLITENICK, M.S. HOOKS & P.W. KALIVAS. 1996. Involvement of the ventral tegmental area in locomotion elicited from the nucleus accumbens or ventral pallidum. J. Pharmacol. Exp. Ther. **277:** 1122–1131.
14. CHURCHILL, L. & P.W. KALIVAS. 1998. Involvement of the mediodorsal thalamus and midbrain extrapyramidal area in opioid-induced locomotionlicted from the nucleus accumbens or ventral pallidum. Behav. Brain Res. In press.
15. KLITENICK, M.A. & P.W. KALIVAS. 1994. Behavioral and neurochemical studies of opioid effects in the pedunculopontine and nucleus mediodorsal thalamus. J. Pharmacol. Exp. Ther. **269:** 437–448.
16. MOGHADDAM, B., B. ADAMS, A. VERMA & D. DALY. 1997. Activation of glutamatergic neurotransmission by ketamine: a novel step in the pathway from NMDA receptor blockade to dopaminergic and cognitive disruptions associated with the prefrontal cortex. J. Neurosci. **17:** 2921–2927.
17. MOGENSON, G.J. & M. WU. 1988. Differential effects on locomotor activity of injections of procaine into mediodorsal thalamus and pedunculopontine nucleus. Brain Res. Bull. **20:** 241–246.
18. SWERDLOW, N.R. & G.F. KOOB. 1987. Lesions of the dorsomedial nucleus of the thalamus, medial prefrontal cortex and pedunculopontine nucleus: Effects on locomotor activity mediated by nucleus accumbens-ventral pallidal circuitry. Brain Res. **412:** 233–243.
19. OYOSHI, T., H. NISHIJO, T. ASAKURA, Y. TAKAMURA & T. ONO. 1996. Emotional and behavioral correlates of mediodorsal thalamic neurons during associative learning in rats. J. Neurosci. **16:** 5812–5829.
20. HUNT, P.R., N. NEAVE, C. SHAW & J.P. AGGLETON. 1994. The effects of lesions to the fornix and dorsomedial thalamus on concurrent discrimination learning by rats. Behav.Brain Res. **62:** 195–205.
21. GAFFAN, D. & E.A. MURRAY. 1990. Amygdalar interaction with the mediodorsal nucleus of the thalamus and the ventromedial prefrontal cortex in stimulus-reward associative learning in the monkey. J. Neurosci. **8:** 3144–3150.
22. NORTH, R.A. 1991. Opioid receptors and ion channels. *In* Neurobiology of Opioids, O. F. X. Almeida & T. S. Shippenberg, Eds. Springer-Verlag. New York.
23. OLIVE, M.F., B. ANTON, P. MICEVYCH, C.J. EVANS & N.T. MAIDMENT. 1997. Presynaptic versus postsynaptic localization of mu and delta opioid receptors in dorsal and ventral striatalpallidal pathways. J. Neurosci. **17:** 7471–7479.

Functional Specificity of Ventral Striatal Compartments in Appetitive Behaviors

ANN E. KELLEY[a]

Department of Psychiatry, University of Wisconsin-Madison Medical School, 6001 Research Park Boulevard, Madison, Wisconsin 53719, USA

ABSTRACT: The nucleus accumbens and its associated circuitry subserve behaviors linked to natural or biological rewards, such as feeding, drinking, sex, exploration, and appetitive learning. We have investigated the functional role of neurotransmitter and intracellular transduction mechanisms in behaviors subserved by the core and shell subsystems within the accumbens. Local infusion of the selective NMDA antagonist, AP-5, into the accumbens core, but not the shell, completely blocked acquisition of a bar-press response for food in hungry rats. This effect was apparent only when infused during the early stages of learning. We have also recently shown that infusion of certain protein kinase inhibitors into the core also impairs learning in the same paradigm. These results suggest that plasticity-related mechanisms within the accumbens core, involving glutamate-linked intracellular second messengers, are important for response-reinforcement learning. In contrast to the core, which primarily connects to somatic motor output systems, the shell is more intimately linked to viscero-endocrine effector systems. We have shown that both AMPA and GABA receptors within the medial shell (but not the core) are critically involved in controlling the brain's feeding pathways, via activation of the lateral hypothalamus (LH). This effect is blocked by local inhibition of the LH in double-cannulae experiments and also strongly and selectively activates Fos expression in the LH. These results provide a newly emerging picture of the differentiated functions of this forebrain region and suggest an integrated role in the elaboration of adaptive motor actions.

INTRODUCTION

In a landmark paper, the Canadian physiological psychologist Gordon Mogenson observed that many of the brain regions involved in emotion or cognition had significant, converging connections to a forebrain structure known as the nucleus accumbens, a prominent part of the ventral striatum.[1] He noted that the nucleus accumbens appeared to be anatomically interposed between two major functional realms, the limbic system and the motor system, perhaps acting to translate thoughts and emotions into movements. The requirement for this integrative function had been noted earlier by Kornhuber,[2] who commented that "movements are parts of actions, and actions have to satisfy the needs of organisms and secure the survival of the species." The thesis of the present review will be that there are two central features of the neural integrative activities of the ventral striatum that are subserved by the two recently defined subterritories of the nucleus accumbens, the core and shell.[3,4] These two

[a]Voice: 608-262-1123; fax: 608-265-3050; aekelley@macc.wisc.edu

functions, which will be elaborated in detail below, constitute the learning of adaptive motor responses and the control of brain feeding circuits (see also a recent review).[5]

Both of these proposed functions have their conceptual and historical roots in a number of theories that attempted to explain motivated behavior and learning. Perhaps the most important of these for the present hypotheses is Thorndike's law of effect, which states that behavioral acts followed by "satisfaction" to the organism would tend to be repeated in the future, whereas behavioral acts followed by negative consequences would diminish in their occurrence.[6] In other words, the law of effect proposes that learning consists of the reinforcing of a connection between a response and a stimulus situation, and this strengthening is dependent on the response being followed by a positive event that is presumably beneficial to the animal in some way. Clark Hull's contribution to learning theory,[7] integrating the concept of drive or biological need with reinforcement and the strengthening of behavior, is also closely related to many current ideas about the nucleus accumbens, more than fifty years later. He proposed that a deprivation state, such as food or water deprivation, energized behavior nonspecifically. This activation increased the probability that an adaptive response would occur. Let us imagine, for example, a very hungry, exploratory rat accidentally bumping into a lever that provides a food pellet (reinforcement). The reduction of drive (and, in Hull's later writings, "drive-stimulus reduction," or reduction of cravings) that results with the reinforcement causes the animal to repeat the response and engage in learning. In Hull's scheme he called the stimulus–response connection "habit" and postulated that drive and habit multiply together to determine the strength of behavior. Hull noted that "... habit strength increases when receptor and effector activities occur in close temporal contiguity, provided their approximately contiguous occurrence is associated with primary or secondary reinforcement" [7] (p. 178). The concept of habit is important, because it has contributed substantially to current thinking about the basal ganglia and learning. As expounded below, this notion may provide a conceptual basis for the neuromolecular events within accumbens associated with response learning.

Another set of historical developments that pertains to the current hypotheses concerning the nucleus accumbens grew out of classical studies on the physiology of motivation. Curt Richter conceived of the idea that motivated behaviors served to maintain the internal homeostatic environment, in coordination with more automatic mechanisms.[8] Thus, motivated behaviors, such as feeding, drinking, nest-building, or temperature-regulating were self-regulatory and highly sensitive to fluctuating internal conditions of the organism. A further significant contribution was the work of Eliot Stellar, who was among the first to develop a truly integrative theory of motivation based on brain-behavior relationships. In his classic papers, he synthesized significant theoretical constructs, such as drive, goal-directed behavior, instinct, sensation, and learning with the current empirical data, forming a broad conceptual framework.[9,10] Although his major focus was on the hypothalamus, Stellar also suggested that "... central neural structures outside of the hypothalamus also contribute excitatory and inhibitory influences to the control of motivation ...." Recent work on the nucleus accumbens, as described below, demonstrates an important role in this regard, with significant functional connections to the hypothalamus.

The anatomical organization of the nucleus accumbens is well-suited to its hypothetical role as a limbic-motor integrator, as elaborated in detail in other chapters in this volume. Within this area there is a convergence of afferents conveying information related to affective and motivational states, arising from limbic structures such as the amygdala, hippocampus, prefrontal cortex, midbrain monoamine systems, and brain stem autonomic centers.[11–15] Moreover, it has extensive connections to skeletal motor and visceral motor output systems.[16–18] Although the nucleus accumbens has long been considered a ventral striatal territory with prominent similarities to the overlying caudate-putamen, in recent years there has been a major anatomical reconceptualization of this structure based on refined anatomical analysis. Analysis of connectivity as well as its histochemical profile indicates that the nucleus accumbens is composed of three major subterritories, which have been termed the core, shell, and rostral pole. The core and shell subregions, which have been most extensively studied, show striking differences in their afferent input and efferent projections.[4,17] For example, although both core and shell receive input from hippocampus, the ventral subiculum projects exclusively to the shell whereas the dorsal subiculum projects to the core. Different regions of prefrontal cortex project to different zones: the prelimbic area projects to core, whereas the infralimbic and piriform cortices project to shell.[12] Specific subcompartments of the amygdala also reach distinct subregions within accumbens core and shell.[19] In terms of outputs, the core subregion connects extensively to classic basal ganglia output structures, such as the ventral pallidum, subthalamic nucleus, and substantia nigra. The shell subregion, by contrast, projects preferentially to subcortical limbic regions, such as the lateral hypothalamus, ventral tegmental area, ventromedial ventral pallidum, and brain stem autonomic centers.

On the basis of these distinctive anatomical profiles, it has been proposed that there may be significant functional specializations of these two subregions and their associated circuitry.[4,17,20] The general notion is that the accumbens core has similarities to the overlying caudate-putamen and may be more allied with voluntary motor functions, whereas the shell has close ties to the "extended amygdala"[3] and its functions are more in the domain of visceral or motivational mechanisms. Evidence is presented in support of this general hypothesis in this paper. Moreover, the hypothesis is further extended to state that the core of accumbens, and particularly NMDA receptors, are critical for instrumental learning, whereas the shell of accumbens, particularly GABAergic and AMPA receptors, are specifically involved in the control of feeding.

GLUTAMATE RECEPTORS WITHIN THE NUCLEUS ACCUMBENS CORE: A FOREBRAIN MECHANISM FOR RESPONSE-REINFORCEMENT LEARNING

Given the long association of the nucleus accumbens with motivation and reward, it is not surprising that many studies have focused on the role of this structure in learning and memory. Earlier studies particularly focused on the role of ventral striatal dopamine (DA) in reward-related learning,[21] and a number of experiments using 6-OHDA lesions or pharmacological manipulations suggested that blockade of DA disrupted learning and enhancement of DA facilitated learning.[22–25] However, it is often difficult to clearly interpret DA manipulations because they nearly always affect response output or performance. Work with an electrolytic or selective excitotoxic has also indicated a role for the nucleus accumbens in learning; for example, such lesions impair acquisition of learning in the Morris water maze,[26] spatial discrimination in a T-maze,[27] and a visual stimulus-response task.[28] Several recent studies employing lidocaine-induced inactivation of the accumbens have provided further evidence for this structure's mediating certain aspects of spatial learning and performance.[29,30] A summary of experiments pertaining to the role of the nucleus accumbens in learning and memory, with particular emphasis on hippocampal input, is provided in a recent review.[31]

Within the framework initiated by Mogenson,[1] much thought has been given over the past decade or so to the role of glutamate-coded inputs to the nucleus accumbens. As in the overlying caudate nucleus, the medium-sized spiny output neurons, which constitute the main cellular component of these structures, receive excitatory input in the form of glutamate.[32,33] Moreover, there are high levels of all glutamate receptor subtypes in the striatum.[34] As noted in the previous section, the area including the nucleus accumbens is particularly distinctive in that it receives strikingly convergent inputs from the hippocampus, prefrontal cortex, amygdala, midbrain, and thalamus, and in turn projects to both somatic and visceral motor output systems. Recently our research has focused on the investigation of functions of the nucleus accumbens and its related circuitry through the study of its glutamatergic innervation. Our first studies showed that blockade of N-methyl-D-aspartate (NMDA) receptors within the core of the accumbens (but not the shell) reduced exploratory locomotion,[35] a result similar to previous work conducted with nonselective glutamate antagonists.[36] We then conducted several studies using NMDA antagonist infusion into accumbens subregions on learning in several spatial tasks. Local infusion of the selective competitive antagonist AP-5 into the core was found to severely disrupt path learning in a spatial food-gathering task.[37] Infusion of the selective AMPA (alpha-amino-3-hydroxy-5-methylisoxazole-4-propionic acid)/kainate antagonist DNQX (6,7-dinitroquinoxaline-2,3-dione) into the core mildly impaired learning, and both drugs had lesser effects when infused into the shell. In a recent study of the effect of striatal infusion of AP-5 in an eight-arm radial arm maze (with four arms baited), blockade of NMDA receptors in the accumbens core, but not the shell, markedly disrupted acquisition of efficient responding.[38] Once the animals had learned the task, however, AP-5 infusion into core had no effect.

Although it was clear that NMDA receptors were involved in spatial learning, we were curious if other forms of learning would be affected by intra-accumbens NMDA blockade. In one series of experiments, the consequences of intra-accumbens infusion of AP-5 on acquisition of a lever-press task for food were investigated.[39] In this task, hungry animals are exposed, in an operant chamber, to two levers, one of which provides a food pellet when pressed, for a 15-minute session on a fixed-ratio 2 schedule. Normal rats learn this task quite rapidly over days. Somewhat to our surprise, rats treated with AP-5 in the core showed no learning whatsoever and only began to learn the task when infusions were no longer given (see FIG. 1). Equivalent infusions in the accumbens shell had little effect on response learning. Parallel experiments examining the effects of these treatments on general motor behavior and feeding indicated that the impairment could not be attributed to a general motor or motivational deficit (TABLE 1). Moreover, AP-5 had no effect once the animals had learned the task, suggesting that as in the spatial learning experiments, NMDA-dependent mechanisms are critical only in the early stages of learning.

TABLE 1. Influence of intra-accumbens AP-5 treatment on feeding and locomotor activity in food-deprived rats (15-minute test)[a]

Accumbens treatment ($n = 8$)	Food intake (g)	Feeding duration (s)	Locomotion
AP-5 (5 nmol)	4.4 ± 0.6	573 ± 49	20 ± 4
Vehicle	4.2 ± 0.8	631 ± 24	18 ± 3

[a]Data represents means ± SEM. Locomotion is frequency of cage crossings. No significant differences between treatments.

These results are among the first demonstrating NMDA-dependent mechanisms in striatal-based learning. Of course, there is much evidence for a major role of basal ganglia structures in motor learning. Several earlier postulates suggested a role for striatal systems in cognitive and affective functions, in addition to their well-known motor functions.[40,41] A considerable array of empirical data supports the contention that both ventral and dorsal striatal regions are important for certain forms of learning. One prominent theory holds that the striatum is crucial for the acquisition of relatively automatic motor "habits," or basic stimulus–response associative learning[42–44] (in contrast to hippocampus and amygdala, which are generally thought to be more involved in contextual or declarative learning, and stimulus-reward learning). In other words, returning to Thorndike's law of effect, a neural mechanism must exist whereby a response followed by satisfaction becomes strengthened, and the probability of its occurrence becomes greatly facilitated in the appropriate stimulus conditions. We

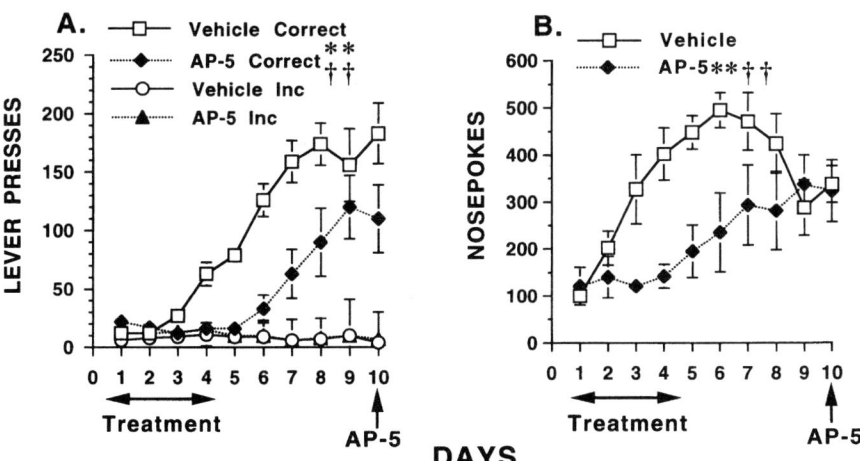

FIGURE 1. Response-reinforcement learning is dependent on NMDA receptor activation in the nucleus accumbens core. **A:** Acquisition of a lever-press response for food over time. **B:** Nose-poking behavior into food tray during learning. Animals were injected in the nucleus accumbens core with the NMDA antagonist, AP-5 (5 nmol bilaterally), or vehicle (saline) before the first four sessions and then were tested without treatment for 5 days. On day 10, all rats (including the vehicle group) received AP-5. Asterisks indicate overall treatment effects in ANOVA analysis; daggers indicate treatment x day interactions. (Kelley et al.[39] With permission from *Proceedings of the Journal of the National Academy of Sciences USA.*)

propose that activation of NMDA receptors in the accumbens core, together with concomitant intracellular molecular events, is such a critical mechanism for adaptive response learning. It should be noted, moreover, that other forms of learning may also be mediated by the accumbens core; for example, it has recently been shown that excitotoxic lesions of the core (but not the shell) impair the learning of anticipatory approach response governed by a pavlovian conditioned stimulus (CS);[45] we have shown a similar impairment with intracore AP-5 infusions.[39] Thus the control of CS–UCS (unconditioned stimulus) over learned behavior may also depend on accumbens core neurons. Also, it is important to emphasize that the accumbens core is not the only region involved in this learning; very recent experiments in our laboratory have indicated that NMDA receptor–dependent plasticity in the amygdala and prefrontal cortex is also required for appetitive instrumental learning.[46]

NEURONAL PLASTICITY IN VENTRAL STRIATUM

There is much empirical evidence to support the hypotheses discussed above, which has emerged relatively recently. Although classic work on neuronal plasticity in relation to learning and memory has focused primarily on the hippocampus, in recent years data have accrued supporting plasticity within the striatum and accumbens, at both the cellular and molecular level. First, striatal neurons are involved in assessing, learning, and responding to stimuli with motivationally significant valence. For example, neurons in the monkey ventral striatum are sensitive to both primary and conditioned rewards.[47–49] Moreover, during acquisition of sensorimotor conditioning in monkeys, in which a cue predicts delivery of juice reward, a progressive increase in the number of tonically active neurons that respond to that cue emerges.[50] Examples of cellular plasticity, such as long-term potentiation and long-term depression, have been demonstrated in both dorsal striatum and accumbens.[51–55] For example, tetanic stimulation of prefrontal efferents induces NMDA-dependent LTP in the nucleus accumbens.[56] A recent study reported simultaneous induction of LTP within the accumbens and prefrontal cortex following stimulation of the fornix-fimbria bundle,[57] suggesting that the accumbens may be part of a distributed network participating in memory formation. Indeed, several recent neural network models incorporate the hippocampal-accumbens pathway as a mechanism for successful selection or "stamping in" of correct locomotor actions.[58,59]

It is important to consider what the role of DA might be in this model. A current influential theory posits that activity in dopaminergic neurons serves as a predictor of reward or stimulus salience.[60] Dopamine neurons alter their firing properties during learning; initially they are activated by primary rewards, but if a stimulus consistently predictive of reward is presented over trials (conditioned stimulus), there is a progressive shift in firing pattern, such that the activation is observed only in response to presentation of the conditioned stimulus, but no longer to the primary reward.[61] Thus, midbrain DA neurons, which project to widespread cortical and striatal areas, are proposed to "construct and distribute information about rewarding events." [60] In relation to the present hypotheses concerning accumbens NMDA receptors, glutamate-dopamine interactions may initiate a cascade of biochemical events that eventually leads to alterations in gene expression, and that would ultimately influence long-term or permanent synaptic changes underlying motor learning. Indeed, several recent theoretical models have been proposed to explain reinforcement learning in corticostriatal systems. These models postulate an interaction of dopaminergic and corticostriatal synapses, and consequent integrated molecular signals, on the dendritic spines of striatal medium-size spiny output neurons.[62–64] Dopaminergic and glutamatergic inputs synapse in close proximity on the same dendritic spine.[65] Activity in spiny neurons is largely dependent on excitatory input from the cortex. Influx of calcium via NMDA receptors in association with dopamine-mediated intracellular changes (such as in the cAMP system) is proposed as essential for the cellular basis of reinforcement. The demonstration of long-term enhancement of synaptic strength when cortical striatal excitation and dopaminergic activation are temporally coordinated supports this notion,[66] and it has also been found that DA selectively enhances NMDA-induced excitations in striatal slices.[67] Thus, it is possible that enhanced dopaminergic activity at a site on the dendritic spine would promote or facilitate the NMDA-mediated synaptic changes necessary for learning. Protein phosphorylation may also play an integral role in this process; for example, we have recently found that intra-accumbens infusions of protein kinase A inhibitors impair response-reinforcement learning.[68] These mechanisms are schematically diagrammed in FIGURE. 2.

Additional evidence for activity-dependent plasticity with the striatum derives from accumulating evidence that drugs of abuse have profound effects on transcrip-

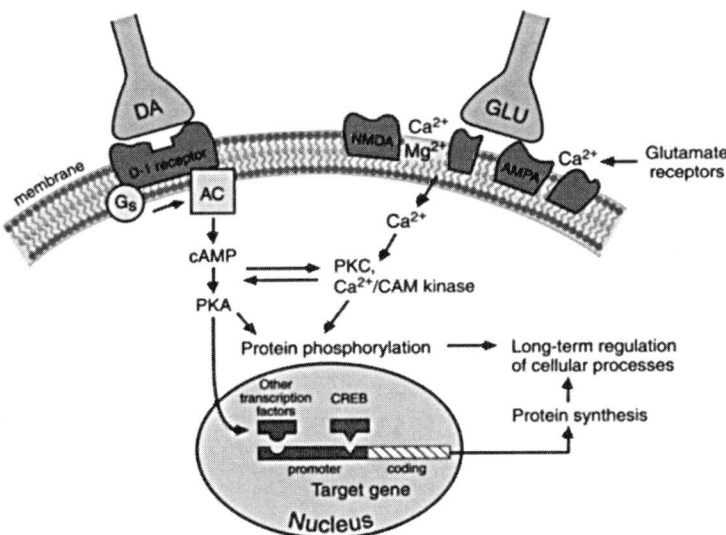

FIGURE 2. Hypothetical events underlying neural plasticity within the dendritic spines of accumbens core medium spiny neurons. Glutamate-DA interactions may initiate a cascade of biochemical events that leads to alterations in signal transduction and gene expression, effecting long-term or permanent synaptic changes underlying motor learning. Dopaminergic inputs from the midbrain and glutamatergic inputs from cortical, limbic, and thalamic regions synapse in close proximity on the same dendritic spine. AC, adenylate cyclase.

tion factors and gene expression. Amphetamine, cocaine, and morphine rapidly induce expression of the nuclear immediate early genes, such as c-*fos*, c-*jun*, *fosB*, *junB*, *Fras*, and *zif/268*,[69–71] and can alter transcription factors, such as the expression of phosphorylated CREB (cyclic AMP response element binding protein), AP-1 binding (protein binding to DNA response elements), and peptide gene expression.[70,71] It is noteworthy that many of these effects appear to be dependent on either NMDA or DA D-1 receptor activation. For example, pretreatment with MK-801, an NMDA antagonist, or the D-1 antagonist, SCH-23390, prevents amphetamine induction of c-*fos* and *zif/268*,[72,73] and the *fos* and *jun* mRNA induction by D-1 agonists or DA in dissociated striatal cultures is blocked by both competitive and noncompetitive NMDA antagonists.[72] Behavioral sensitization to psychostimulants is also prevented by MK-801.[74] Thus, there is intriguing evidence to suggest that plasticity-related neuroadaptations within the ventral striatum and related circuitry may depend on glutamate–dopamine interactions. Most significantly, these neuroadaptations that are concomitants of learning may also underlie the process of addiction. In other words, the neuromolecular effects of addictive drugs appear to mimic the brain's normal mechanisms for ensuring reinforcement learning.

THE NUCLEUS ACCUMBENS SHELL: A CENTRAL INTEGRATOR OF FEEDING

The first suggestion that the shell might be involved in basic motivational drives arose from the theory that it was part of a forebrain system known as the "extended amygdala," which included the central and medial amygdala, and bed nucleus of the stria terminalis,[3,75] and which has prolific outputs to brain stem autonomic and locomotor areas. Recent studies with very discrete injections of retrograde or anterograde tracers show connections, either monosynaptically or indirectly via the pallidum and hypothalamus, to widespread brain stem circuits involved in autonomic arousal, neuroendocrine regulation, consummatory behaviors, pain modulation and defensive behaviors (e.g., central grey, mesopontine tegmentum, nucleus of solitary tract).[17,76]

In the course of our studies on the role of accumbens glutamate in exploratory and spatial behavior, we noticed animals voraciously feeding when they were put back in their home cages, following blockade of AMPA/kainate receptors in the shell with the drug DNQX. This effect was systematically examined, and we reported that blockade of AMPA/kainate receptors within the shell, but not the core, induced marked and prolonged feeding in satiated rats.[77] This feeding has a short onset latency (20–40 s, approximately) and is not elicited by infusion of NMDA antagonists. A detailed mapping study of the ventral and dorsal striatum showed an even greater degree of anatomical specificity; feeding was only elicited from the accumbens shell, and the posterior aspects of the shell were more sensitive than the anterior aspects.[78] This is an interesting pattern because it suggests that cells within the more posterior shell, which is more strongly connected to viscero-endocrine circuits, are preferentially involved in feeding. A study investigating the behavioral specificity of the DNQX effect found that water intake and wood-chip gnawing were not affected; however, palatable sucrose solution intake was increased by the treatment.[79] The feeding response bore remarkable resemblance to electrically induced feeding from

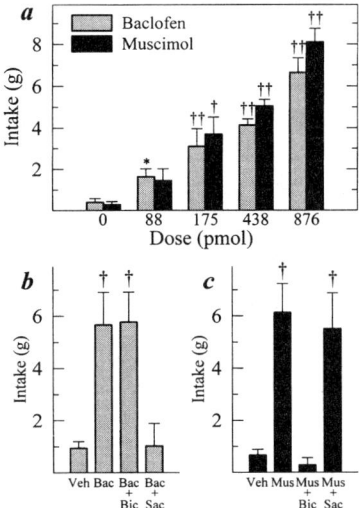

FIGURE 3. GABAergic stimulation of the nucleus accumbens shell induces marked feeding in satiated rats. ***a:*** Bilateral infusion of both the $GABA_A$ agonist, muscimol, and the $GABA_B$ agonist, baclofen, significantly increased feeding in a 30-min session. ***b:*** The baclofen-induced feeding (188 ng balcofen) was eliminated by coadministration of the $GABA_B$ antagonist, saclofen (500 ng), but not by the $GABA_A$ antagonist, bicuculline (75 ng). ***c:*** Conversely, the muscimol-induced feeding (50 ng) was blocked by coadministration of bicuculline but not by saclofen. Symbols indicate significant increases in intake as compared to saline treatment. (Stratford & Kelley.[80] With permission from the *Journal of Neuroscience*.)

the LH, and we tested the hypothesis that activation of the LH is critical for the feeding effect. Indeed, this effect is blocked by concurrent inactivation of the LH with muscimol, suggesting that the ingestive behavior is mediated through activation of cells within the LH. This was a novel demonstration of a specific behavioral role for the accumbens shell and suggested an important functional link between two major brain regions involved in reward, the accumbens and lateral hypothalamus.

If the theory that removal of an excitatory input caused feeding was correct, we speculated that direct inhibition of the cells would also induce feeding. We found that infusion of muscimol, the $GABA_A$ agonist, or baclofen, the $GABA_B$ agonist, both caused intense feeding in satiated rats when infused into the accumbens shell, as shown in FIGURE 3.[80,81] As in DNQX, the effect was also completely specific for feeding (water intake was not affected). A mapping study confirmed the posterior shell as most sensitive to feeding, and a pharmacological double dissociation was shown (the $GABA_A$ effect was blocked by $GABA_A$ antagonists but not by $GABA_B$ antagonists, and vice versa; see FIG. 3). A compound that causes increases in endogenous GABA, gamma-vinyl-GABA, by inhibiting GABA-transaminase, also markedly increased feeding. These findings suggest that the medium spiny neurons within the shell, which contain GABA as their major transmitter, may release GABA to activate normal feeding, which by self-inhibition (through recurrent collaterals) would result in disinhibition of LH or perhaps other downstream cells involved in feeding.

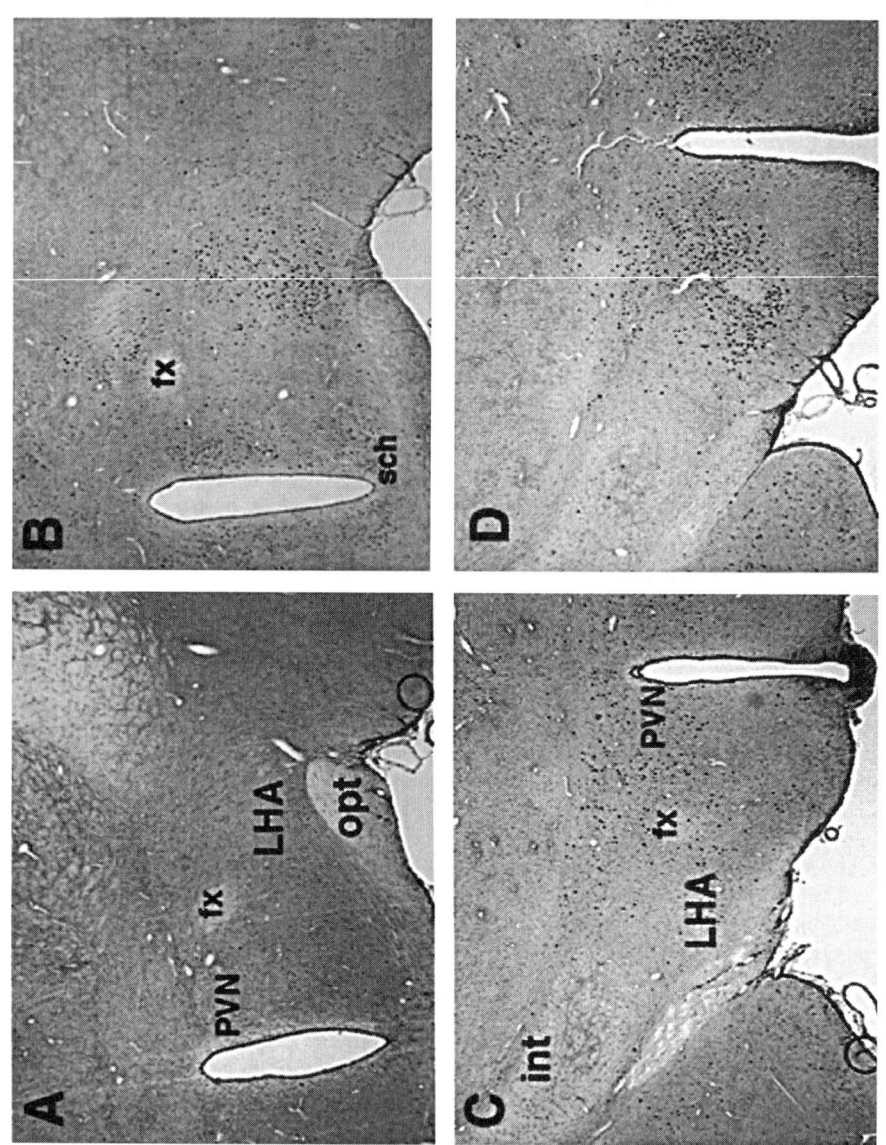

We have recent evidence supporting this hypothesis. Using expression of the immediate early gene c-*fos* as a marker for neuronal activation, we found that intra-shell muscimol markedly activates Fos expression throughout the LH, as shown in FIGURE 4.[82] When LH cells are activated by glutamate agonists, feeding also occurs.[83] Also, the $GABA_B$ effect is interesting because $GABA_B$ receptors are nearly universally presynaptic; thus, if glutamate terminals have presynaptic $GABA_B$ receptors, this could be an additional mechanism by which the glutamate input is attenuated during feeding.

A tentative model regarding the mechanisms underlying the feeding response is proposed, as diagrammed in FIGURE 5. Certain neural inputs may normally exert a tonic excitatory effect on shell neurons, via non-NMDA (AMPA or kainate) receptors. Temporary removal of this excitation with DNQX causes shell neurons to become inactive, thereby disinhibiting intrinsic LH neurons and causing animals to eat. A basic assumption of the model is that neurons arising in the shell exert an inhibitory influence on lateral hypothalamic neurons, via a GABAergic mechanism. Evidence for an inhibitory pathway from medial accumbens to lateral hypothalamus has been demonstrated.[84] However, it should be emphasized that that shell–LH interaction may be mediated via an indirect pathway rather than direct. Additionally, mention should be made of opioid modulation of feeding within the ventral striatum, although it is not the primary focus of this review. We have found that mu opioid stimulation of the nucleus accumbens results in considerable enhancement of food intake, particularly highly palatable foods, such as fat, sucrose, and salt.[85,86] Interestingly, this effect is not specific to the medial shell and is found throughout the ventral (although not dorsal) striatum, with the lateral shell being the most sensitive part.[87] Intra-accumbens opioid injection also activates Fos expression in several hypothalamic regions as well as the nucleus of the solitary tract (unpublished findings), even without food present, suggesting that this forebrain system has direct effects on lower brain stem areas involved in ingestion. These results suggest that opioid peptides within the accumbens shell may play a specific role in palatability and may also interact with the amino acid–coded systems controlling food intake in this region.

INTERACTIONS BETWEEN APPETITIVE AND AVERSIVE STIMULI IN THE ACCUMBENS SHELL

Although our work clearly demonstrates a role for GABAergic accumbens shell neurons in feeding, some puzzling inconsistencies remain. For example, the DA turnover or activation in the shell is very sensitive to a variety of stress proce-

FIGURE 4. Expression of the immediate early gene c-*fos* in the hypothalamus following infusion of the $GABA_A$ agonist muscimol (50 ng) into the nucleus accumbens shell. **A** and **C** are vehicle-treated animals; **B** and **D** are muscimol-treated animals. Food and water were not available following treatment; animals were perfused 90 min following treatment and the brains processed for immunocytochemical detection of Fos protein. Note strong expression in the muscimol-treated rats in the lateral hypothalamus; some expression was also observed in the PVN. PVN, periventricular nucleus of the hypothalamus; fx, fornix; LHA, lateral hypothalamic area; opt, optic tract; sch, suprachiasmatic nucleus; int, internal capsule. (Based on work from Stratford & Kelley[82]).

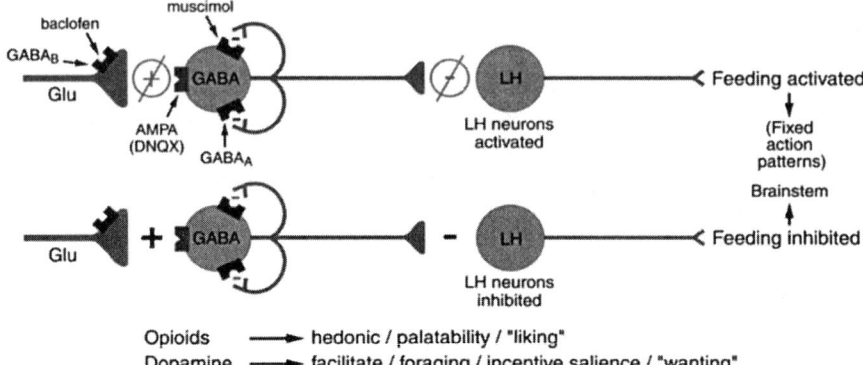

FIGURE 5. Neurotransmitter integration of feeding behavior within shell subregion of nucleus accumbens, as discussed in text. Medium spiny output neurons within the shell contain GABA as their main neurotransmitter; axon collaterals feed back to $GABA_A$ receptors on dendrites in these neurons and also to the dendrites on neighboring neurons (not shown). Cortical and thalamic input reaches spiny neurons via glutamatergic projection; these glutamatergic terminals may contain $GABA_B$ receptors as well. Increased inhibition of these neurons removes the tonic inhibition on lateral hypothalamic (LH) neurons, causing activation of LH neurons and feeding to occur. Blockade of AMPA receptors (via the antagonist DNQX) also lowers activity of shell spiny neurons and results in feeding. It is proposed that phasic glutamate release (perhaps resulting from novel sensory or environmental processing) may overcome GABA-mediate inhibition, cause an override of the feeding signal, and switch behavioral patterning away from feeding if it is adaptive to do so. It is further speculated that opioids within the ventral striatum may modulate palatability ("liking" in the model of Robinson and Berridge[112]), whereas DA has a facility role in promoting motor responses that enable the animal to come in contact with food and signaling incentive state ("wanting" in the Robinson and Berridge model).

dures,[20, 88–91] and expression of c-*fos* is most apparent in shell versus core with exposure to conditioned fear.[92] However, paradoxically, the shell is very sensitive to reward-related effects as well. We have found in our own material that expression of Fos in the shell is activated by both stressful and reinforcing stimuli (unpublished findings). Drugs of abuse tend to activate DA preferentially in the shell compared to the core, [93, 94] and microinjections of D-1 DA antagonists into the shell reduce the reinforcing effects of intravenous cocaine.[95] Certain drugs of abuse are preferentially administered to shell compared with core.[96,97] The shell, therefore, may have a role in regulating both appetitive and aversively motivated behavior. An important question concerns how these two possible functions interact. One interesting conjecture is that there may be distinct neuronal ensembles within the nucleus accumbens, based on analysis of distinct input–output relationships, that suggest even further specialized compartmentalization beyond simply core and shell. Combining tracing techniques with immunohistochemical staining, Wright and colleagues[19,98] have shown that very specific subregions of the amygdaloid complex reach specific subzones within the core and shell of the accumbens and, further, that the output of these zones is very distinct and segregated. Thus, it appears that limbic influences representing appetitive or aversive information could affect "subensembles" within the shell. O'Donnell has proposed that functional thalamo-cortical-striatal neuronal ensembles, encoding information via differential distributions of spatial and temporal activity, could convey specific cognitive information to the nucleus accumbens.[99] Moreover, neurotransmitter influences may regulate the adaptive expression (or suppression) of reward- or stress-related behaviors. The shell is reported to have a substantial noradrenergic innervation,[100] and CRF and its receptors are also dense in this region (see ref. 101). These two systems or their interaction could signal stress- or danger-related information to the nucleus accumbens.

It is of interest to consider the feeding model with regard to appetitive-aversive interactions, and to pose the following question: Why have an accumbens shell if the brain presumably already has several structures that control basic regulatory behaviors (e.g., hypothalamus, extended amygdala, brain stem regions)? Gradual increases in endogenous GABA within the shell (perhaps regulated by circulating humoral factors, such as insulin or leptin) may be associated with increased motivation for food (along with changes in hypothalamic sensing systems). When a threshold level is met, feeding may be triggered, given that food is available. However, imagine a situation where an animal is extremely hungry, finds food, and commences feeding. If a threat arises in the environment, feeding is immediately arrested and the animal engages in appropriate behavior, such as fleeing, freezing, or fighting. Although there may be a considerable energy deficit and the motivation for food is strong, there must exist an immediate and powerful override of neural circuits controlling the feeding behavior. One brain region where such a mechanism could occur is in the accumbens shell. The convergence and rapid processing of glutamate-coded inputs from critical cortical regions processing external stimuli (ventral subiculum, infralimbic prefrontal cortex, amygdala) may be key in this regard. Phasic release of glutamate could reverse the hyperpolarization of the medium spiny neurons induced by GABA, resulting in a major switch in behavioral patterning. The ability to switch between behavioral repertoires has been attributed to the accumbens in other models (see, e.g., refs. 102–104), and such amino acid–coded integration in the shell may strongly influence behavioral selection in response to changing environmental contingencies. Thus the accumbens shell is unique, in that it is influenced by a superimposition of information from both the internal environment and the external world.

Dopamine in the shell does not appear to directly participate in triggering feeding. Although some feeding can be observed following dopaminergic stimulation of this region,[105,106] these small increases in intake are not comparable to that induced by GABAergic agonists or AMPA antagonists. It is generally agreed that DA depletion or antagonism in the accumbens does not affect primary motivation for food. However, in several studies it has been clearly demonstrated that extracellular accumbens DA is increased in hungry animals or rises with feeding.[107–110] What then could be the role for DA in feeding? In accordance with the general hypothesis that DA signals availability of salient, appetitive cues or rewards in the environment, it is likely that availability of food or contexts associated with food stimulates DA, which consequently may have a general activating effect on appetitively motivated behavior. In other words, DA is not specifically involved with controlling feeding circuits, but rather is facilitory, as proposed in many general theories of dopaminergic function.[111–114] Support for this notion is provided by a recent study reporting that extracellular DA increases in the shell of the accumbens when free-feeding animals are presented with a novel, highly palatable food; when the food is not novel, the DA response habituates.[107] It is not yet clear whether DA has distinctive functions with regard to core and shell, and this question has not yet been adequately studied. However, a working hypothesis can be put forward based on the general dissociation of functions expounded in this paper. Because the caudate nucleus and accumbens core are the structures most clearly implicated in response learning, release of DA in these areas may facilitate NMDA receptor–mediated learning. Concurrent release of DA in the accumbens shell may not be involved in learning per se, but rather in signaling incentive salience and promoting motor responses that bring the animal in contact with a potentially rewarding stimulus. In a recent study, we found that the shell was generally much more sensitive to the locomotor-stimulating effects of DA agonists than the core. Therefore DA in the shell may be involved in increasing the initial output of motor responses (that could potentially lead the organism to a rewarding stimulus), whereas DA in the core participates in the stamping in of those responses that led to a satisfactory outcome. In a recent study excitotoxic shell lesions (but not those of the core) abolished the reward-enhancing and locomotor effects of amphetamine.[45] This hypothesis does not exclude the possibility that dopaminergic stimulation of both the shell and core is reinforcing by definition. In other words, it may be that rats would self-administer DA or dopaminergic agonists to both core and shell regions; this experiment has not been carried out to our knowledge.

CONCLUSIONS

Recent detailed anatomical findings have provided convincing evidence for the original major theory concerning the accumbens: that it acts as an integrator of internal and external sensory and motivationally relevant information with effector mechanisms, in order to ensure adaptive motor behavior. New research has allowed refinement of this theory. Our recent work and that of others has supported the general hypothesis that the core region is preferentially aligned with basal ganglia motor functions, whereas the role of the shell lies more in the domain of viscero-endocrine functions. More specifically, it is proposed that the core, and specifically NMDA receptors, mediates response-reinforcement learning. It is proposed that the shell is not involved in motor or response learning per se, but is responsible for integrating basic drives and viscero-endocrine effector mechanisms with cortical and subcortical information processing. This dichotomy leads to a further fundamental question: How are these major functions integrated and coordinated? There is ample evidence provided through detailed analysis of circuitry, particularly with regard to patch-matrix configurations and microcompartmentalizations, that the subregions within the accumbens have extensive cross-talk both locally and through "open" and feed-forward loops.[76,114] Joel and Weiner[115] have suggested the idea of "split" loops with basal ganglia-thalamocortical circuitry, such that information from striatal subregions (limbic, associative, motor) can be integrated in the prefrontal cortex via overlapping projections to substantia nigra, pars reticulata. The shell, which could be considered a "striatal visceral" area, has access to converging input from corticothalamic circuits and additionally has close access to response-learning mechanisms via the core and prefrontal output systems. Further experimentation using integrated and multiple approaches will help to elucidate the intricacies of the brain's motivational network.

ACKNOWLEDGMENTS

Work discussed in this paper has been supported by Grants DA04788 and DA09311 from the National Institute on Drug Abuse.

REFERENCES

1. MOGENSON, G.J., D.L. JONES & C.Y. YIM. 1980. From motivation to action: functional interface between the limbic system and the motor system. Prog. Neurobiol. 14: 69–97.
2. KORNHUBER, H.H. 1974. Cerebral cortex, cerebellum, and basal ganglia: an introduction to their motor functions. In Neurosciences: Third Study Program. F.O. Schmitt & F. G. Worden, Eds.: 267–280. MIT Press. Cambridge.
3. ALHEID, G.F. & L. HEIMER. 1988. New perspectives in basal forebrain organization of special relevance for neuropsychiatric disorders: the striatopallidal, amygdaloid, and corticopetal components of substantia innominata. Neuroscience 27: 1–39.
4. ZAHM, D.S. & J.S. BROG. 1992. On the significance of subterritories in the "accumbens" part of the rat ventral striatum. Neuroscience 50: 751–767.
5. KELLEY, A.E. 1999. Neural integrative activities of nucleus accumbens subregions in relation to motivation and learning. Psychobiology. In press.
6. THORNDIKE, E. 1911. Animal intelligence. Macmillan. New York.
7. HULL, C.L. 1943. Principles of behavior. Appleton. New York.
8. RICHTER, C.P. 1942–1943. Total self-regulatory functions in animals and human beings. Harvey Lect. 37: 63–103.
9. STELLAR, E. 1954. The physiology of motivation. Psychol. Rev. 61: 5–21.
10. STELLAR, E. 1960. Drive and Motivation. In Handbook of Physiology. Sect. 1. Neurophysiology. H.W. Magoun, Ed. Vol. III: 1501–1527. American Physiological Society. Washington, D.C.
11. BECKSTEAD, R.M. 1979. An autoradiographic examination of corticocortical and subcortical projections of the mediodorsal-projection (prefrontal) cortex in rats. J. Comp. Neurol. 84: 43–62.
12. BROG, J.S., A. SALYAPONGSE, A.Y. DEUTCH & D.S. ZAHM. 1993. The patterns of afferent innervation of the core and shell in the "accumbens" part of the rat ventral striatum: immunohistochemical detection of retrogradely transported fluoro-gold. J. Comp Neurol. 338: 255–278.
13. KELLEY, A.E., V.B. DOMESICK & W.J.H. NAUTA. 1982. The amygdalostriatal projection in the rat—an anatomical study by anterograde and retrograde tracing methods. Neuroscience 7: 615–630.
14. KELLEY, A.E. & V.B. DOMESICK. 1982. The distribution of the projection from the hippocampal formation to the nucleus accumbens in the rat: an anterograde- and retrograde-horseradish peroxidase study. Neuroscience 7: 2321–2335.
15. MCDONALD, A.J. 1991. Topographical organization of amygdaloid projections to the caudatoputamen, nucleus accumbens, and related striatal-like areas of the rat brain. Neuroscience 44: 15–33.
16. GROENEWEGEN, H.J. & F.T. RUSSCHEN. 1984. Organization of the efferent projections of the nucleus accumbens to pallidal, hypothalamic, and mesencephalic structures: a tracing and immunohistochemical study in the cat. J. Comp. Neurol. 223: 347–367.
17. HEIMER, L., D.S. ZAHM, L. CHURCHILL, P.W. KALIVAS & C. WOHLTMANN. 1991. Specificity in the projection patterns of accumbal core and shell in the rat. Neuroscience 41: 89–125.

18. NAUTA, W.J.H., G.P. SMITH, R.L.M. FAULL & V.B. DOMESICK. 1978. Efferent connections and nigral afferents of the nucleus accumbens septi in the rat. Neuroscience **3:** 385–401.
19. WRIGHT, C.I., A.V. BEIJER & H.J. GROENEWEGEN. 1996. Basal amygdaloid complex afferents to the rat nucleus accumbens are compartmentally organized. J. Neurosci. **16:** 1877–1893.
20. DEUTCH, A.Y. & D.S. CAMERON. 1992. Pharmacological characterization of dopamine systems in the nucleus accumbens core and shell. Neuroscience **46:** 49–56.
21. BENINGER, R.J. 1983. The role of dopamine in locomotor activity and learning. Brain Res. Rev. **6:** 173–196.
22. ROBBINS, T.W. 1978. The acquisition of responding with conditioned reinforcement: effects of pipradrol, methylphenidate, d-amphetamine, and nomifensine. Psychopharmacology **58:** 79–87.
23. BENINGER, R.J. & A.G. PHILLIPS. 1980. The effect of pimozide on the establishment of conditioned reinforcement. Psychopharmacology **68:** 147–158.
24. TAYLOR, J.R. & T.W. ROBBINS. 1984. Enhanced behavioural control by conditioned reinforcers following microinjections of D-amphetamine into the nucleus accumbens. Psychopharmacology **84:** 405–412.
25. TAYLOR, J.R. & T.W. ROBBINS. 1986. 6-Hydroxydopamine lesions of the nucleus accumbens, but not of the caudate nucleus, attenuate enhanced responding with reward-related stimuli produced by intra-accumbens d-amphetamine. Psychopharmacology **90:** 390–397.
26. SUTHERLAND, R.J. & A.J. RODRIGUEZ. 1989. The role of the fornix/fimbria and some related subcortical structures in place learning and memory. Behav. Brain Res. **32:** 265–277.
27. ANNETT, L.E., A. MCGREGOR & T.W. ROBBINS. 1989. The effects of ibotenic acid lesions of the nucleus accumbens on spatial learning and extinction in the rat. Behav. Brain Res. **31:** 231–242.
28. READING, P.J., S.B. DUNNETT & T.W. ROBBINS. 1991. Dissociable roles of the ventral, medial and lateral striatum on the acquisition and performance of a complex visual stimulus-response habit. Behav. Brain Res. **45:** 147–161.
29. FLORESCO, S.B., J.K. SEAMANS & A.G. PHILLIPS. 1996. Differential effects of lidocaine infusions into the ventral CA1/subiculum or the nucleus accumbens on the acquisition and retention of spatial information. Behav.Brain Res. **81:** 163–172.
30. FLORESCO, S.B., J.K. SEAMANS & A.G. PHILLIPS. 1997. Selective roles for hippocampal, prefrontal cortical, and ventral striatal circuits in radial-arm maze tasks with or without a delay. J. Neurosci. **17:** 1880–1890.
31. SETLOW, B. 1997. The nucleus accumbens and learning and memory. J. Neurosci. Res. **49:** 515–521.
32. MCGEER, P.L., E.G. MCGEER, U. SCHERER & K. SINGH. 1977. A glutamatergic corticostriatal pathway? Brain Res. **128:** 369–373.
33. FONNUM, F. 1984. Glutamate: a neurotransmitter in mammalian brain. J. Neurochem. **42:** 1–10.
34. ALBIN, R.L., R.L. MAKOWIEC, Z.R. HOLLINGSWORTH, L.S. DURE IV, J.B. PENNEY & A.B. YOUNG. 1992. Excitatory amino acid binding sites in the basal ganglia of the rat: a quantitative autoradiographic study. Neuroscience **46:** 35–48.
35. MALDONADO-IRIZARRY, C.S. & A.E. KELLEY. 1994. Differential behavioral effects following microinjection of an NMDA antagonist into nucleus accumbens subregions. Psychopharmacology **166:** 65–72.
36. MOGENSON, G.J. & M. NIELSEN. 1984. Neuropharmacological evidence to suggest that the nucleus accumbens and subpallidal region contribute to exploratory locomotion. Behav. Neural. Biol. **42:** 52–60.
37. MALDONADO-IRIZARRY, C.S. & A.E. KELLEY. 1995. Excitatory amino acid receptors within nucleus accumbens subregions differentially mediate spatial learning in the rat. Behav. Pharmacol. **6:** 527–539.
38. SMITH-ROE, S., K. SADEGHIAN & A.E. KELLEY. 1999. Spatial learning and performance in the radial arm maze is impaired following NMDA receptor blockade in

striatal subregions. Behav. Neurosci. In press.
39. KELLEY, A.E., S. SMITH-ROE & M.R. HOLAHAN. 1997. Response-reinforcement learning is dependent on NMDA receptor activation in the nucleus accumbens core. Proc. Natl. Acad. Sci. USA **94**: 12174–12179.
40. ALEXANDER, G.E., M.R. DELONG & P.L. STRICK. 1986. Parallel organization of functionally segregated circuits linking basal ganglia and cortex. Annu. Rev. Neurosci. **9**: 357–381.
41. DIVAC, I. 1972. Neostriatum and functions of prefrontal cortex. Acta Neurobiol. Exp. (Warsaw) **32**: 461–477.
42. MCDONALD, R.J. & N.M. WHITE. 1993. A triple dissociation of memory systems: hippocampus, amygdala, and dorsal striatum. Behav. Neurosci. **107**: 3–22.
43. MISHKIN, M. & H.L. PETRI. 1984. Memories and habits: some implications for the analysis of learning and retention. *In* Neuropsychology of Memory. N. Butters & L. R. Squire, Eds.: 287–296. Guilford. New York.
44. PACKARD, M.G. & J.L. MCGAUGH. 1992. Double dissociation of fornix and caudate nucleus lesions on acquisition of two water maze tasks: further evidence for multiple memory systems. Behav. Neurosci. **106**: 439–446.
45. PARKINSON, J.A., M.C. OLMSTEAD, L.H. BURNS, T.W. ROBBINS & B.J. EVERITT. 1999. Dissociation in effects of lesions of the nucleus accumbens core and shell in appetitive Pavlovian approach behavior and the potentiation of conditioned reinforcement and locomotor activity by D-amphetamine. J. Neurosci. **19**: 2401–2411.
46. BALDWIN, A.E., M. HOLAHAN, K. SADEGHIAN & A.E. KELLEY. 1999. N-methy-D-aspartate receptor-dependent plasticity within a distr ibuted corticostriatal network mediates response-reinforcement learning. J. Neurosci. Submitted.
47. AOSAKI, T., A.M. GRAYBIEL & M. KIMURA. 1994. Effect of the nigrostriatal dopamine system on acquired neural responses in the striatum of behaving monkeys. Science **265**: 412–415.
48. APICELLA, P., E. SCARNATI, T. LJUNGBERG & W. SCHULTZ. 1992. Neuronal activity in the monkey striatum related to the expectation of predictable environmental events. J. Neurophysiol. **68**: 945–960.
49. BOWMAN, E.M., T.G. AIGNER & B.J. RICHMOND. 1996. Neural signals in the monkey ventral striatum related to motivation for juice and cocaine rewards. J. Neurophysiol. **75**: 1061–1073.
50. AOSAKI, T., H. TSUBOKAWA, A. ISHIDA, K. WATANABE, A.M. GRAYBIEL & M. KIMURA. 1994. Responses of tonically active neurons in the primate's striatum undergo systematic changes during behavioral sensorimotor conditioning. J. Neurosci. **14**: 3969–3984.
51. BOEIJINGA, P.H., A.B. MULDER, C.M. PENNARTZ, I. MANSHANDEN & F.H. LOPES DA SILVA. 1993. Responses of the nucleus accumbens following fornix/fimbria stimulation in the rat. Identification and long-term potentiation of mono- and polysynaptic pathways. Neuroscience **53**: 1049–1058.
52. CALABRESI, P., A. PISANI, N.B. MERCURI & G. BERNARDI. 1996. The corticostriatal projection: from synaptic plasticity to dysfunctions of the basal ganglia [see comments]. Trends Neurosci. **19**: 19–24.
53. KOMBIAN, S.B. & R.C. MALENKA. 1994. Simultaneous LTP of non-NMDA and LTD of NMDA-receptor mediated responses in the nucleus accumbens. Nature **368**: 242–245.
54. LOVINGER, D.M., E.C. TYLER & A. MERRITT. 1993. Short- and long-term synaptic depression in rat neostriatum. J. Neurophysiol. **70**: 1937–1949.
55. UNO, M. & N. OZAWA. 1991. Long-term potentiation of the amygdala-striatal synaptic transmission in the course of development of amygdaloid kindling in cats. Neurosci. Res. **12**: 251–262.
56. PENNARTZ, C.M., R.F. AMEERUN, H.J. GROENEWEGEN & F.H. LOPES DA SILVA. 1993. Synaptic plasticity in an *in vitro* slice preparation of the rat nucleus accumbens. Eur. J. Neurosci. **5**: 107–117.
57. MULDER, A.B., M.P. ARTS & F.H. LOPES DA SILVA. 1997. Short- and long-term plasticity of the hippocampus to nucleus accumbens and prefrontal cortex pathways in the rat, *in vivo*. Eur. J. Neurosci. **9**: 1603–1611.

58. BROWN, M.A. & P.E. SHARP. 1995. Simulation of spatial learning in the Morris water maze by a neural network model of the hippocampal formation and nucleus accumbens. Hippocampus **5:** 171–188.
59. REDISH, A.D. & D.S. TOURETSKY. 1997. Cognitive maps beyond the hippocampus. Hippocampus **7:** 15–35.
60. SCHULTZ, W., P. DAYAN & P.R. MONTAGUE. 1997. A neural substrate of prediction and reward. Science **275:** 1593–1598.
61. SCHULTZ, W., P. APICELLA & T. LJUNGBERG. 1993. Responses of monkey dopamine neurons to reward and conditioned stimuli during successive steps of learning a delayed response task. J. Neurosci. **13:** 900–913.
62. HOUK, J.C., J.L. ADAMS & A.G. BARTO. 1995. A model of how the basal ganglia generate and use neural signals that predict reinforcement. *In* Information Processing in the Basal Ganglia. J. C. Houk, J. L. Davis & D. G. Beiser, Eds.: 249–270. MIT Press. Cambridge, MA.
63. KOTTER, R. 1994. Postsynaptic integration of glutamatergic and dopaminergic signals in the striatum. Prog. Neurobiol. **44:** 163–196.
64. WICKENS, J. & R. KÖTTER. 1995. Cellular models of reinforcement. *In* Information Processing in the Basal Ganglia . J. C. Houk, J. L. Davis & D. G. Beiser, Eds.: 187–214. MIT Press. Cambridge, MA.
65. SMITH, A.D. & J.P. BOLAM. 1990. The neural network of the basal ganglia as revealed by the study of synaptic connections of identified neurones. Trends Neurosci. **13:** 259–265.
66. WICKENS, J.R., A.J. BEGG & G.W. ARBUTHNOTT. 1996. Dopamine reverses the depression of rat corticostriatal synapses which normally follows high-frequency stimulation of cortex *in vitro*. Neuroscience **70:** 1–5.
67. CEPEDA, C., N.A. BUCHWALD & M.S. LEVINE. 1993. Neuromodulatory actions of dopamine in the neostriatum are dependent upon the excitatory amino acid receptor subtypes activated. Proc. Natl. Acad. Sci. USA **90:** 9576–9580.
68. KELLEY, A.E., M.R. HOLAHAN, S. SMITH-ROE & A.E. BALDWIN. 1997. NMDA receptors and intracellular mechanisms within nucleus accumbens core are involved in appetitive learning. Soc. Neurosci. Abst. **23:** 2119.
69. GRAYBIEL, A.M., R. MORATALLA & H.A. ROBERTSON. 1990. Amphetamine and cocaine induce drug-specific activation of the c-fos gene in striosome-matrix compartments and limbic subdivisions of the striatum. Proc. Natl. Acad. Sci. USA **87:** 6912–6916.
70. HOPE, B., B. KOSOFSKY, S.E. HYMAN & E.J. NESTLER. 1992. Regulation of immediate early gene expression and AP-1 binding in the rat nucleus accumbens by chronic cocaine. Proc. Natl. Acad. Sci. USA **89:** 5764–5768.
71. WANG, J.Q., A.J. SMITH & J.F. MCGINTY. 1995. A single injection of amphetamine or methamphetamine induces dynamic alterations in c-fos, zif/268 and preprodynorphin messenger RNA expression in rat forebrain. Neuroscience **68:** 83–95.
72. KONRADI, C., J.C. LEVEQUE & S.E. HYMAN. 1996. Amphetamine and dopamine-induced immediate early gene expression in striatal neurons depends on postsynaptic NMDA receptors and calcium. J. Neurosci. **16:** 4231–4239.
73. WANG, J.Q., J.B. DAUNAIS & J.F. MCGINTY. 1994. NMDA receptors mediate amphetamine-induced upregulation of zif/268 and preprodynorphin mRNA expression in rat striatum. Synapse (NY) **18:** 343–353.
74. WOLF, M.E., F.J. WHITE & X.-T. HU. 1994. MK-801 prevents alterations in the mesoaccumbens dopamine system associated with behavioral sensitization to amphetamine. J. Neurosci. **14:** 1735–1745.
75. HEIMER, L., G.F. ALHEID & D.S. ZAHM. 1993. Basal forebrain organization: an anatomical framework for motor aspects of drive and motivation. *In* Limbic Motor Circuits and Neuropsychiatry. P. W. Kalivas & C. D. Barnes, Eds.: 1–44. CRC Press, Boca Raton, FL.
76. GROENEWEGEN, H.J., C.I. WRIGHT & A.V.J. BEIJER. 1996. The nucleus accumbens: gateway for limbic structures to reach the motor system? Prog. Brain Res. **107:** 485–511.
77. MALDONADO-IRIZARRY, C.S., C.J. SWANSON & A.E. KELLEY. 1995. Glutamate recep-

tors in the nucleus accumbens shell control feeding behavior via the lateral hypothalamus. J. Neurosci. **15:** 6779–6788.
78. KELLEY, A.E. & C.J. SWANSON. 1998. Feeding induced by blockade of AMPA and kainate receptors within the ventral striatum: a microinfusion mapping study. Behav. Brain Res. **89:** 107–113.
79. STRATFORD, T.R., C. J. SWANSON & A.E. KELLEY. 1998. Specific changes in food intake elicited by blockade or activation of glutamate receptors in the nucleus accumbens shell. Behav. Brain Res. **93:** 43–50.
80. STRATFORD, T.R. & A.E. KELLEY. 1997. GABA in the nucleus accumbens shell participates in the central regulation of feeding behavior. J. Neurosci. **17:** 4434–4440.
81. BASSO, A.M. & A.E. KELLEY. 1999. Feeding induced by $GABA_A$ receptor stimulation within nucleus accumbens shell: regional mapping and characterization of macronutrient and taste preference. Behav. Neurosci. **113:** 324–336.
82. STRATFORD, T.R. & A.E. KELLEY. 1997. Feeding elicited by inhibition of neurons in the nucleus accumbens shell depends on activation of neurons in the lateral hypothalamus. Soc. Neurosci. Abstr. **23:** 577.
83. STANLEY, B.G., V.L. WILLET, H.W. DONIAS, L.H. HA & L.C. SPEARS. 1993. The lateral hypothalamus: primary site mediating excitatory amino acid-elicited feeding. Brain Res. **630:** 41–49.
84. MOGENSON, G.J., L.W. SWANSON & M. WU. 1983. Neural projections from nucleus accumbens to globus pallidus, substantia innominata, and lateral preoptic-lateral hypothalamic area: an anatomical and electrophysiological investigation in the rat. J. Neurosci. **3:** 189–202.
85. ZHANG, M. & A.E. KELLEY. 1997. Opiate agonists microinjected into the nucleus accumbens enhance sucrose drinking in rats. Psychopharmacology **132:** 350–360.
86. ZHANG, M., B.A. GOSNELL & A.E. KELLEY. 1998. Intake of high-fat food is selectively enhanced by mu opioid receptor stimulation within the nucleus accumbens. J. Pharmacol. Exp. Ther. **284:** 908–914.
87. ZHANG, M. 1998. Striatal modulation of opioid–induced palatable feeding: anatomical mapping studies. Soc. Neurosci.Abstr. **24:** 706.
88. HORGER, B.A., J.D. ELSWORTH & R.H. ROTH. 1995. Selective increase in dopamine utilization in the shell subdivision of the nucleus accumbens by the benzodiazepine inverse agonist FG 7142. J. Neurochem. **65:** 770–774.
89. KALIVAS, P.W. & P. DUFFY. 1995. Selective activation of dopamine transmission in the shell of the nucleus accumbens by stress. Brain Res. **675:** 325–328.
90. KING, D. & J.M. FINLAY. 1997. Loss of dopamine terminals in the medial prefrontal cortex increased the ratio of DOPAC to DA in tissue of the nucleus accumbens shell: role of stress. Brain Res. **767:** 192–200.
91. TIDEY, J.W. & K.A. MICZEK. 1996. Social defeat stress selectively alters mesocorticolimbic dopamine release: an *in vivo* microdialysis study. Brain Res. **721:** 140–149.
92. BECK, C.H. & H.C. FIBIGER. 1995. Conditioned fear-induced changes in behavior and in the expression of the immediate early gene c-fos: with and without diazepam pretreatment. J. Neurosci. **15:** 709–720.
93. PONTIERI, F.E., G. TANDA & G. DI CHIARA. 1995. Intravenous cocaine, morphine, and amphetmaine preferentially increase extracellular dopamine in the "shell" as compared with the "core" of the rat nucleus accumbens. Proc. Natl. Acad. Sci. USA **92:** 12304–12308.
94. PONTIERI, F.E., G. TANDA, F. ORZI & G. DI CHIARA. 1996. Effects of nicotine on the nucleus accumbens and similarity to those of addictive drugs. Nature **382:** 255–257.
95. CAINE, S., S.C. HEINRICHS, V. COFFIN & G.F. KOOB. 1995. Effects of the dopamine D-1 antagonist SCH 23390 microinjected into the accumbens, amygdala or striatum on cocaine self-administration. Brain Res. **692:** 47–56.
96. CARLEZON, W.A., D.P. DEVINE & R.A. WISE. 1995. Habit-forming actions of nomifensine in nucleus accumbens. Psychopharmacology **122:** 194–197.
97. CARLEZON, W.A. & R.A. WISE. 1996. Rewarding actions of phencyclidine and related drugs in nucleus accumbens shell and frontal cortex. J. Neurosci. **16:** 3112–3122.

98. WRIGHT, C.I. & H.J. GROENEWEGEN. 1996. Pattern of overlap and segregation between insular cortical, intermediodorsal thalamic and basal amygdaloid afferents in the nucleus accumbens. Neuroscience **73:** 359–373.
99. O'DONNELL, P. 1999. Ensemble coding in the nucleus accumbens. Psychobiology. In press.
100. BERRIDGE, C.W., T.L. STRATFORD, S.L. FOOTE & A.E. KELLEY. 1997. Distribution of dopamine-ß-hydroxylase (DBH)-like immunoreactivie fibers within the shell of the nucleus accumbens. Synapse **27:** 230–241.
101. HOLAHAN, M.R., N.H. KALIN & A.E. KELLEY. 1997. Microinfusion of corticotropin-releasing factor into the nucleus accumbens shell results in increased behavioral arousal and oral motor activity. Psychopharmacology **130:** 189–196.
102. EVENDEN, J.L. & M. CARLI. 1985. The effects of 6-hydroxydopamine lesions of the nucleus accumbens and caudate nucleus of rats on feeding in a novel environment. Behav. Brain Res. **15:** 63–70.
103. WEINER, I. 1990. Neural substrates of latent inhibition: the switching model. Psychol. Bull. **108:** 442–461.
104. VAN DEN BOS, R., G.A. CHARRIA ORTIZ & A.R. COOLS. 1992. Injections of the NMDA-antagonist D-2-amino-7-phosphonoheptanoic acid (AP-7) into the nucleus accumbens of rats enhance switching between cue- directed behaviours in a swimming test procedure. Behav. Brain Res. **48:** 165–170.
105. EVANS, K.R. & F.J. VACCARINO. 1990. Amphetamine- and morphine-induced feeding: Evidence for involvement of reward mechanisms. Neurosci. Biobeh. Rev. **14:** 9–22.
106. SWANSON, C.J., S. HEATH, T.R. STRATFORD & A.E. KELLEY. 1997. Differential behavioral responses to dopaminergic stimulation of nucleus accumbens subregions in the rat. Pharmacology, Biochemistry and Behavior **58:** 933–945.
107. BASSAREO, V. 1997. Differential influence of associative and nonassociative learning mechanisms on the responsiveness of prefrontal and accumbal dopamine transmission to food stimuli in rats fed ad libitum. J. Neurosci. **17:** 851–861.
108. HERNANDEZ, L. & B.G. HOEBEL. 1988. Feeding and hypothalamic stimulation increase dopamine turnover in the accumbens. Physiol. Behav. **44:** 599–606.
109. KIYATKIN, E.A. & A. GRATTON. 1994. Electrochemical monitoring of extracellular dopamine in nucleus accumbens of rats lever-pressing for food. Brain Res. **652:** 225–234.
110. WILSON, C., G.G. NOMIKOS, M. COLLU & H.C. FIBIGER. 1995. Dopaminergic correlates of motivated behavior: importance of drive. J. Neurosci. **15:** 5169–5178.
111. ROBBINS, T.W. & B.J. EVERITT. 1996. Neurobehavioural mechanisms of reward and motivation. Curr. Opin. Neurobiol. **6:** 228–236.
112. ROBINSON, T.E. & K.C. BERRIDGE. 1993. The neural basis of drug craving: an incentive-sensitization theory of addiction. Brain Res. Rev. **18:** 247–291.
113. WISE, R. A. & P. P. ROMPRÉ. 1989. Brain dopamine and reward. Ann. Rev. Psychol. **40:** 191–225.
114. PENNARTZ, C.M., H.J. GROENEWEGEN & F.H. LOPES DA SILVA. 1994. The nucleus accumbens as a complex of functionally distinct neuronal ensembles: an integration of behavioural, electrophysiological and anatomical data. Prog. Neurobiol. **42:** 719–761.
115. JOEL, D. & I. WEINER. 1994. The organization of the basal ganglia-thalamocortical circuits: open interconnected rather than closed segregated. Neuroience **63:** 363–379.

Mesolimbic Neuronal Activity across Behavioral States

DONALD J. WOODWARD,[a] JING-YU CHANG, PATRICIA JANAK, ALEXEY AZAROV, AND KRISTIN ANSTROM

Department of Physiology and Pharmacology, Wake Forest University School of Medicine, Medical Center Boulevard, Winston Salem, North Carolina 27157, USA

ABSTRACT: A goal of neurophysiology of the mesolimbic system is to determine the activity patterns within the regions in the prefrontal cortex, ventral neostriatum, and amygdala that regulate behavioral patterns to seek rewards. A new technology has been introduced in which arrays of microwires are implanted in different brain regions while activity patterns of ensembles of neurons are recorded for long periods of time during freely moving behaviors. Multichannel instrumentation and software is used for data acquisition and analysis. An initial hypothesis was that neural signals would be encountered in the nucleus accumbens and associated regions specifically related to reward. However, an initial study of neural activity and behavioral patterns during a simple lever press for intravenous cocaine (1 mg/kg) revealed that phasic excitatory or inhibitory neural activity patterns often appear prior to the reward phase. Individual neurons throughout the mesolimbic system appear to code information specific to sensory and motor events, tones, or lever presses in the chain of tasks leading to all rewards so far studied. Different spatial temporal patterns also appear within the same neural populations, as reward is changed from injected cocaine to heroin, from ingested pure water to ethanol in water or sucrose. Overall, patterns of activity for each neuron are found to shift dynamically during the operant task as changes are made in the target reward. Significant shifts in activity of mesolimbic neurons that are unrelated to specific sensory–motor events also appear during complex sessions, such as during a bout of ethanol consumption to reach satiation or during progressive ratio tasks with increasing difficulty. An emerging hypothesis is that some candidate neural elements in the mesolimbic system code the anticipated reward, whereas others serve internal logic functions of motivation that mediate extinction or resumption of specific goal-directed behaviors.

The mesolimbic system offers unique challenges to the neurophysiologist charged with the goal of understanding the role of distributed neuronal activity in mediating function in this system. Cellular and molecular structures that provide substrates of behavior and accumulated experiences must be played out by the patterns of neural impulses that instantiate actions at each point in time. The concepts we use, termed emotions or motivations, are presumed to become transformed at some stage into temporal-spatial patterns of impulse flow within connected regions

[a]Voice: 336-716-8545; fax: 336-716-8501; wooward@newton.neuro.wfubmc.edu

of the mesolimbic system. The task of the neurophysiologist is to measure this activity over time within the mesolimbic system. The goal is to demonstrate the presence of neural information that encodes internal behaviorial states. The task is to assign new names to mechanisms and processes that seem initially so completely hidden from view across behavioral states.

Traditional experimental design has relied on the ability of the researcher to precisely control the parameters of sensory input or monitor the response of a motor reflex or pattern. However, the mesolimbic system is positioned far from the sensorymotor neural structure and therefore seems intractable to either measurement or control of many variables. Experimental subjects must be allowed to freely behave over long times in different designed contexts so that underlying motivations can be inferred. However, it is not clear at the outset how neural activity should be related to postulated functions of the mesolimbic system.

The concept of "reward" provides an example of this difficulty. At the outset of our studies,[1-4] we postulated that such a construct might be readily observable in terms of well-defined detectable activity patterns. A substantial theoretical background had been suggested[5] that reward evoked by drugs or behavioral circumstance should release dopamine in the nucleus accumbens and cause an excitatory or inhibitory influence on neuronal activity. But should reward be represented by a specific spatial-temporal pattern of neural activity in a zone critical for its control? Similarly, should emotion, affect, motivations, or newer constructs, such as craving, that are now gaining credibility for investigation, be observable directly as simple neuronal activity patterns? Neural activity by single neurons may participate via correlated discharge in larger arrays of complex circuits. These, in turn, may execute logic functions that are linked remotely to the concept of reward. An alternative view is that such function will be found deeply embedded in the patterns of phosphorylation within distributed cellular signaling systems or within patterns of genetic expression. It is likely that these types of cellular and molecular changes are integral to the creation of stable spatial-temporal patterns of firing.

The outlines of the anatomical framework have been emerging to guide the neurophysiologist. The NAS (nucleus accumbens), a substantial component of the "ventral striatum," is a central structure connecting limbic and basal ganglia systems. Abundant afferents exist from the prelimbic cortex.[6-9] The hippocampal formation contributes additional afferents[10,11] as well as the amygdala[12-14] and midline thalamic nuclei[15] and ventral tegmental area (VTA).[15,16] The NAS projects in turn to the ventral pallidus,[18,19] pendunculopontine nucleus, hypothalamus, substantia nigra, and VTA.[18-22] Recent reviews of mesolimbic anatomy have emphasized the interconnections among the medial and lateral frontal cerebral cortex, hippocampus, nucleus accumbens, and amygdala, including the extended amydala, and suggest that these interconnections indicate sharing of their respective processing functions.[8,23] This wealth of anatomical detail encourages a neurophysiological study of all these interconnected regions. This will need to be performed in the future by simultaneous detection of impulse activity to clarify the causal sources of correlated activity.

We felt that the start of an extensive analysis of the patterns of correlated neuronal activity is addressed best by the formulation of a broad exploratory hypothesis, inasmuch as we simply do not know enough at the outset about the candidate mechanisms. Our thesis to guide the start of our work is that the mesolimbic system monitors and weighs conditioned sensory cues in order to compute options for behavior under different behavioral contexts. These neural signals may be used both to regulate immediate ongoing behavior and to affect the strength of associations that govern future behavior. The goal of exploratory work has been to search for temporal patterns of activity within the known anatomical connections across multiple behavioral states, using operant behavior for different reinforcing substances as a means of controlling and exploring context.

EXPERIMENTAL METHODOLOGY

Exploration of conceptual issues in the neurophysiology of the mesolimbic system has been limited mainly by the absence of a means of obtaining adequate numbers of recordings of spike train activity from awake, behaving animals. Until

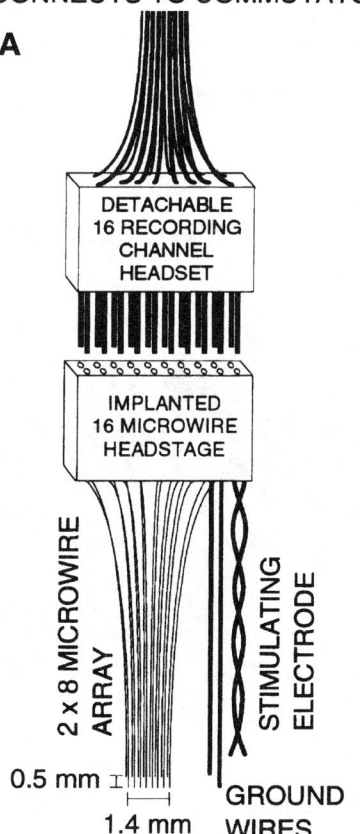

FIGURE 1. Recording probe configuration. **A:** Schematic diagram of the array of 50 micron diameter Teflon-insulated microwires. The array of wires is attached to a strip connector and is embedded in dental acrylic that makes the hat stay on the skull of the animal. A set of surface mount FET headstage followers are mounted in a plug harness. The output ascends through a cable, commutator, and a preamplifier system before signals are processed by a DSP spike sorter system. **B:** A group of up to four arrays of 16 microwires can be recorded from a rat, shown here in a behavioral chamber, for periods of 24 hours while the subject is free to perform operant tasks.

recently the main technique was the use of single movable electrodes in rat or primate. This traditional procedure succeeded well in relatively short-term studies of a few minutes or hours and in situations when the temporal organization of a behavioral event could be controlled. With the introduction, however, of a perfected version of arrays (50 micron, Teflon-coated, stainless steel microwires), it became clear[1,24] that recordings could be obtained from 10 to 50 times more efficiently from recording arrays implanted chronically. Recording groups of spike trains for periods as long as 24 hours or more has become routine. Recording sites can be localized by histological stain after electrolytic deposition of iron. These advances appeared in parallel with the assembly of multichannel FET headstages, preamplifiers, digital signal processors for spike capture and sorting, and tremendous advances in host processor speed and software sophistication to handle the large amounts of data. Fortunately, rodents with attached multiwire cables and plugs readily perform all the complex tasks so far investigated. These include FR1 to FR10 lever press for cocaine; lever press for food, water, sucrose or ethanol solutions; reaction time tasks; progressive ratio tasks for cocaine or water; and spatial delayed match to sample tasks. Motorized commutators allow recordings to be made from up to 64 microwires implanted in a rat brain, with groups of up to 64 or more neurons recorded in different brain regions. Introduction of new microelectronics devices will surely advance these capabilities further in coming years. This field is now at the start of an era. Given effort and patience, long-term spike train recordings can be obtained from localized zones in the mesolimbic system and elsewhere across many behavioral states to define the mechanisms by which coding of information occurs (FIG. 1).

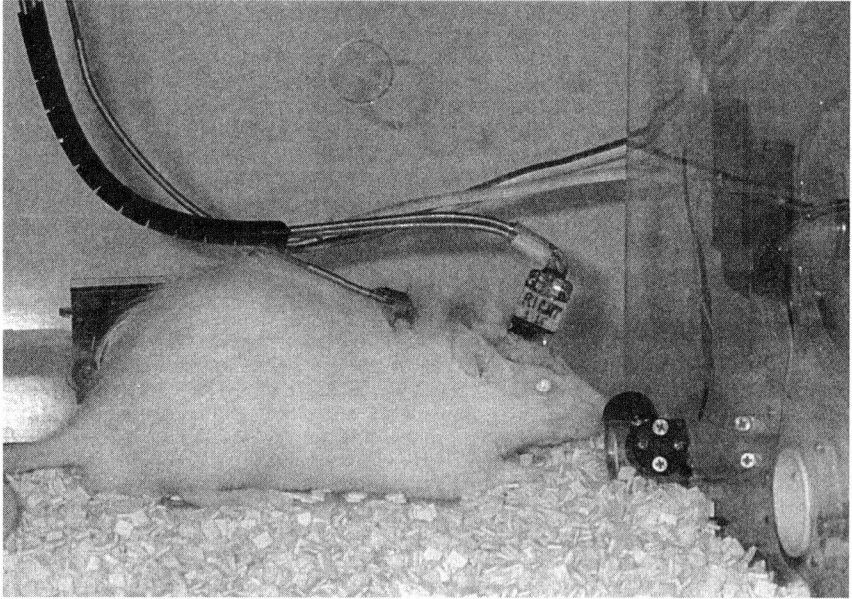

FIGURE 1B. See legend on prior page.

CONTEXT-DEPENDENT ACTIVITY IN DORSAL NEOSTRIATUM

Research on the rodent neostriatum in this laboratory began over a decade ago. Investigations in the dorsal neostriatum revealed[25] a strong influence of novelty and experience in regulating the widespread responses to conditioned auditory cues and also in the background activity during alternate phases of treadmill locomotion and rest. Recordings obtained in the dorsolateral region of the neostriatum[26] demonstrated a topographical mapping of input from body regions defined both by tactile stimulation and responses to movement of the same limb. The results also showed that correlates were not simple obligatory consequences of movement and sensory input but were linked to the specific context in which tactile input and movements occurred. These basic functional features seem applicable to all regions of the neostriatum under different behavioral contexts.

ACTIVITY IN DORSAL AND VENTRAL NEOSTRIATUM DURING TASKS FOR COCAINE

Our initial investigation on activity within the mesolimbic system during "reward" included studies of self-administration of the very strong reinforcer, cocaine. In these studies we recorded the extracellular spike activity of ensembles of nucleus accumbens neurons using microwire arrays during cocaine self-administration.[1–3] In this paradigm, the rat subjects were trained to lever press under a continuous reinforcement schedule for 1 mg/kg iv infusions of cocaine, a dose that led to a reasonably stable repeated motor sequence prior to each lever press. A typical intertrial interval consists of the following sequences of behavior: following an infusion of drug, the rat ceases ambulatory activity for several minutes while engaging in stereotypic behavior; then after 3–4 minutes, the rat begins to move, approaches the lever, raises its head and then its forepaw, presses the lever, returns the forepaw to the floor, receives the next drug infusion, and returns to stereotypic behavior (FIGURES 2 and 3).

This simple FR1 paradigm revealed many fundamental features of activity in the nucleus accumbens in relation to reward. The firing patterns of about half of the neurons do not fluctuate at any point in this sequence, and, hence are not affected by the dramatic changes in either behavioral or pharmacological variables that characterize cocaine self-administration. This was surprising because we predicted that the cocaine should cause a release of dopamine that should bathe the population of nucleus accumbens cells and cause an overall influence on activity in the entire region. The other half of the neurons displayed highly varied patterns of excitatory or inhibitory activity both before and after the lever press. There was not an overall excitation or inhibition inasmuch as equal numbers of reciprocal patterns could be seen. About 10–15% of neurons revealed a phasic excitation or inhibition during the anticipatory events leading up to the lever press. Detailed study of a subset of these neurons with video recording of the behavioral patterns revealed that neurons began or terminated phasic neural responses most often at the onset or termination of segments of movement sequences. These same neurons showed no phasic activation patterns when the rats were placed upon a treadmill, indicating that the cocaine-related responses are not general motor responses. Taken together, the results suggest that the populations of neurons in the nucleus accumbens code each component of the movement se-

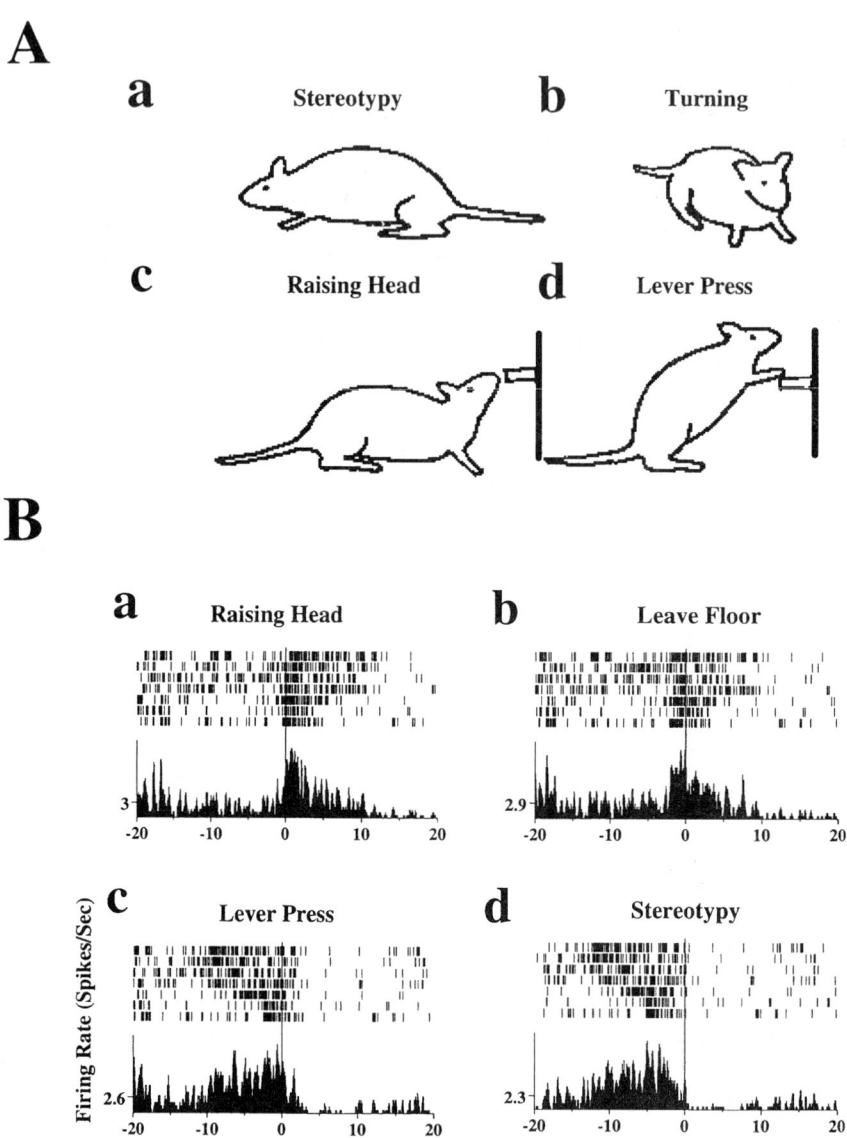

FIGURE 2. The sequence of movements prior to the lever press was captured on video with each frame time synchronized with the times of spike train events. The timing of the behavioral sequence leading up to the lever press (raising head, leave floor, lever press, stereotypy) could be scored from tape (**A**) and displayed along with corresponding spike events centered on 29 behavioral event times. Neurons in the nucleus accumbens and medial prefrontal cortex (shown here for medial prefrontal cortex) revealed onset or termination of activity correlated with the transitions in the behavioral sequence. (Chang et al.[4] With permission from *Synapse (NY)*.)

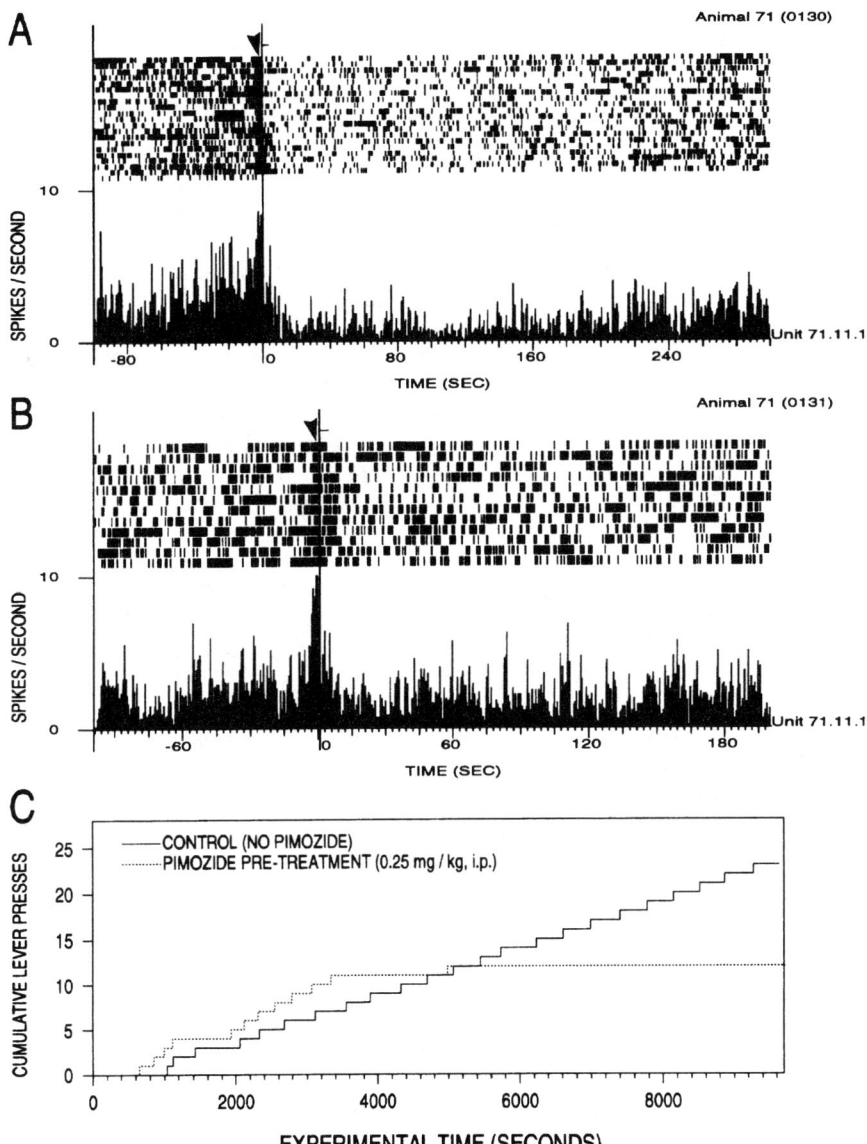

FIGURE 3. A: Neural activity shown as raster histogram displays for typical neurons in rat nucleus accumbens during lever press responding to self-administer 1 mg/kg iv cocaine. Excitatory responses are observed immediately before lever press, followed by a slower rate that decays during the 4- to 5-minute dose intervals. **B:** Administration of the dopamine receptor antagonist, pimozide (0.25 mg/kg ip), caused an initial acceleration and then cessation of lever pressing for cocaine in parallel with an absence of the postcocaine inhibition. **C:** Cumulative lever press plots compare the behavior of controls and rats with pimozide. (Chang et al.[3] With permission from *Neuroscience*.)

quence leading to the reward and that this coding is specific to the context of cocaine self-administration (FIG. 2).[3]

The temporal pattern of self-dosing involves many influences that come into play at different times and conditions. Self-administration of 1 mg/kg cocaine evokes a pattern of bar presses in which the rat self-doses at 3–4 minute intervals. This often occurs after an initial start-up period of rapid lever pressing where that rat builds up blood levels of cocaine until the steady rate in attained. The initial high rate is evidently sustained by the memory of previous drug experiences. The initial lever press is facilitated by a priming dose of cocaine, presumably to trigger the influence of prior experience, but can be retarded by a long-duration presence in the chamber without cocaine, which appears to activate extinction. The direct action of the cocaine is to suppress, for a time, additional lever pressing, but may enhance locomotion, and the rat self-initiates a lever press after the drug effect abates. It is uncertain whether this is due to an immediate aversion to the drug or to an occlusion of a triggering mechanism that drives the lever press behavioral sequence. A subset of neurons reveals a suppression of activity at the injection of cocaine followed by a steady increase and reversal until the time of the next self-initiated lever press.[1,3,27–30] One might postulate that such neuron patterns reflect a threshold mechanism for triggering later behavior.

Passive infusion of cocaine caused a two- to three-minute suppression of activity, similar to that obtained during self-administration of the drug.[2] This effect was blocked by administration of pimozide, a D_2 receptor anatagonist reported to block self-administration of cocaine without impairment of movement. Neuronal recording during administration of pimozide or SCH 23390 (D_2 or D_1 antagonists) evoked a pattern of more rapid lever pressing followed by an abrupt cessation of responding. Significantly, anticipatory activity linked to movement sequences leading to bar press was not altered as long as the behavior of lever pressing was triggered by the rat. This strongly suggests that there is a dopamine-independent, most likely glutamate-driven, phasic activation of NAS neurons that accompanies the details of onset and termination of movement, with dopamine exerting an influence after the completion of the behavior aim to achieve self-administration of reward. The primary influence of dopamine, or its absence, is an altered probability of the subject self-initiating the movement sequence at a much later point in time (FIG. 3).

NEURAL ACTIVITY WITHIN THE PREFRONTAL CORTEX DURING COCAINE SELF-ADMINISTRATION

The medial prefrontal cortex or prelimbic region provides extensive afferent input to the nucleus accumbens and anterior dorsal striatum.[9] Our hypothesis was that signals in this area would be related to the kinds of neural signals found in the ventral striatum. Also, it was postulated that the task of lever pressing, in fact, required the subject to initiate a sequence of individual actions in sequence leading up to a successful lever press. If multiple lever presses were required in an FR2 or 3 and a delay were to be inserted between lever presses, then one might expect the rat to pause between lever presses and to regenerate the neural activity sequence pattern at each stage of the FR series. This hypothesis was confirmed by the discovery that anticipatory activity could be observed prior to each lever press in the FR3 schedule. Longer FR10 schedules without interresponse delays produced a different behavioral response, such that the animals completed the FR requirement by producing a few rapid bar press sequences with occasional pauses. In that case the anticipatory activity assumed a variable pattern; for example, the anticipatory neuronal response in some cases preceded the first lever press, but not the next nine. These anticipatory patterns that were not tightly linked to each of the ten lever presses may represent the initiation of specific phases of the overall behavioral sequence made to obtain the reward.[2]

Both prelimbic cortex and nucleus accumbens have quite similar patterns of activation when recordings are made simultaneously in the two areas. Ten to fifteen percent of neurons in both areas show increased activity during the motor sequence prior to bar press for reward. Roughly equal proportions show decreases prior to bar press. Other responses include increases or decreases in activity after the bar press during the reward administration. About 50% of neurons in any one session in both areas show no change. This general finding also applies to the other mesolimbic regions studied, including the amygdala and the SN reticulata.

SPECIFIC CODING OF DIFFERENT REWARDS

The coding of different rewards may be mediated by different subsets of neurons within the mesolimbic system. Similar types of pre– and post–lever press or nosepoke neuronal activity appear during operant responding for all types of rewards so far studied by various investigators.[3,4,27,28,33,38] Variations in neural activity exist if the animal is required to move to obtain a fluid reward or if the reward is a short transient, such as with a fluid reward, including the taste of water, sucrose, or ethanol, instead of a prolonged drug effect.

Chang *et al.*[33] directly compared neural activity patterns within the nucleus accumbens and prefrontal cortex when rats self-administered both cocaine and heroin in different halves of the same behavioral session. Again, about 50% of neurons in the nucleus accumbens or medial prefrontal cortex showed no modulation of activity during this task, but these were nearly independent populations during self-administration of the two substances. Although substantial proportions of neurons showed changes in spike activity before or after the lever press for iv drug, the anticipatory or post-drug responses of the same neuron to the two drug rewards were the same in only a small fraction (4–6%) of neurons. In some cases where an excitatory response was found prior to the bar press for both of the substances, the video sequence analysis revealed that the neurons became time locked to different events in the movements sequence leading to the reward. Thus it appears that coding properties emerge that are unique to the reinforcer during a session. Distinct coding of visual cues specific to the anticipated reinforcer has been reported in the dorsolateral prefrontal cortex of primates;[35] hence one might postulate that activity specific to the future reinforcer might be widely represented in frontal areas.

This same study by Chang *et al.*[33] found that the baseline firing rates of a population of NAS and prefrontal neurons changed when the reinforcer was changed to cocaine or heroin within the same session. These steady-state changes in firing rates were constant across different days for the same neurons from the same microwires and were also observed during passive administration of the drugs when the timing of a series of drug administrations mimicked that produced during self-administration. Interestingly, differences in both excitatory or inhibitory phasic responses observed before the lever press when the rats were self-administering cocaine versus heroin were noted in cases when no changes appeared in baseline firing rates. Thus the presence of distinct phasic signals related to the specific drug goal does not appear to depend upon changes in baseline firing rates. This type of specific coding for the sequence of sensory-motor or behavioral events for different rewards fits most closely a mechanism that assigns coding nearly randomly from within a common pool of neurons in the system.

CODING DURING OTHER REWARDS, INCLUDING ETHANOL SELF-ADMINISTRATION

An emerging hypothesis is that task components to obtain all reinforcing substances will be represented in the mesolimbic system and that this includes substances that initially may be quite aversive. Self-administration of ethanol in the rodent rarely occurs spontaneously and usually results only after a prolonged training period. The method of "sucrose-fade"[36] includes a period of 12–16 weeks during which 10% sucrose in water is shifted to 10% sucrose and 10% ethanol in water to finally 10% ethanol in water. Most rats acquire a strong motivation to drink the later solution only after this prolonged exposure to the intoxicating actions of ethanol. This is the case with many abused substances, which start with a mixture of adverse and reinforcing qualities. The hypothesis is that neural circuits become modified through, perhaps, a combination of learning and direct pharmacological action, so that a substance such as ethanol can become reinforcing. The major question, of course, is how and where within the mesolimbic system such changes take place and how the changes will be reflected in neural activity patterns.

The ethanol self-administration paradigm that we have used requires the animal to nose poke to start a trial.[37–39] This is followed, in turn, by a variable interval from

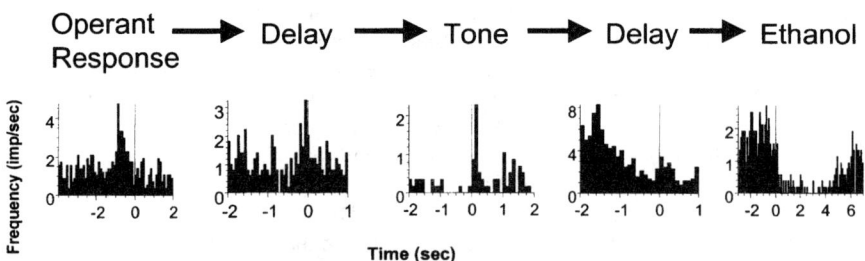

FIGURE 4. Water- and food-sated rats display nose-poke behavior to obtain 10% ethanol. Small subsets of neurons in the nucleus accumbens show responses (impulses/s) specific to temporal components of the paradigm, including the nose poke, variable delay, tone stimulus, fixed delay, and availability and consumption of ethanol in water. (Woodward et al.[24] With permission from *Alcoholism Clinical and Experimental Research*.)

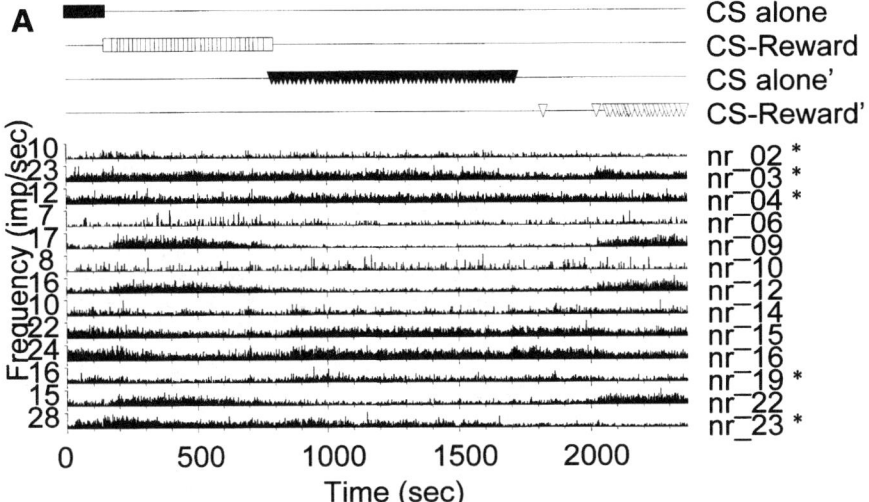

FIGURE 5. Neurons recorded in basolateral amygdala (asterisks) and nucleus accumbens of rat reveal phasic and tonic activity changes during tone-cued behavior to obtain water. In this paradigm the water-deprived rat was repeatedly presented with a 0.5 second tone (CS), a fixed delay of 0.5 s, followed by 0.1 cc of water (Reward). Rats approach the water spout readily upon tone presentation to consume the water. Providing tone alone produced extinction of the spout approach behavior, followed by rapid resumption of drinking behavior when pairing was restored. **A:** Rate strip charts show that mean baseline firing rate rapidly adjusted to cue-reward pairing conditions in the amygdala and nucleus accumbens. Extinction occurred at around 800 s into the session. The tone–water reward pairing resumed at around 2000 seconds. **B:** Perievent histograms and rasters of three neurons (9, 12, and 23) shown in 5A computed around the tone onset for each of the four phases shown in A show rapid changes in response to pairing of tone and reward. The rasters show the spike activity for each neuron for each trial, and the time of the trial is indicated on the y-axis. This result suggests that coordinated distributed activity in the amygdala and accumbens codes for conditioned cues and for reinforcer availability.

0.5 to 2.5 s duration, a 0.5 s tone (2.6 kHz), a fixed delay of 0.5 s, and last by a fluid drop (0.1 cc) made available at a spout. The variable delay prior to the tone was designed to enhance the possibility that the subject would use the predictive information of the tone, inasmuch as the fluid reward is made available at a fixed interval. Ethanol drinking was allowed during a period of one hour daily. During this "bout" a trained rat typically starts the session with behavior driven by memory and the immediate environmental cues. As the small alcohol doses consumed accumulate, the pharmacological actions of ethanol are presumed to sustain the behavior until the doses reached about 0.5–0.9 g/kg ethanol. Finally, the rat becomes visibly slightly uncoordinated in motor actions and spontaneously ceases further consumption. These alcohol doses in humans and the self-imposed limits roughly parallel the amount consumed during normal drinking patterns. The model is somewhat similar to social drinking in humans.

Examination of the neural firing patterns in the nucleus accumbens and the amygdala revealed activity around each node in the behavior, including the nose

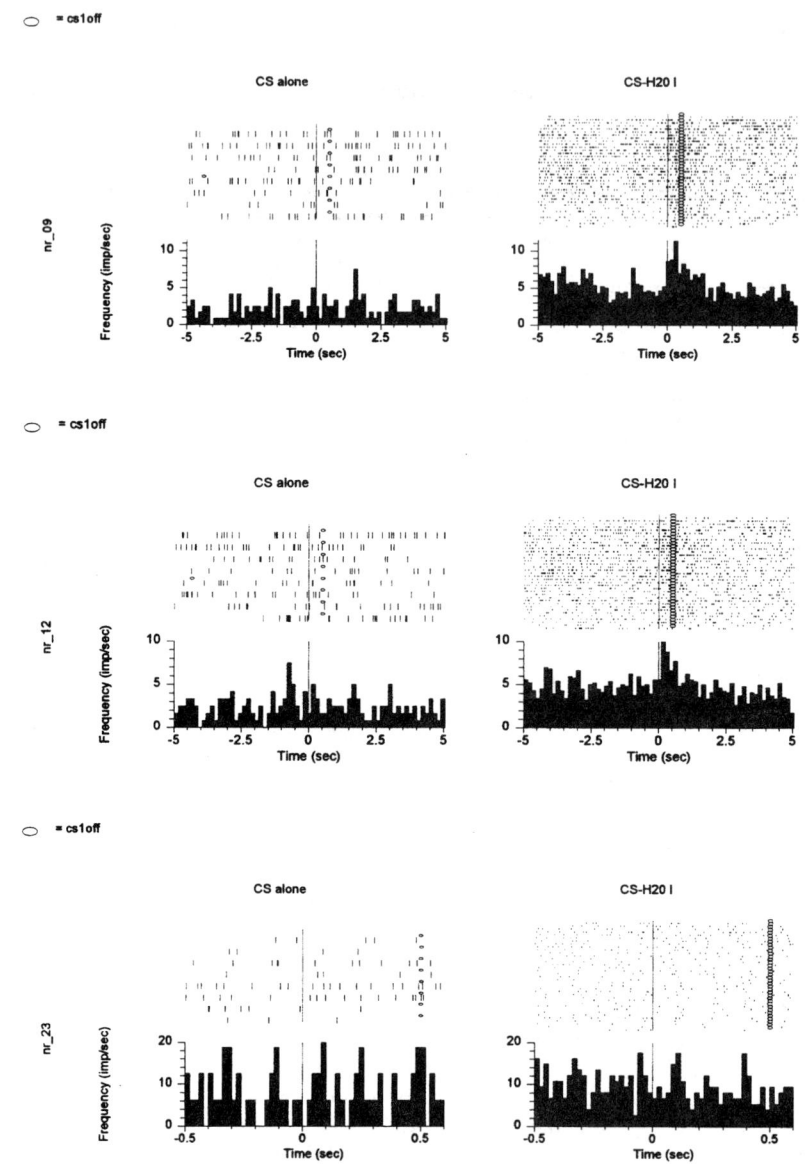

FIGURE 5B. See legend on prior page.

poke, the delays, the tone, and the consumption of the fluid.[38] Thus, as with the other reinforcer substances studied, small subsets of neurons coded each phase of the task (FIG. 4). Unlike previous studies of iv drug administration, there is a clear behavioral component to reinforcer receipt; subjects must locomote to the liquid delivery spout

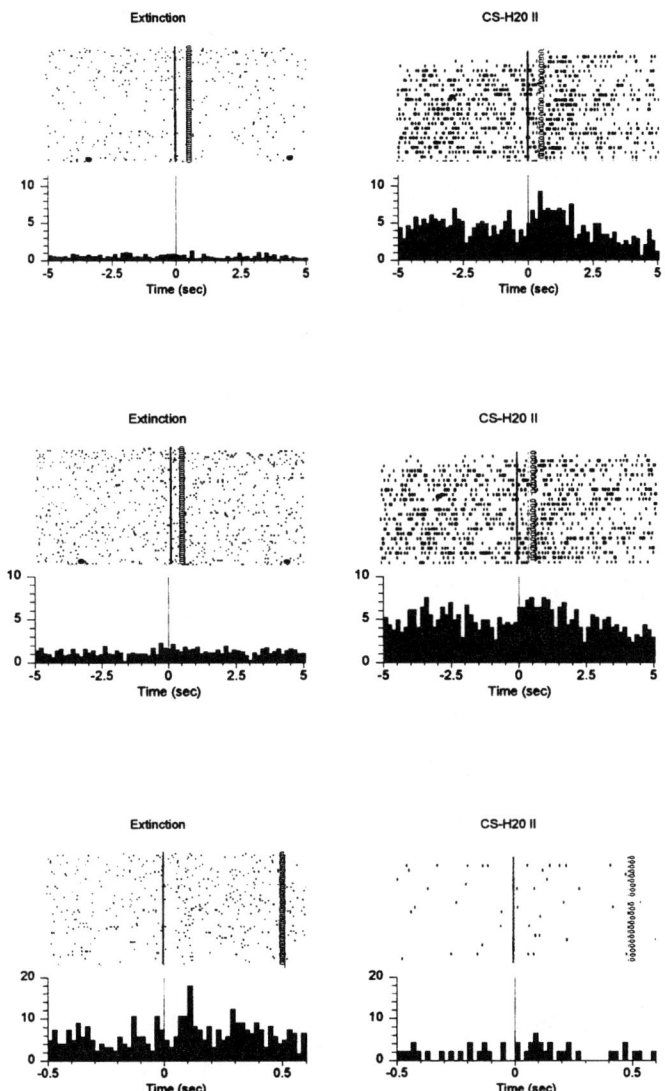

FIGURE 5B. (*Continued*) See legend on prior page.

and consume the ethanol drop. Subsets of neurons were observed that code the consumption of the liquid, often observed as a phasic decrease in activity during licking and swallowing. This reward-related phasic activity may reflect both unconditioned or conditioned responses to the taste and/or tactile sensations or to the motor response because these small orally consumed reinforcer drops cannot induce an immediate pharmacological effect. Rather, considerable numbers of small doses over many trials are required for the pharmacological effect of ethanol to develop. This is unlike the reward from iv cocaine or heroin, where pharmacological effects are established within seconds of the injection. We conclude that a combination of memory and cue processing drives the behavior throughout the gradual increment of systemic ethanol. The transient signals processed within the accumbens and related regions then are available as learning signals to help establish and/or maintain the persistent behavioral context that guides the selection of the appropriate response strategy during the session.

SECONDARY REINFORCING CUES AND CONTEXT CHANGES

The concept has emerged that the neural coding during a task might vary depending on information provided to the animal about the future consequence of reward. Early components of a task may be perceived by the subject as necessary but not sufficient to immediately yield the reward. Cues presented later within the task could permit the subject to anticipate the reward with high certainty. A task of this sort was employed during recording studies in primate ventral striatum[38] for a small cocaine reward per trial (0.05 microgram/kg) or for juice, a less desirable reward. A visual cue dimmed with three successive lever presses so that the monkey could determine that the last in a sequence would yield the reward. The phasic components of neural activity during this cued FR3 task did not vary when cocaine was the reward but changed markedly as the reward trial became certain in the case when the reward was juice.

Our experience with the rat also showed no change in coding during an FR3 sequence when a light was turned on after the second lever press in the FR3 sequence. Thus the results with the rat were similar to those in the primate in that there was no sign of the use of additional information when cocaine, with presumably high motivation, was the source of motivation. One might interpret these results with these protocol designs as inferring that the attentional state or context of coding remained high and constant during the tasks leading to cocaine in both primate and rat.[39,40] Coding changed during the phasic sensory motor sequence when the reward was juice versus cocaine in the primate or when the reward was cocaine versus heroin in the rat.

It is a common finding that a light or tone paired with availability of the reinforcer stabilizes the behavior and prolongs extinction. Phasic responses to such secondary reinforcers are found in the nucleus accumbens.[39] We have found phasic responses to tones in the nucleus accumbens, as well as the basolateral zone of the amygdala, that track the predictive information that water will be provided 0.5 sec after the tone. In addition, baseline firing rates appear to change when reinforcer availability changes (FIG. 5).

Recent studies use a variety of behavioral manipulations to explore the effects of changing reinforcer contexts upon neuronal activity. The first employs a multiple schedule of liquid reinforcer delivery in which responses at a single nose poke produce either 10% ethanol or 10% sucrose for component one of the multiple schedule and water for component two. The two components alternate every few minutes throughout a behavioral session. After a period of learning and adaptation, the rat spontaneously nose pokes to obtain fluid but rapidly changes nose-poke patterns when the fluid is switched from a preferred reinforcer (sucrose or ethanol) to the less preferred water.[41] The activity of a subset of NAS neurons relative to the nose poke and reinforcer comsumption also changes along with the behavior.

In a "progressive ratio" paradigm a rat can be made to nose poke an increasing number of times to obtain the next dose of water or ethanol at a spout or cocaine IV. Behavioral action ceases when the number of nose pokes to obtain the successive reward becomes excessive and presumably frustrating. Changes of mean background firing rates of subsets of neurons can be observed at times when the rat terminates nose-poke behavior. Also, phasic activity of subsets of neurons related to the nose poke for water can be observed to change when an additional reinforcer, cocaine, ethanol, or water, is made available via a second nose-poke device in the chamber.[42] Such results indicate that the context, including the available reinforcer, may regulate computation within this system. These behavioral and neural findings suggest that predictive cue information, and other indicators of behavioral context, propagates widely within the mesolimbic system to control behavior and to affect internal motivational states.

MEMORY FUNCTIONS WITHIN MESOLIMBIC ACTIVITY

The anatomical loop consisting of the medial and lateral prefrontal cortex, nucleus accumbens, ventral pallidum, and thalamus is similar structurally to other prefrontal cortical-basal ganglia loops, wherein working memory has been extensively investigated in primates.[43-45] Our hypothesis is that short- and long-term memory functions will also be evident within meso-cortico-limbic neuronal activity in the rat, provided that a task is structured properly to reveal these functions. Preliminary studies were conducted on mesolimbic activity during performance by a water-deprived rat of a delayed spatial match to sample task. The paradigm was similar to that recently employed by Deadwyler and his associates[46] to study memory function in rat hippocampus. A retractable right or left lever is presented that the rat presses to initiate a trial, and then the rat is required to cross to the opposite side of the chamber and nose poke repeatedly until a variable interval between 10 to 30 s elapses. Two levers are then presented, and to obtain a water reward the rat selects the same (match to sample) lever, or the opposite lever (nonmatch to sample), according to the rule reinforced.

Our finding is that the memory-encoding signals are not confined to the hippocampus but are in fact distributed widely in mesolimbic regions as well.[47-49] Counts of spikes before and after the sample and the match lever presses were binned in 250 ms intervals for 0.5 s before and after the lever press. This allowed a classic discriminant analysis to be performed to classify predictive patterns within the array of variables defined by neuron and time-interval spike counts. Information coding can be found distributed within the activity patterns of populations of cells in medial prefrontal cortex and nucleus accumbens. The population vectors can be shown to predict when a rat is performing a sample versus match phase or a right versus left lever position. Some cells also display elevated activity during the delay between sample and match, with a sensitivity of this delay activity to cannabinoid drug actions[49] that cause a decrease in memory performance.

The trials where errors occur are of particular interest because different patterns of activity appear even during the sample phase that can be used with statistical discriminant analysis to predict the future error behavior at the match phase. The behavior of the rat during a correct versus error trial cannot be readily discerned by the eye. It is clear, however, that neuronal patterns exist within subsets of neurons that correspond to behavioral strategies or internal brain computational contexts that lead to errors. These could be due to an immediate incorrect encoding of the information needed to perform the rule, or match or nonmatch. Such miscoding occurs when the information of the previous match trial segment appears to replace the information of the current trial (proactive memory interference). The error coding could represent a simple predetermination of the subject to select the match lever prior to the sample, and this could be done independently of the presence of a memory trace. The critical finding is the same regions of the mesolimbic system that reveal activity during an operant task for reward also exhibit coding for short-term memory functions, as well as information of choices about future behavior.

COMPUTATION WITHIN MESOLIMBIC CIRCUITS

A picture is beginning to emerge regarding the breadth of neural coding with portions of the mesolimbic system across behavioral tasks. It has become clear that most sensory and motor components of a task sequence are represented in neuronal activity patterns that occur during the operant tasks executed to obtain reinforcement. Samples from populations of neurons in multiple brain regions have revealed that small subsets of neurons, 5–15%, appear to code each segment of a task by phasic changes in excitatory or inhibitory activity. About 50% of neurons in an area typically show little change in activity states across all segments of a task. Moreover, coding during behavioral tasks for different reinforcers appears within different subsets of neurons, depending on the reinforcer. Finally, these regions that exhibit neuronal correlates of behavior also include the capacity to encode traces of memory, as revealed through the influences of previous experience or neural information predictive of future behavior. Specific patterns of activity often do, in fact, appear at the time that the reward is received, but it is difficult to discern the extent to which the activity is due to sensory input or motor pattern information.[50,51] One might speculate that the conceptual mechanism of reward itself may not be readily detected as a specific pattern of activity within particular neurons. The reward process may be carried out by a set of conjunctive conditions at the cellular level that, over time, lead to strengthened and persistent associative computations. Such cellular processes may be out of reach of the techniques of extracellular neuronal recording at this time.

The question arises as to the nature of the neural signals observed; after all, the recordings are obtained at a very high level of the neural axis in regions that are capable of very complex network logic. Are the signals motor or sensory, command, or other types of internal logic signals? What labels can be applied at this early stage of analysis? An experiment showing a single correlation is of marginal value for this problem, and instead a network of correlative findings must be revealed to progress

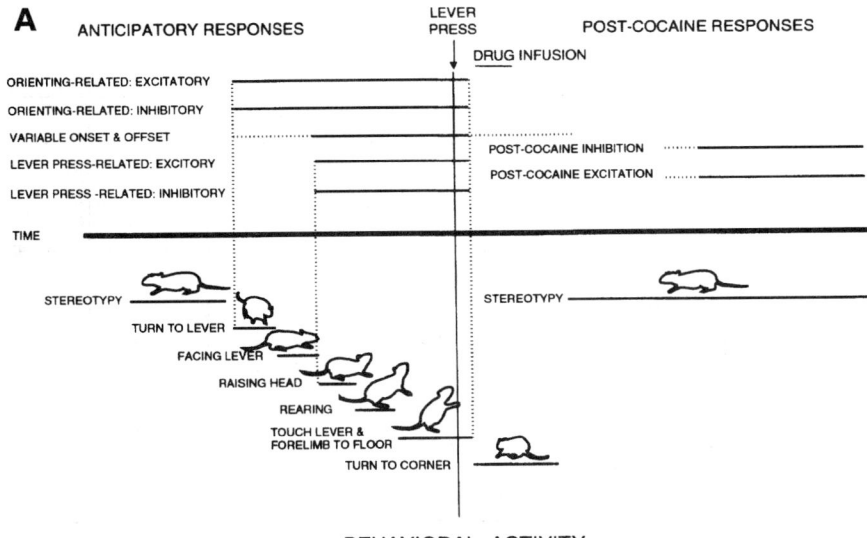

FIGURE 6. Schematic diagrams of response categories of mesolimbic neurons around timing nodes appearing within spontaneous behavior in 6A or in structured paradigms in 6B. **A:** Subsets of neurons revealing onset or termination of activity during the spontaneous sequence of motor events leading to the lever press to obtain self-administered iv cocaine. (Chang et al.[3] With permission from the *Journal of Neuroscience.*) **B:** Subsets of neurons in the cortical-ventral striatal system in primate, as described by Schultz[58] (with permission from MIT Press) reveal anticipatory, cue, delay trigger, delay, and reward specificity during a delayed-response task. These transitions parallel the correlations observed in temporally structured paradigms, as shown in FIG. 5, A and B, and FIG. 6A. These transitions in activity of subsets of neurons suggest a functional role for a sequence of memory-like states. These appear sequentially in time as a result of sensory-motor events in both spontaneous behavior (**A**) and experimenter-paced behavioral sequences (**B**).

from exploratory to causal and confirmatory hypotheses about complex network system functions (FIG. 6).

Our emerging view is that the steady state and phasic signals that appear within subpopulations of mesolimbic neurons reflect a progression of computational processes. Patterns in small ensembles of neurons in the mesolimbic system[8] are created specifically for a given context that is created and persists for varying lengths of time as behavior progresses along a chain of behavioral events. We do not view neural computation in this case to be a continuous process. Distinct transitions can be observed, for example, anticipatory states derived from internal timing or cue-initiated memories. Distinct transitions can be observed for anticipatory states derived from internal timing or memory due to cue- or trigger-initiated states. In traditional delayed-response paradigms[43,45–49,51] the experimenter defines and controls the timing of the cues, triggers, and the availability of reinforcer. A cue is followed by a delay, during which sustained activity is postulated to store a memory for a short time. Our postulate is that the delay period activity, that has been associated with the

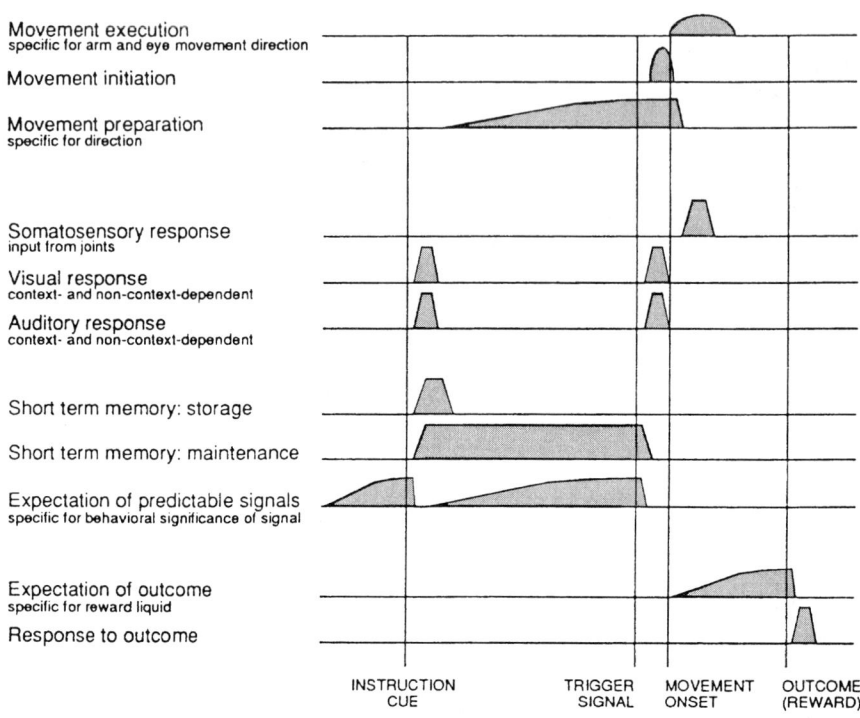

FIGURE 6B. See legend on prior page.

function of "working memory," is, in fact, a very general circuit memory phenomenon to be found in all cortico-striatal looping systems. Local circuit mechanisms, both in cortex and striatum, can contribute to short-term memory;[43,45,53] as a consequence, the same circuit mechanisms may generate much of the activity, as cues are encountered during the task sequence for reward. When the animal initiates a behavioral sequence (perhaps analogous to the progress of human mental calculations or thinking), it is not obvious when the cues, triggers, or transition events appear that are driven by the interaction with the environment or by intrinsic brain computational transitions. It is clear, however, that transitions in neural activity can be found to correlate with distinct nodes in the movement sequences.[3,4] Our conjecture is that much of the activity observed in the mesolimbic system consists of a sequence of short-term memories that are triggered internally or externally and are represented as anticipatory and delay-period states.

The question arises as to how the signals in the mesolimbic system are used, inasmuch as they are removed from primary functions of sensory or motor circuits. One possibility to be explored in future work is that the phasic and steady-state patterns may be part of a system that acts primarily to track the ongoing behavioral events and their consequences, and make comparisons to anticipated outcomes. A function may then be to transmit to other portions of the cortical striatal and amygdala anatomical loops the salient learning signals needed to control future behavioral strategies.[54–58] In this hypothesis neural activity in the mesolimbic system across behavioral states may function as an elaborate learning system that transmits training signals to other parts of the cortex, operates on different time scales, and is posed to react quickly to the emotional valence of the behavioral context.

ACKNOWLEDGMENTS

This work was supported by DA-2338, NIAAA-10980, NSF-DBI-9619063, ONR N00014-96-1-1104, and an Award from the Tourette Syndrome Association to D.J.W.

REFERENCES

1. CHANG, J.Y., S.F. SAWYER, R.-S. LEE, B.N. MADDUX & D.J. WOODWARD. 1990. Activity of neurons in nucleus accumbens during cocaine self-administration in freely moving rats. Neurosci. Abstr. **16:** 252.
2. CHANG, J.Y., J.M. PARIS, S.F. SAWYER, A.B. KIRILLOV & D.J. WOODWARD. 1996. Neuronal spike activity in rat nucleus accumbens during cocaine self-administration under different fixed-ratio schedules. Neuroscience **74:** 483–497.
3. CHANG, J.-Y., S.F. SAWYER, R.-S. LEE & D.J. WOODWARD. 1994. Electrophysiological and pharmacological evidence for the role of the nucleus accumbens in cocaine self-administration in freely moving rats. J. Neurosci. **14:** 1224–1244.
4. CHANG, J.-Y., S.F. SAWYER, J.M. PARIS, A. KIRILLOV & D.J. WOODWARD. 1997. Single neuronal responses in medial prefrontal cortex during cocaine self-administration in freely moving rats. Synapse (NY) **26:** 22–35.
5. WISE, R.A. & M.A. BOZARTH. 1987. A psychomotor stimulant theory of addiction. Psychol. Rev. **94:** 469–492.
6. GROENEWEGEN, H.J., P. ROOM, M.P. WITTER & A.H.M. LOHMAN. 1982. Cortical afferents of the nucleus accumbens in the cat, studied with anterograded and retrograde transport techniques. Neuroscience **7:** 977-995.
7. BROG, J.S., A.Y. DEUTCH & D.S. ZAHM. 1991. Afferent projection to the nucleus accumbens core and shell in the rat. Neurosci. Abst. **17:** 454.
8. PENNARTZ, C.M.A., H.J. GROENEWEGEN & F.H. LOPEZ DA SILVA. 1994. The nucleus accumbens as a complex of functionally distinct neuronal ensembles: an integration of behavioural, electrophysiological and anatomical data. Prog. Neurobiol. **42:** 719–761.
9. BERENDSE, H.W., Y. GALIS-DE GRAFF & H.L. GROENEWEGEN. 1992. Topographical organization and relationship with ventral striatal compartments of prefrontal corticostriatal projections in the rat. J. Comp. Neurol. **316:** 314–347.
10. KELLEY, A. & V.B. DOMESICK. 1982. The distribution of the projection from the hippocampal formation to the nucleus accumbens in the rat: an anterograde- and retrograde-horseradish peroxidase study. Neuroscience **7:** 2321–2335.
11. GROENEWEGEN, H.J., E. VERMEULEN-VAN DER ZEE, A. TE KORTSCHOT & M.P. WITTER. 1987. Organization of the projections from the subiculum to the ventral striatum in the rat. A study using anterograde transport of *Phaseolus vulgaris* leucoagglutinin. Neuroscience **23:** 103–120.
12. KELLY, A., V. DOMESICK & W.J.H. NAUTA. 1982. The amygdalostriatal projection in the rat—an anatomical study by anterograde and retrograde tracing methods. Neurscience **7:** 615–630.
13. ROBINSON, T.G. & P.M. BEART. 1988. Excitant amino acid projections from rat amygdala and thalamus. Brain Res. Bull. **15:** 467–471.

14. MCDONALD, A.J. 1991. Topographical organization of amygdaloid projections to the caudatoputamen, nucleus accumbens and related striatal-like areas of the rat brain. Neuroscience **44:** 15–33.
15. SU, H.S. & M. BENTIVOGLIO. 1990. Thalamic midline cell populations projecting to the nucleus accumbens, amygdala, and hippocampus of the rat. J. Comp. Neurol. **297:** 582–593.
16. ZAHM, D.S. & W.J. HEIMER. 1990. Two transpallidal pathways originating in the rat nucleus accumbens. J. Comp. Neurol. **302:** 437–446.
17. HEIMER, L., D.S. ZAHM & G.F. ALHEID. 1995. Basal ganglia. *In* The Rat Nervous System. G. Paxinos, Ed.: 579–620. Academic Press.
18. NAUTA, W.J.H., G.P. SMITH, R.L.M. FAULL & V.B. DOMESICK. 1978. Efferent connections and nigral afferents of the nucleus accumbens septi in the rat. Neuroscience **3:** 385–401.
19. DOMESICK, V. 1981. Further observation on the anatomy of the nucleus accumbens and caudatoputamen in the rat: similarities and contrasts. *In* Neurobiology of the Nucleus Accumbens. R.B. Chronister & J.F. DeFrance, Eds.: 7–39. Haer Institute for Electrophysiological Research. Brunswick, ME.
20. MOGENSEN, G.L., L.W. SWANSON & M. WU. 1983. Neural projections from nucleus accumbens to globus pallidus, substantia innominata, and lateral preoptic-lateral hypothalamic area: an anatomical and electrophysiological investigation in the rat. J. Neurosci. **3:** 189–202.
21. GROENEWEGEN, H.J. & F.T. RUSSCHEN. 1984. Organization of the efferent projections of the nucleus accumbens, pallidal, hypothalamic, and mesencephalic structures: a tracing and immunohistochemical study in the cat. J. Comp. Neurol. **223:** 347–367.
22. HEIMER, L., D.S. ZAHM, L. CHURCHILL, P.W. KALIVAS & C. WOHLTMANN. 1991. Specificity in the projection patterns of accumbal core and shell in the rat. Neuroscience **41:** 89–125.
23. HEIMER, L. & R.D. WILSON. 1975. The subcortical projections of the allocortex: similarities in the neural association of the hippocampus, the piriform cortex, and the neocortex. *In* Golgi Centennial Symposium, Perspectives in Neurobiology. M. Santini, Ed.: 177–193. Raven. New York.
24. WOODWARD, D.J., P.H. JANAK & J.-Y. CHANG. 1998. Ethanol action on neuronal systems studied with multineuron recording in freely moving animals. Alcoholism Clin. Exp. Res. **22:** 10–22.
25. WEST, M.O., A.J. MICHAEL, S.E. KNOWLES, J.K. CHAPIN & D.J. WOODWARD. 1987. Striatal unit activity and the linkage between sensory and motor events. *In* Basal Ganglia and Behavior: Sensory Aspects of Motor Functioning. J.S. Schneider & T. Lidsky, Eds.: 27–35. Hogrege & Huber. Toronto.
26. WEST, M.O., R.M. CARELLI, M. POMERANTZ, S.M. COHEN, J.P. GARDNER, J.K. CHAPIN & D.J. WOODWARD. 1990. A region in the dorsolateral striatum of rat exhibiting single-unit correlations with specific locomotor limb movements. J. Neurophysiol. **64:** 1233-1246.
27. CARELLI, R.M. & S.A. DEADWYLER. 1997. Cellular mechanisms underlying reinforcement-related processing in the nucleus accumbens: electrophysiological studies in behaving animals. Pharmacol. Biochem. Behav. **57:** 495–504.
28. PEOPLES, L.L., A.J. UZWIAK, F. GEE & M. WEST. 1997. Operant behavior during sessions of intravenous cocaine infusion is necessary and sufficient for phasic firing of single nucleus accumbens neurons. Brain Res. **757:** 280–284.
29. PEOPLES, L., F. GEE, R. BIBI & M.O. WEST. 1998. Phasic firing time locked to cocaine self-infusion and locomotion: dissociable firing patterns of single nucleus accumbens neurons in the rat. J. Neurosci. **18:** 7588–7598.
30. PEOPLES, L.L. & M.O. WEST. 1996. Phasic firing patterns in the rat accumbens correlated with the timing of intravenous cocaine self-administration. J. Neurosci. **16:** 3459–3473.
31. PEOPLES, L.L., A.J. UZWIAK, F.X. GUYETTE & M.O. WEST. 1998. Tonic inhibition of single nucleus accumbens neurons in the rat: a predominant but not exclusive fir-

ing pattern induced by cocaine self-administration sessions. Neuroscience **86:** 13–22.
32. CHANG, J.-Y., L.L. ZHANG, P.H. JANAK & D.J. WOODWARD. 1997. Neuronal responses in prefrontal cortex and nucleus accumbens during heroin self-administration in freely moving rats. Brain Res. **754:** 12–20.
33. CHANG, J-Y, P.H. JANAK & D.J. WOODWARD. 1998. Comparison of mesocorticolimbic neuronal responses during cocaine and heroin self-administration in freely moving rats. J. Neurosci. **18:** 3098–3115.
34. CHEN, L., J.-Y. CHANG & D.J. WOODWARD. 1998. Mesolimbic neuronal responses during nicotine self-administration: comparison with other drugs of abuse. Neurosci. Abstr. **265:** 16.
35. WATANABE, M. 1996. Reward expectancy in primate prefrontal neurons. Nature **382:** 629–632.
36. SAMSON, H.H. 1986 Initiation of ethanol reinforcement using sucrose-substitution procedure in food- and water sated rats. Alcohol Clin Exp Res **10:** 436–442.
37. WOODWARD, D.J., P.H. JANAK & J.-Y. CHANG. 1998. Ethanol action on neuronal systems studied with multineuron recording in freely moving animals. Alcoholism Clin. Exp. Res. **22:** 10–22.
38. JANAK, P.H., J.-Y. CHANG & D.J. WOODWARD. 1999. Neuronal spike activity in the nucleus accumbens of behaving rats during ethanol self-administration. Brain Res. **817:** 172–184.
39. JANAK, P.H. & D.J. WOODWARD. 1997. Neurons recorded from the amygdala and nucleus accumbens of the rat during ethanol self-administration. Neurosci. Abstr. **933:** 18.
40. SHIDARA, M., T. G.AIGNER & B.J. RICHMOND. 1998. Neuronal signals related to progress through a predictable series of trials. J. Neurosci. **18:** 2613–2625.
41. ANSTROM, K.K., P.H. JANAK & D.J. WOODWARD. 1998. An approach to recording neural coding in the mesolimbic reward system during a dual-reward behavioral paradigm. Neurosci. Abstr. **190:** 11.
42. WOODWARD, D.J., A.V. AZAROV & M. ASCHNER. 1998. Behavioral correlations of mesolimbic unit activity during simultaneous intake of ethanol solution and water. Neurosci. Abstr. **190:** 10.
43. WILLIAMS, G.V. & P.S. GOLDMAN-RAKIC. 1995. Modulation of memory fields by dopamine D1 receptors in prefrontal cortex. Nature **376** (6541): 57.
44. GOLDBERG, R.B., J.M. FUSTER & R. ALVAREZ-PELAEZ. 1980. Frontal cell activity during delayed response performance in squirrel monkey. Physiol. Behav. **25:** 425–432.
45. FUSTER, J.M. 1997. Network memory. Trends Neurosci. **20:** 451–459.
46. DEADWYLER, S.A., T BUNN & R.E. HAMPSON. 1996. Hippocampal ensemble activity during spatial delayed-nonmatch-to-sample performance in rats. J. Neurosci. **16:** 354–372.
47. WOODWARD, D.J., J.-Y. CHANG, M.G. LAUBACH & A. KIRILLOV. 1995. Activity patterns in neuron ensembles in cortex and basal ganglia code current and future behavior in a delayed match to sample task in freely moving rats. Am. Coll. Neuropsychopharmacol. Ann. Meeting. Abstract.
48. CHANG, J.-Y., L. CHEN & D.J. WOODWARD. 1999. Neuronal responses in frontal cortex system during delayed matching to sample. Manuscript.
49. CHANG, J.-Y., L. CHEN & D.J. WOODWARD. 1998. Large scale ensemble recording during delayed match to sample task in rats: the effects of delta-9 THC. Neurosci. Abstr. **268:** 3.
50. BOWMAN, E.M., T.G. AIGNER & B.J. RICHMOND. 1996. Neural signals in the monkey ventral striatum related to motivation for juice and cocaine rewards. J. Neurophysiol. **75:** 1061–1073.
51. SCHULTZ, W., P. APICELLA, R. ROMO & E. SCARNATI. 1995. Context-dependent activity in primate striatum reflecting past and future behavioral events. *In* Models of Information Processing in the Basal Ganglia. J.C. Houk, J.L. Davis & D.G. Beiser, Eds.: 11. MIT Press. Cambridge, MA.

52. WOODWARD, D.J., J.-Y. CHANG, M.G. LAUBACH & A. KIRILLOV. 1995. Activity patterns in neuron ensembles in cortex and basal ganglia code current and future behavior in a delayed match to sample task in freely moving rats. Am. Coll. Neuropsychopharmacol. Ann. Meeting Abstract.
53. WOODWARD, D.J., A.B. KIRILLOV, C.D. MYRE & S.F. SAWYER. 1994. Neostriatal circuitry as a scalar memory: modeling and ensemble neuron recording. *In* Models of Information Processing in the Basal Ganglia. A Bradford Book. J.C. Houk, J.L. Davis & D.G. Beiser, Eds.: 316–336. The MIT Press. Cambridge, MA.
54. SHOENBAUM, G, A.A. CHIBA & M. GALLAGHER. 1998. Orbitofrontal cortex and basolateral amygdala encode expected outcomes during learning. Nature: Neuroscience **1:**155–159
55. MURAMOTO, K., T. ONO, H. NISHIJO & M. FUKUDO. 1993. Rat amygdaloid neuron responses during auditory discrimination. Neuroscience **52:** 621–636.
56. NISHIJO, H., T.UWANO, R. TAMURE & O. TAKETOSHI. 1998. Gustatory and multimodal neuronal responses in the amygdala during licking and discrimination of sensory stimuli in awake rats. J. Neurophysiol. **79:** 21–36.
57. WHITELAW, R.B., A. MARKOU, T.W. ROBBINS & B.J. EVERITT. 1996. Excitotoxic lesions of the basolateral amygdala impair the acquisition of cocaine-seeking behavior under a second-order schedule of reinforcement. Psychopharmacology **127:** 213–224.
58. SCHULTZ, W., P. APICELLA, R. ROMO & E. SCARNATI. 1994. Context-dependent activity in primate striatum reflecting past and future behavioral events. In Models of Information Processing in the Basal Ganglia. J.C. Houk, J.L. Davis & D.G. Beiser Eds. MIT Press. Cambridge, MA.

Functional-anatomical Implications of the Nucleus Accumbens Core and Shell Subterritories

DANIEL S. ZAHM[a]

Department of Anatomy and Neurobiology, St. Louis University School of Medicine, 1402 S. Grand Boulevard, St. Louis, Missouri 63104, USA

ABSTRACT: The nucleus accumbens, a major part of the ventral striatum, comprises numerous subterritories and compartments, of which the core and shell appear to be dominant. Shell exhibits greater chemical neuroanatomical diversity than core and is rather directly connected to it by a robust, feed-forward, striatopallido-thalamocortico-striatal pathway. Shell and extended amygdala share afferents, but the two are distinguished by their outputs, strongly toward cortex for shell and descendent toward brain stem effector sites for extended amygdala. Shell responds independently to stimulation by excitatory amino acids and dopamine, which are more mutually permissive in the core. Accordingly, the shell responds to a broad variety of physiological and pharmacological stimuli, including psychomotor and opioid drugs. Whereas locomotion and oro-facial movements are elicitable from the shell, lesions and blockade of EAA transmission in the core reduce locomotion. It is hypothesized that core–shell has a feed-forward functional organization.

INTRODUCTION

Ever since the nucleus accumbens was observed to comprise "core" and "shell" regions,[1,2] there has been great concern as to how this subnuclear organization might contribute to the neural processing of reward–incentive motivation and adaptive motor response. Earlier literature reviews on connectional and histochemical features of the core–shell pattern of organization and some associated functional implications[3–7] have been superseded by a steady stream of recent papers about additional connectional, neurochemical and functional aspects of the core–shell organization. Discussion of this so-called core–shell subterritorial organization, however, should be prefaced with an acknowledgment that the true organization of the nucleus accumbens involves a richly subtle mix of subterritories and compartments that exclusive reference to core–shell organization may cause to be grossly underappreciated. For example, the conspicuously patchy composition of the caudomedial shell that has been elegantly addressed by Groenewegen and his colleagues (e.g., refs. 8 and 9) is one expression of this (FIG. 1). Another expression of it involves the concept of transition,[10–14] in that to the same extent that boundaries between the certain accumbal subterritories show clear definition, they are vague and poorly defined between others. Particularly, between the medial and lateral shell (FIG. 1) and the caudal and rostral part of the accumbens, such boundaries are

---

[a]Voice: 314-577-8280; fax: 314-268-5127; e-mail: zahmds@wpogate.slu.edu

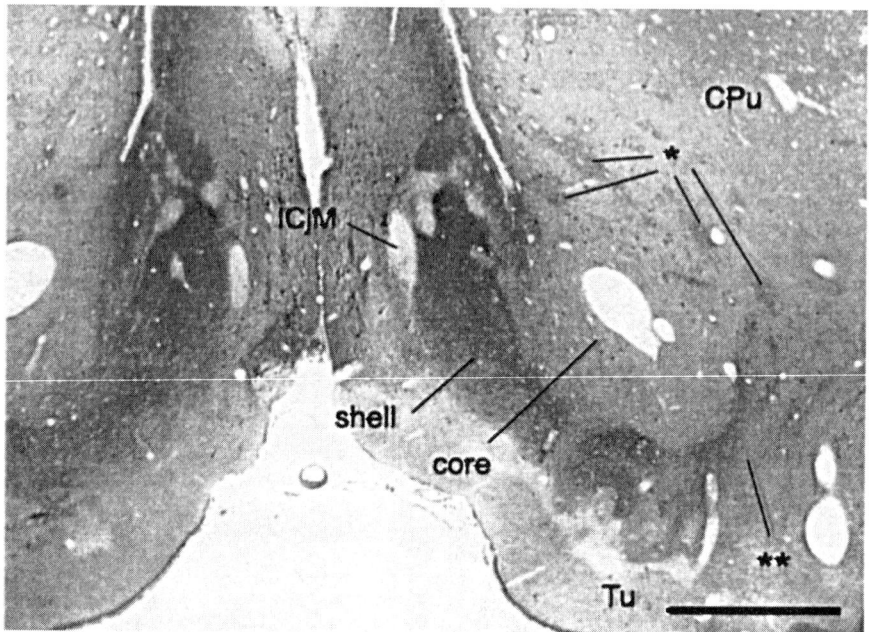

FIGURE 1. Frontal section through the shell and core of the rat nucleus accumbens as exhibited by calretinin (CR) immunoreactivity (ir), which illustrates some salient features observed with a number of markers of the core–shell subterritorial organization. Note that CR-ir is strongest dorsomedially, near the island of Calleja magna (ICjM), adjacent to which marked heterogeneity (patchiness) in the make-up of the shell is apparent. The intensity of CR-ir diminishes in a mediolateral gradient toward the lateralmost parts of the shell where it is nearly gone (**). Although the core is more homogeneous, a number of patches exhibiting CR-ir (*) mark the transition from core to caudate-putamen (CPu). Tu, olfactory tubercle. Scale bar: 1.0 mm.

so transitional and broad as to be virtually nonexistent, leading to controversies regarding, for example, whether the rostral pole is a rostral extension of the shell[15] or a distinct subterritory.[16] Nonetheless, an appreciation of salient patterns of functional-anatomical organization evinced by general consideration of the core and shell is likely to be important to comprehending how the nucleus accumbens functions as a whole.

RECENT CHEMICAL-NEUROANATOMICAL OBSERVATIONS

The previously noted tendency for more neuroactive substances to be represented more strongly in the shell than core[3,4,17] continues to be observed (e.g., 5-HT$_4$ receptors,[18] dopamine D$_3$ receptors,[19] calretinin immunoreactivity,[20] and the cocaine- and amphetamine-regulated transcript and its peptide[21]). Interestingly, a number of substances associated with the extended amygdala are also represented in the caudomedial shell.[10,12–14,22] Whereas the extraordinary richness of some markers of shell, such as, for example, neurotensin, owes to strong expression by neurons residing in the shell and their local dendritic and axonal arbors,[23] other markers reflect neurochemical attributes of afferents (e.g., ref. 2). A variety of drugs elicits expression of the immediate-early gene, Fos, preferentially in the shell.[24–26] In view of all of these observations, it is surprising that intracellularly filled medium spiny neurons in the medial shell are smaller and exhibit fewer and thinner dendrites and fewer dendritic spines than those in the core.[27, 28]

It should be noted, however, that some substances, such as calbindin-D 28 kDa;[29,30] enkephalin;[31,32] and the $GABA_A$[33] receptor are more strongly represented in core than shell. Via the $GABA_A$ receptor, GABA could mediate tonic inhibitory effects that contribute to depressing the metabolism of neuroactive substances in the core. Likewise, the level of dopamine transporter measured by [^{3}H]mazindol binding is greater in the core than shell.[34] Thus, the rate not only of release but also of uptake of dopamine (DA) following medial forebrain bundle stimulation is about three times greater in the core than shell,[34] making it a bit counterintuitive that the basal level of extracellular DA is significantly greater in core than shell.[24,35,36] These data suggest that released dopamine, which is known to suppress the expression of certain peptides (e.g., see ref. 37), might contribute to reducing the neurochemical diversity in the core.

To the contrary, psychomotor and opiate drugs preferentially increase levels of extracellular DA[38,39] and, accordingly, [3H]2-deoxyglucose utilization[40,41] in medial shell more than core of the accumbens. Haloperidol, on the other hand, caused the rate of DA turnover to increase more in core than shell, whereas the atypical antipsychotic clozapine caused equivalent increases in dopamine turnover in the two.[42] Using *in vivo* voltammetric measurements following low and high doses of haloperidol, clozapine, amperozide, risperidone, ritanserin and raclopride, Marcus *et al.*[43] concluded that high 5-HT_2 occupancy favors DA release in shell (clozapine, amperozide, risperidone, and ritanserin), whereas high D_2 receptor occupancy favors DA release in the core (haloperidol and raclopride).

Connectivity

In view of all of these results, it is not surprising that the morphologies,[44] certain neurochemical attributes,[21,45] and vulnerabilities to degeneration[46] of ventral mesencephalic neurons giving rise to the innervation of the shell differ from those of neurons innervating the core. Likewise, the morphologies of DA-containing axons and axon terminals in the core are distinct from those in the shell.[29,47] In general, much of the afferent innervation of the shell derives from cortical and subcortical structures relatively segregated from those projecting strongly to the core, particularly parts of the lateral preoptico-lateral hypothalamic continuum, mesopontine tegmentum, and brain stem that project little if at all to the core.[17]

Likewise, the outputs from the shell and core terminate in distinct structures and subterritories. Shell selectively innervates the ventromedial part (VPm) of the subcommissural ventral pallidum (FIG. 2A)[16, 30, 48, 49] that, in turn, projects to the medial segment of the thalamic mediodorsal nucleus (FIG. 2B and C),[49–52] which has strong reciprocal connections with dorsal prelimbic and agranular insular cortex. These project massively to the core of the nucleus accumbens and adjacent parts of the caudate-putamen.[50, 53] It is noteworthy that this connectional substrate shunts

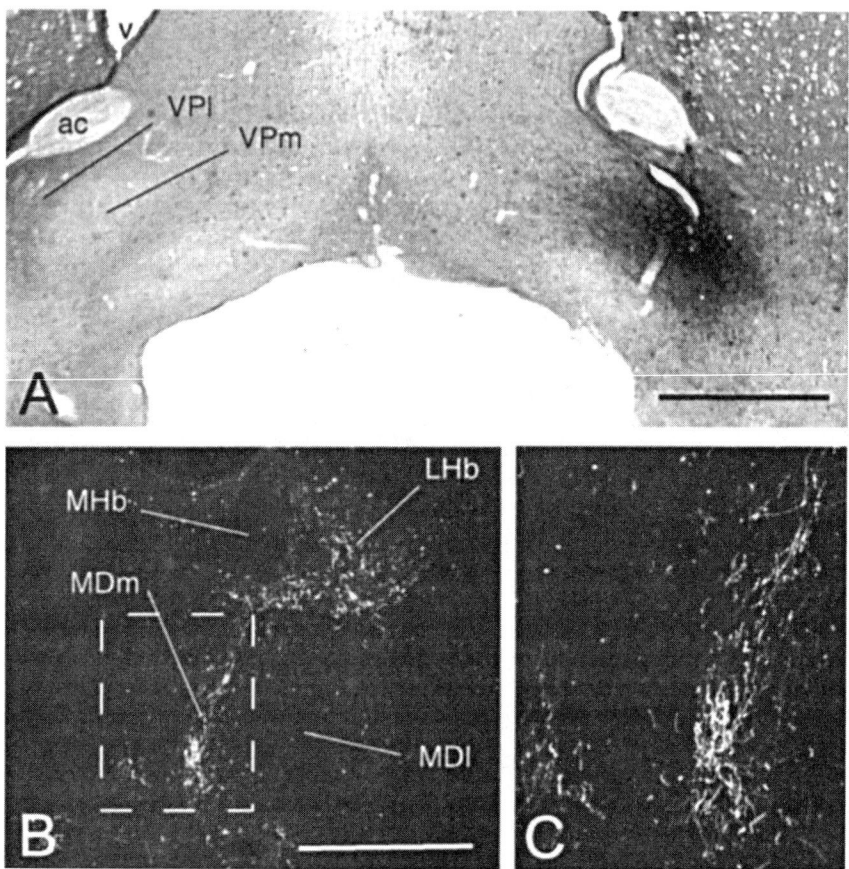

FIGURE 2. Micrographs illustrating the ventral striatopallidothalamocortical projection. The ventromedial part of subcommissural ventral pallidum (VPm), which gives rise to robust ventral pallidothalamic projections exhibits weak calbindin-D 28 kDa (CB) immunoreactivity (ir), indicative of its principal input from the accumbens shell, which also exhibits weak CB-ir. Projections from the core, a structure with strong CB-ir, terminate in VPl, which projects weakly, if at all, to the thalamus. The terminations of the ventral pallidothalamic projection in the medial segment of the mediodorsal nucleus of the thalamus (MDm) are shown in panel **B** and enlarged in **C**. The medial part of MD is strongly reciprocally connected with the dorsal prelimbic and agranular insular cortices (see text for refs.). A weak contralateral projection is shown in the lower left part of the box. VPm also projects to the lateral habenula (LHb). MDl, lateral segment, mediodorsal nucleus; MHb, medial habenula. Scale bars: **A**, 1.0 mm; **B**, 500 µm.

neural information rather directly from the shell to the core of the nucleus accumbens (FIG. 3). [3–7,17,30] Shell also strongly innervates the lateral preoptico-lateral hypothalamic continuum, which together with VPm, projects strongly to the mesencephalic ventral tegmental area of Tsai (VTA),[49,51,54–58] that is itself a third major site of termination of outputs from the shell. To the contrary, the striatopallido-thalamocortical connections of the accumbens core[49] tend to be more reentrant

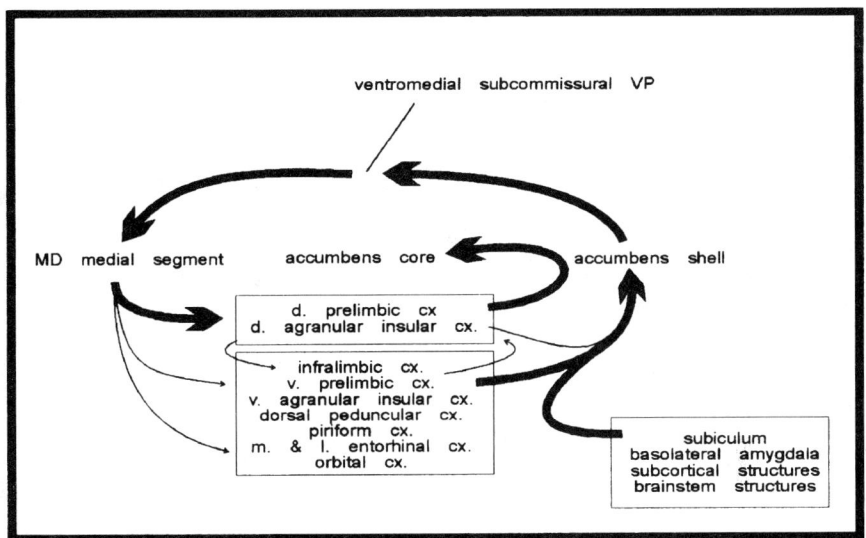

FIGURE 3. Diagram illustrating the prominently feed-forward connectivity by virtue of which the accumbens shell projects relatively directly to the core. See text for details. cx, cortex; MD, mediodorsal; VP, ventral pallidum.

(feedback) in nature (see, e.g., refs. 59–61) in the sense that they begin and end in the dorsal prelimbic and agranular insular cortices (FIG. 4).[62–64]

Core–Shell in Relation to the Central Division of the Extended Amygdala

The rich connectivity of the medial shell with subcortical and brainstem structures, combined with some immunohistochemical and receptor binding observations[10] have elicited the suggestion that the caudomedial shell may represent a rostral extension of the extended amygdala, or, at least, a transitional structure bridging basal ganglia and centromedial amygdaloid patterns of neural organization.[10,13,14,21] Although a survey of afferent connections would tend, although only in part,[65] to support this assessment,[10,13,14,65] consideration of the outputs from the caudomedial shell and central nucleus of the amygdala, a "prototypical" extended amygdaloid structure, reveals substantial differences.[65–68] As noted above, the caudomedial shell projection is strong in the VP, lateral preoptico-lateral hypothalamic continuum and VTA, but distal to this it thins abruptly. To the contrary, the central nucleus projects minimally to these structures, but strongly innervates the bed nucleus of the stria terminalis and associated sublenticular extended amygdala (FIG. 5A), which get little input from accumbens. Central amygdala does project substantially to the lateral hypothalamus but only at levels behind the rostral part of the entopeduncular nucleus, where some overlap with accumbal projections may occur, although even here the pathways appear to be largely distinct (FIG. 5B and C). Although there exists limited innervation of the ventral tegmental area by the central amygdala, its input to the lateral one third of the substantia nigra compacta is substantial. Finally, central amygdaloid projections are robust in the me-

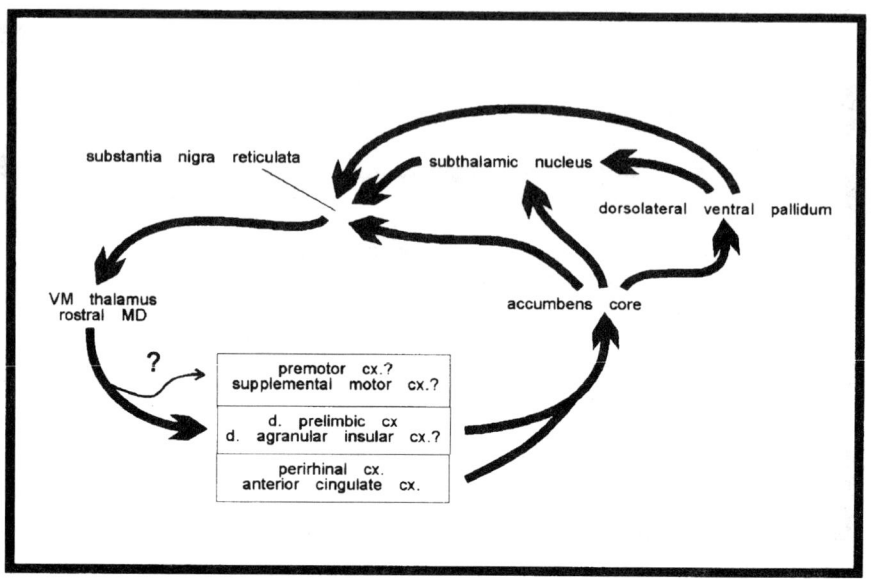

FIGURE 4. Diagram illustrating some cortico-basal ganglia-thalamocortical projections of the accumbens core. At least the relationships involving the dorsal prelimbic cortex would appear to be prominently feedback in nature, according to refs. 62–64. However, it is also clear that some corticostriatal projections, for example, those originating in the perirhinal and, possibly, cingulate cortices feed-forward through these connections. Furthermore, it is likely that the projections from the ventromedial thalamic nucleus (VM) should feed forward to the cortex near or including the pre- and supplemental motor areas (as indicated by ?), although this remains to be shown empirically, at least with regard to parts of the VM connected with the core. See text for more details. cx., cortex; MD, mediodorsal nucleus; VM, ventromedial.

sopontine tegmentum and caudal brain stem sites, such as the reticular formation, parabrachial nucleus, nucleus of the solitary tract and dorsal vagal complex, all of which receive little input from the accumbens. The substantial differences in the output systems of the caudomedial shell of accumbens and central amygdala suggest that the two represent distinct functional-anatomical systems.

SOME RECENT FUNCTIONAL STUDIES

Core–Shell and Reward

Rats will lever press vigorously for injections of PCP, MK-801, and CPP into the shell and frontal cortex and for nomifensine and cocaine into the medial shell,[69] but none of these substances elicit lever pressing for injection into the core. These effects of PCP, MK-801, and CPP are not blocked by sulpiride at doses that antagonize the effects of intrathecal injections of nomifensine,[70] suggesting that the dopaminergic and excitatory amino acid effects are independent. In addition, PCP,

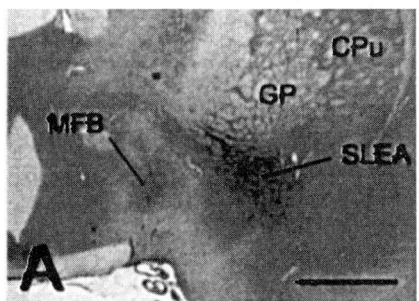
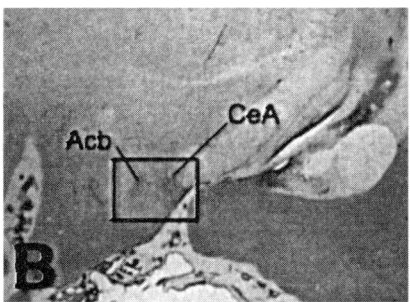
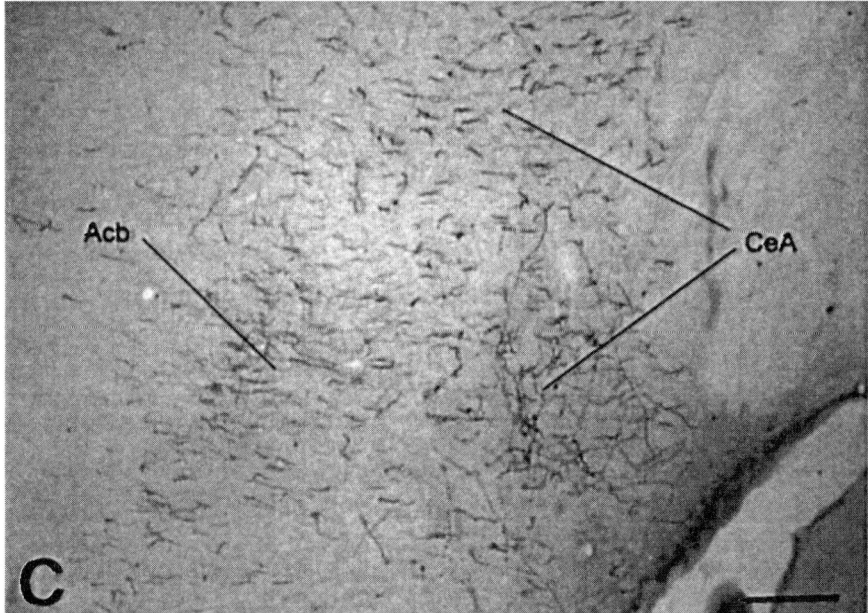

FIGURE 5. Micrographs illustrating the projections of the caudomedial accumbens shell and central amygdaloid nucleus. The two structures in the same brain were injected with different anterogradely transported axonal tracers, which were processed to exhibit different colors. Panel **A** shows a frontal section through the caudate-putamen (CPu), globus pallidus (GP), and sublenticular region. At this level projections from the amygdaloid injection are distributed coextensively with the sublenticular extended amygdala (SLEA), and those from the accumbens shell are restricted to a position corresponding to that of the medial forebrain bundle (MFB). Panel **B** shows a frontal section through the lateral hypothalamus (box), where the projections from the central amygdala (CeA) and caudomedial shell (Acb) are indicated. The boxed area in **B** is shown enlarged in panel **C**. Even in this gray tone micrograph, differences in the character of the anterograde labeling allow fibers from the amygdala (CeA) and accumbens (Acb) to be distinguished. It is apparent that the projections are largely separate at this level. Scale bars: **A** and **B**, 1.0 mm; **C**, 200 μm.

nomifensine, and MK-801 each potentiated lateral hypothalamic self-stimulation when injected into the shell, but not the core.[71] Rebec et al.[72] observed that the initial entry of rats into a novel environment was associated with increased DA in the prefrontal cortex and accumbens shell but not in the accumbens core and caudate-putamen, as measured by *in vivo* voltammetry, nor was an effect observed in any of these structures when the rats reentered the familiar environment.

Core–Shell and Behavioral Sensitization to Psychostimulants

A selective dopamine transporter ligand, [^{125}I]RTI-121, exhibited reduced binding only in the accumbens shell after a period of withdrawal from conditioning administration of cocaine.[73] Concordant findings were generated by Boulay *et al.*,[74] who observed locomotor activity sensitized to administration of cocaine and GBR12783 and decreases in [^{3}H]mazindol binding selectively in the shell, but Sharpe *et al.*[75] reported that after 10 days of recovery following 10 days of cocaine administration [^{3}H]mazindol binding was significantly reduced in medial shell *and* core. However, in agreement with Boulay *et al.*,[74] when Pierce and Kalivas[76] conditioned rats with saline or cocaine and then made injections of amphetamine into the core or shell following short (1–3 days) and longer (20–22 days) periods of withdrawal, they observed locomotor sensitization only at late withdrawal in cocaine-treated rats only after shell injections of amphetamine. Extracellular DA was increased in the shell at both time points and no stimulant effect of SKF-38393 was observed early or late in saline- or cocaine-treated rats.

Movements Elicited from the Accumbens Shell

Koshikawa *et al.*[77] observed that injections of D_1 (SKF 38393) and D_2 (quinpirole) receptor agonists together into shell and, only minimally, core (due probably to spread to shell) resulted in tight contralaterally directed turns. Injected individually, these agonists were ineffective at producing turning, and the effect was attenuated by injection of SCH-23390 (D_1 antagonist) or l-sulpiride (D_2 antagonist). Additional study[78,79] revealed that injections of D1 (SKF 82958) and D3 (7-OH-DPAT) receptor agonists also produced contralateral turns and jaw movements when injected together into shell (see also refs. 80 and 81). Again, the drugs administered individually were ineffective, and the effect was blocked by SCH-23390, l-sulpiride and domperidone, but not PD 128,907 (D_3 antagonist). It was concluded that D_1 and D_2, but not D_3 receptors are involved in the production of these motor effects.

Core–Shell and Dopamine-excitatory Amino Acid Interactions

Injections of AP-5 (NMDA antagonist) into the central (core) accumbens resulted in reductions in locomotion in the periphery and rearing in the center of the test apparatus and attenuated locomotion in the presence of novel objects, whereas shell injections increased locomotion in the presence of novel objects.[82] In related studies, Pulvirenti *et al.*[83] administered cocaine, acutely followed by AP-5, an NMDA antagonist, delivered preferentially into the core or shell. Core injections of AP-5, only at the highest dose, reduced cocaine-induced locomotion. Shell injections, also at the highest dose, very transiently (for less than 10 minutes) reduced locomotion elicited by handling (possibly due to spread to the core). It had been shown earlier that dopamine antagonists injected into the nucleus accumbens attenuate motor activation elicited by accumbal injections of a non-NMDA excitatory amino acid receptor agonist, AMPA,[84,85] which suggests that DA stimulation may be permissive for the locomotor effects of AMPA to be expressed. It was subsequently noted that locomotor stimulatory effects of microinjections of DA in core, shell and ventral pallidum (VP) were equipotent, whereas a significantly more robust locomotor effect was observed with AMPA injected in core as compared to VP and shell.[86] Locomotion elicited by these AMPA injections was abolished following injections of the $GABA_B$ agonist, baclofen, into the ventral tegmental area. In a related experiment, Pierce *et al.*[87] observed following seven consecutive days of conditioning with cocaine that only sensitized rats showed augmented behavioral responses to injections of AMPA in core and shell. Augmentation of extracellular glutamate following a systemic cocaine challenge was seen only in the core and only in rats exhibiting a sensitized locomotor response. This was not blocked by tetrodotoxin and so was thought to reflect nonvesicular release. Interestingly, the motor response to cocaine challenge was attenuated by CNQX in the core.

Core–Shell-Prefrontal Cortex Interactions

Whereas basal extracellular DA concentrations in the core were similar in rats with 6-hydroxydopamine lesions of the mesocortical dopaminergic innervation and sham-operated controls, basal DA overflow in the shell of rats with cortical DA lesions exceeded that of controls.[36] The effects on the core of these cortical DA lesions included attenuations of the amphetamine-stimulated increases in core DA concentration and attenuations of the associated increases in locomotion, suggesting glutamatergic corticostriatal involvement in these effects. Conversely, the amphetamine-induced increase in shell extracellular DA was unaffected by the cortical 6-hydroxydopamine lesion.

Core–Shell and Stress

Tail pressure stress potentiated the cortical DA lesion-induced increase in shell basal DA concentrations but failed to affect DA concentration in the accumbens core in both shams and rats with cortical DA depletion,[36] suggesting that basal and stress-related DA levels in the shell, at least in part, depend on the integrity of the cortical DAergic innervation. Deutch and Cameron[42] also observed that mild immobilization stress increases DA turnover selectively in the shell. Only after protracted periods of immobilization accompanied by strenuous efforts to escape did dopamine levels increase in the core (but possibly due to spread from shell), as has been confirmed with *in vivo* microdialysis.[35]

Core–Shell and Prepulse Inhibition of Acoustic Startle

Prepulse inhibition (PPI) refers to a reduction in the magnitude of the reflex startle response produced in a variety of mammals by exposure to a sudden, noxious auditory stimulus when it is preceded by 30–500 ms with a non-noxious tone. PPI, which is deficient in schizophrenic humans, is disrupted by a variety of drugs having the common characteristic of increasing forebrain dopamine concentration. Wan and Swerdlow[88,89] reported that the reduction in PPI observed following injection of D-amphetamine into the core was attenuated by coadministration of CNQX, an AMPA receptor antagonist, whereas CNQX injected into the accumbens core by itself had no effect on PPI. Nor was the putatively postsynaptic disruption of PPI produced by a D_2 agonist injected directly into the core affected by coadministered CNQX. The reduction in PPI associated with an injection of AMPA into the core was attenuated by haloperidol and dopamine-depleting 6-hydroxydopamine lesions. Alternatively, injections of AMPA, D-amphetamine, and CNQX or NBQX, another AMPA antagonist, into the accumbens shell each reduced PPI by mechanisms that were unaffected either by haloperidol, in the case of AMPA, or CNQX, in the case of D-amphetamine. The authors conclude that the reduction of PPI produced by amphetamine injected into the core is regulated by glutamate acting through AMPA receptors, whereas dopamine and glutamate apparently act independently to reduce PPI in the shell.

Core–Shell and Feeding

Maldonado-Irizarry and Kelley[90] observed that NMDA lesions in the core made rats initially sick and akinetic, but later hyperactive, and that food intake and weight gain were depressed throughout the test period (i.e., beyond the sick period). On the contrary, rats with NMDA lesions of the shell exhibited striking increases in food intake, gained significantly more weight than the sham controls, and were slightly hyperactive in the open field. In related experiments, Maldonado-Irizarry *et al.*[91] injected the AMPA receptor antagonists DNQX, CNQX, or NBQX directly into the core and shell and observed robustly stimulated feeding only following injections into the shell. The NMDA antagonists, AP-5 and MK-801, were ineffective in stimulating food intake following shell injections. Systemic administration of naltrexone had no effect on the response, which, however, was halved by D_1 and D_2 antagonists and blocked by muscimol, a $GABA_A$ receptor agonist, injected into the lateral hypothalamus.

SUMMARY

The neurochemical milieu is of more diverse composition and also more sensitive to a variety of pharmacological and physiological stimuli in the shell than core. The shell appears to possess a "receptive" capacity for current and, possibly, remembered stimulus-reward associations conducted from basal amygdala, hippocampus, hypothalamus, brain stem, and visceral- and olfactory-related cortices. It is possible that it is this capacity that is "high-jacked" by a variety of psychomotor and opiate drugs of abuse.

The existence of a robust and direct striatopallidal-thalamocorticostriatal pathway from the shell to the core suggests that significant coordination of the levels of activity in the two subterritories should exist. Furthermore, the intimate connectional relations of shell and core with the dorsal prelimbic and dorsal agranular insular cortices are consistent with a role for the accumbens in the regulation of cognitive aspects of adaptive responding, possibly involving the gating of response initiation.[92] In view of these striking cortical relationships, it becomes problematic to include even the caudomedial part of the shell with the extended amygdala. To the same extent that accumbens efferents are essentially corticopetal, those of the central division of extended amygdala, of which the central amygdaloid nucleus has been regarded as representative, principally descend to sites in the forebrain, mesopontine tegmentum, and brain stem, with little direct connectional interaction with the cortex, which should be regarded as limiting to their potential contributions to cognitive aspects of adaptive responding.

It is likely that locomotion and orofacial movements observed following stimulation of the shell are subject to additional regulation occurring in the core. Accordingly, blockade of DA or excitatory amino acid neurotransmission in the core results in *reduced* locomotion in a variety of paradigms, just as manipulations that encourage locomotor activation are associated with preferential increases of excitatory amino acids in the core. Interestingly, and in keeping with their psychopharmacological sensitivities, the shell responds independently to stimulation by excitatory amino acids and DA, whereas costimulation by these neuromodulators appears required to elicit responses in the core. Further investigation of the functional interactions of the nucleus accumbens shell and core subterritories with each other and with the prefrontal cortex should enhance our understanding of mechanisms underlying the synthesis of adaptive activities, whether generated in response to internal signals or to stimulus–reward associations elicited by the external environment.

ACKNOWLEDGMENT

The author is indebted to Evelyn Williams for expert technical assistance. The work was supported by USPH Grant NIH NS-23805 and Grants from the American Parkinson Disease Association and the United Parkinson Foundation.

REFERENCES

1. HERKENHAM, M., S. MOON-EDLEY & J. STUART. 1984. Cell clusters in the nucleus accumbens of the rat and the mosaic relationship of opiate receptors, acetylcholinesterase and subcortical afferent terminations. Neuroscience **11:** 561–593.
2. ZABORSZKY, L., G.F. ALHEID, M.C. BEINFELD, L.E. EIDEN, L. HEIMER & M. PALKOVITS. 1985. Cholecystokinin innervation of the ventral striatum: a morphological and radioimmunological study. Neuroscience **14:** 427–453.
3. ZAHM, D.S. & J.S. BROG. 1992. Commentary: On the significance of the core-shell boundary in the rat nucleus accumbens. Neuroscience **50:** 751–767.
4. HEIMER, L., G.F ALHEID & D.S. ZAHM. 1993. Basal forebrain organization: An anatomical framework for motor aspects of drive and motivation. *In* The Mesolimbic Motor Circuit and Its Role in Neuropsychiatric Disorders. P.W. Kalivas & C.D.Barnes, Eds.: 1–44. CRC Press. Boca Raton, FL.
5. HEIMER, L., G.F. ALHEID & D.S. ZAHM. 1995. Basal Ganglia. *In* The Rat Nervous System, 2nd Edition. G. Paxinos, Ed. : 579–628. Academic Press. Sydney.
6. DEUTCH, A.Y., A.J. BOURDELAIS & D.S. ZAHM. The nucleus accumbens core and shell: delineation of extended corticostriatal circuits and their functional attributes. *In* The Mesolimbic Motor Circuit and Its Role in Neuropsychiatric Disorders. P.W. Kalivas & C.D. Barnes, Eds.: 45–88. CRC Press. Boca Raton, FL.
7. KALIVAS, P.W., L. CHURCHILL & M.A. KLITENICK. 1993. The circuitry mediating the translation of motivational stimuli into adaptive motor responses. *In* The Mesolimbic Motor Circuit and Its Role in Neuropsychiatric Disorders. P.W. Kalivas & C.D Barnes, Eds. : 237–288. CRC Press. Boca Raton, FL.
8. WRIGHT, C.I. & H.J. GROENEWEGEN. 1995. Patterns of convergence and segregation in the medial nucleus accumbens of the rat: relationships of prefrontal cortical, midline thalamic and basal amygdaloid afferents. J. Comp. Neurol. **361:** 383–403.

9. WRIGHT, C.I. & H.J. GROENEWEGEN. 1996. Patterns of overlap and segregation between insular cortical, intermediodorsal thalamic and basal amygdaloid afferents in the nucleus accumbens of the rat. Neuroscience **73:** 359–373.
10. ALHEID, G.F. & L. HEIMER. 1988. New perspectives in basal forebrain organization of special relevance for neuropsychiatric disorders: the striatopallidal, amygdaloid and corticopetal components of substantia innominata. Neuroscience **27:** 1–39.
11. HEIMER, L. & G.F. ALHEID. 1991. Piecing together the puzzle of basal forebrain anatomy. *In* The Basal Forebrain: Anatomy to Function. T.C. Napier, P.W. Kalivas & I. Hanin, Eds.: 1–44. Plenum Press. New York.
12. ALHEID, G.F., C. BELTRAMINO, A. BRAUN, R.R. MISELIS, C. FRANCOIS & J.S. DE OLMOS. 1994. Transition areas of the striatopallidal system with the extended amygdala in the rat and primate: observations from histochemistry and experiments with mono- and trans-synaptic tracer. *In* The Basal Ganglia IV. New Ideas and Data on Structure and Function, Advances in Behavioral Biology, Vol. 41. G. Percheron, J.S. McKenzie & J. Feger, Eds.: 95–107. Plenum Press. New York.
13. HEIMER, L., G.F. ALHEID, J.S. DE OLMOS, H.J. GROENEWEGEN, S.N. HABER, R. HARLAN & D.S. ZAHM. 1997. The accumbens: beyond the core-shell dichotomy. J. Neuropsychiatry Clin. Neurosci. **9:** 354–381.
14. HEIMER, L., R.E. HARLAN, G.F. ALHEID, M.M. GARCIA & J. DE OLMOS. 1997. Substantia innominata: a notion which impedes clinical-anatomical correlations in neuropsychiatric disorders. Neuroscience **76:** 957–1006.
15. JONGEN-RELO, A.L., P. VOORN & H.J. GROENEWEGEN. 1994. Immunohistochemical characterization of the shell and core territories of the nucleus accumbens in the rat.. Eur. J. Neurosci. **6:** 1255–1264.
16. ZAHM, D.S. & L. HEIMER. 1993 The efferent projections of the rostral pole of the nucleus accumbens in the rat: Comparison with the core and shell projection patterns. J. Comp. Neurol. **327:** 220–232.
17. BROG, J.S., A. SALYPONGSE, A.Y. DEUTCH & D.S. ZAHM. 1993. The patterns of afferent innervation of the core and shell in the "accumbens" part of the rat ventral striatum: Immunohistochemical detection of retrogradely transported Fluoro-Gold. J. Comp. Neurol. **338:** 255–278.
18. PATEL, S., J. ROBERTS, J. MOORMAN & C. REAVILL. 1995. Localization of serotonin-4 receptors in the striatonigral pathway in rat brain. Neuroscience **69:** 1159–1167.
19. LE MOINE, C. & B. BLOCH. 1996. Expression of the D_3 dopamine receptor in peptidergic neurons of the nucleus accumbens: comparison with the D_1 and D_2 dopamine receptors. Neuroscience **73:** 131–143.
20. TAN, Y., E.S. WILLIAMS & D.S. ZAHM. 1997. Calbindin-D 28kD, but not calretinin, gluR1 or gluR3/2 immunoreactivities in retrogradely labeled ventral mesencephalic neurons following injections of Fluoro-Gold in accumbal subterritories. Soc. Neurosci. Abstr. **23:** 1282.
21. KOYLU, E.O., P.R. COUCEYRO, P.D. LAMBERT & M.J. KUHAR. 1998. Cocaine- and amphetamine-regulated transcript peptide immunohistochemical localization in the rat brain. J. Comp. Neurol. **391:** 115–132.
22. ALHEID, G.F. & L. HEIMER. 1996. Theories of basal forebrain organization and the "emotional motor system." *In* The Emotional Motor System, Progress in Brain Research. G. Holstege, R. Bandler & C.B. Saper, Eds.: **107:** 461–484. Elsevier Science, Amsterdam.
23. ZAHM, D.S., E.S. WILLIAMS, J.E. KRAUSE, M.A. WELCH & D.S. GROSU. 1998. Distinct and interactive effects of d-amphetamine and haloperidol on levels of neurotensin and its mRNA in subterritories in the dorsal and ventral striatum of the rat. J. Comp. Neurol. **400:** 487–503.
24. DEUTCH, A.Y. 1996. Sites and mechanisms of action of antipsychotic drugs as revealed by immediate-early gene expression. *In* Antipsychotics. J.G. Csernansky, Ed. : 117–161. Springer-Verlag. New York.
25. DEUTCH, A.Y., M.C. LEE & M.J. IADAROLA. 1992. Regionally specific effects of atypical antipsychotic drugs on striatal Fos expression: the nucleus accumbens shell as a locus of antipsychotic action. Mol. Cell. Neurosci. **3:** 332–341.

26. ROBERTSON, G.S. & H.C. FIBIGER. 1992. Neuroleptics increase *c-fos* expression in the forebrain: contrasting effects of haloperidol and clozapine. Neuroscience **46**: 315–328.
27. MEREDITH, G.E., R. AGOLIA, M. ARTS, H.J. GROENEWEGEN & D.S. ZAHM. 1992. Morphological differences between projection neurons of the core and shell in the nucleus accumbens of the rat. Neuroscience **50**: 149–162.
28. MEREDITH, G.E., P. YPMA & D.S. ZAHM. 1995. The effects of dopamine depletion on the morphology of medium spiny neurons in the shell and core of the rat nucleus accumbens. J. Neurosci. **15**: 3808–3820.
29. VOORN, P., C.R. GERFEN & H.J. GROENEWEGEN. 1989. Compartmental organization of the ventral striatum of the rat: Immunohistochemical distribution of enkephalin, substance P, dopamine and calcium-binding protein. J. Comp. Neurol. **289**: 189–201.
30. ZAHM, D.S. & L. HEIMER. 1990. Two transpallidal pathways originating in rat nucleus accumbens. J. Comp. Neurol. **302**: 437–446.
31. ROGARD, M., J. CABOCHE, J.-F. JULIEN & M.-J. BESSON. 1993. The rat nucleus accumbens: two levels of complexity in the distribution of glutamic acid decarboxylase (67 kDa) and preproenkephalin messenger RNA. Neurosci. Lett. **155**: 81–86.
32. CABOCHE, J., P. VERNIER, M. ROGARD & M.-J. BESSON. 1993. Haloperidol increases PPE mRNA levels in the caudal part of the nucleus accumbens in the rat. NeuroReport **4**: 551–554.
33. CHURCHILL, L., R.S. CROSS, T.L. PAZDERNICK, S.R. NELSON, D. S. ZAHM, L. HEIMER, R.P. DILTS & P.W. KALIVAS. 1992. Patterns of glucose use after bicuculline-induced convulsions provide a functional marker for the ventral pallidum. Brain Res. **581**: 39–45.
34. JONES, S.R., S.J. O'DELL, J.F. MARSHALL & R.M. WIGHTMAN. 1996. Functional and anatomical evidence for different dopamine dynamics in the core and shell of the nucleus accumbens in slices of rat brain. Synapse **23**: 224–231.
35. KALIVAS, P.W. & P. DUFFY. 1995. Selective activation of dopamine transmission in the shell of the nucleus accumbens by stress. Brain Res. **675**: 325–328.
36. KING, D., M.J. ZIGMOND & J.M. FINLAY. 1997. Effects of dopamine depletion in the medial prefrontal cortex on the stress-induced increase in extracellular dopamine in the nucleus accumbens core and shell. Neuroscience **77**: 141–153.
37. ZAHM, D.S. 1992. Distinct subsets of neurotensin immunoreactive neurons revealed following antagonism of the dopamine-mediated suppression of neurotensin immunoreactivity in the rat striatum. Neuroscience **46**: 335–350.
38. DI CHIARA, G., G. TANDA, R. FRAU & E. CARBONI. 1993. On the preferential release of dopamine in the nucleus accumbens by amphetamine: further evidence obtained by vertically implanted concentric dialysis probes. Psychopharmacology **112**: 389–402.
39. PONTIERI, F.E., G. TANDA & DI CHIARA. 1995. Intravenous cocaine, morphine and amphetamine preferentially increase extracellular dopamine in the "shell" as compared with the "core" of the rat nucleus accumbens. Proc. Natl. Acad. Sci. USA **92**: 12304–12308.
40. ORZI, F., F. PASSARELLI, M. LA RICCIA, R. DI GREZIA & F.E. PONTIERI. 1996. Intravenous morphine increases glucose utilization in the shell of the rat nucleus accumbens. Eur. J. Pharmacol. **302**: 49–51.
41. PONTIERI, F.E., V. COLANGELO, M. LA RICCIA, C. POZZILLI, F. PASSARELLI & F. ORZI. 1994. Psychostimulant drugs increase glucose utilization in the shell of the rat nucleus accumbens. NeuroReport **5**: 2561–2564.
42. DEUTCH, A.Y. & D.S. CAMERON. 1992. Pharmacological characterization of dopamine systems in the nucleus accumbens core and shell. Neuroscience **46**: 49–56.
43. MARCUS, M.M., G.G. NOMIKOS & T.H. SVENSSON. 1996. Differential actions of typical and atypical antipsychotic drugs on dopamine release in the core and shell of the nucleus accumbens. Eur. Neuropharmacol. **6**: 29–38.
44. TAN, Y., J.S. BROG, E.S. WILLIAMS & D.S. ZAHM. 1995. Morphometric analysis of ventral mesencephalic neurons retrogradely labeled with Fluoro-Gold following

injections in the shell, core and rostral pole of the rat nucleus accumbens. Brain Res. **689:** 151–156.
45. TAN, Y., E.S. WILLIAMS & D.S. ZAHM. 1998. Calbindin-D 28kD, but not caretinin, immunoreacitivities in retrogradely labeled ventral mesencephalic neurons following injections of Fluoro-Gold in nucleus accumbens subterritories. Brain Res. In review.
46. ZAHM, D.S. 1991. Compartments in rat dorsal and ventral striatum revealed following injection of 6-hydroxydopamine into the ventral mesencephalon. Brain Res. **552:** 164–169.
47. ZAHM, D.S. 1992. An electron microscopic morphometric comparison of tyrosine hydroxylase immunoreactive innervation in the neostriatum and nucleus accumbens core and shell. Brain Res. **575:** 342–346.
48. HEIMER, L., D.S. ZAHM, L. CHURCHILL, P.W. KALIVAS & C. WOHLTMANN. 1991. Specificity in the projection patterns of accumbal core and shell in the rat. Neuroscience **41:** 89–125.
49. ZAHM, D.S., E.S. WILLIAMS & C. WOHLTMANN. 1996. The ventral striatopallidothalamic projection: IV. Relative contributions from neurochemically distinct pallidal subterritories in the subcommissural region and olfactory tubercle and from adjacent extra pallidal parts of the rostrobasal forebrain. J. Comp. Neurol. **364:** 340–362.
50. GROENEWEGEN, H.J. 1988. Organization of the afferent connections of the mediodorsal thalamic nucleus in the rat, related to the mediodorsal-prefrontal topography. Neuroscience **24:** 379–431.
51. GROENEWEGEN, H.J., H.W. BERENDSE & S.N. HABER. 1993. Organization of the output of the ventral striatopallidal system in the rat: ventral pallidal efferents. Neuroscience **57:** 113–142.
52. O'DONNELL, P., A. LAVIN, L.W. ENQUIST, A.A. GRACE & J.P. CARD. 1997. Interconnected parallel circuits between rat nucleus accumbens and thalamus revealed by retrograde transsynaptic transport of pseudorabies virus. J. Neurosci. **17:** 2143–2167.
53. RAY, J.P. & J.L. PRICE. 1992. The organization of the thalamocortical connections of the mediodorsal thalamic nucleus in the rat, related to the ventral forebrain-prefrontal cortex topography. J. Comp. Neurol. **323:** 167–197.
54. SAPER, C.B., L.W. SWANSON & W.M. COWAN. 1979. An autoradiographic study of the efferent connections of the lateral hypothalamic area in the rat. J. Comp. Neurol. **183:** 689–706.
55. BERK, M.L. & J.A. FINKELSTEIN. 1982. Efferent connections of the lateral hypothalamic area of the rat: an autoradiographic investigation. Brain Res. Bull **8:** 511–526.
56. HABER, S.N., H.J. GROENEWEGEN, E.A. GROVE & W.J.H. NAUTA. 1985. Efferent connections of the ventral pallidum: evidence of a dual striato pallidofugal pathway. J. Comp. Neurol. **235:** 322–335.
57. HABER, S.N., E. LYND-BALTA & S.J. MITCHELL. 1993. The organization of descending ventral pallidal projections in the monkey. J. Comp. Neurol. **329:** 111–128.
58. ZAHM, D.S. 1989. The ventral striatopallidal parts of the basal ganglia in the rat. II. Compartmentation of ventral pallidal efferents. Neuroscience **30:** 33–50.
59. ALEXANDER, G.E., M.D. CRUTCHER & M.R. DELONG. 1990. Basal ganglia-thalamocortical circuits: parallel substrates for motor, oculomotor, "prefrontal" and "limbic" functions. Prog. Brain Res. **85:** 85–146.
60. ALEXANDER, G.E., M.R. DELONG & P.L. STRICK. 1986. Parallel organization of functionally segregated circuits linking basal ganglia and cortex. Annu. Rev. Neurosci **9:** 357–381.
61. GROENEWEGEN, H.J., H.W. BERENDSE, J.G. WOLTERS & A.H.M. LOHMAN. 1991. The anatomical relationship of the prefrontal cortex with the striatopallidal system, the thalamus and the amygdala: Evidence for a parallel organization. *In* Progress in Brain Research. H.B.M. Uylings, C.G. Van Eden, J.P.C. De Bruin, M.A. Corner & M.G.P. Feenstra, Eds.: **85:** 95–118. Elsevier Science Publishers. Amsterdam.

62. DENIAU, J.M., A. MENETREY & A.M. THIERRY. 1994. Indirect nucleus accumbens input to the prefrontal cortex via the substantia nigra par reticulata: a combined anatomical and electrophysiological study in the rat. Neuroscience **61:** 533–545.
63. MAURICE, N., J.M. DENIAU, A. MENETREY, J. GLOWINSKI & A.M. THIERRY. 1997. Position of the ventral pallidum in the rat prefrontal cortex-basal ganglia circuit. Neuroscience **80:** 523–534.
64. MAURICE, N., J.M. DENIAU, A. MENETREY, J. GLOWINSKI & A.M. THIERRY. 1998. Prefrontal cortex-basal gangla circuits of ventral pallidum and subthalamic nucleus. Synapse (NY) **29:** 363–370.
65. ZAHM, D.S. 1998. Is the caudomedial shell of the nucleus accumbens part of the extended amygdala? A consideration of connections. Crit. Rev. Neurobiol. **12:** 245–265.
66. ZAHM, D.S., S. JENSEN, E.S. WILLIAMS & J.R. MARTIN III. 1999. Direct comparison of projections from the central nucleus of the amygdala and nucleus accumbens shell. Eur. J. Neurosci. **11:** 1119–1126.
67. ZAHM, D.S. & E.S. WILLIAMS. 1997. Direct comparison of efferent projections from extended amygdala structures and nucleus accumbens shell. Soc. Neurosci. Abstr. **23:** 1282.
68. ZAHM, D.S., E.S. WILLIAMS, S.L. JENSEN & J.R. MARTIN III. 1998. Shell of accumbens and extended amygdala projections in relation to districts and cell groups in the forebrain and brainstem that exhibit nitric oxide synthase and/or choline acetyltransferase immunoreactivities. Soc. Neurosci. Abstr. **24:** 662.
69. CARLEZON, W.A., JR., D.P. DEVINE & R.A. WISE. 1995. Habit-forming actions of nomifensine in nucleus accumbens. Psychopharmacology **122:** 194–197.
70. CARLEZON, W.A., JR. & R.A. WISE. 1996. Rewarding actions of phencyclidine and related drugs in nucleus accumbens shell and frontal cortex. J. Neurosci. **16:** 3112–3122.
71. CARLEZON, W.A., JR. & R.A. WISE. 1996. Microinjections of phencyclidine (PCP) and related drugs into nucleus accumbens shell potentiate medial forebrain bundle brain stimulation reward. Psychopharmacology **128:** 413–420.
72. REBEC, G.V., C.P. GRABNER, M. JOHNSON, R.C. PIERCE & M.T. BARDO. 1997. Transient increase in catecholaminergic activity in medial prefrontal cortex and nucleus accumbens shell during novelty. Neuroscience **76:** 707–714.
73. PILOTTE, N.S., L.G. SHARPE, S.D. ROUNDTREE & M.J. KUHAR. 1996. Cocaine withdrawal reduces dopamine transporter binding in the shell of the nucleus accumbens. Synapse (NY) **22:** 87–92.
74. BOULAY, D., D. DUTERTE-BOUCHER, I. LEROUX-NICOLLET, L. NAUDON & J. COSTENTIN. 1996. Locomotor sensitization and decrease in [^{3}H]mazindol binding to the dopamine transporter are delayed after chronic treatments by GBR12783 or cocaine. J. Pharmacol. Exp. Ther. **278:** 330–337.
75. SHARPE, L.G., N.S. PILOTTE, W.M. MITCHELL & E.B. DE SOUZA. 1991. Withdrawal of repeated cocaine decreases autoradiographic [^{3}H]mazindol-labelling of dopamine transporter in rat nucleus accumbens. Eur. J. Pharmacol. **203:** 141–144.
76. PIERCE, R.C. & P.W. KALIVAS. 1995. Amphetamine produces sensitized increases in locomotion and extracellular dopamine preferentially in the nucleus accumbens shell of rats administered repeated cocaine. J. Pharmacol. Exp. Ther. **275:** 1019–1029.
77. KOSHIKAWA, N., M. KITAMURA, M. KOBAYASHI & A.R. COOLS. 1996. Contralateral turning elicited by unilateral stimulation of dopamine D_2 and D_1 receptors in the nucleus accumbens of rats is due to stimulation of these receptors in the shell, but not the core, of this nucleus. Psychopharmacology **126:** 185–190.
78. KOSHIKAWA, N., M. KITAMURA, M. KOBAYASHI & A.R. COOLS. 1996. Behavioral effects of 7-OH-DPAT are soley due to stimuation of dopamine D_2 receptors in the shell of the nucleus accumbens: turning behavior. Eur. J. Pharmacol. **308:** 235–241.
79. KOSHIKAWA, N., Y. MIWA, K. ADACHI, M. KOBAYASHI & A.R. COOLS. 1996. Behavioral effects of 7-OH-DPAT are soley due to stimuation of dopamine D_2 receptors

in the shell of the nucleus accumbens: jaw movements. Eur. J. Pharmacol. **308:** 227–234.
80. COOLS, A.R., K. KIKUCHI DE BELTRAN, E.P.M. PRINSSEN & N. KOSHIKAWA. 1993. Differential role of core and shell of the nucleus accumbens in jaw movements of rats. Neurosci. Res. Commun. **13:** 55–61.
81. PRINSSEN, E.P.M., W. BALESTRA, F.F.J. BEMELMANS & A.R. COOLS. 1994. Evidence for a role of the shell of the nucleus accumbens in oral behavior of freely moving rats. J. Neurosci. **14:** 1555–1562.
82. MALDONADO-IRIZARRY, C.S. & A.E. KELLEY. 1994. Differential behavioral effects following microinjection of an NMDA antagonist into the nucleus accumbens subregions. Psychopharmacology **116:** 65–72.
83. PULVIRENTI, L., R. BERRIER, M. KREIFELDT & G.F. KOOB. 1994. Modulation of locomotor activity by NMDA receptors in the nucleus accumbens core and shell regions of the rat. Brain Res. **664:** 231–236.
84. BOLDRY, R.C., D.L. WILLINS, L.J. WALLACE & N.J. URETSKY. 1991. The role of endogenous dopamine in the hypermotility response to intra-accumbens AMPA. Brain Res. **559:** 100–108.
85. WU, M., S.M. BRUDZYNSKI & G.J. MOGENSON. 1993. Functional interaction of dopamine and glutamate in the nucleus accumbens in the regulation of locomotion. Can. J. Physiol. Pharmacol. **71:** 407–413.
86. JOHNSON, K., L. CHURCHILL, M.A. KLITENICK, M.S. HOOKS & P.W. KALIVAS. 1996. Involvement of the ventral tegmental area in locomotion elicited from the nucleus accumbens or ventral pallidum. J. Pharmacol. Exp. Ther. **277:** 1122–1131.
87. PIERCE, R.C., K. BELL, P. DUFFY & P.W. KALIVAS. 1996. Repeated cocaine augments excitatory amino acid transmission in the nucleus accumbens only in rats having developed behavioral sensitization. J. Neurosci. **16:** 1550–1560.
88. WAN, F.-J., M.A. GEYER & N.R. SWERDLOW. 1995. Presynaptic dopamine-glutamate interactions in the nucleus accumbens regulate sensorimotor gating. Psychopharmacology **120:** 433–441.
89. WAN, F.-J. & N.R. SWERDLOW. 1996. Sensorimotor gating in rats is regulated by different dopamine-glutamate interactions in the nucleus accumbens core and shell subregions. Brain Res. **722:** 168–176.
90. MALDONADO-IRIZARRY, C.S. & A.E. KELLEY. 1995. Excitotoxic lesions of the core and shell subregions of the nucleus accumbens differentially disrupt body weight regulation and motor activity in the rat. Brain Res. Bull. **38:** 551–559.
91. MALDONADO-IRIZARRY, C.S., C.J. SWANSON & A.E. KELLEY. 1995. Glutamate receptors in the nucleus accumbens shell control feeding behavior via the lateral hypothalamus. J. Neurosci. **15:** 6779–6788.
92. O'DONNELL, P. & A.A. GRACE. 1995. Synaptic interactions among excitatory afferents to nucleus accumbens neurons: Hippocampal gating of prefrontal cortical input. J. Neurosci. **15:** 3622–3639.

Regulation of Neurotransmitter Interactions in the Ventral Striatum

JACQUELINE F. McGINTY[a]

Department of Anatomy and Cell Biology, East Carolina University, School of Medicine, Greenville, North Carolina 27858-4354, USA

ABSTRACT: Transsynaptic activation of neuronal circuits originating in the basal forebrain contributes to psychostimulant-evoked dopamine and glutamate release and consequent changes in medium spiny neuronal gene expression in the ventral striatum. New evidence from microdialysis studies indicates that amphetamine-induced dopamine and glutamate release *in vivo* is partially calcium dependent. The calcium-dependent component is totally blocked by a kappa opioid receptor agonist, indicating that endogenous opioids may regulate dopamine–glutamate interactions in the ventral striatum. Further, muscarinic receptor blockade increases, and muscarinic receptor stimulation decreases, dialysate glutamate levels in the striatum. Pre- and postsynaptic muscarinic receptors contribute to the ability of the muscarinic antagonist, scopolamine, to augment D_1 receptor-stimulated immediate early and neuropeptide gene expression. Moreover, scopolamine prevents a D_2 antagonist from blocking D_1 agonist-induced gene expression, indicating that activation of cholinergic interneurons contributes to D_1/D_2 interactions in the striatum. Thus, transsynaptic activity and presynaptic muscarinic and kappa opioid receptors regulate dopamine and glutamate interactions that switch on and off multiple intracellular signaling cascades. Changes in immediate early and neuropeptide gene expression that result from activation of these cascades are mediated by such nuclear transcription factors as phosphorylated cyclase response element-binding protein. In addition, a novel signaling pathway involving the RAR/RXR nuclear hormone receptor complex is implicated in the control of dopamine receptor and neuropeptide gene expression in the striatum.

INTRODUCTION

Glutamate and dopamine are the major regulators of medium spiny neurons in the ventral striatum. In turn, presynaptic receptors, including kappa opioid and muscarinic receptors, regulate glutamatergic and dopaminergic transmission. Integration of postsynaptic glutamatergic, dopamine D_1 and D_2, and muscarinic receptor signals triggers changes in gene expression in response to stimuli, such as drugs of abuse, which activate these systems. Although D_1 receptor antagonists block these changes in gene expression, D_2 antagonists also diminish these effects,[1,2] contributing to the idea that both D_1 and D_2 receptors must be activated to increase gene expression in medium spiny neurons.

---

[a]Voice: 252-816-2844; fax: 252-816-2850; mcginty@brody.med.ecu.edu

Stimulation of D_1 dopamine receptors triggers the induction of immediate early genes (IEG) and the phosphorylation of cyclase response element binding protein (CREB) by activating multiple signal transduction cascades in medium spiny neurons. These nuclear transcription factors (nTFs) regulate the expression of target genes, such as preprodynorphin (PPD) and substance P (SP). Recently, a novel signaling pathway using nuclear retinoic acid receptors has been implicated in medium spiny gene expression as well. Changes in the balance among these receptor-activated intracellular pathways may underlie the neuroplasticity that is characeristic of long-term psychostimulant abuse.

REGULATION OF GLUTAMATE RELEASE IN THE STRIATUM

Psychostimulants, like amphetamine and cocaine, not only increase the release of dopamine but increase dialysate levels of glutamate[3–8] and acetylcholine[9] in the dorsal and ventral striatum. In our recent studies, using 2.5 mg/kg, ip amphetamine, the increased dopamine and glutamate levels in ventral striatal dialysates were demonstrated to be partially Ca^{2+} dependent.[8] These data suggest that dopamine released by the initial reversal of its transporter activates transsynaptic pathways in the motive circuit, resulting in action potential- and calcium- dependent glutamate release from ventral striatal terminals arising in the prefrontal cortex, subiculum, amygdala, and/ or thalamus. These terminals express kappa opioid receptors, which are associated with synaptic vesicles.[10] Furthermore, stimulation of kappa opioid receptors with U-69593 has a profound, inhibitory effect on the calcium-dependent component of amphetamine-stimulated glutamate release in addition to its inhibitory effects on dopamine release.[8,11–13] In the dorsal striatum, glutamate evoked by a variety of stimuli is regulated by kappa and delta opioid and muscarinic receptors.[14–16] Thus, transsynaptic as well as intrinsic striatal mechanisms are involved in psychostimulant-induced increases in striatal dopamine and glutamate levels (FIG. 1).

EXCITATORY AMINO ACID RECEPTORS REGULATE PSYCHOSTIMULANT-INDUCED GENE EXPRESSION IN MEDIUM SPINY NEURONS

Ionotropic and metabotropic excitatory amino acid (EAA) receptors regulate the expression of nTFs and neuropeptide mRNAs and their protein levels in the striatum. NMDA receptor antagonists block stimulant-induced Fos protein induction in striatal neurons,[17–21] whereas NMDA agonists induce striatal *c*-fos and/or *zif/268* mRNA expression *in vivo* and *in vitro*.[22–24] The NMDA antagonists, MK-801, CPP, and the kainate/AMPA antagonist, DNQX, attenuate the increases in striatal *zif/268*, preprodynorphin (PPD) and preproenkephalin (PPE) expression induced by acute amphetamine or methamphetamine.[25,26] More recently, the mGluR agonist, ACPD, was demonstrated to increase the constitutive expression of IEG and neuropeptide mRNA in striatal neurons both *in vitro*[24] and *in vivo*.[27,28] Although ACPD has been reported to increase striatal dopamine release,[29] the stimulating effect of the intrastriatal infusion of ACPD on IEG expression in the dorsal striatum was not affected by the dopamine receptor blockade.[28] The nonselective mGluR antagonist, MCPG,

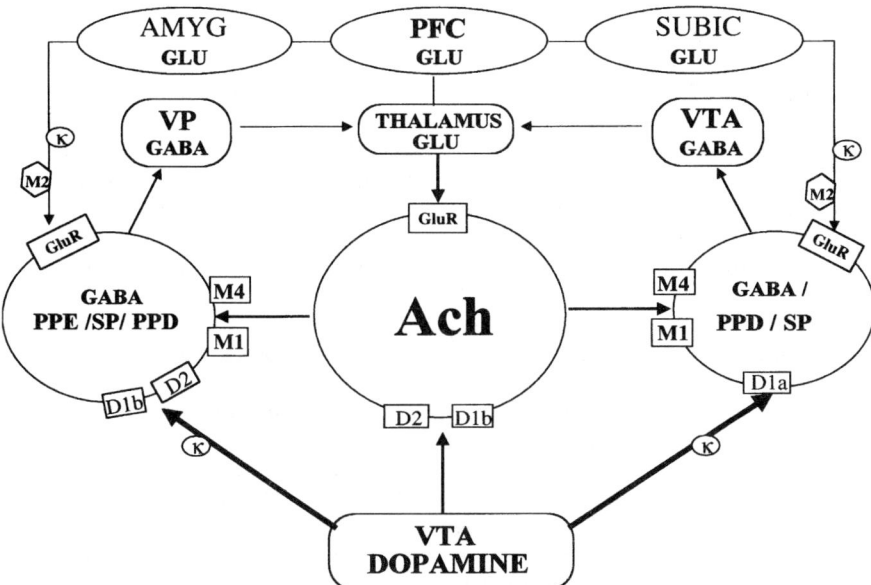

FIGURE 1. Diagram of ventral striatal circuitry. Dopamine from the ventral tegmental area (VTA) and glutamate from the thalamus, amygdala (AMYG), subiculum (SUBIC), and prefrontal cortex (PFC) innervates cholinergic (Ach) and medium spiny (GABA/PPE/SP/PPD or GABA/PPD/SP) neurons. GABA/PPE/SP/PPD neurons primarily project to the ventral pallidum (VP), and GABA/PPD/SP neurons primarily project to the VTA. Muscarinic (presumably M2) and kappa opioid (κ) receptors regulate glutamate release, and kappa receptors regulate dopamine release directly. Cholinergic neurons innervate medium spiny neurons, regulating their gene expression via muscarinic (M4 and M1) receptors, in response to dopaminergic (D1a, D1b, or D2) and glutamatergic stimulation.

markedly attenuated both ACPD- and amphetamine-stimulated gene expression after intrastriatal infuson.[28,30] Thus, EAA receptors of all types are intimately involved in those cellular responses which mediate constitutive and dopamine receptor–stimulated gene expression in the striatum.

MUSCARINIC RECEPTORS REGULATE STRIATAL GENE EXPRESSION

Using *in situ* hybridization, we found that systemic or intrastriatal administration of the nonselective muscarinic receptor antagonist, scopolamine, substantially potentiated the ability of amphetamine or the full D_1 receptor agonist, SKF-82958, to stimulate IEG (*c*-fos and *zif/268*) and peptide gene (PPD and SP) expression in the striatum of intact rats.[31,32] Conversely, oxotremorine attenuated amphetamine-stimulated behavior and PPD and SP gene expression.[31] Thus, it appears that endogenous inhibitory cholinergic tone protects a subpopulation of striatal neurons that express PPD and SP from overexcitation by D_1 receptors and potentially normalizes gene expression after D_1 stimulation. In the dorsal striatum, these are the striatonigral neurons; in the ventral striatum, they are likely to be the accumbens-VTA neurons. Although D_1/muscarinic effects are exerted on the enkephalin-containing striatopallidal neurons in the dorsal striatum (which are opposite those seen on PPD and SP in the striatonigral neurons, see ref. 38), no effects of muscarinic drugs have been detected on preproenkephalin mRNA in the nucleus accumbens.

Based on the information described above, a detailed sequence of events between ventral striatal medium spiny and cholinergic neurons is hypothesized to occur in response to dopamine agonists.[33,34] This sequence (FIG. 1) starts with stimulation of D_1 receptors located on the soma and dendrites of ventral striatal neurons as well as on their terminals in the VTA. Acetylcholine released via this route would bind to presynaptic muscarinic receptors (presumably M2) on glutamatergic terminals and to postsynaptic receptors (presumably M4) on medium spiny neurons and inhibit PPD/SP gene expression by decreasing adenylate cyclase–dependent transcription. At the level of the ventral tegmental area, D_1 receptor stimulation, which facilitates local GABA release, may result in disinhibition of glutamate release in transsynaptic pathways, furthering stimulation of ventral striatal dopamine and acetylcholine release[35] and a compensatory increase in PPD/SP expression. In this manner, the cholinergic neuron would be in a strategic position to serve as a feedforward inhibitor of psychostimulant-induced neuronal activity, as exemplified by scopolamine's ability to enhance D_1-stimulated PPD and SP mRNA expression.

MUSCARINIC RECEPTORS REGULATE D_1/D_2 RECEPTOR INTERACTIONS

The inhibitory influence of cholinergic interneurons on ventral striatal neurons also provides an intrastriatal mechanism for some D_1/D_2 interactions. Even though there is more evidence for colocalization of D_1 and D_2 receptors in medium spiny neurons in the nucleus accumbens than in the caudate-putamen,[36,37] the D_2 contribution to the full expression of D_1-mediated function *in vivo* is likely to include, but perhaps not be limited to, an indirect, transsynaptic mechanism. Inasmuch as D_2 tone is an important inhibitory force on acetylcholine release, it is possible that concomitant stimulation of D_2 receptors, by minimizing acetylcholine release, decreases cholinergic neurotransmission and, thus, synergistically enhances D_1 stimulation of ventral striatal neurons. By contrast, D_2 receptor blockade, by increasing acetylcholine release, would attenuate D_1-stimulated gene expression in these neurons. To support this putative acetylcholine-dependent pathway, we recently found that the D_2-selective antagonist, eticlopride, blocked D_1 agonist-stimulated PPD and SP

FIGURE 2. Retinoic acid alters medium spiny neuronal gene expression in the striatum. *Top*: Vehicle (0.1% DMSO)-treated rats. **A:** The β_2 isoform of the retinoic acid receptor (RAR) mRNA; **B:** the γ isoform of the retinoid X receptor (RXR) mRNA; **C:** preprodynorphin (PPD) mRNA; **D:** substance P (SP) mRNA. *Bottom*: 24 hours after 5 mg/kg, sc *trans*-retinoic acid. **E:** RARβ_2 mRNA; **F:** RXRγ mRNA; **G:** PPD mRNA; **H:** SP mRNA. Note the unique pattern of increase in each mRNA after retinoic acid treatment.

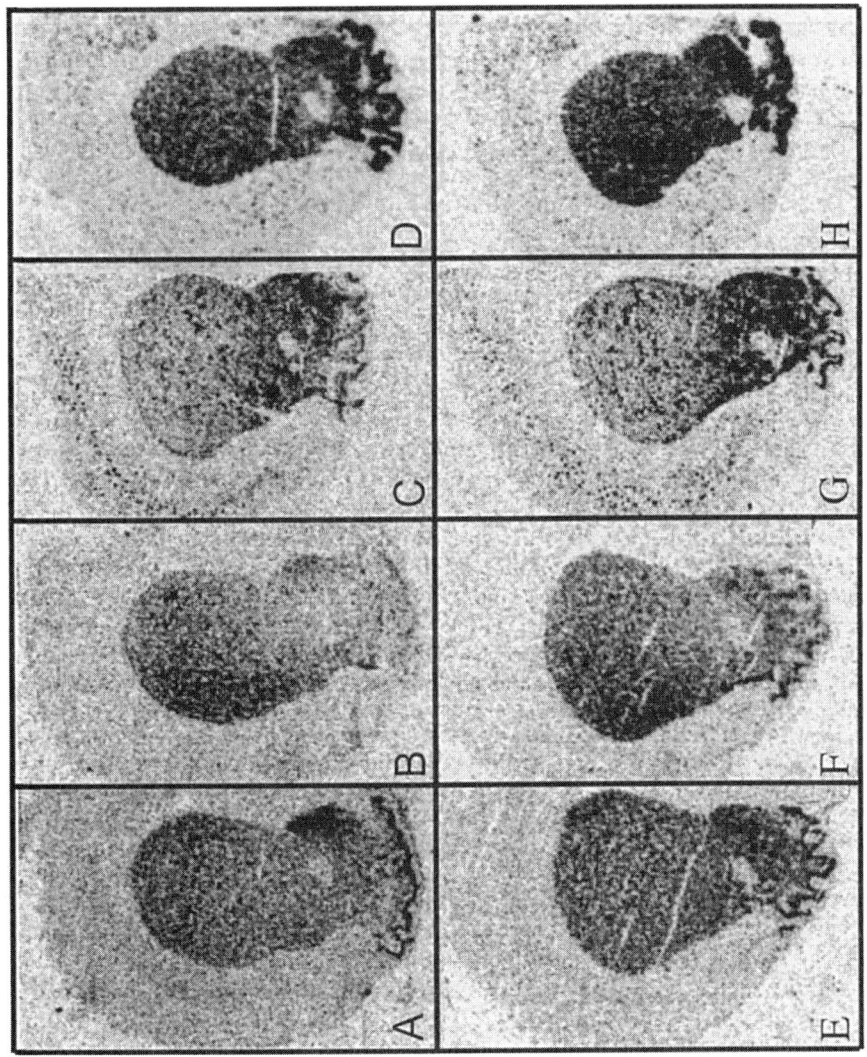

mRNA expression in the rat striatum and that the effect of eticlopride was prevented by scopolamine.[38]

PHOSPHORYLATED-CREB AND RETINOIC ACID RECEPTORS REGULATE MEDIUM SPINY GENE EXPRESSION

Dopamine stimulates gene expression by binding to D_1 receptors which are positively coupled to adenylate cyclase and activating the cAMP-dependent protein kinase A (PKA) pathway. The catalytic portion of PKA translocates to the nucleus and phosphorylates CREB on Ser 133. Phosphorylated (P)-CREB interacts with a CREB binding protein (CBP), and this complex initiates transcription of targets such as *c-fos* and neuropeptide genes (FIG. 3).[39,40] It has recently been demonstrated that CBP acetylates histones, facilitating gene transcription mediated by numerous transcription factors, including P-CREB and the nuclear retinoic acid receptors, RAR and RXR. $RAR\beta_2$ and RXR_γ isoforms are particularly abundant in the nucleus accumbens (FIG. 2), where they are activated by retinoic acid. Furthermore, a class I aldehyde dehydrogenase, which synthesizes retinoic acid from retinaldehyde, is present in the mesostriatal and mesoaccumbal dopaminergic pathways.[41] Linkage to D_2 receptors has been demonstrated by the finding that the D_2 receptor promoter contains a retinoic acid response element (RARE) that binds RAR/RXR heterodimers,[42] and retinoic acid stimulates transcription of the D_2 receptor gene in a pituitary cell line. Finally, in RAR/RXR knockout mice, D_1 and D_2 receptor mRNA was reduced in the medial and ventral striatum, and cocaine was unable to elicit locomotor activity and rearing behaviors in these animals.[43] In our laboratory, treatment of rats with 5 mg/kg sc *trans*-retinoic acid 24 hours before euthanasia induced a robust increase in RXR_γ and $RAR\beta_2$ mRNA, as well as in preprodynorphin and substance P mRNA (FIG. 2). These studies reveal a novel and exciting role for retinoids and their receptors in the regulation of dopamine-responsive gene expression, as diagrammed in FIGURE 3.

GLUTAMATE AND DOPAMINE SYNERGISTICALLY ACTIVATE MULTIPLE KINASE CASCADES

Dopamine and glutamate receptors activate intracellular cAMP and Ca^{2+}-dependent kinase cascades, respectively, which regulate the transcription rate of target genes in striatal neurons. Glutamate, at a concentration insufficient to induce *c-fos* expression by itself, significantly enhances dopamine-stimulated *c-fos* expression in dissociated striatal neurons.[44] This effect appears to be mediated by Ca^{2+}, because the Ca^{2+} ionophore, A23187, mimics the effects of glutamate. Furthermore, the NMDA antagonist, MK801, blocks the ability of dopamine to activate fos induction in striatal cultures,[44] implicating glutamatergic mechanisms in the postsynaptic signaling cascade. Glutamate stimulates gene expression by modifying Ca^{2+}-signaling pathways, which are activated by Ca^{2+} influx primarily through ligand-gated NMDA receptors. Ca^{2+} and Ca^{2+}/calmodulin-dependent protein kinases (CaMK), especially CaMK IV, as demonstrated in dissociated hippocampal cultures,[45] and the MAP kinase/ERK-regulated cascade,[46,47] are the most likely mediators of the glutamate-ini-

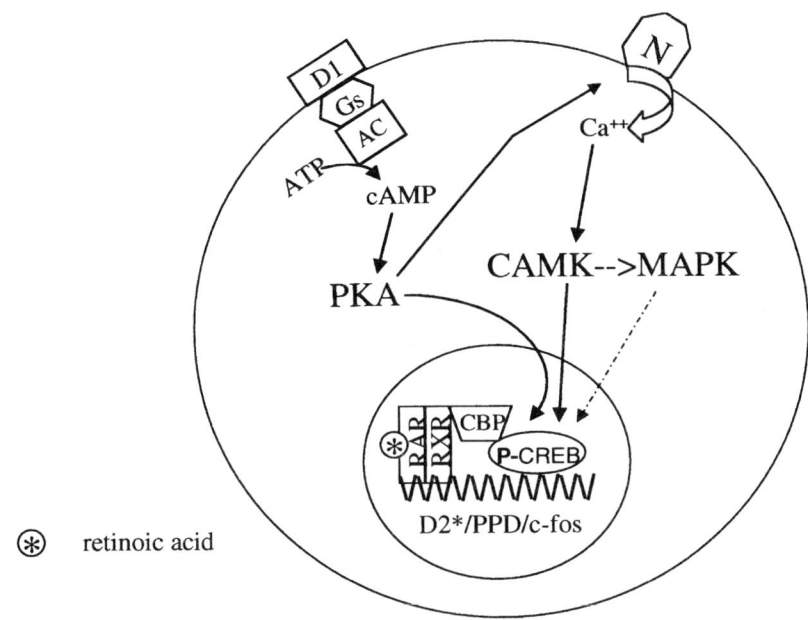

FIGURE 3. Hypothesized intracellular cascades in a generic medium spiny neuron in the ventral striatum. Dopamine D1 receptors are positively coupled to adenylate cyclase (AC) via Gs proteins. D1 receptor stimulation leads to increased cAMP-dependent protein kinase (PKA) activation. The catalytic domain of PKA phosphorylates cytosolic/membrane target proteins, such as NMDA receptors (N) and nuclear targets, such as cyclase response element binding protein (P-CREB). Increased extracellular glutamate levels activate NMDA receptors and cause increased Ca^{2+} influx. Ca^{2+} activates Ca^{2+}-calmodulin-dependent kinases; CAM kinase IV translocates to the nucleus and also phosphorylates CREB. The MAP kinase (MAPK) cascade is also activated and phosphorylates CREB via unidentified intermediates. P-CREB binds to the cyclase response element in a complex that includes CREB-binding protein (CBP) and increases transcription of target genes, such as c-fos and PPD. When activated by retinoic acid, the RAR/RXR dimer also recruits CBP into a complex that regulates D2 (*) receptor transcription.

tiated Ca^{2+}-dependent increase in nuclear gene expression. Interactions between the Ca^{2+} and cAMP signaling pathways may take place at several different levels in order to synergistically facilitate nuclear gene transcription.[47,48] For instance, PKA enhances the activity of voltage-sensitive and NMDA-linked Ca^{2+} channels.[49,50] By contrast, Ca^{2+} influx may interact with Ca^{2+}-dependent adenylate cyclase[51,52] and influence the dephosphorylation of PKA substrates, like the phosphoprotein, DARPP-32, by activating the phosphatase inhibitor, calcineurin.[53] Furthermore, CAM kinases act as positive regulators of ERK/CREB-activated c-fos transcription.[47] The consequences of such interactions may be reflected by changes in the activity of nTFs, such as prolonged CREB phosphorylation after repeated versus acute psychostimulant administration.[40,54]

CONCLUSIONS

Although precise mechanisms of glutamate/dopamine interactions in the regulation of drug actions are far from clear, data so far obtained indicate the existence of both pre- and postsynaptic interactions. Via their presynaptic localization, kappa opioid receptors directly regulate calcium-dependent glutamate release in the nucleus accumbens evoked by amphetamine. By way of their pre- and postsynaptic localization, muscarinic receptors directly regulate glutamate release and the responses of medium spiny neurons to D_1 receptor stimulation. Extensive postsynaptic interactions exist between the receptor-activated intracellular signal transduction pathways. In addition, retinoic acid regulates dopamine receptor and neuropeptide gene expression in medium spiny neurons in the ventral striatum, revealing a novel signal transduction pathway for future investigation. Finally, dopamine and glutamate synergistically augment CREB phosphorylation in response to repeated exposure to psychostimulants, indicating that responses to prolonged drug exposure are encoded at the level of gene expression.

ACKNOWLEDGMENTS

The author thanks current and former members of her laboratory, including James Daunais, Alex Gray, Denise Mayer, Scott Rawls, Jeff Simpson, and John Wang, for their primary contributions to the work described in this review. These studies were supported by DA03982 and DA09256.

REFERENCES

1. DAUNAIS, J.B. & J.F. MCGINTY. 1996. The effects of D_1 or D_2 dopamine receptor blockade on *zif/268* and preprodynorphin gene expression in rat forebrain following a short-term cocaine binge. Mol. Brain Res. **35:** 237–248.
2. WANG, J.Q. & J.F. MCGINTY. 1996. D_1 and D_2 receptor regulation of preproenkephalin and preprodynorphin mRNA in rat striatum following acute injection of amphetamine or methamphetamine. Synapse **22:** 114–122.
3. PIERCE, R.C., K. BELL, P. DUFFY & P.W. KALIVAS. 1996. Repeated cocaine augments excitatory amino acid transmission in the nucleus accumbens only in rats having developed behavioral sensitization. J. Neurosci. **16:** 1550–1560.
4. REID, M.S. & S.P. BERGER. 1996. Evidence for sensitization of cocaine-induced nucleus accumbens glutamate release. NeuroReport **7:** 1325–1329.
5. REID, M.S., K. HSU JR. & S.P. BERGER. 1997. Cocaine and amphetamine preferentially stimulate glutamate release in the limbic system: studies on the involvement of dopamine. Synapse **27:** 95–105.
6. SMITH, J.A., Q. MO, H. GUO, P.M. KUNKO & S.E. ROBINSON. 1995. Cocaine increases extraneuronal levels of aspartate and glutamate in the nucleus accumbens. Brain Res. **683:** 264–269.
7. DALIA, A., N.J. URETSKY & L.J. WALLACE. 1998. Dopaminergic agonists administered into the nucleus accumbens: effects on extracellular glutamate and on locomotor activity. Brain Res. **788:** 111–117.
8. GRAY, A.M., S.M. RAWLS, T.S. SHIPPENBERG & J.F. MCGINTY. The kappa opioid agonist, U-69593, decreases amphetamine-evoked behavior and dialysate levels of dopamine and glutamate in the nucleus accumbens of awake rats. J. Neurochem. In press.

9. GUIX, T., Y.L. HURD & U. UNGERSTEDT. 1992. Amphetamine enhances extracellular concentrations of dopamine and acetylcholine in dorsolateral striatum and nucleus accumbens of freely moving rats. Neurosci. Lett. **138:** 137–140.
10. MESHUL, C.K. & J.F. MCGINTY. Kappa opioid receptor immunoreactivity in nucleus accumbens shell and caudate-putamen is primarily associated with synaptic vesicles in axons. Neuroscience. In press.
11. DI CHIARA, G. & A. IMPERATO. 1988. Opposite effects of mu and kappa opiate agonists on dopamine release in the nucleus accumbens and in the dorsal caudate of freely moving rats. J. Pharmacol. Exp. Ther. **244:** 1067–1080.
12. SPANAGEL, R., A. HERZ & T.S. SHIPPENBERG. 1992. Opposing tonically active endogenous opioid systems modulate the mesolimbic dopaminergic pathway. Proc. Natl. Acad. Sci. USA **89:** 2046–2050.
13. MAISONNEUVE, I.M., S. ARCHER & S.D. GLICK. 1994. U50,488, a kappa opioid receptor agonist, attenuates cocaine-induced increases in extracellular dopamine in the nucleus accumbens of rats. Neurosci. Lett. **181:** 57–60.
14. RAWLS, S.M. & J.F. MCGINTY. 1997. L-*Trans*-pyrrolidine-2,4-dicarboxylic acid-evoked striatal glutamate levels are attenuated by calcium reduction, tetrodotoxin, and glutamate receptor blockade. J.Neurochem. **68:** 1553–1563.
15. RAWLS, S.M. & J.F. MCGINTY. 1998. κ Receptor activation attenuates L-trans-pyrrolidine-2,4-dicarboxylic acid-evoked glutamate levels in the striatum. J. Neurochem. **70:** 626–634.
16. RAWLS, S.M. & J.F. MCGINTY. Delta opioid receptors regulate amphetamine-evoked dialysate glutamate and dopamine levels in the rat striatum. Brain Res. In press.
17. DRAGUNOW, M., B. LOGAN & R. LAVERTY. 1991. 3,4-Methyldioxymethamphetamine induces Fos-like proteins in rat basal ganglia: reversal with MK 801. Eur. J. Pharmacol. **206:** 255–258.
18. SNYDER-KELLER, A.M. 1991. Striatal *c*-fos induction by drugs and stress in neonatally dopamine-depleted rats given nigral transplants: importance of NMDA activation and relevance to sensitization phenomena. Exp. Neurol. **113:** 155–165.
19. TORRES, G. & C. RIVIER. 1993. Cocaine-induced expression of striatal *c*-fos in the rat is inhibited by NMDA receptor antagonists. Brain Res. Bull. **30:** 173–176.
20. OHNO, M., H. YOSHIDA & S. WATANABE. 1994. NMDA receptor-mediated expression of Fos protein in the rat striatum following methamphetamine administration: relation to behavioral sensitization. Brain Res. **665:** 135–140.
21. KEEFE, K.A. & C.R. GERFEN. 1996. D1 dopamine receptor-mediated induction of *zif268* and *c*-fos in the dopamine-depleted striatum: differential regulation and independence from NMDA receptors. J. Comp. Neurol. **367:** 165–176.
22. BERRETTA, S., H.A. ROBERTSON & A.M. GRAYBIEL. 1993. Dopamine and glutamate agonists stimulate neuron-specific expression of Fos-like protein in the striatum. J. Neuroscience **13:** 423–433.
23. PAGE, K.J. & B.J. EVERITT. 1993. Transsynaptic induction of *c*-fos in basal forebrain, diencephalic and midbrain neurons following AMPA-induced activation of the dorsal and ventral striatum. Exp. Brain Res. **93:** 399–411.
24. VACCARINO, F.M., M.D. HAYWARD, E.J. NESTLER, R.S. DUMAN & J.F. TALLMAN. 1992. Differential induction of immediate early genes by excitatory amino acid receptor types in primary cultures of cortical and striatal neurons. Mol. Brain Res. **12:** 233–241.
25. WANG, J.Q., J.B. DAUNAIS & J.F. MCGINTY. 1994. Role of kainate/AMPA receptors in induction of striatal *zif/268* and preprodynorphin mRNA by a single injection of amphetamine. Mol. Brain Res. **27:** 118–126.
26. WANG, J.Q., J.B. DAUNAIS & J.F. MCGINTY. 1994. NMDA receptors mediate amphetamine-induced upregulation of *zif/268* and preprodynorphin mRNA expression in rat striatum. Synapse **18:** 343–353.
27. WANG, J.Q. & J.F. MCGINTY. 1998. Metabotropic glutamate receptor agonist increases neuropeptide mRNA expression in rat striatum. Mol. Brain Res. **54:** 262–269.
28. WANG, J.Q. 1998. Regulation of immediate early gene *c*-fos and *zif/268* mRNA expression in rat striatum by metabotropic glutamate receptor. Mol. Brain Res. **57:** 46–53.

29. VERMA, A. & B. MOGHADDAM. 1998. Regulation of striatal dopamine release by metabotropic glutamate receptors. Synapse (NY) **28:** 220–226.
30. WANG, J.Q. & J.F. MCGINTY. 1996. Intrastriatal injection of the metabotropic glutamate receptor antagonist MCPG attenuates acute amphetamine-stimulated neuropeptide mRNA expression in rat striatum. Neurosci. Lett. **218:** 13–16.
31. WANG, J.Q. & J.F. MCGINTY. 1996. Muscarinic receptors regulate striatal neuropeptide gene expression in normal and amphetamine-treated rats. Neuroscience **75:** 43–56.
32. WANG, J.Q. & J.F. MCGINTY. 1996. Scopolamine augments c-fos and $zif/268$ messenger RNA expression induced by the full D_1 dopamine receptor agonist SKF-82958 in the intact rat striatum. Neuroscience **72:** 601–616.
33. DI CHIARA, G., M. MORELLI & S. CONSOLO. 1994. Modulatory functions of neurotransmitters in the striatum: Ach/dopamine/NMDA interactions. Trends Neurosci. **17:** 228–233.
34. WANG, J.Q. & J.F. MCGINTY. 1996. Glutamatergic and cholinergic regulation of immediate early gene and neuropeptide gene expression in the striatum. In Pharmacological Regulation of Gene Expression in the CNS. K. Merchant, Ed.: 81–113. CRC Press, Inc. Boca Raton.
35. ABERCROMBIE, E.D. & P. DEBOER. 1997. Substantia nigra D_1 receptors and stimulation of striatal cholinergic interneurons by dopamine: a proposed circuit mechanism. J.Neurosci. **17:** 8498–8505.
36. CURRAN, E.J. & S.J. JR. WATSON. 1995. Dopamine receptor mRNA expression patterns by opioid peptide cells in the nucleus accumbens of the rat: a double *in situ* hybridization study. J. Comp. Neurol. **361:** 57–76.
37. LU, X.Y., M.B. GHASEMZADEH & P.W. KALIVAS. 1998. Expression of D_1 receptor, D_2 receptor, substance P and enkephalin messenger RNAs in the neurons projecting from the nucleus accumbens. Neuroscience **82:** 767–780.
38. WANG, J.Q. & J.F. MCGINTY. 1997. The full D_1 dopamine receptor agonist SKF-82958 induces neuropeptide mRNA in the normosensitive striatum of rats: regulation of D_1/D_2 interactions by muscarinic receptors. J. Pharmacol. Exp. Ther. **281:** 972–982.
39. KONRADI, C. & S. HECKERS. 1995. Haloperidol-induced Fos expression in striatum is dependent upon transcription factor cyclic AMP response element binding protein. Neuroscience **65:** 1051–1061.
40. COLE, R.L., C. KONRADI, J. DOUGLASS & S.E. HYMAN. 1995. Neuronal adaptation to amphetamine and dopamine: molecular mechanisms of prodynorphin gene regulation in rat striatum. Neuron **14:** 813–823.
41. MCCAFFREY, P. & U.C. DRAGER. 1994. High levels of a retinoic acid-generating dehydrogenase in the meso-telencephalic dopamine system. Proc. Natl. Acad. Sci. USA **91:** 7772–7776.
42. SAMAD, T.A., W. KREZEL, P. CHAMBON & E. BORELLI. 1997. Regulation of dopaminergic pathways by retinoids: activation of the D2 receptor promoter by members of the retinoic acid receptor-retinoid X receptor family. Proc. Natl. Acad. Sci. USA **94:** 14349–14354.
43. KREZEL, W., N. GHYSELINCK, T.A. SAMAD, V. DUPÉ, P. KASTNER, E. BORRELLI & P. CHAMBON. 1998. Impaired locomotion and dopamine signaling in retinoid receptor mutant mice. Science **279:** 863–867.
44. KONRADI, C., J.C. LEVEQUE & S.E. HYMAN. 1996. Amphetamine and dopamine-induced immediate early gene expression in striatal neurons depends on postsynaptic NMDA receptors and calcium. J. Neurosci. **16:** 4231–4239.
45. BITO, H., K. DEISSEROTH & R.W. TSIEN. 1996. CREB phosphorylation and dephosphorylation: a Ca^{2+}- and stimulus duration-dependent switch for hippocampal gene expression. Cell **87:** 1203–1214.
46. SGAMBATO, V., P. VANHOUTTE, C. PAGÈS, M. ROGARD, R. HIPSKIND, M.-J. BESSON & J. CABOCHE. 1998. *In vivo* expression and regulation of Elk-1, a target of the extracellular-regulated kinase signaling pathway, in the adult rat brain. J. Neuroscience **18:** 214–216.

47. VANHOUTTE, P., J.V. BARNIER, C. PAGÈS, M.-J. BESSON, R. A. HIPSKIND & J. CARBOCHE. 1999. Glutamate induces phosphorylation of ELK-1 and CREB, along with c-fos activation, via an extracellular signal-regulated kinase-dependent pathway in brain slices. Mol. Cell. Biol. **19:** 136–146.
48. GINTY, D.D. 1997. Calcium regulation of gene expression: Isn't that spatial? Neuron **18:** 183–186.
49. ARTALEJO, C.R., M.A. ARIANO, R.L. PERLMAN & A.P. FOX. 1990. Activation of facilitation calcium channels in chromaffin cells by D_1 dopamine receptors through a cAMP/protein kinase A–dependent mechanism. Nature **348:** 239–242.
50. SCULPTOREANU, A., T. SCHEUER & W.A. CATTERALL. 1993. Voltage-dependent potentiation of L-type Ca^{2+} channels due to phosphorylation by cAMP-dependent mechanism. Nature **348:** 239–242.
51. CHETKOVICH, D.M. & J.D. SWEATT. 1993. NMDA receptor activation increases cyclic AMP in area CA1 of the hippocampus via calcium/calmodulin stimulation of adenylyl cyclase. J. Neurochem **61:** 1933–1942.
52. GINTY, D.D., D. GLOWACKA, D.S. BADER, H. HIDAKA & J.A. WAGNER. 1991. Induction of immediate early genes by Ca^{2+} influx requires cAMP-dependent protein kinase in PC12 cells. J. Biol. Chem. **266:** 17454–17458.
53. YAKEL, J.L. 1997. Calcineurin regulation of synaptic function: from ion channels to transmitter release and gene transcription. Trends Pharmacol. Sci. **18:** 124–134.
54. SIMPSON, J.N., J.Q. WANG & J.F. MCGINTY. 1995. Repeated amphetamine administration induces a prolonged augmentation of phosphorylated cyclase response element-binding protein and Fos-related antigen immunoreactivity in rat striatum. Neuroscience **69:** 441–457.

The Synaptic Framework for Chemical Signaling in Nucleus Accumbens

G.E. MEREDITH[a]

*Department of Anatomy, Royal College of Surgeons in Ireland,
123 St. Stephen's Green, Dublin 2, Ireland*

> ABSTRACT: Our knowledge of the organization of the nucleus accumbens has been greatly advanced in the last two decades, but only now are we beginning to understand the complex neural circuitry that underlies the mix of behaviors attributed to this nucleus. Superimposed on the neurochemically defined territories of the shell and core are four or more conduits for information flow. Each of these behaviorally relevant pathways can be characterized by the spatial distribution of inputs to its central unit: the GABAergic projection neuron, a spiny cell that also contains the opioid peptides, enkephalin or dynorphin. In this review, current models of accumbal circuits will be examined and, with the aid of recent anatomical findings, further extended to shed light on how functionally diverse information is processed in this nucleus. However complex, accumbal wiring is not fixed, and, as we will show, psychostimulants, dopamine-deleting lesions, and chronic blockade of dopaminergic receptors can alter the anatomical substrate, synaptology, and neurotrophic factors that govern circuits through the shell and core.

One of the basic principles of neuroscience is that complex behaviors arise from the interconnections of neurons into networks or circuits, but discovering how these networks are organized and understanding the principles that underlie their operation remain among the greatest challenges to modern neuroscience. The ability to perform a task depends upon the basic building blocks of the neural frameworks, especially the synaptic arrangements. However, knowing the cells and their synaptic organization may not be enough, for neural networks with similar connectivity can produce dramatically different activity patterns, and, conversely, similar patterns can be provided by very different networks.[1] Accordingly, synaptic frameworks are also dependent on the neurochemistry and receptor profiles of the projection cells, the types and action of interneurons, and intercellular communication by other means, such as via gap junctions or through the release of gases like nitric oxide.

Our understanding of the organization of the nucleus accumbens has been markedly advanced in the last couple of decades, and new insights have emerged into the neural circuits that underlie the complex behaviors attributed to this part of the brain. It is now thought possible that multiple pathways converge on segregated territories, where they selectively or synergistically activate output neurons, depending on the neuroanatomical substrates and transmitter systems that are brought into play.[2-4]

[a]Voice: 353 1 402 2260/2267; fax: 353 1 402 2355; gmeredit@rcsi.ie

Localizing activity to microcircuits in restricted parts of the accumbens does not imply that the activation of targets is similarly restricted. It is nevertheless important for explaining the mode of drug action on the nucleus. Indeed, some of the most compelling evidence for localizing function comes from experimental studies where lesions or microinjections of drugs, including neurotransmitter or receptor agonists and antagonists, have shown dramatic effects in restricted parts of the nucleus accumbens (see, e.g., refs. 5 and 6).

In this review, accumbal networks will be examined in light of recent findings on their synaptic organization, including the neurochemistry and arrangement of extrinsic inputs and key receptors and local circuit elements. Furthermore, recent data will be presented on how lesions and drugs can alter accumbal circuits structurally and modify their operation.

REGIONAL ORGANIZATION

Thanks to detailed anatomical, neurochemical, and hodological studies of the basal forebrain, beginning some three decades ago, Heimer and colleagues[7-13] have provided us with a structural foundation for systematic investigations of the ventral forebrain, including the nucleus accumbens. These investigators have repeatedly pointed to the heterogenous nature of the accumbens and to the pivotal role it plays in the ventral striatopallidal and extended amygdala systems.[9,10,12] The nucleus accumbens is composed of two large territories that are neurochemically and cytoarchitecturally complex, termed shell and core, and possibly a third division, the rostral pole,[14] which has yet to be distinguished in mammals other than rats.[15] Many different markers, including acetylcholinesterase, immunoreactivity for enkephalin, substance P, cholecystokinin, and calbindin D28k (CaBP), and the distribution of dopamine receptors, are capable of dividing the shell from the core.[8,16-19] These compartments are not homogeneous, and further cytoarchitectonic and chemical subdivisions can be made. For example, in medial parts of the shell, dense concentrations of substance P, dynorphin, and TH overlap enkephalin- or CaBP-poor zones, whereas laterally, moderate immunoreactivity for SP and CaBP are in register with less dense dynorphin and enkephalin.[16,18,20,21] In the core, small rostral and caudal zones are enkephalin and opioid receptor rich, yet CaBP poor.[22] Moreover, sharp regional variations in neurochemistry and in cell and receptor density are aligned with topographically organized terminal fields.[23,24]

There is now a growing body of neurochemical, structural, and connectional evidence to indicate that much of the medial accumbens is segregated, especially at caudal levels, from the more lateral and central parts.[8,9,11,25] This medial sector is currently included in the shell but has much in common with an important part of the basal forebrain, called the extended amygdala (EA).[9] The symptoms of numerous disorders of mood and psyche are thought to arise due to disturbances in the structures belonging to the EA but, presumably, also involve ventral striatal territories.[10,21] Numerous experiments have shown that psychostimulants, neuroleptic drugs, and lesions affect the nucleus accumbens, in general, and the shell or core territory, in particular. Indeed, experimental manipulations usually elicit dramatic responses in either the medial shell or the core but rarely affect both. Therefore, the caudal medial shell should perhaps be recognized as the transitional part of the cen-

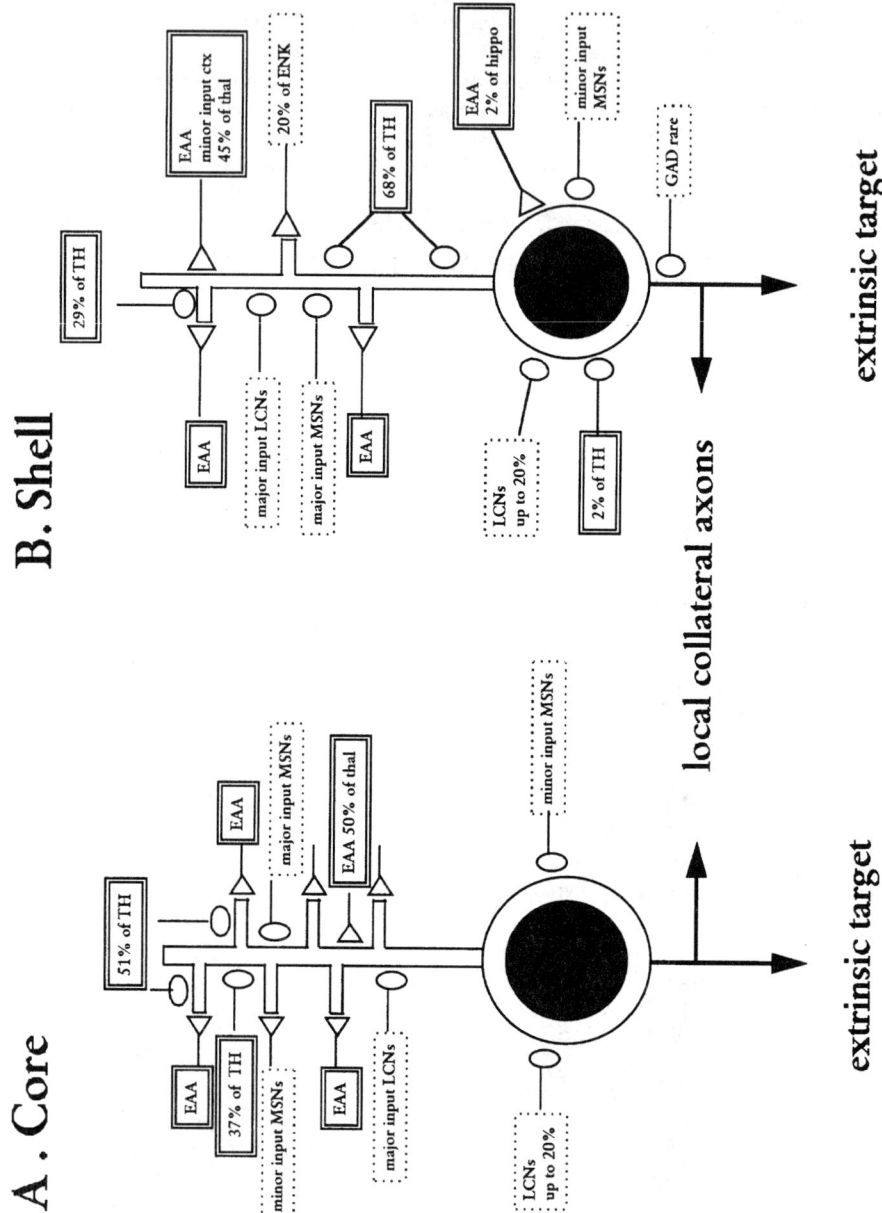

tral division of the EA, or the "transitional EA" as it will be referred to here, and the core, along with other parts of the striatum, as an integral part of the basal ganglia.[9,10,12,13]

CELLULAR FRAMEWORK

In the nucleus accumbens, the principal neurons, also referred to as medium spiny projection neurons, make up approximately 90% of all neurons. They are found throughout the nucleus, and, although some are smaller than their dorsal striatal counterparts (12–18 μm in diameter as compared to 8–20 μm for the accumbens), their appearance is much the same (FIG. 1, A and B).[26–28] Each projection neuron has a large, round, unindented nucleus surrounded by sparse cytoplasm. Dendrites are spine free at proximal segments, that is, up to the first branch point, but are densely covered with spines more distally (FIG. 1, A and B). Each cell has an axon that leaves the soma or a proximal dendrite to arborize locally before projecting out of the accumbens.[28,29] Differences in the "spinyness" of dendrites has been reported between[30] and within[31] shell and core regions (FIG. 1, A and B). Overall, neurons in the caudal medial shell or transitional EA have fewer dendritic branches and significantly lower spine densities than those in the core or in remaining parts of the shell, and, although there is evidence from the dorsal striatum for a second class of projection neuron with low spine density,[32] no such distinction has been made for accumbal neurons as yet. Principal projection neurons contain γ-aminobutyric acid (GABA) as the primary neurotransmitter and immunoreact for CaBP and a variety of neuropeptides, including neurotensin, enkephalin, dynorphin, substance P, and neurokinin B (TABLE 1).[20,29,33–35] Some are also dye coupled, suggesting that they communicate electrotonically.[36]

Local circuit neurons, which make up approximately 10% of all accumbal neurons,[37] vary greatly in size, from 8 μm in diameter for the smallest, calretinin-immunopositive cells, to as large as 35 μm across the greatest diameter for cholinergic cells.[21] These interneurons have nuclear envelopes with deep indentations, dendrites that are almost or completely devoid of spines and are occasionally tortuous or varicose, and axons that arborize locally within the cell's dendritic field.[38,39] They manufacture either acetylcholine, which can be revealed with antibodies against choline acetyltransferase (ChAT) or GABA (TABLE 1).[38] In addition, other peptides, such as vasoactive intestinal peptide (VIP), cholecystokinin, or neurotensin, and the calcium binding protein, CaBP, have been found in neurons that are believed to be interneu-

---

FIGURE 1. Schematic diagrams of the synaptic wiring of typical core (**A**) and caudal medial shell (**B**; transitional EA) neurons in nucleus accumbens. Rectangular boxes surround extrinsic inputs, and dotted lines surround connections that originate locally, either from other medium spiny neurons (MSNs) or local circuit neurons (LCNs). Enkephalin (ENK)-positive terminals end significantly more often on spine necks in the shell than in the core. Excitatory amino acids (EAA) are used by cortical and thalamic (thal) inputs. Tyrosine hydroxylase (TH) represents the presumed dopaminergic input. Note that proximal synapses in the core arise predominately from local neurons (principal and interneurons) and distal connections extrinsically, whereas there is a mixture of inputs to the shell neuron both proximally and distally. GAD, glutamate decarboxylase; hippo, hippocampus.

TABLE 1. Neurochemical and receptor phenotypes of principal and local circuit neurons in nucleus accumbens

Principal Projection Neurons		Local Circuit Neurons			
Medium spiny neurons		ChAT/Ach	parvalbumin	calretinin	NOS/NADPH-diaphorase[38]
GABA[27,29]	GABA[27,29]	D_1 (60%)[46]	GABA[39]	GABA[39]	GABA[39]
ENK[84]	DYN[84]	D_2 (90%)[46]	GAD[39]	GAD[39]	GAD[39]
PPEmRNA[35,84]	Substance P[20,33]	ACHE[27,39]			SS[39]
D_2[83]	PPTmRNA[35,84]				NPY[39]
D_1 (37%)[48]	PPDmRNA[83]				ACHE[39]
D_3[49]	D_1[83]				NMDAR1 [38]
5HT2a(38%)[82]	D_2 (28%)[48]				CaBP[34]
	D_3 (26%)[49]				
	5HT2a (46%)[82]				

Not MSN type specific
CaBP[34]
A2A mRNA[35]
neurokininB (10–15%)[35]
neurotensin[20,35]
NMDA R1[51]
mu-opioid receptor[21]
delta opioid receptor[21]

Abbreviations: Ach, acetylcholine; ACHE, acetylcholinesterase; A2A, adenosine 2A receptor; ChAT, choline acetyltransferase; DYN, dynorphin; ENK, enkephalin; GABA, γ-aminobutyric acid; NADPH, nicotinamide adenine dinucleotide phosphate; NMDAR1, R1 subunit of the *N*-methyl-D-aspartate receptor; PPE, preproenkephalin; PPT, preprotachykinin; SS, somatostatin.

rons.[34,40–42] Whether or not these cells are subtypes of known interneuronal groups or form completely separate populations has yet to be investigated.

The GABAergic interneurons comprise at least three different populations: parvalbumin-, calretinin-, or somatostatin- and neuropeptide Y (NPY)- positive populations. The enzymes, neuronal nitric oxide synthase (NOS) and reduced nicotinamide adenine dinucleotide phosphate-diaphorase (NADPH-diaphorase) are colocalized in the somatostatin/NPY cells, at least in the dorsal striatum.[39] Further in the dorsal striatum, parvalbumin interneurons have been shown to be coupled by gap junctions with other parvalbumen-positive cells along proximal dendrites.[43] In accumbens, most interneurons are distributed homogeneously. However, ChAT-immunoreactive neurons are nearly three times denser in the caudal medial shell than in the core and five times greater than at the rostral pole.[25] Furthermore, parvalbumin cells seem to be less dense medially, especially at caudal levels in the transitional EA, than laterally.[44]

Receptor distribution at the cellular level in the accumbens (TABLE 1) appears to differ little from that in the dorsal striatum. Dopamine D_2 receptor mRNA has been localized to enkephalinergic neurons and most ChAT-immunoreactive cells.[45,46] Recent work[47] has confirmed the presence of D_2 receptors along the plasmalemma of cell bodies and dendrites of both principal and local circuit neurons. The D_1 mRNA is expressed in dynorphinergic neurons and the majority of ChAT-positive cells.[45,46] There is also good evidence that the D_1 and D_2 receptor subtypes are colocalized in just over half of projection neurons, proportions similar to that in the dorsal striatum.[48] In the accumbens, there is a strong territorial difference in receptor profiles.[17] For example, ChAT-positive neurons express significantly lower levels of D_2 mRNA in the caudal shell than elsewhere, and substance P–containing neurons in the shell colocalize the D_1 and D_3 receptors to a greater degree than in the core.[49] Moreover, 60% of the neurons projecting to the ventral tegmental area (VTA) contain the preprotachykinin and D_1 receptor mRNA, and 40% of the cells projecting to the ventral pallidum express preproenkephalin and D_2 receptor mRNA.[50] Inasmuch as the major part of the ventral striatal–VTA projection orginates in the medial shell, it would appear that both D_1 and D_3 receptors are responsible for regulating at least part of the projection neurons there.

Glutamatergic transmission in the nucleus accumbens seems to be mediated by α-amino-3-hydroxy-5-methyl-4-isoxazoleproprionic acid (AMPA)/kainate receptors, although there is evidence that N-methyl-D-aspartate (NMDA) receptors are also responsible for EPSPs in this nucleus.[4,29] Differences in the contributions of these receptor types to excitatory transmission may be regional, inasmuch as NMDA receptors in the shell but not the core, are activated under conditions of reduced GABAergic inhibition.[4,29] In the transitional EA or caudal medial shell, the R1 subunit of the NMDA receptor has been localized primarily to the plasma membranes of dendrites and the somata of principal neurons or interneurons that are NOS immunoreactive (TABLE 1).[51,52]

Identifying the substrate for presynaptic interactions in the accumbens has proved difficult. Pharmacological studies have repeatedly shown that both glutamate and dopamine can act presynaptically, yet ultrastructural investigations have consistently failed to find axo-axonic connections. Recent work has identified the NMDA R1 subunit in axons and terminals that have asymmetrical specializations or contain TH,[51] suggesting that NMDA receptors are capable of presynaptically controlling the release of dopamine or glutamate. Although much less common, the D_2 receptor has also been localized to axon terminals.[47] Presynaptic actions could therefore occur via diffusion-dependent transmission whenever extracellular concentrations of dopamine or glutamate become high enough to activate receptors on terminals in their vicinity (see ref. 29 for further discussion).

SYNAPTIC FRAMEWORK

In the core of the nucleus accumbens, the inputs onto spines and distal dendrites generally arise from extrinsic sources, whereas the synapses situated more proximally on dendrites or perikarya come from intrinsic sources,[21] as schematically illustrated in FIGURE 1A. By contrast, in the caudal medial shell or transitional EA, principal neurons receive a mixture of intrinsic and extrinsic contacts, both distally and proximally (FIG. 1B). An important part of the intrinsic innervation of projection neurons is from other principal cells or from the local circuit neurons (FIGS. 2;

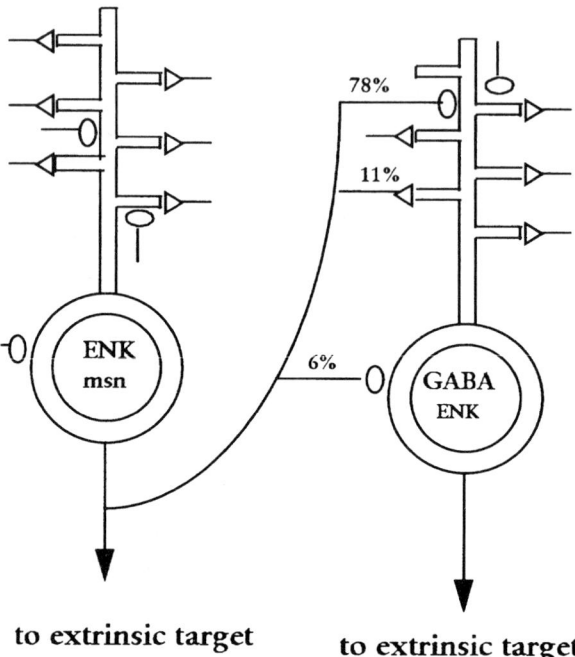

FIGURE 2. Schematic diagram of two principal projection neurons in the core, illustrating their local connections. Local terminals of enkephalinergic (ENK) neurons, which are medium spiny neurons (msn) primarily contact dendrites of other principal cells, some of which contain enkephalin.

3, A and B; and 4A). However, few studies have explicitly noted the regional distribution of terminals of these neurons or the sources of their own synaptic input. Nevertheless, it is known that the four main groups of interneurons provide some input to principal cells, and that parvalbumin- and ChAT- immunopositive neurons receive synaptic input from both extrinsic and intrinsic sources proximally and distally (FIG. 3, A and B).[29,38,44]

In the ventral as in the dorsal parts of the striatum, asymmetrical synaptic specializations occur most commonly at the heads of spines and symmetrical inputs, along dendritic shafts, at the necks of spines, and on perikaryal membranes.[27,29] In both core and shell, the primary asymmetrical input is from excitatory, presumably glutamatergic, axons of cortical and thalamic origins (FIG. 1, A and B). Inputs to both the core and shell arise from the amygdala and prefrontal area.[53,54] The lateral or medial entorhinal areas project primarily to the core, whereas the hippocampal formation innervates neurons primarily in the shell.[21,29] Neurons in both midline and intralaminar thalamic nuclei project topographically to the core and shell, where they presumably make asymmetrical contacts with dendrites and spines.[16,29,32] Other important asymmetrical inputs to the spines of both core and shell principal cells come from terminals containing calretinin or serotonin.[38,55] The calretinin input may be intrinsic, arising from local circuit neurons, or could originate from outside,

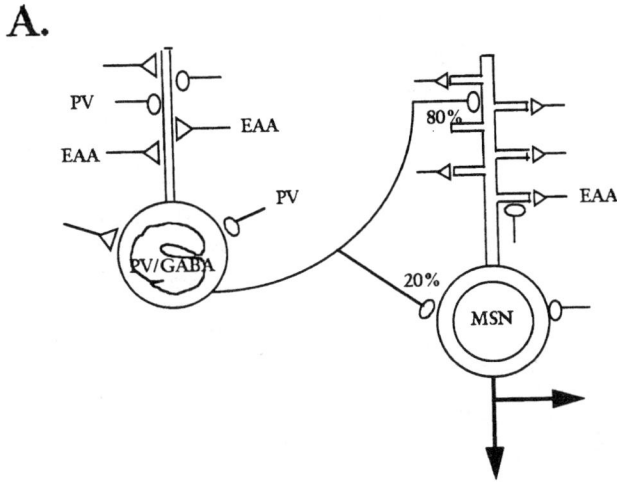

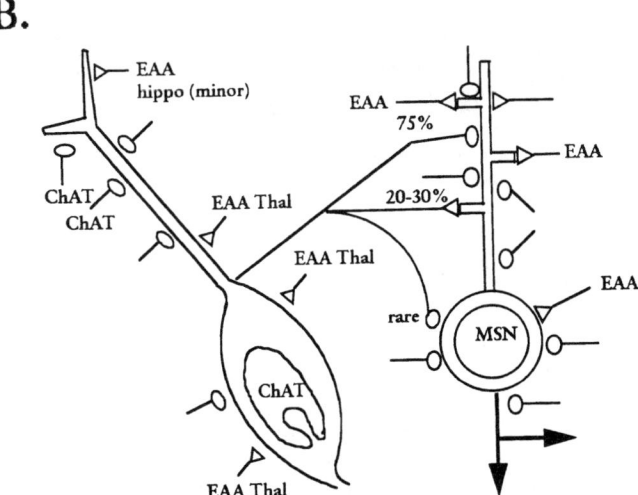

FIGURE 3. A: Schematic diagrams of the connections made by parvalbumin (PV)-positive interneurons. These terminals contact the dendrites and cell bodies of principal projection neurons. Parvalbumin-immunoreactive cells have been shown to be in contact with medium spiny neurons (MSN) that project to the VTA.[44] EAA, excitatory amino acid-positive axons, presumably of cortical origin, terminate on neurons containing PV and on principal cells, that is, medium spiny neurons (MSN). **B:** ChAT-immunoreactive neurons, which are presumably cholinergic, receive cortical inputs (EAA) onto distal small dendrites but thalamic (also EAA) terminals proximally on the cell body or proximal dendrites. ChAT-positive endings contact other ChAT-positive dendrites. The cholinergic interneurons also contact the dendrites of principal projection neurons (MSN).hippo, hippocampus.

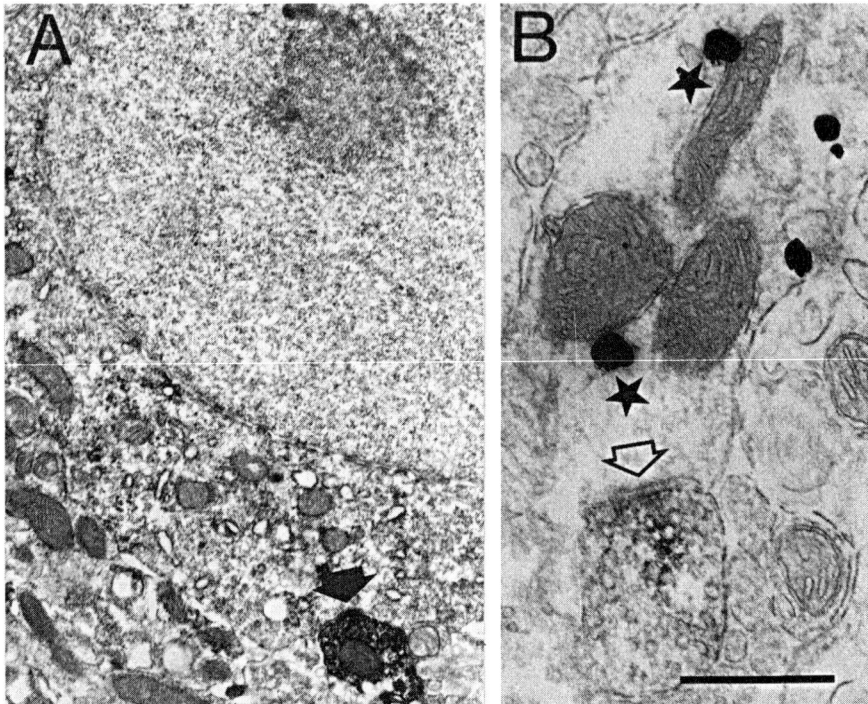

FIGURE 4. A: Electron micrographs illustrating a typical principal neuron with a round, unindented nucleus that is immunolabeled with glutamate decarboxylase (GAD) antibodies. **A:** GAD-positive terminal can be seen making a symmetrial contact with the perikaryal membrane (arrowhead). **B:** Electron micrograph illustrating a terminal immunolabeled for ChAT in contact (open arrowhead) with a dendrite that has been immunoreacted for enkephalin. The enkephalin labeling is silver-enhanced gold, and the granules are marked with stars. The scale bar is 0.5 μm.

inasmuch as projection neurons in certain thalamic and amygdalar regions contain this peptide.[38] Furthermore, extrinsic inputs from dopaminergic centers, or intrinsic contacts such as those containing enkephalin, dynorphin, substance P, somatostatin, ChAT, or neurotensin,[29,33,42,53,56] provide additional but minor asymmetrical axospinous innervations of shell and core principal neurons (FIG. 1, A and B).

Symmetrical synapses in both the shell and the core come onto dendrites and perikarya of projection and interneurons via TH- or dopamine-immunoreactive axons[16,57] that originate in one of the three main dopaminergic cell groups, A8, A9, and A10. The peptides, neurotensin and cholecystokinin, are contained in at least part of these midbrain projections,[9] but cholecystokinin may also be colocalized in fibers from the hippocampal formation.[8] The remaining symmetrical specializations in both territories arise from GABAergic principal cells and certain populations of interneurons. FIGURES 4A and 4B illustrate typical symmetrical inputs from GABAergic and cholinergic terminals onto identified elements of principal neurons. Enkephalinergic, dynorphinergic, and substance P–positive boutons primarily contact dendrites, some of which are proximal segments of other principal neurons, and, infrequently, make axosomatic synapses, which are almost exclusively onto projection neurons.[21,29,33] Among interneurons, the parvalbumin-immunoreactive terminals provide a major input to perikarya and proximal dendrites of principal cells, some of which project to the ventral mesencephalon, but they do not appear to synapse on spines.[38,44] They also form distal contacts with small dendrites and synapse proximally on other parvalbumin cells (FIG. 3A). In the dorsal, and presumably in the ventral, striatum, parvalbumin-immunoreactive neurons receive an extensive innervation from the cortex.[38,44] In the caudal medial shell or transitional EA, fornix stimulation results not only in a monosynaptic EPSP but also in a disynaptic IPSP, which is mediated via both glutamate and GABA.[58] If the parvalbumin-containing interneurons are recipients of this hippocampal input, they would be in a position to provide the inhibitory component and serve as the substrate for feed-forward inhibition (FIG. 3A). Parvalbumin-immunoreactive neurons are relatively sparse in the caudal medial shell,[44] however, and other GABAergic candidates, such as the NOS-immunoreactive interneurons, may be responsible for this action. The NOS-positive cells in the caudal medial shell receive inputs from fibers originating in the VTA[21] and contain the R1 subunit of the NMDA receptor,[52] suggesting that they receive a cortical innervation as well.

In both the shell and core, ChAT- and somatostatin-immunoreactive endings primarily form symmetrical contacts with dendrites (FIG. 4B), but approximately one quarter of the endings terminate on spines. Axosomatic contacts are relatively rare for both types of terminals (FIG. 3B). Nevertheless, when they occur, they are made with both principal and local circuit neurons. Furthermore, ChAT-positive endings contact other ChAT-immunoreactive neurons, and somatostatin-immunoreactive boutons terminate on somatostatin-positive cells. Finally, calretinin-immunoreactive endings establish symmetrical and asymmetrical contacts in equal proportions. They often contact spines and dendrites and, very occasionally, perikarya of accumbal principal neurons.[38] Such synaptic configurations differ from those commonly seen with other local circuit neurons, suggesting that some calretinin-immunoreactive axons could indeed originate elsewhere, outside the nucleus (see above).

Although the regional distributions of accumbal synapses are not completely understood, there are good data that show important differences between the core and transitional EA. In comparison to principal neurons in the core, transitional EA projection neurons have fewer spines,[30] significantly lower levels of dopamine transporter, but more NMDA receptors in axons and terminals.[51,59] In addition, cortical inputs from the amygdala or the prefrontal cortex come almost exclusively onto spines of core principal neurons, whereas 10% of the hippocampal contacts are onto dendrites in the caudal medial shell.[29,54,60,61] In the core, TH-immunoreactive terminals contact distal spine necks and dendrites, but in the transitional EA, they are found more often in contact with dendrites, especially proximal ones, than spines.[29,57,60] These territorial differences in innervation are clearly important for the differential effects of dopamine and glutamate on the output cells and the manner in which dopamine agents mediate feed-forward inhibition and electrotonic coupling.[4,36]

Ultrastructural investigations into thalamic inputs to the core have not been carried out as yet, but these terminals presumably form asymmetrical contacts with spines and dendrites (FIG. 1A), as occurs in the dorsal striatum[32] and in the transitional EA.[29] Among the local axon terminals of principal cells, we find that enkephalin-immunoreactive terminals in the core contact spines almost twice as often as the dynorphin- or substance P–positive terminals[21,33] but form axospinous synapses significantly less than in the transitional extended amygdala.

In the core, cholinergic terminals frequently form symmetrical synaptic specializations with dendrites of principal neurons that contain enkephalin (FIG. 4B); they also appose enkephalin-positive perikarya.[62] In the dorsal striatum, cholinergic neurons receive a dopaminergic input, and acetylcholine release is under dopaminergic control[21,63] However, in the nucleus accumbens, dopamine and acetylcholine can act independently, especially at caudal levels.[64] Although synaptic contacts between dopaminergic and cholinergic elements have not yet been recorded for any part of the accumbens, the pattern of local plexuses of cholinergic fibers in the caudal medial shell matches that of the dopaminergic innervation,[29] and cholinergic neurons contain both D_1 and D_2 receptor mRNA[46] (TABLE 1). Axons from the midline thalamus provide asymmetrical, proximal synapses on cholinergic somata here, but the terminals of principal neurons rarely contact these cells.[29,62]

It is difficult to assess how different afferent inputs to accumbens affect the activity of principal neurons when they are simultaneously active. We know, however, that in convergent arrangements on the same neuron, proximal arrangements can selectively "gate" more distal incoming signals.[3,4,65] There is good physiological but, as yet, no ultrastructural evidence for convergent hippocampal and amygdalar or hippocampal and prefrontal contacts onto the same principal neuron in the transitional EA and in the medial core[66,67] (FIG. 3). The reasons for the discrepancy between anatomical and physiological data are presumably technical, inasmuch as cortical inputs from one source could terminate in only one part of a dendritic field, whereas those from another source end in another dendritic sector, features that potentially pose problems for ultrastructural studies. Because the dendritic trees of principal neurons have as many as 8 primary dendrites in the medial shell and 11 in the core,[30] terminals that are spread out or occur predominately in one dendritic sector can be easily missed. Nevertheless, convergence between cortical and TH-positive inputs have been described ultrastructurally and physiologically.[53,54,65] In the core, prefrontal or amydalar inputs converge with dopaminergic terminals onto the same medium spiny neuron,[53,54] and in the caudal medial shell, hippocampal or amygdalar inputs converge with TH-positive terminals onto the same cell.[53,60]

NEURAL NETWORK ORGANIZATION AND OPERATION

Data on the synaptic arrangements of accumbal circuits are far from complete. Nevertheless, it is now possible to describe the basic organization of shell and core circuits and speculate on their functional significance. Dopamine and glutamate, which come from extrinsic sources, and acetylcholine and GABA from local circuit neurons or from local collaterals of principal projection cells, are all capable of influencing the activity of accumbal principal neurons. Even though the synaptic arrangements of cortical and dopaminergic inputs differ between regions, as illustrated in FIGURE 1, A and B, the dopamine terminals are always found in a position proximal to those with glutamate, and, as such, are effective in gating signals from widely separated cortical areas.

Ever since the discovery that striatal principal neurons had extensive local collaterals, investigators believed that lateral inhibition was a key feature of striatal circuits. Certainly, this type of inhibition must sharpen the responses of principal cells to tonic cortical signals, particularly because principal neurons seem almost exclusively to innervate each other (FIG. 2) often at proximal sites (FIG. 1, A and B). The potential influence of local circuit neurons has been neglected until recently when studies have shown that these cells comprise a larger proportion than previously thought and that they are diverse in both their connections and their actions.[25,34,37-39] All interneuronal types provide some innervation of principal neurons as well as themselves (FIG. 3, A and B), although autaptic synapses have not been described. Feedforward inhibition, which presumably sets the temporal sequence of events, is therefore important for selectively activating extrinsic targets and must involve an interneuron.[4,58] Local circuit neurons, such as those containing parvalbumin or somatostatin and NOS, receive cortical inputs and innervate projection neurons and could therefore serve as feedforward substrates (FIG. 3A). Nitric oxide is likely to have other functions in accumbens as well, inasmuch as it is able to enhance the release of most other transmitters.[39] Cholinergic neurons (FIG. 3B) also seem capable of mediating the action of other transmitters, especially in the transitional EA where cholinergic activity can be initiated by the thalamus, and has been shown to modulate the action of dopamine or GABA.[29,39,64]

The complex activity of neural networks in accumbens are not fixed and can be modified with alterations in neurotransmission, such as those brought about by psychostimulants, neuroleptic drugs, and neuronal toxins. Sustained changes in transmitter activity can lead to the up or down regulation of protein synthesis and eventual alterations in the structural integrity of neurons and their synapses. Circuits ultimately become reordered with profound consequences. For example, neurons may increase or decrease their responsiveness to incoming signals and feedback or feedforward activity could be altered, resulting ultimately in abnormal changes in motor function. At this point, we can only hypothesize about the mechanisms that underlie structural change, but in view of the differences in structural frameworks in the shell and core, the basis for change could differ between territories.

Dendritic spines serve a neuroprotective function by acting as independent calcium compartments that respond to excitatory amino acid inputs rapidly and in a sustained manner.[68] Nevertheless, particularly strong and maintained excitation is associated with neuronal degeneration.[69] In the striatum, dopamine exerts an inhibitory influence over the release of glutamate, and dopamine depletion gives rise to elevations in glutamate.[70] Such increases may be the source of damage to striatal neurons. We know that dopamine-depleting lesions result in the loss of spines from principal neurons in the core and an increase in the tortuosity of the dendritic trees in the caudal medial shell/transitional EA.[71] Such differences in the structural consequences of dopamine depletion provide evidence for the differential properties of shell and core circuits and the necessity to analyze pharmacological and physiological effects on a regional basis. Acute stimulation of dopamine in the shell, but not the core, augments oral movements,[72] and dopamine depletion increases opioid receptor-stimulated motor activity, seemingly at both shell and core sites.[73] Moreover, the blockade of dopamine receptors sensitizes rats to the reinforcing effects of heroin (see ref. 2 for review). Therefore, dopamine-stimulated motor activity, especially in relation to behavioral sensitization, may be site specific and associated with the activation of opioid receptors on principal neurons.

Neuroleptic blockade or psychostimulant administration also affects the structural integrity of accumbal neurons. Recent work has shown increases in the spine density of both shell and core neurons in animals exposed chronically to amphetamine.[74] We would expect such changes to be site specific, inasmuch as there is evidence that repeated, but not acute, cocaine augments levels of GABA, glutamate, and dopamine in the shell but not the core.[75,76] In the shell, dopamine also has the capacity to alter extracellular glutamate, either reducing levels via increased dopamine release or elevating it with D_2 receptor blockade.[77,78] Elevated glutamate could activate NMDA receptors, increase calcium influx, and produce excitotoxic damage, resulting in damage to principal neurons or NOS-immunoreactive interneurons, which also receive dopaminergic inputs[21] and contain the R1 subunit of the NMDA receptor.[52] Recent work has shown that chronic blockade of D_2 receptors with haloperidol dramatically raises levels of opioid peptides in accumbal principal neurons and significantly increases the density of dynorphinergic axospinous contacts in susceptible animals that develop abnormal orofacial movements.[79–80] Increased activation of NMDA receptors may not play a role, inasmuch as recently it has been shown that haloperidol treatment can act in an NMDA-independent manner in the accumbal shell.[81] Calcium-permeable AMPA receptors, however, have an even greater potential to be neurotoxic if activated for prolonged periods,[69,79,81] as could occur with chronic neuroleptic administration.

The mechanisms responsible for these structural changes are only now beginning to come to light. It is clear that a number of different factors could be involved, and further work will be needed to clarify which ones are most important.

ACKNOWLEDGMENTS

I am grateful for the contributions of I.A.J. De Souza, N. Dawson, T. Farrell, and P. Kelleghan to this work. I would also like to thank Dr. S. Totterdell for her comments and contributions. The work was supported by a Health Research Board Grant, 140-97.

REFERENCES

1. GETTING, P.A. 1989. Emerging principles governing the operation of neural networks. *In* Annual Review of Neuroscience. W.M. Cowan, E.M. Shooter, C.F. Stevens & R.F. Thompson, Eds.: **12**: 185–204. Annual Reviews, Inc. Palo Alto, CA.
2. KALIVAS, P.W., L. CHURCHILL & M.A. KLITENICK. 1993. The circuitry mediating the translation of motivational stimuli into adaptive motor responses. *In* Limbic Motor Circuits and Neuropsychiatry. P.W. Kalivas & C.D. Barnes, Eds.: 237–269. CRC Press. Boca Raton, FL.
3. MOGENSON, G.J. *et al.* 1993. From motivation to action: A review of dopaminergic regulation of limbic-nucleus accumbens-ventral pallidum-pedunculopontine nucleus circuitries involved in limbic-motor integration. *In* Limbic Motor Circuits and Neuropsychiatry. P.W. Kalivas & C.D. Barnes, Eds.: 193–236. CRC Press. Boca Raton, FL.

4. PENNARTZ, C.M.A., H.J. GROENEWEGEN & F.H. LOPES DA SILVA. 1994. The nucleus accumbens as a complex of functionally distinct neuronal ensembles: an integration of behavioural, electrophysiological and anatomical data. Prog. Neurobiol. **42:** 719–761.
 5. DEUTCH A.Y. & D.S. CAMERON. 1992. Pharmacological characterization of dopamine systems in the nucleus accumbens core and shell. Neuroscience **46:** 49–56.
 6. KELLEY, A.E., S.L. SMITH-ROE & M.R. HOLAHAN. 1997. Response-reinforcement learning is dependent on N-methyl-D-aspartate receptor activation in the nucleus accumbens core. Proc. Natl. Acad. Sci. USA **94:** 12174–12179.
 7. HEIMER, L. & R.D. WILSON. 1975. The subcortical projections of the allocortex: Similarities in the neural association of the hippocampus, the piriform cortex, and the neocortex. In Golgi Centennial Symposium: Perspectives in Neurobiology. M. Santini, Ed.:177–79. Raven Press. New York.
 8. ZÁBORSZKY, L. et al. 1985. Cholecystokinin innervation of the ventral striatum: a morphological and radioimmunological study. Neuroscience **14:** 427–453.
 9. ALHEID, G.F. & L. HEIMER. 1988. New perspectives in basal forebrain organization of special relevance for neuropsychiatric disorders: the striatopallidal, amygdaloid and corticopetal components of the substantia innominata. Neuroscience **27:** 1–39.
10. HEIMER, L. et al. 1991. "Perestroika" in the basal forebrain: Opening the border between neurology and psychiatry. In Progress in Brain Research. G. Holstege, Ed.: **87:** 109–165. Elsevier Science Publishers, B.V. Amsterdam.
11. HEIMER, L. et al. 1991. Specificity in the projection patterns of accumbal core and shell in the rat. Neuroscience **41:** 89–125.
12. ALHEID, G.F. & L. HEIMER. 1996. Theories of basal forebrain organization and the "emotional motor system." In Progress in Brain Research. G. Holstege, R. Bandler & C.B. Saper, Eds.: **107:** 461–481. Elsevier Science Publishers, B.V. Amsterdam.
13. HEIMER, L., R.E. HARLAN, G.F. ALHEID et al. 1997. Substantia innominata: a notion which impedes clinical-anatomical correlations in neuropsychiatric disorders. Neuroscience **76:** 957–1006.
14. ZAHM, D.S. & L. HEIMER. 1993. Specificity in the efferent projections of the rat nucleus accumbens in the rat: comparison of the rostral pole projection patterns with those of the core and shell. J. Comp. Neurol. **327:** 220–232.
15. MEREDITH G.E. et al. 1996. The shell and core in monkey and human nucleus accumbens identified with antibodies to calbindin-D28k. J. Comp. Neurol. **365:** 628–639.
16. GROENEWEGEN, H.J. et al. 1991. Functional anatomy of the ventral, limbic system-innervated striatum. In The Mesolimbic Dopamine System: From Motivation to Action. P. Willner & J. Scheel-Krüger, Eds : 19–59. John Wiley & Sons. Chichester, U.K.
17. BARDO, M.T. & R.P.HAMMER JR. 1991. Autoradiographic localization of dopamine D1 and D2 receptors in the rat nucleus accumbens: resistance to differential rearing conditions. Neuroscience **45:** 281–290.
18. ZAHM, D.S. & J.S. BROG. 1992. On the significance of subterritories in the "accumbens" part of the rat ventral striatum. Neuroscience **50:** 751–767.
19. JONGEN-RELO, A. L., H.J. GROENEWEGEN & P. VOORN. 1994. Immunohistochemical characterization of the shell and core territories of the nucleus accumbens in the rat. Eur. J. Neurosci. **6:** 1255–1264.
20. ZAHM, D.S. & L. HEIMER. 1988. Ventral striatopallidal parts of the basal ganglia in the rat: I. Neurochemical compartmentation as reflected by the distributions of neurotensin and substance P immunoreactivity. J. Comp. Neurol. **272:** 516–535.
21. MEREDITH, G.E. & S. TOTTERDELL. 1999. The contribution to cognition and reward of shell and core microcircuits in nucleus accumbens. Psychobiology. In press.
22. JONGEN-RELO, A.L., H.J. GROENEWEGEN & P. VOORN. 1993. Evidence for a multicompartmental histochemical organization of the nucleus accumbens in the rat. J. Comp. Neurol. **337:** 267–276.
23. WRIGHT, C.I. & H.J. GROENEWEGEN. 1995. Patterns of convergence and segregation in the medial nucleus accumbens of the rat: relationships of prefrontal cortical, midline thalamic and basal amygdaloid afferents. J. Comp. Neurol. **361:** 383–403.
24. WRIGHT, C.I., A.V.J. BEIJER & H.J. GROENEWEGEN. 1996. Basal amygdaloid complex

afferents to the rat nucleus accumbens are compartmentally organized. J. Neurosci. **16:** 1877–1893.
25. MEREDITH, G.E., B. BLANK & H.J. GROENEWEGEN. 1989. The distribution and compartmental organization of the cholinergic neurons in nucleus accumbens of the rat. Neuroscience **31:** 327–345.
26. HEDREEN, J.C. 1981. Neurons of the nucleus accumbens and other striatal regions in rats. *In* The Neurobiology of the Nucleus Accumbens. R.B. Chronister & J.F. DeFrance Eds.:82–96. The Haer Institute for Electrophysiological Research. Brunswick, ME.
27. BOLAM, J.P. 1984. Synapses of identifed neurons in the neostriatum. *In* Functions of the Basal Ganglia: Ciba Foundation Symposium. D. Evered & M. O'Connor, Eds. **107:**30–47. Pitman. London, U.K.
28. CHANG, H.T. & S.T. KITAI. 1985. Projection neurons of the nucleus accumbens: an intracellular labeling study. Brain Res. **347:** 112–116.
29. MEREDITH, G.E., C. PENNARTZ & H.J. GROENEWEGEN. 1993. The cellular framework for chemical signalling in the nucleus accumbens. *In* Progress in Brain Research. G.W. Arbuthnott & P.C. Emson, Eds.:**99:** 3–24. Elsevier Science Publishers, B.V. Amsterdam.
30. MEREDITH, G.E. *et al.* 1992. Morphological differences between projection neurons of the core and shell in the nucleus accumbens of the rat. Neuroscience **50:** 149–162.
31. O'DONNELL, P. & A.A. GRACE. 1993. Physiological and morphological properties of accumbens core and shell neurons recorded *in vitro*. Synapse **13:** 135–160.
32. DUBE, L., A.D. SMITH & J.P. BOLAM. 1988. Identification of synaptic terminals of thalamic or cortical origin in contact with distinct medium-size spiny neurons in the rat neostriatum. J. Comp. Neurol. **267:** 455–471.
33. PICKEL, V.M., T.H. JOH & J. CHAN. 1988. Substance P in the rat nucleus accumbens: ultrastructural localization in axon teminals and their relation to dopaminergic afferents. Brain Res. **444:** 247–264.
34. HUSSAIN, Z. & S. TOTTERDELL. 1994. Calbindin-D28k immunoreactive neurons form two populations in the rat nucleus accumbens: a compartmental study. Brain Res. **656:** 191–198.
35. HARLAN, R.E. & M.M. GARCIA. 1998. Drugs of abuse and immediate-early genes in the forebrain. Mol. Neurobiol. **16:** 221–267.
36. O'DONNELL, P. & A.A. GRACE. 1993. Dopaminergic modulation of dye coupling between neurons in the core and shell regions of the nucleus accumbens. J. Neurosci. **13:** 3456–3471.
37. THOMAS, E.J., R.R. VAID & S. TOTTERDELL. 1995. An estimate of the proportion of interneurons in the nucleus accumbens [abstract]. Brain Res. Assoc. **12:** 40.
38. HUSSAIN, Z., L.R. JOHNSON & S. TOTTERDELL. 1996. A light and electron microscopic study of NADPH-diaphorase-, calretinin- and parvalbumin-containing neurons in the rat nucleus accumbens. J. Chem. Neuroanat. **10:** 19–39.
39. KAWAGUCHI, Y. *et al.* 1995. Striatal interneurones: chemical, physiological and morphological characterization. Trends Neurosci. **18:** 527–535.
40. TAGAKI, H. *et al.* 1984. The occurrence of cholecystokinin-like immunoreactive neurons in the rat neostriatum: light and electron microscopic analysis. Brain Res. **309:** 346–349.
41. THERIAULT, E. & D.M.D. LANDIS. 1987. Morphology of striatal neurons containing VIP-like immunoreactivity. J. Comp. Neurol. **268:** 29–37.
42. DELLE DONNE, K.T., S.R. SESACK & V.M. PICKEL. 1996. Ultrastructural immunocytochemical localization of neurotensin and the dopamine D2 receptor in the rat nucleus accumbens. J. Comp. Neurol. **371:** 552–566.
43. KITA, H. 1993. GABAergic circuits of the striatum. *In* Progress in Brain Research. G.W. Arbuthnott & P.C. Emson, Eds.:**99:** 51–72. Elsevier Science Publishers, B.V. Amsterdam.
44. BENNETT, B.D. & J.P. BOLAM. 1994. Synaptic input and output of parvalbumin-immunoreactive neurons in the neostriatum of the rat. Neuroscience **62:** 707–719.

45. LE MOINE, C. & B. BLOCH. 1995. D1 and D2 receptor gene expression in the rat striatum: sensitive cRNA probes demonstrate prominent segregation of D1 and D2 mRNAs in distinct neuronal populations of the dorsal and ventral striatum. J. Comp. Neurol. **355:** 418–426.
46. JONGEN-RELO, A.L. et al. 1995. Differential localization of mRNAs encoding dopamine D1 or D2 receptors in cholinergic neurons in the core and shell of the rat nucleus accumbens. Mol. Brain Res. **28:** 169–174.
47. DELLE DONNE, K.T., S.R. SESACK & V.M. PICKEL. 1997. Ultrastructural immunocytochemical localization of the dopamine D2 receptor within GABAergic neurons of the rat striatum. Brain Res. **746:** 239–255.
48. RELO, A.L. 1994. Dopamine Receptors in the Nucleus Accumbens. Ph.D. thesis. Vrije University, Amsterdam.
49. LE MOINE, C. & B. BLOCH. 1996. Expression of the D3 dopamine receptor in peptidergic neurons of the nucleus accumbens: comparison with the D1 and D2 dopamine receptors. Neuroscience **73:** 131–143.
50. LU, X-Y., L. CHURCHILL & P.W. KALIVAS. 1997. Expression of D1 receptor mRNA in projections from the forebrain to the ventral tegmental area. Synapse **25:** 205–214.
51. GRACY, K.N. & V.M. PICKEL. 1996. Ultrastructural immunocytochemical localization of the *N*-methyl-D-aspartate receptor and tyrosine hydroxylase in the shell of the rat nucleus accumbens. Brain Res. **739:** 169–181.
52. GRACY, K.N. & V.M. PICKEL. 1997. Ultrstructural localization and comparative distribution of nitric oxide synthase and *N*-methyl-D-aspartate receptors in the shell of the rat nucleus accumbens. Brain Res. **747:** 259–272.
53. JOHNSON, L. et al. 1994. Input from the amygdala to the rat nucleus accumbens: its relationship with tyrosine hydroxylase immunoreactivity and identified neurons. Neuroscience **61:** 851–865.
54. SESACK, S.R. & V.M. PICKEL. 1992. Prefrontal cortical efferents in the rat synapse on unlabeled neuronal targets of catecholamine terminals in the nucleus accumbens septi and on dopamine neurons in the ventral tegmental area. J. Comp. Neurol. **320:** 145–160.
55. VAN BOCKSTAELE, E. & V.M. PICKEL. 1993. Ultrastructure of serotonin-immunoreactive terminals in the core and shell of the rat nucleus accumbens—cellular substrates for interactions with catecholamine afferents. J. Comp. Neurol. **334:** 603–617.
56. PHELPS, P.E. & J.E. VAUGHN. 1986. Immunocytochemical localization of choline acetyltransferease in rat ventral striatum: A light and electron microscopic study. J. Neurocytol. **15:** 595–617.
57. ZAHM, D.S. 1992. An electron microscopic morphometric comparison of tyrosine hydroxylase-immunoreactive innervation in the neostriatum and nucleus accumbens core and shell. Brain Res. **575:** 751–756.
58. PENNARTZ, C.M.A. & S.T. KITAI. 1991. Hippocampal inputs to identified neurons in an *in vitro* slice preparation of the rat nucleus accumbens: evidence for feed-forward inhibition. J. Neurosci. **11:** 2838–2847.
59. NIRENBERG, M.J. et al. 1997. The dopamine transporter: comparative ultrastructure of dopaminergic axons in limbic and motor compartments of the nucleus accumbens. J. Neurosci. **17:** 6899–6907.
60. TOTTERDELL, S. & A.D. SMITH. 1989. Convergence of hippocampal and dopaminergic input onto identified neurons in the nucleus accumbens of the rat. J. Chem. Neuroanat. **2:** 285–298.
61. JOHNSON, L., R.L.M. AYLWARD & S. TOTTERDELL. 1994. Synaptic organization of the amygdalar input to the nucleus accumbens in the rat. *In* Basal Ganglia IV. G. Percheron, J.S. McKenzie & J.S. Féger, Eds. :109–114. Plenum Press. New York.
62. MEREDITH, G.E. & H.T. CHANG. 1994. Synaptic relationships of enkephalinergic and cholinergic neurons in the nucleus accumbens of the rat. Brain Res. **667:** 67–76.
63. DIMOVA, R. et al. 1993. Ultrastructural features of the choline acetyltransferease-containing neurons and relationships with nigral dopaminergic and cortical afferent pathways in the rat striatum. Neuroscience **53:** 1059–1071.

64. HENSELMANS, J.M.L. & J.C. STOOF. 1991. Regional differences in the regulation of acetylcholine release upon D-2 dopamine and *N*-methyl-D-aspartate receptor activation in rat nucleus accumbens and neostriatum. Brain Res. **566:** 8–12.
65. MOGENSON, G.J., D.L. JONES & C.Y. YIM. 1980. From motivation to action: functional interface between the limbic system and the motor system. Prog. Neurobiol. **14:** 69–97.
66. O'DONNELL, P. & A.A. GRACE. 1995. Synaptic interactions among excitatory afferents to nucleus accumbens neurons: hippocampal gating of prefrontal cortical input. J. Neurosci. **15:** 3622–3639.
67. MULDER, A.B., M.G. HODENPIJL & F.H. LOPES DA SILVA. 1998. Electrophysiology of the hippocampal and amygdaloid projections to the nucleus accumbens of the rat. Convergence, segregation, and interaction of inputs. J. Neurosci. **18:** 5095–5102.
68. SEGAL, M. 1995. Dendritic spines for neuroprotection: a hypothesis. Trends Neurosci. **18:** 468–471.
69. CHOI, D.W. 1988. Glutamate neurotoxicity and diseases of the nervous system. Neuron **1:** 623–634.
70. ZIGMOND, M.J. *et al.* 1990. Compensations after lesions of central dopaminergic neurons: some clinical and basic implications. Trends Neurosci. **13:** 290–296.
71. MEREDITH, G.E., P. YPMA & D.S. ZAHM. 1995. The effects of dopamine depletion on the morphology of medium spiny neurons in the shell and core of the rat nucleus accumbens. J. Neurosci. **15:**3808–3820.
72. PRINSSEN, E.P.M. *et al.* 1994. Evidence for a role of the shell of the nucleus accumbens in oral behavior of freely moving rats. J. Neurosci. **14:** 1555–1562.
73. CHURCHILL, L., B.P. ROQUES & P.W. KALIVAS. 1995. Dopamine depletion augments endogenous opioid-induced locomotion in the nucleus accumbens using both μ1 and δ opioid receptors. Psychopharmacology **120:** 347–355.
74. ROBINSON, T.E. & B. KOLB. 1997. Persistent structural modifications in nucleus accumbens and prefrontal cortex neurons produced by previous experience with amphetamine. J. Neurosci. **17:** 8491–8497.
75. PIERCE, R.C. & P.W. KALIVAS. 1995. Amphetamine produces sensitized increases in locomotion and extracellular dopamine preferentially in the nucleus accumbens shell of rats administered repeated cocaine. J. Pharmacol. Exp. Ther. **275:** 1019–1029.
76. SORG, B.A. *et al.* 1995. Cocaine alters glutamic acid decarboxylase differentially in the nucleus accumbens core and shell. Mol. Brain Res. **29:** 381–386.
77. KALIVAS, P.W. & P. DUFFY. 1995. Selective activation of dopamine transmission in the shell of the nucleus accumbens by stress. Brain Res. **675:** 335–328.
78. SEE, R.E. & M.A. CHAPMAN. 1994. Chronic haloperidol, but not clozapine, produces altered oral movements and increased extracellular glutamate in rats. Eur. J. Pharmacol. **263:** 269–276.
79. EGAN, M.F. *et al.* 1994. Alterations in mRNA levels of D2 receptors and neuropeptides in striatonigral and striatopallidal neurons of rats with neuroleptic-induced dyskinesias. Synapse (NY) **18:** 178–189.
80. MEREDITH, G.E. *et al.* 1997. Ultrastructural changes in dynorphinergic terminals of nucleus accumbens in rats that display neuroleptic-induced vacuous chewing movements [abstract]. Soc. Neurosci. **23:** 399.
81. DE SOUZA, I.E.J. & G.E. MEREDITH. 1999. NMDA receptor blockade attenuates the haloperidol induction of Fos protein in the dorsal but not the ventral sriatum. Synapse (NY) **33:** 1–11.
82. MIJNSTER, M.J. *et al.* 1997. Regional and cellular distribution of serotonin 5-hydroxytraptamine 2a receptor mRNA in the nucleus accumbens, olfactory tubercle, and caudate putamen of the rat. J. Comp. Neurol. **389:** 1–11.
83. GERFEN, C.R., J.F. MCGINTY & W.S. YOUNG. 1991. Dopamine differentially regulates dynorphin, substance P and enkephalin expression in striatal neurons: *in situ* hybridization histochemical analysis. J. Neurosci. **11:** 1016–1031.
84. GERFEN, C.R. & W.S. YOUNG. 1988. Distribution of striatonigral and striatopallidal peptidergic neurons in both patch and matrix compartments: an *in situ* hybridization histochemistry and fluorescent retrograde tracing study. Brain Res. **460:** 161–167.

Modulation of Cell Firing in the Nucleus Accumbens

PATRICIO O'DONNELL,[a,c] JENNIFER GREENE,[a] NINA PABELLO,[a] BARBARA L. LEWIS,[a] AND ANTHONY A. GRACE[b]

[a]*Departments of Pharmacology and Neuroscience and Neurology, Albany Medical College*
[b]*Departments of Neuroscience and Psychiatry, University of Pittsburgh*

ABSTRACT: Pennartz *et al.*[48] have proposed that functions of the nucleus accumbens (NA) are subserved by the activity of ensembles of neurons rather than by an overall neuronal activation. Indeed, the NA is a site of convergence for a large number of inputs from limbic structures that may modulate the flow of prefrontal cortical information and contribute to defining such ensembles, as exemplified in the ability of hippocampal input to gate cortical throughput in the nucleus accumbens. NA neurons exhibit a bistable membrane potential, characterized by a very negative resting membrane potential (down state), periodically interrupted by plateau depolarizations (up state), during which the cells may fire in response to cortical inputs. A dynamic ensemble can be the result of a distributed set of neurons in their up state, determined by the moment-to-moment changes in the spatial distribution of hippocampal inputs responsible for transitions to the up state. Ensembles may change as an adaptation to the contextual information provided by the hippocampal input. Furthermore, for dynamic ensembles to be functionally relevant, the model calls for near synchronous transitions to the up state in a group of neurons. This can be accomplished by the cell-to-cell transfer of information via gap junctions, a mechanism that can allow for a transfer of slow electrical signals, including "up" events between coupled cells. Furthermore, gap junction permeability is tightly modulated by a number of factors, including levels of dopamine and nitric oxide, and cortical inputs, allowing for fine-tuning of this synchronization of up events. The continuous selection of such dynamic ensembles in the NA may be disputed in schizophrenia, resulting in an inappropriate level of activity of thalamocortical systems.

INTRODUCTION

The nucleus accumbens (NAcc) is a unique brain region involved in the adaptation of animals to their environment, with a participation in a variety of functions that are appetitive or aversive in nature.[1] This area is part of the basal forebrain and spans striatal and extended amygdala territories.[2] It has at least two distinct compartments that differ primarily with respect to their input/output organization[3] and in specific neurochemical markers,[4,5] with the core being the NAcc region that has more in common with the dorsal striatum and the shell being the NAcc territory that

---

[c]Address correspondence to Patricio O'Donnell, M.D., Ph.D., Albany Medical College (MC-136), Department of Pharmacology and Neuroscience, 47 New Scotland Avenue, Albany, NY 12208, USA. Voice: 518-262-5904; fax: 518-262-5799; patricio.o'donnell@ccgateway.amc.edu

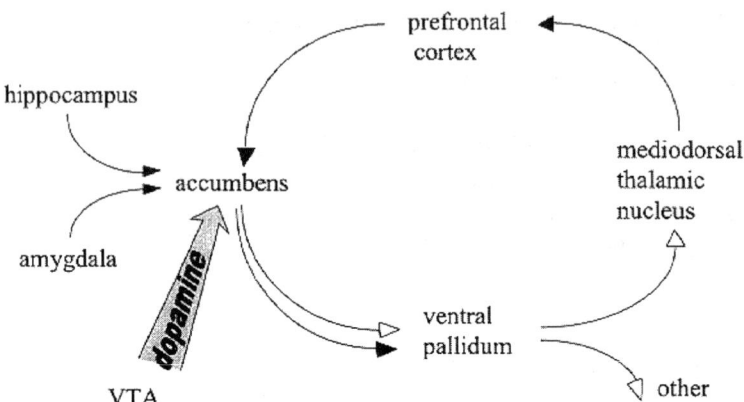

FIGURE 1. Schematic representation of the circuits linking the hippocampus, nucleus accumbens, and prefrontal cortex. The accumbens, as a striatal link within these cortico-subcortical-cortical circuits, projects back to the PFC via its efferents to the ventral pallidum, which, in turn, inhibits specific thalamic nuclei. Open arrows represent GABAergic inhibitory synapses, and filled arrows represent excitatory projections that are mostly glutamatergic, with the exception of the projection from the accumbens to the ventral pallidum that presents substance P.

can be considered a component of the extended amygdala of Heimer and Alheid.[2] The NAcc has been described as participating in feeding mechanisms,[6] sexual behaviors,[7] reward,[8,9] cocaine self-administration,[10,11] stress,[12] spatial learning,[13] antipsychotic drug actions,[14] sensorimotor gating,[15] and probably in the pathophysiology of schizophrenia.[16] As a striatal component within basal ganglia-cortical circuits, the NAcc receives inputs from the prefrontal cortex (PFC) and other "limbic" areas and provides feedback to the PFC[17,18] (FIG. 1). The primary output of the NAcc is directed to the ventral pallidum (VP),[19–22] which among other targets provides an inhibitory input to the thalamocortical system originated in the mediodorsal nucleus (MD) and the reticular thalamic nucleus (RTN) as well.[21,23] Thus, information flowing through this region may be important in gating thalamocortical activity that provides a driving influence to the PFC.

Although a large number of studies have focused on physiological properties of NAcc neurons, several issues related to the information processing taking place in this structure have not been solved. In particular, the interactions among different inputs may be important for the functions in which the NAcc is involved. The NAcc receives afferents from a diverse set of structures involved in higher functions; in addition to the PFC,[24] these include the amygdala,[25,26] hippocampus,[27] and entorhinal cortex.[28,29] The spatial arrangement of these inputs onto their NAcc neuronal targets may determine the functional interactions among these systems. In this regard, anatomical studies have consistently shown that afferents from different sources very rarely overlap within the NAcc.[30] Although this may suggest that different inputs contact distinct populations of neurons in the NAcc, electrophysiological studies have shown a high degree of convergence of synaptic responses on single NAcc neurons evoked by stimulation of these inputs. Extracellular recordings from NAcc neu-

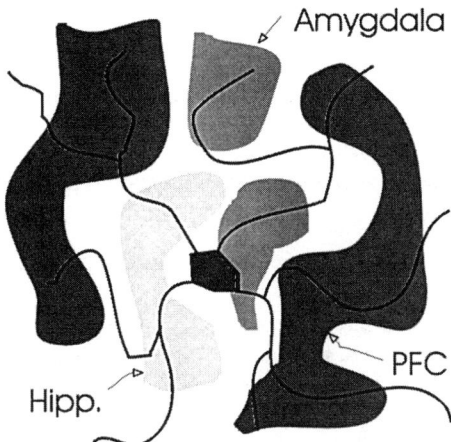

FIGURE 2. Hypothetical arrangement of terminal afferent fields and an accumbens neuron with its dendrites crossing the boundaries of nonoverlapping terminal fields. The areas with different shades of gray indicate hypothetical regions in which afferents from the amygdala, hippocampus (Hipp.) and PFC terminate. The location of synaptic contacts relative to the cell body will determine the impact these afferents will have on cell firing.

rons reported approximately a 10–30% convergence among inputs from the PFC and amygdala or hippocampus.[31] Furthermore, *in vivo* intracellular recordings revealed a much higher proportion of convergence (95%) for the same inputs.[32] This higher convergence observed with intracellular studies may be due to the ability of this technique to detect subthreshold responses that do not elicit action potential discharge. In that study, convergence was measured as the proportion of neurons showing synaptic responses to several afferents in the form of excitatory postsynaptic potentials (EPSP), which are beyond detection with extracellular recording techniques. The apparent discrepancy between anatomical and electrophysiological data, on the other hand, could be explained by the possibility that dendritic trees of NAcc neurons span areas containing terminals from different afferent systems, even if these do not overlap with each other (FIG. 2). In fact, neuroanatomical studies indicating little overlap among terminal fields from different sources did show a close interdigitization of these terminal fields within the NAcc.[30]

This convergence of "limbic" inputs within the NAcc could be involved in blending affective, cognitive, and motor functions within this ventral striatal region. However, the mechanism underlying such a synthesis is still poorly understood. Several models have proposed different views on the integration of information in the NAcc, differing essentially on the issue of whether there is a primary input that is modulated by others or whether all inputs are equally weighed. If the latter is true, the NAcc may behave as a coincidence detector.[33] Regardless of the relative relevance of different inputs, one of the systems affected by this convergence in the NAcc is the thalamic projection to the PFC via the MD. If the PFC input is the signal to be modulated, filtered or reinforced by other inputs, the question of how such influences are exerted remains open. Furthermore, the extensive monoaminergic innervation of the NAcc suggests that dopamine (DA) and other monoamines may play a role in this integration of information. Addressing these and related issues is essential for a more thorough understanding of how basal ganglia loops control prefrontal cortical activity. This approach also offers the possibility of integrating into a single neural system the apparently unrelated brain regions that have been implicated in schizophrenia. Here we will review some recent studies on NAcc physiology using both *in vivo* and *in vitro* recording techniques, focusing on the integration of information in this nucleus and the role of dopamine in its information processing mechanisms.

INTEGRATION OF INFORMATION IN THE NUCLEUS ACCUMBENS

The ability of NAcc neurons to integrate information provided by their inputs is a function of both their afferent organization and their electrophysiological properties. The former is important with respect to assessing the functional relevance of the spatial distribution of inputs to a set of NAcc neurons. Whether a particular set of afferents contacts spines on dendrites located distal from the soma or near the cell body will determine the relative impact these afferents may exert on cell firing. The closer these contacts are to the soma, the stronger will be their effects on membrane potential, resulting in a tighter control over cell activity. NAcc output neurons, the medium-sized densely spiny neurons, receive most of their glutamatergic afferents in the spines located in distal dendrites.[80] However, a fraction of hippocampal, but not PFC, afferents has been shown to contact proximal dendrites and the cell body,[80] positioning them to exert a strong control over cell firing. Furthermore, the electrophysiological properties of individual NAcc neurons are important in determining the relative probabilities that specific individual or groups of inputs will be capable of driving the neuron to firing threshold. NAcc neurons display a characteristic activity pattern in their membrane potential that can underlie complex interactions among afferent synaptic inputs. Most NAcc neurons exhibit a bistable membrane potential; that is, their resting membrane potential, typically very negative (*down state*), is periodically interrupted by plateau depolarizations (*up state*) that are 100–1,000 ms in duration and 10–25 mV in amplitude[32,34] (FIG. 3). These depolariza-

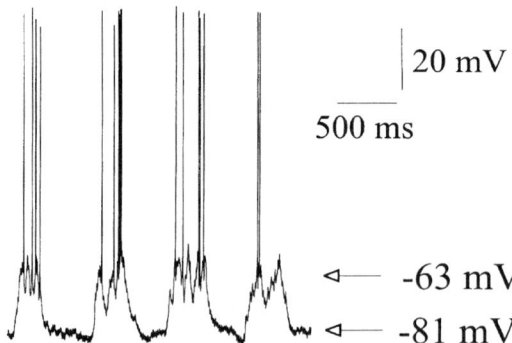

FIGURE 3. Most NAcc neurons exhibit up and down states in their membrane potential. The tracing shows a typical pattern of activity from a bistable neuron. Four up events are shown, and action potential firing is only observed during these events.

tions, or up events, bring the membrane potential of selected neurons close to their firing threshold during a relatively discrete time window. Such bistable membrane potential had been initially observed with *in vivo* intracellular recordings from dorsal striatal neurons as depolarizations underlying bursts of action potentials.[35] Yim and Mogenson[36] reported similar depolarizations in NAcc neurons. Using extracellular recordings, NAcc neurons were found to fire at very slow rates, with occasional bursts of 3 or 4 spikes.[37] It is likely that these bursts correspond to up events in NAcc neurons, because in studies using *in vivo* intracellular recordings, spontaneous action potential firing could only be observed during the up state.[32] The alternations between up and down states may provide a means to selectively gate the transfer of information in NAcc neurons by bringing their membrane potential close to their firing threshold, where afferent inputs are more likely to result in neuronal discharge. Any factor governing the transitions between states will thus have a strong impact on the ability of these neurons to convey to the thalamocortical system the messages they receive from different sources. This control of transitions between states in NAcc neurons can therefore be a very effective means of controlling thalamo-PFC activity.

The resting membrane potential of these neurons, the down state, is maintained at such negative values by a number of factors. A very important one is the inward rectifier K^+ conductance that medium spiny neurons exhibit.[81] As a result of this, any change in membrane potential is very effectively attenuated. However, with sufficient converging and synchronous arrival of glutamatergic excitatory inputs, a strong depolarization may occur. At this point, the inward rectifier current will be shut down, letting the membrane shift to a more depolarized value. This can explain why transitions between states occur abruptly, giving the impression of an all-or-none event rather than a gradual one.

Up events, on the other hand, are dependent on synaptic activation of NAcc cells. This is indicated by the fact that intracellular recordings *in vitro* yield silent neurons with a very negative and stable membrane potential, that lies within the range of the down state observed *in vivo*.[38–40] Furthermore, we have shown that stimulation of the fimbria-fornix system results in transitions to the up state in NAcc neurons.[32] The involvement of this fiber system in driving up events was further supported by *in vivo* intracellular recordings from animals that had received a transection to the fimbria-fornix. In this condition, neurons with a bistable membrane potential could not be detected in the NAcc, although they were still found in the caudate-putamen.[32] Most NAcc neurons recorded in these experiments were silent and exhibited a very negative membrane potential, which was within the range of the down state observed in control animals. Additional recordings were performed in rats before and after administration of the local anesthetic, lidocaine, into the fimbria-fornix. In these cases, up events were temporarily suppressed and returned to control levels approximately 15 to 20 min following the lidocaine injection.[32] Overall, these results indicate that afferents arriving to the NAcc via the fimbria-fornix are important, if not necessary, for the transitions to the up state (FIG. 4). The most likely source of such afferents is the hippocampal formation,[41] particularly the ventral subiculum. It should be noted that these recordings were performed from neurons located in the medial NAcc (either in the shell or the medial core), an area known to receive a dense projection from the ventral subiculum.[27]

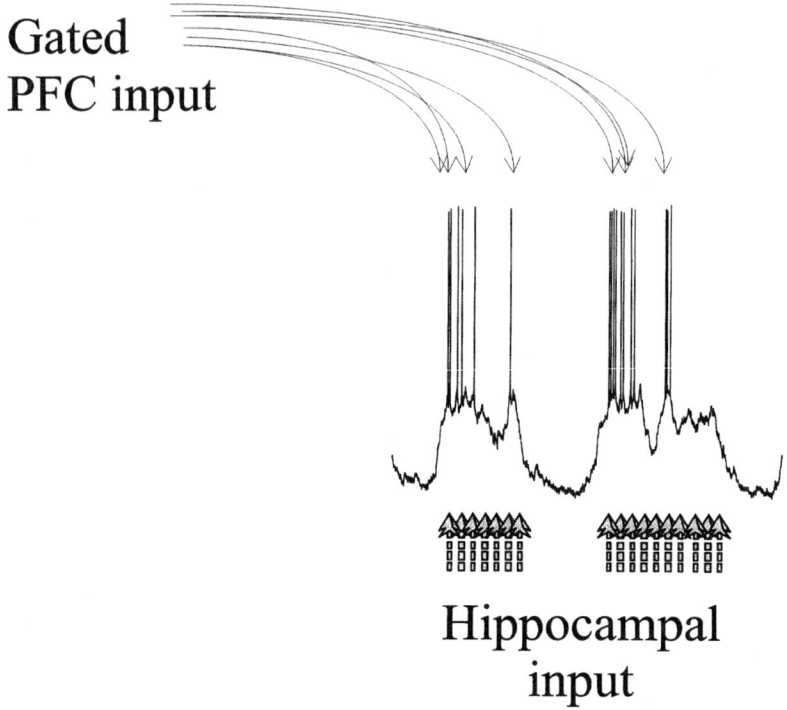

FIGURE 4. Hippocampal gating of prefrontal cortical throughput in NAcc neurons. Tracing from a bistable NAcc neuron, with the vertical arrows indicating the influence of inputs arriving via the fimbria-fornix system that can induce and maintain up events. Because the up state elicited by these inputs brings the membrane potential close to firing threshold, afferent inputs arriving from the PFC (curved arrows) during these periods will easily elicit action potential firing. On the other hand, PFC inputs arriving during the down state will be largely ineffective with respect to action potential firing.

Although synaptic inputs are essential for the presence of up events, the relatively stable membrane potential and the long duration of these events may indicate that certain membrane properties may limit the extent of depolarization, whereas others may contribute to its persistence. Recent studies from striatal medium spiny neurons (which also show up and down states) have described the presence of slowly inactivating K^+ currents (I_A)[42] that may limit the extent of depolarizations, such as those constituting the up state,[43] maintaining the membrane potential during these depolarizations just below firing threshold. In addition, striatal and NAcc neurons exhibit a slow voltage-dependent Na^+ current[44] and slow Ca^{2+} conductances[38,45] that may contribute to the persistence of such depolarizations. As a consequence of the interaction between these forces driving and limiting these depolarizations, up events may take the form of a stable plateau depolarization.

If the subicular afferents are an important factor driving up events in NAcc neurons, then these inputs may have a crucial role in determining the ability of NAcc neurons to trigger action potential discharge in response to other inputs. Indeed, activation of PFC afferents elicits action potential firing only during the up state, independently of whether it occurs spontaneously or is evoked by fornix stimulation.[32] Because the spontaneously occurring up events can be eliminated by transection or local anesthetic application into the fimbria-fornix, it is possible that they are dependent on hippocampal inputs. Thus, this could be envisioned as a gating mechanism, by which the hippocampal afferents are driving a distributed set of NAcc neurons into the up state, allowing them to fire in response to ongoing cortical afferent input activity.

The hippocampal input to the NAcc may also control the activity of the DA innervation of this region. For example, D_2 DA receptors in the NAcc increase two weeks after hippocampal kindling.[46] Moreover, neonatal hippocampal lesions have recently been observed to decrease the DA transporter (DAT) in mesencephalic DA neurons.[47] In short, hippocampal afferents may have a role in the control of the flow of information through the NAcc by a variety of mechanisms.

ENSEMBLE CODING IN THE NUCLEUS ACCUMBENS

Pennartz et al.[48] have proposed that NAcc functions are subserved by the activity of ensembles of neurons rather than by an overall neuronal activation. We believe that this concept can be extended to suggest that ensembles can be dynamic and based on activity states, rather than solely on connectivity patterns.[49] Indeed, the NAcc is a site of convergence for a large number of inputs from limbic structures that may modulate the flow of prefrontal cortical information and contribute to defining such ensembles, as exemplified in the already reviewed ability of hippocampal input to gate cortical throughput in the nucleus accumbens. Thus, a distributed set of neurons in their up state could actually represent an ensemble[49] (FIG. 5). This is similar to what has been described in the hippocampus as "ensemble coding,"[50,51] reflecting the distribution of activity in a population of neurons. Ensembles in the NAcc may change as an adaptation to the contextual information provided by hippocampal inputs[49] or to the affective information provided by the amygdala.[52]

DOPAMINE AND INFORMATION PROCESSING IN THE NUCLEUS ACCUMBENS

The NAcc receives a dense DA innervation[53] that has been shown to play a role in practically every function attributed to this brain region. Despite their importance, our knowledge of the actions of DA is obscured by the inconsistency of results obtained in the attempt to unveil their mechanisms. The concept of DA being a transmitter controlling information processing in the NAcc is beyond doubt. However, there is still considerable confusion regarding the actions of DA at a cellular level. It is common to envision this issue as a debate regarding whether DA is inhibitory or excitatory, with rather uncompelling evidence supporting either possibility. On the other hand, it is being increasingly apparent that this dichotomy is an oversim-

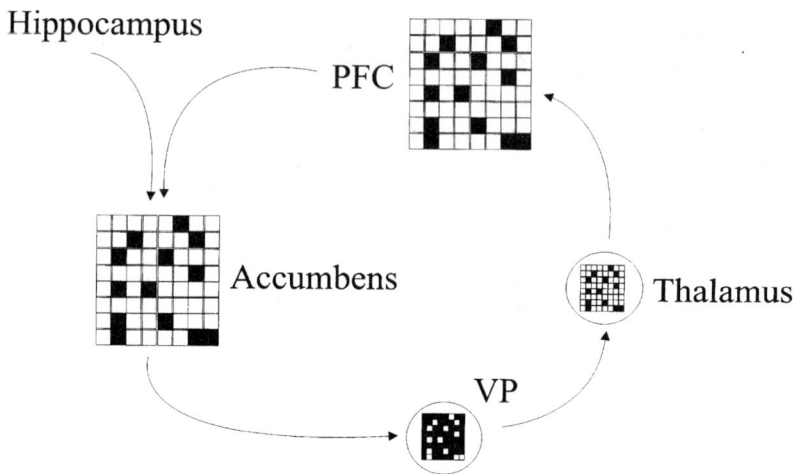

- Unit in the up state
- ☐ Unit in the down state

FIGURE 5. Ensemble coding in the nucleus accumbens. Information processing in the NAcc may be based on a sequence of neuronal ensembles that can be defined by the spatial distribution of neurons in their active, or up, state (black squares in the boxes representing NAcc and PFC neurons). A particular ensemble in the NAcc is determined by PFC afferent inputs and modulated by hippocampal inputs providing contextual and spatial information, and perhaps amygdaloid inputs providing affective information. This distribution of neurons in the up state will determine the activity of neurons in the ventral pallidum (VP) and MD thalamus, which in turn may exert control over activity states in PFC neurons.

plification of the actions of DA. Instead, more recent studies have provided evidence that DA is a modulatory agent that alters the functional impact of other afferent systems. Indeed, such a function may be commonplace for many G protein–linked receptors, which do not exert a direct control over ionic channels on their target neurons. Thus, although DA can be described as neither inhibitory nor excitatory, an alternate possibility could be that it is actually both. DA may have different effects on an individual neuron, depending not only on which receptor subtypes or which afferents it is affecting, but also on the state of the system. For example, DA may exert different actions depending on whether a neuron is in the up or down state of its membrane potential.

Dopaminergic Control of Nucleus Accumbens Cell Excitability

DA has a multiplicity of effects, many of which can affect information processing within the NAcc (FIG. 6). DA actions on NAcc neuron membrane potential are inconsistent, consisting of either depolarizing or hyperpolarizing responses.[54,55] However, a common finding is that action potential firing is more difficult to obtain in the

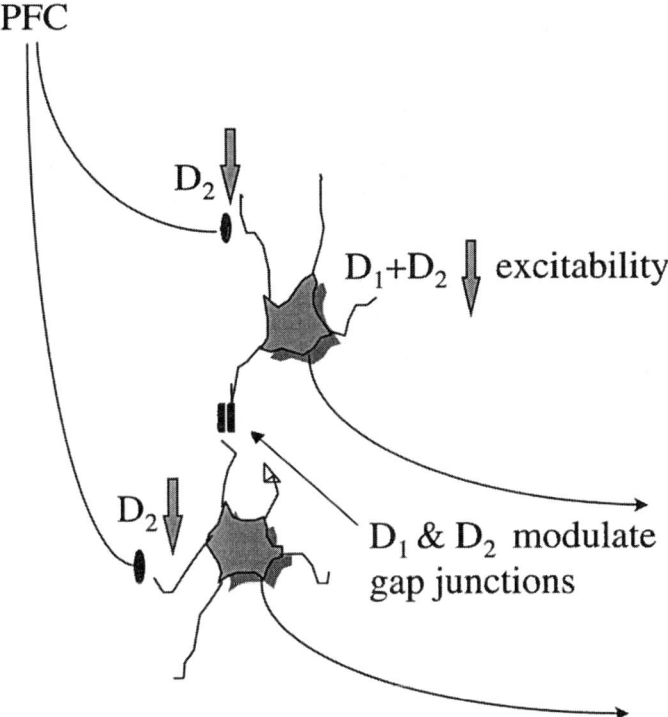

FIGURE 6. Actions of dopamine on information processing within the nucleus accumbens. DA effects with an impact on NAcc cell firing include (a) control of cell excitability mediated by D_1 and D_2 receptor coactivation; (b) presynaptic modulation of glutamatergic afferents via D_2 receptors in the case of PFC afferents and an atypical D_1 receptor in hippocampal afferents; and (c) control of gap junction permeability, with regional differences, including different DA receptor subtypes involved.

presence of DA agonists. *In vitro* studies have shown that the threshold for firing is moved to a more depolarized membrane potential[55,56] and the rheobase (i.e., the minimum amplitude of intracellularly injected current required to elicit an action potential) is increased[56,57] following administration of DA agonists. These results could be interpreted as DA's decreasing cell excitability in the NAcc. Although this may suggest an inhibitory effect, caution should be taken in interpreting these results. First, they are not observed in every cell tested. Second, these involve activation of NAcc neurons by intracellular injection of current; DA may have additional effects on the afferent-mediated activation that may cancel or even reverse any effect due to changes in membrane properties. Also, NAcc neurons recorded in the slice preparation may be the equivalent to a permanent down state, given their lack of spontaneous firing and their very negative membrane potential. In this regard, DA actions observed *in vitro* could provide information relevant to actions on NAcc neurons in the down state.

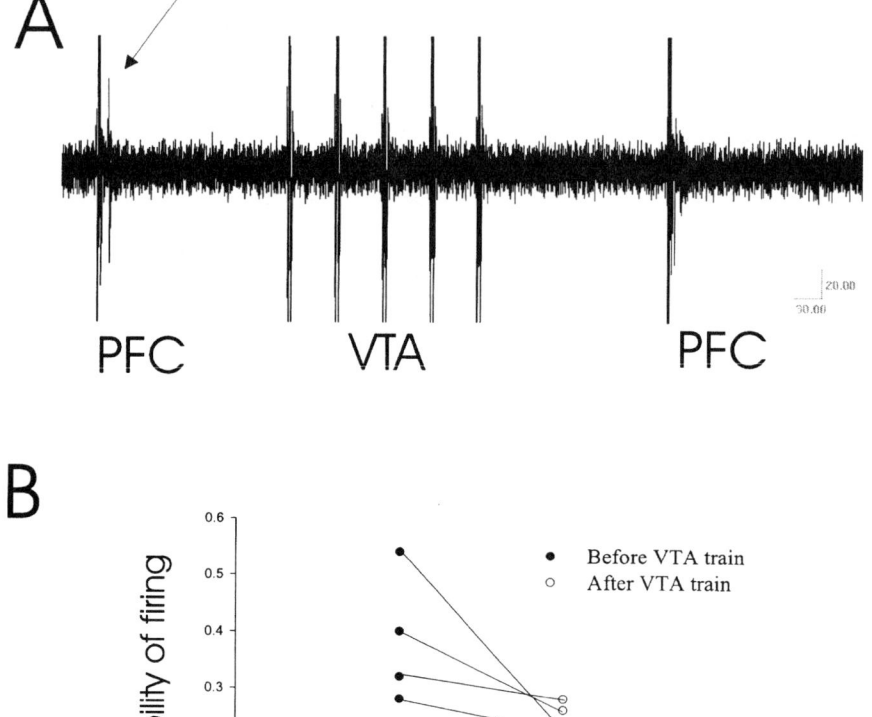

FIGURE 7. VTA stimulation decreases the probability of PFC-evoked action potential firing. **A:** Extracellular recording showing a spike (arrow) in response to a PFC stimulus that is followed by a train of stimuli to the VTA. A second stimulus to the PFC has a reduced probability to evoke action potential firing, as shown in **B**.

Dopamine Actions on Synaptic Responses

Cortical glutamatergic afferents to striatal regions possess presynaptic DA heteroreceptors that modulate glutamate release.[58,59] *In vivo* studies have suggested that DA may exert an inhibition of synaptic responses; in this sense, DA has been described as providing an increase in the signal-to-noise ratio.[60] Stimulation of the ventral tegmental area (VTA), which is the source of DA innervation to the NAcc, as well as the local DA application by iontophoresis, attenuated synaptic responses in NAcc neurons evoked by hippocampal stimulation[61] and amygdala stimulation.[62]

We have also found that VTA stimulation decreases the probability of spike firing elicited by PFC stimulation. During extracellular recordings from 13 NAcc neurons, VTA train stimulation (5 pulses of 0.1 ms, 0.1–1 mA at 20 Hz) was preceded and followed by single shocks to the medial PFC (0.1 ms, 0.1–1 mA). The stimulus intensity of the pretrain PFC stimulation was adjusted to elicit action potential firing in around one half of the trials. In seven of these neurons, the same stimulus intensity delivered after the VTA train stimulation was less likely to elicit spike discharge (FIG. 7). In these neurons, the probability of action potential firing following PFC stimulation was reduced from 0.32 ± 0.05 (mean $\pm$ SEM) to 0.21 ± 0.03 ($p = 0.03$, paired t-test). These results indicate that VTA stimulation may decrease the ability of PFC afferents to elicit synaptic responses that may reach threshold for action potential firing.

Similar experiments were performed using *in vivo* intracellular recordings from NAcc neurons. The amplitudes of PFC-evoked EPSP were compared before and after a train of stimuli was delivered to the VTA. In these experiments, the intensity of cortical stimulation was set to around one half of that needed to evoke an action potential. The ratio between the amplitudes of EPSP evoked by the second (post-VTA train) pulse to the PFC and the EPSP evoked by the first (pretrain) pulse was measured. In four neurons, this ratio was 0.75 ± 0.08 when all the stimuli were delivered during the down state or at very negative membrane potentials (-77.7 ± 11.1 mV), indicating that the amplitude of synaptic responses to PFC afferent stimulation was decreased in NAcc neurons in the down state following a burst of stimuli to the VTA (FIG. 8). The EPSP amplitudes had some variability from cell to cell, but even with this small sample, a paired t-test using raw amplitude values indicated a significant decrease (8.9 ± 2.8 mV before; 6.8 ± 2.2 mV after the train; $p = 0.04$, paired t-test).

In vitro studies in the NAcc shell have shown that D_1 receptor activation decreases synaptic responses to fornix stimulation, presumably by affecting hippocampal afferents.[63] In the core, our electrophysiological studies *in vitro* have shown that activation of D_2, but not D_1, receptors decreases synaptic responses elicited by PFC afferent activation.[64] On the other hand, other studies have reported that D_1 receptors may be involved in the DA-mediated decrease of synaptic responses in the NAcc.[65,66] However, these changes were blocked only by exceedingly high concentrations of the D_1 antagonist, SCH 23390,[66] and could not be affected by manipulations of adenylate cyclase,[65] suggesting that they may involve an atypical D_1

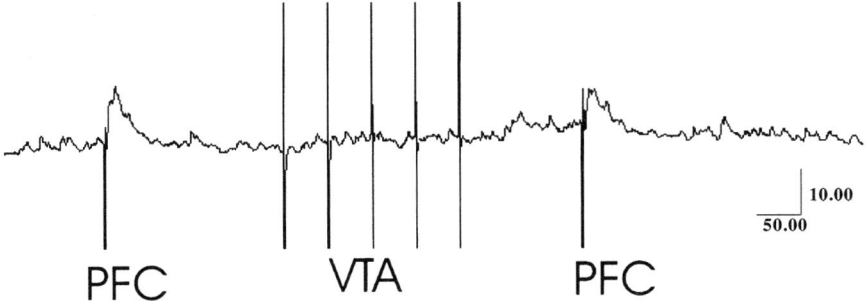

FIGURE 8. *In vivo* intracellular recordings from NAcc neurons using a combination of stimuli similar to that shown in FIG. 7 revealed a decreased amplitude in PFC-evoked EPSP following a train of stimuli to the VTA.

receptor. It now appears that this D_1-like receptor may reduce synaptic responses to hippocampal afferents, but not to cortical afferents[67] that are under D_2 DA control.[64]

Dopamine and Ensemble Coding in the Nucleus Accumbens

Overall, interpreting the net effect of DA on the activity of NAcc neurons presents several paradoxes. For instance, if as some data suggests, DA decreases cell excitability, how is it that DA agonists can be behavioral activators? Some authors have claimed that a general "inhibitory" action of DA could serve as a means to decrease background activity and therefore to increase signal-to-noise ratio.[56,68] In addition, although evidence has shown that DA cells fire "en bloc" upon presentation of behaviorally relevant stimuli,[69] there is also clear data showing that DA neurons exist in functionally distinct cell groups (i.e., motor vs. limbic). An alternative view about DA actions that emphasizes its influence on ensemble coding[49] may circumvent these conflicts. Thus, DA action may vary depending on the membrane potential, even within the same cell.

An elegant series of studies in Michael Levine's laboratory has revealed that D_1 and D_2 receptors may play different roles in the modulation of glutamatergic responses in striatal neurons and that the type of interaction depends on the glutamate receptor subtype involved. Thus, activation of D_1 receptors may enhance NMDA-mediated responses.[70] This is consistent with claims that D_1 receptors may be excitatory in nature.[71] A D_1-NMDA interaction will be substantially different between up and down states. At the very negative membrane potential that characterizes the down state, NMDA receptors are effectively blocked by Mg^{2+}, rendering D_1 receptors ineffective in this action. However, with the membrane depolarization characteristic of the up state, the Mg^{2+} blockade is partially removed, allowing for NMDA responses to be expressed and eventually to be increased by D_1 receptor activation. Thus, a D_1-NMDA interaction may only take place during up events, perhaps contributing to sustaining these depolarizations. Furthermore, D_1 receptors also enhance the activity of L-type Ca^{2+} channels,[45] another effect that may contribute to the sustained depolarization of the up state. On the other hand, activation of D_2 receptors may shunt AMPA-mediated responses. It is during the down state that this modulation can occur without being masked by NMDA activation. Thus, D_2 receptors may effectively attenuate synaptic responses during the down state and contribute to its persistence. In addition, DA can enhance the inwardly rectifying K^+ current that in medium spiny neurons may contribute to holding their membrane potential down. As a consequence, DA actions on glutamatergic transmission could have the effect of stabilizing the current state of the membrane in the neurons affected.

Preliminary data indicate that at least in the PFC, DA can act as a state stabilizer. It may be possible that a similar mechanism exists in the NAcc, although this remains to be studied. As an initial step to address this issue, experiments were performed with VTA stimulation as a means to elicit DA release. In these experiments, neurons were recorded from the PFC, an area that also has neurons with a bistable membrane potential and receives DA innervation from the VTA. *In vivo* intracellular recordings from 17 neurons located in the medial or orbital PFC were performed in anesthetized rats. Immunostaining with Neurobiotin, a marker injected into the cells at the end of the recording session, revealed that these were pyramidal neurons. Nine out of 17 neurons recorded exhibited a bistable membrane potential (down state: −81.3 ±

5.7 mV; up state: −67.1 ± 7.8 mV). Electrical stimulation of the VTA elicited a variety of responses in PFC neurons, depending on whether the neuron was in the up or down state at the time of stimulation. Only neurons with a bistable membrane potential showed responses to VTA stimulation.[78,79] During the up state, the most common response was the permanency of the cell in the up state for more than 100 ms, and during the down state, a brief and small EPSP was followed by a return to the down state (FIG. 9). Stimulation of VTA with a train of pulses elicited similar responses. These results suggest that DA may have different effects depending on the membrane potential of the PFC pyramidal neurons and that in most cases DA may act as a state stabilizer.[78,79]

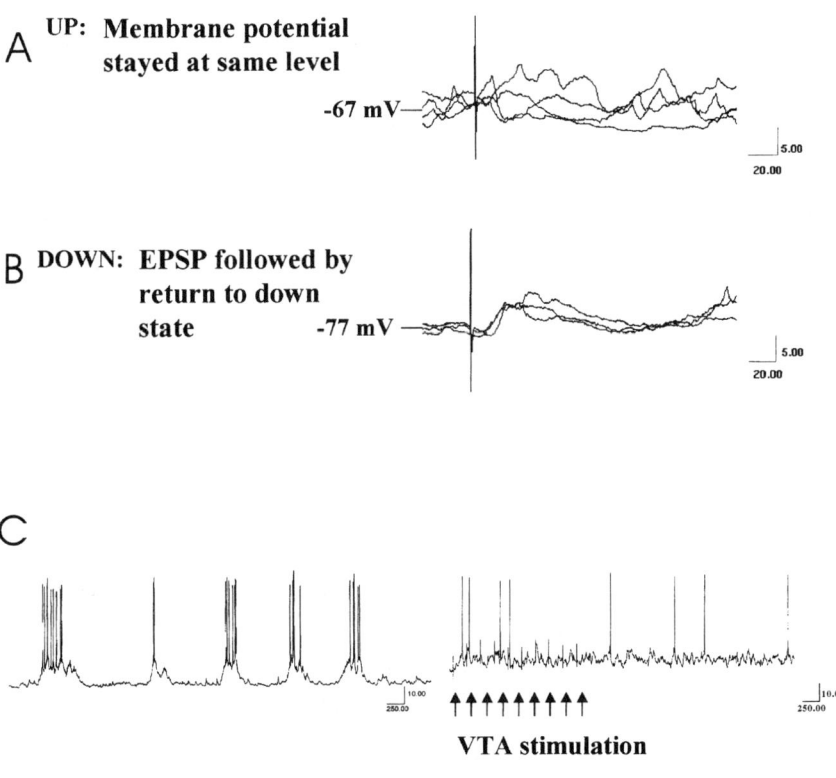

FIGURE 9. In PFC pyramidal neurons, VTA stimulation exhibited a variety of responses. In cells with up and down states in their membrane potential, the most common response was a long-lasting permanence in the state at which the neuron was during VTA stimulation. **A:** Overlay of responses to VTA stimulation obtained from a medial PFC pyramidal cell during the up state. **B:** Overlay of tracings from the same neuron during the down state, showing a brief EPSP followed by a return to the down state. **C:** A train of stimuli to the VTA elicited long-lasting responses; the tracings show the membrane potential from a bistable pyramidal neuron before (left) and during (right) a VTA train stimulation. In this case, the membrane potential stayed in the up state for several seconds.

Since DA is released massively in the striatum and NAcc upon presentation of behaviorally relevant stimuli,[69] this DA message may be interpreted as fixing the state of a distributed set of neurons in these areas; in other words, DA may reinforce a distributed pattern of activation (or ensemble) that may, for example, be associated with appetitive or aversive stimuli.[49] This may be an important mechanism involved in the learning processes in which DA cell firing plays a role. For example, upon successfully learning a task, DA cell activation switches from being reward related to being conditioning-stimulus related.[72] Although highly speculative, this could be interpreted as the DA signal tagging an ensemble that can be associated with obtaining a reward-predicting stimulus and, therefore, reflecting a behavioral pattern that is worth reinforcing.

Gap Junctions and Ensemble Coding

Neuronal ensembles in the NAcc can be defined by a distributed set of neurons in the up state at any given moment. To be functionally meaningful, these up events may require some extent of synchronization. This can be accomplished by the cell-to-cell transfer of information via gap junctions, a mechanism that can allow for a transfer of slow electrical signals, including "up" events, between coupled cells. Furthermore, gap junction permeability is tightly modulated by a number of factors, including dopamine,[73] nitric oxide, and cortical inputs,[74] allowing for fine-tuning of this synchronization of up events.

Although studies attempting to establish the presence of connexin (gap junction protein) or a typical seven-layer electron microscopic image in the brain have not been conclusive regarding their presence in the NAcc, electron microscopy studies have found cell pairings within the NAcc with close membrane appositions (30–90 nm gap) similar to those seen in gap junctions.[75] The difficulties in ascertaining connexins within the NAcc could reflect either a remote site of contact (such as dendrodendritic) or a sparse distribution of connexin channels.

CLINICAL IMPLICATIONS

Current hypotheses of schizophrenia emphasize the presence of temporal lobe (hippocampal) disturbances, hypofrontality, and altered DA systems, among others. The NAcc is a brain region in which each of these systems may interact. Specifically, the convergence of PFC, hippocampal, and DA inputs in this region may provide mechanisms, such as the gating of PFC throughput by limbic afferents, which could become disturbed in schizophrenia. There is also indirect evidence supporting the idea that the hippocampal drive of up events in the NAcc may be affected in schizophrenia. Phencyclidine, perhaps the best pharmacological model of schizophrenia, can reduce the frequency and duration of up events when administered systemically while recording from bistable NAcc neurons.[34] Furthermore, intracellular recordings from NAcc neurons in animals that had received PCP provided a smaller proportion of bistable neurons.[34] These results indicate that this NMDA channel blocker, a psychotomimetic that can reproduce endogenous symptoms in schizophrenics, may exert its action via interfering with the hippocampal gating of up events in NAcc neurons; this could be a neurochemical model that reflects the pathophysiological disturbance caused by a hippocampal deficit in the schizophrenic brain.

The control over the flow of information discussed here can be a means by which a putative developmental hippocampal deficit could cause hypofrontality.[76] Neonatal hippocampal pathology and the consequent disturbance in PFC architecture may result in altered ensemble coding in the NAcc. When coupled with a pathological increase in phasic activity of DA systems,[77] an excessive reinforcement of inappropriate ensembles may arise, thereby giving rise to the positive symptoms of the schizophrenia psychosis.[16]

ACKNOWLEDGMENT

This work was supported by NIH Grant MH57683.

REFERENCES

1. SALAMONE, J.D. 1991. Behavioral pharmacology of dopamine systems: a new synthesis. In The Mesolimbic Dopamine System: From Motivation to Action. P. Willner & J. Scheel-Krüger, Eds.: 599–613. J. Wiley & Sons. New York.
2. HEIMER, L. & G.F. ALHEID. 1991. Piecing together the basal forebrain puzzle. In The Basal Forebrain. Anatomy to Function. T.C. Napier, P.W. Kalivas & I. Hanin, Eds.: 1–42. Plenum. New York.
3. HEIMER, L. et al. 1995. Specificity in the projection patterns of accumbal core and shell in the rat. Neuroscience **41:** 89–125.
4. JONGEN-RÊLO, A.L., P. VOORN & H.J. GROENEWEGEN. 1994. Immunohistochemical characterization of the shell and core territories of the nucleus accumbens in the rat. Eur. J. Neurosci. **6:** 1255–1264.
5. MEREDITH, G.E., C.M.A. PENNARTZ & H.J. GROENEWEGEN. 1993. The cellular framework for chemical signalling in the nucleus accumbens. In Chemical Signaling in the Basal Ganglia. G.W. Arbuthnott & P.C. Emson, Eds. :3–24. Elsevier. Amsterdam.
6. MALDONADO-IRIZARRY, C.S., C.J. SWANSON & A.E. KELLEY. 1995. Glutamate receptors in the nucleus accumbens shell control feeding behavior via the lateral hypothalamus. J. Neurosci. **15:** 6779–6788.
7. DAMSMA, G. et al. 1992. Sexual behavior increases dopamine transmission in the nucleus accumbens and striatum of male rats: comparison with novelty and locomotion. Behav. Neurosci. **106:** 181–191.
8. COLLE, L.M. & R.A. WISE. 1988. Effects of nucleus accumbens amphetamine on lateral hypothalamic brain stimulation reward. Brain Res. **459:** 361–368.
9. SCHULTZ, W. et al. 1992. Neuronal activity in monkey ventral striatum related to the expectation of reward. J. Neurosci. **12:** 4595–4610.
10. CARELLI, R.M. et al. 1993. Firing patterns of nucleus accumbens neurons during cocaine self-administration in rats. Brain Res. **626:** 14–22.
11. PEOPLES, L.L. & M.O. WEST. 1996. Phasic firing of single neurons in the rat nucleus accumbens correlated with the timing of intravenous cocaine self-administration. J. Neurosci. **15:** 3459–3473.
12. ABERCROMBIE, E.A. et al. 1989. Differential effect of stress on in vivo dopamine release in striatum, nucleus accumbens and medial prefrontal cortex. J. Neurochem. **52:** 1655–1658.
13. ANNETT, L.E., A. MCGREGOR & T.W. ROBBINS. 1989. The effects of ibotenic acid lesions of the nucleus accumbens on spatial learning and extinction in the rat. Behav. Brain Res. **31:** 231–242.

14. O'DONNELL, P. & A.A. GRACE. 1996. Basic physiology of antipsychotic drug action. In Handbook of Experimental Pharmacology: Antipsychotics. J.G. Csernansky, Ed.: 163–202. Springer-Verlag. Berlin.
15. WAN, F.-J. & N.R. SWERDLOW. 1996. Sensorimotor gating in rats is regulated by different dopamine-glutamate interactions in the nucleus accumbens core and shell subregions. Brain Res. **722:** 168–176.
16. O'DONNELL, P. & A.A. GRACE. 1998. Dysfunctions in multiple interrelated systems as the neurobiological bases of schizophrenic symptom clusters. Schizophr. Bull. **24:** 267–283.
17. GROENEWEGEN, H.J. & H.W. BERENDSE. 1994. Anatomical relationships between the prefrontal cortex and the basal ganglia in the rat. In Motor and Cognitive Functions of the Prefrontal Cortex. A.-M. Thierry, Ed.: 51–77. Springer-Verlag: Berlin.
18. GROENEWEGEN, H.J., C.I. WRIGHT & A.V.J. BEIJER. 1996. The nucleus accumbens: gateway for limbic structures to reach the motor system? Prog. Brain Res. **107:** 485–511.
19. NAUTA, W.J.H. et al. 1978. Efferent connections and nigral afferents of the nucleus accumbens septi in the rat. Neuroscience **3:** 385–401.
20. ZAHM, D.S., E. WILLIAMS & C. WOHLTMANN. 1996. Ventral striatopallidothalamic projection: IV. Relative involvements of neurochemically distinct subterritories in the ventral pallidum and adjacent parts of the rostroventral forebrain. J. Comp. Neurol. **364:** 340–362.
21. O'DONNELL, P. et al. 1997. Interconnected parallel circuits between rat nucleus accumbens and thalamus revealed by retrograde transynaptic transport of pseudo-rabies virus. J. Neurosci. **17:** 2143–2167.
22. MAURICE, N. et al. 1997. Position of the ventral pallidum in the rat prefrontal cortex-basal ganglia circuit. Neuroscience **80:** 323–334.
23. LAVÍN, A. & A.A. GRACE. 1994. The modulation of mediodorsal and dorsal thalamic nuclei by the ventral pallidum: its role in the regulation of thalamocortical activity in the basal ganglia. Synapse **18:** 104–127.
24. SESACK, S.R. et al. 1989. Topographical organization of the efferent projections of the medial prefrontal cortex in the rat: an anterograde tract-tracing study with Phaseolus vulgaris leucoagglutinin. J. Comp. Neurol. **290:** 213–242.
25. NAUTA, W.J.H. 1979. Expanding borders of the limbic system concept. In Functional Neurosurgery. T. Rasmunssen & P. Marino, Eds.: 7–23. Raven. New York.
26. GROENEWEGEN, H.J., N.E.H.M. BECKER & A.H.M. LOHMAN. 1980. Subcortical afferents of the nucleus accumbens septi in the cat, studied with retrograde axonal transport of horseradish peroxidase and bisbenzimid. Neuroscience **5:** 1903–1916.
27. KELLEY, A.E. & V.B. DOMESICK. 1982. The distribution of the projection from the hippocampal formation to the nucleus accumbens in the rat: an anterograde- and retrograde-horseradish peroxidase study. Neuroscience **7:** 2321–2335.
28. FINCH, D.M. et al. 1995. Neurophysiology and neuropharmacology of projections from entorhinal cortex to striatum in the rat. Brain Res. **670:** 233–247.
29. TOTTERDELL, S. & G.E. MEREDITH. 1997. Topographical organization of projections from the entorhinal cortex to the striatum of the rat. Neuroscience **78:** 715–729.
30. GROENEWEGEN, H.J. et al. 1991. Functional anatomy of the ventral, limbic system-innervated striatum. In The Mesolimbic Dopamine System: From Motivation to Action. P. Willner & J. Scheel-Kruger, Eds.: 19–59. J. Wiley. New York.
31. FINCH, D.M. 1996. Neurophysiology of converging synaptic inputs from the rat prefrontal cortex, amygdala, midline thalamus, and hippocampal formation onto single neurons of the caudate/putamen and nucleus accumbens. Hippocampus **6:** 495–512.
32. O'DONNELL, P. & A.A. GRACE. 1995. Synaptic interactions among excitatory afferents to nucleus accumbens neurons: hippocampal gating of prefrontal cortical input. J. Neurosci. **15:** 3622–3639.
33. PLENZ, D. & A. AERTSEN. 1994. The basal ganglia: "Minimal coherence detection" in cortical activity distributions. In The Basal Ganglia IV. New Ideas and Data on Structure and Function. G. Percheron, J. McKenzie & J. Féger, Eds.: 579–588. Plenum. New York.

34. O'DONNELL, P. & A.A. GRACE. 1998. Phencyclidine interferes with the hippocampal gating of nucleus accumbens neuronal activity *in vivo*. Neuroscience. **87:** 823–830.
35. WILSON, C.J. & P.M. GROVES. 1981. Spontaneous firing patterns of identified spiny neurons in the rat neostriatum. Brain Res. **220:** 67–80.
36. YIM, C.Y. & G.J. MOGENSON. 1988. Neuromodulatory action of dopamine in the nucleus accumbens: an *in vivo* intracellular study. Neuroscience **26:** 403–415.
37. MOGENSON, G.J. & C.Y. YIM. 1981. Electrophysiological and neuropharmacological-behavioral studies of the nucleus accumbens: implications for its role as a limbic-motor interface. *In* The Neurobiology of the Nucleus Accumbens. R.B. Chronister & J.F. DeFrance, Eds.: 210–229. Hauer Institute. Brunswick, ME.
38. O'DONNELL, P. & A.A. GRACE. 1993. Physiological and morphological properties of accumbens core and shell neurons recorded *in vitro*. Synapse **13:** 135–160.
39. CHANG, H.T. & S.T. KITAI. 1986. Intracellular recordings from rat nucleus accumbens neurons in vitro. Brain Res. **366:** 392–396.
40. UCHIMURA, N., E. CHERUBINI & R.A. NORTH. 1989. Inward rectification in rat nucleus accumbens neurons. J. Neurophysiol. **62:** 1280–1286.
41. DEFRANCE, J.F. *et al.* 1985. Characterization of fimbria input to nucleus accumbens. J. Neurophysiol. **54:** 1553–1567.
42. GABEL, L.A. & E.S. NISENBAUM. 1998. Biophysical characterization and functional consequences of a slowly inactivating potassium current in neostriatal neurons. J. Neurophysiol. **79:** 1989–2002.
43. WILSON, C.J. & Y. KAWAGUCHI. 1996. The origins of two-state spontaneous membrane potential fluctuations of neostriatal spiny neurons. J. Neurosci. **16:** 2397–2410.
44. CEPEDA, C. *et al.* 1995. Persistent Na^+ conductance in medium-sized neostriatal neurons: characterization using infrared videomicroscopy and whole cell patch clamp recordings. J. Neurophysiol. **74:** 1343–1348.
45. HERNÁNDEZ-LÓPEZ, S. *et al.* 1997. D_1 receptor activation enhances evoked discharge in neostriatal medium spiny neurons by modulating an L-type Ca^{2+} conductance. J. Neurosci. **17:** 3334–3342.
46. CSERNANSKY, J.G. *et al.* 1988. Mesolimbic dopamine receptor increases two weeks following hippocampal kindling. Brain Res. **449:** 357–360.
47. LIPSKA, B.L. *et al.* 1998. Neonatal damage of the rat ventral hippocampus reduces expression of a dopamine transporter [abstract]. Soc. Neurosci. Abstr. **24:** 356.
48. PENNARTZ, C.M.A., H.J. GROENEWEGEN & F.H. LOPES DA SILVA. 1994. The nucleus accumbens as a complex of functionally distinct neuronal ensembles: an integration of behavioural, electrophysiological and anatomical data. Prog. Neurobiol. **42:** 719–761.
49. O'DONNELL, P. 1998. Ensemble coding in the nucleus accumbens. Psychobiology. In press.
50. DEADWYLER, S.A. & R.E. HAMPSON. 1995. Ensemble activity and behavior: What's the code? Science **270:** 1316–1318.
51. EICHENBAUM, H. *et al.* 1989. The organization of spatial coding in the hippocampus: a study of neural ensemble activity. J. Neurosci. **9:** 2764–2775.
52. GRACE, A.A. & H.M. MOORE. 1996. Gap junction inactivation in the striatum prevents oral stereotypy induced by apomorphine [abstract]. Soc. Neurosci. Abstr. **22:** 405.
53. JOHANSSON, O. & T. HÖKFELT. 1981. Nucleus accumbens: transmitter histochemistry with special reference to peptide-containing neurons. *In* The Neurobiology of the Nucleus Accumbens. R.B. Chronister & J.F. DeFrance, Eds.: 147–171. Hauer Institute. Brunswick, ME.
54. UCHIMURA, N., H. HIGASHI & S. NISHI. 1986. Hyperpolarizing and depolarizing actions of dopamine via D-1 and D-2 receptors on nucleus accumbens neurons. Brain Res. **375:** 368–372.
55. AKAIKE, A. *et al.* 1987. Excitatory and inhibitory effects of dopamine on neural activity of the caudate nucleus neurons *in vitro*. Brain Res. **418:** 262–272.
56. O'DONNELL, P. & A.A. GRACE. 1996. Dopaminergic reduction of excitability in nucleus accumbens neurons recorded *in vitro*. Neuropsychopharmacology **15:** 87–98.

57. ZHANG, X.-F., X.-T. HU & F.J. WHITE. 1998. Whole-cell plasticity in cocaine withdrawal: reduced sodium currents in nucleus accumbens neurons. J. Neurosci. **18:** 488–498.
58. GODUKHIN, O.V., A.D. ZHARIKOVA & A.Y. BUDANSTEV. 1984. Role of presynaptic dopamine receptors in regulation of the glutamatergic neurotransmission in rat neostriatum. Neuroscience **12:** 377–383.
59. FILLOUX, F. et al. 1988. Selective cortical infarction reduces [3H]sulpiride binding in rat caudate-putamen: autoradiographic evidence for presynaptic D_2 receptors on corticostriate terminals. Synapse (NY) **2:** 521–531.
60. DEFRANCE, J.F., R.W. SIKES & R.B. CHRONISTER. 1985. Dopamine action in the nucleus accumbens. J. Neurophysiol. **54:** 1568–1577.
61. YANG, C.R. & G.J. MOGENSON. 1984. Electrophysiological responses of neurones in the accumbens nucleus to hippocampal stimulation and the attenuation of the excitatory responses by the mesolimbic dopaminergic system. Brain Res. **324:** 69–84.
62. YIM, C.Y. & G.J. MOGENSON. 1982. Response of nucleus accumbens neurons to amygdala stimulation and its modification by dopamine. Brain Res. **239:** 401–415.
63. PENNARTZ, C.M.A. et al. 1992. Presynaptic dopamine D_1 receptors attenuate excitatory and inhibitory limbic inputs to the shell region of the rat nucleus accumbens. J. Neurophysiol. **67:** 1325–1334.
64. O'DONNELL, P. & A.A. GRACE. 1994. Tonic D_2-mediated attenuation of cortical excitation in nucleus accumbens neurons recorded in vitro. Brain Res. **634:** 105–112.
65. HARVEY, J. & M.G. LACEY. 1996. Endogenous and exogenous dopamine depress EPSCs in rat nucleus accumbens in vitro via D_1 receptor activation. J. Physiol. **492:** 143–154.
66. NICOLA, S.M., S.B. KOMBIAN & R.C. MALENKA. 1996. Psychostimulants depress excitatory synaptic transmission in the nucleus accumbens via presynaptic D1-like dopamine receptors. J. Neurosci. **16:** 1591–1604.
67. NICOLA, S.M. & R.C. MALENKA. 1998. Modulation of synaptic transmission by dopamine and norepinephrine in ventral but not dorsal striatum. J. Neurophysiol. **79:** 1768–1776.
68. KIYATKIN, E.A. & G.V. REBEC. 1996. Dopaminergic modulation of glutamate-induced excitations of neurons in the neostriatum and nucleus accumbens of awake, unrestrained rats. J. Neurophysiol. **75:** 142–153.
69. SCHULTZ, W. 1992. Activity of dopamine neurons in the behaving primate. Semin. Neurosciences **4:** 129–138.
70. LEVINE, M.S. et al. 1996. Neuromodulatory actions of dopamine on synaptically-evoked neostriatal responses in slices. Synapse **24:** 65–78.
71. GONON, F. 1997. Prolonged and extrasynaptic excitatory action of dopamine mediated by D1 receptors in the rat striatum in vivo. J. Neurosci. **17:** 5972–5978.
72. SCHULTZ, W., P. APICELLA & T. LJUNGBERG. 1993. Responses of monkey dopamine neurons to reward and conditioned stimuli during successive steps of learning a delayed response task. J. Neurosci. **13:** 900–913.
73. O'DONNELL, P. & A.A. GRACE. 1993. Dopaminergic modulation of dye coupling between neurons in the core and shell regions of the nucleus accumbens. J. Neurosci. **13:** 3456–3471.
74. O'DONNELL, P. & A.A. GRACE. 1997. Cortical afferents modulate striatal gap junction permeability via nitric oxide. Neuroscience **76:** 1–5.
75. DOMESICK, V.B. 1981. Further observations on the anatomy of nucleus accumbens and caudatoputamen in the rat: similarities and contrasts. In The Neurobiology of the Nucleus Accumbens. R.B. Chronister & J.F. DeFrance, Eds. Hauer Institute. Brunswick, ME.
76. WEINBERGER, D.R. & B.K. LIPSKA. 1995. Cortical maldevelopment, anti-psychotic drugs, and schizophrenia: a search for common ground. Schizophr. Res. **16:** 87–110.
77. GRACE, A.A. 1991. Phasic versus tonic dopamine release and the modulation of dopamine system responsivity: A hypothesis for the etiology of schizophrenia. Neuroscience **41:** 1–24.

78. O'DONNELL, P. & B.L. LEWIS. 1998. Dopaminergic control of prefrontal cortical activity: effect of VTA stimulation on bistable membrane potential of prefrontal cortical pyramidal neurons. Presented at the "Dopamine 98" meeting. Strasbourg, France. July 25, 1998.
79. LEWIS, B.L. & P. O'DONNELL. 1998. Effects of VTA stimulation of prefrontal cortex neurons recorded *in vivo* [abstract]. Soc. Neurosci. Abstr. **24:** 656.
80. MEREDITH, G.E., F.G. WOUTERLOOD & A. PATTISELANO. 1990 Hippocampal fibers make synaptic contacts with glutamate decarboxylase-immunoreactive neurons in the rat nucleus accumbens. Brain Res. **513:** 329–334.
81. WILSON, C.J. 1995. The contribution of cortical neurons to the firing pattern of striatal spiny neurons. *In* Models of Information Processing in the Basal Ganglia. J.C. Houk, J.L. Davis & D.G. Beiser, Eds.: 29–50. MIT Press. Cambridge, MA.

Opioid Modulation of Ventral Pallidal Inputs

T. CELESTE NAPIER[a] AND IGOR MITROVIC[b]

Department of Pharmacology and Experimental Therapeutics, Neuroscience and Aging Institute, Division for Research on Drugs of Abuse, Loyola University Chicago, Stritch School of Medicine, Maywood, Illinois 60153, USA

ABSTRACT: While the ventral pallidum (VP) is known to be important in relaying information between the nucleus accumbens and target structures, it has become clear that substantial information processing occurs within the VP. We evaluated the possibility that opioid modulation of other transmitters contained in VP afferents is involved in this process. Initially, we demonstrated that opioids hyperpolarized VP neurons *in vitro* and suppressed spontaneous firing *in vivo*. The ability of opioids to modulate other transmitters was determined using microiontophoretically applied ligands and extracellular recordings of VP neurons from chloral hydrate–anesthetized rats. With neurons that responded to iontophoresed opioid agonists, the ejection current was reduced to a level that was below that necessary to alter spontaneous firing. This "subthreshold" current was used to determine the ability of mu opioid receptor (μR) agonists to alter VP responses to endogenous (released by electrical activation of afferents) and exogenous (iontophoretically applied) transmitters. μR agonists decreased the variability and enhanced the acuity (e.g., "signal-to-noise" relationship) of VP responses to activation of glutamatergic inputs from the prefrontal cortex and amygdala. By contrast, μR agonists attenuated both the slow excitatory responses to substance P and GABA-induced inhibitions that resulted from activating the nucleus accumbens. Subthreshold opioids also attenuated inhibitory responses to stimulating midbrain dopaminergic cells. These results suggest that a consequence of opioid transmission in the VP is to negate the influence of some afferents (e.g., midbrain dopamine and accumbal GABA and substance P) while selectively potentiating the efficacy of others (e.g., cortical and amygdaloid glutamate). Interpreted in the context of opiate abuse, μR opioids in the VP may serve to diminish the influence of reinforcement (ventral tegmental area and nucleus accumbens) in the transduction of cognition (prefrontal cortex) and affect (amygdala) into behavior. This may contribute to drug craving that occurs even in the absence of reward.

Since the seminal paper by Heimer and Wilson[1] introducing the concept of the ventral striatopallidal system, the anatomy and the morphology of afferents to the ventral pallidum (VP) have enjoyed considerable attention (see other chapters in this volume). Pioneered by Mogenson,[2] a handful of laboratories now have described the

---

[a]Address for correspondence: T. Celeste Napier, Ph.D., Department of Pharmacology and Experimental Therapeutics, Loyola University Chicago, 2160 South 1st Avenue, Maywood, Illinois 60153. Voice: 708-216-8427; fax: 708-216-6596; cnapier@luc.edu

[b]Current address: Department of Anatomy and W. M. Keck Center for Integrative Neuroscience, University of California San Francisco, San Francisco, CA 94143.

behavioral consequences of activating various transmitter systems in the VP. It is becoming clear that motor behaviors (for a review, see ref. 3), reward,[4-7] and sensory information processing[8,9] are subserved by the VP. The position of the VP at the confluence of motor and limbic systems and its role in the aforementioned behaviors suggest its relevance in the integration of these brain systems and the regulation of motivated behavior. Working from the premise that the integrative function of the VP should have a physiological substrate at the level of the single VP neuron, a primary effort of our laboratory has focused on assessing the interactions among the neurotransmitter systems found in major VP afferents.

The nucleus accumbens region of the ventral striatum (NAc) provides a substantial input to the VP, and this projection contains GABA, substance P, and opioid peptides (for reviews, see refs. 10–12). Excitatory amino acids, most likely glutamate, are contained in VP afferents arising from several cortical regions, including the medial prefrontal cortex and the basolateral nucleus of the amygdala.[13,14] Dopamine-containing projections from both the substantia nigra and ventral tegmental area are also well described (for a review, see ref. 15). Immunohistochemical and receptor binding studies have demonstrated the presence of the receptors for these neurotransmitter systems within the VP (for a review, see ref. 3). In our assessments of afferent interactions, we used various ligands in conjunction with the endogenous transmitter to evaluate the receptor pharmacology of these interactions.

Electrophysiological[16-18] experiments evidence the potent effects of activating the VP mu opioid receptors (μR). Behavioral studies indicate the importance of the μR in motor-[19] and reward-[20,21] related functions. In other brain regions, the μR is known to modulate the effects of activating nonopioid receptors (e.g., refs. 22,23). Thus, we focused on the ability of the μR system to influence the signals generated by various VP afferents.

Before describing μR modulation of VP afferents, it is useful to overview what is known about opioid physiology in the VP. As this series of studies represents the first descriptions of the functional physiology of transmitter-specific inputs to the VP, the physiology of each will be briefly described.

ELECTROPHYSIOLOGICAL RESPONSES OF VP NEURONS TO OPIOID AGONISTS

The firing rate of VP neurons is consistently decreased with systemically administered morphine (threshold = 0.25 mg/kg; ED_{50} = 1 mg/kg iv) in anesthetized rats (FIG. 1).[18] By contrast, morphine (0.4–12.8 mg/kg iv; $ED_{50} \approx$ 1 mg/kg) increases firing of ventral tegmental area neurons,[24,25] and this is thought to be a consequence of opioids hyperpolarizing local inhibitory interneurons.[26] Morphine (2.5 mg/kg iv) increases and decreases in the firing of NAc neurons; these differential effects may be related to neuronal subpopulations.[27,28] The similarity in potency among neurons in the ventral tegmental area-NAc-VP circuit provides for the possibility that morphine-induced changes in the VP may reflect an alteration in VP inputs. Moreover, as 1 mg/kg morphine is reinforcing in rats,[29,30] these results also concur with the concept that changes in neuronal activity in this mesolimbic system are involved in the reinforcing effects of opiate administration. These observations lend behavioral

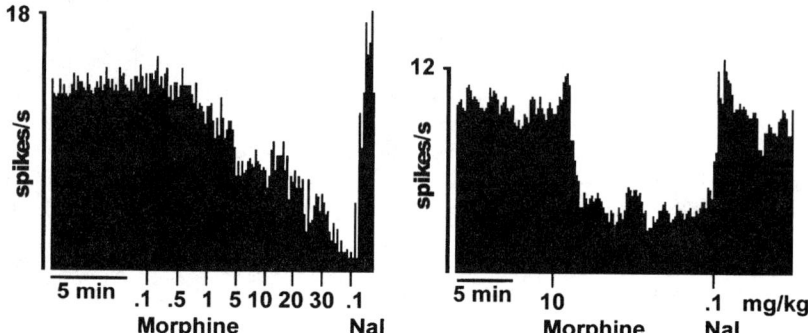

FIGURE 1. Rate histograms illustrating VP neuronal effects of iv-administered morphine and antagonism of these responses by iv naloxone (Nal). Twenty of 22 neurons (91%) tested with iv-administered morphine demonstrated rate changes, with suppression being the most consistent response ($n = 18$). *Left:* A representative cumulative dose-response histogram. These repeated injections produced a dose-related effect with an E_{max} of 73% below control and an ED_{50} of 1 mg/kg iv. *Right:* Suppression observed with a single 10 mg/kg injection of morphine, the magnitude of which was not different from that produced by a cumulative dose of 10 mg/kg (65 ± 5.7% and 59 ± 8.5% below control, respectively). These results verify that an acute desensitization (i.e., tachyphylaxis) did not contribute to the pharmacological profile of the response obtained with rapidly repeated morphine injections. (Napier *et al.*[18] With permission from John Wiley & Sons, Inc.)

relevance to studies on opioid modulation of NAc and ventral tegmental area inputs in the VP (described below).

More recent experiments in our laboratory evaluated morphine-induced effects on VP neurons in forebrain slices using intracellular recording, under current clamp conditions.[31] Bath application of 1–100 μM morphine generally produced a concentration-dependent hyperpolarization and decreased the number of spikes evoked by depolarizing currents (FIG. 2). These studies were conducted without blocking synaptic activity; thus spontaneous postsynaptic potentials (EPSPs and IPSPs) and spiking occurred. Morphine inhibited both. The morphine-induced responses were attenuated by naloxone (1–10 μM; see FIG. 2). Analysis of the change in current/voltage relationships elicited by 10 μM morphine indicated that morphine increased K^+ conductance. As the μR has consistently been shown to open G protein–coupled inwardly rectifying K^+ channels,[32] it is likely that a similar action is involved in morphine-induced effects in VP cells. The opiate effects also could involve μR-mediated inhibition of Ca^{2+} channels[32,33] located on nerve terminals within the VP. Moreover, because these recordings were conducted in sagittal slices that contained both the NAc and VP, it is possible that some of the VP responses resulted from opiate effects on NAc neurons that altered the accumbal inputs to the VP that were left in tact in the slice preparation.

To determine whether the opioid receptors that mediate morphine-induced effects were indeed located within the VP itself, the opiate was applied directly within the vicinity of the recorded neurons using microiontophoresis in *in vivo* electrophysiological experiments. Iontophoretically applied morphine increased and decreased VP cell firing (FIG. 3).[16–18] The responses were blocked by naloxone (FIG. 3), veri-

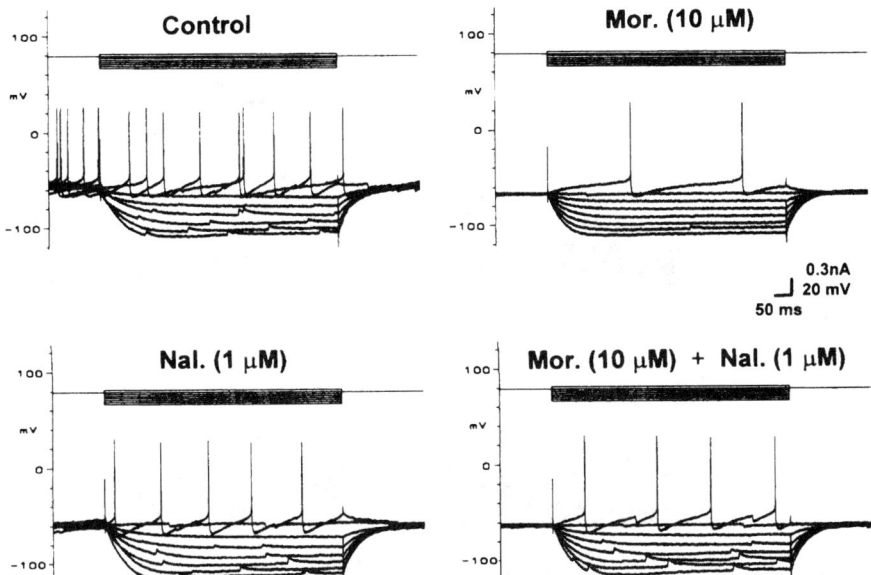

FIGURE 2. Intracellular recordings from a VP neuron demonstrating the effects of morphine (Mor), naloxone (Nal), and their coapplication. During morphine administration (10 μM; upper right panel), the membrane potential was hyperpolarized and the occurrence frequency of postsynaptic potentials and spiking was decreased. These effects lasted for at least 10 minutes (data not shown), and even when naloxone was administered (1 μM, given alone 10 minutes postmorphine; lower left panel), this was not sufficient to return the electrophysiological parameters back to control levels. However, when this concentration of naloxone was subsequently coapplied with morphine, the effects of the agonist were substantially reduced (lower right panel). This reduction was not due to tachyphalaxis, as repeated morphine administration on these cells induced consistent responding (data not shown, but see also FIG. 1).

fying that opioid receptors were involved in both response types. These observations were in contrast to what would be predicted by the results obtained when extra-VP regions were exposed to morphine (as in bath applications with forebrain slices and iv administration *in vivo*). Comparisons of the data obtained with the various routes of opiate administration reveal potential mechanisms that may underlie these response differences: (1) Microiontophoretic application of morphine altered firing in a fewer number of VP neurons as compared to iv administration (e.g., 57–78% vs. 91%, respectively).[16–18,34] This phenomenon would occur if some VP neurons that do not express μR are "downstream" to neurons that do express these receptors. Candidates for these afferent inputs include the NAc, the amygdala, and the ventral tegmental area (e.g., refs. 24, 25, 28, and 35–37). As mentioned previously, the doses of iv morphine tested for the VP also alter neuronal activity in the ventral tegmental area and NAc, which could indirectly alter cell firing in the VP. (2) As suggested for the NAc,[27,28] differences in neuron responses to morphine may reflect different VP populations that are distinguished by the afferent inputs associated with the recorded

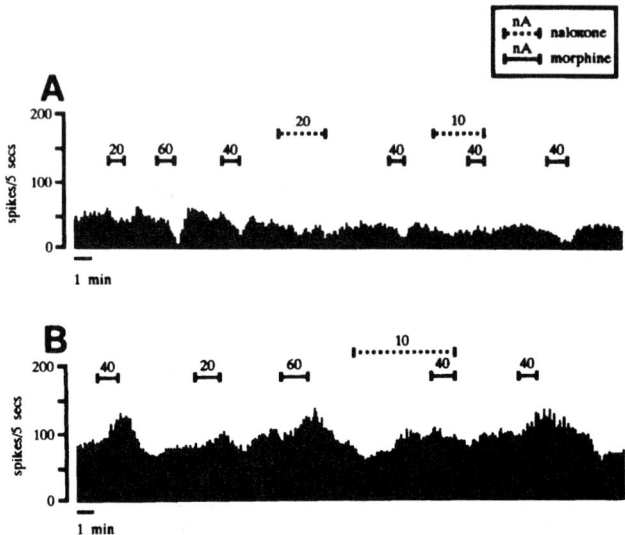

FIGURE 3. Rate histograms illustrating VP neuronal effects of the microiontophoretic application of morphine and antagonism of these responses by naloxone application. The horizontal bars indicate onset and offset of an ejecting current applied to the drug-containing barrel. The numbers above these bars indicate the respective current magnitude in nA. **A:** Morphine-induced inhibition. **B:** A histogram taken from a different VP cell, illustrating morphine-induced increases in firing rate. (Napier et al.[18] With permission from John Wiley & Sons, Inc.)

neuron. We demonstrated that morphine produces an iontophoretic current-dependent, and naloxone-sensitive, increase in neuronal firing rate in 87% of the VP neurons that were evoked by NAc stimulation.[34] This response pattern differed from that obtained with an unbiased sampling of the VP, where roughly equal inhibitory and excitatory effects were observed, and the excited neurons represented 44–59% of the tested cells.[16–18,34] This interpretation is furthered by experiments demonstrating that VP morphine attenuates the inhibitory effects of accumbal GABAergic transmission (discussed below).

Morphine and naloxone demonstrate a high potency for the μR, but both ligands have limited specificity for opioid receptor subtypes and have the potential to activate δR in the concentrations employed by the aforementioned experiments. Consequently, to characterize the particular contribution of μR in VP cell firing, we used microiontophoretic application of ligands with high specificity for the μR, [D-Ala^2,N-Me-Phe^4,Gly-ol^5]-enkephalin (DAMGO), and D-Phe-Cys-Tyr-D-Trp-Orn-Thr-Pen-Thr-NH^2 (CTOP). Iontophoresis of the agonist, DAMGO, altered firing in 59% of the cells tested. In 88% of these, a rate suppression was observed that could be attenuated by the antagonist CTOP[16] (FIG. 4). These experiments verified that μR within the VP is a robust regulator of neuronal activity in this region.

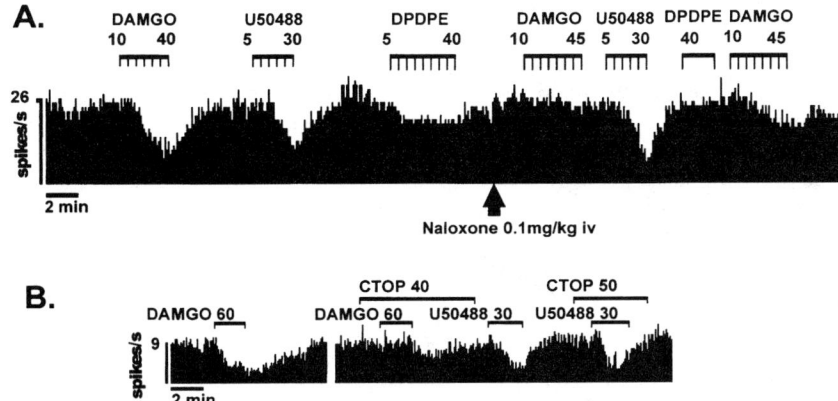

FIGURE 4. Illustrations of the rate-suppressing effects of microiontophoresed opioid receptor–specific agonists. Numbers above the horizontal bars represent the magnitude of ejection current in nA. **A:** A real-time rate histogram of a VP neuron that responded to the μR agonist, DAMGO; the κR agonist, U50488H; and the δR agonist, DPDPE. Ejection currents were applied as a single current level (e.g., 40 nA, DPDPE) and incrementally (5 nA/30 s). Intravenous administration of naloxone in a dose that reverses the effects of iv morphine (refer to FIG. 1) blocked the rate suppression induced by iontophoresed DAMGO and DPDPE, although the effects of U50488H were not altered. The results demonstrate several points about opioid pharmacology in the VP: (1) Naloxone, at this iv dose, likely binds to both μR and δR, but not the κR. (2) The μR occupancy obtained with iontophoresed DAMGO is comparable to that obtained with behaviorally relevant concentrations of iv morphine (in that they both are reversed by the same dose of the competitive antagonist, naloxone). (3) The effects of iv naloxone are quickly reversible (note that the inhibitory response to DAMGO began to recover within minutes after the antagonist treatment). **B:** A rate histogram illustrating the ability of CTOP (a μR antagonist) to antagonize suppression of neuronal activity elicited by DAMGO but not the effects of U50488H. These results illustrate the receptor-subtype selectivity of iontophoresed opioid ligands. (Mitrovic & Napier.[16] With permission from the American Society for Pharmacology and Experimental Therapeutics.)

COMPARISONS BETWEEN MORPHINE AND DAMGO

The consistency of DAMGO to suppress VP cell firing contrasts VP responding to iontophoresis of morphine where rate increases and decreases are observed.[18,34,38] Differences also were observed in the ability of the two agonists to modulate other transmitters; DAMGO almost always potentiated glutamate-evoked excitations, whereas morphine most often attenuated this effect[38] (discussed more thoroughly in upcoming paragraphs). To determine if this response variance could be attributed to morphine and DAMGO altering different populations of cells and/or different opioid receptor subtypes, 19 VP neurons were tested with both agonists.[16] Of these cells, morphine and DAMGO both altered firing in nine, and rate changes were in opposite direction for four. This differential responding was not likely due to differences in the ligand recognition site for the two agonists, for iontophoresis of CTOP antagonized the responses to both morphine and DAMGO. Others have noted variance in responding among µR agonists. For example, activation of µR by DAMGO induces their internalization,[39] but activation by morphine does not.[39,40] On the other hand, morphine elicits µR phosphorylation, while DAMGO does not.[41] Thus, morphine and DAMGO, upon binding to the µR, may initiate dissimilar conformational changes that translate into differential coupling with intracellular effector systems.[39–42] This divergence in receptor-effector coupling could account for different neuronal responses to morphine and DAMGO observed in the VP, and these differences need to be kept in mind when considering the ability of µR agonists to modulate other transmitters.

OPIOID MODULATION OF VENTRAL PALLIDAL AFFERENT TRANSMISSION: TECHNICAL CONSIDERATIONS

The objective of evaluating opioid modulation of the influence of other transmitters within local microcircuits in the VP presents some unique experimental obstacles that dictate the major requirements for the protocol selected. These included the following: (1) A method was required that would allow us to functionally identify the transmitter released by a particular input and to characterize its influence on the recorded VP neuron (which, hitherto, had not been described). (2) To isolate the microcircuits within the VP, a means to ascertain the responses of the recorded VP cell to activation of the µR within the VP itself was needed. These two objectives are best met by using electrophysiological recordings of VP neurons and microiontophoretic application of treatment ligands. (3) A means also was needed to characterize the influence of intra-VP µRs on neurotransmission from an anatomically discrete afferent input. In some brain regions, specific afferent pathways to the recorded cells, for example, the Schaffer collaterals to CA3 pyramidal cells, are anatomically arranged such that they can be discretely activated in slices of hippocampal tissue. In contrast to the hippocampus, afferent inputs to the VP terminate diffusely throughout the VP and do not form discrete bundles. Thus, it was essential that the somatic regions for each respective input be activated. Because these inputs are from anatomically distant brain regions (e.g., the midbrain ventral tegmental area and the forebrain amygdala and NAc), *in vivo* approaches were necessary. To study the pharmacology of the convergence of different afferent systems at the level of the VP neuron requires a protocol to discretely apply receptor-selective agents onto neurons that respond to rapid activation of VP afferents. These criteria are best met using orthodromic activation of the individual input system (via electrical stimulation of the origin of the input) in combination with microiontophoretic application of the treatment ligands. Additionally, by directly comparing VP neuronal responses to exogenously (i.e., microiontophoretically) applied transmitters with responses to endogenously released (via electrical activation of afferent inputs) transmitters, novel information relevant to VP afferent transmission can be suggested. For example, the capacity of the known exogenous transmitter to mimic the effects of the endogenously released substance is used to help identify the endogenous transmitter. Moreover, the ability of a receptor-specific antagonist to attenuate neuronal responding to electrical activation of an afferent input is used to more definitively describe the released transmitter. (This is best accomplished by verifying the ability of the antagonist to attenuate the known exogenous ligand and then using the same ejection current parameters to attenuate the endogenously released transmitter.) Finally, as used in other electrophysiological evaluations of opioid-induced effects (for a review, see ref. 43), contrasting the ability of a μR agonist to influence the presynaptic release of a transmitter, versus influencing the effects of the iontophoretic transmitter (which can act both presynaptically and postsynaptically[32,43]), can indicate whether or not opioid modulation involved the postsynaptic receptor (for additional discussion, see ref. 44).

The objective of evaluating "modulation" also presents its own set of technical considerations. We are interested in the concept that opioids may modify the effects of other transmitters without directly altering the output of a given cell (i.e., its ability to produce action potentials). Thus, we evaluated the effects of opioids using iontophoretic ejection currents that were too low to alter spontaneous firing of VP neurons (termed "subthreshold"). For a detailed discussion of the rationale for the experimental protocol, as well as data analysis and interpretation, the reader is referred to our original papers on opioid modulation of exogenously applied transmitters[17,38] and endogenously released transmitters.[34,44] In sum, the experimental paradigm allowed quantitative assessment of VP opioids to augment or suppress VP responses to both electrical stimulation of afferents or iontophoretically applied transmitter ligands.

μR AGONISTS MODULATING GABAERGIC INPUTS FROM THE NUCLEUS ACCUMBENS

GABA readily inhibited neuronal firing in the VP (FIG. 5).[38,45,46] This effect likely reflects the dense innervation of the VP by NAc GABAergic fibers as well as collaterals from the few GABAergic interneurons that are found within the VP (for reviews, see refs. 10, 11, 47). This anatomical arrangement predicts that an activated NAc would release GABA within the VP to reduce its neuronal activity. In agree-

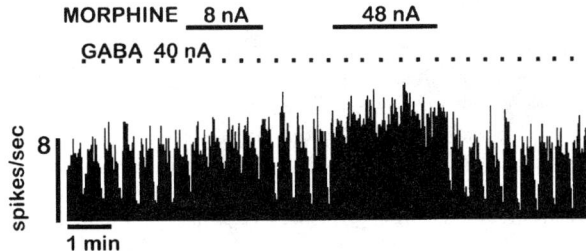

FIGURE 5. This rate histogram illustrates the robust suppression of VP neuron firing that occurs during microiontophoretic applications of GABA and the ability of coapplied morphine to attenuate this response. Iontophoretic applications of morphine are indicated by the long bars located above the histogram. The repetitive, uniform application of GABA (40 nA) is indicated by the dashes above the histogram. Morphine attenuated the effects of GABA when either subthreshold ejection current levels (8 nA) or an ejection current that increased spontaneous firing (48 nA) was coiontophoresed with GABA. (Johnson & Napier.[38] With permission from Elsevier Science.)

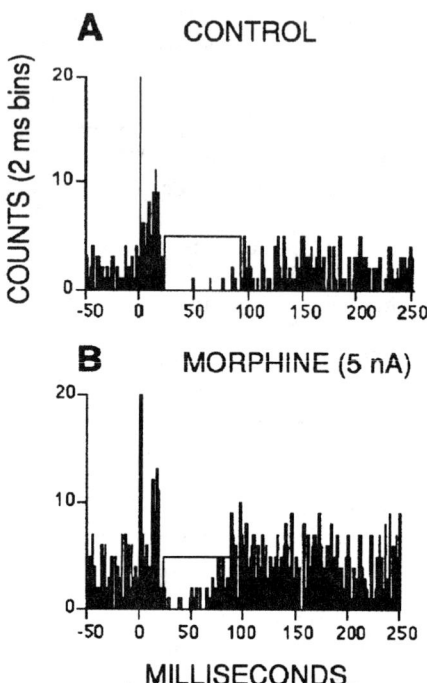

FIGURE 6. Peristimulus histograms illustrating the effects of morphine on the inhibitory component of evoked activity elicited by NAc stimulation. Stimulation is at time 0. Boxed area indicates the onset and duration of the evoked inhibition as defined during control condition. It is important to note that although morphine altered baseline firing in this cell (refer to the prestimulus rate), our statistical evaluations of the evoked response component are weighted to take this into account. (For details of these evaluations, please refer to refs. 34, 44, and 50.) (Chrobak and Napier.[34] With permission from Springer-Verlag.)

ment with previous electrophysiological work by Mogenson and Jones,[48] we observed trans-synaptically mediated decreases in firing following electrical stimulation of the NAc, and these responses were attenuated by the GABA antagonist, bicuculline.[34] The consistent suppression in firing by GABA of the same VP neurons that demonstrated a rapid onset inhibitory response to NAc stimulation, and the ability of bicuculline to attenuate these effects, substantiates the idea that activation of the NAc monosynaptically releases GABA onto VP neurons to decrease their activity.

Like bicuculline, morphine attenuated the decrease in firing evoked by electrically activating the NAc (FIGURES 6B and 7B).[34] Indeed, morphine application resulted in a robust 202% increase in activity that occurred during the inhibitory evoked component, and in a third of the neurons tested, this inhibition was abolished. The onset and duration of the inhibitory component, aside from cases in which it was totally reversed, were not altered by morphine. These observations indicate that morphine attenuates the influence of a single inhibitory transmitter. Evoked responses in the

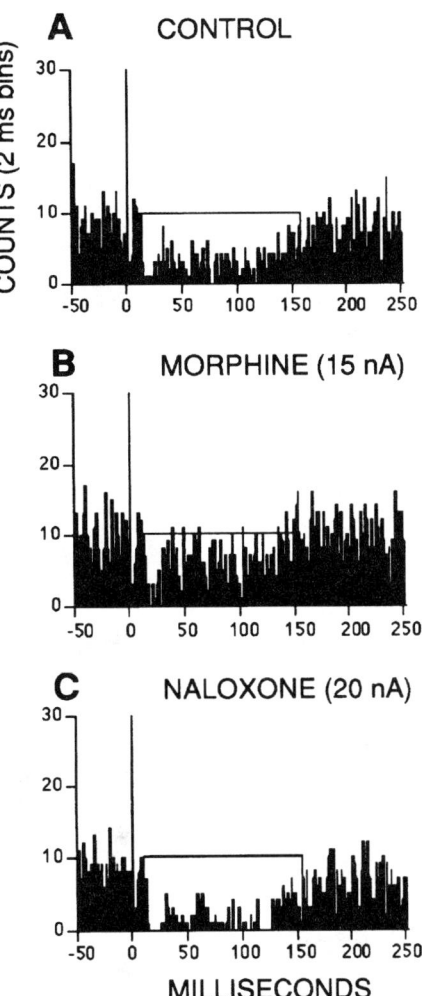

FIGURE 7. Peristimulus histograms illustrating the effects of iontophoretically applied morphine and naloxone on the evoked inhibition of a VP neuron following NAc stimulation (0.8 mA). Stimulation is at time 0. Boxed area indicates onset and duration of inhibition defined during control condition (**A**). Even though spontaneous firing was not altered by the drugs (compare prestimulus rates for all three histograms), morphine (**B**) prominently attenuated the inhibition, whereas naloxone (**C**) enhanced the magnitude of inhibition. (Chrobak and Napier.[34] With permission from Springer-Verlag.)

presence of morphine were opposite to those observed with naloxone; that is, naloxone enhanced NAc-evoked inhibition (FIG. 7c).[34] (This result also indicates that endogenous opioid peptides are tonically released in the chloral hydrate–anesthetized rat preparation.) In sum, it appears that opioid receptor activation is functionally antagonistic to accumbal GABAergic neurotransmission in the VP.

In support of this conclusion, subthreshold ejection currents of morphine (i.e., ejection currents of morphine that were too low to produce a change in spontaneous firing) produced a robust attenuation of the rate-suppressing effect of iontophoretically applied GABA in 44% of the cells tested (FIG. 5).[38] GABAergic effects were enhanced by morphine in 19% and were not altered in 37 percent. Interestingly, the morphine-induced effect on spontaneous activity (i.e., an increase or decrease in spontaneous activity obtained with supra-threshold ejection currents for the opiate) was not a factor in determining morphine's modulatory effects on GABA-evoked responses in the VP (i.e., an attenuation or potentiation of the GABA-induced effects). Thus, the mechanisms that underlie the "direct" effects of morphine may differ from those that allow the opiate to regulate GABA transmission.

µR AGONISTS MODULATE SUBSTANCE P–CONTAINING INPUTS FROM THE NUCLEUS ACCUMBENS

The firing rate of VP neurons was readily enhanced by microiontophoretic applications of substance P or a metabolically stable agonist analogue, DiMeC7.[17,44,49]

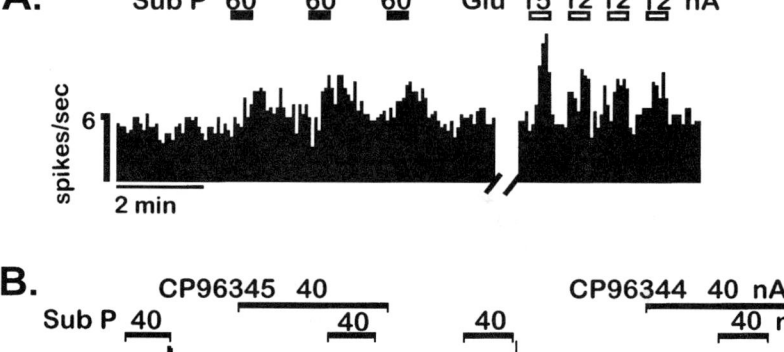

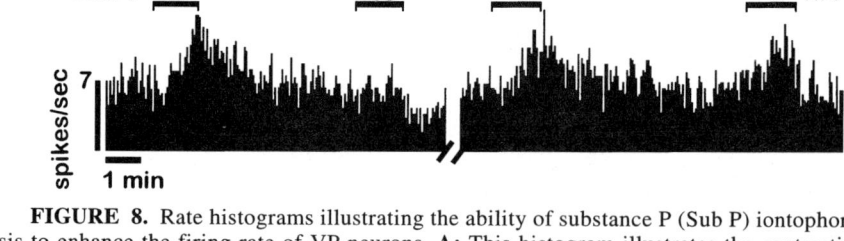

FIGURE 8. Rate histograms illustrating the ability of substance P (Sub P) iontophoresis to enhance the firing rate of VP neurons. **A:** This histogram illustrates the contrasting onset and offset of VP excitations to iontophoresis of Sub P and glutamate (Glu). (Napier *et al.*[49] With permission from Elsevier Science.) **B:** This histogram was obtained from another VP neuron where the tachykinin receptor antagonist, CP96345 (40 nA), blocked the Sub P (40 nA)–evoked increases in firing. By contrast, its inactive enantiomer, CP96344 (40 nA), was unable to alter Sub P–induced effects. (Mitrovic & Napier.[17] With permission from John Wiley & Sons, Inc.)

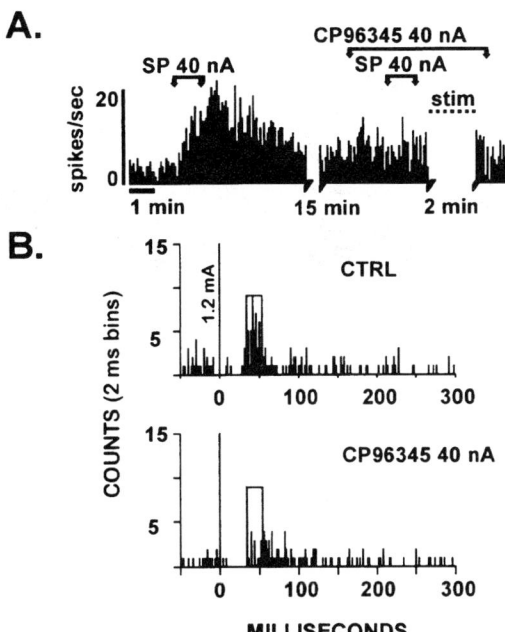

FIGURE 9. Demonstration of the ability of the tachykinin receptor antagonist CP96345 to block the rate increases induced by substance P (SP) iontophoresis and those evoked by NAc stimulation (the same cell is represented in **A** and **B**). **A:** A real time rate histogram illustrating antagonism of SP-induced responses by CP963456. The horizontal bars flanked with arrows indicate onset and offset of the ejections currents. The dashed line (stim) indicates the time period during which the NAc was stimulated. The numbers above the bars indicate the magnitude of the iontophoretic ejection current used to apply the drugs. **B:** Peristimulus time histograms illustrating the ability of C96345 to suppress VP excitatory responses to stimulation of the NAc. The number to the left of the stimulus artifact illustrates the NAc stimulation current. The boxes indicate onset, duration, and peak counts/bin of excitation as defined during the control condition (CTRL). (Mitrovic & Napier.[44] With permission from Elsevier Science.)

Response characteristics were distinguished from glutamate-induced excitations by a slower onset and longer duration of action (FIG. 8A), and by being attenuated by coapplications of the NK1 antagonist, CP96345 (FIGURES 8B and 9A). These response patterns also were observed following electrical activation of the NAc, where the slow rising excitatory responses were reversed by iontophoretic applications of CP96345 onto the VP neuron (FIG. 9B). These experiments verified anatomical descriptions of substance P–containing projections from the NA to the VP[49] and demonstrated the robust excitatory influence that this input has on VP cell firing.

DAMGO microiontophoresis was used to determine if activation of μRs can modulate substance P–mediated excitations in the VP.[17] Because of the long duration of action of substance P, it does not lend itself to evaluations where drug delivery is accomplished using repeated epochs of short duration (as was used for GABA and glutamate). Thus, we evaluated shifts in a substance P ejection current–response

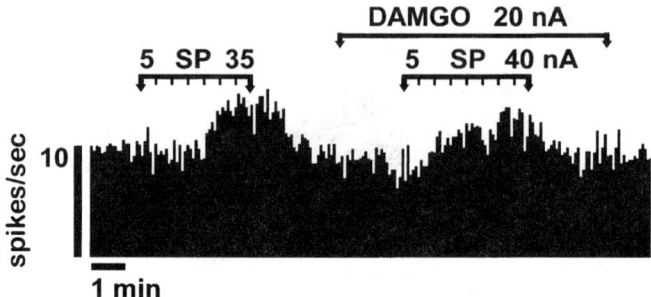

FIGURE 10. Effects of a single ejection current of DAMGO on neuronal responses evoked by incrementally applied substance P. The rate histogram from a VP neuron illustrates that as the ejection current magnitude to the substance P (SP)–containing pipette was increased (applied in 5 nA increments), the magnitude of the rate enhancement increased. The maximal firing rate induced by SP was attenuated by coiontophoresing DAMGO. (Mitrovic & Napier.[17] With permission from John Wiley & Sons, Inc.)

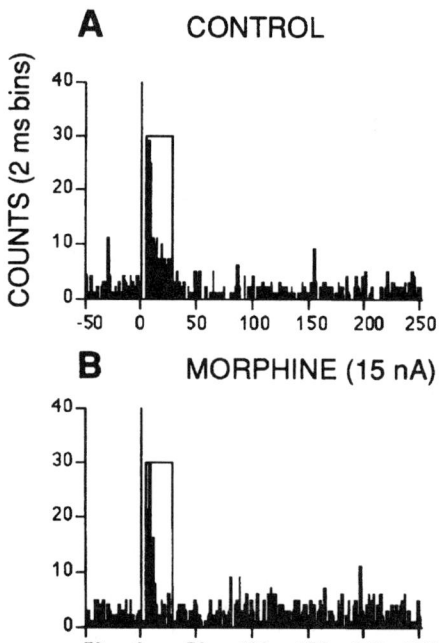

FIGURE 11. Peristimulus time histograms illustrating the effects of morphine application on excitation of a VP neuron following NAc stimulation (1.2 mA). Stimulation is at time 0. Boxed area indicates onset and duration of excitation during control condition. Note that the magnitude of the short latency excitations remained intact during morphine application, whereas the magnitude of the rate increases that occurred several milliseconds after stimulating the NAc were totally blocked by the opiate. (Chrobak & Napier.[34] With permission from Springer-Verlag.)

curve where the tachykinin was applied in continuously incrementing magnitudes of ejection current (see FIG. 10). Coapplication of DAMGO decreased the E_{max} and slope of the substance P ejection current–response curve (E_{max} decreased from $54 \pm 13\%$ to $19 \pm 7\%$ above control, and the slope was decreased from 2.59 ± 0.51 to 1.15 ± 0.19).[17] This effect occurred at subthreshold current levels for opioid. The potency for substance P was not changed by DAMGO ($n = 7$ cells).

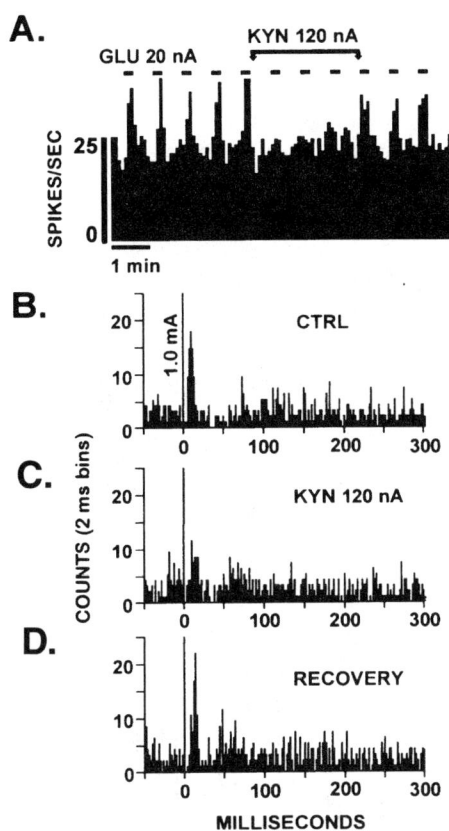

FIGURE 12. Electrophysiological evidence for an excitatory amino acid–containing input from the amygdala to the VP. A: A real-time rate histogram demonstrating that the firing of VP neurons was enhanced by discrete local applications of glutamate (GLU). The ability of the glutamate antagonist, kynurenic acid (KYN), to block this effect verified that the type of receptor acted upon by the agonist was indeed an excitatory amino acid receptor. Note that immediately after the termination of kynurenic iontophoresis, glutamate-evoked responses were reinstated. B, C, and D were taken from the same VP neuron, and these peristimulus time histograms illustrate the rapid onset and short-lived rate increases that were frequently obtained following electrical activation of the amygdala (time 0; 1.0 mA). B: No drug applied (control). C: During iontophoresis of the kynurenic acid at an ejection current that previously blocked exogenously applied glutamate (120 nA). D: After kynurenic acid ejection current was terminated, the response returned to the control state (recovery). The results indicate that activation of the amygdala releases excitatory amino acids within the VP. (Mitrovic & Napier.[44] With permission from Elsevier Science.)

These results agree with our observation that iontophoretically applied morphine attenuates the slow excitatory responses of VP neurons produced by activation of the NAc (FIG. 11).[34] This effect occurred even at ejection current levels for morphine that were subthreshold to those necessary to change spontaneous firing. Thus, μR-acting peptides likely have a modulatory role in the VP that functions to attenuate accumbal-induced excitations of VP neurons that are mediated by substance P.

μR AGONISTS MODULATE GLUTAMATERGIC INPUTS FROM THE AMYGDALA

The VP is contacted by inputs from the amygdala with a substantial portion arising from the basolateral nucleus (e.g., ref. 14). There is good anatomical evidence that this projection largely comprises axons that contain excitatory amino acids.[14] Electrical activation of the basolateral amygdala evokes a rapid onset enhancement of short duration in VP cell firing (FIG. 12).[44,50] Microiontophoresis of glutamate also evokes a rapid excitatory response of short duration[38,44-46] (FIG. 12). The firing

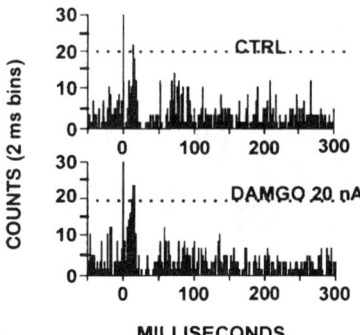

FIGURE 13. Peristimulus time histograms illustrating of ability of subthreshold ejection currents of DAMGO to potentiate the short latency excitatory responses of VP neurons to electrical activation of the amygdala. CTRL, control (no drug application). Note that the initial excitatory response magnitude is slightly enhanced during a 20 nA application of DAMGO (the dashed line is for reference). In the 11 VP neurons tested in this fashion, DAMGO increased amygdala-evoked excitations by 39%, and the opioid potentiated the rate increases induced by iontophoretically applied glutamate (5 cells tested; data not shown). (Mitrovic Napier.[44] With permission from Elsevier Science.)

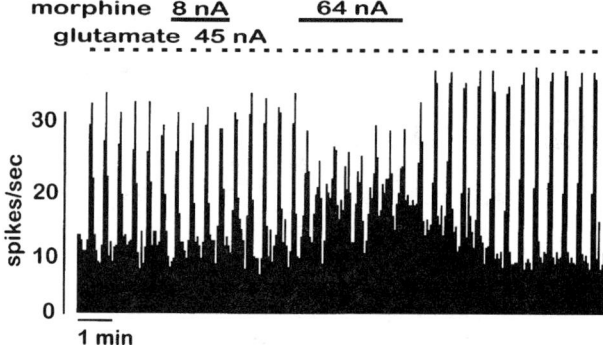

FIGURE 14. A rate histogram demonstrating an attenuation of the relationship between the glutamate-evoked excitatory response and spontaneous firing (i.e., signal-to-noise ratio) when either subthreshold or suprathreshold morphine ejection currents were coiontophoresed with the amino acid. The repetitive, uniform application of the glutamate (45 nA) is indicated by the dashes above the histogram. Iontophoretic applications of morphine are indicated by the long bars located above the histogram. At a subthreshold morphine ejection current (8 nA) (when spontaneous activity is unaffected), the glutamate-evoked activity was slightly attenuated. At a suprathreshold ejection current (64 nA), morphine increased the spontaneous firing rate in this neuron, whereas glutamate-evoked activity was decreased substantially. In this cell, both effects tend to attenuate the relative magnitude of the glutamatergic influence. (Johnson and Napier.[38] With permission from Elsevier Science.)

rate enhancements to both amygdala stimulation and glutamate iontophoresis are readily blocked by iontophoresis of the glutamate antagonist, kynurenic acid (FIG.

12). These studies demonstrate that, as predicted by anatomical evaluations, the basolateral amygdala provides an excitatory (likely glutamatergic) input to the VP, the activation of which produces a rapid and robust enhancement of VP neuronal activity.

The amygdala also inputs the NAc.[14] This anatomical arrangement may provide a mechanism by which the amygdala could increase opioid transmission within the VP. If true, then when the amygdala is activated, firing in both the NAc and the VP would be enhanced; however, by releasing opioids in the VP the NAc would be able to modify these amygdaloid influences on the VP and thus fine-tune communication from the major output of the limbic system. Because of the functional importance of this circuit, we tested the possibility that VP opioids can modulate the effects of amygdala stimulation in the VP.[44] Previous reports of opioids modulating presynaptic release of excitatory amino acid transmission elsewhere in the brain supported the feasibility of the hypothesis.[51,52] As mentioned before, iontophoretically applied DAMGO suppressed spontaneous firing, but interestingly it often potentiated the excitations evoked in VP neurons by electrical stimulation of the amygdala (FIG. 13). This response is in contrast to the attenuation of iontophoretic glutamate-evoked responses often observed with morphine (FIG. 14).[38] These changes were independent of the direction of morphine-induced changes in the spontaneous firing rate. The differences in the modulatory effects of DAMGO and morphine on glutamatergic transmission present some interesting possibilities regarding the signal transduction mechanisms employed by the various μR agonists (discussed above). Regardless of these differences, it is clear that opioid transmission in the VP can wield a powerful modulatory effect on glutamatergic influences that are exerted on this region by the amygdala.

μR AGONISTS MODULATE PUTATIVE GLUTAMATERGIC INPUTS FROM THE CORTEX

Originating largely within the medial prefrontal cortex, an excitatory amino acid-containing projection courses through the NAc to terminate within the VP.[53] This *en passage* projection is activated with electrical stimulation of the NAc and likely is responsible for the non-substance P (i.e., not sensitive to the tachykinin antagonist, CP96345) –evoked excitations of rapid onset and short duration in VP neurons.[34,44] Subthreshold currents of morphine either enhanced or had no effect on firing during this evoked component (FIG. 11).[34] This result is similar to that obtained with subthreshold currents of DAMGO when the opioid is applied during amygdala stimulation (described above), where the glutamate-mediated short latency excitation was potentiated.[44] These responses differed somewhat from those obtained from VP neurons tested with glutamate iontophoresis only. In these cells, subthreshold ejection currents of morphine enhanced the glutamate-evoked response in 44% of the cells, whereas 38% showed an attenuation and 16% did not change.[38] This response distribution suggests that low extracellular concentrations of morphine may elicit very selective modulations of glutamate receptor responding. One possible means by which such an arrangement could exist is if glutamate release from other glutamatergic inputs to the VP (e.g., those arising from the subthalamic nucleus) were more

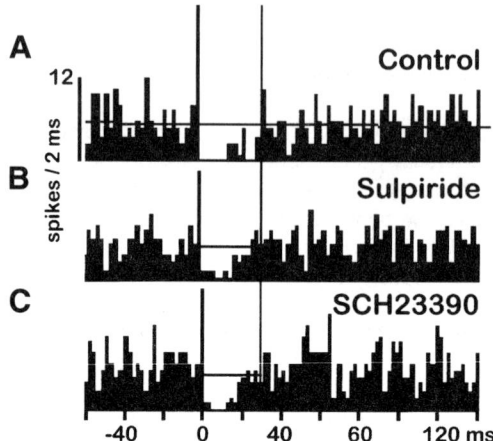

FIGURE 15. Peristimulus histograms of inhibitory responses obtained in the VP following electrical activation of the ventral tegmental area and the ability of dopamine antagonists to attenuate this response. **A:** The inhibitory response evoked by stimulating the ventral tegmental area (time 0; 0.05 mA) is delineated by the bins that fall below the average counts per bin determined in the prestimulus period (horizontal line). Antagonists for the D2-like dopamine receptor, sulpiride, and the D1-like receptor, SCH23390, attenuated this inhibitory response. It is noteworthy that the antagonists only blocked the portion of the inhibitory period that occurred 20 milliseconds after stimulating the midbrain. The rate suppression that occurred more immediately was left in tact. This suggests that other non-dopaminergic mechanisms (and likely non–G protein mediated) may be involved in the rapid inhibitions evoked in the VP following ventral tegmental stimulation (e.g., GABA).

readily attenuated by μR activation. If true, this would allow VP opioids to enhance the throughput of a limbic-oriented drive (from the prefrontal cortex and the amygdala) while attenuating signals from the basal ganglia (i.e., the subthalamic nucleus). Future studies in our laboratory are directed towards testing this hypothesis.

μR AGONISTS MODULATING DOPAMINERGIC INPUTS FROM THE VENTRAL TEGMENTAL AREA

The VP receives a dopaminergic projection that arises from both the substantia nigra and the ventral tegmental area (for a review, see ref. 15), with the latter being the most prevalent and topographically disperse input.[47,54] Electrical activation of these dopaminergic regions readily elicited evoked responses that exhibited an initial inhibition in the activity of the VP neurons (FIG. 15); excitations also were observed.[50,55,56] Iontophoretically applied dopamine produced both increases and decreases in firing rate[45,46,50,57] (e.g., see FIG. 16). Most often, VP neurons that responded to electrical activation of the midbrain demonstrated similar responding to microiontophoretic ejections of dopamine (both with regard to the response direction as well as to the relatively longer duration of the evoked response).[50] VP responses to stimulation of the midbrain and dopamine iontophoresis are attenuated by microiontophoresis of dopaminergic antagonists (FIG. 15), verifying that dopamine

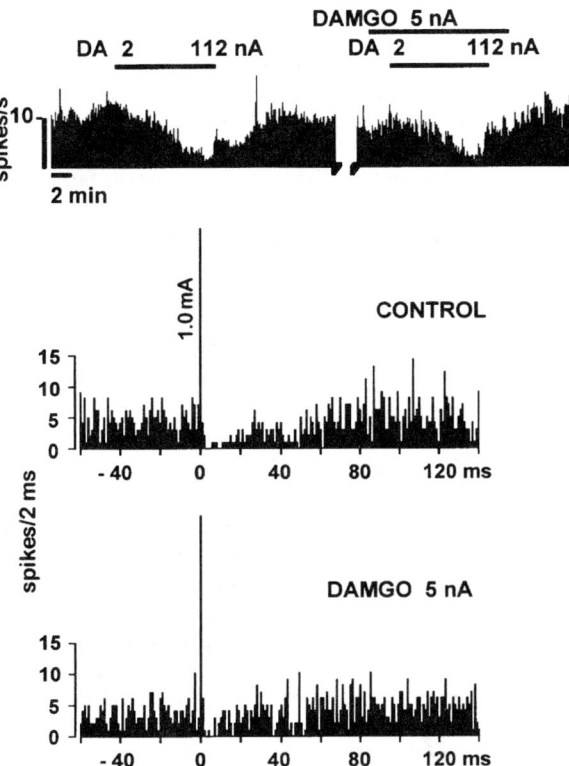

FIGURE 16. Histograms illustrating the ability of DAMGO to attenuate the effects of endogenously released dopamine, but not those of exogenously applied dopamine. *Top:* A real-time histogram illustrating that dopamine (2-112 nA incremented in 30 sec intervals) induced rate suppressions that were not altered by coiontophoresing DAMGO (5 nA). (With larger ejection currents of DAMGO, the firing of this cell was decreased; thus, the cell was sensitive to the μR agonist; data not shown.) When the ejection current–neuronal response relationship was compared with and without subthreshold current levels of DAMGO for the 18 VP cells tested, no difference was obtained in the slope, E_{max}, or the potency indicator for dopamine. *Middle and bottom:* Peristimulus time histograms illustrating the ability of a low ejection current of DAMGO to attenuate ventral tegmental area-evoked (1.0 mA) inhibition.

receptors were being activated by both the endogenously released transmitter as well as iontophoretically applied dopamine. It is noteworthy that the dopamine antagonists were most effective at blocking the later stages of the initial inhibitory response evoked by midbrain stimulation (see FIG. 15 B and C). This observation indicates that another transmitter is responsible for the rapid decreases in firing. We now have preliminary data that suggest a GABAergic involvement in this evoked component (unpublished results). In sum, the profile of the responses evoked by midbrain stimulation, the tendency for iontophoresed dopamine to mimic these responses, and the ability of dopamine antagonists to block both of these effects are consistent with a monosynaptic dopaminergic projection to the VP.

Of the recorded VP neurons that demonstrated an initial inhibitory response to ventral tegmental stimulation, firing in 54% also was decreased by DAMGO.[56] In these cells, subthreshold ejection currents of DAMGO attenuated the inhibitory responses to VTA stimulation (FIG. 16). However, application of DAMGO with these current levels during incremental applications of dopamine failed to alter dopamine-induced rate changes[57] (FIG. 16). Thus, in contrast to the ability of DAMGO to attenuate endogenously released dopamine, the opioid did not influence the efficacy or the potency of exogenously applied dopamine within the VP. The difference in the modulatory efficiency of DAMGO between endogenously released dopamine and exogenously applied dopamine suggests that the opioid modulation of endogenously released dopamine was most likely mediated via a presynaptic µR that influences dopamine release in the VP.

CONCLUSIONS AND SPECULATIONS

This chapter reviews the first characterization of µR-mediated effects on the physiology of VP neurons. The results reveal that bath-applied µR agonists can hyperpolarize VP neurons recorded *in vitro*. As would be predicted from *in vitro* studies, when opiates are given systemically in *in vivo* preparations, VP cell firing often is reduced. When discrete local applications of µR agonists are evaluated for their ability to modulate the effects of other transmitters, however, a variety of responses result. Moreover, the responses vary according to the transmitter and afferent system that is evoked. Nonetheless, it is clear that an important consequence of activating µR in the VP is to modulate the effects of accumbal GABA and substance P, cortical and amygdaloid glutamate, and midbrain dopaminergic inputs on VP activity. When the morphologic arrangement of these inputs, the receptor location, and the signal transduction pathways evoked by activating these receptors are considered in conjunction with our electrophysiological observations, several likely mechanisms become apparent that can account for the observed µR interactions with these other transmitter systems in the VP.

Our data indicate that µR can postsynaptically modulate the effects of substance P, GABA, and glutamate on VP neurons. This scenario assumes (1) that the receptors employed by the respective transmitters would be coexpressed by the recorded neurons, and (2) that some portion of the receptors' signal transduction pathways would overlap.

The µR and its message have been localized within the VP,[58,59] providing strong evidence that VP cells expressed these receptors. Activation of µR is thought to influence target neurons via $G_{i/o}$ GTP binding proteins, which sets into motion several biochemical and electrophysiological events. This includes an inhibition of adenylyl cyclase, leading to decreases in cAMP and cAMP-dependent protein kinases. Moreover, G protein–dependent inwardly rectifying K^+ channels are activated, and voltage-dependent Ca^{2+} channels are inhibited. (For reviews of opioid receptor signal transduction, see refs. 33 and 60-63.) Thus, the influence of other neurotransmitters could be modulated by opioids at the postsynaptic level via an alteration in the phosphorylation state of the numerous proteins that are important in cell function, as well as decreased cell excitability (secondary to effects on K^+ conductance). Numerous studies have demonstrated that VP neurons express receptors for substance P,[64,65] GABA,[66] and glutamate.[67,68] Although the extent of colocalization of μR with these other receptors is not known for VP neurons, our electrophysiological data indicate that coexpression likely occurs in a significant portion of these cells. There is good evidence that sites of overlap in the signal transduction pathway for μR occur with substance P, GABA, and glutamate. For example, in cultured locus caeruleus neurons, substance P closes and met-enkephalin opens a G-protein-linked inwardly rectifying K^+ channel.[69] μRs have been shown to modulate GABA-induced currents in neurons from the mammalian dorsal horn[70] and the snail, *Lymnaea stagnalis*.[71] In spinal trigeminal neurons, activation of μR results in a potentiation of NMDA receptor–mediated glutamate currents via a protein kinase C-dependent mechanism.[72] These studies indicate the prospect that postsynaptic mechanisms may have contributed to the ability of μR agonists to modulate substance P, GABA, and glutamate in the VP.

By acting presynaptically to decrease voltage-dependent Ca^{2+} conductance, it would be predicted that μR agonists could decrease release of the endogenous transmitters. Indeed, evaluations of several brain regions have demonstrated that μR activation alters the release of substance P (e.g., refs. 73 and 74), GABA (e.g., refs. 52 and 75-77), glutamate (e.g., refs. 51, 52, 78), and dopamine (e.g., refs. 79–82). However, as with postsynaptic mechanisms, regional differences in the nature of μR-mediated modulation are demonstrated. Most striking are the biochemical evaluations of local μR influences on dopamine release, where a myriad of responses are reported. Moreover, the variances may reflect controlling factors other than just regional differences. For example, within the striatum, dopamine levels are reported to be enhanced,[79,80,82] decreased,[81,83] or not altered[84] by local μR activation. These responses may be a consequence of differences in the firing state of the dopamine neuron, how much brain area is exposed to the opioid, and the synaptic/extrasynaptic concentration of the ligand. Whereas further study is needed to clarify the exact nature of μR regulation of the release of other transmitters in the VP, μR have been identified on presynaptic elements in this region.[59] In accordance, our electrophysiological findings indicate that, as elsewhere in the brain, a presynaptic modulation of other transmitters is likely important in the integration of afferent inputs in the VP.

Underscoring the concept that VP opioids are important modulators of other transmitters is the observation that opioid agonists, at local concentrations that are below those required to alter spontaneous firing, can substantially regulate the function of other VP inputs. As the VP provides a major output for limbic and basal ganglia systems, this scenario empowers the NAc (the source of VP opioids) with a mechanism to profoundly influence these converging communications. The consequence of this circuit likely involves a fine-tuning of the excitatory drive provided by the excitatory inputs from the cortex and the amygdala. Amgdaloid projections containing excitatory amino acids synapse onto accumbal neurons, thus, it is possible that the amygdala could increase opioid transmission within the VP. If true, activation of the amygdala would enhance firing in both the NAc and the VP; however, by releasing opioids in the VP, the NAc would be able to modify the amygdaloid influences on the VP. Our results indicate that μR agonists decreased the variability and enhanced the acuity (e.g., "signal-to-noise" relationship) of VP responses to activation of glutamatergic inputs from the amygdala. Thus, an activated NAc would effectively fine-tune communication from the limbic system at the level of its major output, that is, the VP.

Recent behavioral studies have greatly advanced our understanding of the functional ramifications of VP opioid transmission. It now is clear that reward[7] and motor behaviors[19,85,86] are influenced by activation of VP µR. Our electrophysiological data are beginning to elucidate the cellular mechanisms that may be directing these behaviors. For example, the differences we observed in VP cell responses to DAMGO and morphine may be of functional relevance; DAMGO-induced effects may represent more closely the function of endogenous neuropeptides, and morphine likely reveals the consequence of heroin use. On a systems level, our results suggest that a consequence of opioid transmission in the VP is to filter out the influence of some afferents (e.g., midbrain dopamine and accumbal GABA and substance P) while selectively potentiating the efficacy of others (e.g., cortical and amygdaloid glutamate). The selective enhancement in the fidelity of a particular afferent to the VP may be a mechanism by which sensorimotor gating is achieved. The VP, NAc, and amygdala are important in the regulation of this function (as measured by a prepulse inhibition paradigm).[8] The VP appears to be especially important in the disruption of the prepulse inhibition mediated by dopaminergic agonists.[87] GABAergic neurotransmission to the VP also is involved in prepulse inhibition,[9] but the role of VP opioids is not known. It is clear, however, that VP opioids (and dopamine) are involved in reward-motivated behaviors.[7,88,89] These behavioral observations in conjunction with our data suggest that disturbances in µR-mediated transmission within the VP would contribute to the disruption of sensorimotor gating as well as to the disruption of motivated behavior. These findings also could be considered in the context of opiate abuse. We recently determined that VP µRs are involved in morphine-induced behavioral sensitization. (The enhanced motor responses normally seen to an acute challenge of morphine following a 72 h after the last of five daily injections of 10 mg/kg ip morphine were blocked if rats received intra-VP injections of CTOP immediately before each of the five daily morphine treatments; unpublished results.) The neuronal plasticity that underlies behavioral sensitization to an acute drug challenge following a period of drug withdrawal may model the changes that induce craving for the drug during its absence in the human opiate abuser. Drug craving can be elicited in abusers by presenting them with drug-use paraphernalia or exposing them to the environment associated with a drug use. This phenomenon clearly has a cognitive component (e.g., associating the paraphernalia and environment with drug-induced hedonia), coupled with a negative affective component (e.g., the discomfort associated with drug withdrawal) that compels the abuser to seek more drug. Our data suggest that activation of the VP µR opioid system may favor VP inputs associated with cognition (prefrontal cortex) and affect (amygdala) over those associated with reward (ventral tegmental area and NAc). Thus, depending upon the specifics of adaptive processes that occur in VP transmission with chronic opiate exposure, the VP µR opioid system may serve to diminish the contribution of reinforcement in the transduction of cognition and affect into behavior. This phenomenon may influence drug craving that occurs even in the absence of reward.

ACKNOWLEDGMENTS

Major contributions to the experimental findings overviewed in this chapter were made by Dr. James Chrobak, Dr. Patricia Johnson, Dr. Jian-Xiang Liao, Dr. Renata Maslowski, and Ms. Fatema Rehman. This research was made possible by the financial support of USPHSG's DA05255, DA05651, and MH45180.

REFERENCES

1. HEIMER, L. & R.D. WILSON. 1975. The subcortical projections of the allocortex: similarities in the neural associations of the hippocampus, the piriform cortex, and the neocortex. In Golgi Centennial Symposium. Proceedings. M. Santini, Ed.: 177–193. Raven Press. New York.
2. MOGENSON, G.J. & C.R. YANG. 1991. The contribution of basal forebrain to limbic-motor integration and the mediation of motivation to action. In The Basal Forebrain: Anatomy to Function. T.C. Napier, P.W. Kalivas & I. Hanin, Eds.: **295**: 267–290. Advances in Experimental Medicine and Biology. Plenun Press. New York.
3. NAPIER, T.C. 1993. Transmitter actions and interactions on pallidal neuronal function. In Limbic Motor Circuits and Neuropsychiatry. P. W. Kalivas & C. D. Barnes, Eds.: 125–153. CRC Press. Boca Raton.
4. PANAGIS, G., E. MILIARESSIS, Y. ANAGNOSTAKIS & C. SPYRAKI. 1995. Ventral pallidum self-stimulation: a moveable electrode mapping study. Behav. Brain Res. **68**: 165–172.
5. WILSON, F.A.W. & E.T. ROLLS. 1990. Neuronal responses related to reinforcement in the primate basal forebrain. Brain Res. **509**: 213–231.
6. MCALONAN, G.M., T.W. ROBBINS & B.J. EVERITT. 1993. Effects of medial dorsal thalamic and ventral pallidal lesions on the acquisition of a conditioned place preference: further evidence for the involvement of the ventral striatopallidal system in reward-related processes. Neuroscience **52**: 605–620.
7. JOHNSON, P.I., J.R. STELLAR & A.D. PAUL. 1993. Regional reward differences within the ventral pallidum are revealed by microinjections of a mu opiate receptor agonist. Neuropharmacology **32**: 1305–1314.
8. KODSI, M.H. & N.R. SWERDLOW. 1995. Prepulse inhibition in the rat is regulated by ventral and caudodorsal striato-pallidal circuitry. Behav. Neurosci. **109**: 912–928.
9. KODSI, M.H. & N.R. SWERDLOW. 1995. Ventral pallidal GABA-A receptors regulate prepulse inhibition of acoustic startle. Brain Res. **684**: 26–35.
10. HEIMER, L., G.F. ALHEID & L. ZABORSZKY. 1985. Basal ganglia. In The Rat Nervous System, Volume 1. Forebrain and Midbrain. G. Paxinos, Ed.: 37–86. Academic Press, Inc. Orlando, Florida.
11. HEIMER, L. & G.F. ALHEID. 1991. Piecing together the puzzle of basal forebrain anatomy. In The Basal Forebrain: Anatomy to Function. T.C. Napier, P.W. Kalivas & I. Hanin, Eds.: **295**: 1–42. Advances in Experimental Medicine and Biology. Plenum Press. New York.
12. ZAHM, D.S. & J.S. BROG. 1992. On the significance of subterritories in the "accumbens" part of the rat ventral striatum. Neuroscience **50**: 751–767.
13. CARNES, K.M., T.A. FULLER & J.L. PRICE. 1990. Sources of presumptive glutamatergic/aspartatergic afferents to the magnocellular basal forebrain in the rat. J. Comp. Neurol. **302**: 824–852.
14. FULLER, T.A., F.T. RUSSCHEN & J.L. PRICE. 1987. Sources of presumptive glutamergic/aspartergic afferents to the rat ventral striatopallidal region. J. Comp. Neurol. **258**: 317–338.
15. NAPIER, T.C., M.B. MUENCH, R.J. MASLOWSKI & G. BATTAGLIA. 1991. Is dopamine a neurotransmitter within the ventral pallidum/substantia innominata? In The Basal Forebrain: Anatomy to Function. T.C. Napier, P.W. Kalivas & I. Hanin. Eds.: **295**:

183–195. Advances in Experimental Medicine and Biology. Plenum Press, New York.
16. MITROVIC, I. & T.C. NAPIER. 1995. Electrophysiological demonstration of μ, δ and k opioid receptors in the ventral pallidum. J. Pharmacol. Exp. Ther. **272:** 1260–1272.
17. MITROVIC, I. & T.C. NAPIER. 1996. Interactions between the *mu* opioid agonist DAMGO and substance P in regulation of the ventral pallidum. Synapse (NY) **23:** 142–151.
18. NAPIER, T.C., J.J. CHROBAK & J. YEW. 1992. Systemic and microiontophoretic administration of morphine differentially effect ventral pallidum/substantia innominata neuronal activity. Synapse (NY) **12:** 214–219.
19. NAPIER, T.C. 1992. Dopamine receptors in the ventral pallidum regulate circling induced by opioids injected into the ventral pallidum. Neuropharmacology **31:** 1127–1136.
20. WISE, R.A. & M.A. BOZARTH. 1982. Action of drugs of abuse on brain reward systems: an update with specific attention to opiates. Pharmacol. Biochem. Behav. **17:** 239–243.
21. UNTERWALD, E.M. & C. KORNETSKY. 1993. Reinforcing effects of opiates–modulation by dopamine. *In* The Neurobiology of Opiates. R. P. Hammer Jr., Ed.: 361–391. CRC Press, Inc. Boca Raton.
22. SPANAGEL, R., A. HERZ & T.S. SHIPPENBERG. 1990. The effects of opioid peptides on dopamine release in the nucleus accumbens: an *in vivo* microdialysis study. J. Neurochem. **55:** 1734–1740.
23. DI CHIARA, G. & A. IMPERATO. 1988. Drugs abused by humans preferentially increase synaptic dopamine concentrations in the mesolimbic system of freely moving rats. Proc. Natl. Acad. Sci. USA **85:** 5274–5278.
24. GYSLING, K. & R.Y. WANG. 1983. Morphine-induced activation of A10 dopamine neurons. Brain Res. **277:** 119–127.
25. MATTHEWS, R.T. & D.C. GERMAN. 1984. Electrophysiological evidence for excitation of rat ventral tegmental area dopamine neurons by morphine. Neuroscience **11:** 617–625.
26. JOHNSON, S.W. & R.A. NORTH. 1992. Opioids excite dopamine neurons by hyperpolarization of local interneurons. J. Neurosci. **12:** 483–488.
27. HAKAN, R.L., C. EYL & S.J. HENRIKSEN. 1994. Neuropharmacology of the nucleus accumbens: systemic morphine effects on single-unit responses evoked by ventral pallidum stimulation. Neuroscience **63:** 85–93.
28. HAKAN, R.L. & S.J. HENRIKSEN. 1987. Systemic opiate administration has heterogenous effects on activity recorded from nucleus accumbnes neurons *in vivo*. Neurosci. Lett. **83:** 307–312.
29. MACKEY, W.B. & D. VAN DER KOOY. 1985. Neuroleptics block the positive reinforcing effects of amphetamine but not of morphine as measured by place conditioning. Pharmacol. Biochem. Behav. **22:** 101–105.
30. MUCHA, R.F. & A. HERZ. 1986. Preference conditioning produced by opioid active and inactive isomers of levorphanol and morphine in rat. Life Sci. **38:** 241–249.
31. LIAO, J.-X. & T.C. NAPIER. 1996. Effects of morphine on rat ventral pallidal neurons recorded *in vitro*. Soc. Neurosci. Abstr. **22:** 1311.
32. NORTH, R.A. 1992. Cellular actions of opiates and cocaine. Ann. N.Y. Acad. Sci. **654:** 1–6.
33. NORTH, R.A. 1993. Opioid actions on membrane ion channels. *In* Handbook of Experimental Pharmacology. 773. Springer-Verlag. Berlin.
34. CHROBAK, J.J. & T.C. NAPIER. 1993. Opioid and GABA modulation of accumbens-evoked ventral pallidal activity. J. Neural Transm. **93:** 123–143.
35. MCCARTHY, P.S., R.J. WALKER & G.N. WOODRUFF. 1977. Depressant actions of enkephalins on neurons in the nucleus accumbens. J. Physiol. **267:** 40P–41P.
36. CHOU, D.T. & S.C. WANG. 1992. Unit activity of amygdala and hippocampal neurons: effects of morphine and benzodiazepines. Brain Res. **126:** 427–440.
37. FREEMAN, J.E. & G.K. AGHAJANIAN. 1999. Opiate and α_2-adrenoceptor responses of rat amygdaloid neurons: co-localization and interactions during withdrawal. J. Neurosci. **5:** 3016–3024.

38. JOHNSON, P.I. & T.C. NAPIER. 1997. Morphine modulation of GABA- and glutamate-induced changes of ventral pallidal neuronal activity. Neuroscience **77:** 187–197.
39. ARDEN, R. J., V. SEGREDO, Z. WANG, J. LAMEH & W. SADEE. 1995. Phosphorylation and agonist-specific intracellular trafficking of an epitope-taged mu-opioid receptor expressed in HEK 293 cells. J. Neurochem. **65:** 1636–1645.
40. KEITH, D., S. MURRAY, P. ZAKI, P. CHU, D. LISSIN, L. KANG, C. EVANS & M. VON ZASTROW. 1996. Morphine activates opioid receptors without causing their rapid internalization. J. Biol. Chem. **271:** 19021–19024.
41. CHAKRABARTI, S., A.M. BABEY, P.Y. LAW, & H.H. LOH. 1996. Cyclic AMP dependent protein kinase induces phosphorylation of morphine-stimulated but not DAMGO-stimulated mu opioid receptors. Soc. Neurosci. Abstr. **22:** 822.
42. JORDAN, B. & L.A. DEVI. 1998. Molecular mechanisms of opioid receptor signal transduction. Br. J. Anaesth. **81:** 12–19.
43. SIMMONS, M. L. & C. CHAVKIN. 1996. Endogenous opioid regulation of hippocampal function. *In* International Review of Neurobiology. R.J. Bradley, R.A. Harris & P. Jenner, Eds.: 145–186. Academic Press. NewYork.
44. MITROVIC, I. & T.C. NAPIER. 1998. Substance P attenuates and DAMGO potentiates amygdala glutamatergic neurotransmission within the ventral pallidum. Brain Res. **792:** 193–206.
45. NAPIER, T.C., P.E. SIMSON & B.S. GIVENS. 1991. Dopamine electrophysiology of ventral pallidal/substantia innominata neurons: comparison with the dorsal globus pallidus. J. Pharmacol. Exp. Ther. **258:** 249–262.
46. JOHNSON, P.I. & T.C. NAPIER. 1997. GABA- and glutamate-evoked responses in the rat ventral pallidum are modulated by dopamine. Eur. J. Neurosci. **9:** 1397–1406.
47. ZABORSZKY, L., W.E. CULLINAN & A. BRAUN. 1991. Afferents to basal forebrain cholinergic projection neurons: an update. *In* The Basal Forebrain: Anatomy to Function. T. C. Napier, P. W. Kalivas & I. Hanin, Eds.: **295:** 43–100. Advances in Experimental Medicine and Biology. Plenum Press. New York and London.
48. JONES, D.L. & G.J. MOGENSON. 1980. Nucleus accumbens to globus pallidus GABA projection: electrophysiological and iontophoretic investigations. Brain Res. **188:** 93–105.
49. NAPIER, T.C., I. MITROVIC, L. CHURCHILL, M.A. KLITENICK, X.Y. LU & P.W. KALIVAS. 1995. Substance P in the ventral pallidum: projection from the ventral striatum, and electrophysiological and behavioral consequences of pallidal substance P. Neuroscience **69:** 59–70.
50. MASLOWSKI-COBUZZI, R.J. & T.C. NAPIER. 1994. Activation of dopaminergic neurons modulates ventral pallidal responses evoked by amygdala stimulation. Neuroscience **62:** 1103–1120.
51. UEDA, M., K. SUGIMOTO, T. OYAMA, Y. KURAISHI & M. SATOH. 1995. Opioidergic inhibition of capsaicin-evoked release of glutamate from rat spinal dorsal horn slices. Neuropharmacology **34:** 303–308.
52. CHIENG, B. & M.J. CHRISTIE. 1994. Inhibition by opioids acting on µ-receptors of GABAergic and glutamatergic postsynaptic potentials in single rat periaqueductal gray neurones *in vitro*. Br. J. Pharmacol. **113:** 303–309.
53. SESACK, S.R. & A. DEUTCH. 1989. Topographical organization of the efferent projections of the medial prefrontal cortex in the rat: an anterograde tract-tracing study with *Phaseolus vulgaris* leucoagglutinin. J. Comp. Neurol. **290:** 213–242.
54. KLITENICK, M.A., A.Y. DEUTCH, L. CHURCHILL & P.W. KALIVAS. 1992. Topography and functional role of dopaminergic projections from the ventral mesencephalic tegmentum to the ventral pallidum. Neuroscience **50:** 371–386.
55. PANG, K., J.M. TEPPER & L. ZABORSZKY. 1998. Morphological and electrophysiological characteristics of noncholinergic basal forebrain neurons. J. Comp. Neurol. **394:** 186–204.
56. MITROVIC, I. & T.C. NAPIER. 1996. Opioid modulation of ventral pallidal responses to activation of dopaminergic projections from the ventral tegmental area. Soc. Neurosci. Abstr. **22:** 1311.
57. MITROVIC, I. & T.C. NAPIER. 1997. Opioid modulation of responses by ventral pallidal neurons to dopmaine. Soc. Neurosci. Abstr. **23:** 2329.

58. MANSOUR, A., C.A. FOX, R.C. THOMPSON, H. AKIL & S.J. WATSON. 1994. μ-Opioid receptor mRNA expression in the rat CNS: comparison to μ-receptor binding. Brain Res. **643:** 245–265.
59. OLIVE, M.F., B. ANTON, P. MICEVYCH, C.J. EVANS & N.T. MAIDMENT. 1997. Presynaptic versus postsynaptic localization of μ and δ opioid receptors in dorsal and ventral striatopallidal pathways. J. Neurosci. **17:** 7471–7479.
60. HARRIS, H.W. & E.J. NESTLER. 1993. Opiate regulation of signal-transduction pathways. *In* The Neurobiology of Opiates. R. P. Hammer Jr., Ed.: 301–332. CRC Press. Boca Raton, Ann Arbor.
61. MIHARA, S. & R.A. NORTH. 1986. Opioids increase potassium conductance in submucous neurones of guinea-pig caecum by activating delta-receptors. Br. J. Pharmacol. **88:** 315–322.
62. KIEFFER, B.L. 1995. Recent advances in molecular recognition and signal transduction of active peptides: receptors for opioid peptides. Cell. Mol. Neurobiol. **15:** 615–635.
63. EVANS, C. 1993. Opioid and Opiate Receptors. *In* Handbook of Receptors and Channels. S. J. Peroutka, Ed.: 251–256. CRC Press. Boca Raton, FL.
64. SHULTS, C.W., R. QUIRION, R.T. JENSEN, T.W. MOODY, T.L. O'DONOHUE & T.N. CHASE. 1982. Autoradiographic localization of substance P receptors using ^{125}I substance P. Peptides **3:** 1073–1075.
65. LIU, H., J.L. BROWN, L. JASMIN, J.E. MAGGIO, S.R. VIGNA, P.W. MANTYH & A.I. BASBAUM. 1994. Synaptic relationship between substance P and the substance P receptor: light and electron microscopic characterization of the mismatch between neuropeptides and their receptors. Proc. Natl. Acad. Sci. USA **91:** 1009–1013.
66. CHURCHILL, L., A. BOURDELAIS, M.C. AUSTIN, S.J. LOLAIT, L.C. MAHAN, A.-M. O'CARROLL & P.W. KALIVAS. 1991. GABA$_A$ receptors containing α_1 and β_2 subunits are mainly localized on neurons in the ventral pallidum. Synapse (NY) **8:** 75–85.
67. PAGE, K.J. & B.J. EVERITT. 1995. The distribution of neurons coexpressing immunoreactivity to AMPA-sensitive glutamate receptor subtypes (GluR1-4) and nerve growth factor receptor in the rat basal forebrain. Eur. J. Neurosci. **7:** 1022–1033.
68. MONAGHAN, D.T. & C.W. COTMAN. 1985. Distribution of N-methyl-D-aspartate-sensitive L-[^{3}H]glutamate-binding sites in rat brain. J. Neurosci. **5:** 2909–2919.
69. VELIMIROVIC, B.M., K. KOYANO, S. NAKAJIMA & Y. NAKAJIMA. 1995. Opposing mechanisms of regulation of a G-protein-coupled inward rectifier K$^+$ channel in rat brain neurons. Proc. Natl. Acad. Sci. USA **92:** 1590–1594.
70. WANG, R.A. & M. RANDIC. 1994. Activation of μ-opioid receptor modulates GABA$_A$ receptor-mediated currents in isolated spinal dorsal horn neurons. Neurosci. Lett. **180:** 109–113.
71. ROZSA, K S., S.S. RUBAKHIN, A. SZUCS & G.B. STEFANO. 1996. Met-enkephalin and morphiceptin modulate a GABA-induced inward current in the CNS of *Lymnaea stagnalis L.* Gen. Pharmacol. **27:** 1337–1345.
72. CHEN, L. & L.-Y.M. HUANG. 1991. Sustained potentiation of NMDA receptor-mediated glutamate responses through activation of protein kinase C by a μ opioid. Neuron **7:** 319–326.
73. SUAREZ-ROCA, H. & W. MAIXNER. 1992. Morphine produces a multiphasic effect on the release of substance P from rat trigeminal nucleus slices by activating different opioid receptor subtypes. Brain Res. **579:** 195–203.
74. SUAREZ-ROCA, H. & W. MAIXNER. 1992. δ-Opioid-receptor activation by [D-Pen^2,D-Pen^5]enkephalin and morphine inhibits substance P release from trigeminal nucleus slices. Eur. J. Pharmacol. **229:** 1–7
75. SUGITA, S. & R.A. NORTH. 1993. Opioid actions on neurons of rat lateral amygdala *in vitro*. Brain Res. **612:** 151–155.
76. LUPICA, C.R. 1995. δ and μ enkephalins inhibit spontaneous GABA-mediated IPSCs via a cyclic AMP-independent mechanism in the rat hippocampus. J. Neurosci. **15:** 737–749.

77. COHEN, G.A., V.A. DOZE & D.V. MADISON. 1992. Opioid inhibition of GABA release from presynaptic terminals of rat hippocampal interneurons. Neuron **9:** 325–335.
78. XIE, C.W., R.A. MORRISETT & D.V. LEWIS. 1992. Mu opioid receptor-mediated modulation of synaptic currents in dentate granule cells of rat hippocampus. J. Neurophysiol. **68:** 1113–1120.
79. MOLEMAN, P., C.F.M. VAN VALKENBURG & J.A. VAN DER KROGT. 1984. Effects of morphine on dopamine metabolism in rat striatum and limbic structures in relation to the activity of dopaminergic neurones. Naunyn-Schmiedeberg's Arch. Pharmakol. **327:** 208–213.
80. DOURMAP, N., A. MICHAEL-TITUS & J. COSTENTIN. 1999. Local enkephalins tonically modulate dopamine release in the striatum: a microdialysis study. Brain Res. **524:** 153–155.
81. SCHLOSSER, B., M.B. KUDERNATSCH, B. SUTOR & G. TEN BRUGGENCATE. 1999. δ, μ and k opioid receptor agonists inhibit dopamine overflow in rat neostriatal slices. Neurosci. Lett. **191:** 126–130.
82. MULDER, A.H., A.N.M. SCHOFFELMEER & J.C. STOOF. 1990. On the role of adenylate cyclase in presynaptic modulation of neurotransmitter release mediated by monoamine and opioid receptors in the brain. *In* Presynaptic Receptors and the Question of Autoregulation of Neurotransmitter Release. Annals of the New York Academy of Sciences. S. Kalsner & T. C. Westfall, Eds.: **604:** 237–249. New York Academy of Sciences. New York.
83. WIDDOWSON, P.S. & R.B. HOLMAN. 1992. Ethanol-induced increase in endogenous dopamine release may involve endogenous opiates. J. Neurochem. **59:** 157–163.
84. WESTFALL, T.C., H. GRANT, L. NAES & M. MELDRUM. 1983. The effect of opioid drugs on the release of dopamine and 5-hydroxytryptamine from rat striatum following activation of nicotinic-cholinergic receptors. Eur. J. Pharmacol. **92:** 35–42.
85. HOFFMAN, D.C., T.E.G. WEST & R.A. WISE. 1991. Ventral pallidal microinjections of receptor-selective opioid agonists produce differential effects on circling and locomotor activity in rats. Brain Res. **550:** 205–212.
86. AUSTIN, M.C. & P.W. KALIVAS. 1990. Enkephalinergic and GABAergic modulation of motor activity in the ventral pallidum. J. Pharmacol. Exp. Ther. **252:** 1370–1377.
87. KRETSCHMER, B.D. & M. KOCH. 1998. The ventral pallidum mediates disruption of prepulse inhibition of the acoustic startle response induced by dopamine agonists, but not by NMDA antagonists. Brain Res. **798:** 204–210.
88. PANAGIS, G. & C. SPYRAKI. 1996. Neuropharmacological evidence for the role of dopamine in ventral pallidum self-stimulation. Psychopharmacology (Berl.) **123:** 280–288.
89. GONG, W.H., D. NEILL & J.B. JUSTICE JR. 1996. Conditioned place preference and locomotor activation produced by injection of psychostimulants into ventral pallidum. Brain Res. **707:** 64–74.

Cross-species Studies of Sensorimotor Gating of the Startle Reflex

NEAL R. SWERDLOW,[a] DAVID L. BRAFF, AND MARK A. GEYER

Department of Psychiatry, University of California, San Diego, La Jolla, California 92093-0804, USA

ABSTRACT: Sensorimotor gating of the startle reflex can be assessed across species, using similar stimuli to elicit comparable response characteristics. As measured by prepulse inhibition (PPI), gating is reduced in patients with some neuropsychiatric disorders, and in rats after manipulations of limbic cortex, striatum, pallidum, or pontine tegmentum. This limbic "CSPP" circuitry can be studied in rats to reveal the neurochemical and neuroanatomical substrates regulating PPI at a high level of resolution. This detailed circuit information is used as a "blueprint" to identify substrates that may lead to PPI deficits in psychiatric-disordered humans. Some human disorders with identifiable, localized lesions in CSPP circuitry, for example, Huntington's disease, provide direct validation for this cross-species model. Studies have begun to assess the pharmacological homology of PPI across species, as an initial step towards translating detailed neural circuit information from rats to humans. These initial studies suggest the possibility that the effects of dopaminergic (DAergic) drugs on PPI (reducing PPI) may be homologous across species; nicotinic drugs may also produce similar effects on PPI across species (increasing PPI). By contrast, the effects of glutamatergic and serotonergic drugs may exhibit disparate effects on PPI across species. The use of DAergic agonists in human studies is complicated by their significant side effects, but new studies demonstrate that several "human friendly" direct DA agonists disrupt PPI in rats and are thus good candidates for further studies of the cross-species homology of the DAergic regulation of PPI. In this manner, PPI can be used to probe the sensitivity of DAergic systems, and perhaps other CSPP elements, across normal and neuropsychiatric-disordered populations.

INTRODUCTION: THE STARTLE REFLEX AND PREPULSE INHIBITION

The startle reflex is a contraction of the skeletal and facial muscles to sudden, relatively intense stimuli, that is usually classified as a defensive response. One major advantage of startle reflex paradigms in psychopathology research is that this reflex can be studied across species. In humans, the eye blink component of startle is typically measured using electromyography (EMG) of the orbicularis oculi muscle. In rats, stabilimeter chambers measure the whole-body flinch elicited by stimuli that are similar to those used in humans. Although the "primary" mammalian acoustic startle circuit[1,2] consists of three synapses linking the auditory nerve with the spinal

---

[a]Address correspondence to Neal R. Swerdlow, M.D., Ph.D., Associate Professor, Department of Psychiatry, 0804, UCSD School of Medicine, 9500 Gilman Drive, La Jolla, CA 92093-0804. Voice: 619-543-6270; fax: 619-543-2493; nswerdlow@ucsd.edu

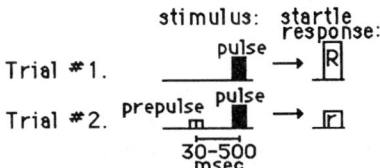

FIGURE 1. Prepulse inhibition is a profound decrease in startle magnitude when the startling pulse is preceded by a weak prepulse. The degree of PPI is expressed as 100−((r/R) × 100).

motor neuron, startle demonstrates several important forms of plasticity, including habituation[3] and fear potentiation,[4] that are regulated by the forebrain. These more complex processes exhibit striking similarities across species, making startle plasticity ideal for translational research. One form of startle plasticity, "prepulse inhibition" (PPI), is the normal suppression of the startle reflex, when the intense startling stimulus is preceded by a weak prestimulus[5] (FIG. 1).

In PPI, a weak sensory event inhibits the motor response to an abrupt, powerful stimulus. PPI is a very robust experimental phenomenon: it occurs when the prepulse and startling stimuli are in the same or different sensory modalities; it occurs in virtually all mammals and primates; it is not a form of conditioning, inasmuch as it occurs on the first exposure to the prepulse and pulse stimuli; and it does not exhibit habituation or extinction over multiple trials. Although the inhibitory effect of the prepulse on startle reactivity is effected within the pons, descending limbic cortico-striato-pallido-pontine circuitry regulates the inhibitory "tone" within the pons and thus determines the degree to which the prepulse inhibits the subsequent startle response (cf. refs. 1, 2, and 6). PPI thus reflects the activation of "hardwired" behavioral gating processes that are regulated by forebrain neural circuitry.

In one conceptual model of PPI,[7] a weak stimulus activates brain-based processes that initially increase and then blunt responsivity to sensory events during a subsequent brief temporal window; the period of "gating" is empirically determined to be approximately 30–500 ms in duration, in both rats and humans[3,5] (FIG. 2). The period of reduced responsivity might momentarily "protect" information contained in the weak stimulus, so that it can be adequately processed, without interference from subsequent stimuli. Whereas PPI is studied under very controlled conditions in the laboratory, under natural circumstances, sensorimotor gating is conceptualized as being continuously active in the waking human nervous system, contributing to our ability to segregate a continuous stream of sensory and cognitive information, and to selectively allocate attentional resources to salient stimuli. The specific characteris-

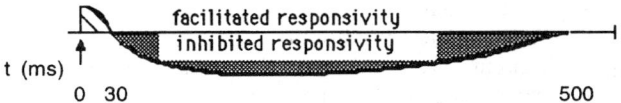

FIGURE 2. A conceptual model of sensorimotor gating, based on findings with PPI: after a weak stimulus (arrow), the behavioral response to subsequent stimuli is facilitated for 0–30 ms and inhibited, or "gated," for 30–500 ms.

tics of an individual's gating processes are viewed to be plastic, shaped by genetic and developmental forces, but also sensitive to changes in the environment, stressors, or the neurochemical and hormonal milieu of the nervous system.[7] A more substantial, pathological breakdown in the gating "window" would be expected to impair the orderly, hierarchical processing of sensory events and result in a flooding of sensory information, with a fragmenting impact on cognition.[8]

PPI IN NEUROPSYCHIATRIC DISORDERS

Interest in PPI as a measure of sensorimotor gating has been stimulated by findings that disorders with known dysfunction in brain substrates that regulate PPI are accompanied by evidence of impaired cognitive or sensorimotor inhibition. Deficient PPI is reported in patients with schizophrenia,[9–12] obsessive compulsive disorder (OCD),[13] Huntington's disease (HD),[14] nocturnal enuresis and attention deficit disorder,[15] and Tourette syndrome.[16] These disorders are all characterized symptomatically by a loss of gating in sensory, motor, or cognitive domains, and by abnormalities in cortico-striato-pallido-pontine circuitry that modulates PPI. Importantly, PPI deficits are not unique to a single form of psychopathology.

PPI may be very valuable for studying the neurobiology of schizophrenia because of the relevance of gating "anatomy" to the pathophysiology of this disorder and because deficits in gating of cognitive and sensory information are clinically important features of this disorder. Schizophrenic patients are impaired in measures of sustained or "voluntary" attention and, clinically, demonstrate an inability to automatically filter or gate irrelevant thoughts and sensory stimuli from intruding into conscious awareness.[8] PPI deficits are seen in schizotypal patients who are not grossly psychotic or receiving antipsychotic medications;[17] thus the relative loss of PPI in schizophrenia spectrum patients does not simply result from gross behavioral impairment or medications. Although we do not know the precise neurobiology of these PPI deficits, studies have revealed abnormalities at several levels of the startle "gating circuitry" in schizophrenic patients, including the hippocampus, nucleus accumbens, striatum, globus pallidus, and thalamus.[18–24]

It has been reported that PPI deficits in schizophrenia patients correlate significantly with perseverative responses on the Wisconsin Card Sorting Task[25] and measures of thought disorder,[26] distractibility,[27] and psychotic symptoms.[28] PPI is also reduced in nonpatient controls who are "psychosis prone,"[29] or who have an MMPI profile associated with specific neuropsychological deficits.[96] Thus, PPI is a measure of sensorimotor gating functions that correlate with, and perhaps contribute to, important determinants of information processing in both patients and nonpatient controls.

The neural substrates that regulate PPI in laboratory animals overlap substantially with brain circuitry that regulates the reinforcing properties of drugs of abuse. Space constraints preclude a complete review of this large field, but there is substantive evidence that the reinforcing properties and withdrawal syndromes associated with psychomotor stimulants, opiates, and ethanol are regulated by specific elements of DAergic and/or serotonergic (5HTergic) circuitry connecting the prefrontal cortex, portions of the extended amygdala, and the ventral pallidum.[31–38] These substrates overlap substantially with brain circuitry that regulates PPI (see below). This overlap in circuitry makes it possible to study neural substrates relevant to drug reinforcement in humans, via measures of PPI. For ethical and logistical reasons, it is much easier to study drug effects on PPI—via dose-response and agonist-antagonist studies, and other standard approaches to pharmacological analyses—compared to measures of drug self-administration or reinforcement, in either normal human or drug-abuse populations. Furthermore, based on the detailed anatomical information from preclinical studies of PPI, it may ultimately be possible to use drug studies with PPI to probe relevant brain circuitry at a very precise level in humans, and to pursue very sophisticated pharmacological strategies for manipulating this circuitry in order to understand the pathophysiology, genetics, and therapeutics of drug addiction. Thus, there are compelling reasons to study the neurochemistry of PPI in humans, to facilitate the cross-species translation of information regarding neural circuitry that has direct relevance to the brain substrates of drug addiction.

CROSS-SPECIES STUDIES OF PPI

Among the neurotransmitters that regulate PPI in laboratory animals, DA appears to exert powerful control, acting at least in part via its effects in the ventral striatum and frontal cortex (cf. refs. 2, and 6). Because of the relevance of this brain circuitry to the pathophysiology of schizophrenia (above) and other disorders, such as Tourette syndrome,[39] and the potential utility of this DAergic regulation of PPI in the development of novel antipsychotics,[40] it is critically important to fully study the DAergic regulation of PPI in cross-species measures of PPI. Consistent with many reports of DAagonist-induced reductions of PPI in rodents, preliminary reports suggest that PPI in normal humans is reduced by the indirect DA agonist, amphetamine,[41] and by the direct DA agonist, bromocriptine.[42] In another study, patients with Parkinson's disease exhibited a loss of PPI after challenge with the direct DA agonist, apomorphine, but not after treatment with L-DOPA.[43] Unfortunately, these initial pharmacologic studies of PPI in humans were variously performed with small samples, using a single dose, or in nonnormative populations, complicating the interpretation of the findings. These studies certainly justify a more thorough assessment of whether manipulations of the DAergic substrates regulating PPI in rats can be extended to human studies and thereby provide critically important information regarding the neural substrates underlying a loss of PPI in clinical populations.

Studies of the regulation of PPI by nicotinic, glutamatergic, and 5HTergic systems underscore the importance of directly verifying cross-species drug effects. In some cases, drug effects are consistent across species, inasmuch as nicotine increases PPI in both rats[44] and humans.[45] By contrast, the noncompetitive NMDA receptor antagonist, ketamine, which consistently disrupts PPI in rats, has been reported to either disrupt,[46] potentiate,[47] or have no effect on PPI in humans.[48] Similarly, although 5HT releasers, such as methylene-dioxy-methamphetamine (MDMA), potently disrupt PPI in rats,[49] preliminary studies suggest that the opposite effects occur in humans.[50] Although methodologic differences in dose, time course, and route of administration might account for cross-species differences in the PPI-modulatory effects of ketamine and MDMA, these issues clearly must be resolved before we can be confident in translating, from rats to humans, information regarding the neural substrates underlying the glutamatergic and 5HTergic regulation of PPI.

It will be extremely valuable to identify neurochemical domains in which information from preclinical studies of PPI can be applied towards understanding human neural circuitry. Based on both animal and preliminary human studies, the DAergic systems appear to be the substrates most likely to exhibit cross-species homology in the regulation of PPI. Animal studies of PPI can assess at a very high level of resolution the functional (i.e., behaviorally consequential) relationships between important neural substrates, such as the interactions between DAergic and glutamatergic systems within subregions of the ventral striatum.[51] Information about these complex physiological systems will complement and greatly enhance the power of existing neuroimaging technologies for understanding detailed neural circuitry in humans.[50] Studies of PPI allow us to understand physiological interactions at a level of neurobehavioral resolution comparable to that obtained with the gill withdrawal reflex of *Aplysia californica*, using behavior and neural substrates that can be directly informative about potentially homologous neural systems in the human brain.

NEURAL SUBSTRATES OF PPI

Studies in rats have revealed that PPI is regulated by sequential and parallel neural connections between limbic cortex (including temporal and medial prefrontal cortex), the ventral striatum, the ventral pallidum, and the pontine tegmentum (cf. refs. 2, 6, 52, and 53). This limbic cortico-striato-pallido-pontine circuitry converges with the primary startle circuit at the level of the nucleus reticularis pontis caudalis (PnC)[54] (FIG. 3). The neurotransmitters active at several levels of this circuitry have also been studied via systemic and central drug infusion studies in rats (see below). Some of this information has already been applied towards predictive models for the development of novel psychopharmacological agents.[6,60,62]

The evidence for specific neurochemical and neuroanatomical substrates regulating PPI, within this limbic CSPP circuitry, has been reviewed in several articles from our group[6,52,53] and from others, particularly Koch and colleagues.[2,55] A complete review of this material would thus be redundant. However, a few specific points are worth emphasizing.

Some of our knowledge of the neural regulation of PPI comes from clinical studies in human populations with known or suspected regions of localized brain dysfunction. Thus, studies of PPI deficits in patients with temporal lobe seizure disorders[56,57] or movement disorders, such as HD[14] or Parkinson's disease (post-apomorphine[43]), yield fairly reliable neural maps for the regulation of PPI in humans. These studies also provide a form of validation for this cross-species model, when these patterns of localized brain dysfunction—recreated in laboratory animals —result in a loss of PPI. PPI deficits in disorders with less understand neuropathologies, such as Tourette disorder,[16] OCD,[13] or nocturnal enuresis,[15] may suggest the regulation of PPI by particular brain systems, such as the basal ganglia (Tourette disorder) or pontine tegmentum (nocturnal enuresis), but these studies do not permit a specific regional localization for the observed loss of PPI.

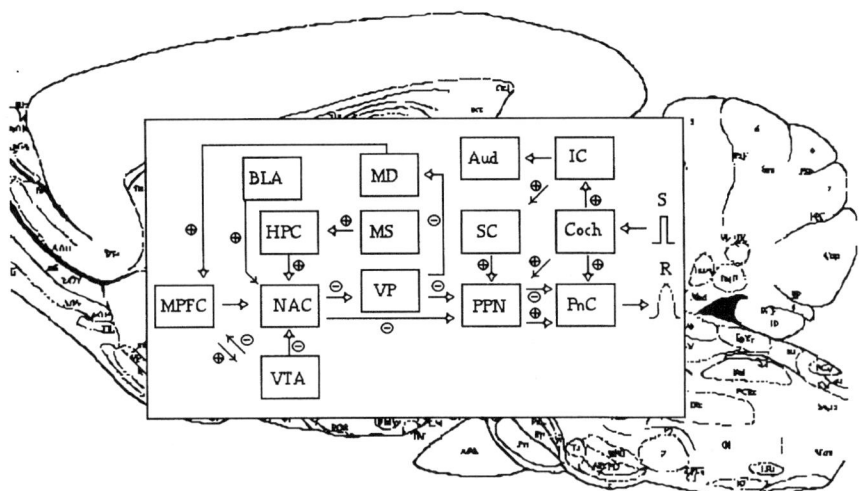

FIGURE 3. Schematic model of neural substrates regulating acoustic startle and PPI in the rat, modified from previous evolving diagrams.[2,52,53] Many connections within this circuitry are omitted, for simplicity of representation. Acoustic stimulus "S" elicits startle response "R" via simple pontine circuitry; prepulse effects on R are mediated via PPN, which is regulated by descending serial and parallel projections from the forebrain. Neurotransmitter identities of excitatory and inhibitory connections can be found within referenced materials. Model is highly schematized, clearly incomplete, and based on work by many groups (e.g., discussed in refs. 1, 2, 30, 55, 58, 59, and 97–108). Aud, auditory cortex; BLA, basolateral amygdala; Coch, cochlea; HPC, hippocampus; IC, inferior colliculus; MPFC, medial prefrontal cortex; MS, medial septal nucleus; NAC, nucleus accumbens; MD, dorsomedial thalamus; PnC, nucleus reticularis pontis caudalis; PPN, pedunculopontine nucleus; SC, superior colliculus; VP, ventral pallidum; VTA, ventral tegmental area.

The process of identifying the neural regulation of PPI in preclinical studies has been driven by several motivating factors. First, investigators wish to localize within specific brain regions the neurochemical substrates responsible for changes in PPI observed after systemic pharmacologic manipulations. For example, these studies have examined the regulation of PPI by forebrain DAergic regions, including the ventral striatum (VS), to attempt to localize the site of action responsible for the PPI-disruptive effects of systemically administered DA agonists[58] or NMDA antagonists,[59] and for the reversal of these effects by antipsychotics.[60–62] One aim of such studies has been to use the apparent *predictive validity* of this measure, for clinical antipsychotic potency,[40] as a basis for exploring substrates that may be responsible for the cross-species parallels in antipsychotic drug effects; the implicit assumption is that such substrates may contribute to the clinical efficacy of antipsychotics.

A second motivation for these studies is to draw on the apparent *construct validity* of this measure, by exploring the regulation of PPI by neural substrates that are implicated in the pathophysiology of specific disorders. Thus, several studies have examined the impact of striatal lesions and effects of striatal neurotoxins on PPI, to understand the basis for the loss of PPI in HD patients.[63,64] Other studies have examined changes in PPI after lesions of the ventral hippocampus or medial prefrontal cortex, based on the suspected involvement of these brain regions in the pathophysiology of schizophrenia[18,21-23] and the reported reduction of PPI in schizophrenia patients. Other models with construct validity for the loss of PPI in schizophrenia patients, using *in utero* (e.g., maternal protein deprivation) or early neonatal (e.g., isolation rearing) manipulations, are now being explored at the level of the underlying neural substrates.[65-67]

A third motivation for these studies is to use PPI as a measure for identifying functional connectivity both within and between critical brain regions, because it is a quantifiable, reliable, and sensitive behavioral measure that is regulated by brain circuitry of interest to a broad band of neuropsychiatric research. Complex interactions between dopamine and glutamate within the accumbens core and shell regions have been explored via this strategy,[61,68,69] as have interactions between the hippocampus, basolateral amygdala and NAC,[70-72] between DA and adenosine,[73] and between DA and several neuropeptides.[74-76] Here, perhaps, is the most important application of this measure—as a tool that can reveal what no microscope can illuminate, what no antibody can label, what no antero- or retrograde transported protein can stain: the ability of specific neural manipulations to modify a behavior of direct relevance to human cognition and brain disorders.

Translating the Dopaminergic Substrates of PPI across Species

Although evidence suggests that the greatest degree of cross-species homology in the neural regulation of PPI is found in DAergic systems, the side effects of many DA agonists in humans are a clear hinderance to cross-species studies of this substrate. The primary tool for such cross-species studies are the DA *agonists*: at baseline states, DA *antagonists* have weak and inconsistent effects on PPI in rats, particularly at doses that do not reduce "pulse alone" startle magnitude.[40,62] Among the different types of DA agonists, indirect agonists, such as amphetamine and cocaine, have potentially problematic psychomotor activating and addicting properties that may limit their utility in human studies and, in rats, produce relatively modest (though statistically reliable) reductions in PPI.[77,78]

The first report of the effects of a direct DA agonist on PPI in rats was published in 1986.[30] In the ensuing 12 years, studies have explored the neurochemical and neuroanatomical substrates mediating the PPI-disruptive effects of DA agonists (cf. refs. 2, 6, and 53). These studies have revealed a clear image of the neural basis—and potential clinical significance—of this DAergic regulation of sensorimotor gating. The DA agonists in these animal studies were chosen for their ability to clearly define neurobiological substrates and not for their applicability to human studies. Direct DA agonists, such as apomorphine, produce a robust disruption of PPI in rats—making them very useful in drug interaction studies[40]—but almost invariably cause intolerable nausea and emesis in humans.[79] Attempts to study the effects of apomorphine on PPI in normal humans have been aborted, due to the emetic effects of this drug, even in the presence of peripheral DA antagonism (M. Stein, M.D., personal communication).

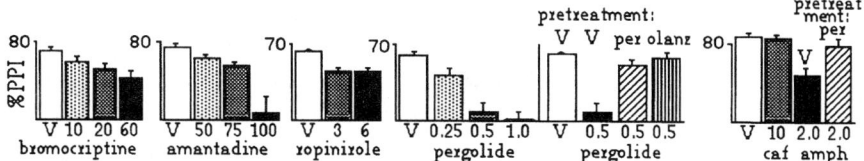

FIGURE 4. Data from ref. 80. Bromocriptine, amantadine, ropinirole, or pergolide cause dose-dependent reductions of PPI in rats. The effects of pergolide are prevented by perphenazine, 0.5 mg/kg (per), or olanzapine, 2.5 mg/kg (olanz). Data are collapsed over time. Amphetamine (but not caffeine) also reduces PPI, and this is prevented by perphenazine. Doses in mg/kg. V, vehicle.

Thus, a critical next step in translating this cross-species model will be to identify pharmacologic tools with tolerable side effects that can be used to effectively probe the DAergic regulation of PPI in humans. Our group recently studied the effects on PPI in rodents of DA agonists that can be effectively administered to humans.[80] Pergolide is a D1/2/3 receptor agonist[81] that has been used to treat both Parkinson's disease and Tourette syndrome.[82] Compared to apomorphine, pergolide produces less nausea and emesis, is better tolerated (even in children[82]), but has not been evaluated for its effects on PPI in clinical studies. Bromocriptine is a direct DA receptor agonist that has been shown previously to reduce PPI in humans - an effect that was antagonized by the D2 receptor antagonist, haloperidol.[42] Bromocriptine also appears to reduce P50 event-related potential (ERP) gating measures in humans.[83] Ropinirole (SKF 101468) is a direct D2 agonist with anti-Parkinsonian properties in humans[84] that also has not yet been studied in humans in the PPI model. Amantadine is an indirect DA agonist and NMDA antagonist[85] that has a variety of clinical applications ranging from anti-Parkinsonian to antiviral. It is well tolerated in humans, with minimal side effects in humans, but its effects on PPI have not been evaluated in humans. In addition, we have previously reported on the PPI-disruptive effects of amphetamine in rats,[77] and there is preliminary evidence that this indirect DA agonist disrupts PPI[41] and related measures of P50 gating in humans.[86]

These "more tolerable" DA agonists, amantadine, bromocriptine, pergolide, and ropinirole, significantly reduce PPI in rats, as seen in FIGURE 4 (from ref. 80). The PPI-disruptive effects of pergolide were blocked by the atypical antipsychotic olanzapine and the typical antipsychotic perphenazine. Interestingly, among these DA agonists, bromocriptine caused only a partial disruption of PPI at doses as high as 60 mg/kg; by contrast, it potently disrupts PPI (effect size approximately 2.0) in humans after an oral total dose of 1.25 mg.[42] As with other cross-species differences in drug effects, it is possible that cross-species differences in bromocriptine potency reflect methodological differences in, for example, drug administration or pharmacodynamics, rather than species-related differences in the DAergic regulation of PPI. Nonetheless, this observation underscores the importance of directly assessing the DAergic regulation of PPI across species, rather than simply assuming that rats and humans will exhibit identical behavioral responses to DAergic challenge in this measure.

SPECIAL ISSUES IN THE CROSS-SPECIES TRANSLATION OF PPI FINDINGS

Several challenges must be addressed as we attempt to translate, from laboratory animals to humans, the neurochemical and neuroanatomical substrates regulating sensorimotor gating.

Sex Differences

Sex differences in PPI have been identified in both humans and rats,[87-89] but their physiological bases are not known. Furthermore, there are some inconsistencies in the literature, with some groups, but not others, reporting a male greater than female PPI difference in both rats[90] and humans.[91] Hormonal regulation of PPI in females has also been reported in both rats[92] and humans,[93] but, again, it is not clear that the physiological bases for these cyclic changes are comparable across species. Thus, one significant challenge facing future cross-species translational studies of PPI will be the need to account for such sex differences and to understand their potential interaction with both pharmacologic probes and disease states.

Measurement and Laterality

Another challenge facing this translational approach relates to methodologic issues in the measurement of PPI. Although many of the stimulus parameters used to assess PPI are identical or nearly identical across species, the hardware used for PPI measures differs greatly across species. Rodent studies of PPI typically measure the whole body flinch response, whereas human studies typically use EMG measures of orbicularis oculi. Until recently, the majority of human startle studies have assessed PPI from only one eye, yielding unilateral measures of startle and PPI. More recently, studies have begun to assess bilateral measures of eyeblink startle and PPI, which affords the opportunity to assess lateralized patterns of sensorimotor gating. The lateralization of the startle pathway, projecting from the PnC to the spinal motor neuron, differs greatly across species, and the degree to which this projection is limited to a contralateral pathway appears to increase along the phylogenetic scale (cf. ref. 53). Thus, another challenge for future studies using this translational approach will be to reconcile the impact of drugs and/or neural manipulations of the whole body flinch response in rats, with the relevant effects on potentially lateralized eyeblink measures of PPI in humans.

Strain-related Effects

A third challenge in the translational analysis of PPI relates to the apparent sensitivity of this measure, and its modification by psychotropic drugs, to slight variations in rat[94,95] and potentially human[17,29,96] strains. We have reported strain differences in the effects of apomorphine and clozapine on PPI in rats,[95] and one recent report suggests that the PPI-disruptive effects of the apomorphine differ significantly even among same-strain rats obtained from different suppliers.[94] Extrapolated across species, such differences in the neurochemical regulation of PPI might be anticipated among clinical populations of different ethnicity or national origin. Differences in PPI among groups with subtle genetic disparities may also underlie patterns of PPI, or of drug sensitivities, that vary significantly with an individual's temperament or personality structure. Obviously, whereas such sensitivity may make this measure particularly valuable for studying the neural basis of complex psychological processes, or cross-cultural/genetic differences, it may also complicate the interpretation of drug effects in a mixed sample of control subjects and, certainly, in comparing such findings across different cultural groups.

SUMMARY

PPI is a quantifiable measure of complex sensorimotor inhibitory processes that are modulated by a well-characterized neural circuit connecting limbic cortical regions and subcortical DAergic systems. This circuit ultimately innervates the primary startle circuit in the pons via subpallidal efferent projections. Abnormal interactions between the limbic cortical and subcortical elements of this circuitry are proposed in several models to underlie the emergence of symptoms in schizophrenia and other major psychiatric disorders. Evidence for the neural regulation of PPI comes largely from studies in rats, although some confirmatory information in humans can be found in PPI deficits among individuals with known or presumed brain lesions. Complex anatomical and neurochemical features of this circuitry have been studied in rats, using PPI as an index of functional circuit "output." To translate this neural circuit information to humans, it will be important to validate basic features of the neurochemical regulation of PPI across species. Critical first steps in this process include the identification of "human-friendly" pharmacologic probes, to assess the similarities and differences of these drugs on PPI in rats versus humans. Initial steps are being taken to accomplish this goal, via drugs acting within dopaminergic, glutamatergic, serotonergic, and nicotinic systems. Many formidable challenges face this translational approach, including the need to assess or control for the potential impact of sex, laterality, and genetic strain on the interpretation of drug effects on PPI in humans and rats. Despite the sensitivity of PPI to such complex variables—indeed, perhaps because of this—it is clear that studies of PPI will permit a cross-species translation of neurobiological information with direct relevance to the pathophysiology of several major neuropsychiatric disorders.

ACKNOWLEDGMENTS

The authors were supported by MH 01436 (N.R.S.), MH 54621 (N.R.S.), MH 53484 (N.R.S.), and MH 42228 (D.L.B., M.A.G., and N.R.S.); and a MIRECC Award from the Veterans Administration (D.L.B. and M.A.G.). N.R.S. was also supported by an Independent Investigator Award from the National Alliance for Research on Schizophrenia and Depression (NARSAD). This review manuscript summarizes findings from many original reports; portions of this manuscript may thus paraphrase or approximate information (e.g., refs. 6 and 53) that has previously been published by the authors.

REFERENCES

1. DAVIS, M. *et al.* 1982. A primary acoustic startle circuit: lesion and stimulation studies. J. Neurosci. **2:** 791–805.
2. KOCH, M. & H-U. SCHNITZLER. 1997. The acoustic startle response in rats: circuits mediating evocation, inhibition and potentiation. Behav. Brain. Res. **89:** 35–49.
3. HOFFMAN, H.S. & J.L. SEARLE. 1968. Acoustic and temporal factors in the evocation of startle. J. Acoust. Soc. Am. **43:** 269–282.
4. BROWN, J.S. *et al.* 1951. Conditioned fear as revealed by magnitude of startle response to an auditory stimulus. J. Exp. Psychol. **41:** 317-328.
5. GRAHAM, F. 1975. The more or less startling effects of weak prestimuli. Psychophysiology **12:** 238–248.
6. SWERDLOW, N.R. & M.A. GEYER. 1998. Using an animal model of deficient sensorimotor gating to study the pathophysiology and new treatments of schizophrenia. Schizophr. Bull. **24:** 285–302.
7. SWERDLOW, N.R. 1996. Cortico-striatal substrates of cognitive, motor and sensory gating: Speculations and implications for psychological function and dysfunction. Adv. Biol. Psychiatry **2:** 179–208.
8. MCGHIE, A. & J. CHAPMAN. 1961. Disorders of attention and perception in early schizophrenia. Br. J. Med. Psychol. **34:** 102–116.
9. BOLINO, F. *et al.* 1994. Sensorimotor gating and habituation evoked by electrocutaneous stimulation in schizophrenia. Biol. Psychiatry **36:** 670–679.
10. BRAFF, D.L. *et al.* 1992. Gating and habituation of the startle reflex in schizophrenic patients. Arch. Gen. Psychiatry **49:** 206–215.
11. BRAFF, D. *et al.* 1978. Prestimulus effects on human startle reflex in normals and schizophrenics. Psychophysiology **15:** 339–343.
12. GRILLON, C. *et al.* 1992. Startle gating deficits occur across prepulse intensities in schizophrenic patients. Biol. Psychiatry **32:** 939–943.
13. SWERDLOW, N.R. *et al.* 1993. A preliminary assessment of sensorimotor gating in patients with obsessive compulsive disorder (OCD). Biol. Psychiatry **33:** 298–301.
14. SWERDLOW, N.R. *et al.* 1995. Impaired prepulse inhibition of acoustic and tactile startle in patients with Huntington's disease. J. Neurol. Neurosurg. Psychiatry **58:** 192–200.
15. ORNITZ, E.M. *et al.* 1992. Prestimulation-induced startle modulation in attention-deficit hyperactivitydisorder and nocturnal enuresis. Psychophysiology **29:** 437-451.
16. CASTELLANOS, F.X. *et al.* 1996. Sensorimotor gating in boys with Tourette's syndrome and ADHD: preliminary results. Biol. Psychiatry **39:** 33–41.
17. CADENHEAD, K.S. *et al.* 1993. Impaired startle prepulse inhibition and habituation in patients with schizotypal personality disorder. Am. J. Psychiatry **150:** 1862–1867.
18. BOGERTS, B. *et al.* 1985. Basal ganglia and limbic system pathology in schizophrenia. A morphometric study of brain volume and shrinkage. Arch. Gen.Psychiatry **42:** 784–791.
19. EARLY, T.S. *et al.* 1987. Left globus pallidus abnormality in newly medicated patients with schizophrenia. Proc. Natl. Acad. Sci. USA **84:** 561–564.
20. PAKKENBERG, B. 1990. Pronounced reduction of total neuron number in mediodorsal thalamic nucleus and nucleus accumbens in schizophrenics. Arch. Gen. Psychiatry **47:** 1023–1029.
21. SILBERSWEIG, D.A. *et al.* 1995. A functional neuroanatomy of hallucinations in schizophrenia. Nature **378:** 176–179.
22. SUDDATH, R.L. *et al.* 1990. Anatomic abnormalities in the brains of monozygotic twins discordant for schizophrenia. N. Engl. J. Med. **322:** 789–794.
23. WEINBERGER, D.R. *et al.* 1992. Evidence for dysfunction of a prefrontal-limbic network in schizophrenia: An MRI and rCBF study of discordant monozygotic twins. Am. J. Psychiatry **149:** 890–897.
24. WONG, D. *et al.* 1986. Positron emission tomography reveals elevated D2 dopamine receptors in drug-naive schizophrenics. Science **234:** 1558–1563.

25. BUTLER, R.W. *et al.* 1991. Wisconsin card sorting deficits and diminished sensorimotor gating in a discrete subgroup of schizophrenic patients. *In* Advances in Neuropsychiatry and Psychopharmacology Vol. 1: Schizophrenia Research. C.A. Tamminga & S.C. Schulz, Eds. : 163–168. Raven Press. New York.
26. PERRY, W. & D.L. BRAFF. 1994. Information-processing deficits and thought disorder in schizophrenia. Am. J. Psychiatry **151:** 363–367.
27. KARPER, L.P. *et al.* 1996. Preliminary evidence of an association between sensorimotor gating and distractibility in psychosis. J. Neuropsychiatry Clin. Neurosci. **8:** 60-66.
28. BRAFF, D.L. *et al.* 1998. Symptom correlates of prepulse inhibition deficits in male schizophrenic patients. Am. J. Psychiatry. In press.
29. CADENHEAD, K.S. *et al.* 1998. Sensorimotor gating deficits in schizophrenic patients and their relatives [abstract]. Biol. Psychiatry **43:** 10S.
30. SWERDLOW, N.R. *et al.* 1986. Central dopamine hyperactivity in rats mimics abnormal acoustic startle in schizophrenics. Biol. Psychiatry **21:** 23–33.
31. HUBNER, C.B. & G.F. KOOB. 1990. The ventral pallidum plays a role in mediating cocaine and heroin self-administration in the rat. Brain Res. **508:** 20–26.
32. IMPERATO, A. & G. DICHIARA. 1986. Preferential stimulation of dopamine release in the nucleus accumbens of freely moving rats by ethanol. J. Pharmacol. Exp. Ther. **239:** 221–225.
33. KOOB, G.F. 1992. Drugs of Abuse: Anatomy, pharmacology, and function of reward pathways. Trends Pharmacol. Sci. **13:** 177–179.
34. KOOB, G.F. *et al.* 1993. The mesocorticolimbic circuit in drug dependence and reward—a role for the extended amygdala? *In* Limbic Motor Circuits and Neuropsychiatry. P.W. Kalivas & C.D. Barnes, Eds.: 289-309. CRC Press. Boca Raton, FL.
35. KOOB, G.F. *et al.* 1977. Effects of d-amphetamine on concurrent self-stimulation of forebrain and brainstem loci. Brain Res. **137:** 109–113.
36. PETTIT, H.O. *et al.* 1984. Destruction of dopamine in the nucleus accumbens selectively attenuates cocaine but not heroin self-administration in rats. Psychopharmacology **84:**167–172.
37. ROBLEDO, P., R. MALDONADO-LOPEZ & G.F. KOOB. 1992. Role of dopamine receptors in the nucleus accumbens in the rewarding properties of cocaine. *In* The Neurobiology of Drug and Alcohol Addiction. P.W. Kalivas & H.H. Samson, Eds.: **654:** 509. New York Academy of Sciences. New York.
38. ROSSETTI, Z.L., F. MELIS, S. CARBONI & G.L. GESSA. 1992. Dramatic depletion of mesolimbic extracellular dopamine after withdrawal from morphine, alcohol or cocaine: a common neurochemical substrate for drug dependence. Ann. N.Y. Acad. Sci. **654:** 513.
39. WOLF, S. *et al.* 1996. Tourette syndrome: Prediction of phenotypic variation in monozygotic twins by caudate nucleus D2 receptor binding. Science **273:** 1225–1227.
40. SWERDLOW, N.R. *et al.* 1994. Assessing the validity of an animal model of sensorimotor gating deficits in schizophrenic patients. Arch. Gen. Psychiatry **51:** 139–154.
41. HUTCHINSON, K.E. & R.M. SWIFT. 1997. Effects of amphetamine on psychophysiological and subjective measures of stimulation in humans. Proc. Soc. Psychophysiological Res.: S45.
42. ABDULJAWAD, K.A.J. *et al.* 1997. Evidence for involvement of D2 dopamine receptors in prepulseinhibition of the startle reflex in man. J. Psychopharmacol. **11:** 69.
43. MORTON, N. *et al.* 1995. The effects of apomorphine and L-DOPA challenge on prepulse inhibition in patients with Parkinson's disease [abstract]. Schizophr. Res. **15:** 181.
44. ACRI, J.B. *et al.* 1994. Nicotine increases sensory gating measured as inhibition of the acoustic startle reflex in rats. Psychopharmacology **114:** 369–374.
45. KUMARI, V. *et al.* 1996. Effect of cigarette smoking on prepulse inhibition of the acoustic startle reflex in healthy male smokers. Psychopharmacology **128:** 54–60.
46. KARPER, L.P. *et al.* 1994. The effect of ketamine on prepulse inhibition and attention [abstract]. Proc. Am. Col. Neuropsychopharmacology.124.

47. DUNCAN, E. *et al.* 1997. Ketamine effects on prepulse inhibition of startle [abstract]. Proc. Am. Col. Neuropsychopharmacology. 299.
48. VAN BERCKEL, R.N.M. *et al.* 1997. The effects of low dose ketamine on sensory gating, neuroendocrine secretion and behavior in healthy human subjects [abstract]. Proc. Am. Col. Neuropsychopharmacology:169.
49. MANSBACH, R.S. *et al.* 1989. Prepulse inhibition of the acoustic startle response is disrupted by *N*-ethyl-3,4-methylenedioxy-amphetamine (MDEA) in the rat. Eur. J. Pharmacol. **167**: 49-55.
50. VOLLENWEIDER, F.X. *et al.* 1997. Effects of MDMA ("Ecstasy") on sensorimotor gating, attention, and mood in healthy volunteers [abstract]. International Congress on the State of the Art in Psychiatry. June 19–21. Basel, Switzerland.: S.28.
51. WAN, F.J. & N.R. SWERDLOW. 1996. Sensorimotor gating in rats is regulated by different dopamine-glutamate interactions in the nucleus accumbens core and shell subregions. Brain. Res. **722**: 168-176.
52. SWERDLOW, N.R. *et al.* 1992. Neural substrates of sensorimotor gating of the startle reflex: a review of recent findings and their implications. J. Psychopharmacol. **6**: 176–190.
53. SWERDLOW, N.R. & M.A. GEYER. 1998. Neurophysiology and neuropharmacology of short lead interval startle modification. *In* Startle Modification: Implications for Neuroscience, Cognitive Science, and Clinical Science. M.E. Dawson *et al.*, Eds. Cambridge University Press. Stanford, CA. In press.
54. KOCH, M. *et al.* 1993. Cholinergic neurons in the pedunculopontine tegmental nucleus are involved in the mediation of prepulse inhibition of acoustic startle response in the rat. Exp. Brain Res. **97**: 71–82.
55. KRETSCHMER, B.D. & M. KOCH. 1998. The ventral pallidum mediates disruption of prepulse inhibition ofthe acoustic startle response induced by dopamine agonists, but not by NMDA antagonists. Brain Res. **798**: 204–210.
56. MORTON, N. *et al.* 1994. Prepulse inhibition in temporal lobe epilepsy [abstract]. Proc. Eur. Behav. Pharmacol. Soc. 191.
57. POURETEMAD, H.R. *et al.* 1998. Impaired sensorimotor gating in patients with non-epileptic seizures. Epilepsy Res. **31**: 1-12.
58. SWERDLOW, N.R. *et al.* 1992. Regionally selective effects of intracerebral dopamine infusion on sensorimotor gating of the startle reflex in rats. Psychopharmacology **108**: 189–195.
59. REIJMERS, L.G. *et al.* 1995. Changes in prepulse inhibition after local administration of NMDA receptor ligands in the core region of the rat nucleus accumbens. Eur. J. Pharmacol. **272** :131–138.
60. BAKSHI, V.P. *et al.* 1994. Clozapine antgaonizes phencyclidine-induced deficits in sensorimotor gating of the startle response. J. Pharmacol. Exp. Ther. **271**: 787–794.
61. HART, S. *et al.* 1998. Localizing haloperidol effects on sensorimotor gating in a predictive model of antipsychotic potency. Pharmacol. Biochem. Behav. **61**: 113–119.
62. SWERDLOW, N.R. *et al.* 1996. Seroquel restores sensorimotor gating in phencyclidine-treated rats. J. Pharmacol. Exp. Ther. **279**: 1290–1299.
63. KODSI, M. & N.R. SWERDLOW. 1995. Prepulse inhibition in the rat is regulated by ventral and caudodorsal striato-pallidal circuitry. Behav. Neurosci. **109**: 912–928.
64. KODSI, M.H. & N.R. SWERDLOW. 1997. Mitochondrial toxin 3-nitropropionic acid produces startle reflex abnormalities and striatal damage in rats that model some features of Huntington's disease. Neurosci. Lett. **231**: 1–5.
65. BARDGETT, M.E. *et al.* 1998. Increased D2-like receptors in the nucleus accumbens, but not the striatum, of prepulse inhibition deficient isolation-reared rats. Soc. Neurosci. **24**: 713.
66. LIN, K-N. *et al.* 1998. Prenatal stress generates adult rats with behavioral and neuroanatomical similarities to human schizophrenics. Soc. Neurosci. **24**: 746.
67. PRINTZ, D.J. *et al.* 1998. Prenatal protein deprivation alters two measures of sensorimotor gating. Soc. Neurosci. **24**: 45.
68. WAN, F.J. *et al.* 1995. Presynaptic dopamine-glutamate interactions in the nucleus accumbens regulate sensorimotor gating. Psychopharmacology **120**: 433–441.

69. WAN, F.J. et al. 1994. Accumbens D2 substrates of sensorimotor gating: assessing anatomical localization. Pharmacol. Biochem. Behav. **49:** 155–263.
70. KLARNER, A. et al. 1998. Induction of Fos-protein in the forebrain and disruption of sensorimotor gating following NMDA infusion into the ventral hippocampus of the rat. Neuroscience **84:** 443–452.
71. WAN, F.J. et al. 1996. The ventral subiculum modulation of prepulse inhibition is not mediated via D2 dopamine or nucleus accumbens non-NMDA glutamate activity. Eur. J. Pharmacol. **314:** 9-18.
72. WAN, F.J. & N.R. SWERDLOW. 1996. The basolateral amygdala regulates sensorimotor gating of acoustic startle in rats. Neuroscience **76:** 715-724.
73. KOCH, M. & W. HAUBER. 1998. Regulation of sensorimotor gating by interactions of dopamine and adenosine in the rat. Behav. Pharmacol. **9:** 23–29.
74. FEIFEL, D. et al. 1997. The effects of intra-accumbens neurotensin on sensorimotor gating. Brain Res. **760:** 80–84.
75. FEIFEL, D. & N. SWERDLOW. 1997. The modulation of sensorimotor gating deficits by mesolimbic cholecystokinin. Neurosci. Lett. **229:** 5-8.
76. KINKEAD, B. et al. 1998. Interaction between the neurotensin receptor antagonist SR142948A and dopamine agonists in prepulse inhibition of the acoustic startle response. Soc. Neurosci. **24:**1926.
77. MANSBACH, R.S. et al. 1988. Dopaminergic stimulation disrupts sensorimotor gating in the rat. Psychopharmacology **94:** 507–514.
78. MARTINEZ, Z.A. et al. 1998. Startle gating deficits during, but not after, sustained exposure to cocaine or phencyclidine [abstract]. Biol. Psychiatry **43:** 14S.
79. CULPIT, G.C. & A.R. TEMPLE. 1984. Gastrointestinal decontamination in the management of the poisoned patient. Emer. Med. Clin. North Am. **2:** 15–28.
80. SWERDLOW, N.R., N. TAAID, J.L. OOSTWEGEL, E. RANDOLPH & M.A. GEYER. 1998. Towards a cross-species pharmacology of sensorimotor gating: effects of amantadine, bromocriptine, pergolide and ropinirole on prepulse inhibition of acoustic startle in rats. Behav. Pharmacol. **9:** 389–396.
81. CLEMENS, J.A. et al. 1993. Dopamine agonist activities of pergolide, its metabolites, and bromocriptine as measured by prolactin inhibition, compulsive turning, and stereotypic behavior. Arzneim. Forsch. **43:** 281-286.
82. LIPINSKI, J.F. et al. 1997. Dopamine agonist treatment of Tourette disorder in children: results of an open-label trial of pergolide. Movement Dis. **12:** 402-407.
83. ADLER, L.E. et al. 1994. Bromocriptine impairs P50 auditory sensory gating in normal control subjects. Biol. Psychiatry **35:** 630.
84. EDEN, R.J. et al. 1991. Preclinical pharmacology of ropinirole (SK&F 101468-A) a novel dopamine D2 agonist. Pharmacol. Biochem. Behav. **38:** 147-154.
85. MIZOGUCHI, K. et al. 1994. Amantadine increases the extracellular dopamine levels in the striatum by re-uptake inhibition and by N-methyl-d-aspartate antagonism. Brain Res. **662:** 255-258.
86. LIGHT, G.A. et al. 1998. P50 suppression in normal subjects after administration of amphetamine. Biol. Psychiatry **43:** 88S-89S.
87. SWERDLOW, N.R. et al. 1993. Men are more inhibited than women by weak prepulses. Biol. Psychiat. **34:** 253–261.
88. SWERDLOW, N.R. et al. 1998. Sex differences in sensorimotor gating of the human startle reflex: All smoke ? Biol Psychiatry. In press.
89. SWERDLOW, N.R. et al. 1995. Lateralized differences in sensorimotor gating of startle for variables of sex and psychosis-proneness [abstract]. Soc. Neurosci. **21:** 746.
90. THOMPSON, T.L. et al. 1998. Sex differences in somatosensory gating: effect of 6-OHDA lesions of the medial prefrontal cortex (MPFC) on prepulse inhibition of acoustic startle. Soc. Neurosci. **24:** 712.
91. DELLA CASA, V.D. et al. 1998. The effects of smoking on acoustic prepulse inhibition in healthy men and women. Psychopharmacology **137:** 362-368.
92. KOCH, M. 1998. Sensorimotor gating changes across the estrous cycle in female rats. Physiol. & Behav. **64:** 625–628.
93. SWERDLOW, N.R. et al. 1997. Changes in sensorimotor inhibition across the menstrual cycle: implications for neuropsychiatric disorders. Biol. Psychiatry **41:** 452–460.

94. RUSH, D.K. & D.E. SELK. 1998. Intra-strain differences in response to apomorphine induced disruption of prepulse inhibition of the startle response. Soc. Neurosci. **24:**2176.
95. SWERDLOW, N.R. et al. 1997. Discrepant findings of clozapine effects on prepulse inhibition of startle: Is it the route or the rats? Neuropsychopharmacology **18:** 50–56.
96. SWERDLOW, N.R. et al. 1995. "Normal" personality correlates of sensorimotor, cognitive and visuo-spatial gating. Biol. Psychiatry **37:** 286–299.
97. FENDT, M. et al. 1994. Sensorimotor gating deficits after lesions of the superior colliculus. NeuroReport **5:** 1725–1728.
98. KOCH, M. & M. BUBSER. 1994. Deficient sensorimotor gating after 6-hydroxydopamine lesion of the ratmedial prefrontal cortex is reversed by haloperidol. Eur. J. Neurosci. **6:** 1837–1845.
99. KOCH, M. 1995. The septohippocampal system is involved in prepulse inhibition of the acoustic startle response in rats [abstract]. Soc. Neurosci. **21:** 1623.
100. KODSI, M.H. & N.R. SWERDLOW. 1997. Regulation of sensorimotor gating by pallidal efferent projections. Brain Res. Bull. **43:** 219-228.
101. KODSI, M.H. & N.R. SWERDLOW. 1995. Ventral pallidal GABA-A receptors regulate prepulse inhibition of aoustic startle. Brain Res. **684:** 26-35.
102. SWERDLOW, N.R. et al. 1990. GABAergic projection from nucleus accumbens to ventral pallidum mediates dopamine-induced sensorimotor gating deficits of acoustic startle in rats. Brain Res. **532:** 146-150.
103. SWERDLOW, N.R. et al. 1990. Schizophrenic-like sensorimotor gating abnormalities in rats following dopamine infusion into the nucleus accumbens. Psychopharmacology **101:** 414–420.
104. SWERDLOW, N.R. & M.A. GEYER. 1993. Prepulse inhibition of acoustic startle in rats after lesions of the pedunculopontine nucleus. Behav. Neurosci. **107:** 104–117.
105. SWERDLOW, N.R. et al. 1995. Increased sensitivity to the gating-disruptive effects of apomorphine after lesions of the medial prefrontal cortex or ventral hippocampus in rats. Psychopharmacology **122:** 27–34.
106. CAINE, S.B. et al. 1992. Hippocampal modulation of acoustic startle and prepulse inhibition in rats. Pharmacol. Biochem. Behav. **43:** 1201–1208.
107. MOGENSON, G.J. 1987. Limbic-motor integration. In Progress in Psychobiology and Physiological Psychology. Vol. **12:** 117–170. Academic Press. New York.
108. SWERDLOW, N.R. & G.F. KOOB. 1987. Dopamine, schizophrenia, mania and depression: toward a unified hypothesis of cortico-striato-pallido-thalamic function. Behav. Brain. Sci. **10:** 197-245.

The Intrinsic Organization of the Central Extended Amygdala

MARTIN D. CASSELL,[a,d] LORIN J. FREEDMAN,[b] AND CHANGJUN SHI[c]

[a]*Department of Anatomy and Cell Biology, University of Iowa, Iowa City, Iowa 52242, USA*
Departments of [b]Neurology and [c]Psychiatry, Emory University, Atlanta, Georgia, USA

ABSTRACT: The central component of the extended amygdala (CEA) comprises the central amygdaloid nucleus (Ce), the dorsal substantia innominata (SI), and the bed nucleus of the stria terminalis (BNST). Anatomical studies have suggested the presence of an intrinsic system of GABAergic neurons that not only connects homologous subareas of the Ce, SI, and BNST but that also acts as an interface between sensory afferents and brain stem–projecting neurons. CEA outputs, with a few exceptions, arise from separate populations of neurons, but all, including GABAergic neurons themselves, are heavily innervated by GABAergic terminals. GABAergic neurons may serve to integrate output activity of the CEA, though GABAergic neurons form a heterogeneous population whose differential intrinsic connections appear related to their peptide content. Afferents from the dysgranular insular cortex and lateral parabrachial complex preferentially innervate GABAergic neurons, suggesting these neurons may also integrate afferent activity. Afferents from the basolateral amygdala (BL) appear to innervate both output neurons and intrinsic GABAergic neurons. Evidence will be presented to show that BL afferents form synaptic complexes with cortical, GABAergic, and TH-immunoreactive terminal boutons on GABAergic dendritic spines. These complexes may be a key element in control of CEA output activity.

INTRODUCTION

Recognizing that the dorsomedial components of the amygdaloid complex are part of an extensive forebrain structure, the extended amygdala,[1] has heralded in a dramatic rethinking of the organization of both the forebrain and, in particular, the vaguely defined amygdaloid complex itself. The realization by Heimer and others that the organization of the neostriatum and globus pallidus (the dorsal striatopallidal system) is replicated in the organization of the structure, neurochemistry, and connections of the nucleus accumbens-ventral pallidum complex (the ventral striatopallidal system) set the stage for the development of the concept that the more caudal (and ventral) forebrain structures comprising the sublenticular substantia innominata, the central and medial amygdaloid nuclei, and the bed nucleus of the stria terminalis may also be part of a distinct forebrain system, the extended amygdala, with strong parallels to the dorsal and ventral striatopallidal systems.[1,2] Though the validity of the concept for the medial amygdaloid nucleus–medial bed nucleus connection as the medial extended amygdala is still subject to dispute, as indeed is the

[d]Voice: 319-335-7753; fax: 319-335-7198; martin-cassell@uiowa.edu

whole concept of the "amygdala,"[3,4] the notion of a central extended amygdala, comprising the central nucleus, substantia innominata, and lateral bed nucleus is now widely accepted.

Despite a considerable body of literature on the connections, neurochemistry, and cellular organization of the CEA, a clear concept of how inputs and outputs interact, how connectional features interact with the chemical architecture, and what type of neural operations are performed by the CEA has yet to emerge. The central problem appears to be the complex relationship between afferents, projection neurons, and neurochemical staining of neurons and neuropil, and between these and the underlying cytoarchitecture. Tentative organizational schemes based on the complimentary patterning of peptide immunoreactivities,[5,6] modality-specific inputs from the parabrachial complex,[7] efferent projections to the brain stem,[8] and the connectivity of intrinsic GABAergic neurons[9,10] have been proposed. However, none has clearly linked the various neuroanatomical and neurochemical features of the CEA into a cohesive framework that has predictive and operational value for understanding its functional role. This chapter does not claim to offer such a cohesive framework but instead focuses on two levels of organization that have experimental support and could form the basis for future investigations of the internal organization of the CEA. The first level concerns the potential compartmental organization of the CEA, and here the cue is taken from the extensive anatomical and histochemical analyses of the compartmental organization of the caudate-putamen/globus pallidus (dorsal striatopallidal) and nucleus accumbens/ventral pallidum (ventral striatopallidal) systems, which have produced such a revolution in understanding the complex organization of the basal ganglia (e.g., refs. 2 and 11–17). The CEA shares fundamental structural and connectional features with the basal ganglia, and the case is made here that by applying the various defining criteria of the compartmental (e.g., patch/striosome-matrix, shell–core) organization of the basal ganglia to the CEA, some principles emerge that can potentially unify the complex organization of its connectional and neurochemical features. The second level of organization focuses on the connections of the striatal-like, GABAergic medium-sized, spiny neurons that appear to be the keystone neuron type in the CEA, and, again, a case will be made that these are essentially striatopallidal in nature.

COMPARTMENTAL ORGANIZATION OF THE CENTRAL EXTENDED AMYGDALA

The rodent CEA consists of several parallel, rostrocaudally oriented columns of neurons that follow a curved (in all three planes) course from the anterior tip of the inferior horn of the lateral ventricle laterally, through the basal forebrain, to the floor of the superior horn of the lateral ventricle medially.[18] Scattered neurons of the CEA also accompany the stria terminalis as it curves posteriorly around the basal ganglia. The dorsal and rostral borders of the rat CEA, respectively, abut against the ventral borders of the caudate-putamen and globus pallidus, and the caudal borders of the nucleus accumbens and ventral pallidum. As noted by Heimer and colleagues, the borders between the caudomedial shell regions of the nucleus accumbens and the CEA blend subtly together and are usually described as transitions rather than clear boundaries.[18,19–21] The argument will be made here that there is probably little transition or change in architecture between the CEA and nucleus accumbens and that the two structures should be viewed as continuous.

The CEA is regionalized, from lateral to medial, into the central amygdaloid nucleus, the sublenticular substantia innominata, and the (dorsolateral) bed nucleus of the stria terminalis. Despite the clear evidence for continuity, both physical and in terms of connectivity and neurochemistry,[1,18] the nomenclature applied to the parallel cell columns is regionally based, with each cell column having a different designation depending on whether it is in the bed nucleus or the central nucleus. This chapter will focus exclusively on the rat central nucleus, though some or all of the organizational principles discussed can be applied to the bed nucleus, and probably to other species too.

In Nissl-stained preparations of the rat central nucleus, four major cell groups have been consistently recognized: using the well-accepted terminology of McDonald,[22] these are designated here the medial (CeM), lateral (CeL), lateral capsular (CeLC), and the intermediate (CeI) subdivisions. Superficially, at least, each division has typical characteristics in terms of neuron size, shape, and chromaffinity,[22,23] and there are no obvious rostrocaudal/mediolateral or other differences in Nissl staining within each subdivision. This cytoarchitectural scheme, however, is, at least grossly, poorly correlated with Ce efferent projections (e.g., ref. 23), specific peptidergic neuron populations,[23] and peptidergic terminal zones (e.g., ref. 6). Some neuron populations projecting to specific brain stem regions overlap two or more cytoarchitectonic zones (e.g., ref. 23); many afferent inputs target specific subregions of particular subdivisions (e.g., ref. 24) without any corresponding distinctive cytoarchitectural features. Correlative studies associating peptides with particular efferent projections[8,25] or morphology[26] have not revealed any clear organizational principles either.

The principal neuron type in the lateral Ce (i.e., CeL, CeI, and CeLC) appears to be a striatal-like GABAergic, medium-sized, densely spinous neuron (see below). This basic feature, together with its heavy dopaminergic and enkephalinergic innervation, unidirectional cortical input, and strong input from the basolateral amygdaloid complex suggests a fundamental affinity between the lateral Ce and the caudate-putamen (CP), core (NAc), and shell (NAs) regions of the nucleus accumbens. Moreover, a subtle continuity between the bed nucleus portion of the CEA and the neurochemically heterogeneous caudomedial shell region of the nucleus accumbens has been repeatedly emphasized (e.g., refs. 1, 16, 18, 20, 21, and 27). In this section, the pattern and organization of some of the principal neurochemical and connectional markers that characterize the compartments of the nucleus accumbens will be reviewed for the central nucleus. Though this involves a comparison of only a proportion of the anatomical features present in both structures, the exercise strongly suggests that the core–shell and multicompartmental organization of the nucleus accumbens is also an organizing principle in the CEA.

The Lateral Capsular Division

As originally designated by McDonald,[22] CeLC encompasses a C-shaped strip along the lateral and dorsal aspects of the Ce. The whole CeLC has a fairly modest cell density, but conspicuous clusters of cells are found at the medial and lateral edges of the dorsal portion. This dorsal portion lying beneath the ventral caudate-putamen (and hence commonly termed the amygdalostriatal transition zone) has generally been excluded from the central nucleus (e.g., refs. 23 and 28), as it possesses little connectional similarities to the rest of the Ce. However, both dorsal and ventral parts of CeLC are heavily immunoreactive for methionine enkephalin (FIG. 1A). This immunoreactivity is unusually coarse in appearance and readily distinguishes CeLC from the caudate-putamen and lateral Ce. The ventral lateral capsular division (vCeLC) contains strong immunoreactivity (FIG. 1, C and D) for substance P and neurotensin,[5] but weak staining for calbindin D28k,[29] dopamine (FIG. 1E), and tyrosine hydroxylase.[30] Both met- and leu-enkephalin immunoreactive neurons are present in vCeLC[23] and are embedded in a fairly strongly immunoreactive neuropil. In leu-enkephalin–stained material, occasional patches of weakly immunoreactive neuropil-containing immunoreactive neurons can be seen (see, e.g., FIG. 7 of ref. 23). Acetylcholinesterase activity appears to be only present in dorsal CeLC, though of lower density than in the adjacent caudate-putamen (FIG. 1F). Discrete patches of intense AChE activity are located, however, in the medial and lateral edges of dCeLC (arrow in FIG. 1F) and appear to be associated with cell clusters. Calbindin D28k immunoreactivity in dCeLC is strong and virtually indistinguishable from that in the caudate-putamen, though two low-density patches are present at the medial and lateral edges.[29] By contrast, tyrosine hydroxylase and dopamine immunoreactivity exhibits a patchy distribution in dCeLC, with prominent patches (arrow in FIG. 1E) again in the medial and lateral edges.[30] Substance P and neurotensin immunoreactivity is weak in dCeLC (FIG. 1, C and D) except for a prominent patch of NT immunoreactive neurons at its lateral edge.

Amygdalar afferents to CeLC arise from the lateral part of the caudal parvocellular basal amygdaloid nucleus (pBAN), which also innervates CeL, and the ventromedial and ventrolateral parts of the lateral nucleus (LN), which only sparsely innervate CeL. The pBAN innervates only the vCeLC (FIG. 2B), whereas both ventral divisions of the lateral nucleus innervate the whole CeLC (FIG. 2A). By comparison, the medial part of the pBAN innervates cell clusters in the (dorsomedial) shell and patches in the core and ventral CP,[31] whereas the ventral LN innervates the ventrolateral shell and core and the ventral and dorsomedial CP (unpublished results). Insular cortical afferents, the principal cortical input to the CEA, tend to avoid CeLC and CeI but heavily innervate CeL (FIG. 2C) and the ventral CP.[32,33] The deep layers of the anterior and posterior periamygdaloid cortices (otherwise referred to as the anterior and posterior basomedial/accessory basal amygdaloid nuclei) heavily target vCeLC (FIG. 2D), with the posterior area projecting additionally to the medial part of dCeLC. Both anterior and posterior deep layers project to the ventral NAs, whereas the posterior projects additionally to the matrix of the NAc.[31] Likewise, prelimbic and infralimbic afferents avoid CeL and CeM but produce a complimentary pattern of termination surrounding the whole Ce. Prelimbic afferents innervate the dorsal CeLC, but terminals and fibers extend into the upper part of vCeLC[34]: infralimbic afferents, which sparsely innervate the caudate-putamen but heavily innervate the dorsomedial NAs, terminate largely ventral to the Ce, though fibers are present in the ventralmost part of CeLC.[35,36] Neocortical projections, on the other hand, avoid dCeLC (FIG. 2E), though heavily innervating adjacent parts of the ventral caudate-putamen.[32,33,37,38]

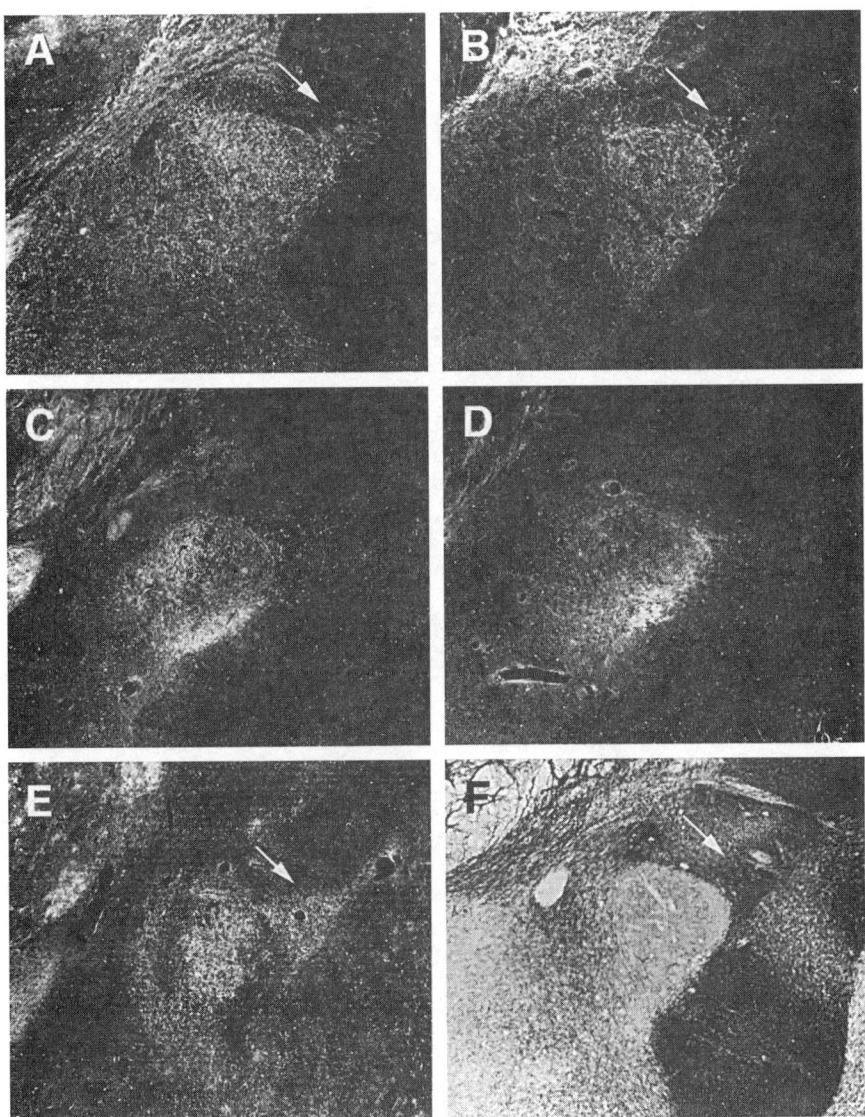

FIGURE 1. Dark (**A–E**) and bright (**F**) field photomicrographs of coronal sections through the approximate midrostrocaudal level of the central nucleus showing the distributions of immunoreactive met-enkephalin (**A**), leu-enkephalin (**B**), neurotensin (**C**), substance P (**D**), dopamine (**E**), and acetylcholinesterase activity (**F**). The immunostained material shows predominantly immunoreactive neuropil. The arrows in panels **A**, **B**, **D**, and **E** indicate the position of a cell cluster in lateral dorsal CeLC. Note the heavy leu-enkephalin, dopamine, and AChE staining here.

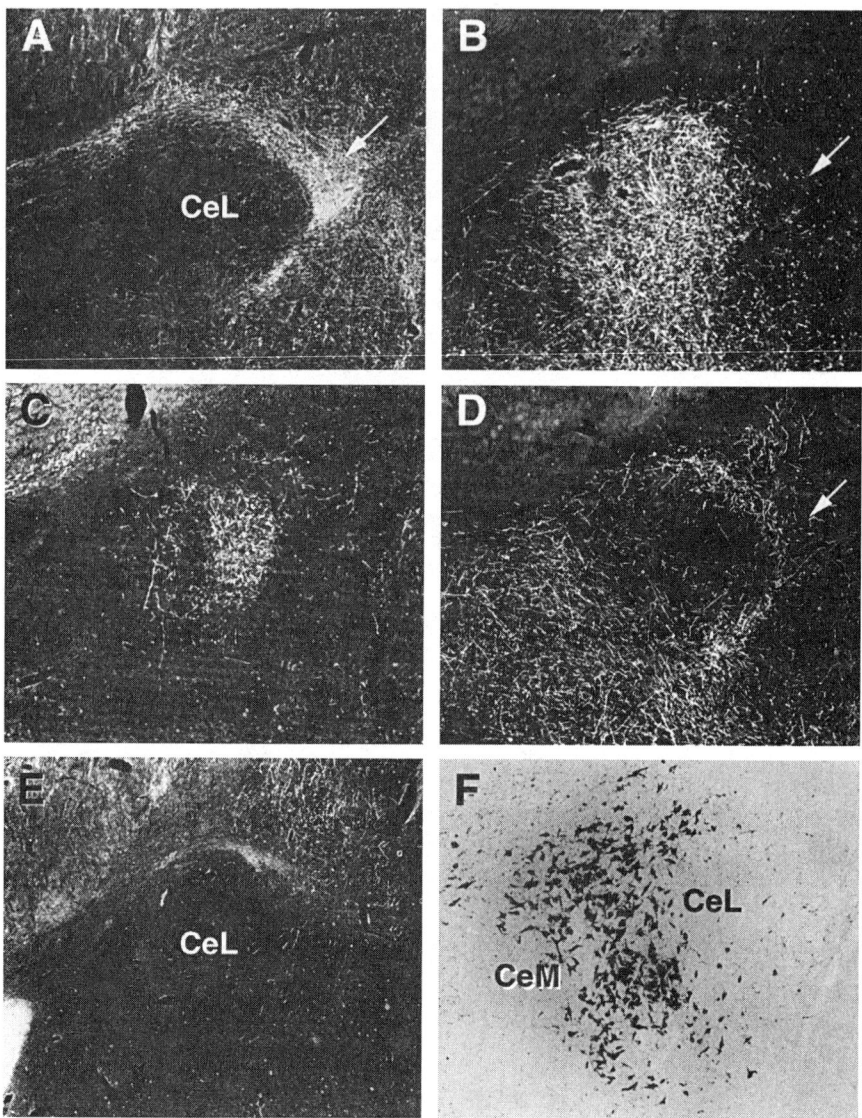

FIGURE 2. Dark (**A–E**) and bright (**F**) field photomicrographs showing the distribution of labeled fibers in the Ce following biocytin injections into the ventral lateral amygdaloid nucleus (**A**), the lateral parvicellular basal amygdaloid nucleus (**B**), the dysgranular posterior insular cortex (**C**), the deep layers of the periamygdaloid cortex (**D**), and the temporal cortical area Te3 (**E**). In **F**, the distribution of neurons in the Ce after HRP injections into the nucleus tractus solitarii is shown. The arrows in panels **A**, **B**, and **D** indicate the lateral cell cluster in dorsal CeLC (see FIG. 1, also). CeL, lateral subdivision; CeM, medial subdivision.

The efferent connections of CeLC have not been studied in detail but appear to be largely intrinsic. Retrograde labeling is found in vCeLC following tracer injections into the lateral BNST,[39] and anterograde tracing indicates that vCeLC innervates CeL and CeM (ref. 40 and unpublished observations). Dorsal CeLC appears to project to the caudal globus pallidus[41] and the pars compacta of the lateral substantia nigra.[42]

Several interesting parallels emerge when the organization of the CeLC is viewed from the perspective of the neurochemical and connectional features that characterize the ventral striatum. The CeLC clearly shares features with both the dorsal and ventral striatum, but in terms of its overall connectional and neurochemical architecture, its closest affiliation appears to be with the shell of the nucleus accumbens. Furthermore, both the dorsal and ventral parts of CeLC, although sharing some features (e.g., met-enkephalin immunoreactivity, lateral nucleus inputs), are quite different in others (e.g., calbindin and AChE staining) and appear to have neurochemical gradients comparable to different parts of the NAs.[13–15] The vCeLC has many, though not all, features in common with the calbindin-poor dorsomedial shell of the accumbens, whereas dCeLC shares features with the calbindin-rich ventrolateral extension of the shell. Finally, the presence of inhomogeneities in some staining patterns (e.g., AChE and enkephalins), particularly in association with cell clusters in dCeLC, suggests the presence of a finer subarchitecture of the kind that has been identified in the nucleus accumbens shell (e.g., ref. 16). Corresponding patches of strong AChE and dopamine immunoreactivity (arrows in FIG. 1, E and F), but low calbindin D28k immunoreactvity, are present in the lateral and medial dCeLC, with the lateral patch associated with clusters of NT and met-enkephalin immunoreactive neurons.

Lateral Subdivision

The lateral subdivision of the central nucleus (CeL) is a cylindrical band of cells many of which are medium-sized spiny neurons immunoreactive to GABA and GAD antisera.[9] GABA neurons in CeL are concentrated caudally and in the central and lateral parts of CeL, with some clustering apparent.[9] GABA is colocalized with neurotensin, somatostatin, and met- and leu-enkephalin in CeL;[43,44] MENK and LENK immunoreactive neurons are concentrated caudally and in central parts of CeL and appear to be clustered within zones of strongly immunoreactive neuropil (FIG. 1, A and B). There is a subtle degree of complimentary patterning between the LENK and MENK immunoreactive neuropil, in that the dense medial zone of MENK immunoreactivity corresponds to a weakly immunoreactive LENK neuropil, and vice verse. A dense area of SP immunoreactivity, continuous with that in vCeLC, is also located in the lateral CeL (FIG. 1D). NT neurons are more numerous rostrally but have a central concentration again in a region of strongly immunoreactive neuropil. The whole of the neuropil of CeL is weakly immunoreactive for calbindin D28k, though a cluster of strongly immunoreactive neurons is present medially.[29]

CeL is conspicuous by its very low level of AChE (FIG.1F) activity, though some regional differences are evident, with a slightly higher density present laterally. TH and DA immunoreactivity is heaviest in the medial and central parts of CeL (FIG. 1E), and a patchy distribution is evident.[30]

Amygdalar afferents to CeL appear to arise exclusively from the caudolateral pBAN and are part of a projection field including vCeLC (FIG. 2B). The projection

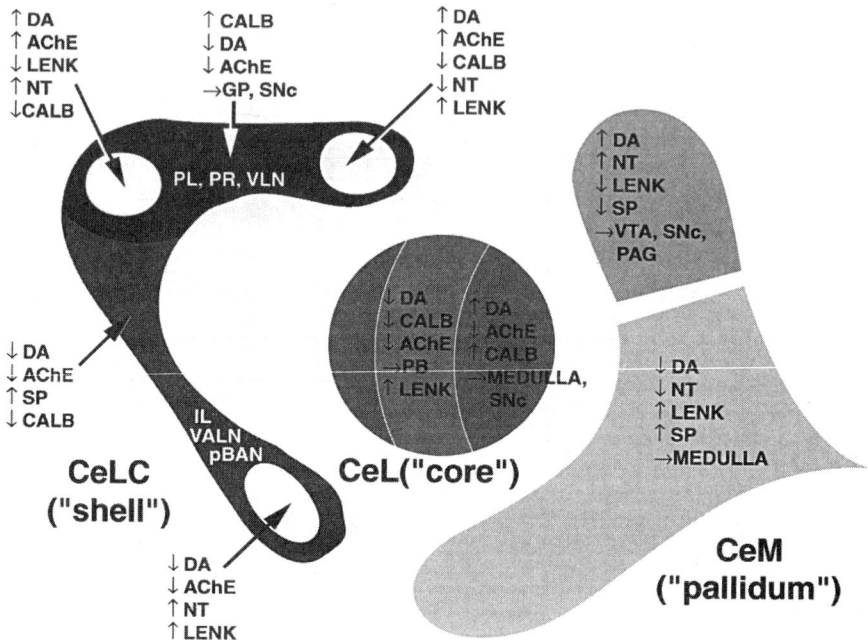

FIGURE 3. Schematic diagram of the subdivisions of the central nucleus in coronal section, summarizing the neurochemical and connectional affiliations of the lateral capsular (CeLC), lateral (CeL), and medial (CeM) subdivisions that suggest a "shell-core-pallidum" arrangement. Additional data taken from refs. 22, 29, 34, and 36.

to lateral CeL appears heaviest. Cortical inputs to CeL arise almost exclusively from the posterior insular cortex, with the dysgranular area targeting CeL (FIG. 2C) and the agranular area targeting both CeL and CeM.[38] Insular projections to the CeL appear to arise largely from layer V, though superficial layers may innervate a narrow strip along the lateral edge of CeL (see FIG. 6, A and B and ref. 38).

The distribution of projection neurons in CeL is complex, with target-specific populations showing partially overlapping medial to lateral trends.[23] Projections to the bed nucleus are concentrated in the central and lateral parts of CeL, with the heaviest concentration caudally, and originate primarily from GABAergic neurons.[9] The lateral and central parts of CeL provide the heaviest input to CeM (ref. 40 and unpublished observations) and, because these projections in part are GABAergic, it has been proposed that these arise as collaterals of GABAergic neurons projecting to the bed nucleus.[10] Projections to the lateral parabrachial nucleus are also concentrated in lateral and central CeL but are concentrated rostrally. These projections are not collaterals of neurons projecting to the bed nucleus[45] and appear to be non-GABAergic.[9] Consistent with its differential neurochemistry (e.g., high DA fiber density and calbindin D28k neurons), the medial part of CeL appears to have a different set of output projections. Injections of retrograde tracers into the dorsal medulla heavily label neurons in CeM (FIG. 2F) but also consistently label a

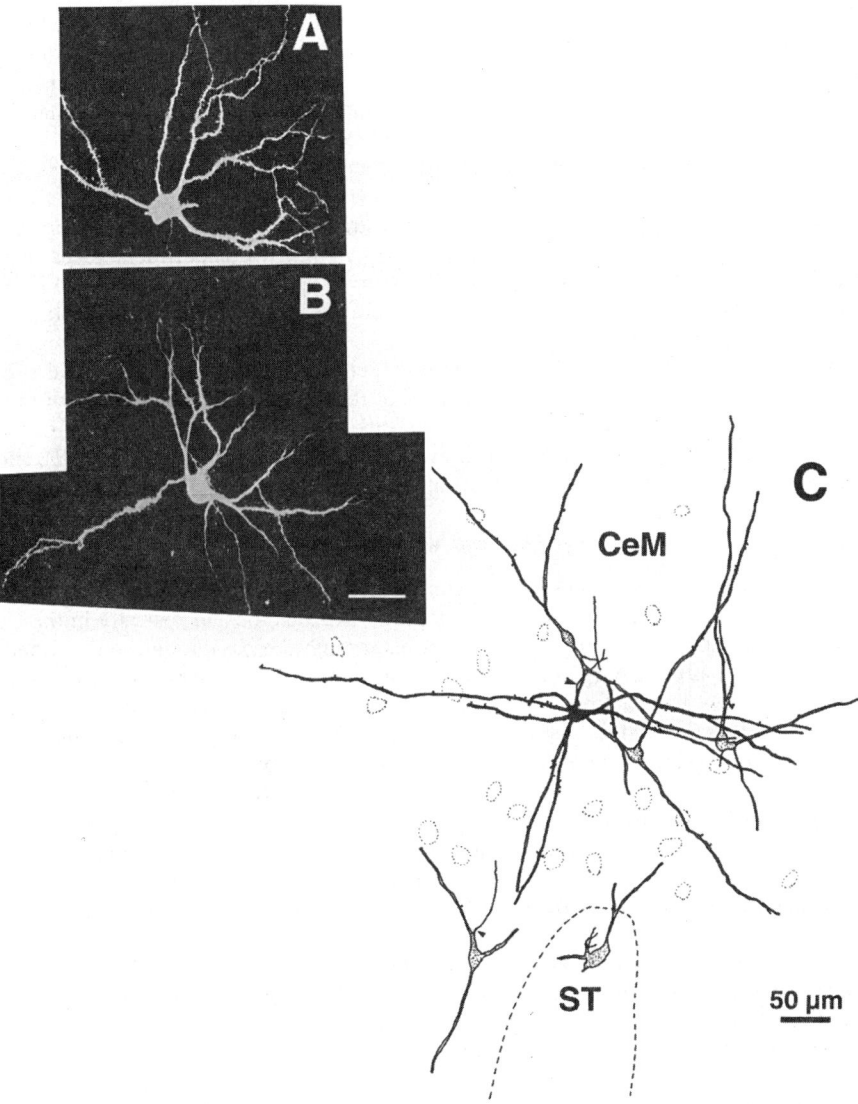

FIGURE 4. Morphological characteristics of neurons from the lateral (**A, B**) and medial (**C**) subdivisions of the central nucleus. **A:** Medium-sized spiny neuron retrogradely labeled by a Fast Blue injection into the bed nucleus and intracellularly injected with Lucifer Yellow. **B:** Intracellularly injected spiny neuron from the medial part of CeL retrogradely labeled after Fast Blue injection into the dorsal medulla. **C:** Golgi preparation of CeM neurons (stippled cells) retrogradely labeled by an HRP injection into the dorsal medulla. The filled cell was not retrogradely labeled. Note the "striatal" appearance of the cells in **A** and **B**, and the "pallidal" appearance of the cells in **C**.

concentrated cluster of cells in the medial CeL.[8,23] Combined intracellular/retrograde labeling indicates that CeL cells projecting to the dorsal medulla are medium-sized spiny neurons (FIG. 4), but these may not be GABAergic. CEA projections to the pars compacta and pars lateralis of the substantia nigra appear to arise from neurons in the medial part of CeL.[23,42] The latter anterograde study also noted that the Ce does not project to the pars reticulata of the substantia nigra.

Taken together, these observations suggest there are a number of key features that must be considered in the organization of CeL (FIG. 3). First, the connectional and neurochemical profile of CeL appears to bear a strong resemblance to that of the core of the nucleus accumbens and the calbindin-poor patch compartment in particular.[15,46] The low AChE activity, patchy DA innervation, clustering of NT and LENK neurons, innervation by deep cortical layers, and presence of neurons projecting to SN pars compacta, but not SN pars reticulata, together with many other features, are consistent with this. Second, there is good evidence for a multicompartmental subarchitecture (FIG. 3) based on combinations of the differential distributions of projection and neurochemically identified neurons, the patch-like appearance in the neuropil of a number of neurochemical markers, including dopamine (FIG. 1E), and regionalization of a number of afferent inputs.

Intermediate and Ventral Subdivisions

The intermediate subdivision of the central nucleus (CeI), first recognized by McDonald,[22] is a thin band of intensely basophilic neurons located rostrally in the Ce between CeL and CeM. CeI possesses neurons resembling medium-sized spiny neurons,[22] as well as GABAergic neurons,[9] neurons projecting to the bed nucleus,[39] and a moderate DA innervation.[30] Although these features suggest similarities with CeL, CeI maintains several distinctive features, including a very strong cell and neuropil calbindin D28k immunoreactivity,[29] projections to the ventromedial[47] and lateral hypothalamus (unpublished observations), and the ventrolateral PAG (ref. 48 and unpublished observations). CeI also appears to lack projections to any other subdivision of the Ce.[40] In these and a number of other respects, CeI resembles the calbindin-rich cell clusters located at the junction between the dorsomedial and ventrolateral compartments of the NAs, which have distinctive projections to the mesencephalon.[11]

The ventral subdivision of the central nucleus (CeV) was tentatively recognized on cytoarchitectural and neurochemical features as a transitional area between CeL and CeM.[23] CeV has a slightly higher AChE activity than CeL (FIG. 1F) but a much lower density of dopaminergic fibers (FIG. 1E and 30). Also, CeV encompasses a calbindin-rich area that is continuous with CeI.[29] Little is known about its connectional features, but it does appear to contain neurons projecting to the bed nucleus and the ventral tegmental area,[23] which would be consistent with it being related, like CeI, to the calbindin-rich clusters in the accumbens shell.

Medial Subdivision

The medial subdivision of the central nucleus is quite distinct from the lateral subdivisions. The principal neuron in CeM appears to be a pyramiform, sparsely spiny neuron very similar to the principal neurons in the globus pallidus, ventral pallidum, and lateral hypothalamus/subthalamic nucleus.[22,49,50] Only a small portion of CeM neurons appear to be GABAergic,[9] these being mostly located caudally. However, neurons in both the medial and lateral central nucleus in primates contain GAD mRNA despite low levels of immunoreactive GABA,[51] and GABAergic projections to the medulla have been reported.[52] Thus, the numbers of GABAergic neurons in CeM may have been underestimated. Like the VP (e.g., ref. 16), the neuropil of CeM is strongly immunoreactive for GABA[9] and met-enkephalin.[5,6] Leucine-enkephalin, SP, and NT immunoreactivity in the neuropil is fairly modest (FIG. 1, C and D), but a heavier patch of labeling for NT and SP is evident in the dorsomedial CeM, particularly at middle and caudal levels. This dorsomedial area of CeM is also related to a dense patch of TH/DA immunoreactivity.[30] Leu-enkephalin immunoreactivity is weak in the dorsomedial part of CeM but of greater intensity in the ventral part. AChE staining in CeM is less dense than in the caudate-putamen but greater than in CeL (FIG. 1F). Calbindin D28k immunoreactivity is moderate in the CeM neuropil, but considerable numbers of immunoreactive neurons are present in CeM, particularly its dorsomedial portion.[29] Neurons in the dorsal part of CeM appear to express D1 receptor mRNA, whereas the ventral part, and CeL, express D2 receptor mRNA.[53]

These data suggest that a preliminary case can be made, on the basis of neurochemical content, for considering the medial subdivision of the central nucleus as being structurally very similar to the ventral pallidum (e.g., ref. 17). Of particular significance is the apparent inhomogeneity in three pallidal markers, substance P, and neurotensin, which are densest in the dorsomedial part of CeM, and LENK, which is denser ventrally, suggesting that division of the ventral pallidum into medial and lateral components[17] may be extended to a dorsomedial and ventrolateral division of CeM.

CeM has widespread projections to diencephalic, mesencephalic, and medullary structures. These projections will not be reviewed in detail, but there are a number of organizational trends that are consistent with the proposed "pallidal-like" nature of CeM. First, CeM innervates many of the same brain stem structures as the ventral pallidum, including the periaqueductal gray (e.g., refs. 48, 54, and 55), midline thalamus,[56,57] the ventral tegmental area, and substantia nigra pars compacta and lateral hypothalamus (e.g., refs. 23, 42, and 58). In fact, tracer injections into these areas give rise to almost continuous populations of neurons that extend across the ventral pallidum, bed nucleus, sublenticular substantia innominata, and central nucleus (e.g., refs. 48 and 59). Two apparent differences, however, include the strong projections of CeM to the dorsal and ventral medulla[8,23,60] and the lack of Ce projections to the mediodorsal thalamic nucleus (e.g., ref. 61). However, it should be noted that tracer injections into the dorsal medulla label an extensive population of forebrain neurons not only in the components of the CEA (FIG. 2F) but in the rostrolateral lateral hypothalamus and caudal parts of the ventral pallidum.[60,62] Second, CeM appears to possess a system of subcortical connections that closely resemble the pallido-mesencephalic and pallido-subthalamic pathways from the ventral pallidum.[55] CeM projects to the lateral ventral tegmental area, lateral substantia nigra pars compacta, and the retrorubral field.[42] In addition, CeM targets the lateral hypothalamic area medial to the subthalamic nucleus.[23,42] This area is also targeted by ventral pallidal afferents (e.g., ref. 55) and projects back to the ventral pallidum and nucleus accumbens.[46] This area, too, is the principal source of "lateral hypothalamic" projections to the central nucleus.[63] Clearly, there appears to be little to distinguish the VP and CeM in the organization of these pallidal projection pathways. Third, projections from CeM tend to arise from separate populations of neurons, though there is no clear evidence for dorsal-ventral preferences in most target-specific populations. Projections to the medial parabrachial complex partly arise as collaterals of neurons projecting to the dorsal medulla,[8] but projections to the bed nucleus, periaqueductal gray, different medullary areas, and lateral hypothalamus appear to arise from separate but largely intermingled populations in CeM (ref. 45 and unpublished observations). Moreover, CeM neurons projecting to the lateral substantia nigra appear to be concentrated in the dorsomedial part of CeM,[23,42] suggesting a further parallel with the medial segment of the ventral pallidum. These findings suggest that functionally distinct circuits may exist in CeM, consistent with the proposed compartmentalized output organization of the VP.[64,65]

Summary and Conclusions (FIGURE 3)

The critical problem in previous attempts to define organizing principles in the CEA has been that the cytoarchitecturally recognizable divisions do not in themselves reflect either the organization of output projections,[23] the distribution of neurochemical markers,[6,23,42] or combinations of both.[25] However, the striatal-like nature of many features of the CEA, together with its well-recognized continuity with the nucleus accumbens,[18,20,27] is strongly suggestive that a clearer picture of the intrinsic organization of the CEA may be obtained by viewing it from the perspective of the organization of the ventral striatopallidal system. This section has thus attempted to identify both connectional and neurochemical features shared by the central nucleus and the nucleus accumbens and ventral pallidum, and, as a corollary, common organizing principles. Though based on a very limited and selective analysis of the anatomical features of both areas, the following tentative conclusions are offered.

First, there appear to be enough common features to suggest that the lateral central nucleus is very similar, in terms of connections and neurochemistry, to the nucleus accumbens, as the medial central nucleus is to the ventral pallidum (FIG. 3). Moreover, the connectional/neurochemical differences between the lateral capsular and lateral subdivisions of the lateral Ce closely parallel differences between the shell and core regions of the nucleus accumbens. Further still, the dorsal and ventral components of the lateral capsular division can be distinguished by the same criteria that distinguish the dorsomedial shell from the ventrolateral shell. The dorsal and ventral parts of the medial Ce also exhibit similar neurochemical features to the medial and lateral segments of the ventral pallidum. Thus, the original cytoarchitectonic parcellation of the Ce by McDonald[22] can be translated, virtually without alteration, into a "shell-core-pallidum" arrangement that offers a much better organizational scheme for understanding the efferent, afferent, and neurochemical features of the central nucleus than either the chemoarchitectural[6] or overlap[23] schemes proposed earlier.

Second, the mosaic-like patterning of many key "striatopallidal" markers, including dopamine, calbindin D28k, enkephalin, and acetylcholinesterase, within these shell, core, and pallidal regions of the Ce suggests the presence of a complex subarchitecture that has close parallels with the multicompartmental organization of the nucleus accumbens and ventral pallidum.[13,14,65] On one end of the scale, these parallels associate the lateral, "core-like" subdivision of the Ce with the patch regions of the NAc rather than with the matrix, and on the other end associate, for example, some dopamine-rich patches with calbindin D28k immunoreactive cell clusters. Although definitive correlative studies still need to be done, future anatomical, as well as functional and pharmacological, studies of the CEA will need to pay careful attention to the organization of its complex intrinsic subarchitecture.

Finally, a shell-core-pallidum scheme offers a useful principle for understanding the CEA as a whole as well as the complex transitions that occur at its borders with the caudomedial shell of the accumbens, and the dorsal striatum, and within the sublenticular substantia innominata.[18,27] Though not explicitly dealt with here, many of the shell-core-pallidum features of the Ce are found in the dorsolateral bed nucleus of the stria terminalis and sublenticular substantia innominata (see refs. 18 and 27 for a review of some of these). In view of the subtle transition between the caudomedial shell and the bed nucleus, some of these features may not be readily apparent in the latter structure, nor may they be exactly the same as in the central nucleus.

THE STRIATO-PALLIDAL-LIKE INTRINSIC CIRCUITRY WITHIN THE CEA

In the previous section, it was argued that the complex intrinsic architecture of the CEA may be best understood by considering it from the perspective of a shell-core-pallidum arrangement that has close parallels with the nucleus accumbens–ventral pallidum complex. An important test of this hypothesis would be to determine whether the anatomy of the intrinsic connections of the nucleus accumbens–ventral pallidum complex, notably the striatopallidal connections, is replicated in the CEA. In this section, the intrinsic connections of the central nucleus, the connections of CEA GABAergic neurons, and the synaptic organization of selected afferents will be reviewed. No attempt has been made to relate the intrinsic connectivity to the complex subarchitecture of the CEA discussed above, and only general principles will be presented. Nonetheless, the data show clearly that the basic intrinsic circuitry of the CEA, the neurons giving rise to these projections (FIG. 4), and the synaptic relationships of some cortical, amygdaloid, and subcortical afferents closely resemble the circuitry found in the caudate-putamen/globus pallidus and nucleus accumbens–ventral pallidum systems.

Intrinsic Connections in the CEA

The intrinsic connections of the central nucleus have only been investigated in detail recently using *Phaseolus vulgaris*-leukoagglutinin (PHA-L).[40] These authors' data are consistent with our own unpublished data obtained from PHA-L, biocytin, and biotinylated dextran-amine (BDA) injections and will be summarized here with additional comments related to our own findings (FIG. 5). Injections into the ventral lateral capsular division heavily label CeM, particularly rostrally. At middle and caudal levels, fibers from vCeLC appear to be concentrated in the dorsomedial part of CeM (see FIG. 5E in ref. 40; unpublished observations). A considerable number of

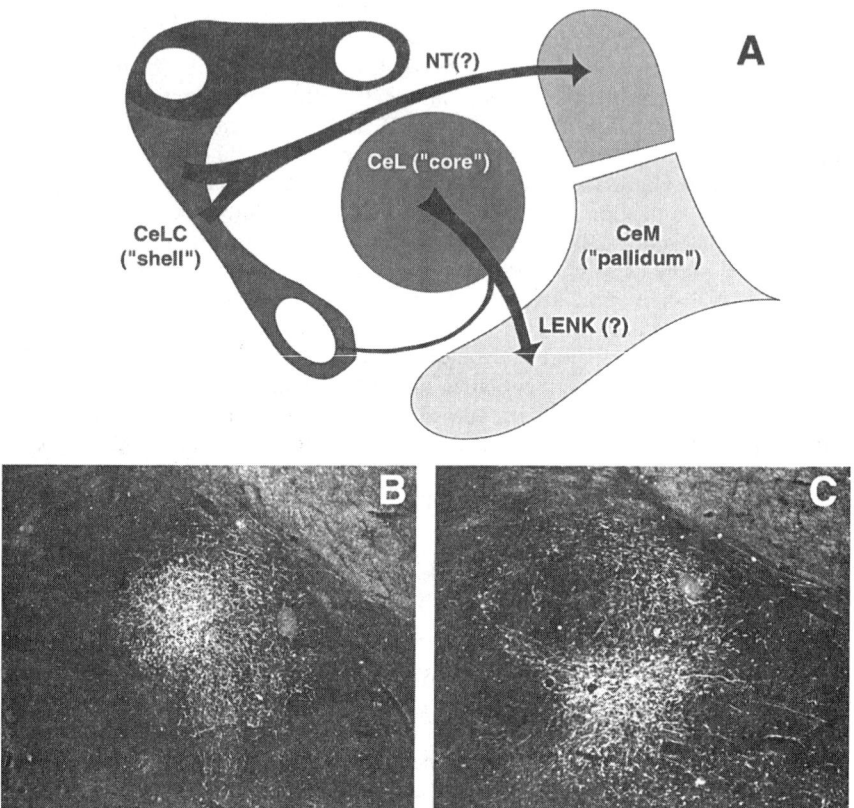

FIGURE 5. Schematic diagram (top) summarizing the intrinsic connections of the lateral capsular (CeLC), lateral (CeL), and medial (CeM) subdivisions of the central nucleus. *Bottom:* Two darkfield micrographs showing the distribution of labeled axons in the central nucleus after biocytin injections into the lateral (left) and the ventral lateral capsular divisions. The diagram also notes a possible neurotensin projection from CeLC to dorsal CeM, and a leucine enkephalin projection from CeL to ventral CeM. Additional data from ref. 40.

fibers remain within vCeLC along its rostrocaudal extent, but none appear to extend into dCeLC. Projections from CeL also targeted CeM but with the heaviest concentration ventrally.[40] The latter authors report moderate projections from CeL to vCeLC; in our material this projection was only seen after injections centered on the lateral part of CeL (unpublished observations). As in the case of CeLC injections, the whole extent of CeL contains labeled fibers after CeL injections. Both CeI and CeM appear to give rise to projections that remain within their own borders but do not appear to project to either CeLC or CeL.[40]

The long intrinsic connections of the CEA, that is, those that connect the central nucleus and bed nucleus, appear to link subdivisions with similar neurochemical and connectional features and mirror intrinsic connections within the Ce. Thus, CeM projects to the posterolateral bed nucleus, and CeL and CeLC project to both the anterolateral and posterolateral bed nucleus.[39] The anterolateral bed nucleus also projects to the posterolateral bed nucleus (unpublished observations), a projection comparable to the CeL to CeM projection. The sublenticular substantia innominata also projects to both the central and bed nuclei,[66] though the suborganization of these projections is unclear.

The organization of intrinsic projections of the CEA suggests that, on at least two levels, these projections closely parallel projections from the nucleus accumbens to the ventral pallidum.[16] First, the core/shell-like lateral subdivisions of the central nucleus (CeLC and CeL) project to the pallidal-like medial subdivision (CeM), and the projection is not reciprocated. Second, the shell-like CeLC projects to the dorsomedial part of CeM, whereas the core-like CeL projects to ventral CeM. This arrangement parallels the respective shell and core accumbens projections to the medial and lateral ventral pallidum (e.g., ref. 16). The projection from the anterolateral bed nucleus to the posterolateral bed nucleus (unpublished observations), which, respectively, have connectional features similar to CeL and CeM, suggests that a similar pattern of connections exists throughout the CEA.

Little is known about the cells of origin of intrinsic projections within the CEA, including those projecting from CeLC/CeL to CeM, though the long intrinsic connections arise in part from GABAergic medium-sized spiny neurons (ref. 9 and FIG. 4A). Considerable circumstantial evidence, however, suggests that it is the GABAergic neurons in the lateral Ce that provide the bulk of the lateral to medial projection. Golgi/intracellular staining of neurons in the central nucleus (refs. 22 and 26; and FIG. 4) suggests that the medium-sized spiny neurons in the lateral Ce can be divided on the basis of axon collateralization into a type with extensive local collaterals but a relatively unbranched axon extending out of CeL, and a type with few local collaterals but extensive branching outside of CeL. This pattern of axon branching is found in medium-sized spiny neurons in the matrix of the caudate-putamen that project to the globus pallidus, entopeduncular nucleus and substantia nigra.[67–69] GABA-immunoreactive terminals in the Ce remain largely unaffected by lesions of the stria terminalis, basolateral amygdala, or ventral amygdalofugal pathway (VAFP), and GABAergic neurons are a medium-sized, spiny type.[9] Though it remains to be shown conclusively, this is strongly suggestive that most, if not all, GABAergic terminals in the Ce are the terminal arrays of the highly branched axons of medium spiny neurons, and that the lateral ("shell/core") to medial ("pallidum") connection and the intra-compartmental connections[40] in the central nucleus are GABAergic.

Peptidergic Intrinsic Connections in the CEA

Neurons in the neostriatum and ventral striatum express a variety of neuropeptides, including substance P, met- and leu-enkephalin, dynorphin, somatostatin, and neurotensin (e.g., refs. 12, 15, and 70–72). Similar peptides are found in neurons in the CEA[1,23,26] and, in particular, neurotensin and the enkephalins are found in medium-sized spiny neurons.[26] Neither leu-enkephalin or met-enkephalin terminal fields in the Ce are appreciably affected by lesions of the stria terminalis, VAFP, or basolateral amygdala (ref. 5 and unpublished observations), suggesting a predominantly intrinsic origin for these peptides. Met- and leu-enkephalin immunoreactive medium-sized spiny neurons in CeL give rise to extensive local collaterals,[26] consis-

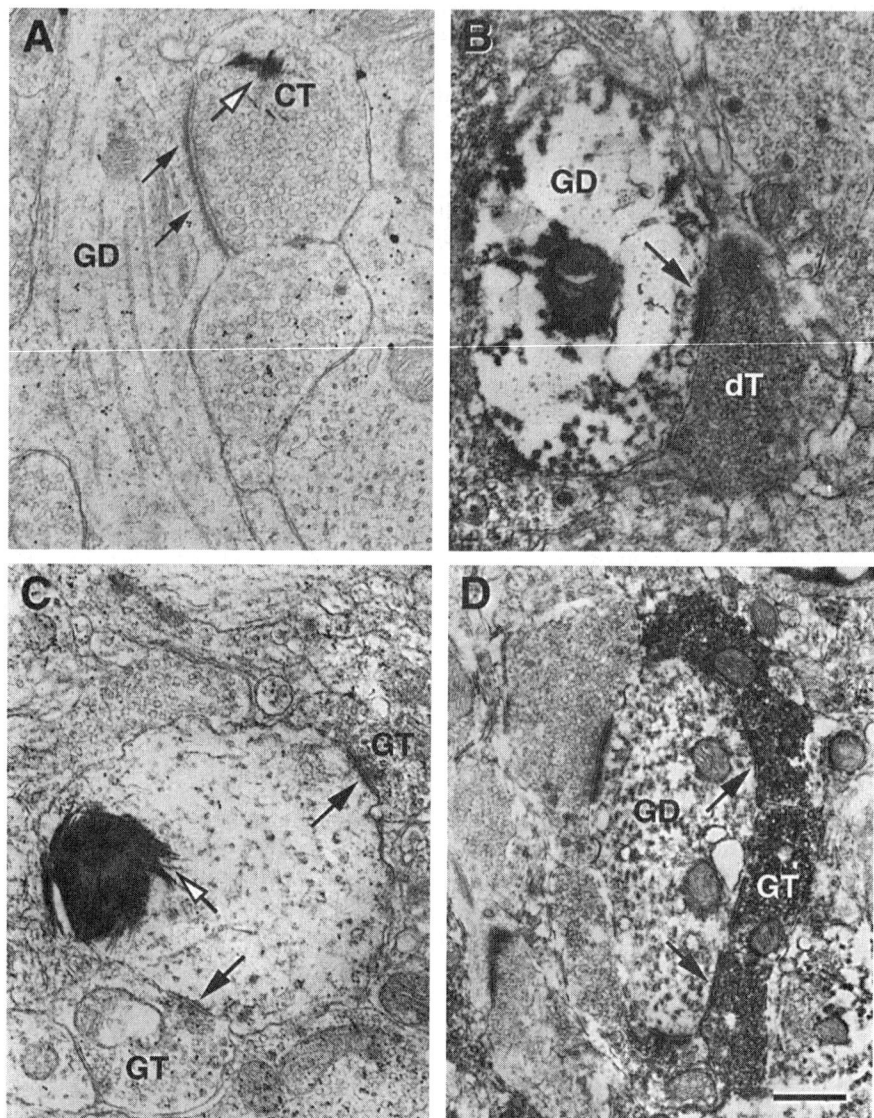

FIGURE 6. Electron micrographs showing striatal-like features of the intrinsic innervation of the CEA. **A:** HRP labeled (white arrow) cortical terminal (CT) from the insular cortex synapses with a GAD-immunoreactive dendrite (GD) labeled with gold particles. Note the asymmetric synapse formed (black arrows). **B:** A degenerating terminal (dT) in the central nucleus produced by a lesion in the parvicellular basal amygdaloid nucleus forms an asymmetric contact with a GD. **C:** Immunogold labeled GABAergic terminals (GT) forming symmetric contacts (black arrows) with a dendritic profile labeled by HRP (white arrow) injected into the dorsal medulla. **D:** GAD immunoreactive terminal (GT) in contact (arrows) with a GD.

tent with an intrinsic origin for these peptides. The moderately dense leu-enkephalin terminal field in the ventral part of CeM may arise from leu-enkephalin neurons in CeL, as this subdivision specifically projects to ventral CeM.[40] Similarly, the moderately dense neurotensin immunoreactive patch in the dorsomedial CeM is unaffected by stria terminalis/VAFP lesions[5] and thus may arise from neurotensin neurons in vCeLC, which projects specifically to this part of CeM.[40] Both these intrinsic pathways, though as yet unconfirmed, closely parallel, in their neurochemical aspects, the core/lateral VP and shell/medial VP projections.[17]

Ce neurons containing corticotropin-releasing factor, substance P, and somatostatin may also contribute local intrinsic connections,[26] though details are currently lacking. Some peptidergic fields show complementary patterning,[5,6] though the relative contributions of intrinsic and extrinsic projections to these fields is largely unknown. Interestingly, the somatostatin immunoreactive terminal field in the lateral Ce actually increases in density following VAFP lesions,[73] suggesting a possible plastic change in an intrinsic system.

Synaptic Interactions in the CEA

A considerable number of studies have examined the ultrastructure of the CEA (e.g., refs. 9, 53, and 73–75), but a comprehensive analysis has yet to be done. This section will therefore focus on two aspects of the ultrastructure of the CEA that have been extensively studied in the basal ganglia: the postsynaptic targets of cortical and basolateral amygdala inputs, and the synaptology of GABAergic, monoaminergic and peptidergic terminals. The main purpose of this focus is to demonstrate that the synaptic organization of these terminal fields in the CEA is remarkably similar to that in the basal ganglia.

Cortical Inputs

Cortical inputs to the caudate-putamen form asymmetric contacts primarily with the dendritic spines and dendritic shafts of the medium-sized, spiny GABAergic neurons (e.g., refs. 76–78). In the nucleus accumbens, entorhinal inputs also appear to preferentially innervate dendritic shafts and spines.[79] The central nucleus receives cortical inputs primarily from the insular cortex. Lesions or tracer injections into the insular cortex result in degeneration or anterograde labeling of terminals forming asymmetric synapses (FIG. 6A) predominantly with the spines and shafts of the dendrites of GABAergic neurons.[10]

Basolateral Amygdala Inputs

Terminals in the nucleus accumbens derived from axons originating in the basolateral amygdala preferentially innervate dendritic spines.[80,81] In one study,[81] over 90% of amygdalar boutons contacted dendritic spines in the NA. Amygdalar terminals contained clear, round vesicles and formed exclusively asymmetric contacts. There are no definitive details of the postsynaptic contacts formed by pBAN or LN afferents in the CEA. Preliminary data (unpublished data) indicate that lesions in the vicinity of the pBAN and posterior basomedial nucleus result in degenerating terminals in contact with dendrites of GABAergic neurons (FIG. 6B).

GABAergic Terminals

The terminal boutons of axons of striatal medium-sized spiny neurons are relatively small (about 1 μm), contain pleomorphic vesicles, form symmetrical synapses, and are GAD/GABA immunoreactive (e.g., refs. 69, 77, and 82). There appears to be little to distinguish boutons derived from local collaterals or projection axons.[76,83] In the ventral pallidum, boutons containing both GABA and met-enkephalin form symmetrical contacts with pallidal neurons.[84] In the CEA, GABAergic terminals form symmetrical synaptic contacts with the perikarya and proximal dendrites of neurons in CeM and posterolateral bed nucleus that project to the dorsal medulla (FIG. 6C), and with neurons in CeL and anterolateral bed nucleus that project to the lateral parabrachial complex.[10] In addition, in CeL, GABAergic terminals form symmetrical contacts with GABA-immunoreactive dendrites (FIG. 6D) and spines.[10]

Somatostatin, neurotensin, and met-enkephalin are largely colocalized with GABA in the CEA.[44] Consistent with this, terminals immunoreactive for these peptides form symmetrical contacts with predominantly dendrites and dendritic spines (refs. 75 and 83; and unpublished observations).

Dopaminergic Terminals

The morphology and types of postsynaptic contacts of putative dopaminergic terminals in both the dorsal and ventral striatum appear essentially similar whether identified using dopamine[85] or tyrosine hydroxylase[78,86–88] antibodies. DA terminals form symmetrical contacts and symmetrical-like appositions preferentially with dendrites and dendritic spines (e.g., ref. 85). There is evidence that synaptic contacts made by cortical boutons are closely related to DA terminals.[87] The ultrastructural features of DA terminals in the central nucleus part of the CEA are similar to those in the striatum.[53,74] DA terminals form symmetrical contacts on dendrites and dendritic spines (though perikaryal contacts are also evident) and appear to innervate GABA, NT, ENK, and somatostatin-synthesizing neurons in all divisions of the central nucleus.[53] Insular cortical lesions produce degenerating terminals at dendritic sites where TH immunoreactive terminals also form contacts (unpublished observations).

Summary (FIGURE 7)

Clearly, in general terms at least, the intrinsic organization of the CEA is remarkably similar to that in both the dorsal and ventral striatum (FIG. 7). The lateral, striatal-like parts of the CEA project to the medial, pallidal-like parts, and GABA, and possibly neurotensin and enkephalin, are transmitters in these projections (FIGURES 5 and 7). Cortical and amygdalar afferents end on GABAergic, medium-sized spiny neurons, with the same dendritic preferences shown by similar terminal endings in the striatum. GABAergic, peptidergic, and dopaminergic terminals show the same types of synaptic specializations and postsynaptic contacts in all three areas. Though an enormous amount of work remains to be done to refine our understanding of the intrinsic organization of the CEA, in terms of the basic internal connectional and neurochemical framework, there appears to be little difference between the dorsal and ventral striatopallidal complexes and the CEA.

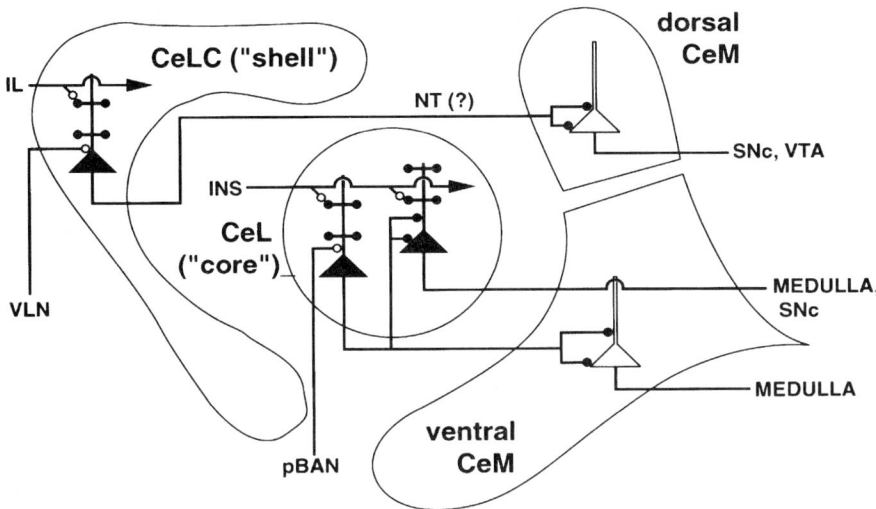

FIGURE 7. Schematic diagram showing the proposed basic intrinsic microcircuitry of the central nucleus. In this scheme, GABAergic medium-sized spiny neurons in CeLC ("shell") and CeL ("core") project to pallidal-like output neurons in CeM. Cortical and basal amygdalar inputs preferentially innervate dendrites and spines of the striatal-like neurons in CeLC and CeL. This circuitry approximates the organization of intrinsic connections in the rest of the basal ganglia.

GENERAL CONCLUSIONS AND COMMENTS

This short review has attempted to bring together a variety of neurochemical and connectional evidence to produce a very basic floor plan of the intrinsic organization of the central extended amygdala. The evidence has been deliberately biased, however, towards neurochemical and connectional features shared by the CEA and the dorsal and ventral striatum. Such bias is not unreasonable given the physical intimacy between the three structures and the nature of the evidence that has been used in progressing both from the dorsal striatopallidal system to the ventral striatopallidal system, and from that system to the central extended amygdala.[1] The case has been made here that the internal anatomy of the CEA appears to be organized along the same lines as the nucleus accumbens–ventral pallidum complex, with a multicompartmental scheme that mirrors both the shell-core-pallidum distinction and the subarchitecture found within these components. The physical continuity between the caudomedial nucleus accumbens and the bed nucleus, and between the accumbens core and subcommissural ventral pallidum and the central nucleus[1,18,27] may not be transitional at all but representative of actual continuities in architecture and subarchitecture between the two structures, an argument supported by the well-recognized extension of many afferents and efferent projection populations across their boundaries.[1,20,21]

If this turns out to be a correct perspective to take, then there are a number of implications for the organization of the forebrain as a whole, and the basal ganglia and amygdaloid complex, in particular. First, a shell-core-pallidum architectural scheme for the CEA makes a fairly compelling argument for including this structure in the basal ganglia macrosystem and excluding it from the amygdaloid complex. The amygdaloid complex is being increasingly criticized as a term that describes a distinct brain entity,[3,4] and the CEA, rather than being viewed as the major output structure of the whole amygdaloid complex,[89] should probably be seen as being one of three major output structures for the basolateral amygdala and for the cortex. Second, the similarities between the basal ganglia and CEA in internal organization should extend to the external connections of the CEA. Some evidence for "direct" and "indirect" CEA output pathways has been alluded to here, but a critical test of the validity of the shell-core-pallidum hypothesis will be determining whether the CEA participates in the type of open/closed loop circuits that are found in both dorsal and ventral striatopallidal systems (e.g., refs. 2 and 90). Finally, the dorsal and ventral striatopallidal systems are increasingly being viewed as major players behind the pathology of several psychiatric disorders, notably schizophrenia (e.g., refs. 91 and 92), and a potential role for the CEA–VTA connection is being increasingly recognized.[93] A clearer understanding of this role, and the involvement of the CEA in stress and anxiety disorders, may come from a recognition that the CEA is a component of the basal ganglia, and its operational organization closely parallels that of the ventral striatopallidal system.

REFERENCES

1. ALHEID, G.F. & L. HEIMER. 1988. New perspectives in basal forebrain organization of special relevance for neuropsychiatric disorders: the striatopallidal, amygdaloid and corticopetal components of substantia innominata. Neuroscience 27: 1–39.
2. GROENEWEGEN, H.J., H.W. BERENDSE, J.G. WOLTERS & A.H.M. LOHMAN. 1990. The anatomical relationship of the prefrontal cortex with the striatopallidal system, the thalamus, and the amygdala; evidence for a parallel organization. Prog. Brain Res. 85: 95–118.
3. CASSELL, M.D. 1998. The amygdala: myth or monolith? Trends Neurosci. 21: 200–201.
4. SWANSON, L.W. & G.D. PETROVICH. 1998. What is the amygdala. Trends Neurosci. 21: 323–331.
5. CASSELL, M.D., N.J. MANKOVICH, T.S. GRAY & T.H. WILLIAMS. 1982. Computer-assisted image analysis of the distribution of peptidergic terminals in the central nucleus of the amygdala. Peptides 3: 283–290.
6. WRAY, S. & G.E. HOFFMAN. 1983. Organization and interrelationship of neuropeptides in the central amygdaloid nucleus of the rat. Peptides 4: 525–541.
7. BERNARD, J.F., M. ALDEN & J.M. BESSON. 1993. The organization of the efferent projections from the pontine parabrachial area to the amygdaloid complex: a *Phaseolus vulgaris* leucoagglutinin (PHA-L) study in the rat. J. Comp. Neurol. 329: 201–229.
8. VEENING, J.G., L.W. SWANSON & P.E. SAWCHENKO. 1984. The organization of projections from the central nucleus of the amygdala to brainstem sites involved in central autonomic regulation: a combined retrograde transport-immunohistochemical study. Brain Res. 303: 337–357.
9. SUN, N. & M.D. CASSELL. 1993. Intrinsic GABAergic neurons in the rat central extended amygdala. J. Comp. Neurol. 330: 381–404.

10. SUN, N., H. YI & M.D. CASSELL. 1994. Evidence for a GABAergic interface between cortical afferents and brainstem projection neurons in the rat central extended amygdala. J. Comp. Neurol. **340:** 43–64.
11. BERENDSE, H. W., H.J. GROENEWEGEN & A.H.M. LOHMAN. 1992. Compartmental distribution of ventral striatal neurons projecting to the mesencephalon in the rat. J. Neurosci. **12:** 2079–2103.
12. GERFEN, C.R. & W.S. YOUNG. 1988. Distribution of striatonigral and striatopallidal peptidergic neurons in both patch and matrix compartments: an in situ hybridization histochemistry and fluorescent retrograde tracing study. Brain Res. **460:** 161–167.
13. JONGEN-RELO, A.L., H.J. GROENEWEGEN & P. VOORN. 1993. Evidence for a multicompartmental histochemical organization of the nucleus accumbens in the rat. J. Comp. Neurol. **337:** 267–276.
14. JONGEN-RELO, A.L., P. VOORN & H.J. GROENEWEGEN. 1994. Immunohistochemical characterization of the shell and core territories of the nucleus accumbens in the rat. Eur. J. Neurosci. **6:** 1255–1264.
15. VOORN, P., C.R. GERFEN & H.J. GROENEWEGEN. 1989. Compartmental organization of the ventral striatum of the rat: immunohistochemical distribution of enkephalin, substance P, dopamine and calcium–binding protein. J. Comp. Neurol. **289:** 189–201.
16. ZAHM, D.S. & J.S. BROG. 1992. On the significance of sub-territories in the "accumbens" part of the rat ventral striatum. Neuroscience **50:** 751–767.
17. ZAHM, D.S. & L. HEIMER. 1988. Ventral striatopallidal parts of the basal ganglia in the rat: I. neurochemical compartmentation as reflected by the distributions of neurotensin and substance P immunoreactivity. J. Comp. Neurol. **272:** 516–535.
18. ALHEID, G.F. C.A. BELTRAMINO, J.S. DE OLMOS, M.S. FORBES, D.J. SWANSON & L. HEIMER. 1998. The neuronal organization of the supracapsular part of the stria terminalis in the rat: the dorsal component of the extended amygdala. Neuroscience **84:** 967–996.
19. HEIMER, L., D.S. ZAHM, L. CHURCHILL, P.W. KALIVAS & C. WOHLTMANN. 1991. Specificity in the projection patterns of accumbens core and shell in the rat. Neuroscience **41:** 89–125.
20. HEIMER, L., G.F. ALHEID, J.S. DE OLMOS, H.J. GROENEWEGEN, S.N. HABER, R.E. HARLAN & D.S. ZAHM. 1997. The accumbens: beyond the core-shell dichotomy. J. Neuropsychiatry Clin. Neurosci. **9:** 354–381.
21. HEIMER, L., R.E. HARLAN, G.F. ALHEID, M.M. GARCIA & J. DEOLMOS. 1997. Substantia innominata: a notion which impedes clinical-anatomical correlations in neuropsychiatric disorders. Neuroscience **76:** 957–1006.
22. MCDONALD, A.J. 1982. Cytoarchitecture of the central amygdaloid nucleus of the rat. J. Comp. Neurol. **208:** 401–418.
23. CASSELL, M.D., T.S. GRAY & J.Z. KISS. 1986. Neuronal architecture in the rat central nucleus of the amygdala; a cytological, hodological and immunocytochemical study. J. Comp. Neurol. **246:** 478–499.
24. GRAY, T.S., M.D. CASSELL & J.Z. KISS. 1984. Distribution of pro-opiomelanocortin-derived peptides and enkephalins in the rat central nucleus of the amygdala. Brain Res. **306:** 354–358.
25. GRAY, T.S. & D.J. MAGNUSSON. 1987. Neuropeptide neuronal efferents from the bed nucleus of the stria terminalis and central amygdaloid nucleus to the dorsal vagal complex in the rat. J. Comp. Neurol. **262:** 365–374.
26. CASSELL, M.D. & T.S. GRAY. 1989. Morphology of peptide-immunoreactive neurons in the rat central nucleus of the amygdala. J. Comp. Neurol. **281:** 320–333.
27. ALHEID, G.F., C.A. BELTRAMINO, A. BRAUN & L. HEIMER. 1994. Transition areas of the striatopallidal system with the extended amygdala in the rat and primate: observations from histochemistry and experiments with mono- and transynaptic tracers. In The Basal Ganglia IV, Vol. 41. G. Percheron, J.S. McKenzie & J. Feger, Eds.: 95–107. Plenum. New York.
28. DE OLMOS, J., G.F. ALHEID & C.A. BELTRAMINO. 1985. Amygdala. In The Rat Nervous System. G. Paxinos, Ed.: Vol. **1:** 223–334. Academic Press. Florida.

29. McDonald, A.J. 1997. Calbindin D28k immunoreactivity in the rat amygdala. J. Comp. Neurol. **383:** 231–244.
30. Freedman, L.J. & M.D. Cassell. 1994. Distribution of dopaminergic fibers in the central division of the extended amygdala of the rat. Brain Res. **633:** 243–252.
31. Wright, C.I., A.V.J. Beijer & H.J. Groenewegen. 1996. Basal amygdaloid complex afferents to the rat nucleus accumbens are compartmentally organized. J. Neurosci. **16:** 1877–1893.
32. Shi, C-J. & M.D. Cassell. 1998. Cascade projections from somatosensory cortex to the rat basolateral amygdala via the parietal insular cortex. J. Comp. Neurol. **399:** 469–482.
33. Shi, C-J. & M.D. Cassell. 1998. Cortical, thalamic, and amygdaloid connections of the anterior and posterior insular cortices. J. Comp. Neurol. **399:** 440–468.
34. Sesack, S.R., A.Y. Deutch, R.H. Roth & B.S. Bunney. 1989. Topographical organization of the efferent connections of the medial prefrontal cortex in the rat: an anterograde tract-tracing study with Phaseolus vulgaris leucoagglutinin. J. Comp. Neurol. **290:** 213–242.
35. Cassell, M.D. & D.J. Wright. 1986. Topography of projections from the medial prefrontal cortex to the amygdala in the rat. Brain Res. Bull. **17:** 321–333.
36. Hurley, K.M., H. Herbert, M.M. Moga & C.B. Saper. 1991. Efferent projections of the infralimbic cortex of the rat. J. Comp. Neurol. **308:** 249–276.
37. McGeorge, A. & R. Faull. 1989. The organization of the projection from the cerebral cortex to the striatum in the rat. Neuroscience **29:** 503–537.
38. Shi, C-J. & M.D. Cassell. 1997. Cortical, thalamic, and amygdaloid projections of rat temporal cortex. J. Comp. Neurol. **382:** 153–175.
39. Sun, N., L. Roberts & M.D. Cassell. 1991. Rat central amygdaloid nucleus projections to the bed nucleus of the stria terminalis. Brain Res. Bull. **27:** 651–662.
40. Jolkonnen, E. & A. Pitkanen. 1998. Intrinsic connections of the rat amygdaloid complex: projections originating in the central nucleus. J. Comp. Neurol. **395:** 53–72.
41. Shammah-Lagnado, S.J., G.F. Alheid & L. Heimer. 1996. Efferent connections of the caudal part of the globus pallidus in the rat. J. Comp. Neurol. **376:** 489–507.
42. Gonzales, C. & M-F. Chesselet. 1990. Amygdalonigral pathway: an anterograde study in the rat with *Phaseolus vulgaris* leucoagglutinin (PHA-L). J. Comp. Neurol. **297:** 182–200.
43. Oertel, W.H., G. Reithmuller, E. Mugnaini, D.E. Schmechel, A. Weindl, C. Gramsch & A. Herz. 1983. Opioid peptide-like immunoreactivity localized in GABAergic neurons of rat neostriatum and central amygdaloid nucleus. Life Sci. **33:** 73–76.
44. Veinante, P., M.E. Stoeckel & M.J. Freund-Mercier. 1997. GABA- and peptide-immunoreactivities co-localize in the rat central extended amygdala. Neuroreport **8:** 2985–2989.
45. Cassell, M.D., N. Sun & L. Roberts. 1990. Distribution patterns of rat central amygdaloid (Ce) efferent neurons. Soc. Neurosci. Abstr. **16:** 125.
46. Groenewegen, H.J. & H.W. Berendse. 1990. Connections of the subthalamic nucleus with ventral striatopallidal parts of the basal ganglia in the rat. J. Comp. Neurol. **294:** 607–622.
47. McDonald, A.J. 1988. Projections of the intermediate subdivision of the central amygdaloid nucleus to the bed nucleus of the stria terminalis and medial diencephalon. Neurosci. Lett. **85:** 285–290.
48. Rizvi, T.A., M. Ennis, M.M. Behbehani & M.T. Shipley. 1991. Connections between the amygdala and the midbrain periaqueductal gray: topography and reciprocity. J. Comp. Neurol. **303:** 121–131.
49. Millhouse, O.E. 1986. Pallidal neurons in the rat. J. Comp. Neurol. **254:** 209–227.
50. Park, M.R., W.M. Falls & S.T. Kitai. 1982 An intracellular HRP study of the rat globus pallidus: I. Responses and light microscopic analysis. J. Comp. Neurol. **211:** 284–294.

51. PITKANEN, A. & D.G. AMARAL. 1994. The distribution of GABAergic cells, fibers, and terminals in the monkey amygdaloid complex: an immunohistochemical and in situ hybridization study. J. Neurosci. **14:** 2200–2224.
52. JIA, H-G., Z-R. RAO & J-W. SHI. 1997. Evidence of ψ-aminobutyric acidergic control over the catecholaminergic projection from the medulla oblongata to the central nucleus of the amygdala. J. Comp. Neurol. **381:** 262–281.
53. ASAN, E. 1997. Interrelationships between tyrosine hydroxylase-immunoreactive dopaminergic afferents and somatostatinergic neurons in the rat central amygdaloid nucleus. Histochem. Cell Biol. **107:** 65–79.
54. BEART, P.M., R.J. SUMMERS, J.A. STEPHENSON, C.J. COOK & M.J. CHRISTIE. 1990. Excitatory amino acid projections to the periaqueductal gray in the rat: a retrograde transport study utilizing D[^{3}H] aspartate and [^{3}H] GABA. Neuroscience **34:** 163–176.
55. HABER, S.N., H.J. GROENEWEGEN, E.A. GROVE & W.J.H. NAUTA. 1985. Efferent connections of the ventral pallidum: evidence of a dual striato-pallidofugal pathway. J. Comp. Neurol. **235:** 322–335.
56. CHEN, S. & H-S. SU. 1990. Afferent connections of the thalamic paraventricular and parataenial nuclei in the rat: a retrograde tracing study with the iontophoretic application of FluorGold. Brain Res. **522:** 1–6.
57. CORNWALL, J. & O.Y. PHILLIPSON. 1988. Afferent projections to the dorsal thalamus of the rat as shown by retrograde lectin transport: II. The midline nuclei. Brain Res. Bull. **21:** 147–161.
58. PHILLIPSON, O.T. 1978. Afferent projections to the ventral tegmental area of Tsai and interfascicular nucleus. A horesradish peroxidase study in the rat. J. Comp. Neurol. **187:** 117–144.
59. BUNNEY, B.S. & G.K. AGHAJANIAN. 1976. The precise localization of nigral afferents in the rat as determined by a retrograde tracing technique. Brain Res. **117:** 423–435.
60. SCHWABER, J,S., B.S. KAPP, G.A. HIGGINS & P.R. RAPP. 1982. Amygdaloid and basal forebrain direct connections with the nucleus of the solitary tract and dorsal motor nucleus. J. Neurosci. **2:** 1424–1438.
61. ZAHM, D.S., E. WILLIAMS & C. WOHLTMANN. 1996. Ventral striatopallidothalamic projection: IV. Relative involvement of neurochemically distinct sub-territories in the ventral pallidum and adjacent parts of the rostroventral forebrain. J. Comp. Neurol. **364:** 340–362.
62. SCHMUED, L.C. 1994. Diagonal ventral forebrain continuum has overlapping telencephalic inputs and brainstem outputs which may represent loci for limbic/autonomic integration. Brain Res. **667:** 175–191.
63. TOUZANI, K., K. TAGHZOUTI & L. VELLEY. 1996. Cellular organization of lateral hypothalamic efferents to the central amygdaloid nucleus of the rat. NeuroReport **7:** 517–520.
64. PENNARTZ, C.M.A., H.J. GROENEWEGEN & F.H. LOPES DA SILVA. 1994. The nucleus accumbens as a complex of functionally distinct neuronal ensembles: an integration of behavioral, electrophysiological and anatomical data. Prog. Neurobiol. **42:** 719–761.
65. ZAHM, D.S. 1989. The ventral striatopallidal parts of the basal ganglia in the rat. II. Compartmentation of ventral pallidal efferents. Neuroscience **30:** 33–50.
66. GROVE, E.A. 1988. Efferent connections of the substantia innominata in the rat. J. Comp. Neurol. **277:** 347–364.
67. KAWAGUCHI, Y., C.J. WILSON & P.C. EMSON. 1990. Projection subtypes of rat neostriatal matrix cells revealed by intracellular injection of biocytin. J. Neurosci. **10:** 3421–3438.
68. MEREDITH, G.E., R. AGOLIA, M.P. M. ARTS, H.J. GROENEWEGEN & D.S. ZAHM. 1992. Morphological differences between projection neurons of the core and shell in the nucleus accumbens of the rat. Neuroscience **50:** 149–162.
69. TOTTERDELL, S., J.P. BOLAM & A.D. SMITH. 1984. Characterization of pallidonigral neurons in the rat by a combination of Golgi-impregnation and retrograde transport

of horseradish peroxidase: their monosynaptic input from the neostriatum. J. Neurocytol. **13:** 593–616.
70. PENNY, G.R., C.J. WILSON & S.T. KITAI. 1988. Relationship of the axonal and dendritic geometry of spiny projection neurons to the compartmental organization of the neostriatum. J. Comp. Neurol. **269:** 275–289.
71. REINER, A. & K.D. ANDERSON. 1990. The patterns of neurotransmitter and neuropeptide co-occurrence among striatal projection neurons: conclusions based on recent findings. Brain Res. Rev. **15:** 251–265.
72. SENGER, B., J.S. BROG & D.S. ZAHM. 1993. Subsets of neurotensin immunoreactive neurons in the rat striatal complex following antagonism of the dopamine D2 receptor: an immunohistochemical double-labeling study using antibodies against Fos. Neuroscience **57:** 649–660.
73. GOTOW, T., T.H. WILLIAMS, J.Y. JEW, M.D. CASSELL, M. PALKOVITS & P.H. HASHIMOTO. 1989. Collateral sprouting of somatostatin-immunoreactive axons after partial deafferentation of the central nucleus of the amygdala. Brain Res. **492:** 326–336.
74. ASAN, E. 1997. Ultrastructural features of tyrosine-hydroxylase-immunoreactive afferents and their targets in the rat amygdala. Cell Tissue Res. **288:** 449–469.
75. GRAY, T.S., M.D. CASSELL & T.H. WILLIAMS. 1982. Synaptology of three peptidergic neuron types in the central nucleus of the amygdala. Peptides **3:** 273–281.
76. BOLAM, J.P. & B. BENNETT. 1995. The microcircuitry of the neostriatum. *In* Molecular and Cellular Mechanisms of Neostriatal Functions. M. Ariano & D.J. Surmeier, Eds.: 1–19. Landes. Austin, Texas.
77. BOLAM, J.P., J.F. POWELL, J-Y WU & A.D. SMITH. 1985. Glutamate decarboxylase-immunoreactive structures in the rat neostriatum: a correlated light and electron microscopic study including a combination of Golgi impreganation with immunocytochemistry. J. Comp. Neurol. **237:** 1–20.
78. BOUYER, J.J., D.M. PARK, T.M. JOH & V.M. PICKEL. 1984a. Chemical and structural analysis of the relation between cortical input and tyrosine hydroxylase-containing terminals in the rat neostriatum. Brain Res. **302:** 267–275.
79. TOTTERDELL, S. & G.E. MEREDITH. 1997. Topographical organization of projections from the entorhinal cortex to the striatum of the rat. Neuroscience **78:** 715–729.
80. JOHNSON, L.R., R.L.M. AYLWARD, Z. HUSSAIN & S. TOTTERDELL. 1994. Input from the amygdala to the rat nucleus accumbens: its relationship with tyrosine hydroxylase immunoreactivity and identified neurons. Neuroscience **61:** 851–865.
81. KITA, H. & S. T. KITAI. 1990. Amygdaloid projections of the frontal cortex and the striatum in the rat. J. Comp. Neurol. **298:** 40–49.
82. ARONIN, N., K. CHASE & M. DIFIGLIA. 1986. Glutamic acid decarboxylase and enkephalin immunoreactive axon terminals in the rat neostriatum synapse with striatonigral neurons. Brain Res. **365:** 151–158.
83. YUNG, K.K.L., A.D. SMITH, A.I. LEVEY & J.P. BOLAM. 1996. Synaptic connections between spiny neurons of the direct and indirect pathways in the neostriatum of the rat: evidence from dopamine receptor and neuropeptide immunostaining. Eur. J. Neurosci. **8:** 861–869.
84. ZAHM, D.S., L. ZABORSKY, V.E. ALONES & L. HEIMER. 1985. Evidence for the coexistence of glutamate decarboxylase and methionine-enkephalin immunoreactivities in axon terminals of rat ventral pallidum. Brain Res. **325:** 317–321.
85. VOORN, P., B. JORRITSMA-BYHAM, C. VAN DIJK & R.M. BUIJS. 1986. The dopaminergic innervation of the ventral striatum in the rat: a light and electronmicroscopical study with antibodies against dopamine. J. Comp. Neurol. **251:** 84–99.
86. ARLUISON, M. M. DIETL & J. THIBAULT. 1984. Ultrastructural morphology of dopaminergic nerve terminals and synapses in the striatum of the rat using tyrosine hydroxylase immunocytochemistry: a topographical study. Brain Res. Bull. **13:** 269–285.
87. BOUYER, J.J., T.M. JOH & V.M. PICKEL. 1984b. Ultrastructural localization of tyrosine hydroxylase in rat nucleus accumbens. J. Comp. Neurol. **227:** 92–103.
88. ZAHM, D.S. 1992. An electron microscopic morphometric comparison of tyrosine hydroxylase innervation in the neostriatum and the nucleus accumbens core and shell. Brain Res. **575:** 341–346.

89. PITKANEN, A,. V. SAVANDER & J.E. LEDOUX. 1997. Organization of intra-amygdaloid circuitries in the rat: an emerging framework for understanding functions of the amygdala . Trends Neurosci. **20:** 517–523.
90. O'DONNELL, P., A. LAVIN, L.W. ENQUIST, A.A. GRACE & J.P. CARD. 1997. Interconnected parallel circuits between rat nucleus accumbens and thalamus revealed by retrograde transynaptic transport of pseudorabies virus. J. Neurosci. **17:** 2143–2167.
91. CARPENTER, W.T. & R.W. BUCHANAN. 1994. Schizophrenia. N. Engl. J. Med. **330:** 681–690.
92. GRAYBIEL, A. M. 1997. The basal ganglia and cognitive pattern generators. Schizophr. Bull. **23:** 459–469.

The Medial Extended Amygdala in Male Reproductive Behavior

A Node in the Mammalian Social Behavior Network

SARAH WINANS NEWMAN[a]

Department of Psychology, Uris Hall, Cornell University, Ithaca, New York 14853, USA

ABSTRACT: Hormonal and chemosensory signals regulate social behaviors in a wide variety of mammals. In the male Syrian hamster, these signals are integrated in nuclei of the medial extended amygdala, where olfactory and vomeronasal system transmission is modulated by populations of androgen- and estrogen-sensitive neurons. Evidence from behavioral changes following lesions and from immediate early gene expression supports the hypothesis that the medial extended amygdala and medial preoptic area belong to a circuit that functions selectively in male sexual behavior. However, accumulated behavioral, neuroanatomical, and neuroendocrine data in hamsters, other rodents, and other mammals indicate that this circuit is embedded in a larger integrated network that controls not only male mating behavior, but female sexual behavior, parental behavior, and various forms of aggression. In this context, perhaps an individual animal's social responses can be more easily understood as a repertoire of closely interrelated, hormone-regulated behaviors, shaped by development and experience and modulated acutely by the environmental signals and the hormonal milieu of the brain.

INTRODUCTION

The concept of the extended amygdala was introduced in the mid 1980s by de Olmos *et al.*[1] and Alheid and Heimer,[2] who subsequently have provided compelling arguments to support this construct.[3] In elucidating the organization of the ventral forebrain they assembled the evidence for parallel rings of cells, extending through the medial and central amygdaloid nuclei, supracapsular and bed nuclei of the stria terminalis (BNST), and the substantia innominata, that are related by shared characteristics in cell morphology, reciprocal neuronal connections, and neurochemical/neurotransmitter identity. The question of whether these discrete rings of cells also share functional identity has been raised, but less evidence has been available to address this hypothesis. Recent studies of male rodent sexual behavior are among those that provide support for functional as well as anatomical continuity, especially with regard to the medial extended amygdala. In the course of these studies, Wood and Newman[4] have argued that the medial extended amygdala is itself composed of two parallel, functionally different circuits of cells, associated with the anterior and posterior divisions of the medial nucleus, respectively, which also can be differentiated

---

[a]Voice: 607-255-1195; fax: 607-255-8433; swn3@cornell.edu

on the basis of connections and neurotransmitters. After reviewing the evidence for functional continuity within these circuits, I will consider these extended amygdala units in a larger framework, an interconnected, gonadal-steroid sensitive network of limbic areas that collectively regulates all social behaviors.

THE MEDIAL EXTENDED AMYGDALA: EVIDENCE FOR ANTERIOR AND POSTERIOR CIRCUITS BASED ON CONNECTIONS, TRANSMITTERS, HORMONE RECEPTORS, AND HORMONE ACTION

Anatomical Continuity within Parallel Circuits

In both the male rat[5] and male Syrian hamster[6,7] the efferents of anterior and posterior regions of the medial amygdala have distinctly different distribution patterns in the BNST. The axons of the anterior dorsal part of the medial amygdaloid nucleus (MeAD) project through the ansa peduncularis (ventral amygdalofugal pathway) and the stria terminalis to a lateral territory in the posterior BNST. In the rat this territory consists of several subgroups of cells for which there is no uniformly accepted terminology (see Alheid et al.[8]). In the hamster we have designated this region the posterointermediate BNST (BNSTpi).[6] By contrast, the posterior dorsal part of the medial nucleus (MePD), and in particular its caudal portion (cMePD), send projections over the same pathways to end in the medial area of the posterior BNST, which we have called the posteromedial subdivision of the BNST (BNSTpm) in the hamster.[6] Recently Coolen and Wood[7] have provided evidence that these connections between MeAD and BNSTpi and between cMePD and BNSTpm in the hamster are not only dense and largely distinct from each other but that they are also bidirectional.

Neurotransmitter/Neuromodulator Continuity within the Posterior-medial Extended Amygdala

In the rat both the MeAD/BNSTpi and cMePD/BNSTpm circuits contain numerous neurons that produce glutamic acid decarboxylase and GABA.[9] A variety of other neurotransmitters and neuromodulators have been localized predominantly within the cMePD/BNSTpm circuit. This selective distribution of neuroactive substances in the posterior circuit, particularly neuropeptides, is also seen in the hamster, but there appear to be a number of species differences. In both rat and hamster the cMePD/BNSTpm system is characterized by numerous substance P neurons[10,11] and more limited populations of enkephalin-producing cells.[10,12] In the rat, arginine vasopressin[13] and cholecystokinin[10,14] cells are also abundant in these nuclei, although they have not been localized here in the hamster brain.[15] By contrast, the hamster has populations of prodynorphin-producing neurons in these nuclei that are not found in the rat[16] and that overlap by at least 50% with the substance P cell population, that is, at least half of the substance P neurons in cMePD and in BNSTpm also contain prodynorphin, and vice versa.[17] A fourth neurochemically distinctive group of cells localized in cMePD and BNSTpm, also found in the hamster but not in the rat brain, is a population of neurons that are immunoreactive for tyrosine hydroxylase (TH) and dopamine.[18] The cells in this caudal MePD circuit differ from TH neurons in MeAD in their dopamine immunoreactivity and in the much larger proportion of the population (75% vs. 30%) that contain androgen receptors.[19]

Gonadal-steroid Receptors and Sexual Dimorphism in the Medial Extended Amygdala

The density of gonadal steroid receptors is also a characteristic that distinguishes the cMePD/BNSTpm from the MeAD/BNSTpi circuit. In the rat, hamster, and other rodents, androgen- and estrogen-receptors are distributed primarily in the cMePD and BNSTpm.[20–24] In the adult rat these cell groups are sexually dimorphic with respect to nuclear volume,[25,26] synaptic organization,[27,28] and neurotransmitters.[13,14,29–31] Furthermore, at least some of these sexually differentiated characteristics can be modulated by hormones in adulthood. Hormone-mediated mRNA or neuropeptide production has been demonstrated in the adult in cholecystokinin cells of this circuit in the rat[10,32,33] and in the substance P neurons in both rat and hamster.[10,11]

In addition, in both of these species, mounting behavior can be restored in castrated males with an implant of testosterone, or its metabolite estradiol, delivered only to the MePD on one side of the brain,[34–36] whereas similar implants in MeAD are ineffective in the hamster.[36] A testosterone implant that delivers hormone to the BNSTpm also reinstates this behavior,[35] but in the hamsters that we have studied to date, the cannulae delivered testosterone to both the BNST and to the adjacent medial preoptic nucleus, where hormone delivery has a well-documented role in restoring male copulation.[37] These data, therefore, do not prove a role for hormones in the BNSTpm alone.

Taken together these observations identify neuroanatomical, neurochemical, and neuroendocrine distinctions between the MeAD/BNSTpi and cMePD/BNSTpm circuits and continuity within the cMePD/BNSTpm circuit in these characteristics. They suggest that the caudal circuit may provide a substrate through which hormone fluctuations over diurnal, estrous, and seasonal breeding cycles modulate reproduction. They also demonstrate that limbic nuclei outside the medial preoptic area provide redundancy in the hormone-sensitive network subserving reproduction.[38,39]

CONTINUITY OF FUNCTION WITHIN THE MEDIAL EXTENDED AMYGDALA CIRCUITS: MALE SEXUAL BEHAVIOR

Lesions of the corticomedial amygdala produce sexual behavior deficits in male rats,[40–44] although the data from these studies do not indicate whether anterior and posterior parts of this amygdalar region, or of the medial nucleus in particular, might have different functions. Further, only one of the laboratories investigating this system, that of Sachs and his colleagues, examined whether the corticomedial amygdala might have functions in common with the BNST.[45,46] After lesions in either amygdala or BNST, these authors found increased intromission frequencies and ejaculation latencies. Thus in the male rat we have limited evidence for continuity of behavioral function in the medial extended amygdala

Early lesion data in hamsters indicated that the MeAD and MePD play very different roles in regulation of male sexual behavior. Males with lesions of MeAD completely failed to mate and showed essentially no chemoinvestigatory behavior with the female.[47,48] By contrast, those with corticomedial lesions that included the caudal half of Me mated to ejaculations. However, the temporal pattern of their mating was altered, and they showed some decrement in chemoinvestigatory behavior.[49] Over several weeks (and in some cases up to two months) of postoperative testing, the latency to ejaculation was consistently increased, primarily as a result of persisting increases in the number of intromissions preceding the first ejaculation and lengthened postejaculatory intervals preceding the second. In addition, these animals showed a decrease of approximately 30% in the rate of anogenital investigation of the female compared to sham-lesioned males. Thus the contrast between behaviors of males with damage to the anterior versus the posterior medial nucleus was striking. Males with MeAD lesions essentially failed to engage in any chemoinvestigatory or copulatory activities, whereas those with lesions, including MePD, showed a modest, although statistically significant, decrease in chemoinvestigation and a lengthening of the copulatory sequence.

Subsequent data from hamsters with lesions of the BNST provided some evidence suggesting that the MeAD/BNSTpi and cMePD/BNSTpm constitute functional as well as anatomical circuits.[50] Conclusions that can be drawn from these data are limited because in these studies no group of males had lesions entirely confined to either BNSTpm or BNSTpi. However, histological analysis of behaviorally different groups revealed interesting differences in the brain areas damaged. A group of males with lesions that overlapped only in the BNSTpm, like males with cMePD damage, showed increased ejaculation latencies and decrements of approximately 50% in two different measures of chemoinvestigatory behavior: anogenital investigation of the female and attraction to female hamster vaginal secretions (FHVS) swabbed on the wall of a clean plastic arena. By contrast, a group of males with lesions that included damage to the BNSTpi as well as the BNSTpm at the level of the anterior commissure showed either no copulatory behavior or only occasional mounts, or, in one case, ejaculations on one test out of four. Further, these males showed essentially no anogenital investigation in mating tests, or response to FHVS in a clean cage. Thus lesions that included the BNSTpi and BNSTpm, but not BNSTpm alone, produced deficits reminiscent of those seen after lesions of MeAD, whereas the smaller lesions centered in the BNSTpm produced the same limited behavioral alterations seen after damage to MePD.

Inasmuch as all of these studies employed electrolytic lesions, they destroyed fibers as well as nuclei and could not provide unambiguous evidence for function of the cell groups in the damaged area. This was a particular problem with regard to the MePD and the BNSTpi, because lesions in either of these areas inevitably damage the stria terminalis, carrying fibers from both the anterior and posterior divisions of the medial amygdala. Additional evidence was needed to test the hypothesis that cell groups within these two circuits of the extended amygdala play different roles in mating behavior.

Subsequent studies from several laboratories, based on c-*fos* gene expression during sexual behavior in male hamsters, have provided important support for this hypothesis. Cells in both MeAD/BNSTpi and cMePD/BNSTpm circuits significantly increase production of Fos protein in response to mating behavior.[22,51] However, the behavioral antecedents of this gene expression differ between the two circuits. Although selected groups of cells in both cMePD and BNSTpm show increased Fos-immunoreactivity correlated with either chemoinvestigation or ejaculations,[52–54] neurons in MeAD and BNSTpi show a generalized and equivalent increase in Fos production after mating and after intermale aggressive encounters.[55] To date no specific motor function or sensory stimulation associated with either mating or agonistic behavior has been correlated with this increase in the MeAD circuit. Furthermore, increased expression of c-*fos* has been observed in MeAD and BNSTpi, not only after mating or aggression in males, but after mating or aggression in female hamsters.[56,57] These findings, in conjunction with the observed elimination of sexual behavior after lesions of MeAD, and after BNST lesions that include BNSTpi, have led us to hypothesize that the MeAD/BNSTpi circuit of the extended amygdala is essential for arousal, or nonspecific activation of social behaviors.[58] This notion is supported by recent observations that tail-pinching male rats, a procedure known to facilitate a variety of social behaviors in the presence of appropriate stimuli, also induces Fos immunoreactivity in this region of the medial amygdala.[59]

By contrast, cell groups within the MePD/BNSTpm circuit of the hamster appear to be activated selectively in response to discrete stimuli or mating events. Exposure of the male hamster to female hamster vaginal secretions in the absence of the female increases Fos production in medial MePD and in the anterodorsal part of BNSTpm or BNSTpm(ad).[52–54] This activity may be both olfactory and vomeronasal in origin, inasmuch as bilateral removal of the vomeronasal organs at day 17 significantly reduces, but does not eliminate, FHVS-mediated activation within these two areas in sexually naive male hamsters.[53] In addition, mating to ejaculations produces a significant increase in Fos-ir in the posterior ventral continuation of BNSTpm [BNSTpm(pv)] and in cMePD,[54] where clusters of labeled cells are apparent with Fos immunocytochemistry when the male nears sexual satiety, regardless of the absolute number of ejaculations exhibited.[60] These densely packed Fos-immunoreactive cells in lateral cMePD have also been observed after copulatory behavior in male gerbils[61] and rats.[62,63]

The data reviewed here on the functions of interconnected, neurochemically related cell groups in the medial amygdala and BNST of the male hamster and other rodents suggest that both anterior and posterior circuits are processing information important for normal mating behavior but that they regulate different aspects of this behavior. Olfactory, vomeronasal, and somatosensory stimuli reaching the MeAD/BNSTpi circuit produce a general behavioral arousal, the readiness to respond to specific signals with appropriate action. Through the cMePD/BNSTpm circuit, hormones maintain cell groups that respond to those discrete signals (e.g., odors of male vs. female, estrous vs. nonestrous, kin vs. nonkin) and other cell groups that determine the pattern of the behavioral response. This formulation of structural and functional unity between cell populations in the amygdala and the BNST supports the concept of the extended amygdala. It also expands the distinction between the central extended amygdala and the medial extended amygdala by suggesting that there is more than one functional extended amygdala circuit within the medial extended amygdala.

Canteras *et al.*[64] and Swanson and Petrovich[9] have objected to the concept of the extended amygdala on a variety of grounds. The latter authors suggest that the amygdala is not an entity but rather an amalgam of dissimilar areas that would more appropriately be reassigned to the cerebral cortex (nuclei of the cortical and basolateral divisions) or to the striatum (the medial and central nuclei). They further suggest that in this framework, the BNST would be recognized as a pallidal element in the forebrain. Heimer et al.[3] disagree with this latter construction. They argue that the patterns of connections between amygdala and BNST, which are reciprocal and equally heavy in both directions, are unlike the predominantly unidirectional projections from striatal to related pallidal elements. Further study, analysis, and scholarly debate are clearly needed before we will reach agreement on a place for the amygdala and BNST in the organization of the forebrain. Whatever that place, the structural and functional continuity of units within the medial amygdala and the BNST will have to be accommodated.

ROLES OF THE MEDIAL EXTENDED AMYGDALA IN OTHER SOCIAL BEHAVIORS

Ascribing discrete components of behavior to the activity of discrete neuroanatomical units is a basic part of the process of delineating functional pathways in the central nervous system. Over the past twenty years, as indicated above, this process has led to the identification of sites in the extended amygdala that play a role in male mating behavior. During this period the same process has been successfully pursued in delineating neural circuits required for, or activated by, other social behaviors in rodents: female sexual behavior,[65-67] aggression,[55-57,68-72] territorial marking,[73,74] and maternal behavior.[75-77] Taken together these studies reveal a dismaying amount of overlap in the circuitry responsible for the behaviors, a result that was largely unexpected. Thus data from studies employing a wide variety of paradigms, including discrete lesions, electrical stimulation, localized hormonal or neuropharmacological manipulations, and immediate early gene expression, have led investigators studying male and female social behaviors to implicate a common group of limbic areas, including nuclear groups within the medial extended amygdala, the lateral septum, the medial preoptic area, the anterior hypothalamus, the ventromedial nucleus and adjacent ventrolateral hypothalamus, and the midbrain periaqueductal gray and adjacent tegmentum.

Together these brain areas influence not only male and female sexual behavior and maternal behavior, but also the reproductive-related behaviors: territorial marking, territorial aggression, and maternal aggression. In fact, the data gathered to date on neural circuits subserving social behaviors force us to consider the possibility that these structures form an integrated social behavior circuit, a network much like the cortical networks that subserve cognitive functions, such as learning and memory or language, but in this case a subcortical limbic network that subserves the entire spectrum of sex-steroid modulated social behaviors. Obviously not every brain structure that plays a role in any one of these behaviors is a candidate member of such a network; that is, there are important additional areas not mentioned in this particular grouping that subserve specific social behavior reflexes or behavior patterns. Nor does this grouping include all of the sexually dimorphic brain areas that integrate endocrine function with social behaviors.[78] Each of the areas illustrated in FIGURE 1 belongs to other functional circuits through connections that they do not share with

The Social Behavior Network

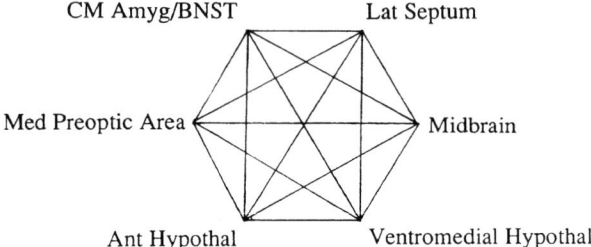

FIGURE 1. Six limbic system areas that are reciprocally interconnected anatomically, each of which is populated with neurons that are sensitive to gonadal steroids and has been implicated in the regulation of more than one mammalian social behavior. Each of these areas is a candidate node for a neuroanatomical network that regulates sexual, aggressive, and parental behaviors in both sexes of mammals.

all members of this basic network. However, all of these areas fulfill several important criteria for nodes in a social behavior network. Each is reciprocally interconnected with all of the others,[7,64,78–87] all are populated with neurons that contain gonadal hormone receptors,[20,23,24] and each of these areas has been identified as an important site of regulation or activation in more than one social behavior. This last point is readily documented by enumerating separate experiments, each demonstrating a role for one or several brain areas in social behavior. Collectively these reports indicate that each area participates in more than one behavior (lateral septum,[54,61,65,71,73] medial extended amygdala,[22,34–36,40–57,60–63,66,67,69,75,88] medial preoptic area,[22,35,37,50–56,61–63,65,75,89,90] anterior hypothalamus,[54,73] ventromedial and ventrolateral hypothalamus,[55,61,65–69,75] midbrain periaqueductal gray, and tegmentum.)[54,55,61–63,65,70,74–77] Only occasionally do these studies analyze the same brain area or areas in the context of more than one type of social behavior[42,55,56,76,77,91,92] or in both females and males,[68,93,94] but these approaches will be particularly useful in exploring the concept of a network with multiple functions.

In what way could a common neuroanatomical network provide a substrate for the broad repertoire we must consider in the category of social behaviors? Again, borrowing an important concept from our colleagues in cognitive neuroscience, we envision that a particular social behavior, for example, male sexual behavior, is an emergent property of the pattern of activity across the network[95] (FIG. 2). It is not an action produced by the "on" or "off" state of any one of the nodes, such as the medial preoptic area, but a sequence of multiple behaviors (e.g., sniffing, mounting, ejaculating, grooming) that is initiated by and emerges from a temporal pattern, and therefore a dynamic pattern, of activity across the network. Initiation and maintenance of male sexual behavior, then, would require activation of the medial preoptic area but in conjunction with particular levels of activation of other areas in the network, and

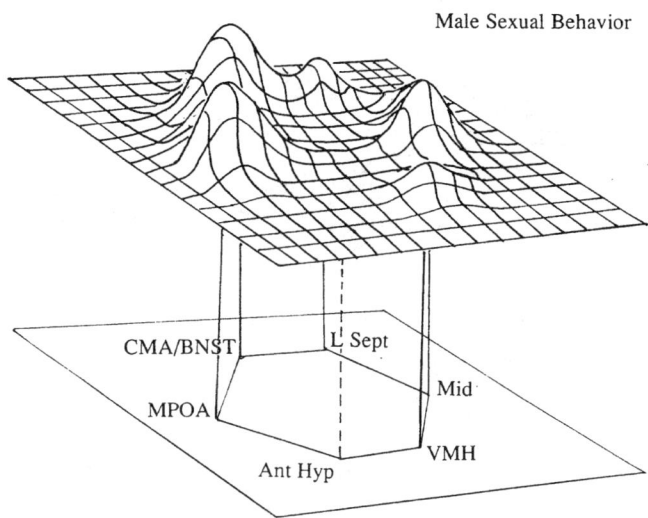

FIGURE 2. A hypothetical representation of the pattern of activity in the mammalian social behavior network at the outset of male sexual behavior. See FIGURE 1 for an explanation of abbreviations.

in the context of a unique temporal pattern of activation across the whole network. Other similar but distinguishable patterns of activity in this same circuit (FIG. 3), arising as a result of changing sensory stimuli or fluctuations in the hormonal milieu, could result in a progression of behaviors flowing seamlessly from one to another, for example, territorial marking and aggressive activities interspersed with copulatory acts to produce the full spectrum of mating behavior observed in a variety of species.

Both the social behaviors that arise from activation of this circuit and the neuronal groups that comprise it share a variety of basic developmental and physiological determinants. Clearly the fundamental developmental determinants are the species and sex of the individual. The species of the animal determines the organization and connections of brain areas and whether they will be responsive to sex steroids, characteristics that are highly conserved in mammals. The species also determines the timing of critical periods for sensitivity to hormones during perinatal development, which is more variable. The genetic sex of the animal determines whether sex steroids will be available to the brain during those critical periods. As a result of steroid action, the network becomes sexually dimorphic with respect to the number of cells and the specific cell types produced in each node. This, in turn, influences the baseline number and types of sex-steroid receptors produced by those cells and the strength of connections between nodes in the network. It is these factors that ultimately regulate the predisposition, but not routinely predictable or exclusive function, of the network to produce particular patterns of activity in a given individual, such as male versus female sexual behavior.

These same factors, sex-steroid sensitivity and neuronal connections, are of course dynamically modulated throughout life by sexual maturation, by experience

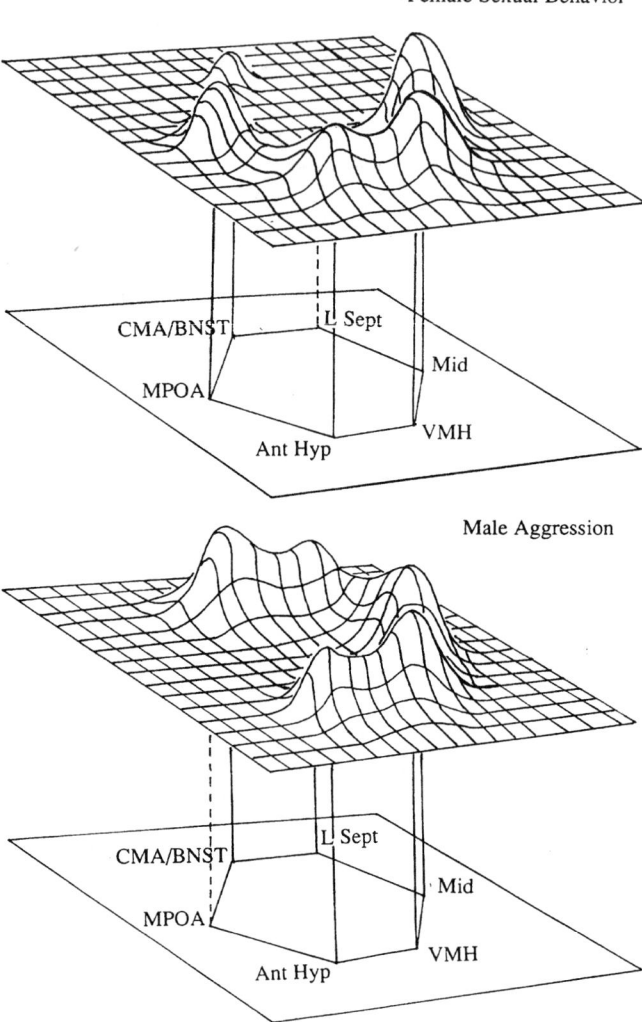

FIGURE 3. Hypothetical representations of the patterns of activity in the mammalian social behavior network at the outset of female sexual behavior and male aggression.

or learning, by reproductive cycles and diurnal cycles, and by disease and aging. On a shorter time frame they are modified by sensory stimuli from other animals by odor, touch, color, motion, and sounds. The pheromones from the female hamster, the flank and vaginal somatosensory stimulation to the female rat, the colorful perineal skin displayed by the female monkey and the estrous call of the female cat all have short-term effects that modify the functioning of the social behavior network in the receiver. At the very least, these stimuli produce immediate changes in synaptic activity in the nodes of the social behavior network. In some cases the effects are long-lasting changes in the strength of synaptic connections. In all mammals, all of the sensory systems have access to the sexually dimorphic social-behavior network, but all sensory modalities are not equally important in eliciting particular behaviors. Coming full circle, the modalities that are the most salient to an individual animal's social responses are determined through evolution by its species and by its sex, in other words, by its genes.

This way of looking at the neural circuits for social behaviors has appealing simplicity. It may appear at first glance to be a useless oversimplification, but it is introduced here as a framework within which to view the data we have collected. It is intended not as an excuse to abandon our efforts to identify behavioral functions attributable to specific cell groups within these areas, but as a way to integrate our findings. It is now clear that male and female courtship behaviors, copulation, attacks, submissiveness, territorial marking, nest building, nursing, guarding of the mate, and protection of the young use overlapping neural pathways. If we are to sustain the "labeled-line" point of view, this social behavior network will have to be teased apart at the level of intermingled cell populations within individual limbic nuclei. We will have to demonstrate minicircuits within this network, each one independently regulating a specific aspect of a particular behavior.

Isn't that what I argued in the first part of this chapter? For example, haven't Coolen et al.,[96] Heeb and Yahr,[61] Kollack-Walker and Newman,[54] and Parfitt and Newman[60] indicated that there are small clusters of neurons embedded within the cMePD of male rats, gerbils, and hamsters that are activated when these animals have ejaculated and are reaching sexual satiety? Can we not conclude that collectively we have identified a unique minicircuit that is involved in timing, and associated with terminating, ejaculatory behavior, an exclusively male-typical behavior? Yes and no. We may be forced to abandon the "exclusively male-typical" point of view when we see the same cell groups activated by vaginocervical stimulation in the female rat, as has clearly been demonstrated by Pfaus et al.,[97] Dudley et al.,[66] and Erskine and Hanrahan.[67] We are led, then, to what may be a more useful hypothesis: that these cells regulate the timing of both male and female sexual behaviors, an aspect of these behaviors that is critical for the successful end point of copulation–pregnancy.[98–101]

The concept of overlapping functions for a single neuroanatomical network is not an original insight. A number of investigators have noted the duality of function, or multiple functions, of areas within this circuit.[56,69,78,91,102,103] However, it clearly will be more difficult to establish that individual cell groups have multiple functions than to pursue the more traditional hypothesis: that there are intermingled labeled-line minicircuits with separate functions in the same brain areas. A first step might be to actively look for evidence of multiple social-behavior functions in studies where identifiable cells groups (e.g., cells in a specific transmitter circuit) are being manipulated or monitored.

For the past thirty years we have struggled to dissect the social behaviors of mammals apart in terms of sensory stimulation, physiological prerequisites, and neuroanatomical substrates. The results of our collective efforts suggest that these behaviors may actually emerge from the activity of a unitary neuroanatomical framework in the central nervous system. We have learned that this network develops and functions under the influence of gonadal hormones, again with a common denominator, estradiol, across species and sexes. Significant differences in the hormonally influenced behaviors emerging from this network, not only across species and sexes, but over time within individuals, arise primarily from the amount of estrogen available to its neurons during development and by the temporal pattern of estrogen availability in adulthood. All of the nodes of this neuroanatomical network are responsive to sex hormones. A greater diversity in this picture of social behaviors appears to be the sensory stimuli that drive them. Clear species and sex differences in the saliency of various sensory systems have evolved through adaptation to different ecological niches, to nocturnal versus diurnal living, and to communal versus noncommunal social systems. However, all sensory systems have access to the limbic network that drives social behaviors in mammals. What we originally viewed as evidence for different social behavior pathways more likely reflects sex and species differences in the weighting of sensory system influences on a common central network. If, in fact, all social behaviors actually emerge from a unitary neuroanatomical framework and shared physiological determinants, our understanding of these behaviors and the neural system that supports them may be greatly advanced by focusing not on differences, but on the common themes arising from our studies of all social behaviors in both sexes and in diverse species.

ACKNOWLEDGMENT

The research was performed in the Department of Anatomy and Cell Biology, University of Michigan, Ann Arbor, MI and supported by Public Health Service grants from NINDS.

REFERENCES

1. DE OLMOS, J.S., G.F. ALHEID & C.A. BELTRAMINO. 1985. Amygdala. *In* The Rat Nervous System. 1st Edition. G. Paxinos, Ed.: 223–334. Academic Press.
2. ALHEID, G.F. & L. HEIMER. 1988. New perspectives in basal forebrain organization of special relevance for neuropsychiatric disorders: the striatopallidal, amygdaloid and corticopetal components of substantia innominata. Neuroscience **27**: 1–39.
3. HEIMER, L., R.E. HARLAN, G.F. ALHEID, M.M. GARCIA & J. DE OLMOS. 1997. Substantia innominata: A notion which impedes clinical-anatomical correlations in neuropsychiatric disorders. Neuroscience **76**: 957–1006.
4. WOOD, R.I. & S.W. NEWMAN. 1995. Hormonal influence on neurons of the mating behavior pathway in male hamsters. *In* Neurobiological Effects of Sex Steroid Hormones. P. E. Micevych & R. P. Hammer, Eds.: 3–39. Cambridge University Press.
5. CANTERAS, N.S., R.B. SIMERLY & L.W. SWANSON. 1995. Organization of the projections from the medial nucleus of the amygdala: A PHAL study in the rat. J. Comp. Neurol. **360**: 213–245.
6. GOMEZ, D.M. & S.W. NEWMAN. 1992. Differential projections of the anterior and posterior regions of the medial amygdaloid nucleus in the Syrian hamster. J. Comp. Neurol. **317**: 195–218.
7. COOLEN, L.M. & R.I. WOOD. 1998. Bidirectional connections of the medial amygdaloid nucleus in the Syrian hamster brain: simultaneous anterograde and retrograde tract tracing. J. Comp. Neurol. **399**: 189–209.

8. ALHEID, G.F., J.S. DE OLMOS & C.A. BELTRAMINO. 1995. Amygdala and extended amygdala. *In* The Rat Nervous System. 2nd Edition. G. Paxinos, Ed.: 495–578. Academic Press.
9. SWANSON, L.W. & G.D. PETROVICH. 1998. What is the amygdala? Trends Neurosci. **21:** 323–331.
10. ECKERSELL, C.B. & P.E. MICEVYCH. 1997. Opiate receptors modulate estrogen-induced cholecystokinin and tachykinin but not enkephalin messenger RNA levels in the limbic system and hypothalamus. Neuroscience **80:** 473–485.
11. SWANN, J.M. & S.W. NEWMAN. 1992. Testosterone regulates substance P within neurons of the medial nucleus of the amygdala, the bed nucleus of the stria terminalis and the medal preoptic area of the male golden hamster. Brain Res. **590:** 18–28.
12. HOLT, A.G. 1997. Immunocytochemical identification of met- and leu-enkephalin positive neurons within mating and agonistic relevant brain nuclei of the male Syrian hamster: modulation by gonadal steroids and social behaviors. Ph.D. Thesis, University of Michigan. Ann Arbor, Michigan.
13. DE VRIES, G.J., R.M. BUIJS, F.W. VAN LEEUWEN, A.R. CAFFE & D.F. SWAAB. 1985. The vasopressinergic innervation of the brain in normal and castrated rats. J. Comp. Neurol. **233:** 236–254.
14. MICEVYCH, P., T. AKESSON & R. ELDE. 1988. Distribution of cholecystokinin- immunoreactive cell bodies in the male and female rat: II. Bed nucleus of the stria terminalis and amygdala. J. Comp. Neurol. **269:** 381–391.
15. ALBERS, H.E., A.C. HENNESSEY & D.C. WHITMAN. 1992. Vasopressin and the regulation of hamster social behavior. Ann. N. Y. Acad. Sci. **652:** 227–242.
16. NEAL, C.R. Jr. & S.W. NEWMAN. 1989. Prodynorphin peptide distribution in the forebrain of the Syrian hamster and rat: A comparative study with antisera against dynorphin A, dynorphin B and the C-terminus of the prodynorphin precursor molecule. J. Comp. Neurol. **288:** 353–386.
17. NEAL, C.R. Jr., J.M. SWANN & S.W. NEWMAN. 1989. The colocalization of substance P and prodynorphin immunoreactivity in neurons of the medial preoptic area, bed nucleus of the stria terminalis and medial nucleus of the amygdala of the Syrian hamster. Brain Res. **496:** 1–13.
18. ASMUS, S.E., A.E. KINCAID & S.W. NEWMAN. 1992. A species-specific population of tyrosine hydroxylase-immunoreactive neurons in the medial amygdaloid nucleus of the Syrian hamster brain. Brain Res. **575:** 199–207.
19. ASMUS, S.E. & S.W. NEWMAN. 1993. Tyrosine hydroxylase neurons in the male hamster chemosensory pathway contain androgen receptors and are influenced by gonadal hormones. J. Comp. Neurol. **331:** 445–457.
20. SIMERLY, R.B., C. CHANG, M. MURAMATSU & L.W. SWANSON. 1990. Distribution of androgen and estrogen receptor mRNA-containing cells in the rat brain: an in situ hybridization study. J. Comp. Neurol. **294:** 76–95.
21. CHEN, T.J. & W.W. TU. 1992. Sex differences in estrogen and androgen receptors in hamster brain. Life Sci. **50:** 1639–1647.
22. WOOD, R.W. & S.W. NEWMAN. 1993. Mating activates androgen receptor-containing neurons in chemosensory pathways of the male Syrian hamster brain. Brain Res. **614:** 65–77.
23. WOOD, R.W. & S.W. NEWMAN. 1995. Androgen and estrogen receptors coexist within individual neurons in the brain of the Syrian hamster. Neuroendocrinology **62:** 487–497.
24. COMMINS, D. & P. YAHR. 1985. Autoradiographic localization of estrogen and androgen receptors in the sexually dimorphic area and other regions of the gerbil brain. J. Comp. Neurol. **231:** 473–489.
25. HINES, M., L.S. ALLEN & R. GORSKI. 1992. Sex differences in subregions of the medial nucleus of the amygdala and the bed nucleus of the stria terminalis of the rat. Brain Res. **579:** 321–326.
26. MIZUKAMI, S., M. NISHIZUKA & Y. ARAI. 1983. Sexual difference in nuclear volume and its ontogeny in the rat amygdala. Exp. Neurol. **79:** 569–575.

27. NISHIZUKA, M. & Y. ARAI. 1981. Sexual dimorphism in synaptic organization in the amygdala and its dependence on neonatal hormone environment. Brain Res. **212:** 31–38.
28. NISHIZUKA, M. & Y. ARAI. 1983. Male-female difference in the intra-amygdaloid input to the medial amygdala. Exp. Brain Res. **52:** 328–332.
29. MALSBURY, C.W. & K. MCKAY. 1987. A sex difference in the pattern of substance P-like immunoreactivity in the bed nucleus of the stria terminalis. Brain Res. **420:** 365–370.
30. MALSBURY, C.W. & K. MCKAY. 1989. Sex difference in the substance P-immunoreactive innervation of the medial nucleus of the amygdala. Brain Res. Bull. **23:** 561–567.
31. VAN LEEUWEN, F.W., A.R. CAFFE & G. J. DE VRIES. 1985. Vasopressin cells in the bed nucleus of the stria terminalis of the rat: sex differences and the influence of androgens. Brain Res. **325:** 391–394.
32. SIMERLY, R.B. & L.W. SWANSON. 1987. Castration reversibly alters levels of cholecystokinin immunoreactivity within cells of three interconnected sexually dimorphic forebrain nuclei in the rat. Proc. Natl. Acad. Sci. USA **84:** 2087–2091.
33. ORO, A.E., R.B. SIMERLY & L.W. SWANSON. 1988. Estrous cycle variations in levels of cholecystokinin immunoreactivity within cells of three interconnected sexually dimorphic forebrain nuclei. Evidence for a regulatory role for estrogen. Neuroendocrinology **47:** 225–235.
34. RASIA-FILHO, A.A., T.M.S. PERES, F.H. CUBILLA-GUTIERREZ & A.B. LUCION. 1991. Effect of estradiol implanted in the corticomedial amygdala on the sexual behavior of castrated male rats. Braz. J. Med. Biol. Res. **24:** 1041–1049.
35. WOOD, R.I. & S.W. NEWMAN. 1995. The medial amygdaloid nucleus and medial preoptic area mediate steroidal control of sexual behavior in the male Syrian hamster. Horm. Behav. **29:** 338–353.
36. WOOD, R.I. 1996. Estradiol, but not dihydrotestosterone, in the medial amygdala facilitates male hamster sex behavior. Physiol. Behav. **59:** 833–841.
37. MEISEL, R.L. & B.D. SACHS. 1994. The physiology of male sexual behavior. *In* The Physiology of Reproduction. 2nd Edition. E. Knobil & J. D. Neill, Eds.: 3–105. Raven Press. New York.
38. WOOD, R.I. 1996. Functions of the steroid-responsive neural network in the control of male hamster sexual behavior. Trends Endocrinol. Metab. **7:** 338–344.
39. WOOD, R.I. 1997. Thinking about networks in the control of male hamster sexual behavior. Horm. Behav. **32:** 40–45.
40. GIANTONIO, G.W., N.L. LUND & A.A. GERALL. 1970. Effect of diencephalic and rhinencephalic lesions on the male rat's sexual behavior. J. Comp. Phsyiol. Psychol. **73:** 38–46.
41. HARRIS, V.S. & B.D. SACHS. 1975. Copulatory behavior in male rats following amygdaloid lesions. Brain Res. **86:** 514–518.
42. MCGREGOR, A. & J. HERBERT. 1992. Differential effects of excitotoxic basolateral and corticomedial lesions of the amygdala on the behavioural and endocrine responses to either sexual or aggression-promoting stimuli in the male rat. Brain Res. **574:** 9–20.
43. Kondo, Y. 1992. Lesions of the medial amygdala produce severe impairment of copulatory behavior in sexually inexperienced male rats. Physiol. & Behav. **51:** 939–943.
44. DE JONGE, F.H., W.P. OLDENBURGER, A.L. LOUWERSE & N.E. VAN DE POLL. 1992. Changes in male copulatory behavior after sexual exciting stimuli: effects of medial amygdala lesions. Physiol. & Behav. **52:** 327–332.
45. EMERY, D.E. & B.D. SACHS. 1976. Copulatory behavior in male rats with lesions in the bed nucleus of the stria terminalis. Physiol. & Behav. **17:** 803–806.
46. VALCOURT, R.J. & B.D. SACHS. 1979. Penile reflexes and copulatory behavior in male rats following lesions in the bed nucleus of the stria terminalis. Brain Res. Bull. **4:** 131–133.

47. LEHMAN, M.N., S.S. WINANS & J.B. POWERS. 1980. Medial nucleus of the amygdala mediates chemosensory control of male hamster sexual behavior. Science **210:** 557–560.
48. LEHMAN, M.N. & S.S. WINANS. 1982. Vomeronasal and olfactory pathways to the amygdala controlling male hamster sexual behavior: autoradiographic and behavioral analyses. Brain Res. **240:** 27–41.
49. LEHMAN, M.N., J.B. POWERS & S.S. WINANS. 1983. Stria terminalis lesions alter the temporal pattern of copulatory behavior in the male golden hamster. Behav. Brain Res. **8:** 109–128.
50. POWERS, J.B., S.W. NEWMAN & M.L. BERGONDY. 1987. MPOA and BNST lesions in male Syrian hamsters: differential effects on copulatory and chemoinvestigatory behaviors. Behav. Brain Res. **23:** 181–195.
51. KOLLACK, S.S. & S.W. NEWMAN. 1992. Mating behavior induces selective expression of Fos protein within the chemosensory pathways of the male Syrian hamster brain. Neurosci. Lett. **143:** 223–228.
52. FIBER, J.M., P. ADAMES & J.M. SWANN. 1993. Pheromones induce c-*fos* in limbic areas regulating male hamster mating behavior. NeuroReport **4:** 871–874.
53. FERNANDEZ-FEWELL, G.D. & M. MEREDITH. 1994. c-Fos expression in vomeronasal pathways of mated or pheromone-stimulated male golden hamsters: contributions from vomeronasal sensory input and expression related to mating performance. J. Neurosci. **14:** 3643–3654.
54. KOLLACK-WALKER, S. & S.W. NEWMAN. 1997. Mating-induced expression of c-*fos* in the male Syrian hamster brain: role of experience, pheromones, and ejaculations. J. Neurobiol. **32:** 481–501.
55. KOLLACK-WALKER, S. & S.W. NEWMAN. 1995. Mating and agonistic behavior produce different patterns of Fos immunolabeling in the male Syrian hamster. Neuroscience **66:** 721–736.
56. JOPPA, M.A., R.L. MEISEL & M.A. GARBER. 1995. c-Fos expression in female hamster brain following sexual and aggressive behaviors. Neuroscience **68:** 783–792.
57. POTEGAL, M., C.F. FERRIS, M. HEBERT, J. MEYERHOFF & L. SKAREDOFF. 1996. Attack priming in female Syrian golden hamsters is associated with a c-*fos*-coupled process within the corticomedial amygdala. Neuroscience **75:** 869–880.
58. NEWMAN, S.W., D B. PARFITT & S. KOLLACK-WALKER. 1997. Mating-induced c-*fos* expression patterns complement and supplement observations after lesions in the male Syrian hamster brain. Ann. N. Y. Acad. Sci. **807:** 239–259.
59. SMITH, W.J., J. STEWART & J.G. PFAUS. 1997. Tail pinch induces Fos immunoreactivity within several regions of the male rat brain: Effects of age. Physiol. and Behav. **61:** 717–723.
60. PARFITT, D.B. & S.W. NEWMAN. 1998. Fos-immunoreactivity within the extended amygdala is correlated with the onset of sexual satiety. Horm. & Behav. **34:** 17–29.
61. HEEB, M.M. & P. YAHR. 1996. c-Fos immunoreactivity in the sexually dimorphic area of the hypothalamus and related brain regions of male gerbils after exposure to sex-related stimuli or performance of specific sexual behaviors. Neuroscience **72:** 1049–1071.
62. BAUM, M.J. & B.J. EVERITT. 1992. Increased expression of c-*fos* in the medial preoptic area after mating in male rats: role of afferent inputs from the medial amygdala and midbrain central tegmental field. Neuroscience **50:** 627–646.
63. COOLEN, L.M., H.J. P.W. PETERS & J.G. VEENING. 1997. Distribution of Fos immunoreactivity following mating versus anogenital investigation in the male rat brain. Neuroscience **77:** 1151–1161.
64. CANTERAS, N.S., R.B. SIMERLY & L.W. SWANSON. 1995. Organization of projections from the medial nucleus of the amygdala: a PHAL study in the rat. J. Comp. Neurol. **360:** 213–245.
65. PFAFF, D.W., S. SCHWARTZ-GIBLIN, M.M. MCCARTHY & L-M. KOW. 1994. Cellular and molecular mechanisms of female reproductive behaviors. *In* The Physiology of Reproduction. 2nd Edition. E. Knobil & J. D. Neill, Eds.: 107–220. Raven Press. New York.

66. DUDLEY, C.A., G. RAJENDREN & R.L. MOSS. 1996. Signal processing in the vomeronasal system: modulation of sexual behavior in the female rat. Crit. Rev. Neurobiol. **10:** 265–290.
67. ERSKINE, M.S. & S.B. HANRAHAN. 1997. Effects of paced mating on c-*fos* gene expression in the female rat brain. J. Neuroendocrinol. **9:** 903–912.
68. KRUK, M.R., C.E. VAN DER LAAN, J. MOS, A.M. VAN DER POEL, W. MEELIS & B. OLIVIER. 1984. Comparison of aggressive behaviour induced by electrical stimulation in the hypothalamus of male and female rats. Prog. Brain Res. **61:** 303–314.
69. LUITEN, P.G.M., J.M. KOOLHAAS, S. DE BOER & S.J. KOOPMANS. 1985. The corticomedial amygdala in the central nervous system organization of agonistic behavior. Brain Res. **332:** 283–297.
70. DEPAULIS, A., K.A. KEAY & R. BANDLER. 1992. Longitudinal neuronal organization of defensive reactions in the midbrain periaqueductal gray region of the rat. Exp. Brain Res. **90:** 307–318.
71. ALBERT, D J. & G.L. CHEW. 1980. The septal forebrain and the inhibitory modulation of attack and defense in the rat. A review. Behav. Neural Biol. **30:** 357–388.
72. ROELING, T.A.P., J.G. VEENING, M.R. KRUK, J.P.W. PETERS, M.E.J. VERMELIS & R. NIEWENHUYS. 1994. Efferent connections of the hypothalamic "aggression area" in the rat. Neuroscience **59:** 1001–1024.
73. FERRIS, C.F., L. GOLD, G.J. DE VRIES & M. POTEGAL. 1990. Evidence for a functional and anatomical relationship between the lateral septum and the hypothalamus in the control of flank marking behavior in golden hamsters. J. Comp. Neurol. **293:** 476–485.
74. HENNESSEY, A.C., D.C. WHITMAN & H.E. ALBERS. 1992. Microinjection of arginine vasopressin into the periaqueductal gray stimulates flank marking in Syrian hamsters (*Mesocricetus auratus*). Brain Res. **569:** 136–140.
75. NUMAN, M. & T.P. SHEEHAN. 1997. Neuroanatomical circuitry for mammalian maternal behavior. Ann. N. Y. Acad. Sci. **807:** 101–125.
76. ROSENBLATT, J.S., E.M. FACTOR & A.D. MAYER. 1994. Relationship between maternal aggression and maternal care in the rat. Aggressive Behav. **20:** 243–255.
77. LONSTEIN, J.S. & J.M. STERN. 1997. Role of the midbrain periaqueductal gray in maternal nurturance and aggression: *c-fos* and electrolytic lesion studies in lactating rats. J. Neurosci. **17:** 3364–3378.
78. SIMERLY, R.B. 1995. Hormonal regulation of limbic and hypothalamic pathways. *In* Neurobiological Effects of Sex Steroid Hormones. P. E. Micevych & R. P. Hammer, Eds.: 85–114. Cambridge University Press.
79. REES, H.D., G.M. SWITZ & R.P. MICHAEL. 1980. The estrogen-sensitive neural system in the brain of female cats. J. Comp. Neurol. **193:** 789–804.
80. COTTINGHAM, S.L. & D.W. PFAFF. 1986. Interconnectedness of steroid hormonebinding neurons: existence and implications. Curr. Top. Neuroendocrinol. **7:** 223–249.
81. SIMERLY, R.B. & L.W. SWANSON. 1988. Projections of the medial preoptic nucleus: a *Phaseolus vulgaris* leucoagglutinin anterograde tract-tracing study in the rat. J. Comp. Neurol. **270:** 209–242.
82. SHIPLEY, M.T., M. ENNIS, T.A. RIZVI & M.M. BEHBEHANI. 1991. Topographic specificity of forebrain inputs to the midbrain periaqueductal gray: evidence for discrete longitudinally organized input columns. *In* The Midbrain Periaqueductal Gray Matter: Functional, Anatomical and Neurochemical Organization. A. Depaulis & R. Bandler, Eds.: 417–448. Plenum. New York.
83. CANTERAS, N.S., R.B. SIMERLY & L.W. SWANSON. 1994. Organization of projections from the ventromedial nucleus of the hypothalamus: a *Phaseolus vulgaris*-leucoagglutinin study in the rat. J. Comp. Neurol. **348:** 41–79.
84. MARAGOS, W.F., S.W. NEWMAN, M.N. LEHMAN & J.B. POWERS. 1989. Neurons of origin and fiber trajectory of amygdalofugal projections to the medial preoptic area in Syrian hamsters. J. Comp. Neurol. **280:** 59–71.
85. RIZVI, T.A., M. ENNIS & M.T. SHIPLEY. 1992. Reciprocal connections between the medial preoptic area and the midbrain periaqueductal gray in rat: A WGA-HRP and PHA-L study. J. Comp. Neurol. **315:** 1–15.

86. RISOLD, P.Y., N.S. CANTERAS & L.W. SWANSON. 1994. Organization of projections from the anterior hypothalamic nucleus: a *Phaseolus vulgaris*-leucoagglutinin study in the rat. J. Comp. Neurol. **348:** 1–40.
87. JAKAB, R.L. & C. LERANTH. 1995. Septum. *In* The Rat Nervous System. 2nd Edition. G. Paxinos, Ed.: 405–442. Academic Press.
88. CHATEAU, D. & Cl. ARON. 1988. Heterotypic sexual behavior in male rats after lesions in different amygdaloid nuclei. Horm. & Behav. **22:** 379–388.
89. POWERS, J.B. & E.S. VALENSTEIN. 1972. Sexual receptivity: facilitation by medial preoptic lesions in female rats. Science **175:** 1003–1005.
90. LISK, R.D. 1962. Diencephalic placement of estradiol and sexual receptivity in the female rat. Am. J. Physiol. **203:** 493–496.
91. NYBY, J. , J.A. MATOCHIK & R.J. BARFIELD. 1992. Intracranial androgenic and estrogenic stimulation of male-typical behaviors in house mice (*Mus domesticus*). Horm. & Behav. **26:** 24–45.
92. MALSBURY, C.W., L.-M. KOW & D.W. PFAFF. 1977. Effects of medial hypothalamic lesions on the lordosis response and other behaviors in female golden hamsters. Physiol. Behav. **19:** 223–237.
93. COOLEN, L.M., H.J.P.W. PETERS & J.G. VEENING. 1996. Fos immunoreactivity in the rat brain following cosummatory elements of sexual behavior: a sex comparison. Brain Res. **738:** 67–82.
94. LEEDY, M.G., & B.L. HART. 1985. Female and male sexual responses in female cats with ventromedial hypothalamic lesions. Behav. Neurosci. **99:** 936–941.
95. MESULAM, M-M. 1990. Large-scale neurocognitive networks and distributed processing for attention, language and memory. Ann. Neurol. **28:** 597–613.
96. COOLEN, L.M., B. OLIVIER, H.J.P.W. PETERS & J.G. VEENING. 1997. Demonstration of ejaculation-induced neural activity in the male rat brain using 5-HT$_{1A}$ agonist 8-OH-DPAT. Physiol. & Behav. **62:** 881–891.
97. PFAUS, J.G., S.P. KLEOPOULOS, C.V. MOBBS, R.B. GIBBS & D.W. PFAFF. 1993. Sexual stimulation activates *c-fos* within estrogen-concentrating regions of the female rat forebrain. Brain Res. **624:** 253–267.
98. ADLER, N.T. 1969. Effects of the male's copulatory behavior on successful pregnancy of the female rat. J. Comp. Physiol. Psychol. **69:** 613–622.
99. LANIER, D.L., D.Q. ESTEP & D.A. DEWSBURY. 1975. Copulatory behavior of golden hamsters: effects on pregnancy. Physiol. & Behav. **15:** 209–212.
100. HUCK, U. & R. LISK. 1985. Determinants of mating success in the golden hamster (*Mesocricetus auratus*): I. Male capacity. J. Comp. Psychol. **99:** 98–107.
101. HUCK, U. & R. LISK. 1985. Determinants of mating success in the golden hamster (*Mesocricetus auratus*): II. Pregnancy initiation. J. Comp. Psychol. **99:** 231–239.
102. BARFIELD, R.J. 1984. Reproductive hormones and aggressive behavior. *In* Biological Perspectives on Aggression. K. J. Flannelly, R. J. Blanchard & D. C. Blanchard, Eds.: 105–134. Alan R. Liss. New York.
103. DE JONGE, F.H. & N.E. VAN DE POLL. 1984. Relationships between sexual and aggressive behavior in male and female rats: effects of gonadal hormones. Prog. Brain Res. **61:** 283–302.

The Extended Amygdala and Salt Appetite

ALAN KIM JOHNSON,[a,c] JOSE DE OLMOS,[b] CINTHIA V. PASTUSKOVAS,[b] ANDREA M. ZARDETTO-SMITH,[a,d] AND LAURA VIVAS[b]

[a]*Departments of Psychology and Pharmacology, and the Cardiovascular Center, University of Iowa, Iowa City, Iowa, USA*

[b]*Instituto de Investigación Médicas, Mercedes y Martín Ferreyra, Córdoba, Argentina*

ABSTRACT: Both chemo- and mechanosensitive receptors are involved in detecting changes in the signals that reflect the status of body fluids and of blood pressure. These receptors are located in the systemic circulatory system and in the sensory circumventricular organs of the brain. Under conditions of body fluid deficit or of marked changes in fluid distribution, multiple inputs derived from these humoral and neural receptors converge on key areas of the brain where the information is integrated. The result of this central processing is the mobilization of homeostatic behaviors (thirst and salt appetite), hormone release, autonomic changes, and cardiovascular adjustments. This review discusses the current understanding of the nature and role of the central and systemic receptors involved in the facilitation and inhibition of thirst and salt appetite and on particular components of the central neural network that receive and process input derived from fluid- and cardiovascular-related sensory systems. Special attention is paid to the structures of the lamina terminalis, the area postrema, the lateral parabrachial nucleus, and their association with the central nucleus of the amygdala and the bed nucleus of the stria terminalis in controlling the behaviors that participate in maintaining body fluid and cardiovascular homeostasis.

INTRODUCTION: PRINCIPLES OF BODY FLUID HOMEOSTASIS

Body fluid and cardiovascular homeostasis requires mechanisms that maintain overall sodium and water balance as well as appropriate regional and compartmental distributions of these substances. In order to maintain consistency of the fluid matrix, the effector actions of several behavioral, autonomic, and endocrine control systems must be coordinated to allow independent adjustments of the rates of intake and loss of both sodium and water. Although a role for water in the regulation of fluid balance is fairly obvious, the contribution of sodium may not be so apparent. Sodium ions do not readily cross cell membranes and are therefore key to determining the distribution of water inside (intracellular fluid compartment) versus outside (extracellular fluid compartment) of cells. That is, the sodium concentration of the extracellular fluid, in large part, determines osmotic gradients that result in the movement of water in and out of cells.

---

[c]Address correspondence to Alan Kim Johnson, Ph.D., Department of Psychology, University of Iowa, 11 Seashore Hall E., Iowa City, IA 52242-1407. Voice: 319-335-2423; fax: 319-335-0191; alan-johnson@uiowa.edu

[d]Current address: Creighton University, School of Pharmacy and Allied Health, Omaha, Nebraska, USA

Under normal physiological conditions, animals eat and drink intermittently. Between the postabsorptive phase, a time when the hydromineral milieu is most likely to be in balance, and the conclusion of the next period of food and water ingestion, internal physiological and behavioral control systems work together to optimize and restore lost body water and sodium. When animals are challenged by environmental (e.g., increased ambient temperature), physiological (e.g., exercise), and pathophysiological (e.g., emesis; diarrhea) conditions, afferent signals are generated that "inform" the central nervous system (CNS) of fluid losses from both the intracellular and the extracellular fluid compartments.

Three Interacting Effector Systems Determine Body Fluid Balance

Hormonal, behavioral, and autonomic mechanisms participate in the intake and loss of sodium and water. Endocrine and sympathetic mechanisms primarily target the kidney to influence the rate of sodium and water loss. Antidiuretic hormone (ADH; also referred to as vasopressin) is a well-established hormonal factor that acts on renal collecting ducts to increase water permeability and reabsorption; aldosterone (ALDO), another well-studied hormone, acts on renal tubules to promote sodium reabsorption. The renal tubules also receive sympathetic innervation, which, when activated, increases the reabsorption of sodium and water. Efferent renal sympathetic nerve activity to the tubules represents the efferent limb of a reflex that responds to increases and decreases in blood volume and blood pressure. Endocrine and autonomic mechanisms interact in the kidney to partially stem sodium and water loss in the face of accruing sodium and water deficits. However, it is only by engaging behavioral mechanisms that the restoration of sodium and water lost to the environment can be achieved ultimately.

Experimental evidence indicates that depletion of either the intracellular or extracellular fluid compartments results in the ingestion of water (i.e., thirst). Depletion of extracellular fluid also produces the mobilization of salt or sodium appetite, characterized by the behaviors involved in the search for and ingestion of salty substances, particularly those containing sodium ions. Salt appetite is well documented in an array of mammals (see refs. 1 and 2 for reviews), including humans,[3,4] and can be elicited by a variety of experimental manipulations, including sodium depletion, hypovolemia, adrenalectomy, and pharmacological doses of ALDO (see TABLE 1). A frequently employed operational definition of salt appetite is a significant increase in the ingestion of concentrated sodium solutions (i.e., usually concentrations > 1.5% NaCl). In the normal fluid-replete state, such concentrated sodium solutions are unpalatable to most mammals. Under experimental conditions that generate a salt appetite where both hypertonic saline and water are present, rats ingest significant amounts of each fluid. The volumes of hypertonic saline and water consumed in such situations are in a ratio that approximates the ingestion of an *isotonic cocktail*. Thus, resolution of an extracellular fluid deficit requires the generation of two discrete behaviors: the consumption of water and the consumption of sodium (often as hypertonic solutions). Current information indicates that extracellular depletion-induced thirst and salt appetite use some of the same afferent signaling mechanisms[5] and up to some point before the final common path for each behavior, many of the same central structures and neurotransmitter systems.[6,7]

TABLE 1. Experimental manipulations commonly employed to induce salt appetite

Primary Salt Appetite
Absolute Sodium Deficit Induced by Depletion
Dietary sodium restriction
Perspiration (exercise in the heat with restoration of water loss without sodium)
Adrenalectomy
Peritoneal dialysis
Natriuretic treatment
Salivary sodium loss
Relative Sodium Deficit
Sequestration of extracellular fluid (e.g., polyethylene glycol (PEG))
Pharmacological Simulation
Combined natriuretic-hypotensive drug (e.g., furosemide + captopril; furosemide + minoxidil)
Aldosterone or deoxycorticosteroid acetate (DOCA)
icv[a] Angiotensin or renin treatment
icv Angiotensin + priming with low-dose aldosterone
α_2-Adrenoceptor antagonist treatment (yohimbine)

[a]icv, intracerebroventricular.

In states when sodium and water are in excess or when there is an alteration of the balance between those substances (i.e., increased sodium/water ratio), one or more hormonal factors (e.g., atrial natriuretic peptide, oxytocin, Na^+/K^+-ATPase inhibitory factor, and probably γ-melanocyte-stimulating hormone) are released (i.e., candidate natriuretic substances) to increase renal water and sodium excretion. In addition reflex autonomic mechanisms acting in the kidney that normally retain sodium and water are actively inhibited. The suppression of reflexes under conditions of body water and sodium excess has a behavioral analogue; both thirst and salt appetite are also, respectively, inhibited in states of water and sodium excess.[8,9]

Activation of facilitory and inhibitory mechanisms that determine the mobilization of thirst- and salt appetite-related behaviors and the patterning of hormonal and autonomic responses involved in the maintenance of body fluid homeostasis necessitates that the CNS receives continuous input about the status of extracellular fluid osmolarity and extracellular fluid volume. Multiple afferent channels signal the brain regarding the disposition of homeostatic end points (e.g., osmolality, blood pressure, and blood volume).

Receptors Located in the Brain and in the Systemic Viscera Detect Humoral Stimuli and Physical Changes That Signal the Status of Body Fluids

There are both chemo- and mechanoreceptors that are sensitive to stimuli that signal fluid and cardiovascular status. These receptors are located in the systemic viscera and in the brain. Experimental increases in the osmolarity of brain extracellular fluid (e.g., by injection of hypertonic cerebrospinal fluid into the cerebral ventricles) activate thirst, vasopressin release, and the sympathetic nervous system to effect an expansion of the intracellular component and to increase blood pressure. These responses are believed to be mediated by hypothetical receptors that sense their own volume and that have traditionally been referred to as *osmoreceptors* in relation to vasopressin release[10] as well as to thirst.[11]

A second major humoral signal that acts on the brain to effect responses consistent with restoration or expansion of body fluids and elevation of blood pressure is the peptide, angiotensin II (ANG II). Systemic administration of exogenous ANG II elevates arterial blood pressure, releases vasopressin and ALDO, and increases the ingestion of water and sodium. Most of these responses are also produced when ANG II is administered directly into the brain.

Although there are many regions in the CNS sensitive to osmotic changes and to ANG II, there are three specific structures lying outside the blood-brain barrier that act as sensors of these humoral signals. These *sensory circumventricular organs* are the subfornical organ (SFO), the organum vasculosum of the lamina terminalis (OVLT), and the area postrema (AP) (see ref. 12). It has been proposed that the *brain renin-angiotensin system* (i.e., a system with its components synthesized *de novo* in the brain) is coupled with the systemic (i.e., renal) renin-angiotensin system through one of the sensory circumventricular organs, the SFO.[13] Thus, it is hypothesized that circulating angiotensin in the mode of a hormone acts on sensory circumventricular organs to activate brain neural pathways. These brain interneurons, in turn, release intracellular stores of brain angiotensin from their axon terminals to function in a manner analogous to other neurotransmitters/neuromodulators.[6,12,14]

In recent years, there has been considerable attention paid to mineralocorticoid receptors located in the brain and their contribution to salt appetite.[15] Mineralocorticoids (e.g., ALDO) when given in pharmacological doses[16] or in more physiological concentrations in conjunction with ANG II,[17] generate salt appetite. The facilitory interaction of low doses of ALDO and ANG II in the brain has been referred to as the *synergy hypothesis*.[15]

The receptors identified as most pertinent to sensing extracellular volume (or blood volume) and arterial blood pressure are located in the periphery. The great veins and atria (i.e., the low pressure side of the circulation) contain receptors that are sensitive to stretch. These receptors generate nerve traffic to the CNS in proportion to distention of the walls of the great veins (e.g., superior vena cava) and atria. Similar stretch receptors located in the aortic arch and carotid sinus sense changes in arterial blood pressure. Outputs from these receptors change as a function of arterial blood pressure.

Information from low (also referred to as cardiopulmonary receptors and as blood volume receptors) and high (also referred to as arterial baroreceptors) pressure receptors reaches the CNS by the IXth and Xth cranial nerves. When pressure and/or volume falls below their normal operating points, nerve activity declines and generates reflex release of vasopressin and activation of the sympathetic nervous system and, ultimately, behaviors leading to increased salt and water intake. There is evidence indicating that input from systemic baroreceptors "synergizes" with the central action of ANG II to generate thirst and sodium appetite.[5,18] When blood pressure and blood volume increase above "normal" levels, vasopressin secretion, sympathetic outflow, and the behaviors of water and sodium ingestion are actively inhibited.

A Visceral Neuraxis Comprises the Network That Receives and Processes Information Related to Body Fluid Balance

Cranial nerves (IX and X) enter the CNS and synapse primarily in the nucleus of the tractus solitarius (NTS). Input sensed by circumventricular organs (SFO; OVLT; AP) is carried by efferent nerves emanating from these structures into the brain neuropil. Many brain nuclei and pathways that process information derived from systemic receptors and from the sensory circumventricular organ have been identified by employing both functional and neuronal tract-tracing techniques. The result has been the delineation of a *visceral neural network* that carries and integrates information pertinent to the control of fluid balance. Presumably, every structure and pathway in the brain can potentially influence information processing in the visceral neuraxis. However, there are certain regions that have been found to be especially critical for maintaining normal cellular and extracellular volume and blood pressure. Most notable among these brain regions are (1) the sensory circumventricular organs (i.e., SFO, OVLT and AP), (2) the NTS, (3) caudal and rostral ventrolateral medulla, (4) parabrachial nucleus (PBN), (5) the median preoptic nucleus (MePO; periventricular preoptic nuclei), (6) parvocellular hypothalamic paraventricular nucleus, (7) magnocellular paraventricular nucleus, (8) supraoptic nucleus, (9) amygdala (particularly the central (CeA) and medial (MeA) nuclei of the amygdala), (10) bed nucleus of the stria terminalis (BST), (11) lateral hypothalamus, and (12) the interomediolateral cell column of the spinal cord. Multiple reciprocal pathways employing diverse neurotransmitters/neuromodulators connect these structures and provide ample capacity for the types of feedforward and feedback loops required for parallel, distributed processing of fluid-related information.

Many of the neurotransmitters/neuromodulators associated with the visceral fluid-control network are known. These include (1) glutamate, (2) GABA, (3) acetylcholine, (4) norepinephrine, (5) epinephrine, (6) serotonin, (7) renin-angiotensin, (8) vasopressin, (9) oxytocin, and (10) corticotrophin-releasing hormone. Whereas some of these neurochemical systems may be associated with specific subcomponents of the visceral neuraxis (i.e., local processing), others appear to be more widely dispersed. The brain norepinephrine and renin-angiotensin systems are broadly distributed in the CNS and are associated with most of the structures constituting the visceral neuraxis. A reasonable body of experimental evidence indicates that these two brain neurochemical systems are among the most important aspects of the neural substrate that, when activated in critical areas, mobilize effector systems that expand extracellular volume.[6,14,18]

In addition to facilitory mechanisms, it is probable that there are inhibitory counterparts represented in the central fluid regulatory network. It is reasonable to hypothesize that, when activated, this counterposed subsystem acts to retard overexpansion of the extracellular fluid compartment. Evidence indicates that such inhibition involves brain oxytocin,[9] serotonin,[18–20] tachykinin,[21] cholecystokinin,[22] and/or bombesin[23] pathways.

The Neural Pathways Carrying Humoral and Neural Sensory Signals Important for Salt Appetite Converge on the Amygdala

Acquisition, verification, and consumption are crucial behaviors that comprise the expression of a salt appetite. These responses require the central integration of sensory information derived from several different types of sensory receptors and systems. Visceral afferent signals must communicate the body's need for sodium to the brain. Telereceptive systems (depending upon species, it is olfaction and/or vision) are engaged for identification of potential sources of the ion in the external environment, and taste mechanisms assess potential sources when in close proximity

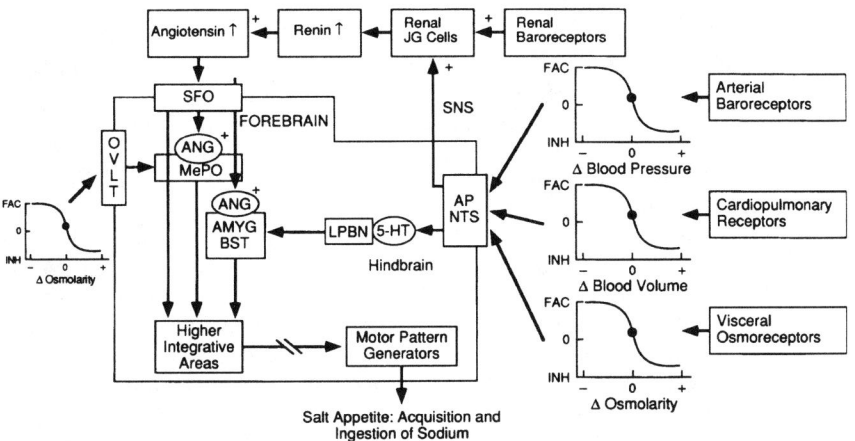

FIGURE 1. Diagram depicting the nature of neural and hormonal inputs into the brain of viscerally derived information and the central neural pathways that mediate sensory integration of signals for the generation of sodium ingestion (salt appetite). Both inhibitory and excitatory input from the periphery derives from arterial and cardiopulmonary baroreceptors and probably systemic osmo-/Na$^+$-receptors. Information carried in afferent visceral nerves projects mainly to the nucleus of the tractus solitarius (NTS). Circulating angiotensin (ANG) acts in the form of ANG II on the subfornical organ (SFO). Information reflecting input to the SFO is carried in efferent pathways, some of which are likely to use ANG in the mode of a neurotransmitter, to forebrain structures such as the median preoptic nucleus (MePO). Changes in extracellular osmolarity influences activity of cells in or near the organum vasculosum of the lamina terminalis (OVLT). The OVLT also projects to the MePO. A hindbrain inhibitory pathway originating in the area postrema (AP) and medial NTS ascends to the lateral parabrachial nucleus (LPBN). This projection uses serotonin (5-HT) as a neurotransmitter. This inhibitory system prevents excessive sodium and water intake, thereby limiting excessive expansion of blood volume. The amygdala (AMYG) and bed nucleus of the stria terminalis (BST) receive input from both the SFO and the LPBN. JG, juxtaglomerular; SNS, sympathetic nervous system; FAC, facilition; INH, inhibition.

and determine the rate and duration of sodium consumption. Different types of sensory input enter the CNS over distinct afferent channels. Signals in the central component of each sensory system are processed within their own networks and progress through the neuraxis to ultimately converge with one another at points critical for determining the seeking, sampling, consumption, and satiation phases associated with salt appetite.

Essentially all levels of the nervous system are involved in the expression of salt appetite. Midcollicular transection abolishes oral responses associated with sodium deprivation,[24] whereas responses to oral glucose elicited by systemic glucoprivation are not disrupted by this lesion.[25] Both the forebrain and hindbrain house receptive target tissues for humoral signaling molecules and the portals of entry of sensory nerves. Over recent years, significant progress has been made in several laboratories in identifying forebrain and hindbrain components of the visceral neural network subserving salt appetite (FIG. 1). Systemically derived information has immediate access to some key forebrain areas implicated in salt appetite. Substances that cannot readily cross the blood-brain barrier can act on the two sensory circumventricular organs associated with the lamina terminalis, which is the ependymal layer that forms the rostral wall of the third cerebral ventricle. The SFO is situated in the dorsal aspect of the third ventricle, whereas the OVLT lies along the ventral part of the lamina terminalis. As in the case of endocrine and autonomic reflexes and drinking behavior (thirst), the forebrain sensory circumventricular organs, SFO and OVLT, have also been implicated as targets for angiotensin's natriorexigenic actions. In addition, because the osmotic status of extracellular fluid is likely to facilitate (via hypo-osmolarity) or inhibit (via hyperosmolarity) salt appetite, putative osmoreceptors in the SFO and OVLT probably contribute to this process. Both the SFO and OVLT project to the MePO, which lies between them and is located inside the blood-brain barrier. The MePO is an important integrative node processing both angiotensin-derived and osmotic-related information to then influence activity in many of the control systems influencing body fluid homeostasis.[26] Studies have implicated both the ventral MePO[27,28] as well as the ventral MePO and OVLT, which are key structures contained in periventricular lesions of the anteroventral third ventricle (i.e., AV3V; ref. 29), in the control of salt appetite. Efferents from the lamina terminalis, particularly the SFO, project to the CeA, MeA, and BST.[30,31]

Mineralocorticoids, such as ALDO, another class of humoral stimulus related to salt appetite, have ready access to the brain, in general. Such steroidal hormones are lipid soluble, and their effects depend upon availability of functional receptors located in brain target tissues.[32]

In contrast to the facilatory actions of angiotensin, hypo-osmolality and mineralocorticoid binding in the forebrain, recent studies have described a hindbrain system that keeps ingestive behaviors (i.e., water and sodium intake), which contribute to expanding extracellular fluid volume, in check. This inhibitory system involves the neural circuitry of the AP and the medial portion of the nucleus of the tractus solitarius (AP/mNTS) and the lateral PBN (see ref. 18 for review). Ablation of the AP/mNTS markedly increases the intake of the concentrated sodium chloride solution both in chronic[33] and acute[34] experimental testing situations. A major constituent of a neural pathway projecting from the AP/mNTS to the lateral PBN[35–37] contains serotonin.[38] Bilateral injections of serotonin antagonists directly into the lateral PBN markedly enhance both water and concentrated NaCl solution intake to numerous dipsogenic and natriorexigenic challenges.[19,20,39–41] The lateral PBN appears to be an integrative region involved in processing viscerally derived information from regions such as cardiopulmonary baroreceptors,[42] and such processing requires the presence of lateral PBN cell bodies.[43]

The efferents from the lateral PBN that are involved in the control of salt appetite have not yet been specified. However, there are major ascending projections from the lateral PBN to the CeA.[44] As such, the amygdala appears to be ideally positioned to receive both blood-borne angiotensin-related information arising from the structures of the lamina terminalis (i.e., the SFO) as well as visceral baroreceptor-derived input via the PBN (see FIG. 1). In addition, the amygdala receives somatic sensory information (e.g., somatosensory, taste, and olfaction). In light of this convergence of multiple types of visceral and somatic sensory inputs, the amygdala has long been recognized to be a likely candidate contributing to the control of such complex behaviors as those associated with salt appetite.

THE IMPLICATION OF COMPONENTS OF THE EXTENDED AMYGDALA (ExA) IN SALT APPETITE

Recent analyses[45–47] have reaffirmed the concept initially proposed by Johnston[48] that the amygdala and the BST were once a single structure that became separated in mammals by development of the internal capsule. This has given rise to the concept of the ExA, which is formed by what appears as a continuum of structures, including mainly the CeA and MeA nuclei and their extensions in the lateral and medial divisions of the bed nucleus of the stria terminalis (BSTL and BSTM, respectively; refs. 45, 46, and 49). Cytochemoarchitectural, tract tracing, and immunocytochemical studies indicate that the BSTL-CeA and the region of the BSTM-MeA have structural, hodological, and neurochemical similarities. This supports the idea that these are corresponding areas that are interrelated and likely to have similar functions. In light of the need for integrating multiple somatic and visceral sensory inputs necessary for the generation of salt appetite, the ExA becomes a primary subcortical candidate for this function. Earlier studies investigating the amygdala in salt appetite showed that extensive damage to large parts of the amygdala[50,51] or transection of the ventral amygdalofungal pathway[52] decreased experimentally induced sodium intake. More recent studies have been directed at a more precise determination of the nuclei or components of the ExA that are necessary for full expression of salt appetite. The MeA and the CeA have been the major components of the amygdala that have been studied recently.

Electrolytic damage to the MeA impairs or abolishes mineralocorticoid-induced salt appetite while not affecting intake that is induced by adrenalectomy or by acute sodium depletion.[53,54] These latter types of salt appetite are apparently not dependent upon elevated mineralocorticoid actions but require the central actions of ANG II. Recent evidence indicates that cells rather than fibers of passage within the MeA are essential for this steroid-induced salt appetite, because cell body damage produced by ibotenic acid in this nucleus impairs ALDO-induced salt intake without interfering with sodium depletion-induced or angiotensin-dependent salt appetites.[55] The selective impairments induced by MeA lesions do not seem to result from interrupting connections between the amygdala and the ventral forebrain through the stria terminalis.[56] Adrenal steroid implants (ALDO or deoxycorticosterone acetate (DOCA)) in the MeA produce a rapid arousal of specific sodium intake, and central administration of mineralocorticoid antagonist (RU28318) or mineralocorticoid receptor antisense inhibits salt appetite stimulated by systemic ALDO or DOCA, but not by adrenalectomy.[57,58]

Studies indicate that lesions of the CeA markedly attenuate *ad libitum* sodium intake and greatly impair salt appetite induced by DOCA, sodium depletion, systemic yohimbine treatment, and icv ANG II.[59,60] The impairment of salt intake in rats with lesions of the CeA does not appear to be the result of disordered gustatory function because rats with such lesions discriminate between different tastes. That is, the animals demonstrate different responses to taste stimuli as a function of their internal states, but they do not increase sodium intake.[61,62] Similar to CeA lesions, ablation of the BST also significantly attenuates salt appetite induced by various methods.[60,63]

In addition to lesion studies, pharmacological studies employing intracranial injections have also investigated the role of neurotransmitters/modulators in salt appetite. Tachykinins delivered into the MeA inhibit renin-angiotensin-associated forms of salt appetite.[21] Also bilateral injections of the same peptide into the BSTM inhibits salt appetite by studies involving bilateral injections of the tachykinin, eledoisin, into the posterior portion of the BSTM, which blocks sodium intake in response to a variety of salt-appetite-inducing protocols.[64]

Recent studies from our laboratories investigating the BST and amygdaloid counterparts of the ExA have employed both lesions of the CeA and the BST Fos-immunoreactivity (Fos-ir). The ablation studies[60] investigated salt appetite in rats with CeA and with BST lesions maintained and tested under near-identical experimental conditions.

Electrolytic Lesions of the CeA and of the BST Provide Functional Evidence of Involvement of the ExA in Salt Appetite

The role of components of the ExA was investigated by making bilateral electrolytic lesions in either the CeA or the BST.[60] In two comparable experiments, male Sprague-Dawley rats were first pretested for drinking responses to hypertonic saline and to systemically administered ANG II and for salt appetite induced by two different experimental manipulations. One type of rapid onset experimental salt appetite was induced by sc administration of yohimbine (3 mg/kg), and the intake of 2% NaCl was recorded over a 3-h test period. Both systemic and central treatment with this α_2-adrenergic receptor antagonist produces copious salt intake with a short latency. Neither the circulating renin-angiotensin system nor circulating ALDO is necessary for yohimbine-induced salt appetite. The second type of sodium appetite was induced by depleting the animal of sodium by administration of sc furosemide (10 mg/kg given twice over a 2-h interval) and then maintenance for 24 h in a sodium-free environment (i.e., access only to water and sodium-deficient food). Following the conclusion of the depletion/deprivation period, animals were given access to 2% NaCl, and the intake was studied over the course of 3 hours.

In each experiment, lesion groups (i.e., either CeA lesions or BST lesions) and sham-lesion (control) groups were formed. Four weeks after surgery, animals were once again tested for drinking (thirst) to ANG II and to hypertonic saline, and for the intake of 2% NaCl induced by yohimbine treatment and by furosemide plus 24 h in a sodium-free environment. Six out of 15 animals regained drinking within one week postsurgery and had bilateral BST lesions that were reasonably restricted to the nuclei and bilaterally complete (that is, with gliosis and/or necrosis destroying at least two thirds of the rostral caudal extent of each BST). These rats were defined as the BST-lesion group (FIG. 2). Five of 22 animals regained drinking within a week and had CeA lesions that were reasonably restricted to the nuclei and that were bilaterally complete (that is, had gliosis and/or necrosis throughout a minimum of two thirds of the rostral caudal extent of each nucleus). These rats constituted the CeA lesion group (FIG. 3).

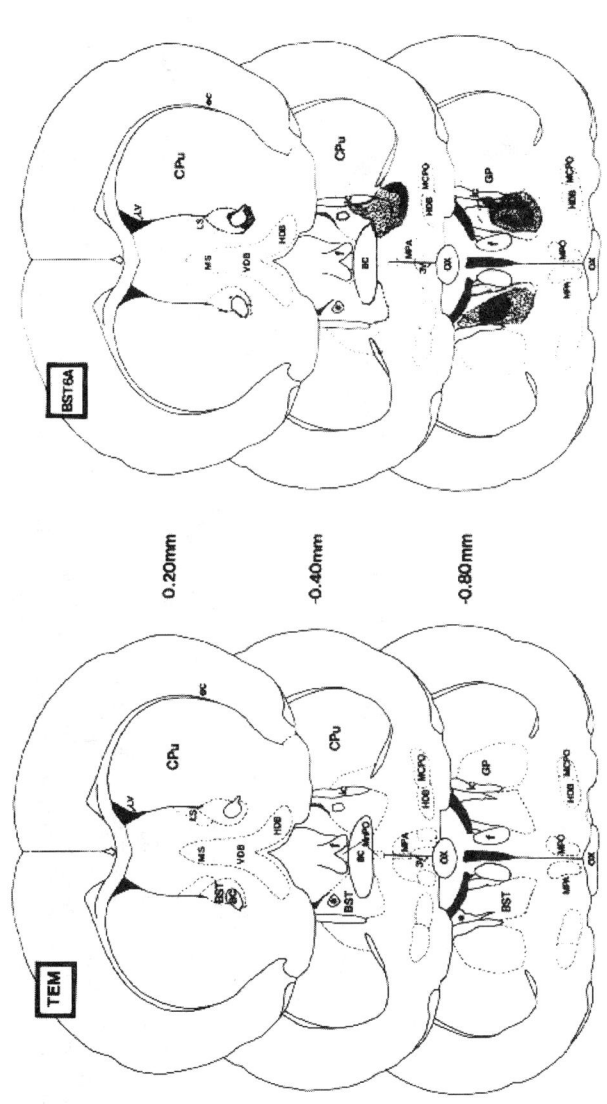

FIGURE 2. *Right:* Camera lucida drawings showing the rostral-caudal extent of an example of a lesion judged as complete (through at least two thirds of the extent of the nucleus) bilateral lesions of the bed nucleus of the stria terminalis (BST). The template (TEM, *left*) shows the three levels of the BST (adapted from Paxinos and Watson[77]), at which the extent of the lesion in each case was characterized. The distance from bregma is denoted to the right of each level of the TEM. Black denotes complete ablation, heavy stippling represents heavy necrosis, and fine stippling indicates the extent of gliosis and/or light necrosis. The asterisk denotes the stria terminalis. (Adapted from Zardetto-Smith *et al.*[60]) 3V, third ventricle; ac, anterior commissure; CPu, caudate putamen; ec, external capsule; f, fornix; GP, globus pallidus; HDB, nucleus of the horizontal limb of the diagonal band; ic, internal capsule; LS, lateral septal nucleus; LV, lateral ventricle; MCPO, magnocellular preoptic nucleus; MnPO, median preoptic nucleus; MPA, medial preoptic area; MPO, medial preoptic nucleus; MS, medial septal nucleus; OX, optic chiasm; VDB, nucleus, vertical limb of the diagonal band.

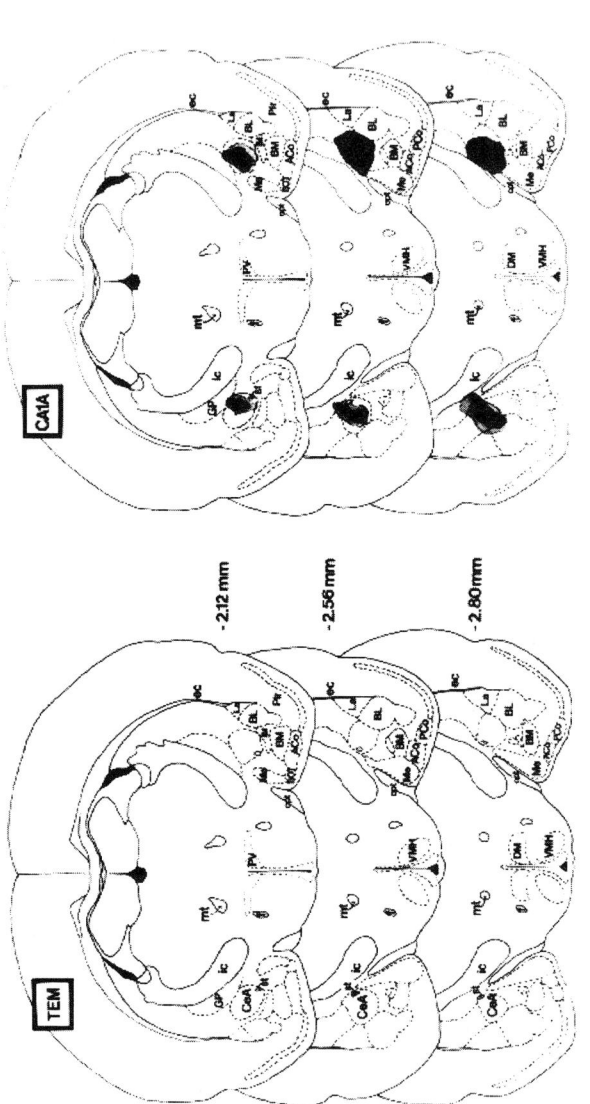

FIGURE 3. *Right:* Camera lucida drawings showing the rostral-caudal extent of an example of a lesion judged as complete (through at least two thirds of the extent of the nucleus) bilateral lesions of the central nucleus of the amygdala (CeA). The template (TEM, *left*) shows the three levels of the CeA (adapted from Paxinos and Watson[77]), at which the extent of the lesion in each case was characterized. The distance from bregma is denoted to the right of each level of the TEM. Black denotes complete ablation, heavy stippling represents heavy necrosis, and fine stippling indicates the extent of the gliosis and/or light necrosis. (Adapted from Zardetto-Smith *et al.*[60]) ACo, anterior cortical amygdaloid nucleus; BL, basolateral amygdaloid nucleus; BM, basomedial amygdaloid nucleus; BOT, bed nucleus accessory olfactory tract; DM, dorsomedial hypothalamic nucleus; ec, external capsule; f, fornix; GP, globus pallidus; ic, internal capsule; IM, intercalated amygdaloid nucleus, main; La, lateral amygdaloid nucleus; Me, medial amygdaloid nucleus; mt, mammillothalamic tract; opt, optic tract; PCO, posterior cortical amygdaloid nucleus; Pir, piriform cortex; PV, paraventricular hypothalamic nucleus; st, stria terminalis; VMH, ventromedial hypothalamic nucleus.

TABLE 2. Effects of bed nucleus of the stria terminalis (BST) or central nucleus of the amygdala (CeA) lesions on water intake in response to sc hypertonic saline (6% NaCl)

Group	Water intake (mL ± SEM)	
	Before surgery	After surgery
BST sham lesion ($n = 6$)	6.2 ± 0.9	4.8 ± 1.3
BST lesion ($n = 6$)	6.8 ± 1.1	6.2 ± 1.2
CeA sham lesion ($n = 10$)	3.4 ± 0.6	4.8 ± 0.9
CeA lesion ($n = 5$)	4.2 ± 1.3	4.2 ± 1.1

When postoperative testing began four weeks after surgery, both the BST-lesion and the CeA-lesion animals had significantly attenuated NaCl intake to both of the salt appetite-inducing experimental challenges (FIGURES 4 and 5). Importantly, the impairments in ingestive behavior were specific to salt appetite. That is, animals with BST or CeA lesions both drank comparable amounts of water in comparison to their respective control groups in response to either hypertonic saline or systemic ANG II administration (TABLES 2 and 3). Taken together, these parallel experiments demonstrate that both BST and CeA lesions reliably produce reductions in salt ap-

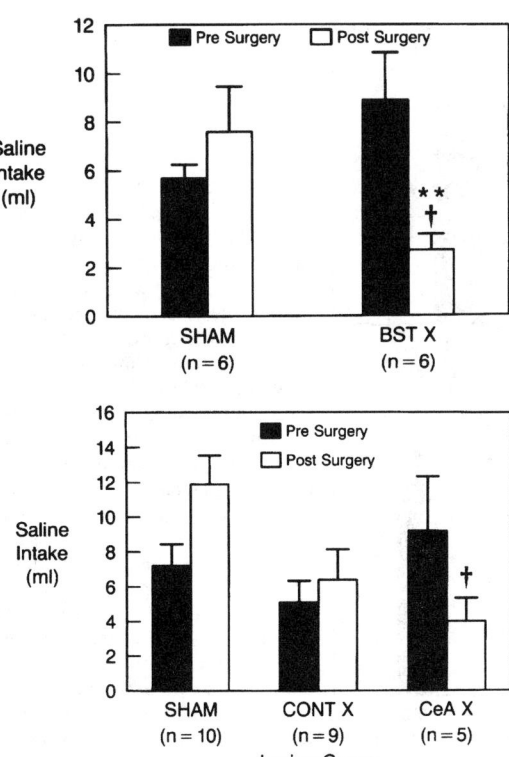

FIGURE 4. Pre- and postsurgery averages of cumulative 3 h 2% NaCl intake in response to sc yohimbine (3 mg/kg) in rats with lesions of the bed nucleus of the stria terminalis (BST X; *upper*) or central nucleus of the amygdala (CeA X; *lower*) and their respective sham-lesion control groups, or, in the case of the CeA experiment, also a control lesion group (i.e., misplaced lesions; CONT X). Values represent the combined data from two separate trials, pre- and post-surgery. Follow-up statistical tests indicated statistical differences (†) between the postsurgery intakes of complete lesion groups versus the postsurgery intakes of their respective control groups and (**) between the postsurgery versus presurgery intakes in the BST X groups. (Adapted from Zardetto-Smith et al.[60])

TABLE 3. Effects of bed nucleus of the stria terminalis (BST) or central nucleus of the amygdala (CeA) lesions on water intake in response to sc angiotensin II

Group	Water intake (mL ± SEM)	
	Before surgery	After surgery
BST sham lesion ($n = 6$)	3.7 ± 0.2	2.1 ± 0.6
BST lesion ($n = 6$)	2.7 ± 0.3	1.5 ± 0.8
CeA sham lesion ($n = 10$)	3.7 ± 0.6	3.3 ± 1.1
CeA lesion ($n = 5$)	5.1 ± 1.3	3.3 ± 1.0

petite to two different types of natriorexigenic stimuli. Neither of the bilateral lesions completely abolished salt appetite to the challenges. The reductions in the different salt appetite produced by each lesion were on the order of 50 to 65% of control intakes. This is perhaps not surprising and may indicate that the BST and CeA make roughly equal contributions to these forms of experimentally induced salt appetite.

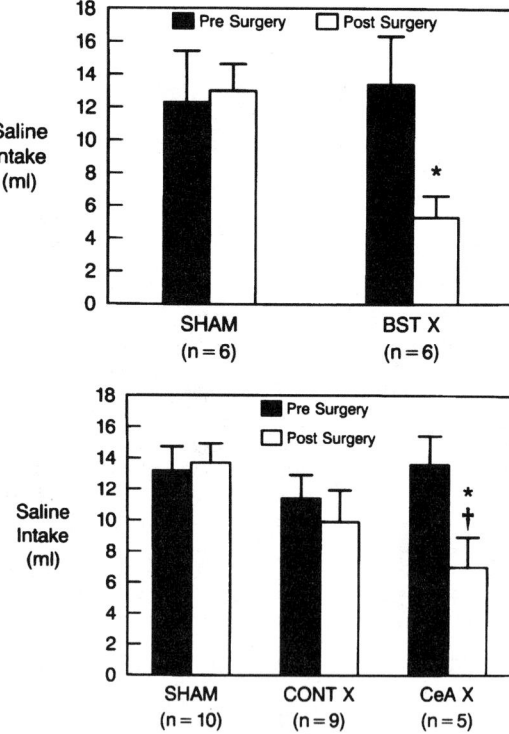

FIGURE 5. Pre- and postsurgery averages of cumulative 3 h 2% NaCl intakes following sodium depletion by furosemide diuresis in rats with complete, bilateral lesions of the bed nucleus of the stria terminalis (BST X; *upper*) or central nucleus of the amygdala (CeA X; *lower*) and their sham-lesion control groups, and, in the case of the CeA experiment, also a control lesion group (i.e., misplaced lesions; CONT X). Values represent the combined data from two separate trials both pre- and postsurgery. Planned follow-up statistical tests indicated statistical difference (∗) between pre- and postsurgery intakes and (†) between postsurgery intakes between lesion groups and their respective sham-lesion control groups. (Adapted from Zardetto-Smith *et al.*[60])

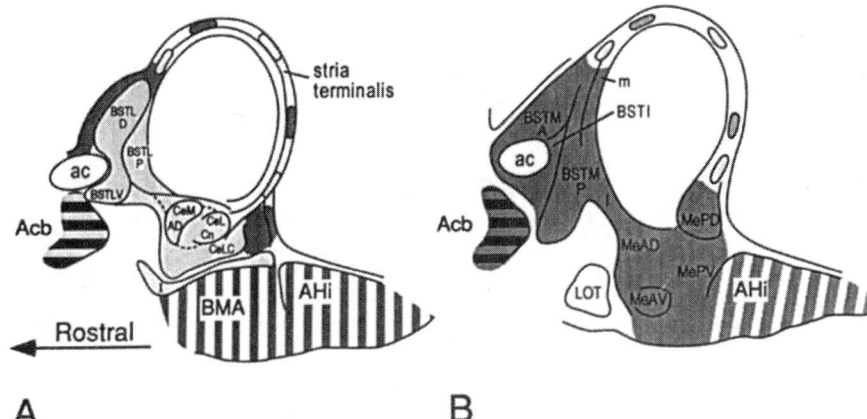

FIGURE 6. Schematic view of the central division (**A**) and medial division (**B**) of the extended amygdala (ExA). The ExA basically comprises two ring-like cell columns, central and medial. The former encompasses the central amygdaloid nucleus (CeA), central sublenticular extended amygdala, the interstitial nucleus of the posterior limb of the anterior commissure, the lateral division of the bed nucleus of the stria terminalis (BSTL), and the supracapsular extension of it. The second comprises the medial nucleus of the amygdala (MeA), the small-celled superficial sectors of the anterior amygdaloid area, medial sublenticular extended amygdala, and the medial part of the bed nucleus of stria terminalis (BSTM) and its supracapsular extension. On the basis of morphological and chemical characteristics and connectivity, both major divisions of the ExA can be further subdivided into external, intermediate, and medial cell subcolumns, which in turn can also be subdivided into dorsal supracapsular and ventral sublenticular tiers. ac, anterior commissure; Acb, accumbens; AHi, amygdalohippocampal area; BMA, basomedial amygdaloid nucleus; BSTi, intermediate division of the bed nucleus of stria terminalis; BSTLD, dorsal part of the lateral division of the bed nucleus of stria terminalis; BSTLP, posterior part of the lateral division of the bed nucleus of stria terminalis; BSTLV, ventral part of the lateral division of the bed nucleus of the stria terminalis; BSTMA, anterior part of the medial division of the bed nucleus of the stria terminalis; BSTMP, posterior part of the medial division of the bed nucleus of the stria terminalis; CeLC, central amygdaloid nuclei, capsular subdivision of the lateral division; CeLCn, central subdivision of the lateral part of the central amygdaloid nucleus; CeMAD, anterior dorsal subdivision of the lateral part of the central amygdaloid nucleus; I, intercalate mass; LOT, nucleus of the lateral olfactory tract; m, medial subdura of the supracapsular subdivision of the bed nucleus of the stria terminalis; MeAD, anterodorsal median amygdala; MeAV, anterior ventral median amygdala; MePD, posterior dorsal medial amygdala; MePV, medial amygdaloid, posterior ventral.

C-fos *Is Activated in the ExA by Salt Appetite-inducing Sodium Depletion*

The assessment of immediate early gene (IEG) activity is a powerful new tool used to identify components of neural systems activated under physiological states, such as those that accompany salt appetite. The IEG, c-*fos*, or its protein product, Fos, are widely used as markers of neural activity. One method employs immunocytochemistry for Fos protein so that the number of ir cells present under experimental versus control conditions serves as an index of neural activation. We[65,66] have recently used this technique to study activation of components of the ExA activated by

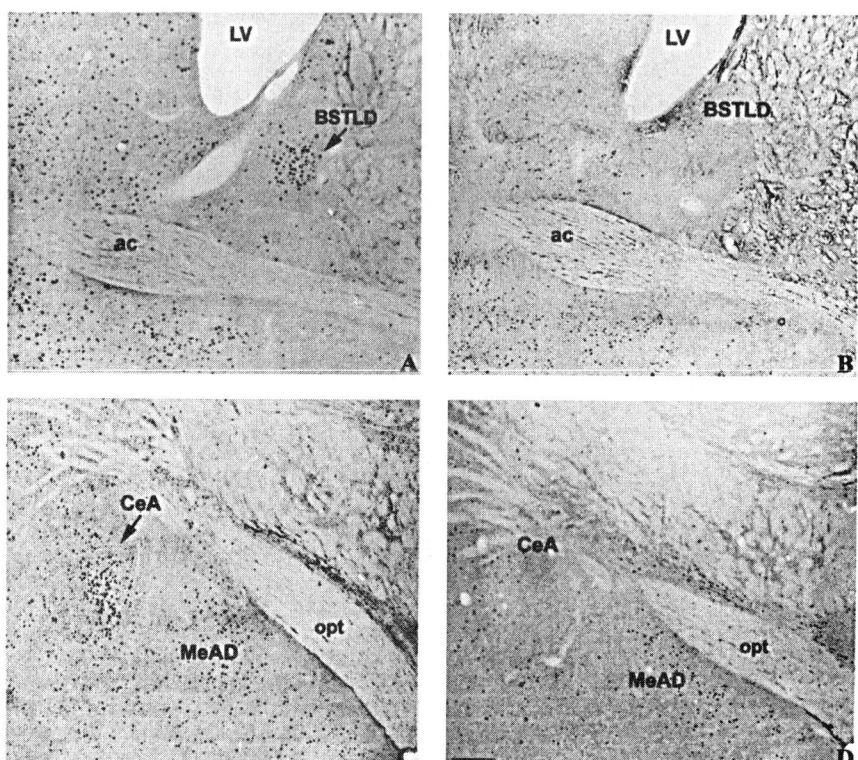

FIGURE 7. Photomicrographs of coronal sections of the lateral division of the bed nucleus of the stria terminalis (BSTLD) and central nucleus of the amygdala (CeA), showing Fos-ir neurons stimulated by sodium depletion induced by peritoneal dialysis in experimental (**A** and **C**) and control rats (**B** and **D**). Calibration mark of 100 μm (**D**) applies to all photomicrographs. ac, anterior commissure; LV, lateral ventricle; MeAD, anterodorsal part of the medial amygdaloid nucleus; opt, optic tract.

sodium depletion induced by peritoneal dialysis (PD). The technique of PD, which has been described previously[67] was used in the present studies. Briefly a 5% glucose solution (37°C) in a volume equivalent to 10% of the rat's body weight is first injected into the peritoneal cavity. One hour later, ascitic fluid containing approximately 0.8 mEq/100 g body weight of sodium is removed from the peritoneal cavity with a needle. The animals are then housed with distilled water but no food. Typically, rats subjected to this protocol with a 24-h delay in access to 2% saline solution consume on the order of 4 mL/100 g body weight of hypertonic NaCl solution within 1 h, whereas nondialyzed control animals take in only approximately 0.5 mL/100 g body weight.

In the present experiment, rats received either PD or a control procedure (i.e., insertion of a needle without delivery or removal of fluid) and were sacrificed 4 h later. Previous work[68] has shown that 4 h after PD, there is a maximal drop in plasma and

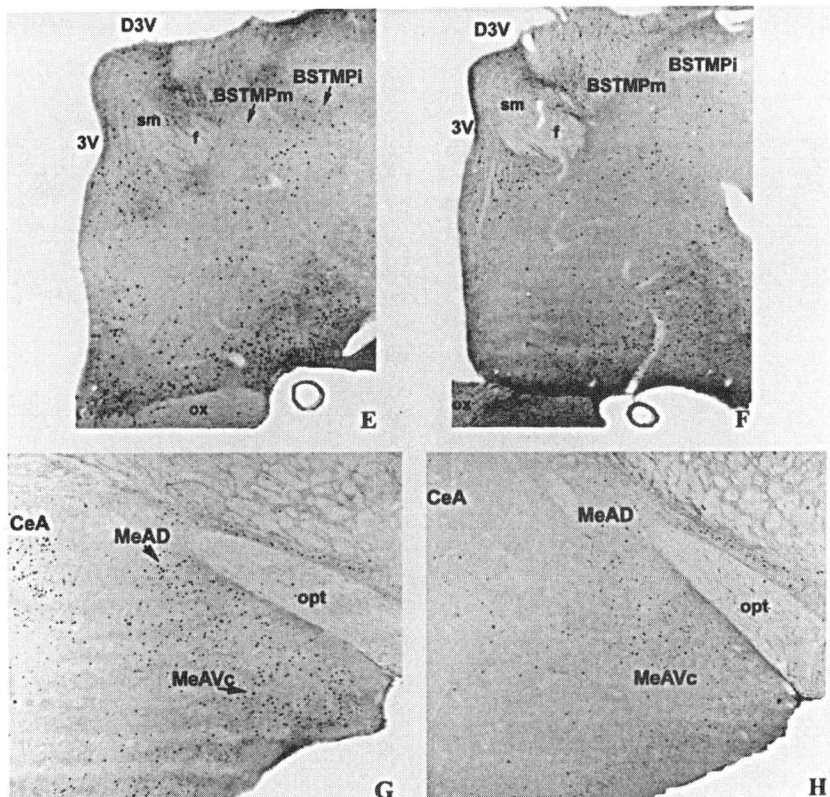

FIGURE 8. Photomicrographs of coronal sections of the medial division of the bed nucleus of the stria terminalis (BSTM) and medial nucleus of the amygdala (MeA), showing the Fos-ir neurons stimulated by sodium depletion induced by peritoneal dialysis. In plates **E** and **F**, the pattern of Fos-ir cell nuclei is observed within the intermediate subnucleus of the posteromedial BST (BSTMPi) in experimental and control rats. An absence of c-*fos* expression along the medial subnucleus of the posteromedial BST (BSTMPm) is also apparent. Plates **G** and **H** show Fos-ir neurons within the anterodorsal and caudoventral subdivision of the MeA (MeAD and MeAVc) in experimental and control groups. Calibration mark of 100 μm (**H**) applies to all photomicrographs. 3V, third ventricle; CeA, central amydaloid nucleus; DV3, dorsal third ventricle; f, fornix; opt, optic tract; sm, stria medullaris.

cerebrospinal fluid sodium concentrations and a major increase in c-*fos* expression in the circumventricular organs of the lamina terminalis. The brains of the experimental and control animals were collected and processed for Fos-ir (see ref. 69 for a description of methods), and the components of the ExA were analyzed.

Body sodium depletion induced by PD produced a pattern of highly localized and intense Fos-ir cells within specific portions of the central and medial division of the ExA (see FIG. 6; and refs. 65 and 66). Compared with the control groups, the largest

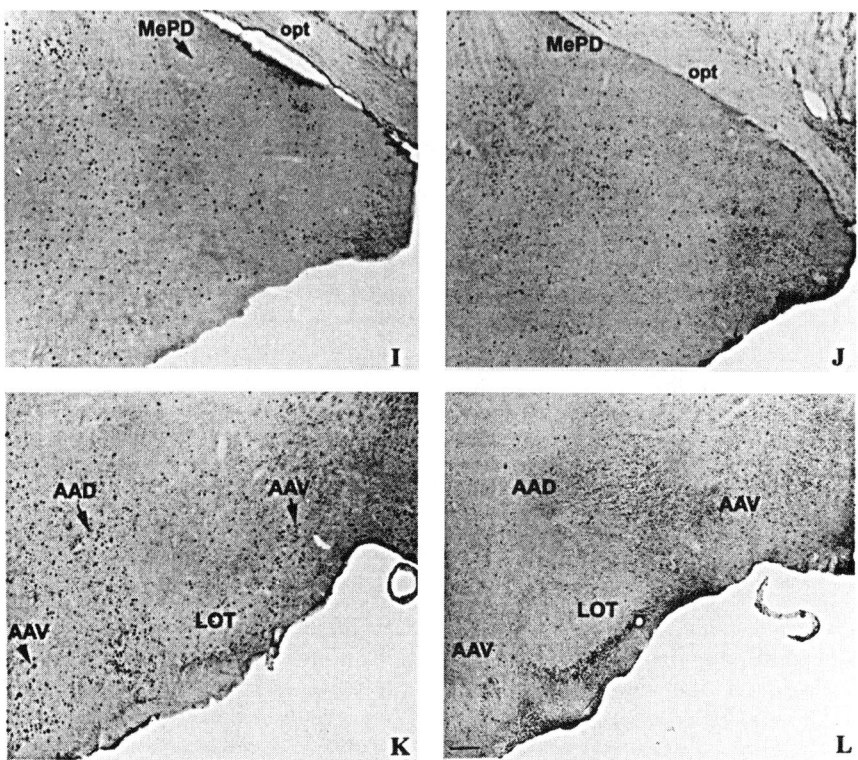

FIGURE 9. Photomicrographs of coronal sections through the posterodorsal medial amygdaloid nucleus (MePD) and the anterior amygdala area. Plates **I** and **J** show the absence of significant changes of c-*fos* expression in the MePD in the experimental and control groups, respectively. In plates **K** and **L**, a significant increase of Fos activation in the AA of sodium-depleted animals can be observed. This finding is consistent with the recent proposal that the AA should be included as part of the medial ExA. Calibration mark of 100 μm (**L**) applies to all photomicrographs. AAD, dorsal part of the anterior amygdala area; AAV, ventral part of the anterior amygdala area; LOT, nucleus of the lateral olfactory tract; opt, optic tract.

increase in c-*fos* activation was found in the central ExA division, specifically in the central subdivision of the lateral part of the central amygdaloid nucleus (CeLCn) and its continuation in the dorsal part of the lateral bed nucleus of the stria terminalis (BSTLD; FIG. 7). Along the medial division of the ExA complex, there was activation of the corresponding part of the MeA and the BSTM, which more precisely can be defined as the anterodorsal and caudoventral part of the anterior MeA (MeAD, MeAVc) and the intermediate, medium-celled subdivision of the posterior part of the medial bed nucleus (BSTMPi; FIG. 8). Consistent with its recent inclusion as part of the medial ExA,[70] the anterior amygdala area (AA) also displayed a significant increase in Fos-ir (FIG. 9). By contrast, the remaining subnucleus of the medial and central ExA complex showed no significant changes in Fos-ir, suggesting that cells within this continuum have other functions. Neither the medial and lateral capsular

CeA subdivisions (CeM, CeLC) nor medial and lateral parts of the interstitial nucleus of the posterior limb of the anterior commissure (IPAC, IPACM, and IPACL, respectively) showed significant changes in Fos-ir induced by sodium depletion. Similarly Fos-ir in the other subdivisions of the medial ExA, like the medial, small-celled subdivision of the BSTPM and its extension in the posterodorsal MeA, did not differ from control animals (FIGURES 8 and 9, respectively).

The present study shows that there are specific groups of cells within the different subdivisions of the ExA that express c-*fos* after an acute sodium depletion.[65,66] Because c-*fos* expression following a salt appetite–inducing procedure probably identifies individual cellular components of functional neural networks[65,68,71,72] activated as a result of a specific physiological state, the presence of sodium depletion–induced Fos-ir neurons in the ExA provides further evidence that the ExA is involved in the regulation of sodium balance. The results of these experiments provide initial evidence that neuronal activation of specific ExA cells is produced by body sodium deficit that normally would result in the consumption of concentrated NaCl (i.e., a salt appetite).

In light of the rather confined localization of the FOS-ir positive cells in selected subpopulations of neurons scattered along nuclear subdivisions of both the central and medial main divisions of the ExA, these findings provide functional anatomical support for the hypothesis proposed by de Olmos et al.[46] (see also ref. 45) of the presence of a neuronal continuum stretching from the CeA and MeA to the BSTL and BSTM. In the present experimental material, the central ExA cells associated with sodium depletion appear to be confined to the central subdivisions of the CeA and the dorsolateral subdivision of the BST, whereas in the medial ExA, Fos-ir cells were confined to the MeAD and MeAVc sectors of MeA, the superficial small-celled AA, the medial sublenticular extended amygdala, and the anterior and posterior intermedial medium-celled BST. Fos-ir cells were almost completely absent in the posterior subdivisions of MeA and in the medial small-celled and lateral large-celled subdivisions of the BSTM. The Fos-positive labeling patterns of the present study appear to be far more restricted than those activated along the medial ExA in male rats exposed to an array of sexual stimuli.[73] Therefore, the functional/morphological findings of the present study suggest that the elements activated during sodium depletion may constitute a neuronal group independent from other medial ExA cells that are probably involved with other functions.

The results of this Fos study are consistent with previous reports showing that ablation of the medial or central ExA alter both angiotensin and mineralocorticoid-induced salt appetite.[52–55,57,59,60,63] The fact that no other subdivision of the central and medial ExA showed significant changes in the c-*fos* expression induced by sodium depletion suggests a specific activation of confined groups along the lateral ExA (central subdivision) and medial ExA (medial subdivision). These are locations where ANG II and ALDO appear to act to induce sodium intake.[2] The medial ExA is one of the regions of the brain with the highest uptake of ALDO;[74,75] thus it is a likely site where ALDO exerts its action to induce salt appetite.[53–55,57,58] ANG II-ir is found in the central ExA,[30] and the CeA contains angiotensinergic projections as well as mineralocorticoid receptors. This region has been postulated as a possible site of interaction between ANG II and ALDO, which can act synergistically to induce salt appetite.[17,76]

SUMMARY AND CONCLUSIONS

The maintenance of body fluid and cardiovascular homeostasis requires the integrative capacity of the CNS. The brain receives multiple types of visceral and somatic sensory input that allows computed "decisions" to be made that activate both reflexes and behaviors for optimizing fluid distribution and restoring balance. One of the key sets of behaviors that is necessary for recovering normal fluid balance are those that lead to the acquisition and consumption of sodium ions.

Progress has been made over recent years that indicates that the brain receives hormonal input from factors normally excluded by the blood-brain barrier (e.g., peptides such as ANG II) through sensory circumventricular organs. Afferent input from the viscera accesses the central neuraxis through the NTS. Information from such humoral and neural afferent inputs converges at various sites in the brain. One key area where this confluence takes place is in components of the ExA. Recent experimental evidence from several laboratories indicates that lesions of specific components of the ExA produce response deficits to various forms of an experimentally induced salt appetite. The present paper reviews studies in which lesions of the CeA and of the BST are shown to reduce salt appetite produced by both rapid onset and sodium depletion experimental models of salt appetite by approximately the same degree. Such findings are consistent with other studies using the Fos-ir method to detect neuronal populations within the ExA that were activated during sodium depletion. Taken together, both the functional and anatomical findings reported here provide support for the concept of the extended amygdala.

ACKNOWLEDGMENTS

This research was in part supported by Grants from the National Heart, Lung, and Blood Institute, HL14388 and HL57472; NASA NAG5-6171; the Office of Naval Research, N00014-97-1-0145; and a Fogarty International Research Collaboration Award, TW00965.

REFERENCES

1. DENTON, D. 1982. The Hunger for Salt. Springer-Verlag. New York.
2. SCHULKIN, J. 1991. Sodium Hunger: The Search for a Salty Taste. Cambridge University Press. New York.
3. NADEL, E.R., G.W. MACK & A. TAKAMATA. 1993. Thermoregulation, exercise, and thirst: interrelationships in humans. *In* Perspectives in Exercise Science and Sports Medicine, Vol. 6, Exercise, Heat, and Thermoregulation. C.V. Gisolfi, D.R. Lamb & E.R. Nadel, Eds.: 225–256. Brown & Benchmark. Dubuque.
4. TAKAMATA, A., G.W. MACK, C.M. GILLEN & E.R. NADEL. 1994. Sodium appetite, thirst, and body fluid regulation in humans during rehydration without sodium replacement. Am. J. Physiol. **266:** R1493–1502.
5. JOHNSON, A.K. & R.L. THUNHORST. 1995. Sensory mechanisms in the behavioral control of body fluid balance: thirst and salt appetite. *In* Progress in Psychobiology and Physiological Psychology. S.J. Fluharty, A.R. Morrison, J.M. Sprague & E. Stellar, Eds.: 145–176. Academic Press, Inc. New York.

6. JOHNSON, A.K. 1990. Brain mechanisms in the control of body fluid homeostasis. *In* Perspectives in Exercise Science and Sports Medicine: Fluid Homeostasis During Exercise. C.V. Gisolfi & D.R. Lamb, Eds.: 347–419. Benchmark Press. Dubuque.
7. ZARDETTO-SMITH, A.M., R.L. THUNHORST, M.Z. CICHA & A.K. JOHNSON. 1993. Afferent signaling and forebrain mechanisms in the behavioral control of extracellular fluid volume. *In* The Neurohypophysis: A Window on Brain Function. W.G. North, A.M. Moses & L. Share, Eds.: **689:** 161–176. Annals of the New York Academy of Sciences. New York.
8. FITZSIMONS, J.T. 1979. The Physiology of Thirst and Sodium Appetite. Cambridge University Press. United Kingdom.
9. STRICKER, E.M. & J.G. VERBALIS. 1990. Sodium appetite. *In* Handbook of Behavioral Neurobiology. Neurobiology of Food and Fluid Intake. E.M. Stricker, Ed.: **10:** 387–419. Plenum Press. New York.
10. VERNEY E.B. 1947. The antidiuretic hormone and the factors which determine its release. Proc. R. Soc. Lond. **135B:** 25–106.
11. WOLF, A.V. 1950. Osmometric analysis of thirst in man and dog. Am. J. Physiol. **161:**75–86.
12. JOHNSON, A.K. & P.M. GROSS. 1993. Sensory circumventricular organs and brain homeostatic pathways. FASEB J. **7:** 678–686.
13. JOHNSON, A.K. 1985. The periventricular anteroventral third ventricle (AV3V): Its relationship with the subfornical organ and neural systems involved in maintaining body fluid homeostasis. Brain Res. Bull. **15:** 595–601.
14. JOHNSON, A.K. & G.L. EDWARDS. 1991. Central projections of osmotic and hypovolaemic signals in homeostatic thirst. *In* Thirst. D.J. Ramsay & D.A. Booth, Eds.: 149–175. Springer-Verlag. New York.
15. EPSTEIN, A.N. 1982. Mineralocorticoids and cerebral angiotensin may act together to produce sodium appetite. Peptides **3:** 493–494.
16. WOLF, G. 1964. Sodium appetite elicited by aldosterone. Psychon. Sci. **I:** 211–212.
17. FLUHARTY, S.J. & A.N. EPSTEIN. 1983. Sodium appetite elicited by intracerebroventricular infusion of angiotensin II in the rat: Synergistic interaction with mineralocorticoid. Behav. Neurosci. **97:** 746–758.
18. JOHNSON, A. K. & R.L. THUNHORST. 1997. The neuroendocrinology of thirst and salt appetite: Visceral sensory signals and mechanisms of central integration. Front. Neuroendocrinol. **18:** 292–353.
19. MENANI, J.V. & A.K. JOHNSON. 1995. Lateral parabrachial serotonergic mechanisms: angiotensin-induced pressor and drinking responses. Am. J. Physiol. **269:** R1044–R1049.
20. MENANI, J.V., R.L. THUNHORST & A.K. JOHNSON. 1996. Lateral parabrachial nucleus and serotonergic mechanisms in the control of salt appetite in rats. Am. J. Physiol. **270:** R162–R168.
21. MASSI, M., L. GENTILI, M. PERFUMI, G. DE CARO & J. SCHULKIN. 1990. Inhibition of salt appetite in the rat following injection of tachykinins into the medial amygdala. Brain Res. **513:** 1–7.
22. MENANI, J.V. & A.K. JOHNSON. 1998. Cholecystokinin actions in the parabrachial nucleus: Effects on thirst and salt appetite. Am. J. Physiol. **275:** R1431–R1437.
23. DE CARO, G., C. POLIDORI, J.V. MENANI & A.K. JOHNSON. 1998. Bombesin affects the central nervous system to produce sodium intake inhibition in rats. Physiol. & Behav. **63:** 15–23.
24. GRILL, H.J., J. SCHULKIN & F.W. FLYNN. 1986. Sodium homeostasis in chronic decerebrate rats. Behav. Neurosci. **100:** 536–543.
25. FLYNN, F.W. & H.J. GRILL. 1983. Insulin elicits ingestion in decerebrate rats. Science **221:** 188–190.
26. JOHNSON, A.K., J.T. CUNNINGHAM & R.L. THUNHORST. 1996. Integrative role of the lamina terminalis in the regulation of cardiovascular and body fluid homeostasis. Clin. Exp. Pharmacol. Physiol. **23:** 183–191.
27. FITTS, D.A., D.S. TJEPKES & R.O. BRIGHT. 1990. Salt appetite and lesions of the ventral part of the ventral median preoptic nucleus. Behav. Neurosci. **104:** 818–827.

28. FITTS, D.A. 1991. Effects of lesions of the ventral median preoptic nucleus or subfornical organ on drinking and salt appetite after deoxycorticosterone acetate or yohimbine. Behav. Neurosci. **105(5):** 721–726.
29. DE LUCA, JR., L.A., O. GALAVERNA, J. SCHULKIN, S-Z YAO & A.N. EPSTEIN. 1992. The anteroventral wall of the third ventricle and the angiotensinergic component of need-induced sodium intake in the rat. Brain Res. Bull. **28:** 73–87.
30. LIND, R.W. & D. GANTEN. 1990. Angiotensin. *In* The Handbook of Chemical Neuroanatomy, Neuropeptides in the CNS. A. Bjorklund, T. Hokfelt & M.J. Kuhar, Eds.: **9:** 165–286. Elsevier. New York.
31. MISELIS, R.R., M.L. WEISS & R.E. SHAPIRO. 1987. Modulation of the visceral neuraxis. *In* Circumventricular Organs and Body Fluids, Volume III. P.M. Gross, Ed.: 143–162. CRC Press. Boca Raton.
32. MCEWEN B.S., R. DEKLOET & W. ROSTENE. 1986. Adrenal steroid receptors and actions in the nervous system. Physiol. Rev. **66:** 1121–1188.
33. CONTRERAS, R.J. & P.W. STETSON. 1981. Changes in salt intake after lesions of the area postrema and the nucleus of the solitary tract in rats. Brain Res. **211:** 355–366.
34. EDWARDS, G.L., T.G. BELTZ, J.D. POWER & A.K. JOHNSON. 1993. Rapid onset "need-free" sodium appetite after lesions of the dorsomedial medulla. Am. J. Physiol. **264:** R1242–R1247.
35. SHAPIRO, R.E. & R.R. MISELIS. 1985. The central neural connections of the area postrema of the rat. J. Comp. Neurol. **234:** 344–364.
36. CUNNINGHAM, JR., E.T., R.R. MISELIS & P.E. SAWCHENKO. 1994. The relationship of efferent projections from the area postrema to vagal motor and brain stem catecholamine-containing cell groups: an axonal transport and immunohistochemical study in the rat. Neuroscience **58(3):** 635–648.
37. VAN DER KOOY, D. & L.Y. KODA. 1983. Organization of the projections of a circumventricular organ: the area postrema in the rat. J. Comp. Neurol. **219:** 328–338.
38. LANÇA, A.J. & D. VAN DER KOOY. 1985. A serotonin-containing pathway from the area postrema to the parabrachial nucleus in the rat. Neuroscience **14:** 1117–1126.
39. MENANI, J.V., D.S.A. COLOMBARI, T.G. BELTZ, R.L. THUNHORST & A.K. JOHNSON. 1998. Salt appetite: interaction of forebrain angiotensinergic and hindbrain serotonergic mechanisms. Brain Res. **801:** 29–35.
40. COLOMBARI, D.S.A., J.V. MENANI & A.K. JOHNSON. 1996. Forebrain angiotensin type 1 receptors and parabrachial serotonin in the control of NaCl and water intake. Am. J. Physiol. **271:** R1470–R1476.
41. MENANI, J.V., L.A. DE LUCA JR. & A.K. JOHNSON. 1998. Lateral parabrachial nucleus serotonergic mechanisms and salt appetite induced by sodium depletion. Am. J. Physiol. **274:** R555–R560.
42. OHMAN, L.E. & A.K. JOHNSON. 1995. Role of lateral parabrachial nucleus in the inhibition of water intake produced by right atrial stretch. Brain Res. **695:** 275–278.
43. EDWARDS, G.L. & A.K. JOHNSON. 1991. Enhanced drinking after excitotoxic lesions of the parabrachial nucleus in the rat. Am. J. Physiol. **261:** R1039–R1044.
44. TAKEUCHI, Y., J.H. MCLEAN & D.A. HOPKINS. 1982. Reciprocal connections between the amygdala and parabrachial nuclei: Ultrastructural demonstration by degeneration and axonal transport of horseradish peroxidase in the cat. Brain Res. **239:** 583–588.
45. ALHEID, G.F., J. DE OLMOS & C.A. BELTRAMINO. 1995. Amygdala and extended amygdala. *In* The Rat Nervous System, 2nd Edition. G. Paxinos, Ed.: 495–578. Academic Press. San Diego.
46. DEOLMOS, J., G.F. ALHEID & C.A. BELATRIMINO. 1985. Amygdala. *In* The Rat Nervous System, Vol. 1. Forebrain and Midbrain. G. Paxinos, Ed.: 223–334. Academic Press. Orlando.
47. PRICE, J.L., F.T. RUSSCHEN & D.G. AMARAL. 1987. The limbic region III: The amygdaloid complex. *In* Handbook of Chemical Neuroanatomy, Vol. 5: Integrated Systems of the CNS, Part 1. A. Björklund, T. Hökfelt & L.W. Swanson, Eds.: 279–388. Elsevier. Amsterdam.

48. JOHNSTON, J.B. 1923. Further contributions to the study of the evolution of the forebrain. J. Comp. Neurol. **35:** 337–481.
49. DEOLMOS, J.S. 1990. Amygdala. *In* The Human Nervous System. G. Paxinos. Ed.: 583–710. Academic Press. Marrickville, NSW, Australia.
50. GENTIL, C.G., J. ANTUNES-RODRIGUES, A. NEGRO-VILAR & M.R. COVIAN. 1968. Role of amygdaloid complex in sodium chloride and water intake in the rat. Physiol. Behav. **3:** 981–985.
51. COX, J.R., C.E. CRUZ & J. RUGER. 1978. Effects of total amygdalectomy upon salt regulation in rats. Brain Res. Bull. **3:** 431–435.
52. CHIARAVIGLIO, E. 1971. Amygdaloid modulation of sodium chloride and water intake in the rat. J. Comp. Physiol. Psychol. **76:** 401–407.
53. NITABACH, M.N., J. SCHULKIN & A.N. EPSTEIN. 1989. The medial amygdala is a part of a mineralocorticoid-sensitive circuit controlling NaCl intake in the rat. Behav. Brain Res. **35:** 127–134.
54. SCHULKIN, J., J. MARINI & A.N. EPSTEIN. 1989. A role for the medial region of the amygdala in mineralocorticoid-induced salt hunger. Behav.Neurosci.**103:** 178–185.
55. ZHANG, D.M., A.N. EPSTEIN & J. SHULKIN. 1993. Medial region of the amygdala: involvement in adrenal-steroid-induced salt appetite. Brain Res. **600:** 20–26.
56. BLACK, R.M., H.P. WEINGARTEN, A.N. EPSTEIN, R. MAKI & J. SCHULKIN. 1992. Transection of the stria terminalis without damage to the medial amygdala does not alter behavioural sodium regulation in rats. Acta Neurobiol. Exp. **52:** 9–15.
57. REILLY, J.J., D.B. MAMANI, J. SCHULKIN, B. SLOTNIK, B.S. MCEWEN & R.R. SAKAI. 1993. Adrenal steroid implants into amygdala arouse sodium intake in the rat [Abstract]. Soc. Neurosci. Abstr. **19:** 582.
58. SAKAI R.R., L.Y. MA, D.M. ZHANG, B.S. MCEWEN & S.J. FLUHARTY. 1996. Intracerebral administration of mineralocorticoid receptor antisense oligonucleotides attenuate adrenal steroid-induced salt appetite in rats. Neuroendocrinology **64:** 425–429.
59. GALAVERNA, O., L.A. DE LUCA JR., J. SCHULKIN, S-Z YAO & A.N. EPSTEIN. 1992. Deficits in NaCl ingestion after damage to the central nucleus of the amygdala in the rat. Brain Res. Bull. **28:** 89–98.
60. ZARDETTO-SMITH, A.M., T.G. BELTZ & A.K. JOHNSON. 1994. Role of the central nucleus of the amygdala and bed nucleus of the stria terminalis in experimentally-induced salt appetite. Brain Res. **645:** 123–134.
61. GALAVERNA, O.G., R.J. SEELEY, K.C. BERRIDGE, H.J. GRILL, A.N. EPSTEIN & J. SCHULKIN. 1993. Lesions of the central nucleus of the amygdala. I: Effects on taste reactivity, taste aversion learning and sodium appetite. Behav. Brain Res. **59:** 11–17.
62. SEELEY, R.J., O. GALAVERNA, J. SCHULKIN, A.N. EPSTEIN & H.J. GRILL. 1993. Lesions of the central nucleus of the amygdala. II: Effects on intraoral NaCl intake. Behav. Brain Res. **59:** 19–25.
63. REILLY, J.J., R. MAKI, J. NARDOZZI & J. SCHULKIN. 1994. The effects of lesions of the bed nucleus of the stria terminalis on sodium appetite. Acta Neurobiol. Exp. **54:** 253–257.
64. POMPEI, P., S.J. TAYEBATY, G. DE CARO, J. SCHULKIN & M. MASSI. 1991. Bed nucleus of the stria terminalis: site for the antinatriorexic action of tachykinins in the rat. Pharmacol. Biochem. Behav. **40:** 977–981.
65. PASTUSKOVAS, C., L. VIVAS & J. DE OLMOS. 1997. Expresión de c-fos en la division lateral de la amigdala extendida (AEx) de ratas sujetas a una depleción aguda de sodio corporal. Rev. Fac. Med. Caracas N: 1, **20:** 108.
66. PASTUSKOVAS, C., L. VIVAS & J. DE OLMOS. 1998. Role of the medial extended amygdala (MExA) on sodium appetite in rats [Abstract]. Appetite. In press.
67. FERREYRA, M.D. & E. CHIARAVIGLIO. 1977. Changes in volemia and natremia and onset of sodium appetite in sodium depleted rats. Physiol. Behav. **19:** 197–201.
68. VIVAS L., C.V. PASTUSKOVAS & L. TONELLI. 1995. Sodium depletion induces Fos inmunoreactivity in the circumventricular organs of the lamina terminalis. Brain Res. **679:** 34–41.

69. PASTUSKOVAS, C. & L. VIVAS. 1997. Effect of intravenous captopril on c-*fos* expression induced by sodium depletion in neurons of the lamina terminalis. Brain Res. Bull. **44:** 233–236.
70. HEIMER, L., J.S. DE OLMOS, G.F. ALHEID, J. PEARSON, N. SAKAMOTO, J. MARKSTEINER & R.C. SWITZER. 1999. The Human Basal Forebrain, Part II, 3. Extended Amygdala. *In* Handbook of Chemical Neuroanatomy. Vol. 15: The Primate Nervous System. Part III. F.E. Bloom, A. Björklund & T. Hökfelt, Eds.: Elsevier Science B.V.
71. LANE, J.M., J. HERBERT & J.T. FITZSIMONS. 1997. Increased sodium appetite stimulates c-fos expression in the organum vasculosum of the lamina terminalis. Neuroscience **78:** 1167–1176.
72. THUNHORST R.L., Z. XU, M.Z. CICHA, A.M. ZARDETTO-SMITH & A.K. JOHNSON. 1998. Fos expression in rat brain during depletion-induced thirst and salt appetite. Am. J. Physiol. **274:** R1807–1814.
73. BAUM, M.J. & B.J. EVERITT. 1992. Increased expression of c-fos in the medial preoptic area after mating in male rats: role of afferent inputs from the medial amygdala and midbrain central tegmental field. Neuroscience **50:** 627–646.
74. DE NICOLA A.F., C. GRILLO & S. GONZALEZ. 1992. Physiological, biochemical and molecular mechanisms of salt appetite control by mineralocorticoid action in brain. Brazilian J. Med. Biol. Res. **25:** 1153–1162.
75. MCEWEN, B.S., L.T. LAMBDIN, T.C. RAINBOW & A.F. DE NICOLA. 1986. Aldosterone: effects on salt appetite in adrenalectomized rats. Neuroendocrinology **43:** 38–43.
76. THORTON, S.N. & S. NICOLAIDIS. 1994. Long term mineralocorticoid-induced changes in rat neuron properties plus interaction of aldosterone and ANG II. Am. J. Physiol. **266:** R564–R571.
77. PAXINOS, G. & C. WATSON. 1986. The Rat Brain in Stereotaxic Coordinates. Academic Press. New York.

The Extended Amygdala: Are the Central Nucleus of the Amygdala and the Bed Nucleus of the Stria Terminalis Differentially Involved in Fear versus Anxiety?

MICHAEL DAVIS[a] AND CHANGJUN SHI

Emory University School of Medicine, Department of Psychiatry, 1639 Pierce Drive, Suite 4000, Room 4311, Atlanta, Georgia 30322, USA

ABSTRACT: Although there is a close correspondence between fear and anxiety, and the study of fear in animals has been extremely valuable for understanding the neural basis of anxiety, it is also clear that a richer animal model of human anxiety disorders would include measures of both stimulus-specific fear and something less stimulus specific, more akin to anxiety. Patients with posttraumatic stress syndrome seem to show normal fear reactions but abnormal anxiety measured with the acoustic startle reflex. Studies in rats, also using the startle reflex, indicate that highly processed explicit cue information (lights, tones) activates the central nucleus of the amygdala, which projects to and modulates the acoustic startle pathway in the brain stem. Less explicit information, such as that produced by exposure to a threating environment or by intraventricular administration of corticotropin-releasing hormone, may activate another part of the extended amygdala, the bed nucleus of the stria terminalis, which also projects to the startle pathway. Because this information may be less specific and of long duration, activation of the bed nucleus of the stria terminalis may mediate anxiety, whereas activation of the central nucleus of the amygdala may mediate stimulus-specific fear.

INTRODUCTION

Over the last several years, our laboratory has been studying how a simple reflex, the acoustic startle reflex, can be modified by treatments that produce a pattern of behavioral reactions seen during states of fear and anxiety in people. Recent data now suggest that different parts of the extended amygdala may be involved when different methods are used to produce emotional behavior. This has led us to suggest that different parts of the extended amygdala may be involved in fear versus anxiety, which could have significant clinical implications.

THE FEAR-POTENTIATED STARTLE EFFECT

When the startle reflex is elicited by a loud sound 3-4 seconds after a light has been turned on, there is no systematic change in the amplitude of the startle reflex.

[a]Voice: 404-727-3591; fax: 404-727-3436; mdavis4@emory.edu

However, if the day before, or even a month before, the light had come on 3-4 s before a shock for a few times, startle would have been potentiated when elicited after the light came on. This fear-potentiated startle effect, first described by Brown,[4] only occurs following prior light-shock pairings and not when lights and shocks have been presented in an unpaired or "random" relationship,[9] indicating its dependence on prior pavlovian fear conditioning. When the eyeblink component of the startle reflex is measured in humans, fear-potentiated startle can be produced using very similar conditioning procedures to those we use in rodents.[18] If the light is presented over and over again, without further light-shock pairings, it no longer increases startle,[12] indicative of extinction of prior fear conditioning. This effect probably indicates that the light produces a state of fear that increases reflexive behavior, because drugs like diazepam or buspirone, which reduce fear in humans, block the increase in startle in the presence of the light but do not systematically alter startle in the absence of the light when appropriate doses are used.

THE LIGHT-ENHANCED STARTLE EFFECT

When the startle reflex is elicited by a loud sound 5–20 min after a bright light has been turned on, there is an increase in the startle reflex.[38] This effect also is significantly decreased by drugs like buspirone[38] or chlordiazepoxide (Walker and Davis, unpublished observations). This may indicate an unconditioned anxiogenic effect of bright light that enhances startle, consistent with several other behavioral measures[7,15] (see ref. 40 for a review). Recently, we have found that humans show a significant increase of startle amplitude (i.e., of the eyeblink response) in the dark.[20] The species difference may reflect fear of the light in a nocturnal species (rats) compared to fear of the dark in a diurnal species (humans). When the lights are suddenly turned off, many people feel more anxious, especially if they had been afraid of the dark when they were young.[20] In patients with posttraumatic stress disorder, startle is increased in the dark to a greater degree than that seen in combat controls.[19] These individuals report that the darkness makes them think of being back at their guard post in Vietnam and anxious about being hit by an incoming mortar.

As far as we can tell, light-enhanced startle in rats does not depend on prior conditioning. Moreover, at least in rats, this method of increasing startle does not extinguish because it does not decrease in magnitude either within or across several test sessions.[38] Hence, this method of increasing startle seems to reflect an unconditioned, rather than a conditioned, anxiogenic effect. It is less certain whether dark-enhanced startle in people results from prior conditioning, although explicit conditioning in the laboratory is not required to see this phenomenon.

THE ROLE OF THE AMYGDALA IN FEAR-POTENTIATED STARTLE

Like other measures of fear, there is a great deal of evidence that the amygdala is critically involved in both the acquisition and expression of fear-potentiated startle (cf. ref. 8). Lesions of the central nucleus of the amygdala (CeA) block the expression of fear-potentiated startle using either a visual[23] or auditory conditioned stimulus.[5,22] Blockade of glutamate receptors in the CeA via local infusion of a non-NMDA glutamate receptor antagonist has a similar effect.[25] The CeA projects directly to the nucleus reticularis pontis caudalis,[33] a critical part of the acoustic startle pathway,[31] and lesions at several points along this pathway blocked the expression of fear-potentiated startle.[21] Both conditioned fear and sensitization of startle by footshocks appear to ultimately modulate startle at the level of the nucleus reticularis pontis caudalis.[2,3,26] Selective destruction of cell bodies via local infusion of neurotoxic doses of NMDA into the lateral and basolateral nuclei caused a complete blockade of fear-potentiated startle when the lesions were made either before or after training.[35] All animals had sparing of the CeA. This blockade of fear-potentiated startle did not seem to result from a disruption of vision, and other studies found that NMDA-induced lesions of these amygdaloid nuclei also blocked fear-potentiated startle using an auditory conditioned stimulus.[5] These results are consistent with other work that indicates that the lateral nucleus of the amygdala provides a critical link for relaying auditory information involved in fear conditioning to the amygdala.[27]

Because the CeA projects directly to the nucleus reticularis pontis caudalis[33] and lesions at several points along this pathway blocked the expression of fear-potentiated startle,[21] we suggested that this direct pathway may mediate both fear potentiated startle and sensitization of startle produced by prior footshocks.[21,24] However, those studies only used electrolytic lesions of the amygdalofugal pathway at several levels, including the ventrolateral central gray, so that obligatory synapses at points along this pathway could not be ruled out.[21] Recent data now suggest that a synapse between the amygdala and the central gray may be required for both fear-potentiated startle and shock sensitization, because fiber-sparing chemical lesions of the central gray have been reported to block both phenomena.[14,16]

DIFFERENTIAL EFFECTS OF INACTIVATION OF THE AMYGDALA VERSUS THE BED NUCLEUS OF THE STRIA TERMINALIS ON FEAR-POTENTIATED STARTLE VERSUS LIGHT-ENHANCED STARTLE

Because, as mentioned above, local infusion of glutamate antagonists into the CeA completely blocks the expression of fear-potentiated startle,[25] we wondered whether this treatment would also block light-enhanced startle. As a control, we measured the effects of local infusion of glutamate antagonists into the bed nucleus of the stria terminalis (BNST). This is considered to be part of the so-called extended amygdala because it is highly similar to the CeA in terms of its transmitter content, cell morphology, and efferent connections.[1] However, lesions of the BNST fail to block either fear-potentiated startle[21] or conditioned freezing using an explicit cue,[28] suggesting that it may not be involved in explicit cue conditioning. On the other hand, several ongoing studies in our laboratory suggested that the BNST might be involved in elevations of startle that were more long lasting than the increase in startle observed in explicit cue conditioning. For example, lesions of the BNST blocked long-term sensitization of the startle reflex[17] or the excitatory effect of the peptide corticotropin-releasing hormone on startle[30] (see below).

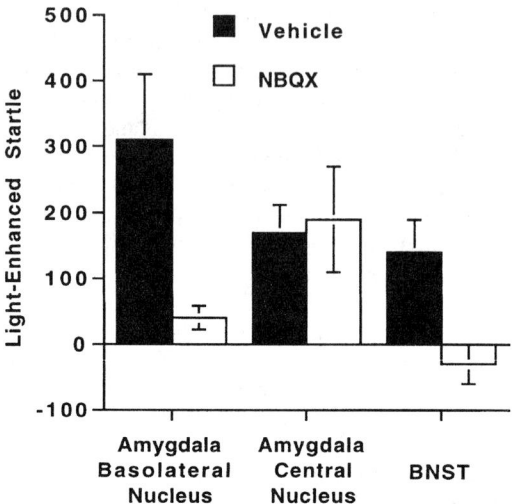

FIGURE 1. Glutamate inactivation of basolateral amygdala or BNST but not central amygdala blocks light-enhanced startle. Mean change in startle amplitude from the dark phase to the light phase (light-enhanced startle) after infusion of the glutamate antagonist NBQX or its vehicle into either the basolateral nucleus of the amygdala, the central nucleus of the amygdala, or the lateral bed nucleus of the stria terminalis.

To evaluate the role of the BNST versus the amygdala in light-enhanced startle, animals were implanted with bilateral cannulas in either the BNST, the basolateral complex of the amygdala (i.e., the lateral and basolateral nuclei), or the CeA.[39] One week later animals were tested for light-enhanced startle shortly following bilateral infusion of the glutamate antagonist, NBQX, into the different brain areas. FIGURE 1 shows the results. Local inactivation of either the basolateral nucleus of the amygdala or the BNST significantly decreased light-enhanced startle. Other studies showed that this could not be attributed to a general depressant effect on baseline startle. To our surprise, however, infusion of the glutamate antagonist into the CeA had no effect.

These data indicate an important role for both the lateral/basolateral amygdala complex and the BNST in light-enhanced startle. It is possible, however, that the cannulas in the CeA were misplaced and that this accounted for the lack of an effect of inactivation of the central nucleus on light-enhanced startle. To evaluate this, the rats used in the light-enhanced startle experiment were trained and tested for fear-potentiated startle after infusion of NBQX into either the amygdala or BNST. FIGURE 2 shows that, consistent with previous results, infusion of the glutamate antagonist into the CeA completely blocked the expression of fear-potentiated startle. This was also true after an infusion of NBQX into the basolateral nucleus of the amygdala. By contrast, infusion of NBQX into the BNST had no effect on fear-potentiated startle. These data indicate, therefore, that the location of the cannulas in the CeA was adequate to allow infusion of NBQX to totally block fear-potentiated startle. Hence, the ineffectiveness of NBQX infused into the CeA to block light-en-

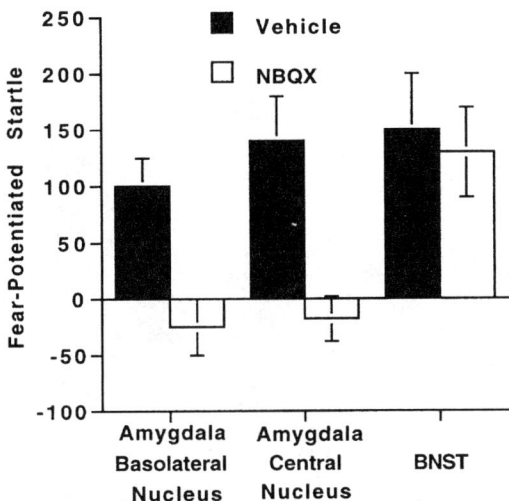

FIGURE 2. Glutamate inactivation of basolateral or central amygdala, but not BNST, blocks fear-potentiated startle. Mean change in startle amplitude on the light–noise versus the noise alone trials (fear-potentiated startle) after infusion of the glutamate antagonist NBQX or its vehicle into either the basolateral nucleus of the amygdala, the central nucleus of the amygdala, or the lateral bed nucleus of the stria terminalis.

hanced startle cannot be attributed to misplaced cannulas. Moreover, these data show a double dissociation between inactivation of glutamate receptors in the CeA versus the BNST in relationship to fear-potentiated versus light-enhanced startle.

PROJECTIONS FROM THE BASOLATERAL NUCLEUS OF THE AMYGDALA TO THE CEA VERSUS THE LATERAL BNST

At this time it is certainly not clear why the CeA and the BNST seem to play different roles in relationship to fear-potentiated startle versus light-enhanced startle. Both effects are produced by exposure to the very same light using exactly the same response measure. Both are sensitive to anxiolytic compounds. One difference is that fear-potentiated startle is a phasic event, where the light facilitates startle almost immediately after it is turned on, but then this effect subsides quickly, once the light is turned off.[11] Light-enhanced startle takes more time to develop and lasts for a much longer period of time once the light goes off.[38] Perhaps, therefore, sustained increases in startle require the BNST and not the CeA. However, local infusion of NBQX into the CeA also decreases contextual fear-potentiated startle (startle amplitude facilitation caused by returning the animal to the box where it previously was shocked; McNish and Davis, unpublished observations). Like light-enhanced startle, context conditioning represents a sustained way to increase startle because animals continue to show elevated levels of startle even after being in the fearful context for many min-

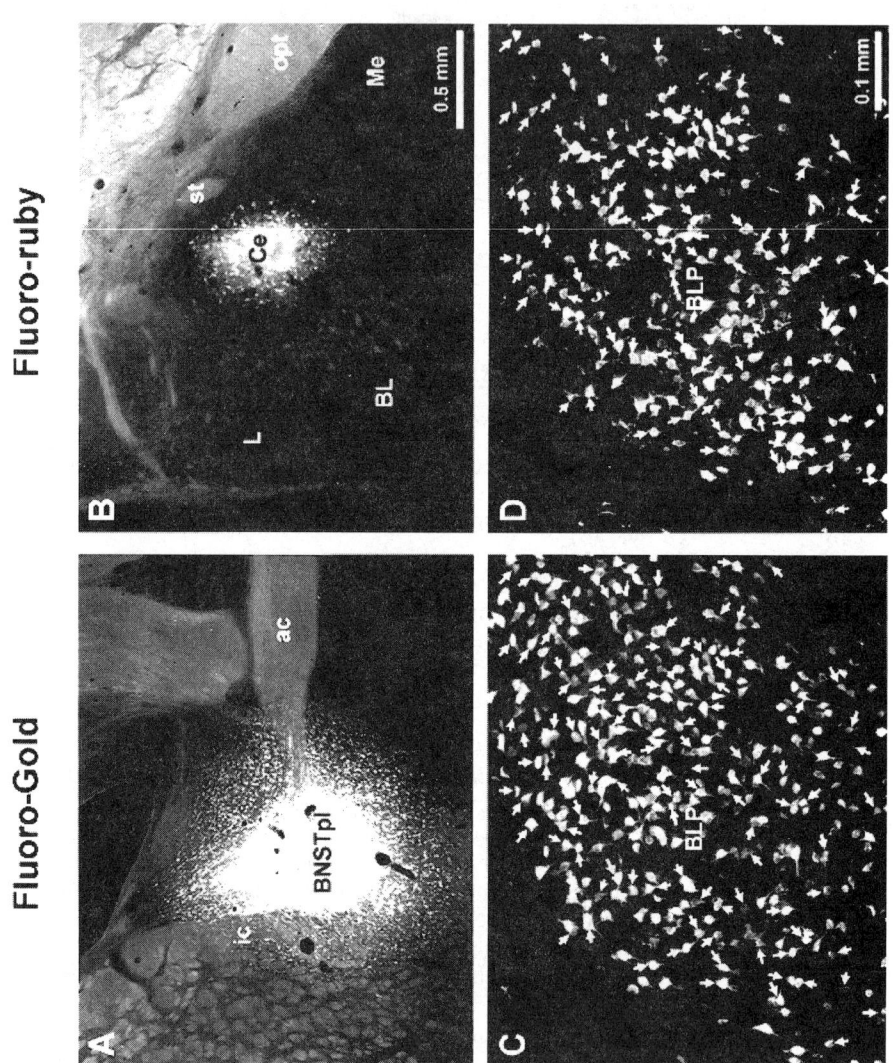

utes. These data would suggest that the CeA is still necessary for tonic increases in startle.

A major difference between fear-potentiated startle, be it in the presence of an explicit cue or a context, and light-enhanced startle is that fear-potentiated startle depends on prior conditioning, whereas light-enhanced startle does not. Perhaps, therefore, the CeA is especially important when stimuli have been paired with shock, whereas the BNST responds to stimuli that are anxiogenic but not by virtue of being paired with shock.

Considerable data now indicate that the basolateral complex of the amygdala (lateral, basolateral, and basomedial nuclei) is important for the acquisition of fear-potentiated startle when aversive shocks are used. Local infusion of NMDA antagonists into the basolateral amygdala blocks the acquisition but not the expression of fear-potentiated startle.[6,32] Fanselow and Kim[13] found that local infusion of an NMDA antagonist into the basolateral amygdala blocked the acquisition of conditioned freezing, whereas infusion into the CeA did not. We have found similar effects using fear-potentiated startle (Walker and Davis, unpublished observations). These and other data suggest that the association between a conditioned stimulus and footshock may occur in the basolateral amygdala, which then projects to the CeA to affect various behaviors. Perhaps, therefore, neurons in the basolateral amygdala that project to the CeA also receive inputs from pain pathways (cf. ref. 36), whereas neurons in the basolateral amygdala that project to the BNST do not. This could explain why connections between the basolateral amygdala and the CeA are involved in conditioned fear, whereas connections between the basolateral amygdala and BNST are not.

To begin to explore this question, each rat was infused with two different retrograde tracers, one into the CeA and the other in the lateral division of the BNST. Histological examination of their brains indicated that many cells in the posterior division of the basolateral nucleus of the amygdala project to both the CeA and the BNST. Importantly, however, there were also a large number of cells that were not double labeled (FIG. 3). This indicates that some cells in the basolateral nucleus of the amygdala project to the CeA and not the BNST and other cells in the basolateral nucleus project to BNST but not the CeA. This conclusion has been confirmed using anterograde tracers with axon reconstruction. Perhaps, therefore, only those cells that uniquely project to the CeA receive afferent pain information necessary for the acquisition of conditioned effects. Although this will be difficult to demonstrate, it provides a way to think about the different roles played by the CeA versus the BNST in fear-potentiated versus light-enhanced startle.

FIGURE 3. A: Photomicrograph of a deposit of Fluoro-Gold in the posterolateral BNST. **B:** Photomicrograph of a deposit of Fluoro-ruby in the CeA. **C:** Neurons labeled with Fluro-Gold in the posterior region of the basolateral amygdala following infusion of Fluoro-Gold in the posterolateral BNST. Arrows indicate cells that were also labeled with Fluoro-ruby infused into the CeA. **D:** Neurons labeled with Fluoro-ruby in the posterior region of the basolateral amygdala following infusion of Fluoro-ruby in the CeA. Arrows indicate cells that were also labeled with Fluoro-Gold infused into the posterolateral BNST.

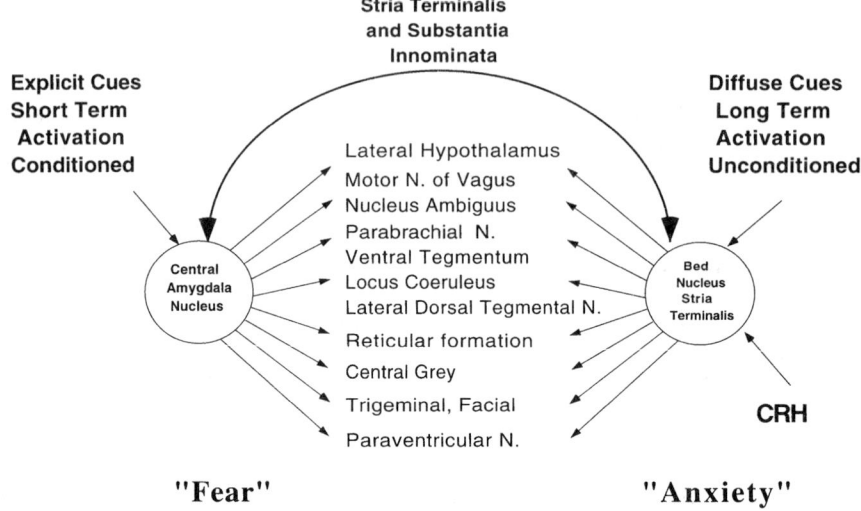

FIGURE 4. Hypothetical schematic suggesting that the central nucleus of the amygdala and the bed nucleus of the stria terminalis may be differentially involved in fear versus anxiety, respectively. Both brain areas have highly similar hypothalamic and brain-stem targets known to be involved in specific signs and symptoms of fear and anxiety. However, the stress peptide CRH appears to act on receptors in the bed nucleus of the stria terminalis rather than the amygdala, at least in terms of an increase in the startle reflex. Furthermore, the bed nucleus of the stria terminalis seems to be involved in the anxiogenic effects of a very bright light presented for a long period of time but not when that very same light has previously been paired with a shock. Just the opposite is the case for the central nucleus of the amygdala, which is critical for fear conditioning using explicit cues, such as a light or tone paired with aversive stimulation (i.e., conditioned fear).

DIFFERENTIAL ROLES OF THE BNST AND THE CEA IN FEAR VERSUS ANXIETY

We have found a clear distinction between the CeA and the BNST in relationship to fear-potentiated startle versus light-enhanced startle. Other work has shown that the peptide, corticotropin-releasing hormone (CRH), increases startle after intraventricular administration by acting on receptors in the BNST and not in the amygdala.[29,30] Because the facilitatory effect of CRH on startle appears to be anxiogenic, given that it is blocked by anxiolytic compounds, such as chordiazepoxide,[37] but does not require conditioning, provides further evidence for a role of the BNST in unconditioned anxiogenic effects. We suggest that the BNST may be a system that responds to signals more akin to anxiety than those akin to fear, whereas the CeA is clearly involved in fear and perhaps not as much in anxiety (FIG. 4). Both these structures have very similar efferent connections to various hypothalamic and brain-stem target areas known to be involved in specific signs and symptoms of fear and anxiety (cf. ref. 8). Both receive highly processed sensory information from the basolateral nucleus of the amygdala and hence are in a position to respond to emotionally significant stimuli. Corticotropin-releasing hormone is known to be released during periods of stress or anxiety, some of which may come from corticotropin-releasing hormone–containing neurons in the CeA that project to and act on receptors in the BNST.[34] Thus, phasic activation of the amygdala by certain stressors could lead to a long-term activation of the BNST via corticotropin-releasing hormone. Assuming that phasic activation is like fear, whereas sustained activation of similar structures is like anxiety, would suggest differential roles of the amygdala versus the BNST in fear versus anxiety, respectively. Because of the potential clinical implications of this distinction, further investigation of the functional similarities and differences between these two parts of the extended amygdala is currently under way.

ACKNOWLEDGMENTS

Research reported in this chapter was supported by NIMH Grants MH-57250 and MH-47840; Research Scientist Development Award MH-00004; a grant from the Air Force Office of Scientific Research; and the State of Connecticut.

REFERENCES

1. ALHEID, G., J.S. DE OLMOS & C.A. BELTRAMINO. 1995. Amygdala and extended amygdala. *In* The Rat Nervous System. G. Paxinos, Ed.: 495–578. Academic Press. New York.
2. BERG, W.K. & M. DAVIS. 1985. Associative learning modifies startle reflexes at the lateral lemniscus. Behav. Neurosci. **99:** 191–199.
3. BOULIS, N. & M. DAVIS. 1989. Footshock-induced sensitization of electrically elicited startle reflexes. Behav. Neurosci. **103:** 504–508.
4. BROWN, J. S., H.I. KALISH & I.E. FARBER. 1951. Conditional fear as revealed by magnitude of startle response to an auditory stimulus. J. Exp. Psychol. **41:** 317–328.
5. CAMPEAU, S. & M. DAVIS. 1995. Involvement of the central nucleus and basolateral complex of the amygdala in fear conditioning measured with fear-potentiated startle in rats trained concurrently with auditory and visual conditioned stimuli. J. Neurosci. **15:** 2301–2311.
6. CAMPEAU, S., M.J.D. MISERENDINO & M. DAVIS. 1992. Intra-amygdala infusion of the *N*-methyl-D-aspartate receptor antagonist AP5 blocks acquisition but not expression of fear-potentiated startle to an auditory conditioned stimulus. Behav. Neurosci. **106:** 569–574.
7. CRAWLEY, J.N. 1981. Neuropharmacologic specificity of a simple animal model for the behavioral actions of benzodiazepines. Pharmacol. Biochem. Behav. **15:** 695–699.
8. DAVIS, M. 1992. The role of the amygdala in conditioned fear. *In* The Amygdala: Eurobiological Aspects of Emotion, Memory and Mental Dysfunction. J. Aggleton, Ed.: 255–305. John Wiley & Sons, Inc. New York.
9. DAVIS, M. & D.I. ASTRACHAN. 1978. Conditioned fear and startle magnitude: effects of different footshock or backshock intensities used in training. J. Exp. Psychol. Anim. Behav. Processes **4:** 95–103.
10. DAVIS, M., W.A. FALLS, S. CAMPEAU & M. KIM. 1993. Fear-potentiated startle: a neural and pharmacological analysis. Behav. Brain Res. **58:** 175–198.
11. DAVIS, M., L.S. SCHLESINGER & C.A. SORENSON. 1989. Temporal specificity of fear-conditioning: effects of different conditioned stimulus-unconditioned stimulus intervals on the fear-potentiated startle effect. J. Exp. Psychol. Anim. Behav. Processes **15:** 295–310.

12. FALLS, W.A., M.J.D. MISERENDINO & M. DAVIS. 1992. Extinction of fear-potentiated startle: blockade by infusion of an NMDA antagonist into the amygdala. J. Neurosci. **12:** 854–863.
13. FANSELOW, M.S. & J.J. KIM. 1994. Acquisition of contextual Pavlovian fear conditioning is blocked by application of an NMDA receptor antagonist D,L-2-amino-5-phosphonovaleric acid to the basolateral amygdala. Behav. Neurosci. **108:** 210–212.
14. FENDT, M., M. KOCH & H.-U. SCHNITZLER. 1996. Lesions of the central gray block conditioned fear as measured with the potentiated startle paradigm. Behav. Brain Res. **74:** 127–134.
15. FILE, S.E. 1980. The use of social interaction as a method for detecting anxiolytic activity of chlordiazepoxide-like drugs. J. Neurosci. Methods **2:** 219–238.
16. FRANKLIN, P.W. & J.S. YEOMANS. 1995. Fear-potentiated startle and electrically evoked startle mediated by synapses in rostrolateral midbrain. Behav. Neurosci. **109:** 669–680.
17. GEWIRTZ, J.C., K.A. MCNISH & M. DAVIS. 1998. Lesions of the bed nucleus of the stria terminalis block sensitization of the acoustic startle reflex produced by repeated stress, but not fear-potentiated startle. Prog. Neuro-Psychopharmacol. Biol. Psychology **22:** 625–648.
18. GRILLON, C. & M. DAVIS. 1997. Fear-potentiated startle conditioning in humans: effects of explicit and contextual cue conditioning following paired vs. unpaired training. Psychophysiology **34:** 451–458.
19. GRILLON, C., C.A. MORGAN, M. DAVIS & S.M. SOUTHWICK. 1998. Effects of darkness on acoustic startle in Vietnam veterans with PTSD. Am. J. Psychiat. **155:** 812–817.
20. GRILLON, C., M. PELLOWSKI, K.R. MERIKANGAS & M. DAVIS. 1997. Darkness facilitates the acoustic startle reflex in humans. Biol. Psychiatry **42:** 461–471.
21. HITCHCOCK, J.M. & M. DAVIS. 1991. The efferent pathway of the amygdala involved in conditioned fear as measured with the fear-potentiated startle paradigm. Behav. Neurosci. **105:** 826–842.
22. HITCHCOCK, J.M. & M. DAVIS. 1987. Fear-potentiated startle using an auditory conditioned stimulus: effect of lesions of the amygdala. Physiol. & Behav. **39:** 403–408.
23. HITCHCOCK, J.M. & M. DAVIS. 1986. Lesions of the amygdala, but not of the cerebellum or red nucleus, block conditioned fear as measured with the potentiated startle paradigm. Behav. Neurosci. **100:** 11–22.
24. HITCHCOCK, J.M., C.B. SANANES & M. DAVIS. 1989. Sensitization of the startle reflex by footshock: blockade by lesions of the central nucleus of the amygdala or its efferent pathway to the brainstem. Behav. Neurosci. **103:** 509–518.
25. KIM, M., S. CAMPEAU, W.A. FALLS & M. DAVIS. 1993. Infusion of the non-NMDA receptor antagonist CNQX into the amygdala blocks the expression of fear-potentiated startle. Behav. Neural Biol. **59:** 5–8.
26. KRASE, W., M. KOCH & H.U. SCHNITZLER. 1994. Substance P is involved in the sensitization of the acoustic startle response by footshock in rats. Behav. Brain Res. **63:** 81–88.
27. LEDOUX, J.E., P. CICCHETTI, A. XAGORARIS & L.M. ROMANSKI. 1990. The lateral amygdaloid nucleus, sensory interface of the amygdala in fear conditioning. J. Neurosci. **10:** 1062–1069.
28. LEDOUX, J.E., J. IWATA, P. CICCHETTI & D.J. REIS. 1988. Different projections of the central amygdaloid nucleus mediate autonomic and behavioral correlates of conditioned fear. J. Neurosci. **8:** 2517–2529.
29. LEE, Y. & M. DAVIS. 1996. The role of bed nucleus of the stria terminalis in CRH-enhanced startle: an animal model of anxiety. Soc. Neurosci. Abstr. **22:** 465.
30. LEE, Y. & M. DAVIS. 1997. Role of the hippocampus, bed nucleus of the stria terminalis and amygdala in the excitatory effect of corticotropin releasing (CRH) hormone on the acoustic startle reflex. J. Neurosci. **17:** 6434–6446.
31. LEE, Y., D.E. LOPEZ, E.G. MELONI & M. DAVIS. 1996. A primary acoustic startle circuit: obligatory role of cochlear root neurons and the nucleus reticularis pontis caudalis. J. Neurosci. **16:** 3775–3789.

32. MISERENDINO, M.J.D., C.B. SANANES, K.R. MELIA & M. DAVIS. 1990. Blocking of acquisition but not expression of conditioned fear-potentiated startle by NMDA antagonists in the amygdala. Nature **345:** 716–718.
33. ROSEN, J.B., J.M. HITCHCOCK, C.B. SANANES, M.J.D. MISERENDINO & M. DAVIS. 1991. A direct projection from the central nucleus of the amygdala to the acoustic startle pathway: anterograde and retrograde tracing studies. Behav. Neurosci. **105:** 817–825.
34. SAKANAKA, M., T. SHIBASAKI & K. LEDERIS. 1986. Distribution and efferent projections of corticotropin-releasing factor-like immunoreactivity in the rat amygdaloid complex. Brain Res. **382:** 213–238.
35. SANANES, C.B. & M. DAVIS. 1992. N-Methyl-D-aspartate lesions of the lateral and basolateral nuclei of the amygdala block fear-potentiated startle and shock sensitization of startle. Behav. Neurosci. **106:** 72–80.
36. SHI, C.-J. & M. DAVIS. 1999. Pain pathways involved in fear conditioning measured with fear-potentiated startle: lesion studies. J. Neurosci. In press.
37. SWERDLOW, N.R., M.A. GEYER, W.W. VALE & G.F. KOOB. 1986. Corticotropin-releasing factor potentiates acoustic startle in rats: blockade by chlordiazepoxide. Psychopharmacology **88:** 147–152.
38. WALKER, D.L. & M. DAVIS. 1997. Anxiogenic effects of high illumination levels assessed with the acoustic startle paradigm. Biol. Psychiatry **42:** 461–471.
39. WALKER, D.L. & M. DAVIS. 1997. Double dissociation between the involvement of the bed nucleus of the stria terminalis and the central nucleus of the amygdala in light- enhanced versus fear-potentiated startle. J. Neurosci. **17:** 9375–9383.
40. WALSH, R.N. & R.A. CUMMINS. 1976. The open-field test: a critical review. Psychol. Bull. **83:** 482–504.

Brain and Sexual Behavior

KNUT LARSSON[a,c] AND SVEN AHLENIUS[b]

[a]*Department of Psychology, University of, Göteborg, Box 500, SE-405 30, Göteborg, Sweden*

[b]*Department of Physiology and Pharmacology, Karolinska Institute, S-171 77 Stockholm, Sweden*

> ABSTRACT: This chapter will give personal accounts of the neural basis of male rat sexual behavior from two somewhat different perspectives, one tilted towards neuroanatomy (K.L.), and one tilted towards monoaminergic pharmacology (S.A.). Both perspectives were strongly influenced by the Zeitgeist, the former imperceptibly merging into the latter as relations between the neural substrate for monoaminergic neurotransmission was elucidated.[1]

THE NEUROANATOMICAL PERSPECTIVE

Introduction

In the late 1940s, when I began my graduate studies, psychology and physiology still had not met as scientific disciplines. Animal behavior was studied in the American laboratories of psychology but not in its relation with physiological processes. Hull[2] and Skinner,[3] the leading behaviorists at the time, both framed models of operant and instrumental conditioning. Hull conceptualized physiological processes as intervening variables without making any attempts to define and characterize them further. Skinner was equally certain that concepts like intervening variable were unjustified and even scientifically unsound, specifying stimulus-response relationships as all that was needed.

In Europe, the behavior of mammals was studied systematically by the ethological school with leaders like von Frisch, Lorentz, and Tinbergen as towering figures. The ethologists assumed inborn "instincts" as organizers of behavior. By instincts[4] was meant inherent, species-typical behavior patterns that were assumed to have developed under the pressure of evolution like the morphological and physiological features of the species.

The behaviorists and the ethologists differed in methods and outlook on science. The behaviorists formulated problems that allowed the use of animals to answer research questions in behavioristic terms and gave a methodology that would permit fine-grained analysis of the behavior. A main contribution of the ethologists was observation of animal behavior in the wild as part of the animal's normal life and their emphases on the evolutionary perspective. The behaviorists considered individual experience as the main organizer of behavior, whereas the ethologists focused on species variations determined by the genome. In one respect, however, the approach to behavior of the two schools was similar. Both thought that the behavioral analysis

---

[c]Voice: +46-31-7731641; fax: +46-31-7734628; knut.larsson@psy.gu.se

was a prerequisite to obtaining a complete explanation of the behavior. None was concerned with the role of the brain in the regulation of behavior, or, for that matter, of the importance of any measures relating molar and molecular event. None anticipated the explosive rise of physiological psychology, nor the development of behavioral neuroscience soon to come.

I had from my early school days been curious about animal behavior and its physiological bases, but when I entered the university in the midst of the 1940s, psychology did not even exist as a separate subject in the Swedish universities. I wanted to approach animal behavior in a way that allowed me to study behavioral and physiological variables in their interaction. I happened to hear that in Norway there was an anatomist, Alf Brodal, and a neurophysiologist, Birger Kaada, who both tried to relate anatomy, physiology, and behavior to each other. So I went to Oslo. At the Anatomical Institute in Oslo, where both these researchers worked, I was given the task of studying the female mouse estrous cycle. This study became a revelation for me. Sitting at night in the animal room and looking at the behavior of the mice, I felt I was looking down directly into nature itself. I observed each fourth day, how the female mouse, within a matter of an hour, entered a state of receptivity when her rejection of the male was turned into acceptance. The behavioral cyclicity was a reflection of endocrine, morphological, and neuronal changes, controlled by the brain. Brodal, once a student of Judson Herrick, gave me the attractive book of his teacher, *The Brain of Rats and Man*, together with his own writings on the limbic brain.[5] Kaada, who had done his Ph.D. studies during the war with John Fulton at Yale university, gave me his work on electrical recordings from the brain.[6] These experiences made me decide to study reproductive behavior, which, in such a wonderful way, twins hormonal, neural, and behavioral influences.

Some years later, now with a doctoral degree in male rat sexual behavior completed, I met Lennart Heimer, who just had ended his medical studies and had even written an introductory textbook on neuroanatomy for medical students, the first Swedish book of this kind. Joined by our common interest in brain and behavior, we began to work together looking for brain correlates of sexual behavior. I will, to begin, outline the main lines of this work. Questions proposed during the course of these studies prepared for later studies that were oriented towards neurotransmitters possibly involved in sexual behavior. These problems will be dealt with in the second part of this report.

Central Neural Control of Male Rat Sexual Behavior

As a background for the experiments to be described below, FIGURE 1 depicts male rat sexual behavior.[7] When exposed to a receptive female, the experienced male approaches her and mounts her. After repeated mounts and intromissions, ejaculatory behavior is elicited. The ejaculation is followed by a refractory period when the male is sexually unresponsive. After 4–5 minutes, he resumes pursuance and mounting of the female. Mounts, intromissions, and ejaculations can be easily recognized, counted, and expressed in terms of frequency and latency of their first appearance. It is assumed that the intromissions cause a rising sexual excitation cumulating in ejaculation.

When Lennart and I begun our studies in the beginning of the 1960s, little was known about the role of the brain in the regulation of sexual behavior. Removal of large parts of the cerebral cortex, independently of their localization, disrupted cop-

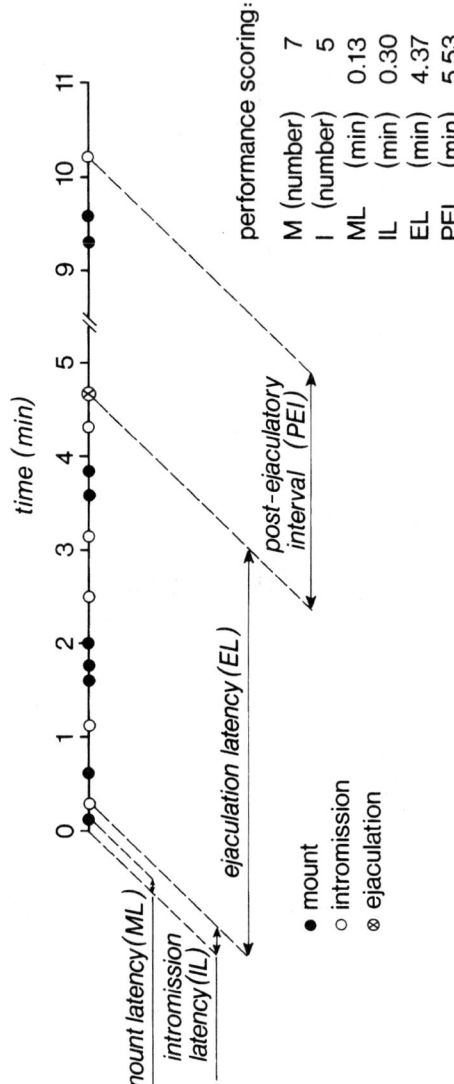

FIGURE 1. Schematic presentation of the male rat copulatory performance.[7]

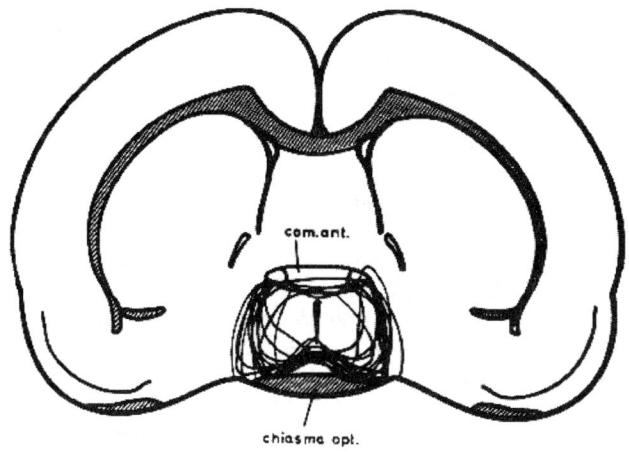

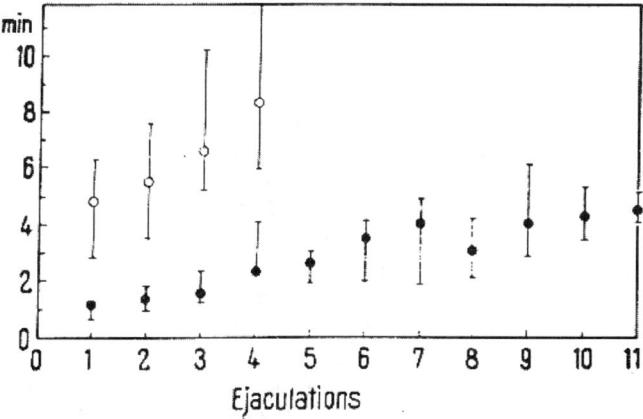

FIGURE 2. *Top*: Outline of individual lesions in the medial preoptic-anterior hypothalamic continuum that eliminated mating behavior.[15] *Bottom*: The figure demonstrates the reduction of the postejaculatory intervals and the accompanying increase in ejaculation frequency in one male rat subjected to lesions at the junction of the diencephalon and mesencephalon. The behavior was observed during three subsequent 60-min tests. Filled circles represent the median values of the postejaculatory intervals recorded during these tests. Vertical lines represent maximal and minimal values. Open circles represent the corresponding performances of a group of 31 intact males.

ulation in males of several species.[8] Later studies[9] showed, however, that lesions in the medial-frontal cortex abolished mating in some rats, whereas lesions in the more posterior regions, including the cingulate gyrus, had little or no effects on mating, suggesting different roles of frontal and posterior parts of the rat cortex. It was not until the end of the 1940s that stereotaxic surgery was introduced into the laboratory, allowing investigators to place discrete lesions within the depths of the brain.[10] It was reported that electrolytic lesions in the hypothalamus impaired male rat sexual behavior without causing any apparent hormonal deficits.[11,12] The subcortical lesions performed in these studies were, however, too large to admit localization of the behavioral impairment to any specific group of cells. Therefore, Lennart and I decided, as a first task, to locate the neural circuits essential for the sexual behavior. For this we needed a stereotaxic instrument. We built such an instrument, with the help of Victor Kuikka, the skillful technician of the anatomy department.[13]

Not knowing where to begin, in the anterior or the posterior end of the brain, we decided to start in the rostral end of the brain stem to continue forward. We made two interesting findings (FIG. 2). First, extensive lesions in the junction of the diencephalon and mesencephalon made them hypersexual.[14] The males ejaculated after only a few intromissions, within a very short time, and showed abnormally shortened PEIs. Within an hour, some males had ejaculated a dozen times compared to three or four times normally. Our second finding pertained to lesions in the area of the medial preoptic nucleus and the anterior hypothalamus (MPOA). Extensive lesions in this area abolished sexual behavior seemingly permanently; minor lesions in this area, independent of location, caused only a temporary impairment of the behavior.[15] Both these findings led us to suggest two neural mechanisms regulating male rat sexual behavior, one involving subcortical structures in the caudal diencephalon and anterior mesencephalon, exerting an inhibitory influence upon mating, and another mechanism located in the MPOA, mediating sexual arousal and controlling the motoric aspects of mating.

The medial preoptic-anterior hypothalamic continuum occupies a strategic position in the limbic system (FIG. 2). Its lateral zone is an interstitial nucleus of the medial forebrain bundle, a polysynaptic fiber system that provides a major reciprocal link between the medial basal telencephalon rostrally and the midbrain tegmentum caudally. It is located outside the main stream of the medial forebrain bundle, but it is known to receive numerous short fibers from the lateral zone, making its functional state likely to be influenced by impulses arriving in the hypothalamic region by way of the medial forebrain bundle.[16] Such impulses are supposed to originate from visceral and somatic sensory structures of the lower brain stem, from the hippocampus, cingulate cortex, septal area, and amygdaloid complex. Of equal relevance should be axons to the medial forebrain bundle arising from olfactory structures, such as the piriform cortex, the olfactory tubercle, and the olfactory lobes.[17]

Besides its more diffuse afferent connections from the lateral hypothalamic zones, the MPOA receives a component of the stria terminalis, a major fiber system originating in the amygdaloid complex.[18] The stria terminalis, in part at least, originates from the cortico-medial subdivision of the amygdala, a region known to receive numerous fibers directly from the accessory olfactory lobes.[19] The position of this intermediate area between what was then called the limbic and olfactory telencephalon on the one hand, the midbrain tegmentum on the other hand, and bordering the gonadotrophic mechanisms of the tuberal hypothalamus was compatible with our finding that this region is important for the regulation of mating. Considering the highly heterogeneous, multimodal afferent relationships, among which the olfactory modality appeared to be particularly strongly represented, we decided to focus on the role of the olfactory system and moved, thereafter, in the posterior direction, being interfered with by lesions at various levels of the limbic system. Failing any good

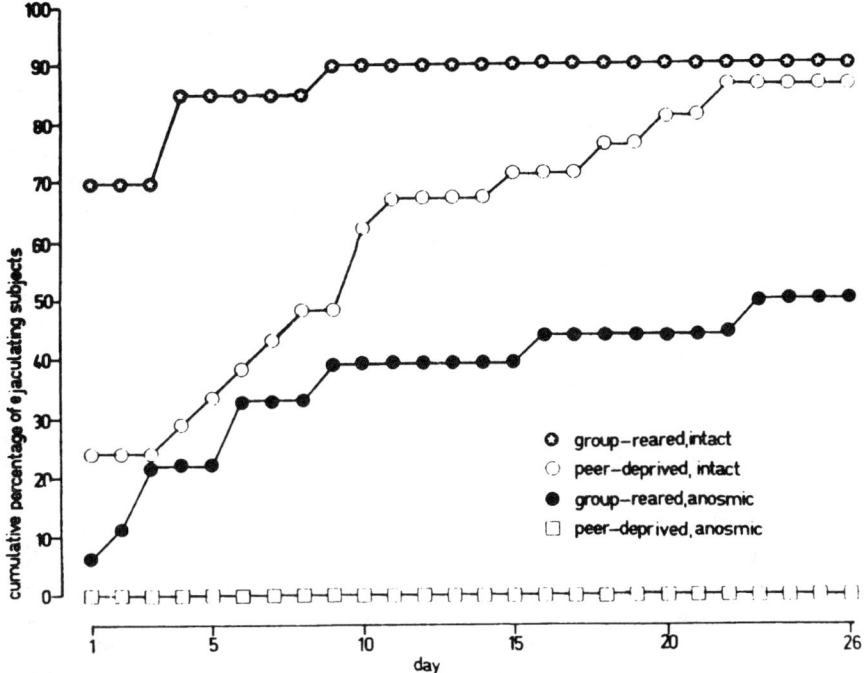

FIGURE 3. Cumulative percentage of male rats showing ejaculation in 26 daily mating tests following surgical destruction of the main olfactory lobes or sham operation at 30 days of age. Peer-deprived rats were reared in single cages from 10 days of age until the end of testing. Group-reared rats lived together with two female litter mates.

anatomical guidance, Lennart started to study the basal forebrain using various silver-impregnation techniques. Soon he had developed a technique of his own, later to be published as the Fink-Heimer technique.[20]

Electrolytic lesions of the main olfactory bulb, or surgical section of the lateral olfactory tract, impaired, but did not prevent, the occurrence of sexual behavior.[21] Further work was undertaken involving destruction of the main olfactory bulb or sectioning of the lateral olfactory tract. Again, we found a striking variation of the behavioral effects obtained, suggesting a role for factors other than olfaction, as such (FIG. 3). We soon discovered that sexual experience was one of these disturbing factors: those males that were sexually naive when made anosmic rarely ever started to mate. The sexually experienced males, by contrast, showed relatively small effects of anosmia.[22–24]

The observation of the importance of experience for sexual behavior came as a complete surprise to us. From the considerable literature on sex and olfaction existing at that time, we were made to believe that odoiferous signals were mainly coupled with preprogrammed behaviors. Our observation, however, pointed at a powerful role of olfactory memory. More recent work has confirmed these observations, and, in addition, indicated the importance of the vomeronasal organ and the accessory olfactory lobe in such a mechanism.[25] It appears that the sense of olfaction is particularly well suited for storing emotionally important memories.[26]

After these studies were concluded, Lennart went to Walle Nauta at MIT to continue his neuroanatomical work, which he had begun in Sweden. This research was going to result in this conceptual remodeling of the basal forebrain that we are discussing here. As I have tried to show you, this research program was guided by a need to find ways to explore the role of the brain in behavior, and reproductive funtions, in particular. The work subsequently performed by Lennart and his associates has shown the role of a collection of structures, including the nucleus accumbens, olfactory tubercle, septum, diagonal band nuclei, and bed nucleus of stria terminalis as well as the extensive territory beneath the temporal limb of the anterior commissure, which long was referred to as the substantia innominata.[27] Of special importance to reproductive funtions is the ventral striatopallidal system, the extended amygdala, and the areas of transition between these two systems.[18] The concept of a critical role of the MPOA in mammalian sexual behavior has been confirmed in all mammals studied.[27] The MPOA, the bed nucleus of stria terminals, and the medial nucleus of the amygdala are reciprocally connected anatomically, and the medial nucleus of the amygdala receives direct projections from the main and accessory olfactory lobes.[29,30] An additional input from the main olfactory lobe is received by afferents from the cortical nucleus of the amygdala.[30] Pathways linking the cortiocomedial amygdala with the bed nucleus of stria terminalis may convey impulses generated by chemosensory receptors of the olfactory systems promoting sexual arousal. This applies in various degrees, to all mammals, including humans. In view of the major importance of gonadal hormones for sexual behavior, it should be noted that all of these areas are densely packed with gonadal hormone receptors.[28] These receptors are closely associated with enzymatic systems that process the prehormones to active agents.[31–33]

THE MONOAMINERGIC PERSPECTIVE

Introduction

Returning to the early 1960s, Arvid Carlsson, Åke Hillarp, and their students in the pharmacology department close to our laboratory in Göteborg were studying another aspect of brain physiology, namely neurotransmitters. Dopamine (DA) and 5-hydroxytryptamine (5-HT) had just been discovered as having functions of their own as neurotransmitters. The neurons producing these substances could be visualized by the histofluorescent methods, then newly reported. We looked upon the pictures of the rat brain offered to us, showing skies of neurons, in deep green, transferring catecholamines, and, in bright yellow, neurons using 5-hydroxytryptamine. The neurons were longer than had ever been seen, stretching out between the brain stem and the forebrain.[34–39] Naturally, we were eager to know more about the function of these neuronal systems.

Dopamine

Dopamine (DA) is involved in all aspects of sexual behavior, including sexual arousal, copulation, and penile reflexes.[40] Exposing the male rat to a receptive female, we found a selective increase in the synthesis of DA in the nucleus accumbens.[41] Further studies indicated that this increase is characteristic of sexually naive rats and does not occur in experienced ones, suggesting a role of DA in the novelty aspect of sexual stimulation rather than sexual activity, as such.[42]

Dopaminergic projections from the substantia nigra and ventral tegmentum pass to the ventral striatum and nucleus accumbens, respectively.[43] DA activity is reduced after localized lesions are produced by treatments with a neurotoxin, 6-hydroxydopamine. Further, systemic treatment with both DA D_2 and mixed DA $D_{1/2}$ receptor antagonists in these areas reduces the level of sexual arousal as assessed by prolonged mount and intromission latencies and PEIs, without accompanying alterations of the copulatory activity.[44–50]

The administration of a variety of DA agonists enhances the copulatory activity, and this effect is reversed by treatment with DA D_2 receptor antagonists, as evidenced by a reduction of the ejaculation latency.[51–54] The MPOA is the only site of action identified for the stimulatory effect of DA in copulatory activity. Such dopamine receptor agonists as apomorphine, quinpirole, and lisuride stimulate copulation, penile erection, and seminal emission; their effects are reversed by DA receptor antagonists. The stimulatory effect on penile erection requires the presence of testosterone and appears to be mediated postsynaptically.[55] The stimulation of penile erection originates in the paraventricular nucleus, because injection of DA agents in this nucleus induces penile erection combined with yawning,[56,57] an effect probably mediated by a release of oxytocin.[58]

Noradrenaline

The noradrenergic system originates in the locus caeruleus and innervates the entire forebrain. It stimulates sexual activity probably in an indirect way but has an inhibitory role on penile erection.[59–61] Lesions of the locus caeruleus, inhibition of noradrenaline (NA) synthesis, and inhibition of NA release by α_2-andrenoceptor agonists are all agents causing a prolongation of ML, IL, and PEI.[62] Yohimbine, an α_2-adrenoceptor antagonist, has repeatedly been reported to be effective in stimulating sexual activity, presumably because the NA cell bodies in the nucleus caeruleus are under tonic α_2-adrenoceptor influence.[59,60,63]

5-Hydroxytryptamine

Central brain serotonergic systems were long considered to inhibit the neural mechanisms regulating male and female sexual behavior. This contention was based on (1) the observation that a decrease in brain serotonin facilitates ejaculation in rats, as evidenced by a decrease in the number of intromissions to ejaculation and a shortening of the ejaculation latency and (2) the observation that an increase in availability of synaptic 5-HT inhibited the behavior, as evidenced by an increased number of intromissions and a prolonged ejaculation latency (see ref. 7). A behavioral facilitation was produced by the inhibition of tryptophan hydroxylase by treatment with *p*-chlorophenylalanine,[64,65] selective destruction of brain serotonergic neurons by 5,7-dihydroxytryptamine,[66] or electrolytic lesions of serotonergic projections from the raphe nucleas to the MPOA.[67]

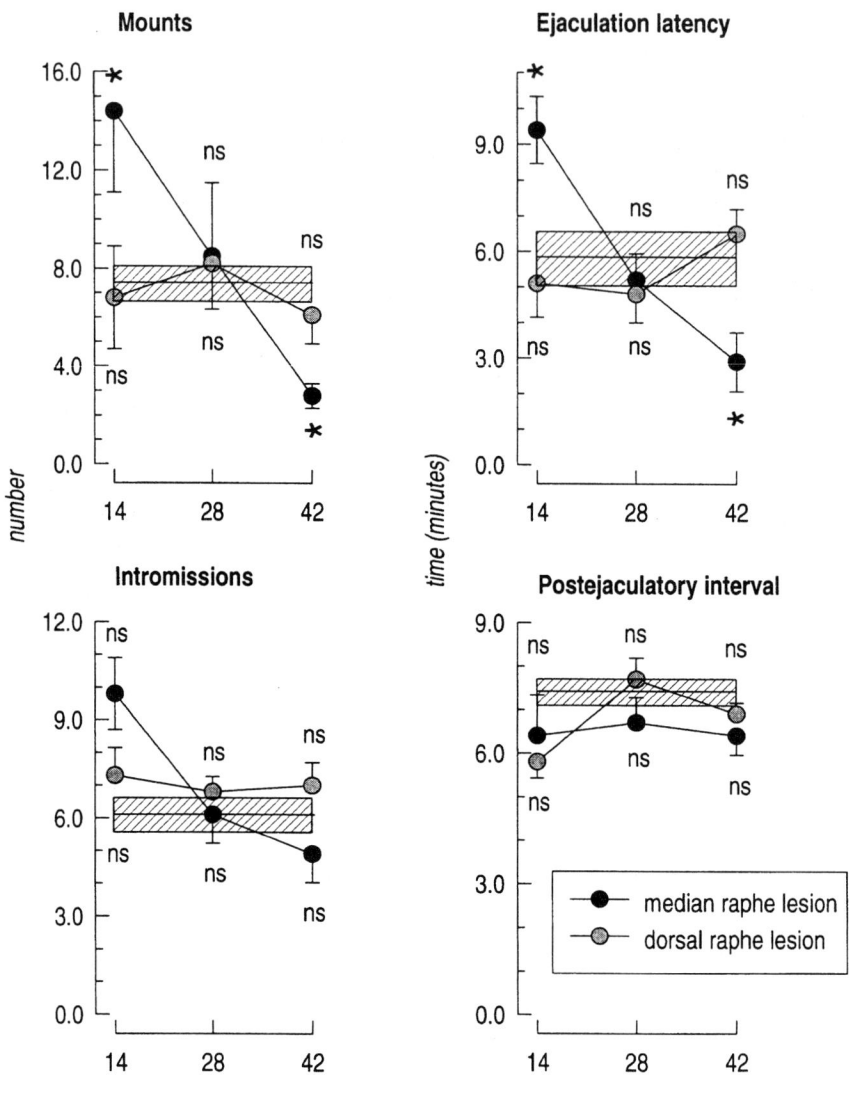

FIGURE 4. Effects of median and dorsal raphe electrolytic lesions on male rat copulatory behavior. The FIGURE shows medians ± semi-interquartile range. Sham-lesioned controls from two groups were pooled and are shown by the shaded area. Statistical comparisons with sham-lesioned controls were performed by means of the Mann-Whitney U-test, as shown in the FIGURE. ns, $p > 0.05$; *$p < 0.05$. For further details see Ahlenius and Larsson.[6]

The major sources of serotonergic innervation of the forebrain are the dorsal (DR) and median (MR) raphe nuclei.[68] A study was undertaken of the effects on masculine sexual behavior of lesions aimed specifically either at the median or the dorsal raphe nuclei.[7] In parallel experiments we checked the specificity of the lesions by examining the 5-HT decrease in target areas. The MR lesions produced a relatively greater decrease in septal than in neostriatal 5-HT content: the DR lesions produced the opposite pattern. The MR lesions caused a marked facilitation of sexual behavior, as evidenced by a decrease in the number of intromissions to ejaculation and a shortening of the ejaculation latency and of the postejaculatory intervals. No changes in the mating behavior were observed after DR lesions (FIG. 4). These results receive further support from pharmacological studies.[69]

In our efforts to characterize the role of the serotonergic transmitter systems in the regulation of sexual behavior, we were given access to a new substance, 8-OH-2-(di-*n*-propylamino)tetralin (8-OH-DPAT). This substance was developed at the Department of Pharmacology, University of Göteborg, and at the Department of Organic Pharmaceutical Chemistry, University of Uppsala, and was characterized as a 5-HT receptor agonist.[70] We expected that this compound would inhibit the behavior. Instead we found that 8-OH-DPAT produced a drastic facilitation of the ejaculation reflex. The number of intromissions was lowered and the time to ejaculation shortened. Sometimes the male ejaculated after one single intromission, resulting in an *ejaculatio precox*-like effect[7] (FIG. 5).

This highly specialized 5-HT receptor agonist we had received in our hands was soon shown to have high affinity to a subtype of receptor named the $5-HT_{1A}$ receptor.[71] It had been known earlier that certain β-blocking agents, like propranolol and pindolol, could antagonize behaviors involving the 5-HT receptor. These compounds, having selective affinities to $5-HT_{1A}$ receptors, antagonized the facilitation of the ejaculation reflex induced by 8-OH-DPAT. Recently another, more selective $5-HT_{1A}$ receptor blocker, WAY-100635, was found to have the same effect. These and other observations suggest that 8-OH-DPAT exerts its dramatic effect upon male rat sexual behavior by stimulating $5-HT_{1A}$ receptors in the brain. Several other compounds with high affinity for the $5-HT_{1A}$ receptor, including buspirone, flesinoxan, and FG 5893, have later been shown to share the effects of 8-OH-DPAT on ejaculation behavior.[72,73]

In order to examine a possible site of action for these effects, we locally applied 8-OH-DPAT to two sites in the ventral forebrain and also onto cell bodies of origin in the DR and MR. Infusion of 8-OH-DPAT in the MR accelerated the rate of copulation, possibly by stimulating $5-HT_{1A}$ somatodendritic autoreceptors, thereby causing an inhibition of neuronal 5-HT activity.[69,74] No facilitation was produced by infusing 8-OH-DPAT into the DR. The median raphe injections decreased 5-HT synthesis in the nucleus accumbens, the ventromedial striatum, and the amygdala, as well as in the hippocampus and the septum. Also the DR injections of 8-OH-DPAT produced a decreased 5-HT synthesis in the forebrain, but the effects were most pronounced in the dorsolateral striatum and the globus pallidus. Summarizing these observations, we conclude that the MR belongs to a midbrain neural system, inhibitory to sexual behavior.

Also experiments with 5-HT clearly demonstrated region-selective effects. Local application of 5-HT into the nucleus accumbens inhibited sexual behavior, whereas local application into striatal areas ventral or dorsal to this site produced no effects.[69] The local application of 5-HT onto serotonergic somatodendritic autoreceptors in the DR and the MR facilitated the behavior.[75]

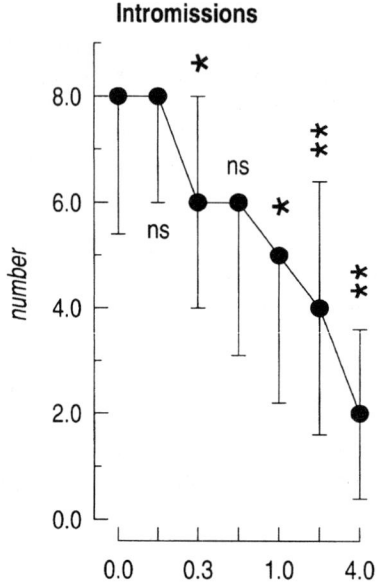

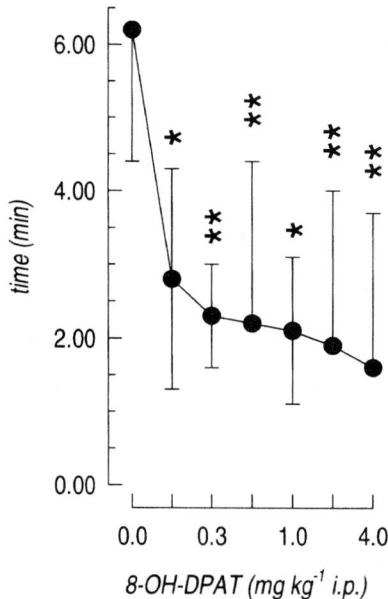

FIGURE 5. Facilitation of male rat ejaculatory behavior by the administration of the 5-HT$_{1A}$ receptor agonist, 8-OH-DPAT. The FIGURE shows medians ± semi-interquartile range based on repeated observations of the same animals in a changeover design. Statistical analysis was performed by means of the Friedman two-way ANOVA, followed by the Wilcoxon matched-pairs signed-ranks t-test, for comparisons with saline-treated controls, as shown in the FIGURE. ns, $p > 0.05$; *$p < 0.05$; **$p < 0.01$. For further details see Ahlenius et al.[86]

If activation of 5-HT_{1A} receptors mediate a facilitatory influence on sexual behavior, the inhibitory influence obtained after treatment with 5-HTP must be a consequence of stimulation of other receptors. One of them may be the 5-HT_{1B} receptor. Several pharmacological agents selectively stimulate this receptor, resulting in an increase in the number of intromissions and prolongation of the response latencies.[76] Another class of 5-HT receptors is the 5-HT_2 receptor. Treatment with DOI, a selective $5\text{-HT}_{2A/C}$ receptor agonist, inhibits male sexual behavior, an effect that is blocked by selective $5\text{-HT}_2/5\text{-HT}_{1C}$ antagonists, like ritanserin and ketanserin.[77] Unlike the effects produced by the various 5-HT_1-selective receptors, this last effect does not seem to be an effect specific to the ejaculation behavior and may not even be specifically associated with sexual behavior. This raises the problem of possible differences between 5-HT_{2A} and 5-HT_{2C} receptors. New and selective pharmacological tools will probable soon be available to clarify the role of different 5-HT_2 receptors in male sexual behavior.

Treatment with 5-HTP presumably results in an increased release of 5-HT at all serotonergic synapses. In a series of recent studies, we asked whether treatment with selective serotonin antagonists even influences the inhibitory effects produced by 5-HTP. By antagonizing the effect of 5-HTP on the 5-HT_{1A}, receptor we would receive a potentiation of the inhibitory influence produced by 5-HTP. Male rats were injected with 5-HTP combined with benserazide, and thereafter treated with either WAY-100635 (5-HT_{1A} receptor antagonist), isamoltane (5-HT_{1B} receptor antagonist), or ritanserine ($5\text{-HT}_{2A/C}$ receptor antagonist). We found that WAY-100635 potentiated the effects of 5-HTP, whereas isamoltane blocked these effects. The ejaculation pattern remained unaffected by ritanserin. These results support the hypothesis that 5-HTP stimulates as well 5-HT_{1A} as 5-HT_{1B} receptors, the net effect of 5-HTP representing a balance between activation of these two receptor types.[78]

It is worth noting that the drug effects on male rat ejaculatory behavior reported here are very different from their effects on penile erections. Thus, 8-OH-DPAT, which facilitates ejaculatory behavior, inhibits penile erections.[79,80] Furthermore, the nonselective 5-HT_{1B} receptor agonist, 1-(3'-chlorophenyl)-piperazine (mCPP), induces penile erections (ref. 81, cf. ref. 82), whereas the 5-HT_{1B} receptor agonist, anpirtoline, inhibits ejaculatory behavior.[83] Finally, stimulation of 5-HT_{2C} receptors (formerly the 5-HT_{1C} receptor) induces penile erections.[82–85]

CONCLUDING REMARKS

Let us trace our journey together. In the beginning, the problem was to find an approach to behavior that would reasonably well lend itself to an analysis of underlying biological mechanisms. Reproductive behavior, turned out to be eminently suited for this purpose: essential for the survival of the species, shaped along with other morphological and physiological features of the species, yet not of critical importance for survival of the individual. Furthermore, it is a behavior dependent upon the senses and hormonal regulation, intricately linked to brain functions. Few neuroanatomists or psychologists in the late 1950s thought about behavior in these terms. After the first fumbling attempts to find the brain structures involved in the control of male rat sexual behavior, we discovered how little was known of the neural organization of the brain, not least of which were those circuits that controlled reproduction. From a different perspective, this surely was a challenge for Lennart Heimer to devote himself to in-depth studies on the neural organization of the basal forebrain. The new conceptualization he has brought to this brain territory has been a great gift to all investigators in the fields of psychoactive and emotional behavior, including behavioral functions related to reproduction. The parallel discoveries of monoaminergic neurons connecting mesencephalic and lower brain stem structures with all other parts of the nervous system was revolutionary. Coupling these insights with the wiring and neuroanatomical delineation of structures in the basal forebrain not only shed new light on relations between brain and behavior, but also opened the possibility of exploring brain functions with pharmacological probes. Anatomy and pharmacology became two sides of the same coin.

REFERENCES

1. CARLSSON, A. 1987. Perspectives on the discovery of central monoaminergic neurotransmission. Annu. Rev. Neurosci. **10**: 19–40.
2. HULL, C.L. 1943. Principles of behavior. Appleton-Century-Crofts. New York.
3. SKINNER, B. 1938. The behavior of the organisms. Appleton-Century. New York.
4. TINBERGEN, N. 1951. The study of instinct. Oxford University Press. New York.
5. HERRICK, J. S. 1926. Brains of rats and men. University of Chicago Press. Chicago.
6. KAADA, B. 1951. Somato-motor, autonomic and electrocorticographic responses to stimulation of "Rhinencephalic" and other structures in primates, cat and dog. A study of responses from the limbic, subcallosal, orbito-insular, piriform and temporal cortex, hippocampus-fornix and amygdala. Acta Physiol. Scand. 24, suppl. 283.
7. AHLENIUS, S. & K. LARSSON. 1991. Physiological and pharmacological implications of specific effects by $5-HT_{1A}$ agonists on rat sexual behavior. In $5-HT_{1A}$ agonists, $5-HT_3$ antagonists and benzodiazepines: Their comparative behavioural pharmacology. R.J. Rodgers & S.J. Cooper, Eds.: 281–315. John Wiley & Sons. Chichester.
8. BEACH, F.A. 1940. Effects of cortical lesions upon the copulatory behavior. J Comp. Psychol. **29**: 193–245.
9. LARSSON, K. 1964. Mating behavior in male rats after cerebral cortex ablation. II Effects of lesions in the frontal lobes compared to lesions in the posterior half of the hemispheres. J. Exp. Zool. **155**: 203–214.
10. HILLARP, N-Å, H. OLIVECRONA & W. SILFVERSKIÖLD. 1954. Evidence for the participation of the preoptic area in male mating behaviour. Experientia **10**: 224.
11. BROOKHART, J.H. & F.L. DAY. 1941. Reduction of sexual behavior in male guinea pigs by hypothalamic lesions. Am. J. Physiol. **133**: 551–554.
12. SOULAIRAC, A. & M-L. SOULAIRAC. 1956. Effets de lésions hypothalamiques sur le comportement sexuel et le tractus génital du rat mâle. Ann. Endocrinol. (Paris) **17**: 731–745.
13. HEIMER, L., V. KUIKKA, K. LARSSON & E. A. NORDSTRÖM. 1971. A head for stereotaxic operations of small laboratory animals. Physiol. Behav. **7**: 263–264.
14. HEIMER, L. & K. LARSSON. 1964. Drastic changes in the mating behavior of male rats following lesions in the junction of diencephalon and mesencephalon. Experientia **20**: 460.
15. HEIMER, L. & K. LARSSON. 1966/67. Impairment of mating behavior in male rats following lesions in the preoptic-anterior hypothalamic continuum. Brain Res. **3**: 248–263.
16. HEIMER, L., G. ALHEID & L. ZABORSZKY. 1985. Basal ganglia. In The rat nervous system. G. Paxinos, Ed. Vol. **1**: 37–86. Academic Press.
17. SWITZER, R.C., J. DE OLMOS & L. HEIMER. 1985. Olfactory system. In The rat nervous system G. Paxinos, Ed. Vol. **1**: 1–36. Academic Press.
18. ALHEID, G.F. & L. HEIMER. 1996. Theories of basal forebrain organization and the

"emotional motor system." *In* Progress in Brain Research. G Holstege, R. Bandler & C.B. Saper, Eds. Vol. l07: 461–484. Elsevier.
19. LUSKIN, M.B. & J.I. PRICE. 1983. The topographic organization of associational fibers of the olfactory system in the rat including centrifugal fibers of the olfactory bulb. J. Comp. Neurol. **216:** 264–291.
20. FINK, R.P. & L. HEIMER. 1967. Two methods for selective silver impregnation of degenerating axons and their synaptic endings in the central nervous system. Brain Res. **4:** 369–374.
21. HEIMER, L. & K. LARSSON. 1967. Mating behavior of male rats after olfactory bulb lesions. Physiol. Behav. **2:** 207–209.
22. LARSSON, K. 1969. Failure of gonadal and gonadotrophic hormones to compensate for an impaired sexual function of anosmic male rats. Physiol. Behav. **4:** 33–737.
23. WILHELMSSON, M. & K. LARSSON. 1973. The development of sexual behavior in anosmic male rats reared under various social conditions. Physiol. Behav. **11:** 227–232.
24. LARSSON, K. 1975. Sexual impairment of inexperienced male rats following pre- and postpuberal olfactory bulbectomy. Physiol. Behav. **14:** 195–199.
25. EDWARDS, D.A., K. T. GRIFFIS & TARDIVEL, C. 1990. Olfactory bulb removal: effects on sexual behavior and partner preference in male rats. Physiol. Behav. **48:** 447–450.
26. ROSENBLATT, J.S. 1983. Olfaction mediates developmental transitions in the altricial newborns of selected species of mammals. Dev. Psychol. **16:** 347–375.
27. HEIMER, L., R.E. HARLAN, G.F. ALHEID, M.M. GARCIA & J. DE OLMOS. 1997. Substantia innominata: a notion which impedes clinical-anatomical correlations in neuropsychiatric disorders. Neuoscience **4:** 957–1006.
28. MEISEL, R.L. & B.D. SACHS. 1994. The physiology of male sexual behaviors *In* The Physiology of Reproduction. E. Knobil & J.D. Neill, Eds.: 3–105. Raven Press. New York.
29. LEHMAN, M.N., S.S. WINANS & J.B. POWERS. 1982. Vomeronasal and olfactory pathways to the amygdala controlling male sexual behavior: autoradiographic and behavioral analysis. Brain Res. **240:** 27–41.
30. SCALIA, F. & S.S. WINANS. 1975. The differential projections of the olfactory bulb and accessory olfactory bulb in mammals. J. Comp. Neurol. **161:** 31–56.
31. SAR, M. & W.E. STUMPF. 1973. Autoradiographic localization of radioactivity in the rat brain after the injection of 1,2-^{3}H-testosterone. Endocrinology **92:** 251–256.
32. KIERNIESKY, N.C. & A.R. GERALL. 1973. Effects of testosterone propionate implants in the brain on the sexual behavior and peripheral tissue of the male rat. Physiol. Behav. **11:** 633–640.
33. WOOD, R.I. & S.W. NEWMAN. 1995. Hormonal influences on neurons of the mating behavior pathway in male hamsters. *In* Neurobiological Effects of Sex Steroid Hormones. P. Micevychre & R. Hammar, Eds.: 3–39. Cambridge University Press. Cambridge.
34. DAHLSTRÖM, A. & K. FUXE. 1964. Evidence for the existence of monoamine-containing neurons in the central nervous system. Acta Physiol. Scand. **62:** 1–55.
35. ANDÉN, N-E., A. DAHLSTRÖM, K. FUXE & K. LARSSON. 1965. Further evidence for the presence of nigro-neostriatal dopamine neurons in the rat. Am. J. Anat. **116:** 329–333.
36. ANDÉN, N-E., A. DAHLSTRÖM, K. FUXE & K. LARSSON, 1965. Mapping out of catecholamine and 5-hydroxytryptamine neurons innervating the telencephalon and diencephalon. Life Sci. **4:** 1275–1279.
37. ANDÉN, N-E., A. DAHLSTRÖM, K. FUXE & K. LARSSON. 1966. Functional role of the nigro-neostriatal dopamine neurons. Acta Pharmacol. Toxicol. **24:** 263–274.
38. ANDÉN, N-E., A. DAHLSTRÖM, K. FUXE, K. LARSSON, L. OLSON & U. UNGERSTEDT. 1966. Ascending monoamine neurons to the telencephalon and diencephalon. Acta Physiol. Scand. **67:** 313–326.
39. ANDÉN, N-E., K. FUXE & K. LARSSON. 1966. Effect of large mesencephalic-diencephalic lesions on the noradrenalin, dopamine and 5-hydroxytryptamine neurons of the central nervous system. Experientia **22:** 842–843.

40. HULL, E.M. 1995. Dopaminergic influences on male rat sexual behavior. *In* Neurobiological Effects of Sex Steroid Hormones. P.E. Micevych & R. Hammar, Eds.: 234–253. Cambridge University Press. Cambridge.
41. AHLENIUS, S., A. CARLSSON, V. HILLEGART, S. HJORT & K. LARSSON. 1987. Region-selective activation of brain monoamine synthesis by sexual activity in the male rat. Eur. J. Pharmacol. **144:** 77–82.
42. AHLENIUS, S., V. HILLEGART & K. LARSSON. 1991. Motivation and performance: Region-selective changes in forebrain monoamine synthesis due to sexual activity in rats. *In* Behavioral Biology: Neuroendocrine Axes. T. Archer & S. Hansen, Eds.: 93–103. Lawrence Erlbaum Associates. Hillsdale.
43. BECKSTEAD, R.M., V.B. DOMESICK & W.J.H. NAUTA. 1979. Efferent connections of the substantia nigra and ventral tegmental area in the rat. Brain Res. **175:** 191–217.
44. MCINTOSH, T.K. & R.J. BARFIELD. 1984. Brain monoaminergic control of male reproductive behavior. III. Norepinephrine and the post-ejaculatory refractory period. Behav. Brain Res. **12:** 275–281.
45. BRACKET, N.L., P.M. IUVONE & D.A. EDWARDS. 1986. Midbrain lesions, dopamine and male sexual behavior. Behav. Brain Res. **20:** 231–240.
46. PFAUS, G. & A.G. PHILIPS. 1989. Differential effects of dopamine receptor antagonists on sexual behaviour of male rats. Psychopharmacology (Berlin) **98:** 363–368.
47. EVERITT, B.J. 1990. Sexual motivation: a neural and behavioural analysis of the mechanisms underlying appetite and copulatory responses of male rats. Neurosci. Biobehav. Rev. **14:** 217–232.
48. CAGIANO, R., R.J. BARFIELD, N.R. WHITE, E.T. PLEIM & V. CUOMO. 1989. Mediation of rat postejaculatory 22 kHz ultrasonic vocalization by dopamine D_2 receptors. Pharmacol. Biochem. Behav. **34:** 53–58.
49. AGMO, A. & Z. PICKER. 1990. Catecholamines and the initiation of sexual behavior in male rats without sexual experience. Pharmacol. Biochem. Behav. **35:** 327–334.
50. HULL, E.M., T.J. BAZZETT, R.K. WARNER, R.C. EATON & J.T. THOMSON. 1990. Dopamine receptors in the ventral tegmental area modulate male sexual behavior in rats. Brain Res. **512:** 1–6.
51. GRAY, G.D., H.N. DAVIS & D.A DEWSBURY. 1974. Effects of L-dopa on the heterosexual copulatory behaviour of male rats. Eur. J. Pharmacol. **27:** 367–370.
52. TAGLIAMONTE, A., W. FRATTA, F. DEL FIACCO & G.L. GESSA. 1974. Possible stimulatory role of brain dopamine in the copulatory behavior of male rats. Pharmacol. Biochem. Behav. **2:** 257–260.
53. AHLENIUS, S. & K. LARSSON. 1984. Apomorphine and haloperidol-induced effects on male rat sexual behavior: no evidence for actions due to stimulation of central dopamine autoreceptors. Pharmacol. Biochem. Behav. **21:** 463–466.
54. CLARK, J.T. & E.R. SMITH. 1986. Failure of pimozide and metergoline to antagonize the RDS-127-induced facilitation of ejaculatory behavior. Physiol. Behav. **37:** 47–52.
55. BERENDSEN, H.H.G. & A.J. GOWER. 1986. Opiate-androgen interactions in drug-induced yawning and penile erections in the rat. Neuroendocrinology **42:** 185–190.
56. MELIS, M.R., A. ARGIOLAS & G.L. GESSA. 1987. Apomorphine-induced penile-erection and yawning: site of action in the brain. Brain Res. **415:** 98–107.
57. HOLMGREN, B., R. URBA-HOLMGREN, N. TRUCIOS, M. ZERMENO & J.R. EGUIBAR. 1985. Association of spontaneous and dopaminergic-induced yawning and penile erections in the rat. Pharmacol. Biochem. Behav. **22:** 31–35.
58. ARGIOLAS, A. 1992. Oxytocin stimulation of penile erection. Pharmacology, Site, and Mechanism of Action. Ann. N. Y. Acad. Sci. **652:** 194–203.
59. CLARK, J.T., E.R. SMITH & J.M. DAVIDSON. 1984. Enhancement of sexual motivation in male rats by yohimbine. Science **225:** 847–849.
60. CLARK, J.T., E.R. SMITH & J.M. DAVIDSON. 1985. Evidence for the modulation of sexual behavior by α-andrenoceptors in male rats. Neuroendocrinology **41:** 36–43.
61. STEFANICK, M.L., E.R. SMITH, D.A. SZUMOWSKI & J.M. DAVIDSON. 1983. Reproductive physiology and behavior in the male rat following acute and chronic peripheral adrenergic depletion by guanethidine. Pharmacol. Biochem. Behav. **23:** 55–63.
62. HANSEN, S. & S.B. ROSS. 1983. Role of descending monoaminergic neurons in the

control of sexual behavior: effects of intrathecal infusions of 6-hydroxydopamine and 5,7-dihydroxytryptamine. Brain Res. **268:** 285–290.
63. QUINTIN BUDA, M., G. HILAVIC, C. BARDELAY, M. GHIGNONE & J.F. PIEJOL. 1986. Catecholamine metabolism in the rat locus coeruleus as studied by *in vivo* differential pulse voltammetry. III. Evidence for the existence of an alpha-2-adrenergic tonic inhibition in behaving rats. Brain Res. **375:** 235–245.
64. LARSSON, K., S. AHLENIUS, H. ERIKSSON, K. MODIGH & P. SÖDERSTEN. 1971. Mating behavior in the male rat treated with *p*-chlorophenylalanine methyl ester alone and in combination with pargyline. Psychopharmacologia **21:** 13–16.
65. MALMNÄS, W. 1973. Monoaminergic influence on testosterone-activating copulatory behavior in the castrated male rats. Acta Physiol. Scand. Suppl. **395:** 1–128.
66. LARSSON, K., K. FUXE, B.J. EVERITT, M. HOLMGREN & P. SÖDERSTEN. 1978. Sexual behavior in male rats after intracerebral injection of 5,7-dihydroxytryptamine. Brain Res. **141:** 293–303.
67. MCINTOSH, T.K. & R.J. BARFIELD. 1984. Brain monoaminergic control of male reproductive behavior. I. Serotonin and the postejaculatory refractory behavior. Behav. Brain Res. **12:** 255–265.
68. TÖRK, I. 1985. Raphe nuclei and serotonin containing systems. *In* The Rat Nervous System. G. Paxinos, Ed.: Vol 2: 43–78.
69. HILLEGAART, V., S. AHLENIUS & K. LARSSON. 1991. Region selective inhibition of male rat sexual behaviour and motor performance by localized forebrain 5-HT injections: a comparison with effects produced by 8-OH-DPAT. Behav. Brain Res. **42:** 169–180.
70. HJORTH, S., A. CARLSSON, P. LINDBERG, D. SANCHEZ, H. WIKSTRÖM, L-E. ARVIDSSON, U. HACKSELL & J.L.G NILSSON. 1982. 8-Hydroxy-2-(di-*n*-propylamino)tetralin, 8-OH-DPAT, a potent and selective simplified ergot congener with central 5-HT-receptor stimulating activity. J. Neural Transm. **55:** 169–188.
71. MIDDLEMISS, D.N. & J.R. FOZARD. 1983. 8-Hydroxy-2-(di-*n*-propylamino) tetralin discriminates between subtypes of the 5-HT$_{1A}$ recognition site. Eur. J. Pharmacol. **90:** 151–153.
72. AHLENIUS, S. & K. LARSSON. 1989. Antagonism by pindolol, but not betaxolol, of 8-OH-DPAT-induced facilitation of male rat sexual behavior. J. Neural. Transm. **77:** 163–170.
73. ANDERSSON, G. & K. LARSSON. 1994. Effects of FG 5893, a new compound with 5-HT$_{1A}$ agonistic and 5-HT$_2$ antagonistic properties, on male rat's sexual behavior. Eur. J. Pharmacol. **255:** 131–137.
74. HILLEGAART, V., S. HJORTH & S. AHLENIUS. 1990. Effects of 5-HT and 8-OH-DPAT on forebrain monoamine synthesis after local application into the median and dorsal raphe nuclei of the rat. J. Neural Transm. (Gen. Sect.) **81:** 131–145.
75. HILLEGAART, V., S. AHLENIUS & . K. LARSSON. 1989. Effects of local application of 5-HT into the median and dorsal raphe nuclei on male rat sexual and motor behavior. Behav. Brain Res. **33:** 279–286.
76. FERNÁNDEZ-GUASTI, A., A. ESCALANTE & A. ÅGMO. 1989. Inhibitory action of various 5-HT$_{1B}$ receptor agonists on rat masculine sexual behaviour. Pharmacol. Biochem. Behav. **34:** 811–816.
77. KLINT, T., I.L. DAHLGREN & K. LARSSON. 1992. The selective 5-HT$_2$ receptor antagonist amperozide attenuates 1-(2,5-dimethoxy-4-iodophenyl)-2-aminopropane-induced inhibition of male rat sexual behavior. Eur. J. Pharmacol. **212:** 241–246.
78. AHLENIUS, S. & K. LARSSON. 1998. Evidence for an involvement of 5-HT$_{1B}$ receptors in the inhibition of male rat ejaculatory behavior produced by 5-HTP. Psychopharmacology **137:** 374–382.
79. MATHES, C.W., E.R. SMITH, B.R. POPA & M. DAVIDSON. 1990. Effects of intrathecal and systemic administration of buspirone on genital reflexes and mating behavior in male rats. Pharmacol. Biochem. Behav. **36:** 63–68.
80. FINBERG, J.P. & Y. VARDI. 1990. Inhibitory effect of 5-hydroxytryptamine on penile erectile function in the rat. Br. J. Pharmacol. **101:** 698–702.
81. BERENDSEN, H.H.G. & C.L.E. BROEKKAMP. 1987. Drug-induced penile erections in rats: indications of serotonin-1$_B$ mediation. Eur. J. Pharmacol. **135:** 279–287.

82. BERENDSEN, H.H.G., F. JENCK & C.L.E. BROEKKAMP. 1990. Involvement of 5-HT$_{1C}$ receptors in drug-induced penile erections in rats. Psychopharmacology **101:** 57–61.
83. HILLEGAART, V. & S. AHLENIUS. 1998. Facilitation and inhibition of male rat ejaculatory behavior by the respective 5-HT$_{1A}$ and 5-HT$_{1B}$ receptor agonists 8-OH-DPAT and anpirtoline, as evidenced by use of the corresponding new and selective receptor antagonists NAD-299 and NAS-181. Br. J. Pharmacol. **125:** 1733–1743.
84. STANCAMPIANO, R., M.R. MELIS & A. ARGIOLAS. 1994. Penile erection and yawning induced by 5-HT$_{1C}$ receptor agonists in male rats: relationship with dopaminergic and oxytocinergic transmission. Eur. J. Pharmacol. **261:** 149–155.
85. MILLAN, M.J. & S. PERRIN-MONNEYRON. 1997. Potentiation of fluoxetine-induced penile erections by combined blockade of 5-HT$_{1A}$ and 5-HT$_{1B}$ receptors. Eur. J. Pharmacol. **321:** R11–R13.
86. AHLENIUS, S., K. LARSSON, L. SVENSSON, S. HJORTH, A. CARLSSON, P. LINDBERG, H. WIKSTRÖM, D. SANCHEZ, L-E. ARVIDSSON, U. HACKSELL & J.G.L. NILSSON. 1981. Effects of a new type of 5-HT receptor agonist on male rat sexual behavior. Pharmacol. Biochem. Behav. **15:** 785–792.

Cortical Afferents to the Extended Amygdala

ALEXANDER J. McDONALD,[a,d] SARA J. SHAMMAH-LAGNADO,[b]
CHANGJUN SHI,[c] AND MICHAEL DAVIS[c]

[a]Department of Cell Biology and Neuroscience, University of South Carolina
School of Medicine, Columbia, South Carolina 29208, USA
[b]Department of Physiology and Biophysics, University of São Paulo,
Institute of Biomedical Science, São Paulo, SP 05508, Brazil
[c]Department of Psychiatry and Behavioral Science,
Emory University School of Medicine, Atlanta, Georgia 30322, USA

ABSTRACT: The projections of the cerebral cortex to the extended amygdala were studied in the rat using anterograde and retrograde tract-tracing techniques. Most cortical areas with strong projections to the extended amygdala preferentially targeted either the medial extended amygdala (including the medial amygdalar nucleus, ventromedial substantia innominata, and the medial part of the bed nucleus the stria terminalis) or the central extended amygdala (including the central amygdalar nucleus, dorsolateral substantia innominata, and the lateral part of the bed nucleus of the stria terminalis). Some cortical areas, however, had equal projections to both medial and central portions. The main areas projecting preferentially to the medial extended amygdala were the ventral subiculum, infralimbic cortex, ventral agranular insular area, and the rostral part of the ventrolateral entorhinal area. The main areas projecting preferentially to the central extended amygdala were the prefrontal cortex, viscerosensory and somatosensory portions of the insular cortex, and the amygdalopiriform transitional area. It is suggested that these cortical inputs may be important for cognitive, mnemonic, and affective aspects of emotional and motivated behavior.

ABBREVIATIONS: AA, anterior amygdaloid area; AB, accessory basal nucleus; ac, anterior commissure; ACd, dorsal anterior cingulate cortex; ACv, ventral anterior cingulate cortex; AHA, amygdalohippocampal area; AId, dorsal agranular insular cortex; AIp, posterior agranular insular cortex; AIv, ventral agranular insular cortex; Apir, amygdalopiriform transitional area; ASt, amygdalostriatal transitional area; BAOT, bed nucleus of the accessory olfactory tract; Bmg, magnocellular basal nucleus; Bpc, parvicellular basal nucleus; BSTia, bed nucleus of the stria terminalis, intra-amygdaloid subdivision; BSTLd, lateral bed nucleus of the stria terminalis, dorsal subdivision; BSTLj, lateral bed nucleus of the stria terminalis, juxtacapsular subdivision; BSTLp, lateral bed nucleus of the stria terminalis, posterior subdivision; BSTLs, lateral bed nucleus of the stria terminalis, supracapsular subdivision; BSTLv, lateral bed nucleus of the stria terminalis, ventral subdivision; BSTM, medial bed nucleus of the stria terminalis; BSTMa, medial bed nucleus of the stria terminalis, anterior subdivision; BSTMpi, medial bed nucleus of the stria terminalis, posterior intermediate subdivision; BSTMpl, medial bed nucleus of the stria terminalis, posterior lateral subdivision; BSTMpm, medial bed nucleus of the stria

---

[d]Voice: 803-733-3378; fax: 803-733-3212; mcdonald@dcsmserver.med.sc.edu

terminalis, posterior medial subdivision; BSTMv, medial bed nucleus of the stria terminalis, ventral subdivision; cAIp, posterior agranular insular cortex, caudal portion; cERC, entorhinal cortex, caudal portion; CI, central nucleus, intermediate subdivision; CL, central nucleus, lateral subdivision; CLC, central nucleus, lateral capsular subdivision; CM, central nucleus, medial subdivision; Coa, cortical nucleus, anterior subdivision; CP, caudatoputamen; CXA, central extended amygdala; DI, dysgranular insular cortex; DIg, dysgranular insular cortex, gustatory portion; DIv, dysgranular insular cortex, visceral portion; DPC, dorsal peduncular cortex; End, endopiriform nucleus, dorsal subdivision; Env, endopiriform nucleus, ventral subdivision; ERC, entorhinal cortex; fx, fornix; GI, granular insular cortex; GP, globus pallidus; ic, internal capsule; Ic, intercalated nucleus; IL, infralimbic cortex; IPAC, interstitial nucleus of the posterior limb of the anterior commissure; Ld, lateral nucleus, dorsolateral subdivision; LH, lateral hypothalamus; LPO, lateral preoptic area; Lv, lateral nucleus, ventromedial subdivision; Mad, medial nucleus, anterodorsal subdivision; Mav, medial nucleus, anteroventral subdivision; Mpd, medial nucleus, posterodorsal subdivision; Mpv, medial nucleus, posteroventral subdivision; MCPO, magnocellular preoptic nucleus; MPO, medial preoptic nucleus; MXA, medial extended amygdala; NLOT, nucleus of the lateral olfactory tract; NXA, nonextended amygdala; Oc1, primary occipital cortex; Oc2, secondary occipital cortex; oc, optic chiasm; ot, optic tract; PAC, periamygdaloid cortex; PaRh, parietal rhinal cortex; PC, piriform cortex; PL, prelimbic cortex; PRC, perirhinal cortex; PRCd, perirhinal cortex, dorsal portion; PRCv, perirhinal cortex, ventral portion; PrCl, lateral precentral cortex; PrCm, medial precentral cortex; PT, paratenial thalamic nucleus; PV, parietal ventral area; rAIp, rostral posterior agranular insular area; rDLEA, rostral dorsolateral entorhinal area; Rt, reticular thalamic nucleus; rVLEA, rostral ventrolateral entorhinal area; S, subiculum; SI, substantia innominata; SIb, substantia innominata, basal subdivision; SId, substantia innominata, dorsal subdivision; SIv, substantia innominata, ventral subdivision; SI, primary somatosensory area; SII, secondary somatosensory area; sm, stria medullaris; st, stria terminalis; Subv, ventral subiculum; Te1, rat temporal cortex, area 1; Te2, rat temporal cortex, area 2; Te2D, rat temporal cortex, area 2, dorsal portion; Te3, rat temporal cortex, area 3; Te3R, rat temporal cortex, area 3, rostral portion; TT, tenia tecta; Tu, olfactory tubercle; VLEA, ventrolateral entorhinal area; VMEA, ventromedial entorhinal area; VP, ventral pallidum.

INTRODUCTION

Anatomical and histochemical studies conducted by Lennart Heimer and his colleagues during the last 20 years have demonstrated that concealed within the seemingly disorganized array of neurons in the basal forebrain, there exist discrete, functionally specific components that constitute important links in separate descending cortical pathways.[1-3] One of these components is the "extended amygdala," which consists of the centromedial amygdala, the bed nucleus of the stria terminalis (BST), and several structures that extend between these two regions. This complex forms a key component of the "emotional motor system," a critical substrate for emotion and motivated behavior.[4]

In all mammals, including humans, the most complex inputs to the amygdala originate from the cerebral cortex, especially from higher-order association areas.[5] Although it is known that several areas send robust inputs to the extended amygdala, there have been no comprehensive studies of these projections. In the investigations described below, these inputs have been studied in the rat using anterograde and retrograde tract-tracing techniques. The anterograde studies used *Phaseolus vulgaris* leukoagglutinin (PHA-L) as an anterograde tracer. PHA-L injections were made into virtually all cortical regions known to project to the amygdala. Retrograde studies, which were only conducted on the central extended amygdala, used cholera toxin B subunit or fluorescent dyes (Fluoro-gold and dextran-rhodamine) as retrograde tracers.

There is evidence from anatomical, histochemical, and functional studies that the extended amygdala can be divided into central and medial parts. The central portion of the extended amygdala (CXA) consists of the central amygdalar nucleus, lateral part of the BST (BSTL), dorsolateral portions of the sublenticular substantia innominata (SId), interstitial nucleus of the posterior limb of the anterior commissure (IPAC), and the "lateral pocket" of the supracapsular portion of the BST (BSTLs; discontinuous clusters of neurons located along the course of the lateral part of the stria terminalis). The medial portion of the extended amygdala (MXA) consists of the medial amygdalar nucleus, medial part of the BST (BSTM), ventromedial portions of the sublenticular substantia innominata (SIv), and the "medial pocket" of the supracapsular portion of the BST (BSTMs; scattered neurons located along the course of the medial part of the stria terminalis). In the studies described below the subdivisions of the BST, SI, and medial amygdalar nucleus recognized by Alheid and coworkers[3] were, with some modifications, used to describe projections to these regions. In general, the central nuclear region was subdivided according to the description by McDonald.[6] However, on the basis of immunohistochemical and connectional studies, the rostrodorsal portion of the lateral capsular subdivision of the central nucleus (CLC) is considered to represent a caudal part of the IPAC, whereas the caudodorsal CLC is considered to represent a portion of the amygdalostriatal transitional area (ASt). Only the ventral part of the CLC, as originally described, will be termed the CLC (i.e., the portion located adjacent to the medial border of the basal nucleus).

The results of the PHA-L anterograde studies will be described first, followed by the retrograde tract-tracing findings. Only ipsilateral projections will be described. Significant contralateral corticoamygdalar projections were seen from some cortical areas (e.g., frontal, insular, and temporal) but not others (e.g., entorhinal, subicular, and amygdalopiriform). Contralateral projections to the central extended amygdala generally mirror those seen ipsilaterally but usually are lighter. By contrast, no significant contralateral projection to the medial extended amygdala was observed.

FRONTAL PROJECTIONS TO THE EXTENDED AMYGDALA

The frontal cortex of the rat consists of medial, orbital, and lateral portions (FIG. 1). The medial and lateral portions are the main sources of amygdalar afferents. The amygdalopetal medial frontal cortex consists of six areas arranged from ventral

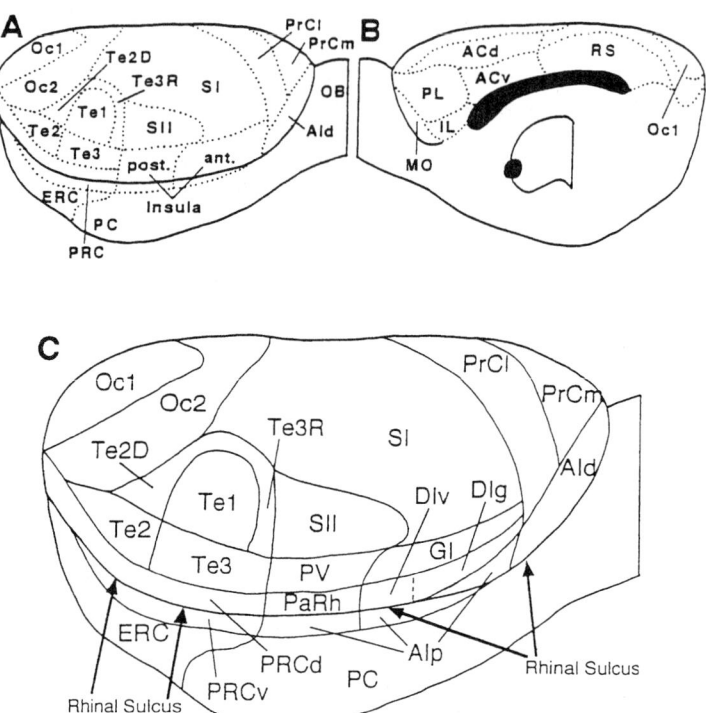

FIGURE 1. Anatomy of the rat cerebral cortex. Major cortical areas are illustrated on the lateral (**A**) and medial (**B**) surfaces of the cerebral hemisphere. Details of the insular region are shown in **C** (see text).

to dorsal: the dorsal peduncular, infralimbic, prelimbic, anterior dorsal cingulate, and the medial precentral areas. The amygdalopetal lateral frontal cortex consists of two rostral insular areas: the dorsal and ventral agranular insular areas.

Infralimbic Cortex (IL)

The efferents resulting from injections of PHA-L into the anterior and central part of the IL (FIG. 2) mainly target the MXA. These IL projections innervate a continuous terminal field that involves, from rostral to caudal, the BSTM, SIv, and the medial nucleus (FIG. 3). The projections to the BST target the anterior (BSTMa), ventral (BSTMv), and posterolateral (BSTMpl) parts of the BSTM (FIG. 3, A and B). Most of the fibers in the BSTL and SId do not exhibit axonal varicosities and thus appear to be passing through these regions without forming synaptic connections. There are also projections to the basal part of the SI (FIG. 3A). Efferents to the medial nucleus terminate in all subdivisions of the nucleus, with the exception of its posterodorsal subdivision (FIG. 3, E–G). There are also projections to the intra-amygdaloid part of the BST (BSTia). Although some fibers pass through the central amygdalar nucleus, axonal terminations are only seen in its lateral capsular subdivision (CLC) (FIG. 3E). The latter terminal field is continuous with a projection to the

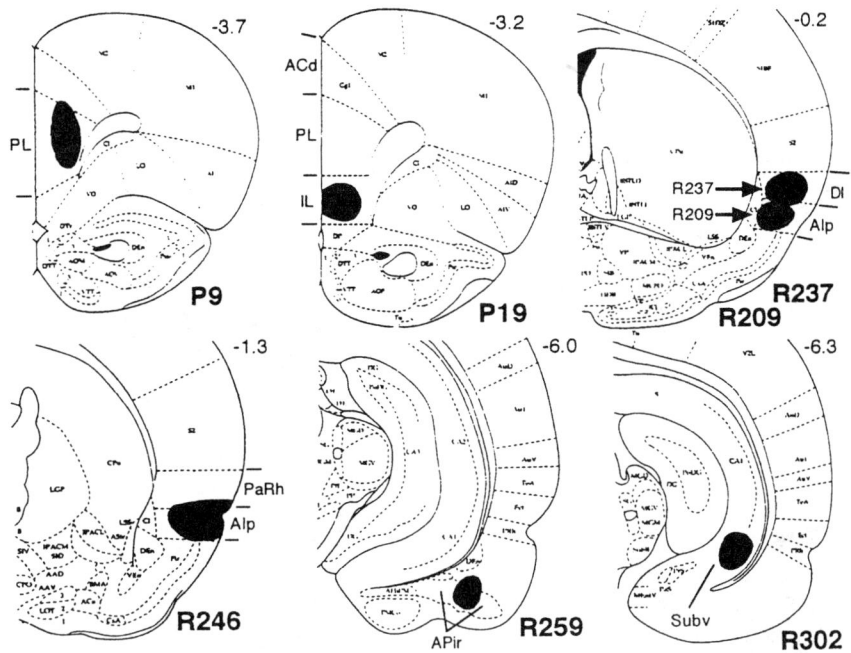

FIGURE 2. Locations of the PHA-L injection sites in the cases mapped in FIGURES 3–9. Black area indicates the effective injection site (i.e., the region containing labeled perikarya that give rise to the observed projection). Numbers in the upper right corner of each section indicate its anteroposterior level in relation to bregma (as illustrated in the atlas by Paxinos and Watson[13]).

amygdalostriatal transitional region (ASt) (FIG. 3F). The IL projects to the rostral part of the interstitial nucleus of the posterior limb of the anterior commissure (IP-AC) at the level of the anterior commissure, but this projection mainly targets its ventral edge (FIG. 3, A and B). This projection is not present at levels caudal to the BST.

The caudal pole of the IL has efferents that are similar to those of the anterocentral IL, but additional light to moderate projections are seen to portions of the CXA, including the BSTL and the medial (CM) and intermediate (CI) subdivisions of the central amygdalar nucleus. The projections to the dorsal (BSTLd) and juxtacapsular (BSTLj) subdivisions of the BSTL are light, whereas the projections to the ventral (BSTLv) and posterior (BSTLp) subdivisions are moderate. The terminal field in the CI continues caudally into the medial half of the lateral subdivision of the central nucleus (CL), but there are very few fibers in the lateral half of the CL. In addition, projections to the BSTia are particularly strong with injections into the caudal part of the IL.

Dorsal Peduncular Cortex (DPC)

The DPC is located just ventral to the IL. It has projections that are similar to those of the IL projections, but the efferents to the BSTM are very light.

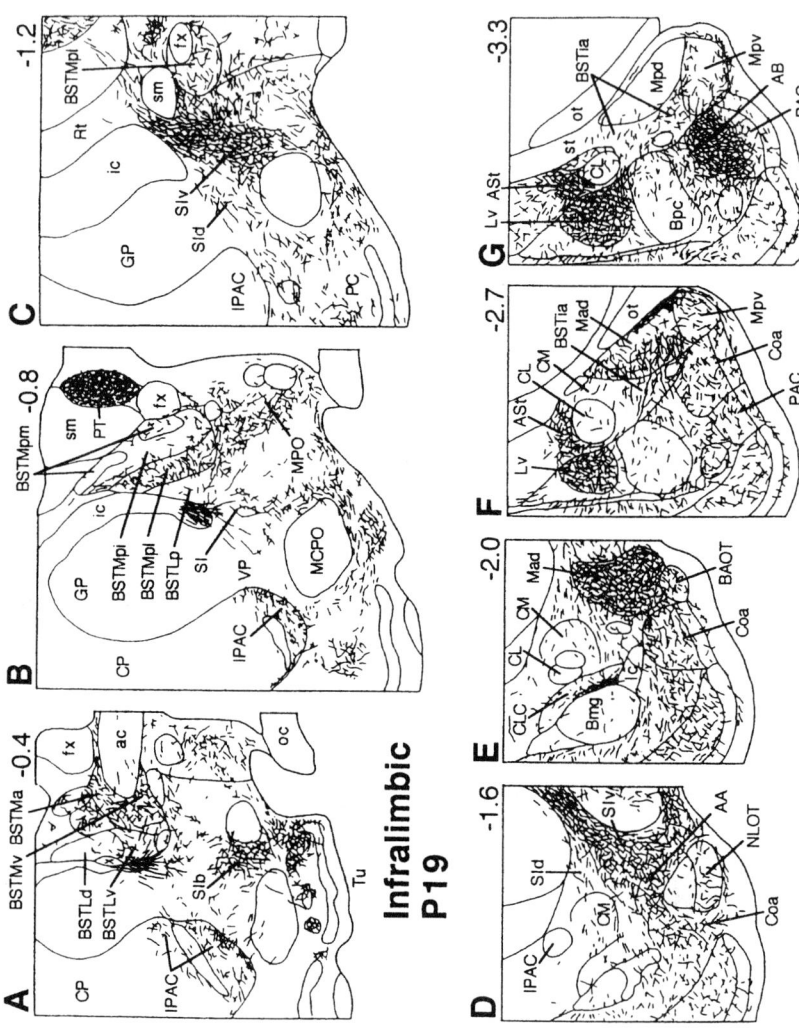

FIGURE 3. Drawing of coronal sections arranged from rostral (A) to caudal (G), illustrating the distribution of labeled axons following a PHA-L injection into the infralimbic frontal cortex (case P19, see FIG. 2). Only levels that contain the extended amygdala are drawn.

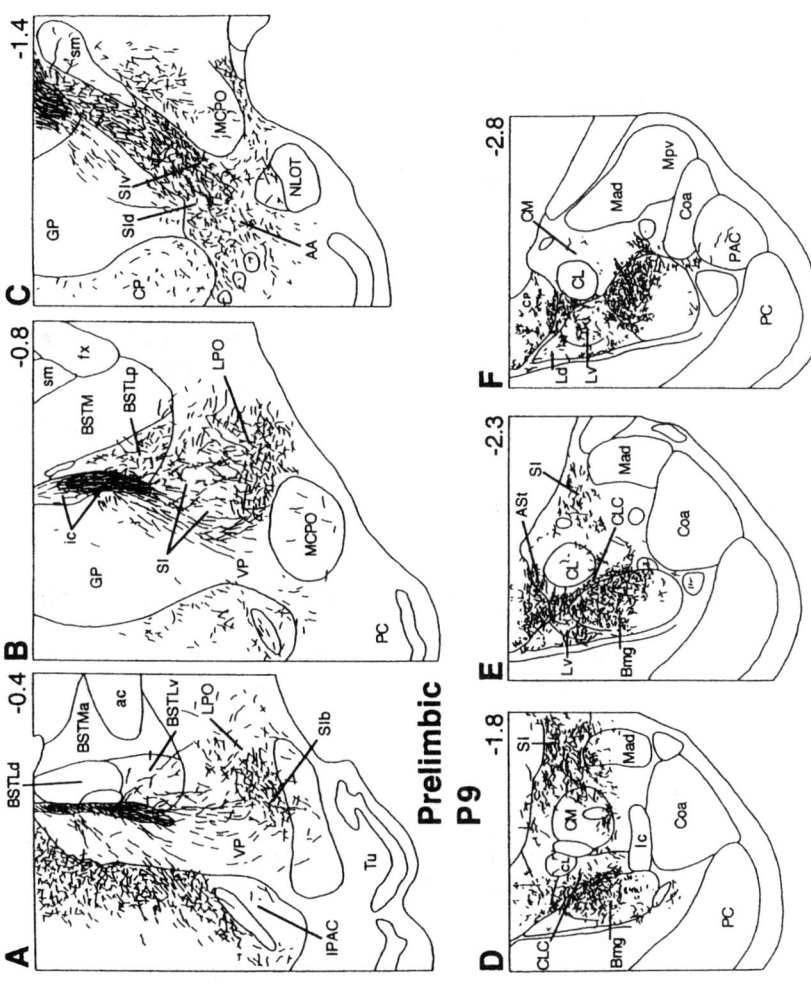

FIGURE 4. Drawing of coronal sections arranged from rostral (A) to caudal (F), illustrating the distribution of labeled axons following a PHA-L injection into the prelimbic frontal cortex (case P9, see FIG. 2). Only levels that contain the extended amygdala are drawn.

Prelimbic Cortex (PL)

The PL sends efferents to restricted regions of the extended amygdala (FIG. 4). There are no projections to the BSTM or anterior parts of the BSTL (BSTLd, BSTLj) and only very weak projections to the BSTLv. However, the PL sends strong to moderate projections to the BSTLp that continue caudally into the SI (FIG. 4, B–E). The efferents to the latter area appear to involve both the SId and SIv. Although the terminal field in the SI can be followed caudally to the amygdala proper, there are no significant projections to the medial or central nuclei, with the exception of a light projection to the CLC (FIG. 4, D and E). The PL has projections to the IPAC region that mainly target the region just dorsal to the posterior limb of the anterior commissure (FIG. 4A). These projections are greatly attenuated at levels caudal to the BST.

Medial Precentral (PrCm) and the Dorsal Anterior Cingulate (ACd) Areas

The PrCm and ACd have no projection to the extended amygdala with the exception of a light projection to the CLC.

Dorsal Agranular Insular Cortex (AId)

The AId has light projections to a more or less continuous sagittally oriented zone that includes, from rostral to caudal, the BSTLv, BSTLp, SId, and the medial subdivision of the central nucleus (CM). There is also a light to moderate projection to the IPAC. At the level of the rostral third of the magnocellular basal nucleus, the terminal field in IPAC merges with terminal fields in the rostrodorsal part of the CLC, the lateral rim of the rostral CL, and the rostral part of the CM. There is no significant projection to the middle and caudal thirds of the central nucleus.

Ventral Agranular Insular Cortex (AIv)

The AIv has a strong projection to the rostral part of the CLC. Although there are many fibers that course through the anterodorsal subdivision of the medial nucleus (Mad) and the SIv, only some of these bear axonal varicosities. Thus, these regions receive only a light to moderate projection from the AIv. There are no projections to any part of the BST.

INSULAR PROJECTIONS TO THE EXTENDED AMYGDALA

The most rostral insular regions in the rat (i.e., AId and AIv) are generally considered to represent the lateral prefrontal cortex (see above). The rat insular region that is located caudal to the lateral prefrontal cortex contains gustatory, visceral, and somatosensory representations. Anatomical and physiological studies suggest that the anterior three fifths of this nonprefrontal insular region (between bregma levels +2.5 and −1.0), which will be termed the "anterior insular cortex" (FIG. 1A), is involved in gustatory and general visceral functions.[5,7–9] The posterior two fifths of the caudal insular region (between bregma levels −1.0 and −3.5), which will be termed the "posterior insular cortex" (FIG. 1A), is primarily involved in somesthesis.[5,10,11]

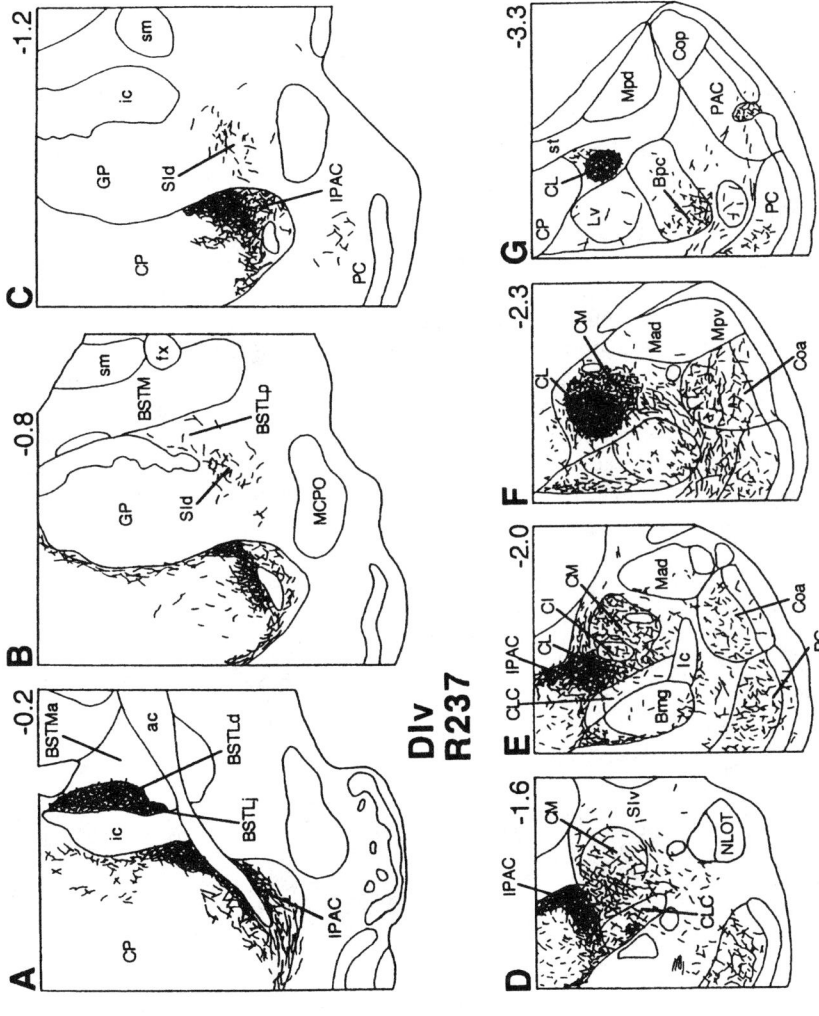

FIGURE 5. Drawing of coronal sections arranged from rostral (A) to caudal (G), illustrating the distribution of labeled axons following a PHA-L injection into the viscerosensory portion of the dysgranular insular cortex (case R237, see FIG. 2). Only levels that contain the extended amygdala are drawn.

Anterior Insular Cortex

The anterior insular region comprises three zones arranged from dorsal to ventral: (1) granular anterior insular cortex (GI), (2) dysgranular anterior insular cortex (DI), and (3) the rostral part of the posterior agranular insular cortex (AIp) (FIG. 1C). Only the DI and AIp have significant projections to the amygdala. Kosar *et al.*[7] have shown that the primary gustatory cortex is located in the rostral part of the DI. This cortical area, located between bregma +2.5 and bregma +0.2, will be termed the "gustatory DI" (DIg of FIG. 1C). The caudal part of the DI contains neurons that are responsive to general visceral sensory stimulation.[8] This cortical area, located between bregma +0.2 and bregma −1.0, will be termed the "visceral DI" (DIv of FIG. 1C). Viscerosensory areas in the GI have little or no projection to the amygdala. The AIp located adjacent to the DI receives afferents from the overlying gustatory/visceral receptive cortices and the piriform cortex.[5,9,12]

The DI region has robust projections to the extended amygdala. The projections from the gustatory (DIg) and visceral (DIv) areas of DI were similar. These areas targeted the CXA but not the MXA. The DI has strong projections to the BSTLd and BSTLj at the level of the anterior commissure (FIG. 5A). These terminal fields are continuous laterally with a terminal field in the rostral part of IPAC. There is also a light projection to the BSTLp that is continuous caudolaterally with a projection to the SId (FIGURE 5, B and C). The latter terminal field is continuous with a projection to the medial part of the central nucleus (FIG. 5D). The terminal field in the IPAC, which was particularly dense in its medial portion, can be followed caudally to the rostral pole of the amygdala, where it extends ventrally to become continuous with

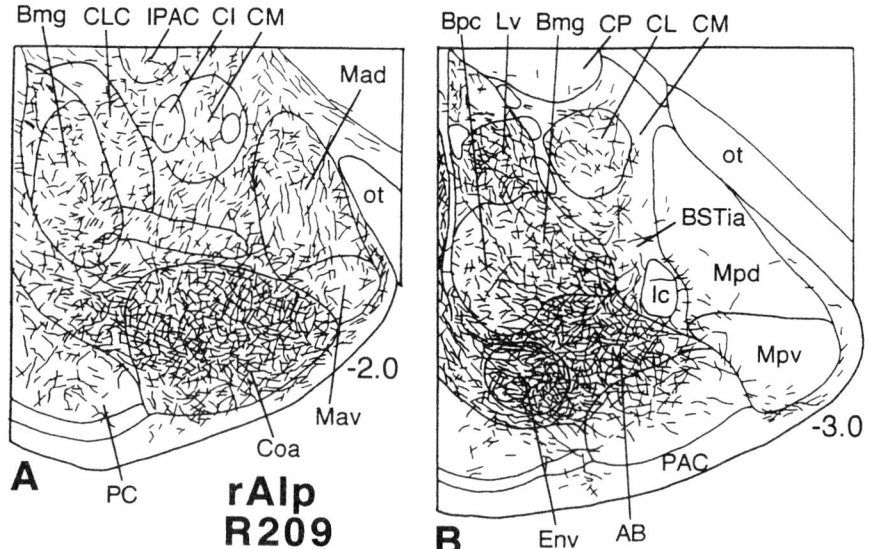

FIGURE 6. Drawing of coronal sections arranged from rostral (**A**) to caudal (**B**), illustrating the distribution of labeled axons in the rostral amygdala following a PHA-L injection into the rostral half of the posterior agranular insular cortex (case R209, see FIG. 2).

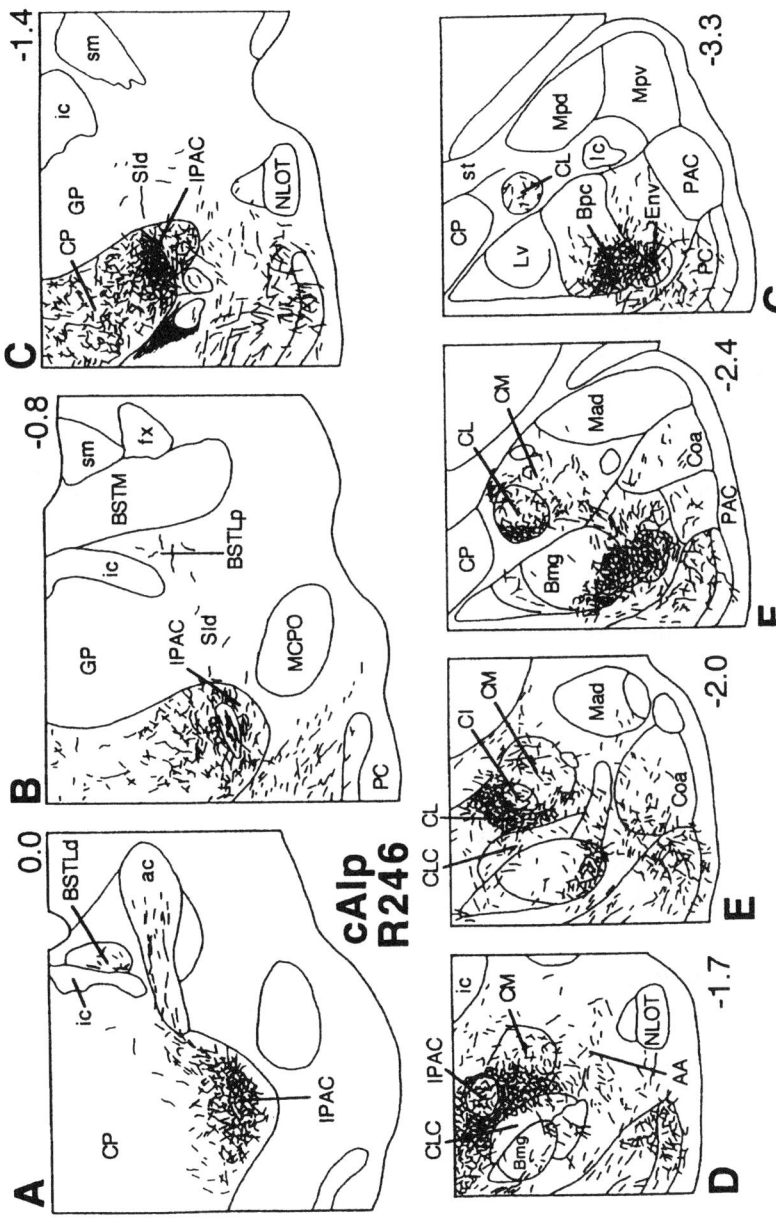

FIGURE 7. Drawing of coronal sections arranged from rostral (A) to caudal (G), illustrating the distribution of labeled axons following a PHA-L injection into the caudal half of the posterior agranular insular cortex (case R246, see FIG. 2). Only levels that contain the extended amygdala are drawn.

a very dense terminal field in the CL (FIG. 5E). There are also projections to the CI and CM at this level, but these projections are lighter than the CL projection. The projections to the CL and CM extend as far caudal as the caudal pole of the central nucleus. There is also a light projection to the rostral pole of the CLC (FIG. 5D) and a strong projection to the lateral pocket of the supracapsular division of the BST (BSTLs).

The portion of AIp located ventral to the DI has projections to widespread portions of the extended amygdala that are light and diffuse (FIG. 6). There are a small number of fibers scattered throughout all portions of the lateral and medial BST. However, there are never more than 5–10 fibers in each subdivision in each section. There are similar diffuse projections to the SId and SIv, rostral portions of the medial nucleus (Mad and Mav), and to all portions of the central nucleus (FIG. 6). Finally, there is a projection to the IPAC that mainly targets the ventral edge of this region, similar to the projection from the infralimbic cortex.

Posterior Insular Cortex

The posterior insular region comprises three zones arranged from dorsal to ventral: (1) the parietal ventral cortex (PV), (2) parietal rhinal cortex (PaRh), and (3) the caudal part of the posterior agranular insular cortex (AIp) (FIG. 1C). These areas extend from bregma −1.0 to −3.5.[5,11] They are replaced caudally by perirhinal and temporal cortical areas. The caudal half of PaRh and AIp (bregma −1.8 to −3.5) corresponds to a region formerly considered to be the anterior part of the perirhinal cortex.[13] However, the connections of this region suggest that it is actually part of the somatosensory insula.[5,11] The AIp located adjacent to PaRh receives afferents from the piriform cortex and from overlying somatosensory receptive cortices.[5,11,12] Amygdalar projections arise mainly from the PaRh, located on the dorsal bank of the rhinal fissure, and from the ventrally adjacent AIp, located on the ventral bank of the rhinal fissure.

The PaRh projections to the extended amygdala mainly terminate in the CLC. By contrast, the projections of the ventrally adjacent AIp tend to avoid the CLC. At the level of the BST, the AIp has very light projections to the BSTLd and BSTLp, but strong projections to the IPAC (FIGURE 7, A–C). At more caudal levels the terminal field in IPAC is continuous with a terminal field that occupies the lateral half of the CL (FIGURE 7, D–F). There are also light projections to the CM.

TEMPORAL AND PERIRHINAL PROJECTIONS TO THE EXTENDED AMYGDALA

The perirhinal cortex (PRC) occupies the banks of the rhinal fissure from about the bregma −3.5 level to the caudal pole of the hemisphere[5,11] (FIG. 1). The temporal association areas (Te2 and Te3) are located dorsally adjacent to the PRC throughout most of its rostrocaudal extent. Te2 and Te3 are visual and auditory association areas, whereas the PRC appears to be polymodal, receiving projections from visual, auditory, somatosensory, and olfactory cortical areas.[5] The only portion of the extended amygdalar region targeted by the temporal association areas is the ASt. The PRC has moderate projections to the ASt and the CLC. In addition, light to moderate

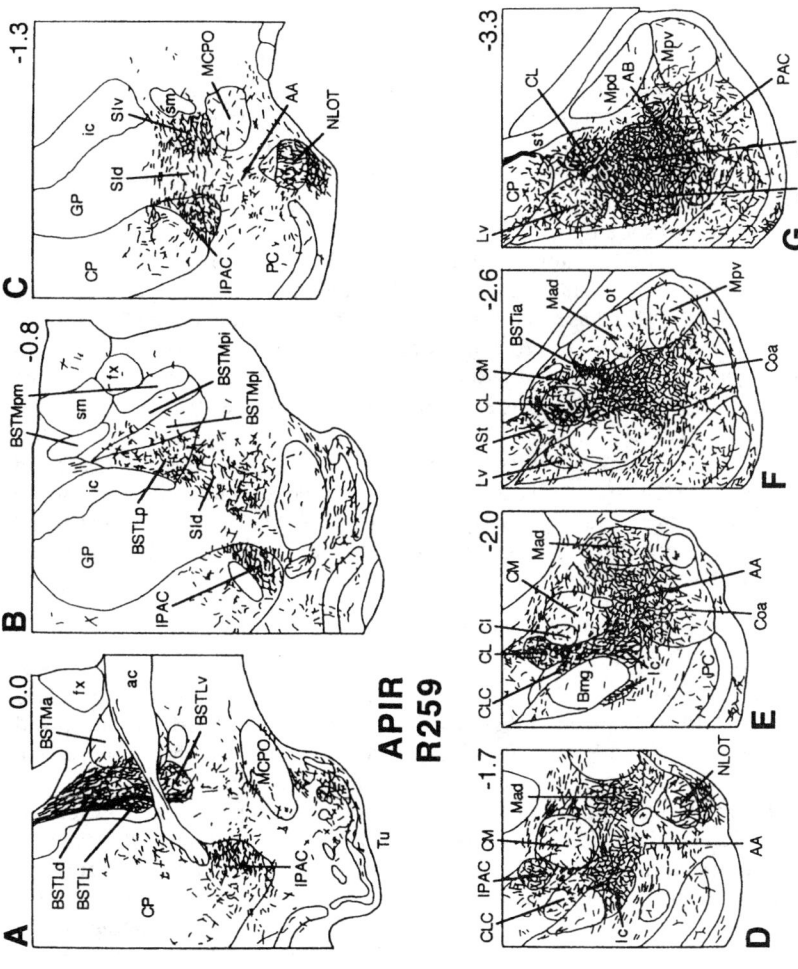

FIGURE 8. Drawing of coronal sections arranged from rostral (A) to caudal (G), illustrating the distribution of labeled axons following a PHA-L injection into the amygdalopiriform transitional area (case R259, see FIG. 2). Only levels that contain the extended amygdala are drawn.

projections to the Mad were seen in some PRC cases. Some fibers from the PRC run through the IPAC, but few appear to terminate there.

ENTORHINAL, PIRIFORM, AND AMYGDALOPIRIFORM TRANSITIONAL AREA PROJECTIONS TO THE EXTENDED AMYGDALA

Entorhinal Cortex

The entorhinal projection to the amygdala arises mainly from the lateral entorhinal cortex (ERC). The lateral ERC consists of three fields arranged from medial to lateral: the (1) ventromedial entorhinal area (VMEA), (2) ventrolateral entorhinal area (VLEA), and (3) dorsolateral entorhinal area (DLEA). Only the rostral fourth of the ERC has significant projections to the extended amygdala. Projections from its caudal three fourths are light.

All three areas in the caudal three fourths of the ERC have very modest projections to the extended amygdala. Thus, the VMEA and VLEA have a light projection to the Mad, and the VLEA has an additional moderate projection to the CLC and the ASt. The DLEA has only light projections to the latter areas. There were light to moderate projections to the ventral part of the rostral IPAC (i.e., ventral to the posterior limb of the anterior commissure) from the DLEA and the VLEA.

In rostral DLEA cases, there were light to moderate projections to both the CXA (CL, CLC, BSTL, and the ventral part of the rostral IPAC) and the MXA (Mad and Mpv). By contrast, the rostral VLEA had light to moderate projections mainly to portions of the MXA (including the Mad, and the BSTM [BSTMa, BSTMv, and BSTMpl]). There were also moderate projections to the CLC. Although many fibers ran through the rostral IPAC, few terminated in this region.

Amygdalopiriform Transitional Area (APir)

The APir is located at the caudal pole of the parvicellular basal amygdalar nucleus, the caudomedial corner of the piriform cortex, and the rostral pole of the DLEA/VLEA border. A PHA-L injection that involved the APir, as well as adjacent rostral portions of the DLEA and VLEA (FIG. 2), produced a very robust projection to the extended amygdala, especially to the CXA (FIG. 8). There were light projections to the CM, CI, and the ASt and strong projections to the ventral part of the CLC and to the CL, especially its lateral half (FIGURE 8, D–G). At the rostral pole of the central nucleus, the terminal field in the CL was continuous with a terminal field that occupied the ventromedial part of the IPAC (FIGURE 8, D and E). At the level of the BST, the terminal field in the IPAC extended dorsomedially to become continuous with a terminal field that extended through all subdivisions of the BSTL (FIGURE 8, A and B). There were also efferents to the BSTL that ran through the lateral part of the stria terminalis. Some of these strial fibers provided an innervation of the lateral pocket of the supracapsular part of the BST (BSTLs). In addition there was a projection that extended through and terminated in the SI (SIv and to a lesser extent SId). At rostral levels this SI projection was continuous with the terminal field in the BSTLp. Finally, there was also a light projection to the BSTMpl and a moderate projection to the medial nucleus (especially Mad). The latter projections were stronger with in-

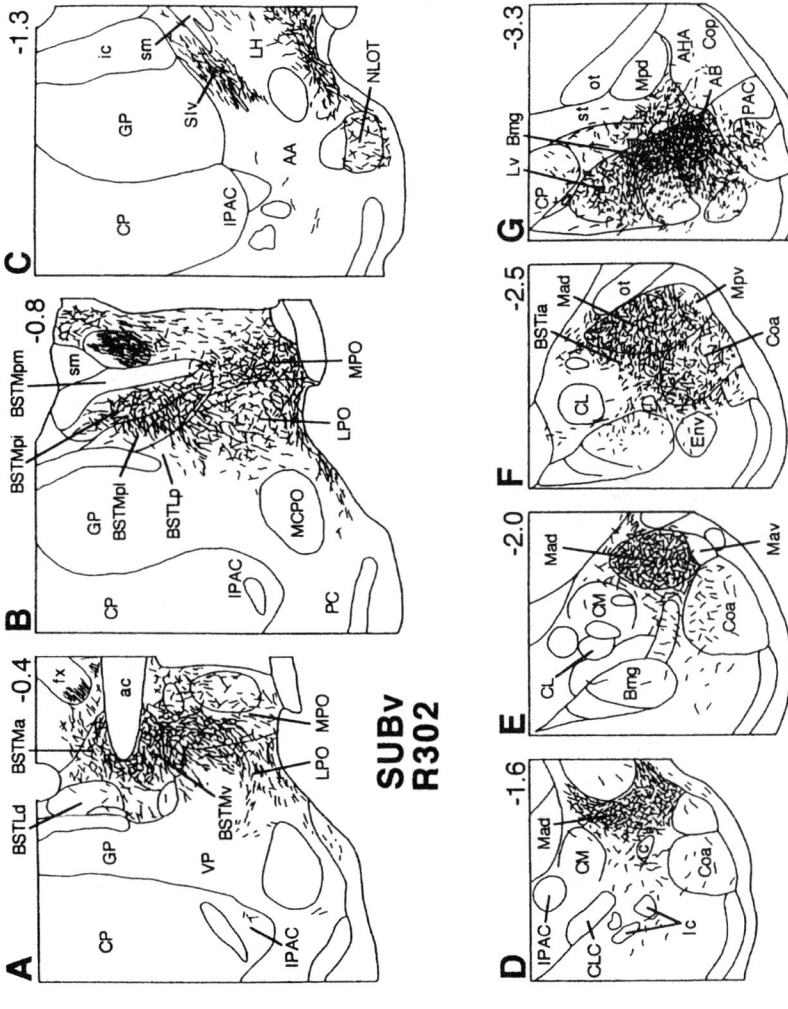

FIGURE 9. Drawing of coronal sections arranged from rostral (**A**) to caudal (**G**), illustrating the distribution of labeled axons following a PHA-L injection into the ventral subiculum (case R302, see FIG. 2). Only levels that contain the extended amygdala are drawn.

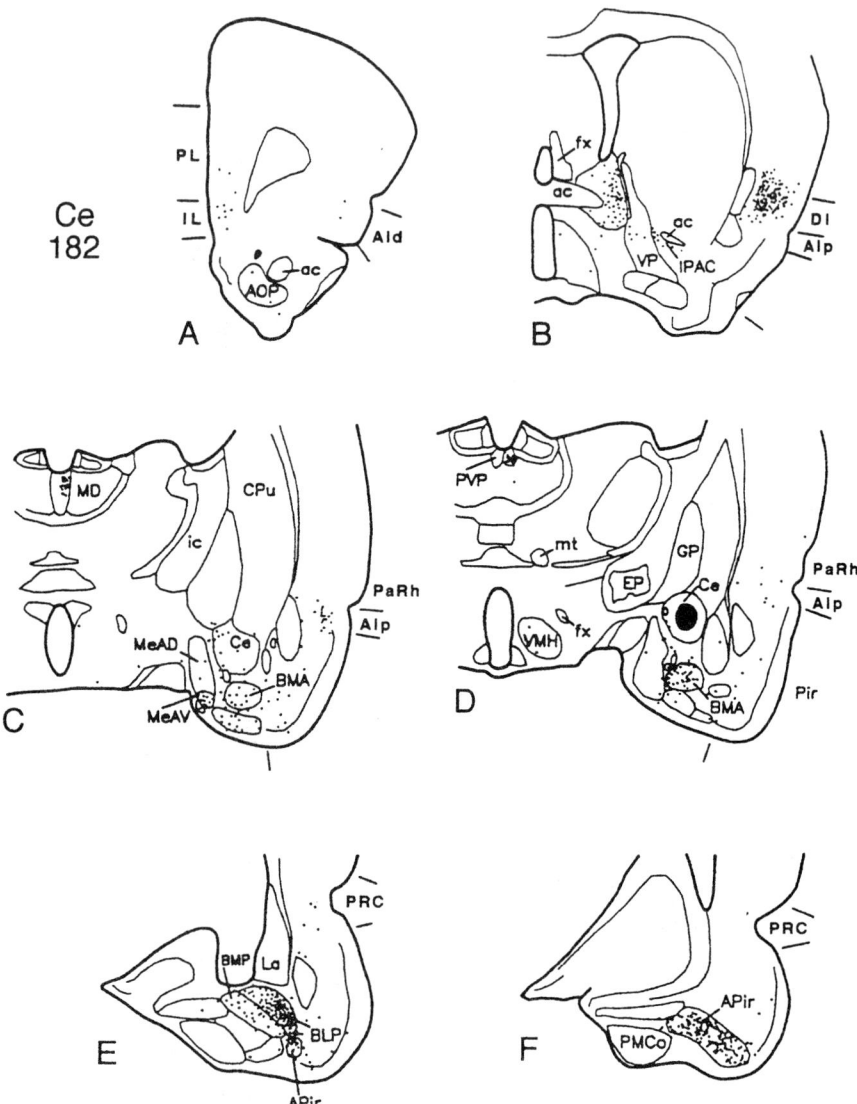

FIGURE 10. Drawing of coronal sections arranged from rostral (**A**) to caudal (**F**), illustrating the distribution of retrogradely labeled neurons following an injection of cholera toxin B subunit into the lateral subdivision of the central nucleus. Each dot represents two labeled neurons. The black area indicates the center of the injection site (**D**).

jections of PHA-L confined to the medial part of APir but were still considerably less dense than those to the CXA.

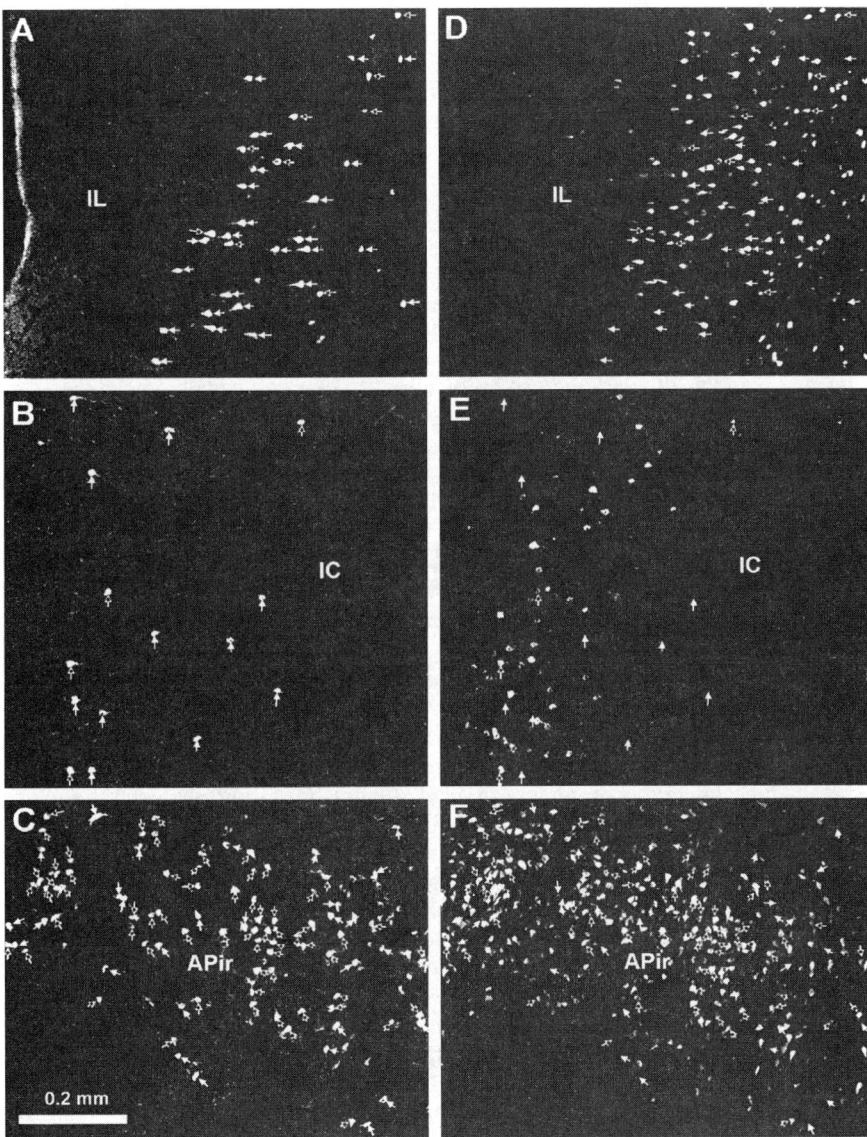

FIGURE 11. Fluorescence photomicrographs of retrogradely labeled neurons in the infralimbic cortex (**A, D**), anterior insular cortex (**B, E**), and APir (**C, F**). Photomicrographs A–C show neurons labeled by a small injection of dextran-rhodamine (DR) into the medial part of the central nucleus (using filters for DR). Photomicrographs **D–F** show neurons labeled in the same three sections by a large injection of Fluoro-gold (FG) into the BSTL/BSTM (using filters for FG). Solid arrows in **A–C** indicate neurons that are single labeled for DR (their positions are shown by solid arrows in **D–F**). Open arrows indicate neurons that contain both DR and FG (i. e., that project to both the central nucleus and the BST).

Piriform Cortex (PC)

With injections of PHA-L into central portions of the PC and the adjacent dorsal endopiriform nucleus at the level of the rostral amygdala, limited projections to the central and medial extended amygdala were seen. There were light to moderate projections to the CLC, CL, Mad, and SIv and strong projections to the ventral part of the rostral IPAC. In addition, a few scattered fibers were seen in the BSTM.

HIPPOCAMPAL PROJECTIONS TO THE EXTENDED AMYGDALA

Hippocampal projections to the amygdala arise from the ventral portions of the subiculum and the adjacent CA1. The CA1 appeared to send no efferents to the extended amygdala, although there are projections to other amygdalar nuclei. By contrast, PHA-L injections into the ventral subiculum (FIG. 2), all of which were centered in its lateral half, produced robust anterograde label throughout the medial extended amygdala (FIG. 9). These projections terminated in a continuous field that included the BSTM (BSTMa, BSTMv, BSTMpl, and BSTMpi), the SIv, the medial amygdalar nucleus (mainly Mad), and the BSTia (FIGURE 9, A–F). There was also a light projection to the BSTL (BSTLv and BSTLp) and the most medial portion of the ASt located adjacent to the CL.

RETROGRADE TRACT-TRACING EXPERIMENTS

Retrograde tract-tracing experiments were mainly confined to the central extended amygdala. Injections of cholera toxin B subunit (CTb) into the central nucleus produced significant numbers of retrogradely labeled cells in several cortical areas, including the infralimbic cortex (IL), dysgranular portions of the anterior (gustatory/visceral) insular cortex (DIg and DIv), agranular portions of the posterior insular cortex (i.e., the caudal part of AIp), and the amygdalopiriform transitional area (APir) (FIG. 10). Injections of different color fluorescent dyes (Fluoro-gold and dextran-rhodamine) into the central nucleus and the BST (involving the BSTL and, to a lesser extent, the BSTM) produced similar retrograde labeling in the cortex, including many double-labeled cells in the caudal IL, DI/AIp, and APir (FIG. 11). The latter findings indicate that many neurons in these cortical areas have axons that branch to innervate both the central nucleus and the BSTL.

Injections of CTb into the ventral and medial parts of the IPAC produce more extensive retrograde labeling than that seen with the central nucleus injections (FIG. 12). Labeled areas included most portions of the prefrontal cortex, the mesocortex along the entire rostrocaudal extent of the rhinal fissure, the piriform cortex and amygdalopiriform transitional area, the medial and lateral ERC, and the subiculum. Thus, the ventromedial IPAC receives projections from all of the cortical areas that innervate the central nucleus, as well as from additional areas that were primarily located along the more caudal portions of the rhinal sulcus (PaRh, PRC, and the temporal association areas) and in the hippocampal region (ERC and subiculum).

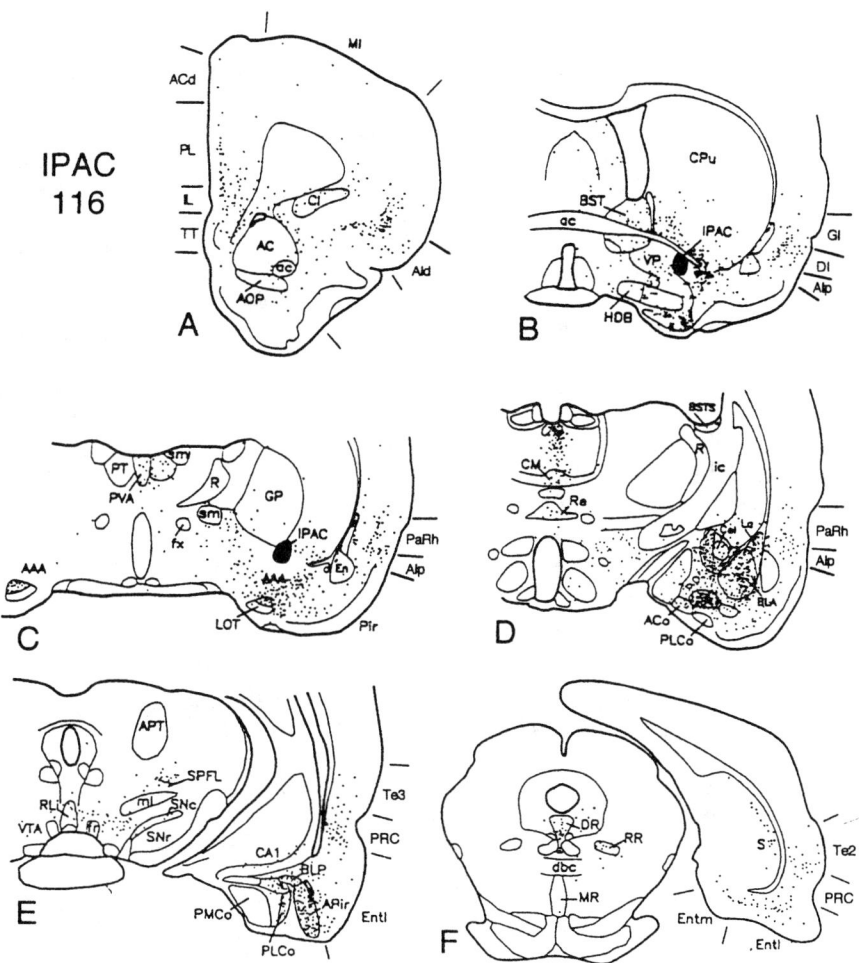

FIGURE 12. Drawing of coronal sections arranged from rostral (**A**) to caudal (**F**), illustrating the distribution of retrogradely labeled neurons following an injection of cholera toxin B subunit into the interstitial nucleus of the posterior limb of the anterior commissure (IPAC). Each dot represents two labeled neurons. The black area indicates the center of the injection site (**B** and **C**).

DISCUSSION

The results of the PHA-L anterograde experiments are displayed in TABLE 1, which groups the principal targets of cortical afferents to the extended amygdalar region into three regions arranged from medial to lateral: the (1) medial extended amygdala (MXA), (2) central extended amygdala (CXA), and (3) a region that may not be a portion of either the CXA or MXA (i.e., it may be a nonextended amygdalar region, NXA), consisting of the CLC and the ASt. The MXA and CXA appear to have components that extend from the amygdala proper to the bed nucleus of the stria terminalis, whereas this does not appear to be true of the structures in the NXA (see below).

The cortical areas in TABLE 1 have been grouped into four types on the basis of their extended amygdalar targets. Group 1 areas project mainly to the CXA. Group 2 areas project mainly to the MXA. Group 3 areas have roughly equal projections to the CXA and MXA. Group 4 areas have no significant projections to the CXA or MXA but do have projections to the NXA (CLC and/or the ASt). The latter nuclei also receive significant inputs from the cortical areas in groups 1–3. The results of the retrograde tracing experiments, which were performed on structures in the CXA (central nucleus, BSTL, and IPAC) are, in general, consistent with the anterograde findings.

One of the most interesting findings is that cortical areas with robust projections to the extended amygdala preferentially target either the CXA or the MXA. Another noteworthy finding is that many cortical areas that target the CXA or MXA have projections that terminate in the two poles of the extended amygdala (centromedial amygdala and the BST), as well as in the "corridors" that bridge these regions. Moreover, the double-labeling retrograde studies indicate that individual cortical neurons may have axons that branch to innervate both poles of the CXA. It remains to be determined whether neurons in cortical areas that innervate the MXA do the same.

CORTICAL AREAS THAT PREFERENTIALLY TARGET THE MEDIAL EXTENDED AMYGDALA

The main cortical areas projecting to the MXA are the ventral subiculum (Subv), infralimbic (IL) and dorsal peduncular (DPC) cortices, rostral portions of the VLEA (rVLEA), and the AIv (TABLE 1). Consistent with the concept of the extended amygdala, these cortical areas tend to project in a continuous manner to two or three adjacent portions of the medial extended amygdala, including the medial amygdalar nucleus (particularly its anterodorsal subdivision, Mad), the ventromedial part of the substantia innominata (SIv), and the medial part of the BST (BSTM).

Ventral Subiculum and VLEA

The ventral subiculum and VLEA are interconnected portions of the hippocampal region. In the present study, PHA-L injections into the ventral subiculum produced a robust, continuous terminal field that involved the BSTM (BSTMa, BSTMv, BSTMpl, BSTMpi), the SIv, the medial amygdalar nucleus (mainly Mad), and the adjacent BSTia. The only fibers associated with the central extended amygdalar region were a few axons located in the BSTL, a moderately dense terminal field located adjacent to the ventral edge of the medial subdivision of the central nucleus (CM), and a light projection to the caudal pole of the ASt.

In general, these findings are consistent with previous anterograde[5,14–16] and retrograde[17] tract-tracing studies in the rat. Although it has been reported that there is a strong projection of the ventral subiculum to the caudal pole of the CL,[15] this may actually represent a projection to the caudal part of the ASt, which appears to extend medially to wrap around the caudal pole of the CL at this level (personal observations). Cullinan and coworkers[16] reported projections from the ventral subiculum to the CM and the BSTL that were much stronger than those seen in the present study. This may indicate that the projections from the ventral subiculum to the extended amygdala exhibit a topographical organization.

In the present study the rostral VLEA was found to have light to moderate projections to the MXA, including the Mad, SIv, and the BSTM (BSTMa, BSTMv, and BSTMpl). The projections to the Mad were reported previously.[18] In addition, the caudal three fourths of the VLEA was found to have a light projection to the Mad. These projections of the VLEA to the MXA are interesting considering that the VLEA is the main entorhinal target of the ventral subiculum,[19] which also has significant projections to the MXA.

Infralimbic Cortex (IL), Dorsal Peduncular Cortex (DPC), and AIv

The IL, DPC, and AIv are ventral frontal regions that receive prominent olfactory inputs. IL and DPC have projections to the MXA that include the medial nucleus (Mad, Mpv), the SIv, and the BSTM (BSTMa, BSTMv, and BSTMpl). In addition, caudal portions of the IL have moderate projections to portions of the central extended amygdala, including the BSTL and medial portions of the central nucleus (CM and CI) (see below). AIv has projections to the medial nucleus and the SIv but not to the BSTM.

With injections into central and caudal portions of the IL/DPC region, Hurley *et al.*[20] found projections to the centromedial amygdala and SI that were similar to our findings. However, they reported that the projections to the BST mainly targeted its "lateral and ventrolateral" portions. Because their injections generally involved caudal portions of the IL, it is not surprising that moderately dense terminal fields were seen in the BSTL. However, in all of our cases it was clear that the main target in the BST was the BSTM. Although Hurley *et al.*[20] did not provide illustrations of terminal fields in posterior portions of the BST, it is possible that the BSTMpl may have been considered to represent part of their ventrolateral BST. In another PHA-L study of IL efferents,[21] all cases exhibited a terminal field located just caudal to the anterior commissure that extended in a ventromedial direction from the lateral ventricle towards the medial preoptic area (and thus appears to correspond to the BSTMpl). The failure of BSTM retrograde tracer injections to label neurons in the IL/DPC region[20] could be explained if the injections only involved the most medial portions of the BSTMp (i.e., BSTMpi and BSTMpm), which did not exhibit labeled axons in our IL and DPC cases. Finally, the projections of the IL to the "lateral division of the central nucleus" reported by Takagishi and Chiba[21] appear to have terminated mainly in the CLC (see their FIG. 7A). Thus, it appears that the main projection of the IL and DPC is to the MXA, although caudal portions of IL have additional projections to portions of the CXA.

Functional Aspects of the Cortical Afferents to the MXA

It is of considerable interest that cortical areas that project to the MXA send fibers to all portions of this extended nuclear complex with the exception of the Mpd and

TABLE 1. Main projections of different cortical areas to nuclei of the bed nucleus of the stria terminalis, substantia innominata, and centromedial amygdaloid region as seen in PHA-L experiments[a]

Group	Area	Modality	NXA			CXA						MXA	
			CLC	ASt	IPAC	CL	CM	Sld	BSTLp,v	BSTLd,j	Mad/Mpv	SIv	BSTM
1	DI	Visc/Gust	•	•	•••	•••	•••	•	•	•••			
	PaRh	Somatic	••		••								
	cAIp	Olf/Somatic	•	•	•••	••	•		•	•			
	AId	Polymodal	•	•	•	•	•	•	•				
	PL	Polymodal	•	•	•			••	••				
	APir	Olfactory	•••	•	•••	•••	•	•••	•••	•••	••		
2	Subv	Polymodal		•					•		••	••	•••
	IL/DPC	Olf/Poly	••	••	•		•		•		••	••	•••
	rVLEA	Polymodal	••	••							••	•	••
	Alv	Olf/Poly	••	•								•	
3	PC/End	Olfactory	••		••	•						•	
	rDLEA	Polymodal	••		••	•			•	•	••	•	
	rAIp	Polymodal	•				••		•	•	••	•	
4	cERC	Polymodal	••	••							•		
	PRC	Polymodal	••	••	•						•		
	Te3,2	Aud/Visl		••									
	ACd	Polymodal	•										

[a] NOTATION: •••, strong projections; ••, moderate projections; •, light projections. NXA, nonextended amygdala; CXA, central extended amygdala; MXA, medial extended amygdala.

the BSTMpm. These nontargeted portions of the MXA share cytoarchitectural, histochemical, connectional, and functional characteristics[3,22] and are considered to represent homologous components of the MXA. Likewise, the portions of the MXA that are targeted by cortical afferents (including the Mad, Mpv, SIv, BSTMpl, BSTMa, and BSTMv) are tightly interconnected and have similar extrinsic connections, but have only sparse connections with the Mpd/BSTMpm system.[3,22] Although both subsystems of the MXA send robust projections to the medial preoptic-hypothalamic region, there is evidence that the main role of the projections from the Mpd/BSTMpm is the regulation of hormonal release by the anterior pituitary, whereas the main role of the MXA structures targeted by cortical afferents is the generation of social behaviors, including reproductive and agonistic (defensive/aggressive) behaviors.[22]

The MXA receives direct vomeronasal inputs from the accessory olfactory bulb and indirect vomeronasal inputs from the posterior cortical amygdalar nucleus.[17,23–26] This complex also receives direct olfactory inputs from the main olfactory bulb and indirect olfactory inputs from the anterior cortical amygdalar nucleus (Coa) and the periamygdaloid cortex (PAC).[17,23–26] In light of the olfactory connections of the MXA, it is of interest that the frontal cortical areas that have strong projections to the MXA (infralimbic, dorsal peduncular, and ventral agranular insular cortices) also receive robust projections from the primary olfactory cortex (including the piriform cortex, Coa, and PAC).[12,14] However, in addition to these olfactory inputs, the infralimbic cortex receives presumed polymodal inputs from the basolateral amygdala,[14] the ventral subiculum,[27] and the lateral entorhinal and perirhinal cortices (McDonald, personal observations). Thus, the IL may be a higher-order olfactory area that integrates olfactory information with polymodal nonolfactory inputs. These complex stimulus representations may be important for cognitive, affective, and mnemonic functions. The projections of the IL to the MXA may allow this olfactory/polymodal information to influence social behavior and other behaviors regulated by the MXA.

The other main cortical regions with strong projections to the MXE are the ventral subiculum and rostral VLEA of the hippocampal region. These areas presumably transmit complex polymodal information (that has been processed by the trisynaptic circuit of the hippocampus) to the MXE. Inasmuch as the hippocampus is known to be involved in mnemonic activities, these inputs to the MXE may be important for social learning processes mediated by the MXE.[28] The IL inputs to the MXE may also play a role in social learning because lesions that involve IL and adjacent areas of the medial prefrontal cortex have been shown to disrupt extinction of emotional learning.[29]

In addition, it has been suggested that the projection of the ventral subiculum to the BSTM may allow the hippocampal region to influence the activity of the hypothalamic-pituitary-adrenal axis. Fibers labeled by PHA-L injections into the ventral subiculum formed apparent appositions with neurons in the BSTM that were retrogradely labeled by Fluoro-gold injections into the paraventricular hypothalamic nucleus (PVN).[16] The latter nucleus regulates the secretion of adrenocorticotropic hormone via its release of corticotropin-releasing hormone in the median eminence. In addition, because the medial amygdalar nucleus also projects to the PVN,[30] this portion of the MXC may have a similar function.

CORTICAL AREAS THAT PREFERENTIALLY TARGET THE CENTRAL EXTENDED AMYGDALA

The main cortical areas that have strong projections to the central extended amygdala (CXA) are the prefrontal cortex (PL, AId, and the caudal part of IL), the insular cortex (DI of the anterior insula, and PaRh and the adjacent AIp of the posterior insula), and the amygdalopiriform transitional region (APir) (TABLE 1). Consistent with the concept of the extended amygdala, these cortical areas tend to project in a continuous manner to two or three adjacent portions of the CXA, including the central nucleus, the substantia innominata (primarily its dorsolateral portion, SId), and the lateral part of the BST (BSTL).

Prefrontal Cortex

The prelimbic cortex had a strong projection to the substantia innominata that was continuous with a moderate projection to the BSTLp, but no terminating fibers were seen in the CL and CM. Although the projection to the SI seemed to include both the SId (a CXA structure) and the SIv (a MXA structure), no other MXA nuclei were targeted by these projections. The AId had very light projections to the CXA that included the BSTLp, SId, and the rostral pole of the central nucleus. In general, these findings are consistent with previous studies of prefrontal cortical projections.[9,17,31,32]

In addition to strong projections to the MXA, the caudal portions of the IL have additional moderate projections to portions of the CXA, including the BSTL and medial portions of the central nucleus (CM and CI). Similar projections were also seen by Hurley et al.[20] Moreover, retrograde tract-tracing studies conducted by Hurley et al.[20] suggest that both the IL and the ventrally adjacent dorsal peduncular cortex contribute to projections to the BSTL and the medial central nuclear region. This is consistent with the finding that lesions that involve the tenia tecta and dorsally adjacent dorsal peduncular cortex produce degenerated axon terminals in the central nucleus that synapse with dendritic shafts and spines.[17]

Insular Cortex

The insular projection to the CXA arises primarily from the gustatory and viscerosensory dysgranular insular areas of the anterior insular cortex (DIg and DIv) and the somatosensory posterior insular cortex (PaRh and the caudal AIp). The caudal AIp also receives olfactory input from the primary olfactory cortex.[5] In general, these findings are consistent with previous studies of insulo-amygdalar connections.[9,11,33–35]

The projection of the DI to the CXA is complimentary to that exhibited by the prefrontal cortex (PFC). Thus, whereas the DI has robust projections to the BSTLd, BSTLj, CL, CM, and the supracapsular portion of the BSTL (BSTLs), these CXA areas receive little or no projection from the PFC. Likewise, the DI projections to the main CXA targets of the PFC (BSTLp and SI) are relatively light. It is also of interest that the dense terminal field in the BSTLd seen with DI injections is continuous with the dense terminal field in the IPAC, which, in turn, is continuous with the dense terminal field in the CL. Both the BSTLd and the CL are characterized by principal neurons that closely resemble the medium-sized spiny neurons of the striatum.[6,36]

In addition, the BSTLs, another target of the DI, contains similar medium spiny neurons (personal observations). By contrast, the principal neurons of the BSTLp, SId, and CM are characterized by principal neurons that have fewer dendritic branches and a lower spine density.[6,36] Thus, both connectional and cytoarchitectural data suggest that there are at least two sets of homologous nuclei in the CXA (see also ref. 3).

The projection of the somatosensory posterior insula targets a subset of the CXA structures innervated by the DI. Thus, the projections to IPAC and the far lateral part of CL are very dense, whereas the projections to other portions of the DI projection field are lighter than that exhibited by DI. It is of interest that the caudal AIp projection to CL mainly targets its lateral half. The medial half, which appears to merge with the CI rostrally, was less densely labeled.

Amygdalopiriform Transitional Area (APir)

The APir had robust projections to several parts of the CXA, including the SId, the central nucleus, and all portions of the BSTL. Similar to the caudal AIp, the projection to the medial half of CL was lighter than that to its lateral half. Not surprisingly, APir contained many retrogradely labeled cells with injections of retrograde tracers into the central nucleus and BST. These findings corroborate and extend the work of Ottersen[17] who previously observed robust retrograde labeling in the APir with injections of tracers into the central nucleus. Unlike other cortical areas with strong projections to the CXA, the APir also had a significant projection to the MXA that targeted the Mad and the SIv.

Functional Aspects of the Cortical Afferents to the CXA

It is now well established that the central amygdalar nucleus plays a very important role in the generation of somatomotor, autonomic, neuroendocrine, and arousal components of emotional responses during fear conditioning and stress.[37–39] These responses are produced by the projections of the central nucleus to several functionally distinct regions in the basal forebrain, lateral hypothalamus and brain stem.[23,39] The SId and BSTL have projections that are similar to those of the central nucleus, and injections of retrograde tracers into brain stem targets of these CXA nuclei produce retrograde labeling that extends in a fairly continuous fashion throughout the central nucleus, SId, and lateral BST.[40,41] Although these anatomical findings suggest that the functions of the BSTL and SId might be identical to those of the central nucleus, recent studies suggest that whereas the central nucleus is critical for conditioned fear, but not unconditioned fear, the opposite is true for the BSTL.[42]

In addition to the cortical afferents described in the present account, the CXA receives important inputs from the basolateral amygdala, thalamus, and brain stem.[23] The results of the present study indicate that all cortical areas that project to the CXA also have projections to the basolateral amygdala. Whereas the projections of the basolateral amygdala to the CXA appear to be essential for certain aspects of conditioned and unconditioned fear,[37,39,42] the functions of the direct projections of the prefrontal, insular, and APir cortical areas to the CXA have not been determined.

The prefrontal areas that project to the CXA (PL and AId) are higher-order sensorimotor areas that receive polymodal inputs from the basolateral amygdala,[14] and the perirhinal and entorhinal cortices (personal observations). The strong projection of the PL to the SId and SIv suggests that these inputs may be targeting a specific structure found mainly in SI (e.g., the corticopetal cholinergic neurons of the nucleus basalis), in addition to neurons of the extended amygdala.

The anterior insular and posterior insular regions apparently transmit gustatory/visceral and somatosensory information, respectively, to the CXA.[5,9,11] It is of interest that the brain stem projections to the CXA (from the parabrachial nucleus and nucleus tractus solitarius) transmit information from these same sensory modalities.[43–45] Most of the somatosensory information from the parabrachial nucleus,[43-45] and perhaps from the posterior insula,[46] is nociceptive. These direct nociceptive inputs to the CXA may be important for generating stress-related responses to painful stimuli, and may be critical for aspects of aversive conditioning that are not dependent on the basolateral amygdala.[47]

Emotion and stress are both characterized by robust visceral activity (e.g., changes in heart rate, blood pressure, and gastrointestinal activity) and somatomotor activity (e.g., muscle tension). Feedback regarding these bodily changes may be important for the regulation, maintenance, and interpretation of ongoing emotional responses.[48] This viscerosensory and somatosensory feedback could be transmitted to the CXA via its cortical and subcortical afferents. Whereas the feedback provided to the CXA from the brain stem may be important for reflexive adjustments of various components of ongoing emotional responses, it is possible that the feedback provided to the CXA from the viscerosensory and somatosensory portions of the insular cortex might be more important for higher cognitive aspects of emotion, perhaps contributing to the conscious experience of emotional feelings.[49] The latter projections also appear to be able to regulate visceral function, inasmuch as it has been shown that electrical stimulation of the visceral insular cortex affects the activity of central nucleus neurons that project to the brain stem.[50]

APir, which receives inputs from the olfactory tract, merges with the caudolateral aspect of the parvicellular basal nucleus. Similar to the parvicellular basal nucleus,[51] the APir has strong projections to the CXA. However, like many primary olfactory areas, it also has projections to the MXA. The anatomical relationships of APir suggest that it may be a source of olfactory inputs to the central nucleus in olfactory heart-rate conditioning.[52]

CORTICAL AREAS THAT TARGET BOTH THE CENTRAL AND MEDIAL EXTENDED AMYGDALA

Three cortical areas appear to target the CXA and MXA equally: (1) the piriform cortex and associated dorsal endopiriform nucleus (PC/End), (2) the rostral part of the DLEA (rDLEA), and (3) the rostral half of the AIp (rAIp) (TABLE 1). Some of these projections have been reported in previous studies.[5,18,53] All three of these cortical areas receive prominent olfactory inputs, but the DLEA and AIp also receive additional nonolfactory projections as well.[5] The dorsal endopiriform nucleus receives olfactory inputs from the overlying PC and is sometimes considered to represent a deeper portion of the PC. Previous autoradiographic studies suggest that the projections to the medial nucleus from the piriform region probably originate only from the endopiriform nucleus.[25]

CORTICAL AREAS THAT TARGET THE CLC AND ASt, BUT NOT OTHER PORTIONS OF THE EXTENDED AMYGDALA

Four cortical regions appear to target the CLC and ASt without sending significant projections to other parts of the extended amygdala: (1) the caudal three fourths of the lateral entorhinal cortex (cERC), (2) the perirhinal cortex (PRC), (3) the temporal association areas (Te3 and Te2), and (4) the dorsal anterior cingulate and medial precentral cortices (ACd/PrCm). These projections have all been reported in previous studies.[5,18,31,53] The finding that there are several cortical areas with projections to the CLC and/or ASt that do not target any portion of the SI or BST suggests that the CLC and ASt may not have homologues in the latter regions and, by definition, may not constitute portions of the extended amygdala. Likewise, although portions of the parabrachial nucleus that target the CM and CL also target their homologues in the BSTL, portions of the parabrachial nucleus with projections to the CLC send no significant projections to the BST.[43,44]

All four cortical regions with projections confined to the CLC and ASt are bimodal or polymodal association areas.[5] The CLC/ASt also receives diverse sensory information from almost every other cortical area that projects to the main body of the CXA and MXA, particularly the cortical areas that target the MXA. This may allow nociceptive inputs from the parabrachial nucleus to be associated with diverse higher-order multisensory inputs in the CLC.[44]

CONCLUSIONS

This study indicates that distinct cortical areas project to specific subsets of homologous structures in the extended amygdala, with varying degrees of overlap. These projections appear to constitute the first link in multiple corticofugal pathways that transmit information through the extended amygdala. Similar to the corticofugal pathways associated with the striatum, each of the pathways associated with the extended amygdala may have a specific function. Cortical networks mediating interactions among various cortical areas may generate specific behaviors at different times by activating distinct cortico-extended-amygdalar pathways. It remains to be seen whether the anatomical organization of these projections is similar in other species, including primates.

ACKNOWLEDGMENTS

This work was supported by NIH Grant NS19733 (A.J.M.), Grant FAPESP 96/7794-5 (S.J.S.), and NIMH Grants MH-25642, MH-47840, and MH-57250 (M.D.).

REFERENCES

1. HEIMER, L., J. DE OLMOS, G.F. ALHEID & L. ZÁBORSKY. 1991. "Perestroika" in the basal forebrain: opening the border between neurology and psychiatry. Prog. Brain Res. **87:** 109–165.

2. HEIMER, L., R.E. HARLAN, G.F. ALHEID, M.M. GARCIA & J. DE OLMOS. 1997. Substantia innominata: A notion which impedes clinical anatomical correlations in neuropsychiatric disorders. Neuroscience **76:** 957–1006.
3. ALHEID, G.F., J.S. DE OLMOS & C.A. BELTRAMINO. 1995. Amygdala and extended amygdala. *In* The Rat Nervous System. G. Paxinos, Ed.: 495–578. Academic Press. Orlando, FL.
4. HOLSTEGE, G. 1992. The emotional motor system. Eur. J. Morphol. **30:** 67–79.
5. MCDONALD, A.J. 1998. Cortical pathways to the mammalian amygdala. Prog. Neurobiol. **55:** 257–332.
6. MCDONALD, A.J. 1982. Cytoarchitecture of the central amygdaloid nucleus of the rat. J. Comp. Neurol. **208:** 401–418.
7. KOSAR, E., H.J. GRILL & R. NORGREN. 1986. Gustatory cortex in the rat. I: Physiological properties and cytoarchitecture. Brain Res. **379:** 329–341.
8. CECHETTO, D.F. & C.B. SAPER. 1987. Evidence for a viscerotopic sensory representation in the cortex and thalamus in the rat. J. Comp. Neurol. **262:** 27–45.
9. SHI, C-J. & M.D. CASSELL. 1998. Cortical, thalamic, and amygdaloid connections of the anterior and posterior insular cortices. J. Comp. Neurol. **399:** 440–468.
10. FABRI, M. & H. BURTON. 1991. Ipsilateral cortical connections of primary somatic sensory cortex in rats. J. Comp. Neurol. **311:** 405–424.
11. SHI, C-J. & M.D. CASSELL. 1998. Cascade projections from somatosensory cortex to the rat basolateral amygdala via the parietal insular cortex. J. Comp. Neurol. **399:** 469–491.
12. LUSKIN, M.B. & J.L. PRICE. 1983. The topographic organization of association fibers of the olfactory system in the rat, including centrifugal fibers to the olfactory bulb. J. Comp. Neurol. **216:** 264–291.
13. PAXINOS, G. & C. WATSON. 1986. The Rat Brain in Stereotaxic Coordinates. Academic Press. New York.
14. KRETTEK, J.E. & J.L. PRICE. 1977. Projections of the amygdaloid complex to the cerebral cortex and thalamus in the rat and cat. J. Comp. Neurol. **172:** 687–722.
15. CANTERAS, N.S. & L.W. SWANSON. 1992. Projections of the ventral subiculum to the amygdala, septum, and hypothalamus: a PHAL anterograde tract-tracing study in the rat. J. Comp. Neurol. **324:** 180–194.
16. CULLINAN, W.E., J.P. HERMAN & S.J. WATSON. 1993. Ventral subicular interaction with the hypothalamic paraventricular nucleus: evidence for a relay in the bed nucleus of the stria terminalis. J. Comp. Neurol. **332:** 1–20.
17. OTTERSEN, O.P. 1982. Connections of the amygdala of the rat. IV. Corticoamygdaloid and intraamygdaloid connections as studied with axonal transport of horseradish peroxidase. J. Comp. Neurol. **205:** 30–48.
18. MCDONALD, A.J. & F. MASCAGNI. 1997. Projections of the lateral entorhinal cortex to the amygdala: a *Phaseolus vulgaris* leucoagglutinin study in the rat. Neuroscience **77:** 445–460.
19. WITTER, M.O., H.J. GROENEWEGEN, F.H. LOPES DA SILVA & A.H.M. LOHMAN. 1989. Functional organization of the extrinsic and intrinsic circuitry of the parahippocampal region. Prog. Neurobiol. **33:** 161–253.
20. HURLEY, K.M., H. HERBERT, M.M. MOGA & C.B. SAPER. 1991. Efferent projections of the infralimbic cortex of the rat. J. Comp. Neurol. **308:** 249–276.
21. TAKAGISHI, M. & C. CHIBA. 1991. Efferent projections of the infralimbic (area 25) region of the medial prefrontal cortex in the rat: an anterograde tracer PHA-L study. Brain Res. **566:** 26–39.
22. CANTERAS, N.S., R.B. SIMERLY & L.W. SWANSON. 1995. Organization of projections from the medial nucleus of the amygdala: a PHAL study in the rat. J. Comp. Neurol. **360:** 231–245.
23. DE OLMOS, J.S., G.F ALHEID & C.A. BERTRAMINO. 1985. Amygdala. *In* The Rat Nervous System. G. Paxinos. Ed.: 223–334. Academic Press. Orlando.

24. KRETTEK, J.E. & J.L. PRICE. 1978. Amygdaloid projections to subcortical structures within the basal forebrain and brainstem in the rat and cat. J. Comp. Neurol. **178:** 225–254.
25. KRETTEK, J.E. & J.L. PRICE. 1978. A description of the amygdaloid complex in the rat and cat with observations on intra-amygdaloid axonal connections. J. Comp. Neurol. **178:** 255–280.
26. SCALIA, F. & S.S. WINANS. 1975. The different projections of the olfactory bulb and accessory olfactory bulb in mammals. J. Comp. Neurol. **161:** 31–56.
27. SWANSON, L.W. & W.M. COWAN. 1977. An autoradiographic study of the organization of the efferent connections of the hippocampal formation in the rat. J. Comp. Neurol. **172:** 49–84.
28. LUITEN, P.G.M., J.M. KOOLHAAS, S. DE BOER & S.J. KOOPMANS. 1985. The corticomedial amygdala in the central nervous system organization of agonistic behavior. Brain Res. **332:** 283–297.
29. MORGAN, M.A., L.M. ROMANSKI AND J.E. LEDOUX. 1993. Extinction of emotional learning: contribution of medial prefrontal cortex. Neurosci. Lett. **163:** 109–113.
30. GRAY, T.S., E.C. CARNEY & J.M. MANGUSSON. 1989. Direct projections from the central amydaloid nucleus to the hypothalamic paraventricular nucleus: possible role in stress-induced adrenocorticotropin release. Neuroendocrinology **50:** 433–446.
31. MCDONALD, A.J., F. MASCAGNI & L. GUO. 1996. Projections of the medial and lateral prefrontal cortices to the amygdala: a *Phaseolus vulgaris* leucoagglutinin study in the rat. Neuroscience **71:** 55–75.
32. SESACK, S.R., A.Y. DEUTCH, R.H. ROTH & B.S. BUNNEY. 1989. Topographical organization of the efferent projections of the medial prefrontal cortex in the rat: an anterograde tract-tracing study with *Phaseolus vulgaris* leucoagglutinin. J. Comp. Neurol. **209:** 213–242.
33. MCDONALD, A.J. & T.R. JACKSON. 1987. Amygdaloid connections with posterior insular and temporal cortical areas in the rat. J. Comp. Neurol. **262:** 59–77.
34. SAPER, C.B. 1982. Convergence of autonomic and limbic connections in the insular cortex of the rat. J. Comp. Neurol. **210:** 163–173.
35. YASUI, Y., C.D. BREDER, C.B. SAPER & D.F. CECHETTO. 1991. Autonomic responses and efferent pathways from the insular cortex in the rat. J. Comp. Neurol. **303:** 355–374.
36. MCDONALD, A.J. 1983. Neurons of the bed nucleus of the stria terminalis: a Golgi study in the rat. Brain Res. Bull. **10:** 11–120.
37. DAVIS, M. 1992. The role of the amygdala in conditioned fear. *In* The Amygdala: Neurobiological Aspects of Emotion, Memory, and Mental Dysfunction. J.P. Aggleton, Ed.: 255–306. Wiley-Liss. New York.
38. GALLAGHER, M. & P.C. HOLLAND. 1992. Understanding the function of the central nucleus: is simple conditioning enough? *In* The Amygdala: Neurobiological Aspects of Emotion, Memory, and Mental Dusfunction. J.G. Aggleton, Ed.: 307–321. Wiley-Liss. New York.
39. LEDOUX, J.E. 1992. Emotion and the amygdala. *In* The Amygdala: Neurobiological aspects of Emotion, Memory, and Mental Dysfunction. J. P. Aggleton, Ed. 339–351. Wiley-Liss. New York.
40. HOLSTEGE, G., L. MEINERS & T. TAN. 1985. Projections of the bed nucleus of the stria terminalis to the mesencephalon, pons and medulla oblongata in the cat. Exp. Brain Res. **58:** 379–391.
41. SCHWABER, J.S., B.S. KAPP & G. HIGGINS. 1980. The origin and extent of direct amygdala projections to the region of the dorsal motor nucleus of the vagus and the nucleus of the solitary tract. Neurosci. Lett. **20:** 15–20.

42. WALKER, D.L. & M. DAVIS. 1997. Double dissociation between the involvement of the bed nucleus of the stria terminalis and the central nucleus of the amgydala in startle increases produced by conditioned versus unconditioned fear. J. Neurosci. **17:** 9375–9383.
43. ALDEN, M., J-M. BESSON & J-F. BERNARD. 1994. Organization of the efferent projections from the pontine parabrachial area to the bed nucleus of the stria terminalis and neighboring regions: a PHA-L study in the rat. J. Comp. Neurol. **341:** 289–314.
44. BERNARD, J.F., M. ALDEN & J.M. BESSON. 1993. The organization of the efferent projections from the pontine parabrachial area to the amygdaloid complex: a *Phaseolus vulgaris* leucoagglutinin (PHA-L) study in the rat. J. Comp. Neurol. **329:** 201–229.
45. RICARDO, J.A. & E.T. KOH. 1978. Anatomical evidence of direct projections from the nucleus of the solitary tract to the hypothalamus, amygdala and other forebrain structures in the rat. Brain Res. **153:** 1–26.
46. BARNETT, E.M., G.D. EVANS, N. SUN, S. PERLMAN & M.D. CASSELL. 1995. Anterograde tracing of trigeminal afferent pathways from the murine tooth pulp to cortex using herpes simplex virus type 1. J. Neurosci. **15:** 2972–2984.
47. KILLCROSS, S., T.W. ROBBINS & B.J. EVERITT. 1997. Different types of fear-conditioned behavior mediated by separate nuclei within the amygdala. Nature **388:** 377–380.
48. LEDOUX, J. 1996. The Emotional Brain. Simon and Schuster. New York.
49. JAMES, W. 1884. What is emotion? Mind **19:** 188–205.
50. PASCOE, J.P. & B.S. KAPP. 1987. Responses of amygdaloid central nucleus neurons to stimulation of the insular cortex in awake rabbits. Neuroscience **21:** 471–485.
51. MCDONALD, A.J. 1991. Topographical organization of amygdaloid projections to the caudatoputamen, nucleus accumbens, and related striatal-like areas of the rat brain. Neuroscience **44:** 15–33.
52. SANANES, C.B. & B.A. CAMPBELL. 1989. A role of the central nucleus of the amygdala in olfactory heart rate conditioning. Behav. Neurosci. **103:** 519–525.
53. MASCAGNI, F., A.J. MCDONALD & J.R. COLEMAN. 1993. Cortico-amygdaloid and cortico-cortical projections of the rat temporal cortex: a *Phaseolus vulgaris* leucoagglutinin study. Neuroscience **57:** 697–715.

The Basal Forebrain Corticopetal System Revisited

L. ZABORSZKY,[a,f] K. PANG,[b] J. SOMOGYI,[c] Z. NADASDY,[d] AND I. KALLO[e]

[a]*Center for Molecular and Behavioral Neuroscience, Newark, New Jersey*
[b]*Department of Psychology, Bowling Green State University, Bowling Green, Ohio*
[c]*Flinders University, Faculty of Health Sciences, Bedford Park, Australia*
[d]*Center for Neural Computation, The Hebrew University, Jerusalem, Israel*
[e]*Department of Anatomy, King's College London, United Kingdom*

ABSTRACT: The medial septum, diagonal bands, ventral pallidum, substantia innominata, globus pallidus, and internal capsule contain a heterogeneous population of neurons, including cholinergic and noncholinergic (mostly GABA containing), corticopetal projection neurons, and interneurons. This highly complex brain region, which constitutes a significant part of the basal forebrain has been implicated in attention, motivation, learning, as well as in a number of neuropsychiatric disorders, such as Alzheimer's disease, Parkinson's disease, and schizophrenia. Part of the difficulty in understanding the functions of the basal forebrain, as well as the aberrant information-processing characteristics of these disease states lies in the fact that the organizational principles of this brain area remained largely elusive. On the basis of new anatomical data, it is proposed that a large part of the basal forebrain corticopetal system be organized into longitudinal bands. Considering the topographic organization of cortical afferents to different divisions of the prefrontal cortex and a similar topographic projection of these prefrontal areas to basal forebrain regions, it is suggested that several functionally segregated cortico-prefronto-basal forebrain-cortical circuits exist. It is envisaged that such specific "triangular" circuits could amplify selective attentional processing in posterior sensory cortical areas.

INTRODUCTION

The term *basal forebrain* (BF) refers to a heterogeneous collection of structures located close to the medial and ventral surfaces of the cerebral hemispheres. Part of the difficulty in understanding the function of the basal forebrain lies in the anatomical complexity of the region. Using the latest tracing and immunocytochemical techniques, Lennart Heimer[1–6] was among the first to parcel the "unnamed" substance of Reil[7] into functional–anatomical compartments, including the ventral pallidum, the core/shell of the nucleus accumbens and the "extended amygdala." Basal forebrain areas, including the medial septum/vertical limb of the diagonal band (MS/VDB), horizontal limb of the diagonal band (HDB), sublenticular substantia innominata, and peripallidal regions contain cell types different in transmitter content,

---

[f]Address for correspondence: Laszlo Zaborszky, M.D., Ph.D., Center for Molecular and Behavioral Neuroscience, Rutgers Univeristy, 197 University Ave., Newark, NJ 07102, USA. Voice: 973-353-1080 ext. 3181; fax: 973-353-1272; zaborszk@axon.rutgers.edu

morphology, and projection pattern.[8–12] Among these different neuronal populations, the cholinergic corticopetal projection neurons have received particular attention due to their prominent loss in Alzheimer's and related disorders.[13] However, cholinergic projection neurons represent only a fraction of the total cell population in these forebrain areas, which also contain various GABAergic and peptidergic neurons.

CHOLINERGIC NEURONS

Mesulam[14] proposed the Ch nomenclature to designate different groups of cholinergic neurons. The human basal forebrain-Ch complex extends from the level of the olfactory tubercle to that of the rostral level of the lateral geniculate body, spanning a rostrocaudal length of 19 millimeters. It attains its greatest mediolateral width of 18 mm within the substantia innominata. The constituent neurons of the BF-Ch complex can be subdivided into four regions: the Ch1 and Ch2 regions (corresponding to the MS/VDB complex), the Ch3 region (HDB), and the Ch4 region. The latter region, also termed the nucleus basalis of Meynert, can be further subdivided into six sectors that occupy its anteromedial (Ch4am), anterolateral (Ch4al), anterointermediate (Ch4ai), intermediodorsal (Ch4id), intermedioventral (Ch4ai), and posterior (Ch4p) regions. Applying a three-dimensional sampling design, Vogels *et al.*[15] estimated the total number of neurons within the human Ch complex to be 1.2 million in each hemisphere. The number of cholinergic neurons were estimated earlier by Arendt *et al.*[16] to be about 220,000 on each side. Experimental neuroanatomical studies in the monkey[17] have shown that different cortical regions receive their major input from individual sectors of the BF-Ch complex. Thus, neurons within the MS/VDB complex (Ch1/Ch2) provide the major cholinergic innervation of the hippocampus, and cholinergic cells within the HDB (Ch3) project to the olfactory bulb. The Ch4am provides the major source of input to medial cortical areas, including the cingulate gyrus; Ch4al to frontoparietal opercular areas and the amygdala; Ch4i to lateral (pre)frontal, posterior parietal, peristriate, inferotemporal, parahippocampal, and orbitoinsular regions; and Ch4p to superior temporal and temporopolar regions.

The number of cholinergic neurons in one hemisphere of the rat brain has been estimated to be between 18,000–20,000.[10] Tracing studies in rodents established that cholinergic neurons in the BF innervate the entire cortex, including the hippocampus and amygdala according to a rough mediolateral and anteroposterior topography.[12,18–25] The dendrites of cholinergic neurons extend in an apparent random fashion for several hundred microns and often constitute overlapping fields (FIG. 1).

FIGURE 1. Composite map illustrating the distribution of cholinergic neurons and their initial (about 150 μ) dendrites. This map was generated from seven sections stained for choline acetyltransferase, using the Neurolucida software package. For better visualization only the outlines and the corpus callosum are indicated. Anterior view. **A:** low magnification; **B:** enlargement from **A**. Note that orientation of the dendrites shows systematic shift along the rostrocaudal continuum of cholinergic cells. MS/VDB, medial septum/vertical limb of the diagonal band; HDB, horizontal limb of the diagonal band; GP, globus pallidus; ic, internal capsule; SI, substantia innominata. From the unpublished material of J. Somogyi and Zaborszky.

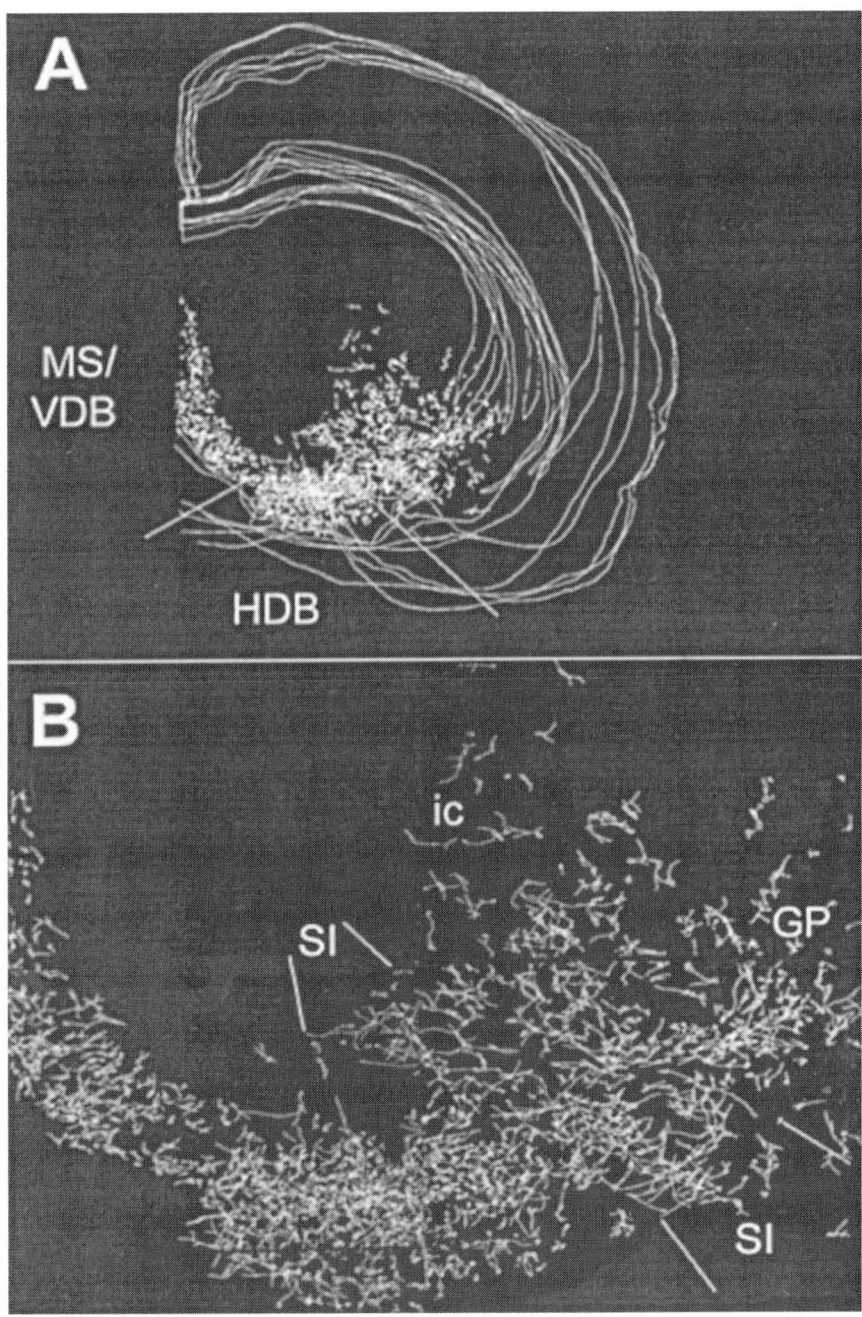

However, using a computerized mapping system, the primary and secondary dendrites tend to show characteristic orientation according their location in the BF (J. Somogyi and Zaborszky, in preparation).

The density of cholinergic cells is not uniform; they often form clusters consisting of 3–15 tightly packed cell bodies. Computational studies (Zaborszky, Nadasdy, Somogyi, in preparation) suggest that the density of these clusters is unexpected based upon random distribution. Moreover, it appears that in the monkey a proportionally larger population of cholinergic cells is located in such clusters than in rodents (FIG. 2). At present, it is not known whether or not the diffusely located cholinergic cells and the clusters project to different or similar layers in the cortex. Their separate projection would explain, in part, how the BF can participate in both general (e.g., arousal) and more specific functions, including sensory processing or selective attention (see below).

GABAergic NEURONS

It was earlier suggested that in both rodents[20] and monkeys[26] about 90% of the neurons that project to the neocortex are cholinergic, although this ratio would be smaller for septohippocampal cells (50–70%). More recent studies in rats,[27] however, questioned the validity of such data, showing that the proportion of cholinergic cells in some areas of the substantia innominata may be as low as 10%, and that cholinergic projection neurons make up only about half of the total projection to the somatosensory and prefrontal cortices.[28,29] In a quantitative study,[10] it was calculated that the total number of GABAergic neurons in one side of the basal forebrain is 38,579, as compared to 18,236 cholinergic neurons, which would suggest, on the average, a 2:1 ratio for GABAergic/cholinergic neurons. Using calbindin (CB), calretinin (CR), and parvalbumin (PV) as markers for different classes of GABAergic neurons, we[30] found a much higher GABAergic/cholinergic ratio of 3.8:1 (FIG. 4). Individual structures show different ratios. In the MS/VDB, HDB, ventral pallidum, and the internal capsule the total GABAergic/cholinergic ratio is 3–4:1; however, in the globus pallidus and the extended amygdala (bed nucleus of stria terminals and substantia innominata), an even higher ratio of 8:1 is found. Although at this point it is unclear what proportion of the above defined different GABAergic populations par-

---

FIGURE 2. Scaling of three-dimensional density distribution of cholinergic cells across species. The total volume in which cholinergic cells are located has been divided both in one rat (upper) (4.35 × 7.18 × 3.40 mm) and in one monkey (lower picture) (16.8 × 16.3 × 0.75 mm) into one hundred equal cubes. Red dots represent cubes that contain at least 1 cholinergic cell (total cell number: rat = 15,777; monkey = 5,736). Asterisks symbolize cubes that contain 3–8 cells in the rat and 6–14 neurons in the monkey. These cubes altogether contain the most dense upper 20% of cells in each animal. The number of such cubes in rat (904) is much higher than in monkey (153). Distances in the coordinate system are in μ. Note the different scaling factor in the two-coordinate system. In the monkey (*Macaca mulatta*) we used an antibody against the low-affinity NGF receptor for a cholinergic marker, which is colocalized in 90–95% of the cholinergic neurons.

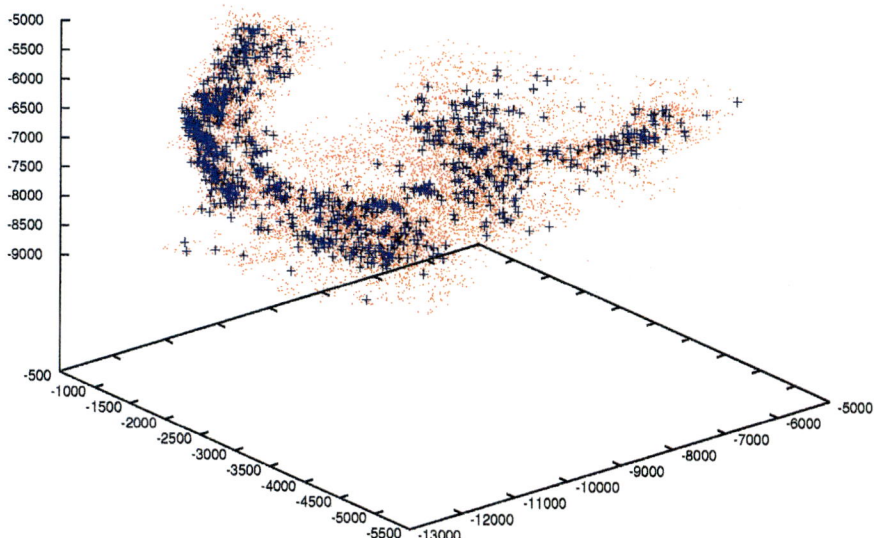

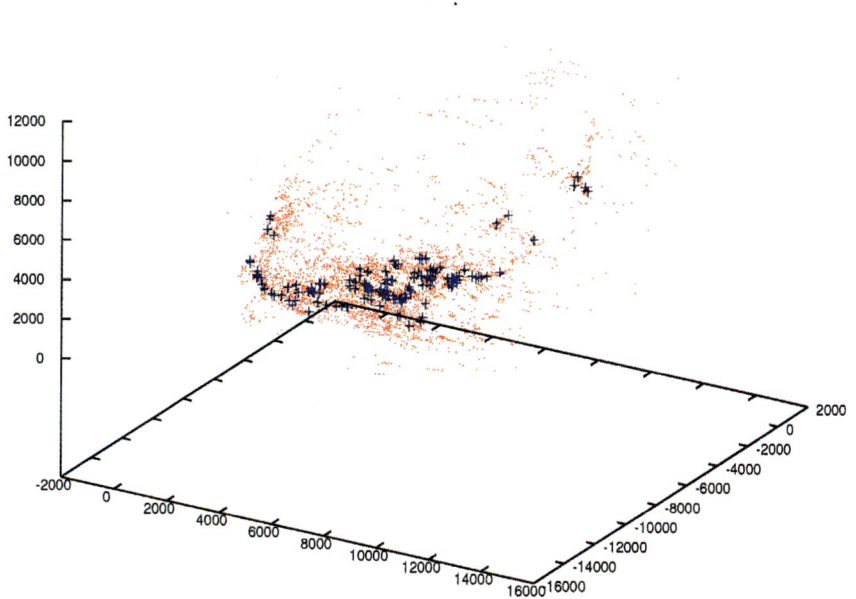

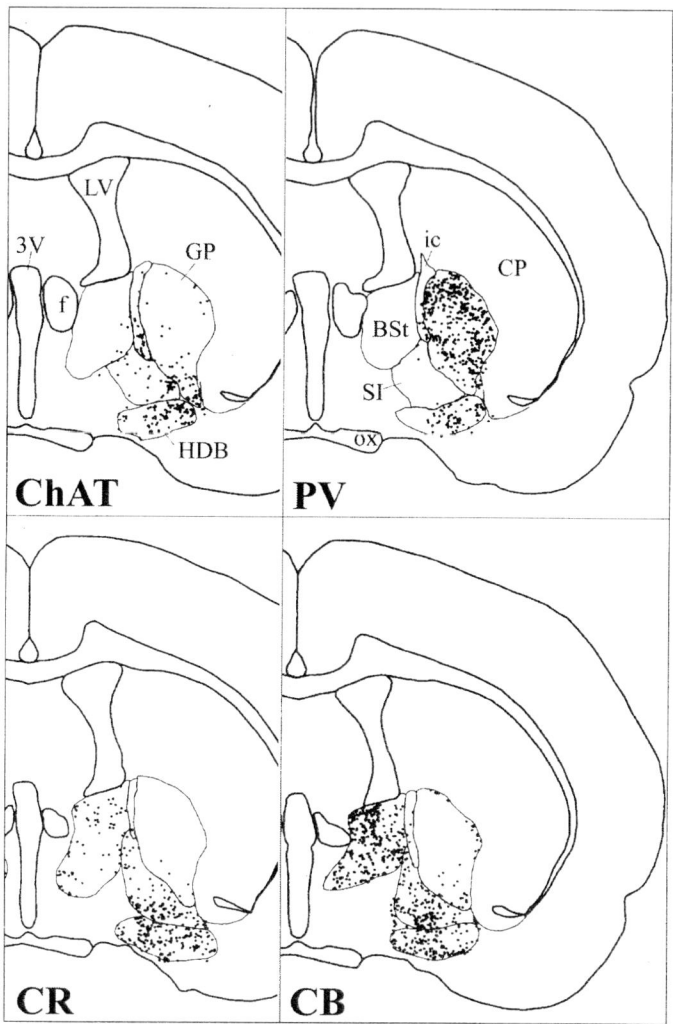

FIGURE 3. Distribution of cholinergic- (ChAT), parvalbumin- (PV), calretinin- (CR) and calbindin- (CB) containing neurons in adjacent sections, alternately stained for these four markers. Each dot represents one cell body. The approximate distances of the sections from the bregma are indicated in parentheses: ChAT (−0.82 mm), PV (0.88 mm), CR (−0.76 mm), and CB (−0.69 mm). 3V, third ventricle.

ticipate in the cortical projections, our preliminary studies suggest that at least a portion of CB, CR, and PV neurons indeed project to various cortical areas (FIGURES 7–9).

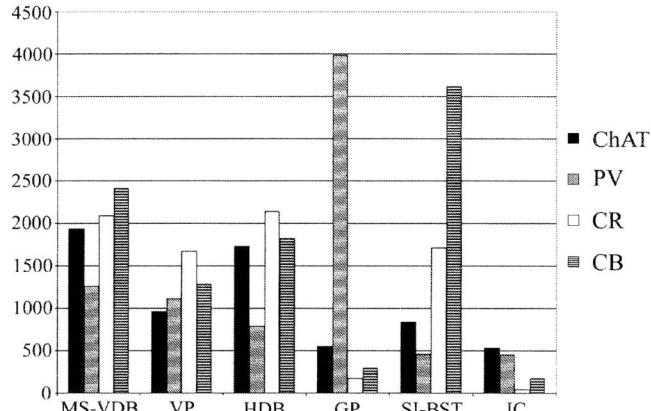

FIGURE 4. Quantitative comparison of the four markers (ChAT, PV, CR, and CB) in different basal forebrain structures. Ordinate indicates cell number counted in both sides in each structure using 48 alternately stained sections. Note the different numerical values for these four cell populations in the individual forebrain regions. VP, ventral pallidum; IC, internal capsule; BST, bed nucleus of the stria terminalis.

ASPECTS OF ORGANIZATION IN THE BASAL FOREBRAIN

Spatial Relations among Different Transmitter-specific Neurons

As FIGURES 3 and 4 suggest, the four cell types show heterogeneous distribution across different structures. However, looking from a three-dimensional perspective, these four cell types seem to construct longitudinal, obliquely (lateromedially) oriented, partially overlapping bands, or columns (FIG. 5). In the caudal two thirds of the basal forebrain, the lateromedial order of cells is PV-ChAT[g] -CR-CB, whereas in the septum[31] this pattern is clearly reversed. Located most medially are the parvalbumin cells, and most laterally are the calbindin neurons. Cholinergic and calretinin cells are deposited in between. If this reverse-banded pattern is confirmed, this would suggest that the different cell "columns" should be twisted in the area of the HDB. Interestingly, evidence that this "twisted pattern" in the longitudinal organization of the basal forebrain may exist is clearly visible from our study, showing how the mediolateral portions of the hypothalamus innervate different lateromedially located cholinergic cells in the septum.[32]

Projection Pattern

Because most of the studies used only a few sections to map the distribution of retrogradely labeled cells, it remains to be tested in systematic three-dimensional re-

---

[g]For visualizing cholinergic neurons in rats, we used an antibody against choline acetyltransferase.[61]

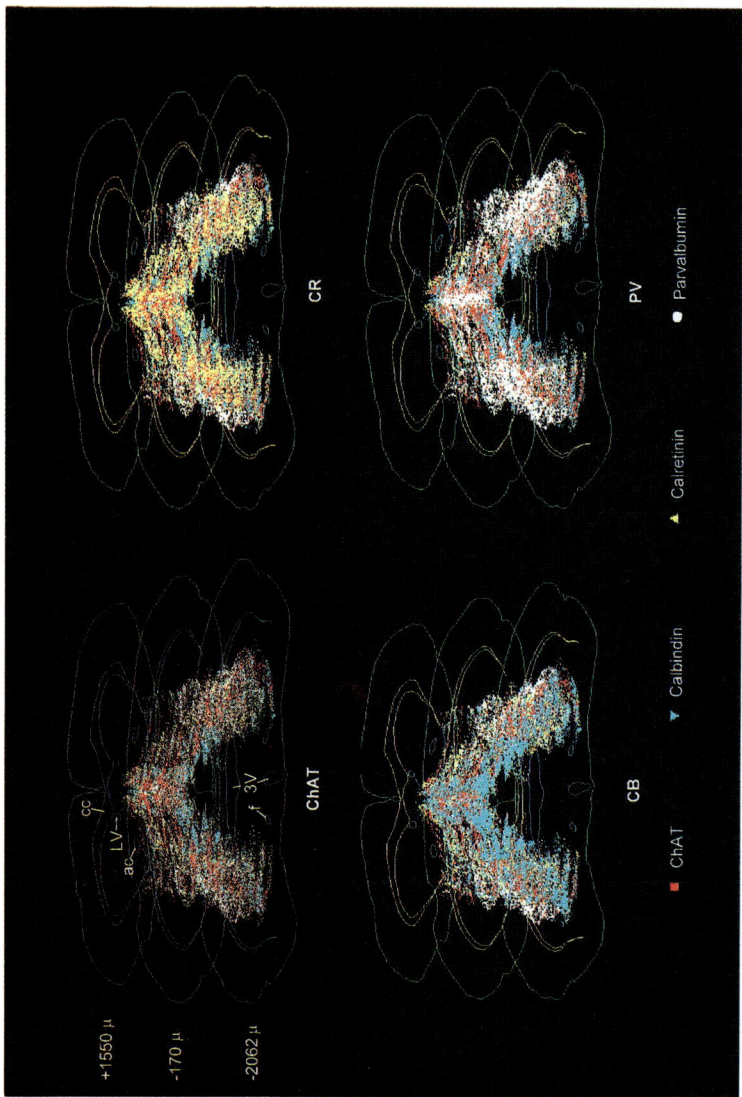

FIGURE 5. Three-dimensional spatial relational distribution of ChAT, PV, CR, and CB cells in the basal forebrain. The viewpoint of the model is from below, and most of the outlines are removed for clarity. The three sections with their approximate location to the bregma is for orientation. Because the symbols representing the different cell types are not transparent, in order to appreciate their real position, the four models show four different renderings, placing one type of symbol on the top.

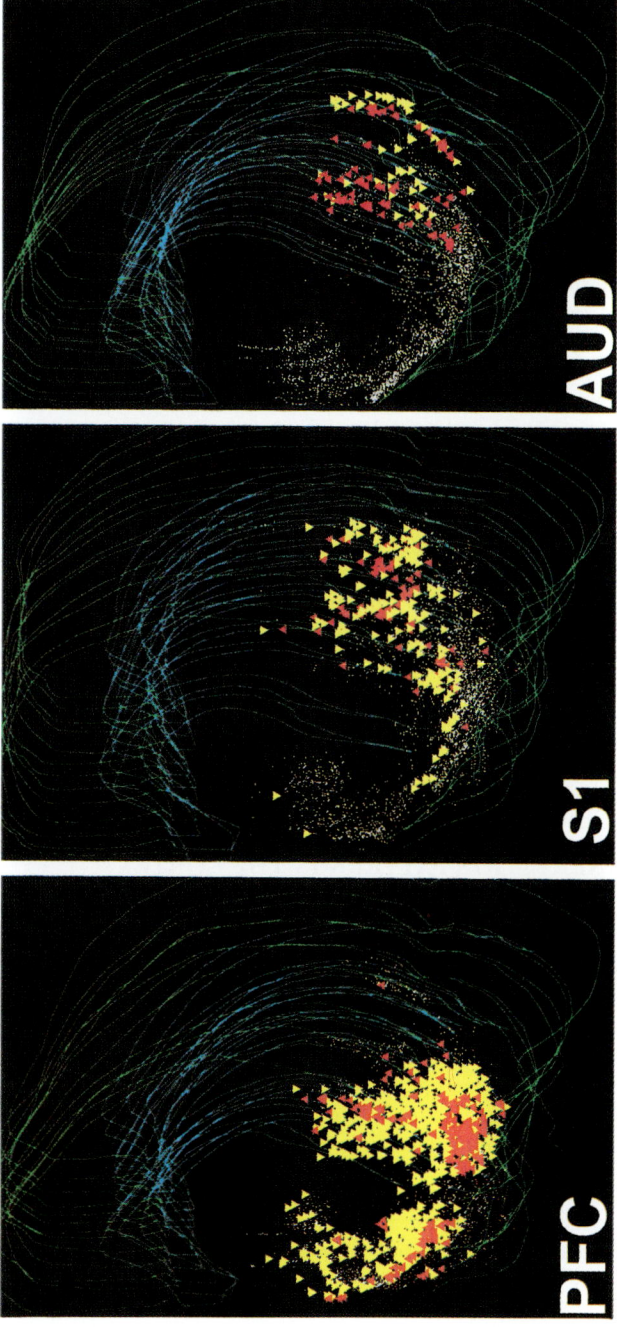

FIGURE 6. Comparative distribution of basal forebrain cells projecting to the prefrontal cortex (PFC), the primary somatosensory cortex (S1), and the auditory cortex (AUD). These maps were generated from 12 sections from three brains using the retrograde tracer Fluoro-Gold deposited in these cortical areas. Only the outlines and the corpus callosum are shown. Lateral view: left is rostral, right is caudal. White dots label the presence of cholinergic neurons, yellow down triangles symbolize retrograde noncholinergic cells, and the red up triangles mark the location of cholinergic projection neurons. Note that the center of gravity of S1 projection neurons is slightly more rostral than that for auditory projection neurons.

construction studies whether or not corticopetal projection neurons in the BF are also organized according to rostrocaudal "bands," and how these bands relate to functionally or developmentally different cortical areas. According to a partial reconstruction of the neurons projecting to the prefrontal cortex and different sensory areas in rats, it is apparent (FIG. 6) that occasional retrograde-labeled cells are distributed along bands in the whole rostrocaudal extent of the BF. The majority of projection neurons are confined, however, to specific regions of the BF. For example, the largest proportion of cells projecting to the auditory cortex are located around 2.5–2.8 mm behind the bregma, whereas the bulk of the neurons innervating the somatosensory (S1) cortex are located between 1.6–2.0 mm behind the bregma. On the other hand, the prefrontal cortex seems to receive projections from extended portions of the basal forebrain (FIG. 6). Comparing different cases or using double labeling, however, suggests that neurons projecting to functionally different cortical areas (e.g. somatosensory/versus visual) are segregated only by a narrow space of 50–200 µ from each other in extended portions of the BF.

Powell and his coworkers[33] proposed that different cortical areas receive their input from longitudinally curved, partially overlapping bands of cells in the basal forebrain. They also noticed that functionally interrelated areas of the prefrontal, sensory or motor areas of the cortex receive their projections from partially overlapping areas from the BF. Data from anterograde and retrograde studies and the distribution pattern of ChAT-PV-CR-CB suggests that a large part of the BF is organized into longitudinally oriented bands. This would be an extension of the original notion of Niewenhuys et al.[34] that the different fiber components in the medial forebrain bundle retain their three-dimensional spatial relationship across the entire length of the forebrain. Of course, the consequence of these data would be that neurons in these twisted parallel bands may have a separate input–output pattern and, thus, may participate in different functions.

INNERVATION PATTERN IN THE CORTEX

Cholinergic Innervation

According to immunohistochemical and biochemical studies, the cholinergic innervation is heterogeneous across various cortical areas and different species. For example, in humans,[35] the cholinergic innervation of the primary sensory, unimodal and heteromodal association areas are lighter than that of paralimbic and limbic areas. Within unimodal association areas, the density of cholinergic axons and varicosities is significantly lower in the upstream (parasensory) sectors than in downstream sectors. Within paralimbic regions, the nonisocortical sectors have a higher density

---

FIGURE 7. Parvalbumin-containing cells projecting to the prefrontal cortex. **A:** Three Fluoro-Gold–labeled cells. **B:** Two of the retrogradely labeled cells are positive for parvalbumin (arrows). Lower inset shows the location of the photomicrograph (star). CP, caudate putamen; LV, lateral ventricle; ox, optic chiasm; ac, anterior commissure; HDB, horizontal limb of the diagonal band. Scale bar: 50 µ.

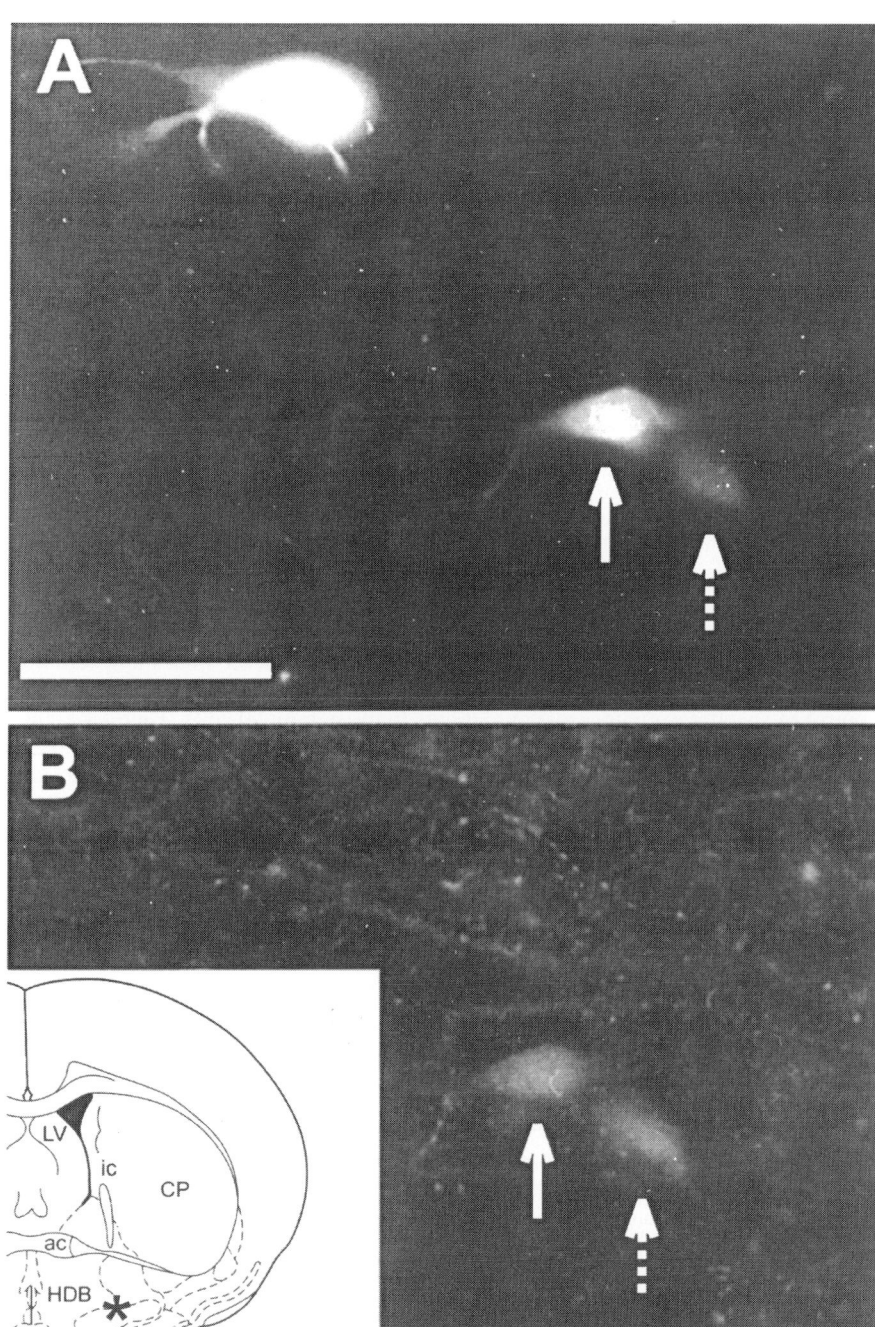

of cholinergic innervation than in the isocortical sectors. The highest density of cholinergic axons was encountered in such core limbic structures as the hippocampus and amygdala. A similar trend can be observed in the rhesus monkey[36] and rat cortices.[37]

Cholinergic varicosities are present in all cortical layers[38] and a varying proportion of them were reported to form clearly identifiable synapses (15% in rat parietal cortex,[39] 44% in monkey prefrontal cortex,[40] and 67% in human temporal cortex[41]), innervating pyramidal, spiny stellate, and GABAergic neurons. There are marked laminar variations in the density of cholinergic synapses and the identity of their postsynaptic targets. For example, the proportion of GABA-positive postsynaptic elements are highest in layer IV and lowest in layers V–VI in the visual cortex.[42] Due to distribution on various postsynaptic neurons that, in turn, may have different cholinergic receptors and specific intracortical connections, cholinergic activation may have a complex effect in cortical information processing. For example, acetylcholine (ACh) has been shown to excite layer V low-threshold spike (LTS) GABAergic cells through nicotinic receptors, whereas it elicites hyperpolarization in fast-spiking (FS) GABAergic neurons in the same layer through muscarinic receptors.[43] Axons of LTS cells mainly distribute vertically to upper layers (I–III), and those of FS cells are primarily confined to layer V pyramidal neurons. Activation of the cholinergic system could thus reduce, in the least, some forms of intralaminar inhibition (via FS cells) and together, with direct muscarinic depolarization of layer V pyramidal cells,[44] increase pyramidal to pyramidal recurrent excitation and thus enhance the transfer of information between cortical columns. By contrast, nicotinic excitation of LTS cells would promote intracolumnar inhibition and enhance the inhibitory control of specific excitatory synaptic inputs to the pyramidal cells. Therefore, cholinergic activation may change the direction of information flow within cortical circuits, which may be important in enhanced response selectivity in cortical sensory processing that is observed during arousal or attention.[45–49]

GABAergic Innervation Pattern

GABAergic projection neurons in the basal forebrain seem to exclusively innervate various inhibitory neurons in the cortex.[50] Because these GABAergic axons establish multiple contacts with inhibitory neurons, it is assumed that they can control a large population of principal cells. A recent electrophysiological study[51] lends some credence to this assumption.

Because no individual corticopetal cholinergic or GABAergic axons have been identified thus far, their spatial distribution in a cortical column is unclear. Interestingly, the distribution of muscarinic and $GABA_A$ receptors in the visual cortex show segregated but partially overlapping columns (Zilles, personal communication). If these receptor distributions reflect the spatial arrangement of cholinergic and GABAergic axons arising from the BF, one can hypothesize that the somewhat segregated cholinergic and noncholinergic columns in the BF (see FIG. 6, AUD) would relate to separate cortical modules. This would further strengthen the idea that a subpopulation of BF neurons and specific cortical areas are interlinked through selective circuitries.

SYNAPTIC INPUT TO THE BASAL FOREBRAIN

Cholinergic and other BF neurons are located in the way station for several ascending and descending pathways and thus may receive diverse input. For example, light microscopic tracer studies in rodents, carnivores, and nonhuman primates[52–60] suggest that basal forebrain areas receive input from nonisocortical paralimbic cortical areas (orbitofrontal–prefrontal, temporopolar, insular, parahippocampal, and cingulate), the amygdala, the hypothalamus, and various brain stem cell groups. Indeed, electron microscopic studies in the rat confirmed the presence of synaptic input to BF cholinergic neurons from the amygdala, dorsal and ventral striatum, hypothalamus, locus caeruleus, and midbrain dopaminergic cell groups.[61–69] Furthermore, based upon electron microscopic double-labeling studies in rats, it has been found that cholinergic neurons in the ventral pallidum receive a massive GABAergic input.[70] Additionally, cholinergic neurons receive restricted input from enkephalin,[71,72] somatostatin,[73] NPY,[73] substance P,[74] cholinergic,[75] CGRP,[76] and galanin[130] axon terminals. In a recent electron microscopic study in the monkey,[77] the presence of GABAergic, cholinergic, and catecholaminergic synapses on cholinergic neurons was confirmed, indicating a similarity in the afferent organization of cholinergic neurons between rodents and primates.

Because the painstaking electron microscopic studies confirmed most of what previous light microscopic studies suggested, it was a surprise that glutamatergic axons from the prefrontal cortex seem to terminate exclusively on noncholinergic neurons, including parvalbumin-containing GABAergic cells,[78] indicating some selectivity in the innervation pattern of BF neurons. Parvalbumin-containing neurons in the BF also receive dopaminergic input from the ventral tegmental area[79] and synaptic input from the mesopontine tegmentum (FIGURES 10 and 11). The transmitter character of this latter input is currently under investigation.

COMPARTMENTS IN THE BASAL FOREBRAIN

Although the noradrenergic and dopaminergic axons contact cholinergic neurons in extensive portions of the BF, the majority of afferents (cortical, striatal, peptidergic) appear to have a preferential distribution on subsets of BF neurons, as discussed in earlier reviews.[80,81] Thus, the emerging view is that different subsets of BF neurons may receive different combinations of afferents according to their location in the BF. If this afferent topography would be retained in their efferent channels to the cortex, it would imply that subdivisions of the BF modulate selective cortical areas through certain restricted inputs.

Immuno- and histochemical studies also support the notion that BF neurons are neurochemically compartmentalized.[82–89] However, it is unclear how the chemical signature of the neurons relates to their input–output pattern.

The suggestion that various noncholinergic neurons may participate in different circuitries and thus contribute to functional compartments in the BF is implicated by our preliminary electrophysiological studies. FIGURE 12 shows the location of nine morphologically identified noncholinergic neurons in the BF that were examined for their response to substantia nigra–ventral tegmental area (SN-VTA) or locus caer-

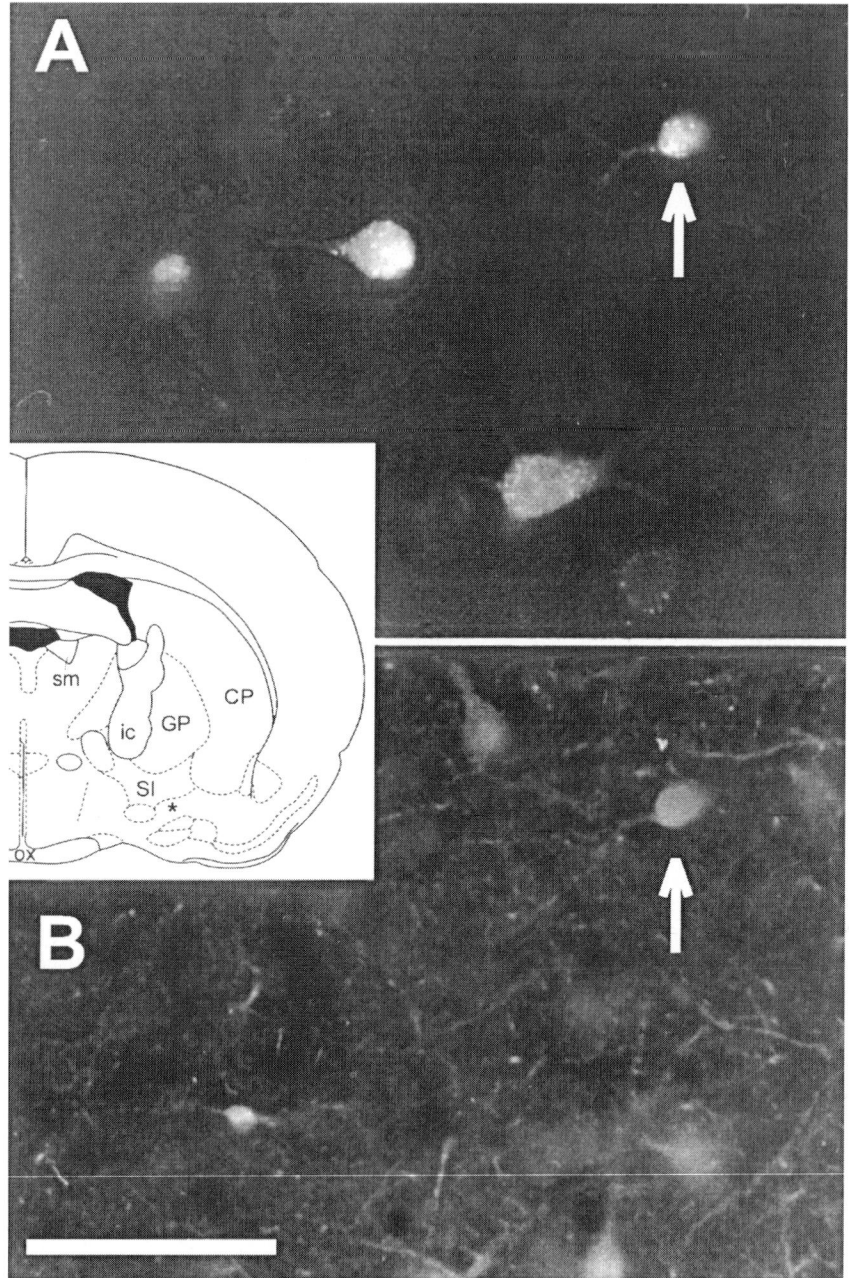

FIGURE 8. Calbindin-containing neurons projecting to the prefrontal cortex from the anterior amygdaloid area. **A:** Fluoro-Gold–labeled retrograde cells. Arrows point to a neuron that is also positive for calbindin (**B**). GP, globus pallidus; SI, substantia innominata; sm, stria medullaris. Scale bar: 50 μ.

TABLE 1. Electrophysiology and morphology of noncholinergic BF cells

ID #	Location	SN	LC	Spontaneous activity	ChAT	Axon morphology
1	VP	↑	—	random, 16.7 Hz		profuse local arborizations
2	VP	↑	—	regular, 46.2 Hz	—	profuse local arborizations with basket-like terminals
3	SI	↓↑	—	bursty, 35.1 Hz		rich local arborizations
4	vGP	↓	↓	regular, 24 Hz		long axon, few collaterals
5	SI	↑↓↑	↓↑	regular, 22 Hz	—	few local collaterals
6	SI	↑↑	↑↑	regular, 14 Hz	—	projection neuron
7	SI	↑↓↑		random, 3.8 Hz	—	axon with few collaterals
8	SI	↑↓	↑↑↓	bursty, 5 Hz	—	projection neuron
9	SI	—	—	random, 11 Hz	—	long axon, moderate collaterals

SN, substania nigra; LC, locus caeruleus; ChAT, choline acetyltransferase; SI, substantia innominata; vGP, ventral globus pallidus; VP, ventral pallidum. For SN and LC columns, ↑, excitation, ↓, inhibition, —, no response at 2 µA stimulation.

uleus (LC) stimulation. These neurons expressed different patterns of spontaneous activity and a wide range of firing rates. Stimulation of the SN or LC resulted in complex responses (TABLE 1). The morphology and axonal arborization pattern of these neurons were also heterogeneous. From this small pool of recorded neurons, it is apparent that SN-VTA stimulation elicits responses from both projection neurons (identified antidromically from the cortex or having long projection axons without local collaterals) and putative interneurons (having rich local axonal arborizations with no noticeably long axons). Interestingly, none of the three interneurons (#1–3, FIG. 12 and TABLE 1) responded to LC stimulation. Whether noradrenergic input in the BF would indeed affect primarily projection neurons whereas the dopaminergic system could influence both local and projection neurons remains to be established in much larger samples.

Careful monitoring of the behavioral effect of selective lesions indeed suggests that compartments of the basal forebrain, together with specific cortical areas, may participate in different cognitive operations.[90] For example, the septohippocampal projection may be involved in short-term spatial (working) memory processes; the diagonal band-cingulate cortex cholinergic projection impacts on the ability to use response rules through conditional discrimination, the nucleus basalis-neocortical projection is involved in visual attention, and the nucleus basalis-amygdala cholinergic projection may have a role in the retention of affective conditioning (also see chapters of Sarter, Everitt, and Gallagher, this volume). It is unclear, however, whether or not these functional compartments are organized according to "traditional" borders or along longitudinally oriented bands, as would be predicted based upon previous sections in this chapter.

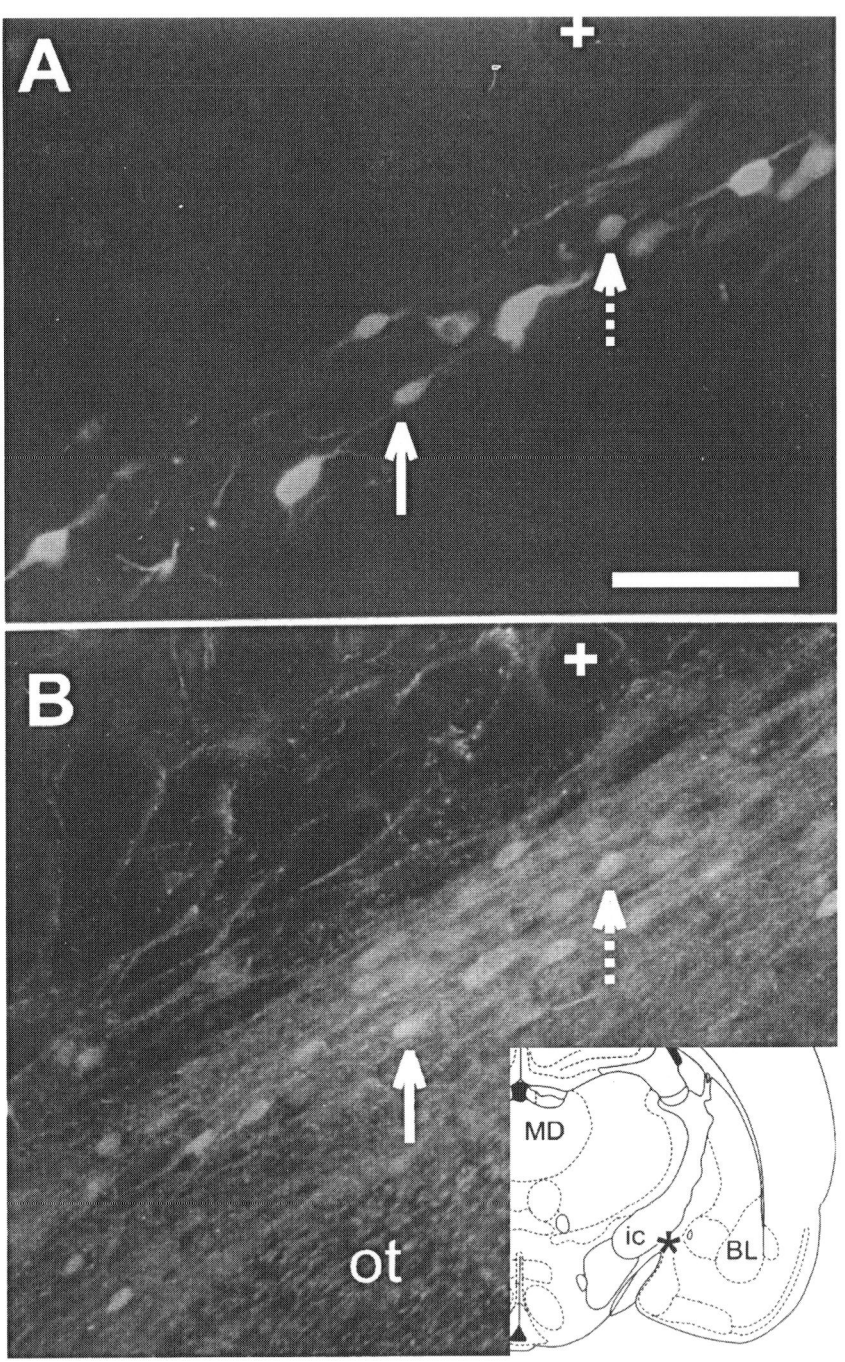

ATTENTION AND BASAL FOREBRAIN

Recent studies in rats and monkeys using more specific lesioning of the basal forebrain cholinergic neurons indicate that the cholinergic projection neurons may not be required for learning, per se, but rather they may be important for specific aspects of attention.[91,92] For example, monkeys with ibotenic acid lesions in the substantia innominata showed enhanced sensitivity to disruptive effects of invalid trials in a visuospatial attention-shift paradigm.[92] This lesion effect is strikingly similar to deficits of Alzheimer patients on this task.[93] Similarly, rats with 192-saporin lesions showed impaired choice accuracy and stimulus discriminability in a visual attention task.[94] Using a cross-modal divided-attention paradigm, immuonolesions of the cholinergic system increased the response latencies under the condition of modality uncertainty.[95] The impairments in two-choice[96] or multiple-choice[97] reaction time tasks in rodents, after blocking the central cholinergic neurotransmission, also suggests that the BF is involved in some form of bottom-up attentional processes. Finally, immunolesions in a different part of the basal forebrain[98] suggest that pathways via the BF affect top–down attentional processes. More recently, PET neuroimaging studies in a human auditory vigilance test showed rCBF changes in the BF, indicating that this brain region is involved in arousal and/or attentional networks.[99]

BASAL FOREBRAIN IN CORTICAL PLASTICITY

BF stimulation delivered before the presentation of a sensory stimulus (within 200 ms) facilitates the evoked responses in the somatosensory or auditory cortices in anesthetized and awake animals.[100–103] This facilitatory cortical effect could also be elicited by local cortical administration of ACh and blocked by muscarinic antagonists[102,104] or local application of the immunotoxin 192-saporin.[105] BF lesions prevent cortical receptive field reorganization after peripheral deafferentation,[106,107] and electrical stimulation in the BF elicits change in the representational cortical map.[108] PET studies in human subjects during auditory discrimination classical conditioning tasks are in accordance with animal studies of experience-dependent plasticity, showing that rCBF of the auditory cortex positively covaried with activity in the BF, amygdala, and orbitofrontal cortex.[109] These results support the notion that the BF cholinergic projection to the cortex is an important factor in learning-induced synaptic plasticity in the cortex.

FIGURE 9. Calretinin-containing (CR) neurons projecting to the auditory cortex. **A:** Row of retrogradely labeled cells in the narrow zone between the optic tract (ot) and the internal capsule. **B:** Two of the CR-containing neurons (arrows) are retrogradely labeled in **A**. Lower right inset shows the location of the micrographs. + sign label the same vessel. MD, mediodorsal nucleus of the thalamus; BL, basolateral amygdaloid nucleus; ic, internal capsule. Scale bar: 100 μ.

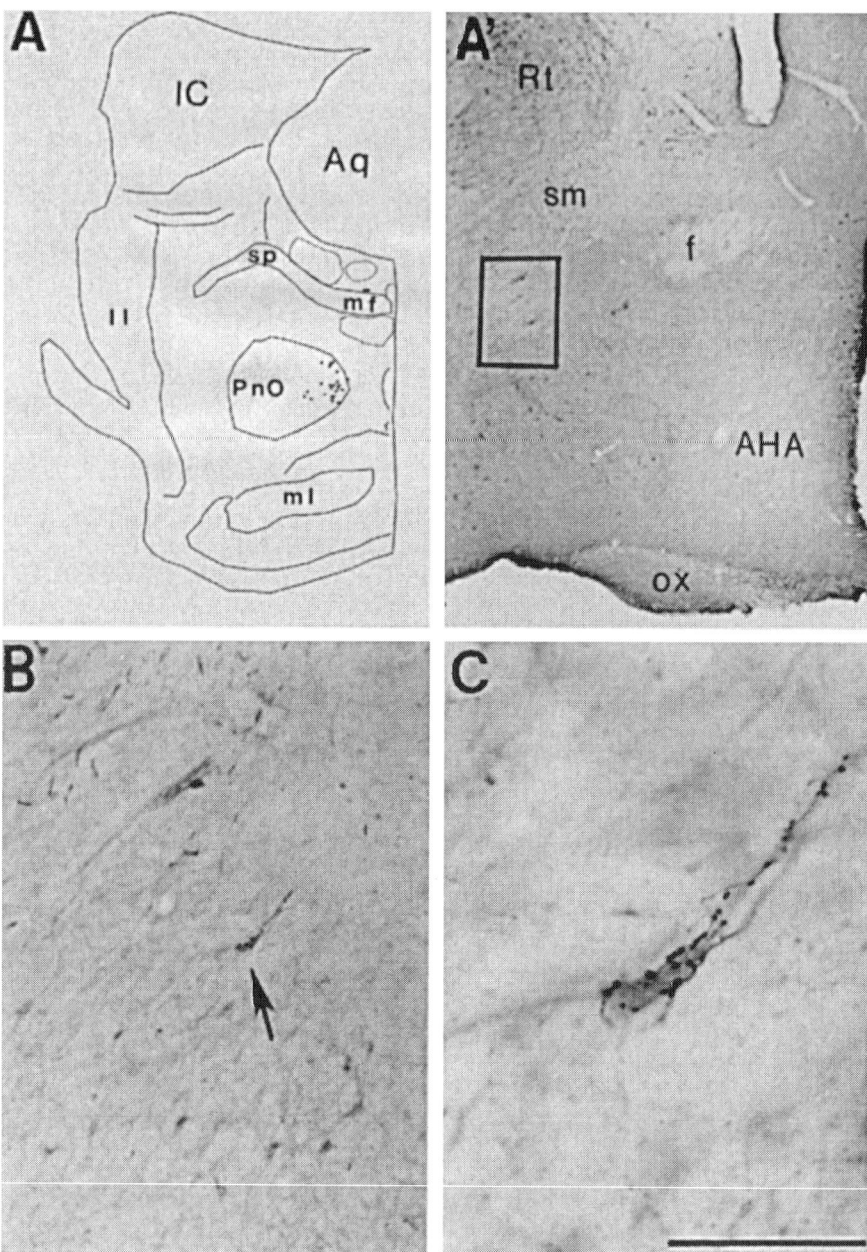

FIGURE 10. Ascending input from the pontine reticular formation to parvalbumin-containing (PV) basal forebrain neuron. **A:** PHA-L–labeled neurons in the oral part of the pontine reticular nucleus (PnO). Aq, aqueductus cerebri; ll, lateral lemniscus, ml, medial lemniscus; IC, inferior colliculus; mf, medial longitudinal fascicle; sp, superior cerebellar peduncle. **A':** Box is shown with higher magnification in **B**. Rt, reticular thalamic nucleus; sm, stria medullaris; f, fornix; AHA, anterior hypothalamic area; ox, optic chiasm. **B:** Arrow points to a PV cell in the substantia innominata. **C:** The PV-containing neuron is enwrapped by PHA-L–labeled varicosities. Scale bar: 50 μ.

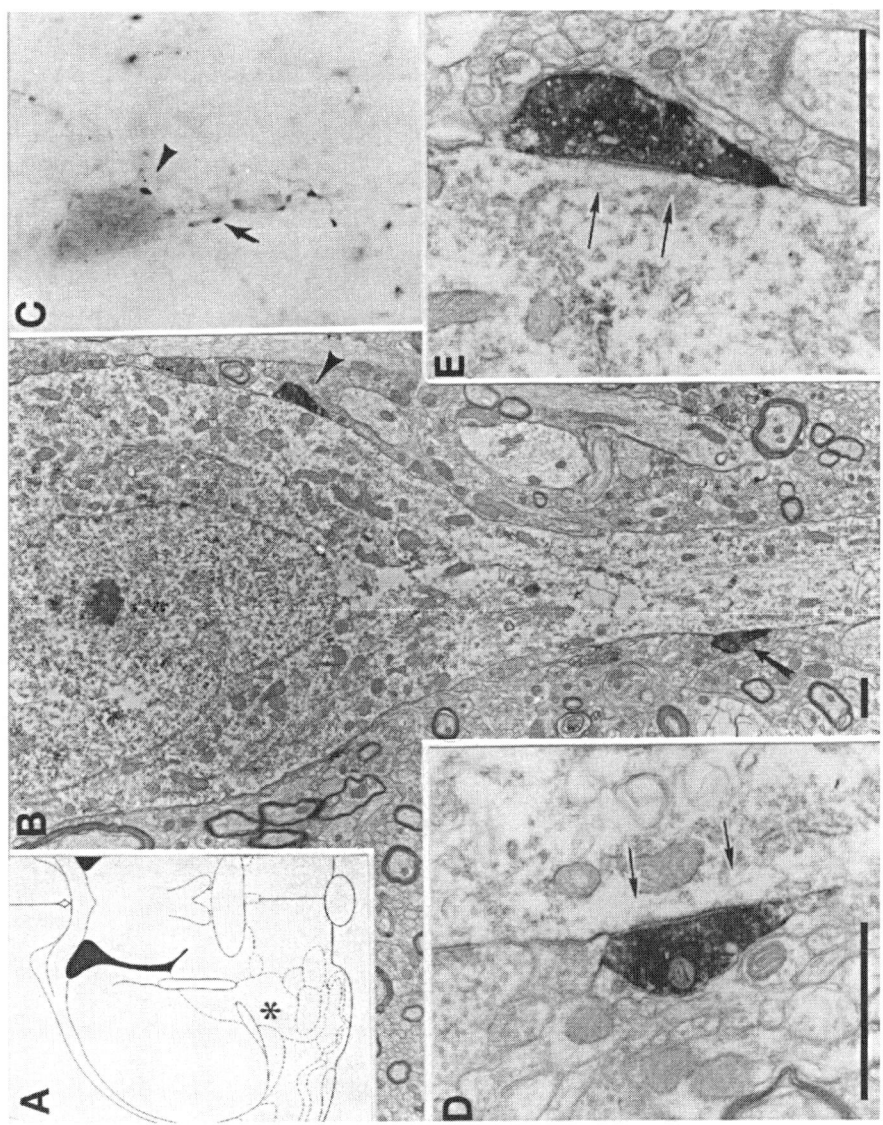

SPECIFIC CIRCUITS VIA THE BASAL FOREBRAIN

Based upon clinical, imaging, and anatomical studies, several networks are suggested as basic to attentional construction.[110–114] The obligatory components of such circuits are posterior thalamocortical areas involved in perceptual categorization, and anterior (prefrontal, cingulate) cortical areas involved in working memory and planning for action. Given the significance of the BF in mediating tonic cortical cholinergic activation upon electrical stimulation of the midbrain reticular formation,[115–117] it is no surprise to find increased rCBF in basal forebrain areas during attentional tasks. It is possible that BF activation would cause a global enhancement of cortical ACh release and that the observed cortical plasticity is due to synaptic modifications through interaction of specific thalamic, "diffuse" cholinergic and local cortical mechanisms.[100,118] However, such a general cholinergic mechanism could hardly explain why only the responses to a specific stimulus are selectively enhanced. The emerging organizational plan of the BF, as described above, implies that BF circuits may participate in modality-specific (selective) attention and cortical plasticity. According to this model, the enhancement of a sensory representation in the task-relevant sensory cortical area depends on activation of specific sensory cortex-prefrontal-BF-sensory cortex reentrant circuits that mediate the behavioral relevance of the situation.

The schematic diagram of FIGURE 13 is based on electron microscopic data using the strict criteria of correlating neurochemically identified neurons and synapses as well as assumptions derived from the putative organizational principles of the BF. The following points deserve discussion.

Brain Stem Pathways Leading to Activation of BF Neurons

Unexpected or salient stimuli characteristically results in phasic activation of locus caeruleus units.[119] The locus caeruleus, via its input to the BF,[65] may send a "warning signal" to the forebrain. Basal forebrain neurons, through their input from the mesopontine tegmentum (FIGURES 10 and 11), may also receive broadly tuned sensory-related information. Considering the conduction velocity of these brain stem axons,[120] it is likely that BF units may be activated as early as 12–14 ms after delivery of the sensory stimulus.[115,121] Given the diffuse distribution of noradrenergic inputs to the BF, one could assume that this input would result in only a slight global increase of cortical ACh efflux.

Information Processing in the Cortex

Attention effects on single-unit discharges are usually observed well after the initial arrival of the thalamo-cortical sensory afferent volleys. For example, auditory

---

FIGURE 11. Synaptic input from the brain stem to a PV-containing neuron in the ventral pallidum (**A:** asterisk). **B:** Low magnifcation overview of a PV-containing neuron. Arrows point to PHA-L–labeled synaptic terminals. **C:** High-magnification light micrograph of the PV-containing neuron depicted in **B**. Arrows point to PHA-L–labeled varicosities originating from the injection site in the brain stem (FIG. 10A). **D** and **E:** High-magnification electron micrographs of the left and right synaptic boutons from **B**. Arrows point to the postsynaptic site. Scale bars: 1 μ. (*Figure 11 is on preceding page.*)

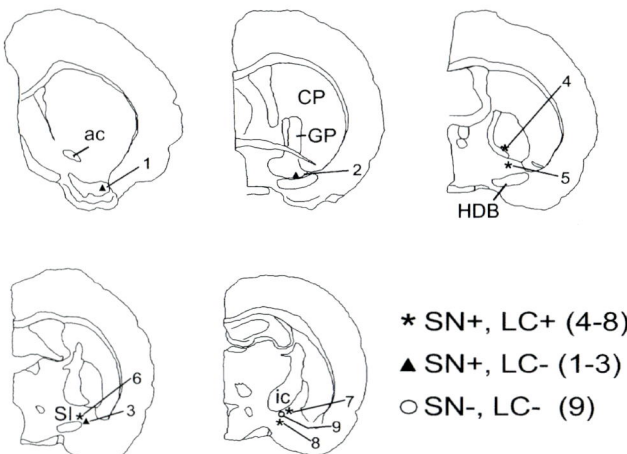

FIGURE 12. Rostrocaudal series of schematic coronal sections depicting the locations of juxtacellularly labeled noncholinergic basal forebrain neurons that were tested for responses after substantia nigra (SN) or locus caeruleus (LC) stimulation using 2 µA. Cell #4–8 responded both to SN and LC stimulation, whereas cell #1–3 responded only to SN stimulation. Cell #9 did not respond to either stimulation. From the unpublished material of Pang, Tepper, and Záborszky.

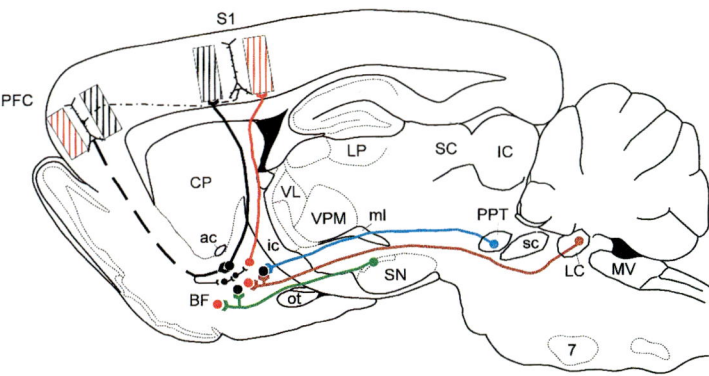

FIGURE 13. Hypothetical circuitry between prefrontal (PFC) and specific somatosensory (S1) cortical areas via GABAergic local and projection neurons of the basal forebrain. Cholinergic and noncholinergic neurons in the basal forebrain receive identified synaptic input from the locus caeruleus (LC, brown), the substantia nigra (SN, green) and the mesopontine tegmentum (PPT, blue). The projection target of these BF neurons was not determined. The innervation territory of GABAergic and cholinergic axons in the PFC and S1 are indicated schematically as nonoverlapping black (GABA) and red (cholinergic) columns. The axons of pyramidal cells in the S1 cortex (hyphenated line) innervate a pyramidal neuron in the PFC. IC, inferior colliculus; LP, lateral posterior thalamic nucleus (n); ml, medial lemniscus; MV, medial vestibular n.; PPT, peduculopontine tegmental n.; SC, superior colliculus; sc, superior cerebellar peduncle; VL, ventrolateral thalamic n.; VPM, ventral posteromedial n.; 7, facial n. To prepare this drawing, we used figure 84 from the atlas of Paxinos and Watson.[129]

and somatosensory inputs arrive at the primary cortex in 10–15 ms, but attention-related modulations occur 40–60 ms or even later.[122] From the sensory cortex information flow proceeds via hierarchical and parallel routes[123,124] and could eventually reach the prefrontal cortex within 10–15 ms after somatosensory (S1) stimulation (Nunez, personal communication).

Origin of Late Components of the Event-related Potentials

Selective somatosensory responses can also be observed in the BF 25 ms after stimulation of the prefrontal cortex (Nunez, personal communication). BF stimulation provoked bursts in sensory cortex 40–60 ms after the end of the stimulus,[51] which is also associated with increased ACh efflux in the appropriate cortical area. Thus, the proposed reentrant circuitry could explain the timeline of attention-related evoked potentials in the sensory cortex, and the prefrontal input could amplify computations in a particular sensory area that initially performed the computation, a common observation in human imaging studies during attention tasks.[110]

Topographically Organized Parallel Circuits

Attention in different sensory modalities is characterized by a special pattern of rCBF increase in the prefrontal cortex. Perception of different modalities gave rise to differently located activations in the prefrontal cortex of humans,[113] which is compatible with the presence of separate modality-specific sensory areas in the prefrontal cortex of monkeys.[125] Partially overlapping sensory areas has also been shown in the rat prefrontal cortex.[123] Inasmuch as different subdivisions of the prefrontal cortex project topographically to the BF,[58] this projection via the longitudinally oriented cell bands of the BF could feed back to functionally segregated posterior sensory areas. It is envisaged that if the cell clusters in the BF receive prominent prefrontal input, they would be in a powerful position in amplifying selective cortical processing. This more selective cortical activation would be against the low-level global cortical activation induced through noradrenergic input to the diffusely located scattered corticopetal cells. It is expected that several cortico-prefrontal-BF-cortical circuits exist and are somewhat similar to the better-known parallel forebrain circuits that involve the prefrontal cortex, the basal ganglia, and the thalamus.[126]

CONCLUDING REMARKS

Recent anatomical as well as electrophysiological data[127,128] contributed substantially to our understanding of the operational features of single basal forebrain cells. However, further investigation of the functions of the basal forebrain as a system requires the appreciation of the precise spatial relation of the different transmitter-specific neurons and their input–output characteristics. We suggest that the working memory and executive (prefrontal, cingulate) cortical areas work in close association with the basal forebrain in funneling towards the respective posterior cortical areas the "energetic factors" (arousal) and the affective state (amygdala) necessary for coordinating distributed cognitive operations. There are a lot of aspects in the proposed triangular amplification circuit (especially the precise local BF circuitry) that have to be considered hypothetical, but it appears to be consistent with what we know from the neurobiology and psychology of attention and cortical plasticity, respectively, and could serve as a basis for further testing.

ACKNOWLEDGMENT

This research was supported by NIH Grant No. NS23945. Special thanks are due to Mr. Derek Buhl, Mrs. E. Rommer, Mr. S. Poobalasingham, and Mr. B. Lynch for expert technical assistance.

REFERENCES

1. HEIMER, L. & R.D. WILSON. 1975. The subcortical projections of the allocortex; similarities in the neural associations of the hippocampus, the piriform cortex and the neocortex. In Golgi Centennial Symposium Proceedings. M. Santini, Ed.: 177–193. Raven Press. New York.
2. HEIMER, L., R.D. SWITZER & G.W. VAN HOESEN. 1982. Ventral striatum and ventral pallidum. Components of the motor system? Trends Neurosci. **5:** 83–87.
3. HEIMER L., G.F. ALHEID & L. ZABORSZKY. 1985. The basal ganglia. In The Rat Nervous System, Vol. 1. Forebrain and Midbrain. G. Paxinos, Ed.: 37–86. Academic Press. Sydney.
4. HEIMER L., G.F. ALHEID & L. ZABORSZKY. 1989. Substantia innominata and basal forebrain. In Neuroscience Year. G. Adelman, Ed.: 21–24. Birkhauser. Boston.
5. HEIMER L, J. DE OLMOS, G.F. ALHEID & L. ZABORSZKY. 1991. "Perestroika" in the basal forebrain: opening the border between neurology and psychiatry. Prog. Brain Res. **87:** 109–165.
6. ZABORSZKY L., G.F. ALHEID, M.C. BEINFELD, L.E. EIDEN, L. HEIMER & M. PALKOVITS. 1985. Cholecystokinin innervation of the ventral striatum: a morphological and radioimmunological study. Neuroscience **14:** 427–453.
7. REIL, J.C. 1809. Untersuchungen uber den Bau des grossen Gehirn in Menschen. Arch. Psysiol. (Halle) **9:** 136–208.
8. BRAUER, K., A. SCHOBER, J.R. WOLFF, E. WINKELMAN, H. LUPPA, H.-J. LUTH & H. BOTTCHER. 1991. Morphology of neurons in the rat basal forebrain nuclei: comparison between NADPH-diaphorase histochemistry and immunohistochemistry of glutamic acid decarboxylase, choline acetyltransferase, somatostatin and parvalbumin. J. Hirnforsch. **32:** 1–17.
9. DINOPOULOS, A., J.G. PARNAVELAS, H.B.M. UYLINGS & C.G. VAN EDEN. 1988. Morphology of neurons in the basal forebrain nuclei of the rat: a Golgi study. J. Comp. Neurol. **272:** 461–474.
10. GRITTI, L., L. MAINVILLE, & B.E. JONES. 1993. Codistribution of GABA-with acetylcholine-synthesizing neurons in the basal forebrain of the rat. J. Comp. Neurol. **329:** 438–457.
11. WALKER, L. C., V.E. KOLIATSOS, C.A. KITT, R.T. RICHARDSON, A. ROKAEUS &. D.L. PRICE. 1989. Peptidergic neurons in the basal forebrain magnocellular complex of the rhesus monkey. J. Comp. Neurol. **280:** 272–282.
12. ZABORSZKY, L., J. CARLSEN, H.R. BRASHEAR & L. HEIMER. 1986. Cholinergic and GABAergic afferents to the olfactory bulb in the rat with special emphasis on the projection neurons in the nucleus of the horizontal limb of the diagonal band. J. Comp. Neurol. **243:** 488–509.
13. PRICE, D.L., P.J. WHITEHOUSE & R.G STRUBLE. 1986. Cellular pathology in Alzheimer's and Parkinson's diseases. Trends Neurosci. **9:** 29–33.
14. MESULAM, M.M., E.J. MUFSON, B.H. WAINER & A.I. LEVEY. 1983. Central cholinergic pathways in the rat: an overview based on an alternative nomenclature (Ch1-Ch6). Neuroscience **10:** 1185–1201.

15. VOGELS, O.J.M., C.A.J. BROERE, H.J. TER LAAK, H.J. TEN DONKELAAR, R. NIEUWENHUYS & B.P.M. SCHULTE. 1990. Cell loss and shrinkage in the nucleus basalis Meynert complex in Alzheimer's disease. Neurobiol. Aging **11:** 3–13.
16. ARENDT, T., V. BIGL., A. TENNSTEDT & A. ARENDT. 1985. Neuronal loss in different parts of the nucleus basalis is related to neuritic plaque formation in cortical target areas in Alzheimer's disease. Neuroscience **14:** 1–14.
17. MESULAM, M.M., E.J. MUFSON, A.I. LEVEY & B.H. WAINER. 1983. Cholinergic innervation of cortex by the basal forebrain: cytochemistry and cortical connections of the septal area, diagonal band nuclei, nucleus basalis (substantia innominata), and hypothalamus in the rhesus monkey. J. Comp. Neurol. **214:** 170–197.
18. SOFRONIEW, M.V., F. ECKENSTEIN, H. THOENEN & A.C. CUELLO. 1982. Topography of choline acetyltransferase-containing neurons in the forebrain of the rat. Neurosci. Lett. **33:** 7–12.
19. ARMSTRONG, D.M., C.B. SAPER, A.I. LEVEY, B.H. WAINER & R.D. TERRY. 1983. Distribution of cholinergic neurons in the rat brain demonstrated by immunohistochemical localization of choline acetyltransferase. J. Comp. Neurol. **216:** 53–68.
20. RYE, D.B., B.H. WAINER, M.-M. MESULAM, E.J. MUFSON & C.B. SAPER. 1984. Cortical projections arising from the basal forebrain: a study of cholinergic and noncholinergic components combining retrograde tracing and immunohistochemical localization of choline acetyltransferase. Neuroscience **13:** 627–643.
21. WOOLF, N.J., F. ECKENSTEIN & L.L. BUTCHER. 1984. Cholinergic systems in the rat brain. I. Projections to the limbic telencephalon. Brain Res. Bull. **13:** 751–784.
22. AMARAL, D.G. & J. KURZ. 1985. An analysis of the origins of the cholinergic and non- cholinergic septal projections to the hippocampal formation in the rat. J. Comp. Neurol. **240:** 37–59.
23. CARLSEN, J., L. ZÁBORSZKY & L. HEIMER. 1985. Cholinergic projections from the basal forebrain to the basolateral amygdaloid complex: a combined retrograde fluorescent and immunohistochemical study. J. Comp. Neurol. **234:** 155–167.
24. LUITEN, P.G.M., R.P.A. GAYKEMA, J. TRABER & D.G. SPENCER. 1987. Cortical projection patterns of magnocellular basal nucleus subdivisions as revealed by anterogradely transported *Phaseolus vulgaris* leucoaagglutinin. Brain Res. **413:** 229–250.
25. GAYKEMA, R.P.A., P.G.M. LUITEN, C. NYAKAS & J. TRABER. 1990. Cortical projection patterns of the medial septum-diagonal band complex. J. Comp. Neurol. **293:** 103–124.
26. MESULAM, M.M., E.J. MUFSON & B.H. WAINER. 1986. Three-dimensional representation and cortical projection topography of the nucleus basalis (Ch4) in the macaque: concurrent demonstration of choline acetyltransferase and retrograde transport with a stabilized tetramethylbenzidine method for HRP. Brain Res. **367:** 301–308.
27. PANG, K., J.M. TEPPER & L. ZABORSZKY. 1998. Morphological and electrophysiological characteristics of non-cholinergic basal forebrain neurons. J. Comp. Neurol. **394:** 186–204.
28. LYNCH, B., D. OROSZ & L. ZABORSZKY. 1996. Basal forebrain corticopetal system: 3-D computer graphic reconstruction. Soc. Neurosci. Abstr. **22:** 1256.
29. GRITTI, I., L. MAINVILLE, M. MANCIA & B. JONES. 1997. GABAergic and other non-cholinergic basal forebrain neurons, together with cholinergic neurons, project to the mesocortex and isocortex in the rat. J. Comp. Neurol. **383:** 163–177.
30. POOBALASINGHAM, S., K. PANG & L. ZABORSZKY. 1996. Distribution of neurons containing different type of calcium binding proteins in the cholinergic basal forebrain. Soc. Neurosci. Absrt. **22:** 1255.
31. KISS, J., Z. MAGLOCZKY, J. SOMOGYI & T.F. FREUND. 1997. Distribution of calretinin containing neurons relative to other neurochemically identified cell types in the medial septum of the rat. Neuroscience **78:** 399–410.
32. CULLINAN, W.E. & L. ZABORSZKY. 1991. Organization of ascending hypothalamic projections to the rostral forebrain with special reference to the innervation of cholinergic projection neurons. J. Comp. Neurol. **306:** 631–667.
33. PEARSON, R.C.A., K.C. GATTER, P. BRODAL & T.P.S. POWELL. 1983. The projection of the basal nucleus of Meynert upon the neocortex in the monkey. Brain Res. **259:** 132–136.

34. NIEUWENHUYS, R., L.M.G. GEERAEDTS & J.G. VEENING. 1982. The medial forebrain bundle of the rat. I. General information. J. Comp. Neurol. **206:** 49–81.
35. MESULAM, M.-M., L.B. HERSH, D.C. MASH & C. GEULA. 1992. Differential cholinergic innervation within functional subdivisions of the human cerebral cortex: a choline acetyltransferase study. J. Comp. Neurol. **318:** 316–328.
36. MESULAM, M.M., L., VOLICER, J.K. MARQUIS, E.J. MUFSON & R.C. GREEN. 1986. Systematic regional differences in the cholinergic innervation of the primate cerebral cortex: distribution of enzyme activities and some behavioral implications. Ann. Neurol. **19:** 144–151.
37. LYSAKOWSKI, A., B.H. WAINER, G.C. BRUCE & L.B. HERSH. 1988. An atlas of the regional and laminar distribution of choline acetyltransferase immunoreactivity in rat cerebral cortex. Neuroscience **28:** 291–336.
38. HOUSER, C.R., G.D. CRAWFORD, P.M. SALVATERRA & J.E. VAUGHN. 1985. Immunocytochemical localization of choline acetyltransferase in rat cerebral cortex: a study of cholinergic neurons and synapses. J. Comp. Neurol. **234:** 17–34.
39. UMBRIACO, D., K.C. WATKINS, L. DESCARRIES, C. COZZARI & B.K. HARTMAN. 1994. Ultrastructural and morphometric features of the acetylcholine innervation in adult rat parietal cortex: An electron microscopic study in serial sections. J. Comp. Neurol. **348:** 351–373.
40. MRZLJAK, L., M. PAPPY, C. LERANTH & P.S. GOLDMAN-RAKIC. 1995. Cholinergic synaptic circuitry in the macaque prefrontal cortex. J. Comp. Neurol. **357:** 603–617.
41. SMILEY, J.F., F. MORRELL & M.M. MESULAM. 1997. Cholinergic synapses in human cerebral cortex: an ultrastructural study in serial sections. Exp. Neurol. **144:** 361–368.
42. BEAULIEU, C. & P. SOMOGYI. 1991. Enrichment of cholinergic synaptic terminals on GABAergic neurons and coexistence of immunoreactive GABA and choline acetyltransferase in the same synaptic terminals in the striate cortex of the cat. J. Comp. Neurol. **304:** 666–680.
43. XIANG, Z., J.R. HUGUENARD & D.A. PRINCE. 1998. Cholinergic switching within neocortical inhibitory networks. Science **281:** 985–988.
44. MCCORMICK, D.A. 1993. Action of acetylcholine in the cerebral cortex and thalamus and implications for function. Prog. Brain Res. **98:** 303–308.
45. LIVINGSTON, M.S. & D.H. HUBEL. 1981. Effects of sleep and arousal on the processing of visual information in the cat. Nature **291:** 554–561.
46. LEWANDOWSKI, M.H., C.M. MULLER & W. SINGER. 1993. Reticular facilitation of cat visual cortical responses is mediated by nicotinic and muscarinic cholinergic mechanisms. Exp. Brain Res. **96:** 1–7.
47. MULLER, C.M., M.H. LEWANDOWSKI & W. SINGER. 1993. Structures mediating cholinergic reticular facilitation of cortical responses in the cat: effects of lesions in immunocytochemically characterized projections. Exp. Brain Res. **96:** 8–18.
48. MUNK, M.H.J., P.R. ROELSEMA, P. KONIG, A.K. ENGEL & W. SINGER. 1996. Role of reticular activation in the modulation of intracortical synchronization. Science **272:** 271–274.
49. SILLITO, A.M. 1993. The cholinergic modulatory system: an evaluation of its functional roles. Prog. Brain Res. **98:** 371–378.
50. FREUND, T.F. & A.I. GULYAS. 1991. GABAergic interneurons containing calbindin D28k or somatostatin are major targets of GABAergic basal forebrain afferents in the rat neocortex. J. Comp. Neurol. **314:** 187–199.
51. JIMENEZ-CAPDEVILLE, M.E., R.W. DYKES & A.A. MYASNIKOV. 1997. Differential control of cortical activity by the basal forebrain in rats: a role for both cholinergic and inhibitory influences. J. Comp. Neurol. **381:** 53–67.
52. JONES, E.G., H. BURTON, C.B. SAPER & L. SWANSON. 1976. Midbrain, diencephalic and cortical relationships of the basal nucleus of Meynert and associated structures in primates. J. Comp. Neurol. **167:** 385–420.
53. MESULAM, M.M. & E.J. MUFSON. 1984. Neural inputs into the nucleus basalis of the substantia innominata (Ch4) in the rhesus monkey. Brain **107:** 253–274.
54. RUSSCHEN, F.T., D.G. AMARAL & J.L. PRICE. 1985. The afferent connections of the substantia innominata in the monkey, *Macaca fascicularis*. J. Comp. Neurol. **242:** 1–27.

55. IRLE, E.H. & J. MARKOWITSCH. 1986. Afferent connections of the substantia innominata/ basal nucleus of Meynert in carnivores and primates. J. Hirnforsch. **27:** 343–367.
56. GROVE, E.A., V.B. DOMESICK & W.J.H. NAUTA. 1986. Light microscopic evidence of striatal input to intrapallidal neurons of cholinergic cell group Ch4 in the rat: a study employing the anterograde tracer *Phaseolus vulgaris* leucoagglutinin (PHAL). Brain Res. **367:** 379–384.
57. SEMBA, K., P.B. REINER, E.G. MCGEER & H.C. FIBIGER. 1988. Brainstem afferents to the magnocellular basal forebrain studied by axonal transport, immunohistochemistry, and electrophysiology in the rat. J. Comp. Neurol. **267:** 433–453.
58. SESACK, S. R., A. Y. DEUTCH, R. H. ROTH & B. S. BUNNEY. 1989. Topographical organization of the efferent projections of the medial prefrontal cortex in the rat: An anterograde tract-tracing study with *Phaseolus vulgaris* leucoagglutinin. J. Comp. Neurol. **290:** 213–242.
59. JONES, B.E & A.C. CUELLO. 1989. Afferents to the basal forebrain cholinergic cell area from the pontomesencephalic-catecholamine, serotonin, and acetylcholine-neurons. Neuroscience **31:** 37–61.
60. HURLEY, K.M., H. HERBERT, M.M. MOGA & C.B. SAPER. 1991. Efferent projections of the infralimbic cortex of the rat. J. Comp. Neurol. **308:** 249–276.
61. ZABORSZKY, L., C. LERANTH & L. HEIMER. 1984. Ultrastructural evidence of amydalofugal axons terminating on cholinergic cells of the rostral forebrain. Neurosci. Lett. **52:** 219–225.
62. ZABORSZKY, L. & W.E. CULLINAN. 1989. Hypothalamic axons terminate on forebrain cholinergic neurons: an ultrastructural doublelabeling study using PHAL tracing and ChAT immunochemistry. Brain Res. **479:** 177–184.
63. CULLINAN, W.E. & L. ZABORSZKY. 1991. Organization of ascending hypothalamic projections to the rostral forebrain with special reference to the innervation of cholinergic projection neurons. J. Comp. Neurol. **306:** 631–667.
64. ZABORSZKY, L. & W.E CULLINAN. 1992. Projections from the nucleus accumbens to cholinergic neurons of the ventral pallidum: a correlated light and electron microscopic double-immunolabeling study in rat. Brain Res. **570:** 92–101.
65. ZABORSZKY, L., W.E. CULLINAN & V.N. LUINE. 1993. Catecholaminergic-cholinergic interaction in the basal forebrain. Prog. Brain Res. **98:** 31–49.
66. ZABORSZKY, L. & W. E CULLINAN. 1996. Direct catecholaminergic-cholinergic interactions in the basal forebrain. I. Dopamine-β-hydroxylase- and tyrosine hydroxylase input to cholinergic neurons. J. Comp. Neurol. **374:** 535–554.
67. GAYKEMA, R.P.A. & L. ZABORSZKY. 1996. Direct catecholaminergic-cholinergic interactions in the basal forebrain. II. Substantia nigra and ventral tegmental area projections to cholinergic neurons. J. Comp. Neurol. **374:** 555–577.
68. RODRIGO, J., P. FERNANDEZ, M.L. BENTURA, J.M. DE VELASCO, J. SERRANO, O. UTTENTHAL & R. MARTINEZ-MURILLO. 1998. Distribution of catecholaminergic afferent fibres in the rat globus pallidus and their relations with cholinergic neurons. J. Chem. Neuroanat. **15:** 1–20.
69. HENDERSON, Z. 1997. The projection from the striatum to the nucleus basalis in the rat: an electron microscopic study. Neuroscience **78:** 943–955.
70. ZABORSZKY L., L. HEIMER, F. ECKENSTEIN & C. LERANTH. 1986. GABAergic input to cholinergic forebrain neurons: an ultrastructural study using retrograde tracing of HRP and double immunolabeling. J. Comp. Neurol. **250:** 282–295.
71. CHANG, H.T., G.R. PENNY & S.T. KITAI. 1987. Enkephalinergic-cholinergic interaction in the rat globus pallidus: a pre-embedding double-labeling immunocytochemistry study. Brain Res. **426:** 197–203.
72. MARTINEZ-MURILLO, R. BLASCO, I. ALAVREZ, F.J. VILLALBA, R. SOLANO, M.L. MONTERO-CABALLERO & J. RODRIGO. 1988. Distribution of enkephalin-immunoreactive nerve fibers and terminals in the region of the nucleus basalis magnocellularis of the rat: a light and electron microscopic study. J. Neurocytol. **17:** 361–376.
73. ZABORSZKY, L. 1989. Afferent connections of the forebrain cholinergic projection neurons with special reference to monoaminergic and peptidergic fibers. *In* Central Cholinergic Synaptic Transmission. M. Frotscher & U. Misgeld, Eds.: 12–22. Birkhauser. Basel.

74. BOLAM, J.P., C.A. INGHAM, P.N. IZZO, A.I. LEVEY, D.B. RYE, A.D. SMITH & B.H. WAINER. 1986. Substance P–containing terminals in synaptic contact with cholinergic neurons in the neostriatum and basal forebrain; a double immunocytochemical study in the rat. Brain Res. **397:** 279–289.
75. MARTINEZ-MURILLO, R., R.M. VILLALBA & J. RODRIGO. 1990. Immunocytochemical localization of cholinergic terminals in the region of the nucleus basalis magnocellularis of the rat: a correlated light and electron microscopic study. Neuroscience **36:** 361–376.
76. CSILLIK, B., P. RAKIC & E. KNYIHAR-CSILLIK. 1998. Peptidergic innervation and the nicotinic acetylcholine receptor in the primate basal nucleus. Eur. J. Neurosci. **10:** 573–585.
77. SMILEY, J.F. & M.-M. MESULAM. 1998. Cholinergic neurons of the nucleus basalis of Meynert receive cholinergic, catecholaminergic and GABAergic synapses: an electron microscopic investigation in the monkey. Neuroscience **88:** 241–254.
78. ZABORSZKY, L., R.P. GAYKEMA, D.J. SWANSON & W.E. CULLINAN. 1997. Cortical input to the basal forebrain. Neuroscience **79:** 1051–1078.
79. GAYKEMA, R.P.A. & L. ZABORSZKY. 1997. Parvalbumin-containing neurons in the basal forebrain receive direct input from the substantia nigra-ventral tegmental area. Brain Res. **478:** 375–381.
80. ZABORSZKY, L., W.E. CULLINAN & A. BRAUN. 1991. Afferents to basal forebrain cholinergic projection neurons: an update. *In* Basal Forebrain: Anatomy to Function. T. C. Napier, P.W. Kaliwas & I. Hanin, Eds.: 43–100. Plenum Press. New York.
81. ZABORSZKY, L. 1992. Synaptic organization of basal forebrain cholinergic projection neurons. *In* Neurotransmitter Interactions and Cognitive Functions. E.D. Levin, M. Decker & L. Butcher, Eds.: 27–65. Birkhauser. Boston.
82. BENZING, W.C., J.H. KORDOWER & E.J. MUFSON. 1993. Galanin immunoreactivity within the primate basal forebrain: evolutionary change between monkeys and apes. J. Comp. Neurol. **336:** 31–39.
83. BURGUNDER, J.M. & W.S. YOUNG III. 1989. Neurons with neurokinin B mRNA in the rat magnocellular basal nucleus: distribution, projection and colocalization studies. J. Chem. Neuroanat. **2:** 239–251.
84. DING, Y.Q., R. SHIGEMOTO, M. TAKADA, H. OHISHI, S. NAKANISHI & N. MIZUNO. 1996. Localization of the neuromedin K receptor (NK_3) in the central nervous system of the rat. J. Comp. Neurol. **364:** 290–310.
85. GEULA, C., C.R. SCHATZ & M.-M. MESULAM. 1993. Differential localization of NADH-diaphorase and calbindin-D_{28k} within the cholinergic neurons of the basal forebrain, striatum and brainstem in the rat, monkey, baboon and human. Neuroscience **54:** 461–476.
86. PLANAS, B., P.E. KOLB, M.A. RASKIND & M.A. MILLER. 1995. Vasopressin and galanin mRNAs coexist in the nucleus of the horizontal diagonal band: a novel site of vasopressin gene expression. J. Comp. Neurol. **361:** 48–56.
87. RANCE, N.E., W.S. YOUNG III & N.T. MCMULLEN. 1994. Topography of neurons expressing luteinizing hormone-releasing hormone gene transcripts in the human hypothalamus and basal forebrain. J. Comp. Neurol. **339:** 573–586.
88. SOBREVIELA, T., S. JAFFAR & E.J. MUFSON. 1998. Tyrosine kinase A, galanin and nitric oxide synthase within basal forebrain neurons in the rat. Neuroscience **87:** 447–461.
89. SUGAYA, K. & M. MCKINNEY. 1994. Nitric oxide synthase gene expression in cholinergic neurons in the rat brain examined by combined immunocytochemistry and *in situ* hybridization histochemistry. Mol. Brain Res. **23:** 111–125.
90. EVERITT, B.J. & T.W. ROBBINS. 1997. Central cholinergic systems and cognition. Annu. Rev. Psychol. **48:** 649–684.
91. DUNNETT, S.B., B.J. EVERITT & T.W. ROBBINS. 1991. The basal forebrain-cortical cholinergic system: interpreting the functional consequences of excitotoxic lesions. Trends Neurosci. **14:** 494–501.
92. VOYTKO, M.L., D.S. OLTON, R.T. RICHARDSON, L.K. GORMAN, J.R. TOBIN & D.L. PRICE. 1994. Basal forebrain lesions in monkeys disrupt attention but not learning and memory. J. Neurosci. **14:** 167–186.

93. PARASURAMAN, R., P.M. GREENWOOD, J.V. HAXBY & C.L. GRADY. 1992. Visuospatial attention in dementia of the Alzheimer type. Brain **115:** 711–733.
94. STOEHR, J.D., S.L. MOBLEY, D. ROICE, R. BROOKS, L.M. BAKER, R.G. WILEY & G.L. WENK. 1997. The effects of selective cholinergic basal forebrain lesions and aging upon expectancy in the rat. Neurobiol. Learn. Mem. **67:** 214–227.
95. TURCHI, J. & M. SARTER. 1997. Cortical acetylcholine and processing capacity: effects of cortical cholinergic deafferentation on crossmodal divided attention in rats. Cogn. Brain Res. **6:** 147–158.
96. PANG, K., M.J. WILLIAMS, H. EGETH & D.S. OLTON. 1993. Nucleus basalis magnocellularis and attention: effects of muscimol infusions. Behav. Neurosci. **107:** 1031–1038.
97. MUIR, J.L., B.J. EVERITT & T.W. ROBBINS. 1994. AMPA-induced excitotoxic lesions of the basal forebrain: a significant role for the cortical cholinergic system in attentional function. J. Neurosci. **14:** 2313–2326.
98. BAXTER, G.M & M. GALLAGHER. 1997. Cognitive effects of selective loss of basal forebrain cholinergic neurons: implications for cholinergic therapies of Alzheimer's disease. *In* Pharmacological Treatment of Alzheimer's Disease: Molecular and Neurobiological Foundations. J.E. Brioni & M.W. Decker, Eds.: 87–103. Wiley-Liss, Inc. New York.
99. PAUS, T., R.J. ZATORRE, N. HOFLE, Z. CARAMANOS, J. GOTMAN, M. PETRIDES & A.C. EVANS. 1997. Time-related changes in neural systems underlying attention and arousal during the performance of an auditory vigilance task. J. Cogn. Neurosci **9:** 392–408.
100. BAKIN, J.S. & N.W. WEINBERGER. 1996. Induction of a physiological memory in the cerebral cortex by stimulation of the nucleus basalis. Proc. Natl. Acad. Sci. USA **93:** 11219–11224.
101. EDELINE, J.-M., B. HARS *et al.* 1994. Transient and prolonged facilitation of tone-evoked responses induced by basal forebrain stimulations in the rat auditory cortex. Exp. Brain Res. **97:** 373–386.
102. METHERATE, R. & J.H. ASHE. 1991. Basal forebrain stimulation modifies auditory cortex responsiveness by an action at muscarinic receptors. Brain Res. **559:** 163–167.
103. TREMBLAY, N., R.A. WARREN & R.W. DYKES. 1990. Electrophysiological studies of acetylcholine and the role of the basal forebrain in the somatosensory cortex of the cat. II. Cortical neurons excited by somatic stimuli. J. Neurophysiol. **64:** 1212–1222.
104. MAALOUF, M., A.A. MIASNIKOV & R.W. DYKES. 1998. Blockade of cholinergic receptors in rat barrel cortex prevents long-term changes in the evoked potential during sensory preconditioning. J. Neurophysiol. **80:** 529–545.
105. SACHDEV, R.N.S., S.M. LU, R.G. WILEY & F.F. EBNER. 1998. Role of the basal forebrain cholinergic projection in somatosensory cortical plasticity. J. Neurophysiol. **79:** 3216–3228.
106. BASKERVILLE, K.A., J.B. SCHWEITZER & P. HERRON. 1997. Effects of cholinergic depletion on experience-dependent plasticity in the cortex of the rat. Neuroscience **80:** 1159–1169.
107. JULIANO, S.L., W. MA M.F. BEAR & D. ESLIN. 1990. Cholinergic manipulation alters stimulus-evoked metabolic activity in cat somatosensory cortex. J. Comp. Neurol. **297:** 106–120.
108. KILGARD, M.P. & M.M. MERZENICH. 1998. Cortical map reorganization enabled by nucleus basalis activity. Science **279:** 1714–1718.
109. MORRIS, J.S., K.J. FRISTON & R.J. DOLAN. 1998. Experience-dependent modulation of tonotopic neural responses in human auditor cortex. Proc. R. Soc. Lond. B. **265:** 649–657.
110. POSNER, M.I. & M.E. RAICHLE. 1997. Images of Mind. Scientific American Library. New York.
111. LABERGE, D. 1995. Attentional Processing. Harvard University Press. Cambridge, MA. p. 262.
112. HEILMAN, K.H., R.T. WATSON & E. VALENSTEIN. 1993. Neglect and related disorders. *In* Clinical Neuropsychology. K.M. Heilman & E. Valenstein, Eds.: 279–336. Oxford University Press. New York.

113. ROLAND, P.E. 1994. Brain Activation. Wiley-Liss. New York. p. 589.
114. MESULAM, M-M. 1990. Large-scale neurocognitive networks and distributed processing for attention, language, and memory. Ann. Neurol. **28:** 597–613.
115. DETARI, L., K. SEMBA & D.D. RASMUSSON. 1997. Responses of cortical EEG-related basal forebrain neurons to brainstem and sensory stimulation in urethane-anaesthetized rats. Eur. J. Neurosci. **9:** 1153–1161.
116. JONES, B.E. & M. MUHLETALER. 1999. Cholinergic and GABAergic neurons of the basal forebrain: Role in cortical activation. *In* Handbook of Behavioral State Control. R. Lydic & A.A. Baghdoyan, Eds.: 213–233. CRC Press. Boca Raton, FL.
117. STERIADE, M., E.G. JONES & D.A. MCCORMICK. 1997. Thalamus. Vol. 1. Organization and Function. Elsevier. Amsterdam. p. 959.
118. SARTER, M. & J.P. BRUNO. 1997. Cognitive functions of cortical acetylcholine: toward a unifying hypothesis. Brain Res. Rev. **23:** 28–46.
119. ASTON-JONES, G., J. RAJKOWSKI, P. KUBIAK & T. ALEXINSKY. 1994. Locus coeruleus neurons in monkey are selectively activated by attended cues in a vigilance task. J. Neurosci. **14:** 4467–4480.
120. FAIERS, A.A. & G.J. MOGENSON. 1976. Electrophysiological identification of neurons in locus coeruleus. Exp. Neurol. **53:** 254–266.
121. MAHO, C., B. HARS, J-M. EDELINE & E. HENNEVIN. 1995. Conditioned changes in the basal forebrain: relations with learning-induced cortical plasticity. Psychobiology **23:** 10–25.
122. WOODS, D.L. 1990. The physiological basis of selective attention: implications of event-related potential studies. *In* Event-Related Brain Potentials: Issues and Interdisciplinary Vantages. J. W. Rohrbaugh, R. Johnson & R. Parasuraman, Eds.: 178–209. Oxford University Press. New York.
123. VAN EDEN, C.G., V.A.F. LAMME & H.B.M. UYLINGS. 1991. Heterotopic cortical afferents to the medial prefrontal cortex in the rat. A combined retrograde and anterograde tracer study. Eur. J. Neurosci. **4:** 77–97.
124. FELLEMAN, D.J. & D.C. VAN ESSEN. 1991. Distributed hierarchical processing in the primate cerebral cortex. Cereb. Cortex **1:** 1–47.
125. PANDYA, D.N. & E.H. YETERIAN. 1985. Architecture and connections of cortical association areas. *In* Cerebral Cortex. Vol. 4. A. Peters & E.G. Jones, Eds.: 3–61. Plenum Press. New York.
126. ALEXANDER, G.E. & M.D. CRUTCHER. 1990. Functional architecture of basal ganglia circuits: neural substrates of parallel processing. Trends Neurosci. **13:** 266–271.
127. MOMIYAMA, T. & J.A. SIM. 1996. Modulation of inhibitory transmission by dopamine in rat basal forebrain nuclei: activation of presynaptic D1-like dopaminergic receptors. J. Neurosci. **16:** 7505–7512.
128. ALONSO, A. 1999. Intrinsic electroresponsiveness of basal forebrain cholinergic and non-cholinergic neurons. *In* Handbook of Behavioral State Control. R. Lydic & A.A. Baghdoyan, Eds.: 297–309. CRC Press. Boca Raton, FL.
129. PAXINOS, G. & C. WATSON. 1998. The Rat Brain in Stereotaxic Coordinates. Academic Press. San Diego, CA.
130. HENDERSON, Z. & N. MORRIS. 1997. Galanin-immunoreactive synaptic terminals on basal forebrain neurons in the rat. J. Comp. Neurol. **383:** 82–93.

Basal Forebrain Afferent Projections Modulating Cortical Acetylcholine, Attention, and Implications for Neuropsychiatric Disorders

MARTIN SARTER,[a] JOHN P. BRUNO, AND JANITA TURCHI

The Ohio State University, Department of Psychology and Neuroscience Program, Columbus, Ohio 43210, USA

ABSTRACT: Cortical acetylcholine (ACh) mediates the detection, selection, and processing of stimuli and associations, and the allocation of processing resources for these attentional functions. For example, loss of cortical cholinergic inputs impairs the performance of rats in tasks designed to assess sustained or divided attention. Intrabasalis infusions of benzodiazepine receptor (BZR) agonists block increases in cortical ACh efflux and impair attentional abilities. Studies on the regulation of cortical ACh efflux by nucleus accumbens (NAC) dopamine (DA) demonstrate that increases in cortical ACh efflux are attenuated by intra-accumbens administration of D1 and, more potently, D2 receptor antagonists. These and other data support the hypothesis that NAC DA, via GABAergic projections to the basal forebrain, controls the excitability of basal forebrain cholinergic neurons. As increases in NAC DA have been hypothesized to represent a major neuronal mediator of schizophrenia and the compulsive use of addictive drugs, the data predict that the abnormal regulation of cortical ACh release represents a crucial neuronal mechanism mediating the cognitive components of these psychopathological disorders.

LENNART HEIMER'S CALL FOR *PERESTROIKA* IN THE BASAL FOREBRAIN HEARD

... it is reasonable to suggest that pathological changes in the medial temporal lobe structures, which seem to be significantly involved in at least some patients with Alzheimer's disease and schizophrenia, can disturb the physiology or change the anatomical circuits in the ventral striatopallidal system, extended amygdala, and the magnocellular corticopetal forebrain system with subsequent disruption of a number of areas ranging from motor functions, basic drives like eating, drinking, and sexual behavior, to personality changes involving stress, mood, and higher cognitive functions .... (Heimer *et al.*[1])

Obviously, this view by Lennart Heimer and colleagues contrasts strikingly with the predominating perspectives in biological psychiatry and neurology that aim at the attribution of different behavioral abnormalities to different neuronal substrates. The idea that the same basal forebrain circuits contribute to the mediation of symptoms as discordant as dementia or psychosis runs counter to the widespread belief

---

[a]Address correspondence to Martin Sarter, The Ohio State University, Department of Psychology, 27 Townshend Hall, 1885 Neil Avenue, Columbus, OH 43210. Voice: 614-292-1751; fax: 614-688-4723; sarter.2@osu.edu

that, for example, the neuronal basis of the positive versus negative symptoms of schizophrenia can and should be dissociated.[2] Heimer *et al.* identify the "unfortunate dichotomy between neurology and psychiatry" (p. 150) as the basis of these opposed views, specifically the focus of neurology on disease defined by traditional anatomical concepts (such as "basal ganglia disorders" or "subcortical dementia") that contrasts with the clinical nosology-dominated conceptualizations in psychiatry (such as "hallucinations" or "anhedonia"). Heimer *et al.* hope that modern functional neuroanatomy opens the borders between the two areas (hence the term *perestroika*) and that such a process fosters the plausibility of theories suggesting that aberrations in major forebrain circuits contribute to the development of behaviorally diverse disorders.

The results of the research by Heimer and colleagues and their conceptual derivations[1,3,4] provide compelling support for their brand of *perestroika*. However, amending the traditional boundaries between neurological and psychiatric research approaches requires a crucial step that is implied in Heimer's discussion: the removal of clinical nosology as a research guiding principle. To the extent that research focuses on the identification of different neuronal substrates for clinical symptoms that are likely to interact (e.g., the various symptoms of schizophrenia), it will remain difficult to conceive how a particular region (such as the basal forebrain) could be involved in disorders that clinically (nosologically) are considered unrelated (e.g., schizophrenia vs. dementia). Moreover, clinical nosology is unlikely to be isomorphic with neuronal information processing; for example, "emotional flattening" is unlikely to represent a unit of neuronal information processing.[5,6] Therefore, to be successful, Heimer's *perestroika* first requires theories about fundamental processing dysfunctions that may give rise to potentially diverse clinical symptoms; second, research must be designed to determine the specific neuronal aberrations that mediate such fundamental cognitive dysfunctions and their escalating heterogeneous clinical manifestations.

As discussed elsewhere,[7–10] heterogeneous disorders, such as schizophrenia, dementia, generalized anxiety disorder, and compulsive addictive drug use are linked to alterations in basal forebrain neuronal mechanisms (as suggested by Heimer—see the above-written quote). This proposal is based theoretically on the importance of attentional dysfunctions in the development of these disorders and the crucial role of basal forebrain corticopetal cholinergic neurons in the mediation of such attentional functions. Pathological processes, and resultant abnormalities in the regulation of the excitability of cholinergic neurons, mediate impairments in early steps of the detection, selection, and processing of stimuli and associations, and consequently diminish the allocation of processing resources. In the long term, such attentional dysfunctions are thought to give rise to major cognitive disorders. A general, critical component of this hypothesis refers to the bidirectional nature of attentional impairments, ranging from the overprocessing of selected stimuli to the inability to detect and select relevant stimuli, that are mediated via pathological increases and decreases, respectively, in the excitability of cortical cholinergic inputs.

Below, we will first describe briefly the attentional functions of cortical cholinergic inputs, the available evidence concerning transsynaptic regulation of the excitability of this system, and the consequences for attentional functions. Finally, dysfunctions in the afferent regulation of cortical cholinergic inputs will be hypothesized to contribute essentially to the development of major psychiatric disorders. As will be evident, our combined behavioral and neurochemical research has been largely motivated by, and conceptually depends upon, the work by Lennart Heimer. We would certainly like to think of the results of our experiments as advancing his call for *perestroika*.

ATTENTIONAL FUNCTIONS OF CORTICAL ACETYLCHOLINE: EVIDENCE AND UNSETTLED QUESTIONS

The evidence in support of the rather specific functions of cortical ACh in the detection, selection, and processing of stimuli and associations has been extensively reviewed.[8,11] This evidence strongly indicates a close relationship between specific reductions in the density of cortical cholinergic inputs and the performance of animals in tasks designed to assess sustained, selective, and divided attention, whereas performance in more conventional tests of learning and memory is less consistent or not affected.[12–16] The overall significance of the behavioral evidence in support of the attentional functions of cortical ACh is limited by the dominance of experiments demonstrating impairments as a result of lesions. Although some initial studies have suggested relationships between demands on attentional functions and cortical ACh efflux, as well as ACh-mediated neuronal activity,[17,18] and have demonstrated that, conversely, changes in ACh efflux are not correlated with performance in basic operant schedules,[19] critical evidence concerning the mediation of attentional functions by the intact cholinergic system remains lacking. As discussed elsewhere, such studies entail exceptionally intricate experimental and technical concerns, as well as interpretative complexities.[20]

Two additional major issues concerning the determination of the attentional functions of cortical ACh require study. First, whereas the attentional impairments following manipulations of the cholinergic system are robust and persistent, and whereas these impairments are theoretically predicted to result in massive declines in learning and memory,[21] such attention-dependent consequences of manipulations of the cholinergic system have not been systematically studied; furthermore, experimental paradigms for that purpose may not be readily available. The extent to which attentional impairments due to the damage of cortical cholinergic inputs escalate into impairments in the acquisition of new information, and retrieval of complex associations, is of critical importance for discussing adequately the clinical significance of changes in this neuronal system (see below).

A second experimental approach, that may also require the development of new conceptual and experimental research avenues, concerns the interactions between the ascending "arousal"-mediating catecholaminergic and cholinergic afferents from the brain stem[22–25] and the mediation of attentional functions by the basal forebrain-cortical cholinergic projections. Despite efforts to reconceptualize the rather global construct, arousal,[26] its heuristic limitations may be blamed, in part, for the rather circumscribed understanding of the behavioral or cognitive functions that are mediated via interactions between brain stem inputs and cortical cholinergic afferents (see the discussion in ref. 27). Although it may seem obvious that these ascending systems generally modulate the excitability of basal forebrain efferent projections,[28] it will be important to specify the behavioral/cognitive functions that depend on such interactions and their exact implications for the ACh-mediated attentional functions. Concerning the ascending noradrenergic projections, data and concepts are accumulating and thus allow a brief illustration of the nature of such interactions. For example, performance in a sustained attention task does not depend on the integrity of ascending noradrenergic projections,[29] unless optimization of such performance is triggered by urgent (e.g., aversive) stimuli.[30] Presumably, the effects of such a stressor are mediated via sympathoexcitatory inputs to the locus caeruleus (LC)[31] whose noradrenergic projections stimulate basal forebrain cholinergic neurons via α_1 receptors,[32] thereby biasing cortical information processing toward such stimuli.[33] Data from studies on the effects of infusions of the α_1 agonist phenylephrine into the basal forebrain (Fadel, Sarter, and Bruno, unpublished results; see FIG. 1)

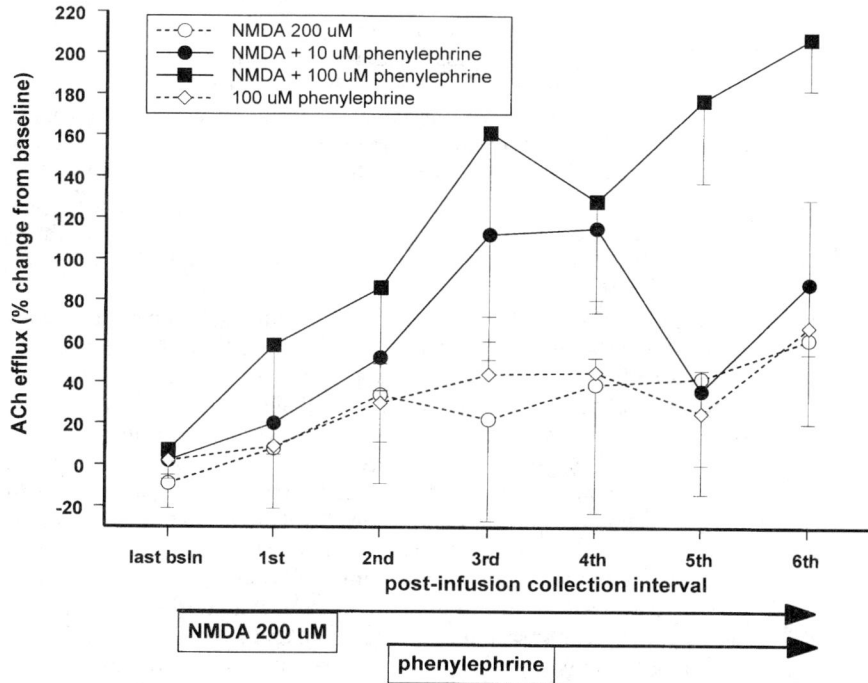

FIGURE 1. Interactions between the effects of infusions of NMDA and phenylephrine (PP) into the basal forebrain on cortical (medial prefrontal) acetylcholine (ACh) efflux. NMDA and phenylephrine were perfused through a probe situated in the area of the nucleus basalis/substantia innominata. The animals were extensively handled and adapted to the experimental environment and manipulations but remained otherwise unchallenged. Infusions of NMDA alone or PP alone did not affect cortical ACh efflux. The combined infusion of both compounds potently increased ACh efflux. These data suggest that noradrenergic stimulation via α_1 receptors suffices to remove the voltage-dependent channel block by Mg^{2+} and thus allows telencephalic glutamatergic inputs to this region to stimulate cholinergic neurons (Fadel, Sarter, and Bruno; unpublished results).

further illuminate the nature of the modulatory effects of noradrenaline in the basal forebrain. Although phenylephrine alone did not affect medial prefrontal ACh efflux, it interacted synergistically with the effects of infusions of NMDA to increase cortical ACh efflux (see FIG. 1). These data allow the speculation that increases in activity in noradrenergic afferents to basal forebrain cholinergic neurons permit the telencephalic glutamatergic afferents to stimulate cholinergic neurons via NMDA receptors. Other data from our laboratory demonstrate that, once cholinergic neurons are stimulated, blockade of α_1 receptors remains ineffective (Fadel, Sarter, and Bruno, unpublished results). In functional terms, these findings provide support for the hypothesis that activation of this brain stem afferent projection can contribute to the onset of processing via telencephalic–basal forebrain circuits (see also ref. 34), but that, thereafter, processing may no longer depend on noradrenergic activity.

In sum, the attentional functions mediated via cortical cholinergic inputs have been well characterized. Whereas the modulation of this neuronal system by brain stem ascending inputs and the functional implications have remained less clear, data, such as those summarized above, will result in more specific and testable hypotheses about the nature of the activating influences mediated via cholinergic and catecholaminergic inputs from brain stem areas. As will be discussed next, the role of telencephalic afferents to basal forebrain cholinergic neurons has been more extensively studied in recent years, and the information from this research bears directly on major models about the neuronal basis of neuropsychiatric disorders.

GABAergic MODULATION OF ACTIVATED CORTICAL ACH EFFLUX

Basal forebrain neurons, including the cholinergic neurons, receive direct contacts from GABAergic afferents.[35,36] Although it is believed that the majority of these GABAergic afferents arise in the nucleus accumbens (NAC),[37] the extent to which basal forebrain GABAergic interneurons or collaterals of GABAergic corticopetal neurons contribute to this innervation remains unsettled. Our studies on the modulation of cortical ACh efflux via basal forebrain GABAergic inputs focused on the effects of benzodiazepine receptor (BZR) agonists and inverse agonists to yield experimental findings that depend on endogenously released GABA. A series of studies (for review, see ref. 38) demonstrated that, although basal cortical ACh efflux is not affected by the systemic or intrabasalis administration of BZR ligands, activated ACh efflux (produced by the presentation of a conditioned stimulus for reward[39]) is attenuated by administration of an agonist and augmented by BZR inverse agonists. These findings suggest that the effects of BZR ligands can serve to probe the functions of cortical ACh, as effects would only be expected in behavioral situations that activate this system (it is important to reiterate that this statement does not generalize to the effects of direct $GABA_A$-receptor agonists or antagonists[38]). Indeed, similar to the effects of cholinergic lesions,[15,16] infusions of a BZR agonist into the basal forebrain were found to impair the performance of rats tested in a sustained-attention[40] and a divided-attention task.[41] However, infusions of such a compound in animals, performing a conditional discrimination task known to not require the integrity of the cholinergic system,[19,42] produced no effects,[43] thus supporting the usefulness of BZR ligands for assessing the functions of cholinergic projections of the basal forebrain.

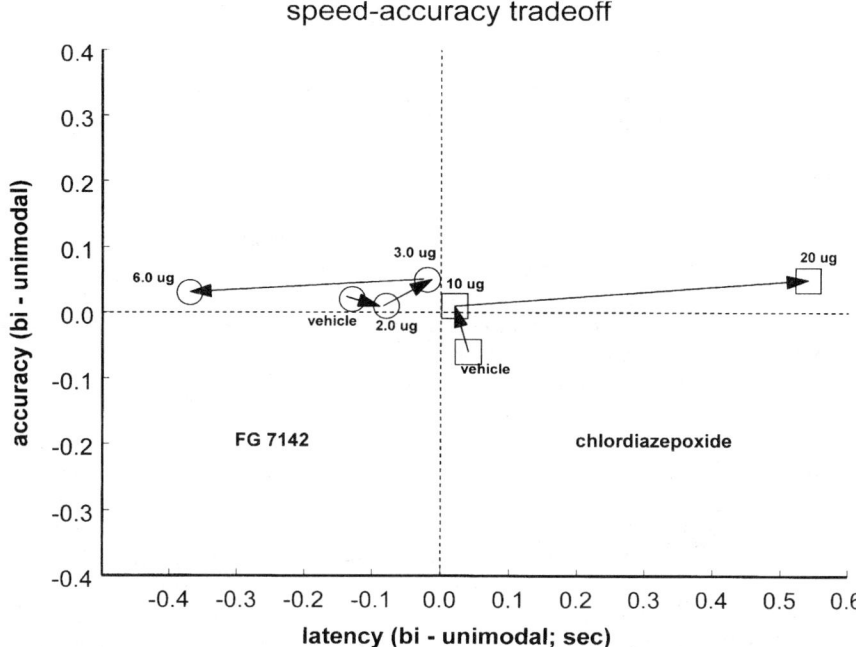

FIGURE 2. Effects of infusions of the BZR agonist, chlordiazepoxide (CDP: 0, 10, 20 μg/0.5 μL/hemisphere), or of the BZR partial-inverse agonist, FG 7142 (FG: 0, 2, 3, 6 μg/ 0.5 μL/hemisphere; FG was complexed with cyclodextrin, as described in ref. 49), into the basal forebrain of intact rats performing a cross-modal divided-attention task (L.A.H. Miner, J. Hanje & M. Sarter, unpublished results; for details about the task, see refs. 16 and 41). The ordinate of the FIGURE depicts the difference between the response latencies between unimodal blocks of trials and the bimodal (random order of visual and auditory conditioned stimuli) block of trials. The abscissa depicts the differences between unimodal and bimodal response accuracy values (expressed in angular transformed percent data). In absolute terms, response accuracy was high in both uni- and bimodal blocks of trials (>80% correct responses) and remained stable across all treatment conditions. Infusions of the highest dose of CDP selectively increased the response latencies in the bimodal component of the task while not affecting response accuracy, indicating an increase in speed–accuracy trade-off. Conversely, the highest dose of FG shortened the response latencies selectively in the bimodal block of trials. The selectivity of the effects of the BZR ligands is speculated to be due to their bidirectional modulation of activated cortical ACh release, as performance in unimodal blocks of trials does not depend on the integrity of cortical cholinergic inputs (see text).

The attentional effects of infusions of BZR inverse agonists into the basal forebrain are of particular importance for the discussion of clinical relevance (see below). The selective increase in the number of false alarms observed following infusions of the BZR inverse agonist β-CCM into the basal forebrain[40] was interpreted as reflecting the pathological overprocessing of the stimulus situation due to drug-induced augmentation of activity in cortical cholinergic inputs; however, the precise extent to which these effects were mediated by this mechanism remains unclear. It is important to note that in addition to the possibly more obvious attentional impairments produced by loss of inhibition of corticopetal cholinergic neurons, abnormal over(re)activity of these neurons is also predicted to impair attentional functions, albeit yielding a very different type of impairment characterized by hyperattentional performance.

Whereas infusions of BZR inverse agonists into the basal forebrain produce a hyperattentional impairment in rats performing a sustained-attention task, infusions of the BZR partial inverse agonist FG 7142 (FG) resulted in a decrease in the speed-accuracy trade-off in rats performing a cross-modal divided-attention task (FIG. 2). The effects of FG suggested a facilitation of performance, as the drug exclusively facilitated response latencies in the bimodal condition of the task (FIG. 2), thus excluding main effects on the motor components of the response. Such exclusive effects of BZR ligands on the bimodal part of the task were expected as the task's unimodal components consist of simple conditional visual and auditory discriminations; as stressed above, simple conditional discriminations do not depend on cortical ACh, and the effects of BZR ligands are hypothesized to be due to their effects on activated ACh efflux.

The BZR inverse agonist–induced impairment in sustained attention and the facilitation of divided-attention performance may not necessarily represent conflicting results. Although one would normally expect that hypervigilant impairments entail costs in terms of processing capacity, it is important to note that the cross-modal divided-attention task does not tax stimulus detection and selection processes but rather exclusively taxes the capacity available to process competing cross-modal propositional rules. Thus, to the extent these findings can be attributed to disinhibitory effects on basal forebrain cholinergic neurons,[16,38] they suggest that disinhibition of corticopetal cholinergic projections detrimentally affects the early stages of stimulus detection and discrimination, while processing capacity allocation benefits from a disinhibited cholinergic system. Such attentional effects of infusions of BZR inverse agonists into the basal forebrain may be relevant for predicting the possibility that, in humans, the systemic administration of weak or selective[44] BZR inverse agonists[45] or, to a more limited extent,[44] of more traditional cholinomimetics, such as cholinesterase inhibitors,[46,47] may improve aspects of processing efficiency. However, it is more likely that the cortical cholinergic hyperactivity-associated impairments in the ability to select appropriate stimuli and associations for processing will escalate into major cognitive impairments, as an overprocessing of irrelevant stimuli and associations in the long term limits the influence of previous experience to guide attentional processing[48] (see below).

DOPAMINERGIC MODULATION OF CORTICAL ACH VIA ACCUMBENS EFFERENTS TO THE BASAL FOREBRAIN

As already mentioned above, the majority of GABAergic projections to the basal forebrain originate in the nucleus accumbens, and most of the cholinergic neurons in this area receive accumbens input.[35–37,50,51] The possible contributions of basal forebrain intrinsic GABAergic neurons and of GABAergic afferents from the amygdala[52] to the direct GABA-cholinergic contacts in the basal forebrain are unclear. As basal forebrain GABAergic mechanisms control the excitability of corticopetal cholinergic neurons (see above), the question about the ability of the NAC, via the GABAergic projections to the basal forebrain, to modulate cortical ACh arises (this discussion ignores the likely existence of parallel peptidergic and other projections from the NAC to the basal forebrain). Several lines of evidence support the hypothesis that increases in NAC dopamine receptor stimulation decreases the GABAergic output to the basal forebrain, thereby disinhibiting cortical ACh efflux. For example, Bourdelais and Kalivas[53,54] showed that systemic administration of amphetamine and apomorphine decreases GABA release in the basal forebrain, and that 6-OHDA lesions of the NAC produced more robust effects of apomorphine. The latter result was considered due to supersensitive dopamine (DA) receptors in the deafferented NAC. Furthermore, infusions of the DA receptor antagonists, SCH 23390 and raclopride, into the NAC increased basal forebrain GABA release,[55] thus supporting the inhibitory control of the GABAergic projection to the basal forebrain by NAC DA receptors. Numerous behavioral experiments support the functional significance of the NAC DA–basal forebrain GABAergic interaction. For instance, Swerdlow et al.[56] demonstrated that the effects of infusions of DA into the NAC on the acoustic startle response is blocked by infusions of a $GABA_A$ agonist into the basal forebrain (see also refs. 57 and 58).

Although earlier studies noticed the close correlations between increases in NAC DA and cortical ACh release in response to aversive events,[59] evidence directly supporting the modulation of cortical ACh efflux by NAC DA receptors modulating cortical ACh is more scarce. The potent increase in cortical ACh efflux following the systemic administration of amphetamine[60] was attributed to the effects of amphetamine on the forebrain, including NAC DA release, as 6-OHDA lesions attenuated the increases in ACh efflux and as local cortical dopaminergic mechanisms do not seem to contribute to the effects of amphetamine on cortical ACh efflux.[61] However, recent data by Darracq et al.,[62] as well as from our own laboratory (presented by M. Arnold et al. at this meeting), strongly indicate that the effects of systemic amphetamine on NAC efferent networks, including cortical ACh efflux and associated functions, cannot be fully explained by the effects of amphetamine on NAC DA efflux. Our data indicate that intra-accumbens infusions of amphetamine (250 μM) result in up to a 15-fold higher DA release in the NAC than systemic amphetamine (2 mg/kg), whereas the systemic dose increases cortical ACh efflux 2-fold over the increase resulting from the intra-accumbens administration (Arnold, Nelson, Sarter & Bruno, unpublished results). This dissociation may underlie the differential effects of intra-accumbens and systemic amphetamine on latent inhibition,[63] particularly if it can be shown that NAC DA release-sensitizing pretreatment with systemic amphetamine[64] diminishes the dissociations summarized above.

More direct evidence supporting the role of NAC DA receptors in the modulation of cortical ACh was generated by a study that assessed the effects of intra-accumbens infusions of D_1 and D_2 receptor antagonists on the increases in cortical ACh produced by systemic administration of the BZR partial inverse agonist FG 7142 (FG).[65,66] Intra-accumbens infusions of haloperidol and the D_2 antagonist, sulpiride, potently attenuated the FG-induced increases in cortical ACh efflux, whereas infusions of the D_1-antagonist, SCH 23390, into the NAC remained less effective. Furthermore, intracortical infusions of these DA receptor antagonists did not affect cortical ACh efflux. Although the interpretation of these data are complicated by the multiple effects of FG, including increases in mesolimbic DA release,[67,68] they document the potent role of NAC DA receptors in the regulation of increases in cortical ACh efflux under certain conditions. Moreover, the potent effects of sulpiride and haloperidol suggest that the effects of FG may prove interesting as a model of the aberrations in mesolimbic-efferent networks in schizophrenia[68] (see below), particularly as these data contrast with the relatively low potency of systemically administered D_2 receptor antagonists in attenuating the increases in ACh efflux that result from systemic administrations of amphetamine.[60] Future studies need to determine whether stimulation of D_1 and/or D_2 receptors in the NAC disinhibit basal forebrain cholinergic corticopetal projections and, if so, whether this effect is mediated via reductions in the GABAergic inhibition of these neurons.

ABERRATIONS IN THE TRANSSYNAPTIC MODULATION OF CORTICAL ACH EFFLUX AS CRUCIAL NEURONAL MECHANISMS GIVING RISE TO MAJOR NEUROPSYCHIATRIC DISORDERS

The available evidence permits the following two general hypotheses: (1) cortical cholinergic inputs are critically involved in the mediation of the ability to detect, select, and process stimuli and associations, and (2) the excitability of basal forebrain corticopetal cholinergic projections is modulated by NAC DA receptors, predominantly via the GABAergic efferent projections to the basal forebrain.

The clinical implications of these hypotheses are straightforward and profound (see ref. 9 for a more detailed discussion of the clinical relevance of these hypotheses). First, to the extent that the manifestation of schizophrenic symptoms is mediated, neuronally, via increases in mesolimbic dopaminergic transmission (e.g., see ref. 69), the available data predict that disinhibition of corticopetal cholinergic neurons represents an associated efferent consequence. Functionally, it is hypothesized that hyperattentional impairments may be considered a central cognitive component in the development and escalation of the cognitive dysfunctions that eventually manifest as schizophrenic symptoms (for more details, see refs. 7 and 9).

The notion that similar considerations apply to the investigation of the neuronal and cognitive bases of compulsive addictive drug use fosters interesting discussion about the possible relationships between the cognitive dysfunctions mediating the manifestation of schizophrenic symptoms and repeated addictive drug seeking and consuming behavior. The sensitization of mesolimbic dopaminergic systems has been considered central to the manifestation of addictive behavior,[70,71] and sensitization-induced biases in the processing of stimuli[72] associated with repeated addictive drug use has been proposed to play a critical role in the manifestation of compulsive addictive drug–seeking and drug-taking behavior[73] (see FIG. 3). Again, disinhibition of cortical cholinergic inputs are predicted to be associated with sensitized mesolimbic dopaminergic transmission, and the biased attentional processing of drug-related stimuli is hypothesized to be primarily mediated via those over(re)active inputs.[9] Similar hypotheses have been developed concerning other neuropsychiatric disorders characterized by a strong bias toward the processing of selected groups of stimuli and contexts, such as generalized anxiety disorder and panic attacks.[33]

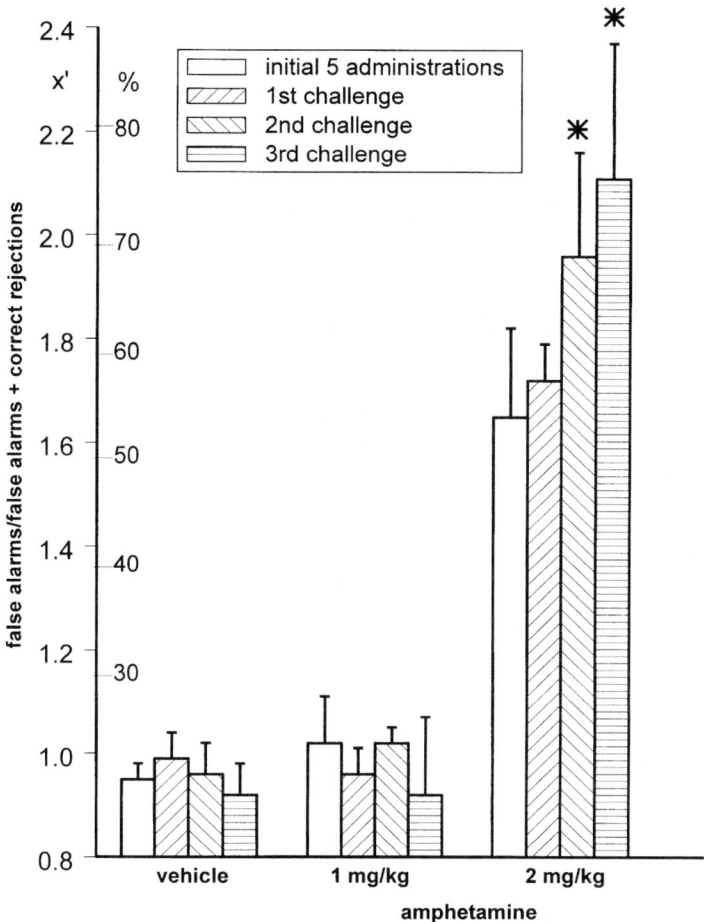

FIGURE 3. Effects of repeated systemic administration of amphetamine on sustained attention performance in rats (adapted from Deller & Sarter[72]). This experiment aimed at the development of a model of the hyperattentional dysfunctions that result from psychostimulant-induced sensitization[73] and that are hypothesized to be mediated via disinhibition of cortical cholinergic inputs consequent to sensitization-induced increases in NAC dopaminergic transmission (see text). Rats were trained in a task that required the detection of signals and the correct rejection of blanks (for details, see ref. 15). Amphetamine was initially administered every other day for a total of 5 days (or sessions). Subsequent "challenge" doses were administered 7, 13, and 19 days following the initial "sensitization" treatment. FIGURE 3 depicts the effects on the relative number of false alarms, that is, "claims for hits while no signals were presented." The left group of bars indicates that, in vehicle-treated animals, the false-alarm rate remained under 30%. Following the administration of 2 mg/kg, the relative number of false alarms increased dramatically toward the end of the initial treatment period (open bars depict the average number of false alarms following the five initial administrations). The magnitude of this effect further increased significantly (stars) after the second and third challenge administrations, yielding over 70% false alarms. It is speculated that this "overprocessing" of the stimulus situation may model aspects of the attentional dysfunctions mediated via disinhibition of cortical cholinergic inputs.

It should not come as a surprise that the most rostral cortical input systems, innervated by major telencephalic, limbic, and paralimbic networks, are involved in the manifestation of major symptoms of heterogeneous neuropsychiatric disorders. It is possible that aberrations in the afferent networks of basal forebrain cholinergic neurons unavoidably affect the excitability of cortical cholinergic inputs. Furthermore, cortical cholinergic inputs mediate the early steps of information processing that, if functioning improperly over long periods of time, evolve into major cognitive disorders. It is important to note that hypoactivity of cortical cholinergic inputs, including loss and degeneration of cholinergic neurons, mediates impairments in attentional functions that are fundamentally different than the hyperattentional impairments mediated via disinhibited cortical cholinergic inputs[7–9] (see also the important discussion about the misleading interpretation of the effects of acutely and systemically administered cholinergic drugs in schizophrenic patients in refs. 8 and 9).

In conclusion, accumulating evidence details the afferent networks of the basal forebrain, the transsynaptic regulation of the excitability of corticopetal cholinergic neurons arising from that area, and the involvement of these circuits in the manifestation of major neuropsychiatric disorders. Moreover, the neuropharmacological and cognitive elements underlying the assumption that seemingly heterogeneous symptoms may be mediated via diverse aberrations in the transsynaptic interactions in these circuits have become increasingly apparent in recent years. Lennart Heimer's call for *perestroika* in the basal forebrain[1] continues to echo loud and clear.

ACKNOWLEDGMENTS

The authors' research was supported in part by PHS Grants NS32938, MH57436, and NS37026, and a Research Scientist Development Award to M.S. (MH01072).

REFERENCES

1. HEIMER, L., J. DE OLMOS, G.F. ALHEID & L. ZABORSZKY. 1991. "Perestroika" in the basal forebrain: opening the border between neurology and psychiatry. Prog. Brain Res. **87:** 109–165.
2. TANDON, R. & J.F. GREDEN. 1989. Cholinergic hyperactivity and negative schizophrenic symptoms. Arch. Gen. Psychiatry **46:** 745–753.
3. ALHEID, G.F. & L. HEIMER. 1988. New perspectives in basal forebrain organization of special relevance for neuropsychiatric disorders: the striatopallidal, amygdaloid, and corticopetal components of substantia innominata. Neuroscience **27:** 1–39.
4. ALHEID, G.F. & L. HEIMER. 1996. Theories of basal forebrain organization and the "emotional motor system." Prog. Brain Res. **107:** 461–484.
5. SARTER, M. & J.P. BRUNO. 1997. Dopamine's role. Science **278:** 1549–1550.
6. SARTER, M., G.G. BERNTSON & J.T. CACIOPPO. 1996. Brain imaging and cognitive neuroscience: toward strong inference in attributing function to structure. Am. Psychol. **51:** 13–21.
7. SARTER, M. 1994. Neuronal mechanisms of the attentional dysfunctions in senile dementia and schizophrenia: two sides of the same coin? Psychopharmacology **114:** 539–550.
8. SARTER, M. & J.P. BRUNO. 1997. Cognitive functions of cortical acetylcholine: toward a unifying hypothesis. Brain Res. Rev. **23:** 28–46.

9. SARTER, M. & J.P. BRUNO. 1999. Abnormal regulation of corticopetal cholinergic neurons and impaired information processing in neuropsychiatric disorders. Trends Neurosci. **22:** 67–74.
10. SARTER, M. & J.P. BRUNO. 1998. Cortical acetylcholine, reality distortion, schizophrenia and Lewy body dementia: too much or too little acetylcholine? Brain Cogn. **38:** 297–316.
11. EVERITT, B.J. & T.W. ROBBINS. 1997. Central cholinergic systems and cognition. Annu. Rev. Psychol. **48:** 649–684.
12. TORRES, E.M., T.A. PERRY, A. BLOKLAND, S. WILKINSON, R.G. WILEY, D.A. LAPPIS & S.B. DUNNETT. 1994. Behavioral, histochemical and biochemical consequences of selective immunolesions in discrete regions of the basal forebrain cholinergic system. Neuroscience **63:** 95–122.
13. MUIR, J.L., B.J. EVERITT & T.W. ROBBINS. 1994. AMPA-induced excitotoxic lesions of the basal forebrain: a significant role for the cortical cholinergic system in attentional function. J. Neurosci. **14:** 2313–2326.
14. CHIBA, A.A., D.J. BUCCI, P.C. HOLLAND & M. GALLAGHER. 1995. Basal forebrain cholinergic lesions disrupt increments but not decrements in conditioned stimulus processing. J. Neurosci. **15:** 7315–7322.
15. MCGAUGHY, J., T. KAISER & M. SARTER. 1996. Behavioral vigilance following infusions of 192 IgG-saporin into the basal forebrain: selectivity of the behavioral impairment and relation to cortical AChE-positive fiber density. Behav. Neurosci. **110:** 247–265.
16. TURCHI, J. & M. SARTER. 1997. Cortical acetylcholine and processing capacity: effects of cortical cholinergic deafferentation on crossmodal divided attention in rats. Cogn. Brain Res. **6:** 147–158.
17. SARTER, M., J.P. BRUNO, B. GIVENS, H. MOORE, J. MCGAUGHY & K. MCMAHON. 1996. Neuronal mechanisms mediating drug-induced cognition enhancement: cognitive activity as a necessary intervening variable. Cogn. Brain Res. **3:** 329–343.
18. GILL, T.M., D.M. KENT, M. SARTER & B. GIVENS. 1997. Behavioral correlates of neural activity recorded from the rodent medial prefrontal cortex during sustained visual attention. Soc. Neurosci. Abstr. **23:** 716.10.
19. HIMMELHEBER, A.M., M. SARTER & J.P. BRUNO. 1997. Operant performance and cortical acetylcholine release: role of response rate, reward density, and non-contingent stimuli. Cogn. Brain Res. **6:** 23–36.
20. BRUNO, J.P., M. SARTER, M. ARNOLD & A.M. HIMMELHEBER. 1999. In vivo neurochemical correlates of cognitive processes: methodological and conceptual challenges. Rev. Neurosci. **10:** 25–48.
21. COWAN, N. 1995. Attention and memory. An integrated framework. Oxford University Press. New York.
22. SEMBA, K., P.B. RAINER, E.G. MCGEER & H.C. FIBIGER. 1989. Brainstem afferents to the magnocellular basal forebrain studies by axonal transport, immunohistochemistry, and electrophysiology in the rat. J. Comp. Neurol. **267:** 433–453.
23. ZABORSZKY, L., W.E. CULLINAN & V.N. LUINE. 1993. Catecholaminergic-cholinergic interaction in the basal forebrain. Prog. Brain Res. **98:** 31–49.
24. JONES, B.E. & A.C. CUELLO. 1989. Afferents to the basal forebrain cholinergic cell area from pontomesencephalic-catecholamine, serotonin, and acetylcholine-neurons. Neuroscience **31:** 37–61.
25. CONSOLO, S., R. BERTORELLI, G.L. FORLONI & L.L. BUTCHER. 1990. Cholinergic neurons of the pontomesencephalic tegmentum release acetylcholine in the basal nuclear complex of freely moving rats. Neuroscience **37:** 717–723.
26. STERIADE, M. & G. BUZSAKI. 1990. Parallel activation of thalamic and cortical neurons by brainstem and basal forebrain cholinergic systems. In Brain Cholinergic Systems. M. Steriade & D. Biesold, Eds.: 3–62. Oxford University Press. Oxford.
27. ROBBINS, T.W. & B.J. EVERITT. 1995. Arousal systems and attention. In The Cognitive Neurosciences. M. Gazzaniga, Ed.: 703–720. MIT Press. Cambridge, MA.
28. MESULAM, M-M. 1995. Cholinergic pathways and the ascending reticular activating system of the human brain. Ann. N.Y. Acad. Sci. **757:** 169–179.
29. MCGAUGHY, J., M. SANDSTROM, S. RULAND, J.P. BRUNO & M. SARTER. 1997. Lack of

effects of lesions of the dorsal noradrenergic bundle on behavioral vigilance. Behav. Neurosci. **111:** 646–652.
30. CARLI, M., T.W. ROBBINS, J.L. EVENDEN & B.J. EVERITT. 1983. Effects of lesions of ascending noradrenergic neurones on performance of a 5-choice serial reaction task in rats: implications for theories of dorsal noradrenergic bundle function based on selective attention and arousal. Behav. Brain Res. **9:** 361–380.
31. ASTON-JONES, G., J. RAJKWOSKI, P. KUBIAK, R.J. VALENTINO & M.T. SHIPLEY. 1996. Role of the locus coeruleus in emotional activation. Prog. Brain Res. **107:** 379–402.
32. FORT, P., A. KHATEB, A. PEGNA, M. MÜHLETHALER & B.E. JONES. 1995. Noradrenergic modulation of cholinergic nucleus basalis neurons demonstrated by in vitro pharmacological and immunohistochemical evidence in the guinea pig brain. Eur. J. Neurosci. **7:** 1502–1511.
33. BERNTSON, G.G., M. SARTER & J.T. CACIOPPO. 1998. Anxiety and cardiovascular reactivity: the basal forebrain cholinergic system. Behav. Brain Res. **94:** 225–248.
34. CAPE, E.G. & B.E. JONES. 1998. Differential modulation of high frequency γ-electroencephalogram activity and sleep-wake state by noradrenaline and serotonin microinjections into the region of cholinergic basalis neurons. J. Neurosci. **18:** 2653–2666.
35. ZABORSZKY, L., L. HEIMER, F. ECKENSTEIN & C. LERANTH. 1986. GABAergic input to cholinergic forebrain neurons: an ultrastructural study using retrograde tracing of HRP and double immunolabeling. J. Comp. Neurol. **250:** 282–295.
36. INGHAM, C.A., J.P. BOLAM & A.D. SMITH. 1988. GABA-immunoreactive synaptic boutons in the rat basal forebrain: comparison of neurons that project to the neocortex with pallidosubthalamic neurons. J. Comp. Neurol. **273:** 263–282
37. MOGENSON, G.J., L.W. SWANSON & M. WU. 1983. Neural projections from nucleus accumbens to globus pallidus, substantia innominata, and lateral preoptic-lateral hypothalamic area: an anatomical and electrophysiological investigation in the rat. J. Neurosci. **3:** 189–202.
38. SARTER, M. & J.P. BRUNO. 1994. Cognitive functions of cortical ACh [acetylcholine]: lessons from studies on the trans-synaptic modulation of activated efflux. Trends Neurosci. **17:** 217–221.
39. INGLIS, F.M., J.C. DAY & H.C. FIBIGER. 1994. Enhanced acetylcholine release in hippocampus and cortex during the anticipation and consumption of a palatable meal. Neuroscience **62:** 1049–1056.
40. HOLLEY, L.A., J. TURCHI, C. APPLE & M. SARTER. 1995. Dissociation between the attentional effects of infusions of a benzodiazepine receptor agonist and an inverse agonist into the basal forebrain. Psychopharmacology **120:** 99–108.
41. McGAUGHY, J., J. TURCHI & M. SARTER. 1994. Crossmodal divided attention in rats: effects of chlordiazepoxide and scopolamine. Psychopharmacology **115:** 213–220.
42. EVENDEN, J.L., H.M. MARSTON, G.H. JONES, V. GIARDINI, L. LENARD, B.J. EVERITT & T.W. ROBBINS. 1989. Effects of excitotoxic lesions of the substantia innominata, ventral and dorsal globus pallidus on visual discrimination acquisition, performance and reversal in the rat. Behav. Brain Res. **32:** 129–149.
43. DUDCHENKO, P. & M. SARTER. 1992. Failure of chlordiazepoxide to reproduce the behavioral effects of muscimol administered into the basal forebrain. Behav Brain Res. **47:** 202–205.
44. SARTER, M., J.P. BRUNO & P. DUDCHENKO. 1990. Activating the damaged basal forebrain cholinergic system: tonic stimulation versus signal amplification. Psychopharmacology **101:** 1–17.
45. DUKA, T., V. EDELMANN, B. SCHÜTT & R. DOROW. 1988. β-carbolines as tools in memory research. Human data with the β-carboline ZK 93426. In Benzodiazepine Receptor Ligands, Memory and Information Processing. I. Hindmarch, H. Ott & T. Roth, Eds.: 246–251. Springer. New York.
46. FURLEY, M.L., P. PETRINI, J.V. HAXBY, G.E. ALEXANDER, H.C. LEE, J. VAN METER, C.L. GRADY, U. SHETTY, S.I. RAPOPORT, M.B. SCHAPIRO & U. FREO. 1997. Cholinergic stimulation alters performance and task-specific regional cerebral blood flow during working memory. Proc. Natl. Acad. Sci. USA **94:** 6512–6516.
47. SAHAKIAN, B.J., A.M. OWEN, N.J. MORANT, S.E. EAGGER, S. BODDINGTON, L. CRAY-

TON, H.A. CROCKFORD, M. CROOKS, K. HILL & R. LEVY. 1993. Further analysis of the cognitive effects of tetrahydroaminoacridine (THA) in Alzheimer's disease: assessment of attentional and mnemonic function using CANTAB. Psychopharmacology **110:** 395–401.
48. GRAY, J.A. 1998. Integrating schizophrenia. Schizophr. Bull. **24:** 249–266.
49. SMITH, C.G., R.J. BENINGER, P.E. MALLET, K. JHAMANDAS & R. BOEGMAN. 1994. Basal forebrain injections of the benzodiazepine partial inverse agonist F 7142 enhance memory of rats in the double Y-maze. Brain Res. **666:** 61–67.
50. ZABORSZKY, L., W.E. CULLINAN & A. BRAUN. 1991. Afferents to basal forebrain cholinergic projection neurons: an update. *In* The Basal Forebrain. Anatomy to Function. T.C. Napier, P.W. Kalivas & I. Hanin, Eds.: 43–100. Plenum Press. New York.
51. ZABORSZKY, L. & W.E. CULLINAN. 1992. Projections from the nucleus accumbens to cholinergic neurons of the ventral pallidum: a correlated light and electron microscopic double-immunolabeling study in the rat. Brain Res. **570:** 92–101.
52. PARÉ, D. & Y. SMITH. 1994. GABAergic projections from the intercalated cell masses of the amygdala to the basal forebrain in cats. J. Comp. Neurol. **344:** 33–49.
53. BOURDELAIS, A. & P. KALIVAS. 1990. Amphetamine lowers extracellular GABA concentrations in the ventral pallidum. Brain Res. **516:** 132–136.
54. BOURDELAIS, A. & P. KALIVAS. 1992. Apomorphine decreases extracellular GABA in the ventral pallidum of rats with 6-OHDA lesions in the nucleus accumbens. Brain Res. **577:** 306–311.
55. FERRÉ, S., W.T. CONNOR, P. SNAPRUD, U. UNGERSTEDT & K. FUXE. 1994. Antagonistic interaction between adenosine A_{2A} receptors and dopamine D_2 receptors in the ventral striopallidal system. Implications for the treatment of schizophrenia. Neuroscience **63:** 765–773.
56. SWERDLOW, N.R., D.L. BRAFF & M.A. GEYER. 1990. GABAergic projection from the nucleus accumbens to ventral pallidum mediates dopamine-induced sensorimotor gating deficits of acoustic startle in rats. Brain Res. **532:** 146–150.
57. HOOKS, M.S. & P.W. KALIVAS. 1995. The role of mesoaccumbens-pallidal circuitry in novelty-induced behavioral activation. Neuroscience **64:** 587–597.
58. SHREVE, P.E. & N.J. URETSKY. 1988. Effect of GABAergic transmission in the subpallidal region on the hypermotility response to the administration of excitatory amino acids and picrotoxin into the nucleus accumbens. Neuropharmacology **12:** 1271–1277.
59. IMPERATO, A., S. PUGLISI-ALLEGRA, M.G. SCROCCO, P. CASOLINI, S. BACCHI & L. ANGELUCCI. 1992. Cortical and limbic dopamine and acetylcholine release as neurochemical correlates of emotional arousal in both aversive and non-aversive environmental changes. Neurochem. Int. **20:** 265S–270S.
60. DAY, J. & H.C. FIBIGER. 1992. Dopaminergic regulation of cortical acetylcholine release. Synapse **12:** 281–286.
61. DAY, J., C.S. THAM & H.C. FIBIGER. 1994. Dopamine depletion attenuates amphetamine- induced increases in cortical ACh release. Eur. J. Pharmacol. **263:** 285–292.
62. DARRACQ, L., G. BLANC, J. GLOWINKSI & J.P. TASSIN. 1998. Importance of the noradrenaline-dopamine coupling in the locomotor activating effects of D-amphetamine. J. Neurosci. **18:** 2729–2739.
63. KILLCROSS, A.S. & T.W. ROBBINS. 1993. Differential effects of intra-accumbens and systemic amphetamine on latent inhibition using an on-baseline, within-subject conditioned suppression paradigm. Psychopharmacology **110:** 479–489.
64. ROBINSON, R.E. & J.B. BECKER. 1986. Enduring changes in brain and behavior produced by chronic amphetamine administration: a review and evaluation of animal models of amphetamine psychosis. Brain Res. Rev. **11:** 157–198.
65. MOORE, H., S. STUCKMAN, M. SARTER & J.P. BRUNO. 1995. Stimulation of cortical acetylcholine efflux by FG 7142 measured with repeated microdialysis sampling. Synapse **21:** 324–331.
66. MOORE, H., J. FADEL, M. SARTER & J.P. BRUNO. 1999. Role of accumbens and cortical dopamine receptors in the regulation of cortical acetylcholine release. Neuroscience. **88:** 811–822.

67. HORGER, B.A., J.D. ELSWORTH & R.H. ROTH. 1995. Selective increase in dopamine utilization in the shell subdivision of the nucleus accumbens by the benzodiazepine inverse agonist FG 7142. J. Neurochem. **65:** 770–774.
68. MURPHY, B.L., A.F.T. ARNSTEN, P.S. GOLDMAN-RAKIC & R.H. ROTH. 1996. Increased dopamine turnover in the prefrontal cortex impairs spatial working memory performance in rats and monkeys. Proc. Natl. Acad. Sci. USA **93:** 1325–1329.
69. GRAY, J.A., M.H. JOSEPH, D.R. HEMSLEY, A.M.J. YOUNG, E.C. WARBURTON, P. BOULENGUEZ, G.A. GRIGORYAN, S.L. PETERS, J.N.P. RAWLINS, C.T. TAIB, B.K. YEE, H. CASSADAY, I. WEINER, G. GAL, O. GUSAK, D. JOEL, E. SHADACH, U. SHALEV, R. TARRASCH & J. FELDON. 1995. The role of mesolimbic dopaminergic and retrohippocampal afferents to the nucleus accumbens in latent inhibition: implications for schizophrenia. Behav. Brain Res. **71:** 19–31.
70. KALIVAS, P. & J. STEWART. 1991. Dopamine transmission in the initiation and expression of drug- and stress-induced sensitization of motor activity. Brain Res. Rev. **16:** 223–244.
71. DICHIARA, G. 1998. A motivational learning hypothesis of the role of mesolimbic dopamine in compulsive drug use. J. Psychopharmacol. **12:** 54–67.
72. DELLER, T. & M. SARTER. 1998. Effects of repeated administration of amphetamine on behavioral vigilance: evidence for "sensitized" attentional impairments. Psychopharmacology **137:** 410–414.
73. ROBINSON, T.E. & K.C. BERRIDGE. 1993. The neural basis of drug craving: an incentive-sensitization theory of addiction. Brain Res. Rev. **18:** 247–291.

Prefrontal Cortical Networks Related to Visceral Function and Mood

JOSEPH L. PRICE[a]

Department of Anatomy and Neurobiology, Washington University School of Medicine, St. Louis, Missouri 63110, USA

ABSTRACT: At least twenty-two architectonic areas can be distinguished within the orbital and medial prefrontal cortex (OMPFC). Although each of these areas has a distinct structure and connections, they can be grouped into two "networks," defined by cortico-cortical connections that primarily interconnect areas within each network. The networks also have different connections to the striatum, medial thalamus, and other brain regions. The orbital network consists of most of the areas in the orbital cortex. It receives several sensory inputs (olfactory, gustatory, visceral afferent, somatic sensory, and visual) that appear to be related to feeding. It also receives many limbic inputs from the amygdala, entorhinal and perirhinal cortex, and subiculum, including a specific projection from the ventrolateral part of the basal amygdaloid nucleus. The orbital network may therefore serve as a substrate to integrate viscerosensory information with affective signals. The medial network consists of areas on the medial frontal surface together with a few select areas in the orbital cortex. These areas have few direct sensory inputs, and their limbic inputs are somewhat different than those to the orbital network (e.g., from the ventromedial part of the basal amygdaloid nucleus). However, they provide the major output from the OMPFC to the hypothalamus and brain stem (especially the periaqueductal gray). The medial network may therefore serve as a visceromotor system to provide frontal cortical influence over autonomic and endocrine function. Connections between the networks presumably allow information flow from viscerosensory to visceromotor systems. In addition to a probable role in eating behavior, this system appears to be involved in guiding behavior and regulation of mood. Lesions of the ventromedial prefrontal cortex result in sociopathic behavior and difficulty in making appropriate choices, whereas functional imaging studies indicate that subjects with unipolar and bipolar depression have abnormal activity in medial and orbital prefrontal areas. Many of these areas also show volume changes and decreased glial number and density in mood-disordered subjects.

ABBREVIATIONS: AIP, G, Iai, Ial, Iam, Iapm, SI, SII, 9, 10m, 10o, 11l, 11m, 12l, 12m, 12o, 12r, 13a, 13b, 13l, 13m, 14c, 14r, 24, 25, 32, 45, 46, 47l, 47m: architectonic areas; AON: anterior olfactory nucleus; PC: piriform cortex; v,dVPMpc: central and dorsal laminae of the ventroposterior medial nucleus of the thalamus, pars parvicellular; dl, l, vlPAG: dorsolateral, lateral, or ventrolateral column of periaqueductal gray; d, l, m Hypothal: dorsal, lateral, and medial parts of the hypothalamus.

---

[a]Address for correspondence: Joseph L. Price, Department of Anatomy and Neurobiology, Washington University School of Medicine, 660 S. Euclid Avenue, St. Louis, MO 63110. Voice: 314-362-3587; fax: 314-747-115; pricej@thalamus.wustl.edu

INTRODUCTION

The cortical connections of the amygdala, and other limbic areas, are primarily directed to the orbital and medial prefrontal cortex (OMPFC) and a contiguous, more caudal, strip of cortex that extends through the ventral insula and along the rhinal sulcus. This paper will consider the areas in the OMPFC that interact not only with the amygdala but also with related structures in the medial thalamus and ventromedial basal ganglia. These areas form a circuit that appears to be involved in such functions as stimulus–reward association, reward-guided behavior, and determination of mood.

ARCHITECTONIC AREAS IN THE OMPFC

The OMPFC is a complex region, containing agranular, dysgranular, and granular regions. Walker[1] recognized seven architectonic areas within the OMPFC (areas 10, 11, 12, 13, 14, 25, and 24). A recent analysis of the OMPFC with several different staining methods (e.g., Nissl, myelin, acetylcholinesterase, and Timm methods, as well as several immunohistochemical stains) identified further subdivisions of these areas, resulting in at least 22 distinct architectonic areas[2] (FIG. 1). The caudal part of the orbital surface is occupied by a rostral extension of the agranular insular, which was subdivided into five areas, Iam, Iai, Ial, Iapm, and Iapl. Dorsolateral to these areas is the primary gustatory cortex (G). More rostrally, dysgranular areas 12, 13, and 14 were subdivided into areas 12r, 12l, 12m, 12o, 13a, 13b, 13m, 13l, 14r, and 14c. Near the rostral pole of the cortex, areas 10 and 11 were subdivided into areas 10m, 10o, 11m, and 11l. Of these, area 10m extends primarily onto the medial wall of the hemisphere, where areas 24, 25, and 32 were also recognized. Although these are similar to the areas delineated by Brodmann,[3] his area 24 has been further subdivided into 24a, 24b, and 24c.

CORTICO-CORTICAL NETWORKS WITHIN THE OMPFC

This architectonic analysis provides the basis for demonstration of the connections of the OMPFC with small injections of retrograde and anterograde tracers into restricted cortical areas. The cortico-cortical connections defined in these experiments show that the areas within the OMPFC can be divided into distinct cortico-cortical networks, which provide separation of sensory and visceromotor functions within the OMPFC (FIG. 1). These networks, which have been termed the "orbital" and "medial" prefrontal networks,[4] also have different connections with the

---

FIGURE 1. A: Architectonic areas within the OMPFC, as defined from staining patterns with nine different stains.[4] **B:** Cortico-cortical connections that define the "orbital prefrontal network." Note also the sensory inputs to areas in the caudal and lateral parts of this network. **C:** Cortico-cortical connections that define the "medial prefrontal network." Areas of this network also provide visceromotor outputs to the hypothalamus and periaqueductal gray (PAG).[4]

PRICE: PREFRONTAL CORTICAL NETWORKS

A. Architectonic Areas

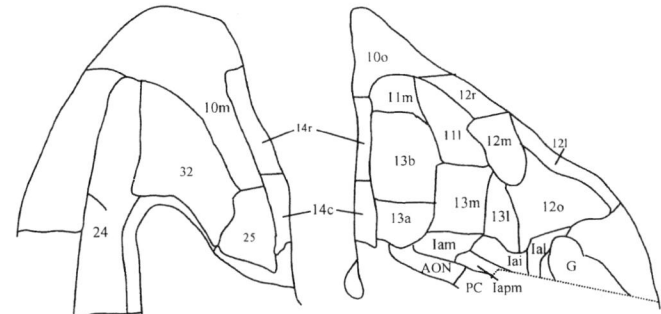

B. Orbital Prefrontal Network

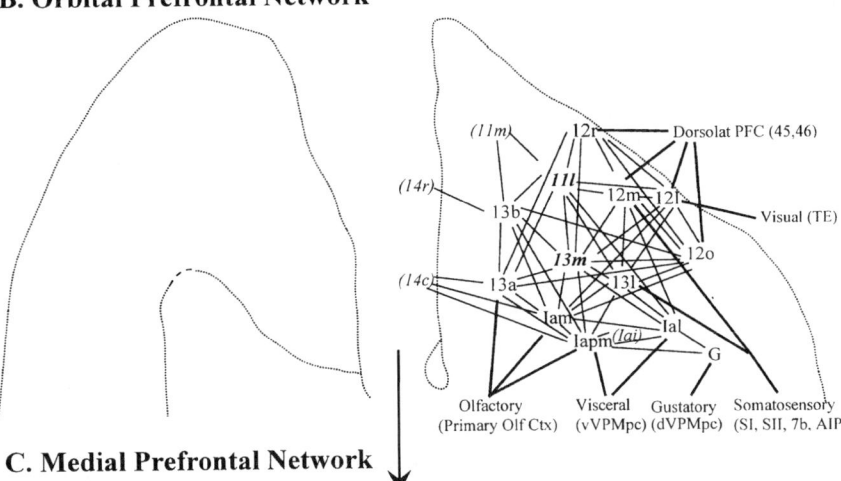

C. Medial Prefrontal Network

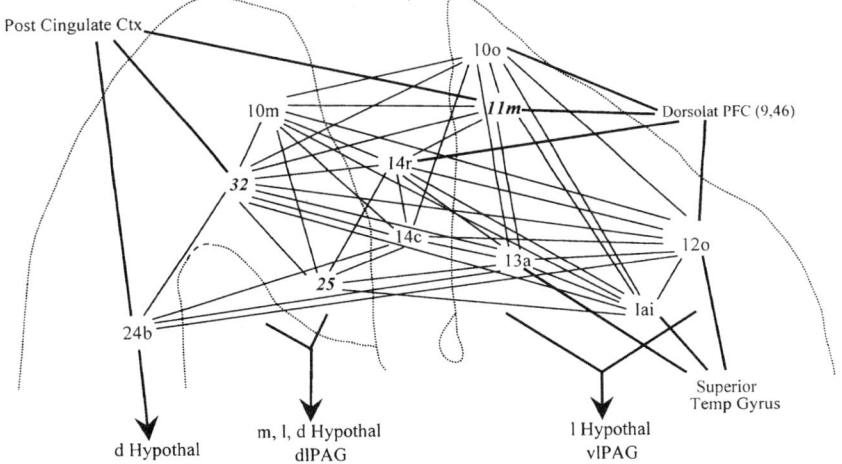

amygdala and other limbic structures, as well as the medial thalamus and the basal ganglia.[5-7]

The orbital prefrontal network was demonstrated with tracer injections into most of the orbital cortical areas. These label connections with other orbital areas, but few with the medial surface of the hemisphere[4] (FIG. 1). Strikingly, there are fewer connections with the orbital area Iai, indicating that the orbital network includes most, but not all, of the orbital areas. As discussed below, there are indications that it may be involved in sensory or viscerosensory integration.

Injections of tracers into the areas on the medial wall of the hemisphere demonstrate the medial prefrontal network.[4] In these cases most of the labeled connections are with other medial areas (10m, 24, 25, and 32) (FIG. 1). There are few connections with areas in the orbital cortex, except for areas 12o and Iai, which are substantially connected to the medial areas. Because areas 12o and Iai have relatively few connections within the orbital network, they can be recognized as parts of the medial network. As described below, the medial network is the source of most of the outputs to visceral control structures in the hypothalamus and brain stem.

Several areas around the ventromedial corner of the hemisphere (areas 14c, 14r, 13a, and 11m) have connections to both networks. Although they have been previously included in the medial network,[4] they also have some connections with the orbital network areas. These areas may serve as connecting links between the two networks.

LIMBIC CONNECTIONS OF THE OMPFC

Both the medial and orbital networks are directly connected with many limbic and limbic-related structures, including the amygdala, the hippocampal formation, the entorhinal cortex, the perirhinal cortex, and the temporal polar cortex[6] (FIG. 2). The most substantial limbic projections are to the posteromedial orbital cortex and the posterior medial cortex, although there are also projections from the amygdala to the lateral orbital cortex. Most, although not all, of these projections are reciprocated by projections from the cortex back to the limbic structures. These substantial limbic connections suggest that the OMPFC is involved in affective as well as sensory functions.

The amygdaloid projections to the OMPFC originate predominantly in the basal nucleus, although there are also projections from the accessory basal and lateral nuclei. In each experiment, cells labeled from localized injections of retrograde tracers into the OMPFC tend to be clustered together in the amygdala. Within the basal nucleus, three separate projection systems can be recognized. Cells in the ventromedial part of the basal nucleus project primarily to areas within the orbital prefrontal network described above, whereas cells in the ventrolateral part of the basal nucleus project mainly to areas in the medial.[6] Return projections from the cortical areas reciprocate the amygdalocortical projections. These two projection systems give further support for the distinction between the orbital and medial networks within the OMPFC.

In addition, cells in the dorsal, magnocellular part of the basal nucleus project to area 12l, and anterograde tracer injections in this area show that it projects back to the same region of the basal nucleus and to the adjacent part of the lateral amygdaloid nucleus.[6] These same parts of the basal and lateral nuclei are also interconnected with the visual areas in the inferior temporal and occipital cortex, (including V1, V2, V4, MT, and MST8), and, as described below, area 12l itself receives visual-related inputs from the inferior temporal cortex. The amygdaloid connections with area 12l can therefore be recognized as part of a system relating the amygdala with visual areas.

The hippocampal input to the OMPFC arises primarily from the rostral part of the subiculum and from a strip of cells along the border between the subiculum and the field CA1.[6,9] These are the same areas that have reciprocal connections with the amygdala.[10,11] The caudal pole of the subiculum has few if any such connections, indicating that there is a rostrocaudal functional division within the hippocampal formation.

SENSORY INPUTS TO THE OMPFC

There are a number of sensory inputs to the OMPFC, all of which are directed to areas within the orbital network[12,13] (FIG. 1). These include inputs from olfactory, gustatory/visceral, visual, and somatic sensory systems, most of which appear to represent sensations associated with food. Olfaction and taste are obviously important components of food sensation, together contributing to the conjoint sensation of flavor. Even the somatic sensory inputs appear to be derived from cortical areas related to the hand and face, that is, body areas that are involved in feeding. The visual inputs may provide information about the appearance of food. The orbital cortex is the first part of the brain where these modalites are represented together.

The sensory inputs are initially directed towards specific areas in the posterior and lateral orbital cortex. The olfactory inputs are derived from the primary olfactory cortex areas (e.g., the anterior olfactory nucleus and piriform cortex) and terminate predominantly in agranular insular areas, Iam and Iapm12 (FIG. 1). Gustatory and visceral inputs reach the OMPFC through a thalamic relay in the "parvicellular" part of the ventroposterior medial nucleus (VPMpc), which, in turn, receives ascending inputs from the nucleus of the solitary tract (NTS).[13,14] This projection system appears to provide parallel pathways for gustatory and other, nongustatory visceral afferent information, through relays in the dorsal and ventral laminae of the VPMpc. More dorsal cells in the VPMpc receive input principally from the rostral, gustatory part of NTS and project to the gustatory cortex, whereas ventral cells in the VPMpc receive input from the caudal, visceral part of NTS and project to areas Ial and Iapm.[13,15]

Visual and somatic sensory inputs to the orbital cortex appear to originate in sensory-association cortical areas[13,16] (FIG. 1). The most lateral orbital area, 12l, along with area 45 on the ventrolateral convexity, receives inputs from visual association area TE in the inferior temporal cortex.[13,17] By contrast, area 12m, adjacent to area 12l, receives little input from the inferior temporal cortex but instead is connected to somatic sensory-related areas, including face- and hand-related parts of the first and second somatic sensory cortex, and parietal area 7b.[13]

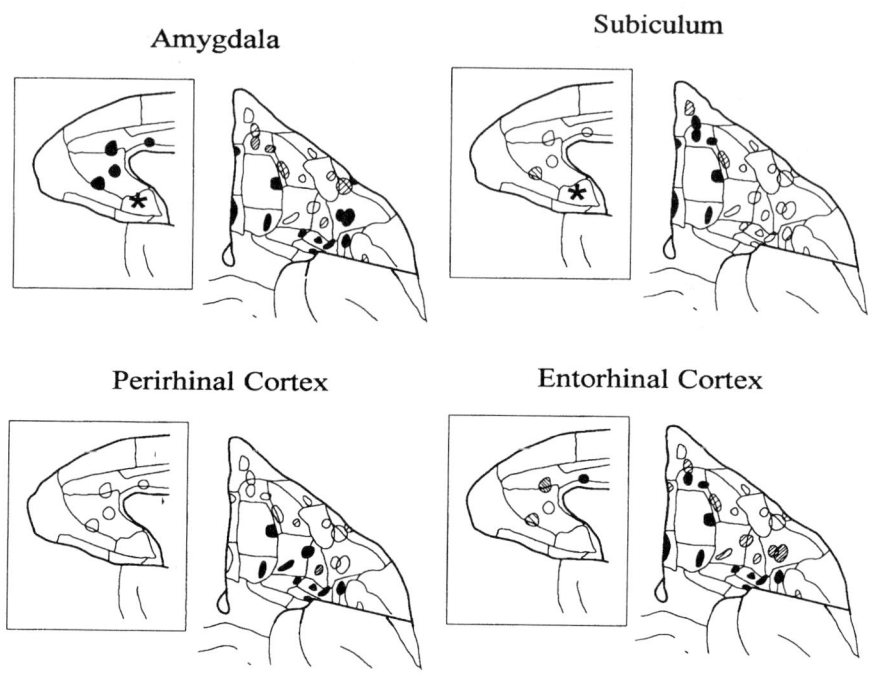

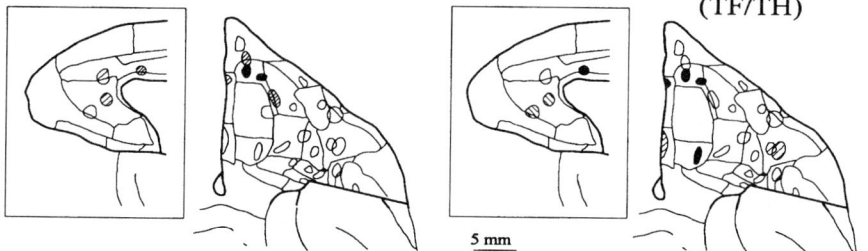

FIGURE 2. Maps illustrating the pattern of input to the OMPFC from several limbic areas. The oval outlines on each map represent the retrograde tracer injection site. The filled outlines indicate injections that labeled many cells in the amgydala, subiculum, or other limbic structures. Cross-hatched outlines indicate injections that labeled a few cells in each structure, and open outlines indicate injections that did not label any cells in that structure. The asterisks indicate areas on the posterior medial wall where injections were not available but where other studies indicate received inputs from the amygdala and subiculum.[6]

The cortico-cortical connections within the orbital network appear to provide a system for the integration of these several modalities with each other and with the limbic inputs from the amygdala, hippocampus and parahippocampal gyrus (FIGS. 1 and 2). Indeed, this is supported by neurophysiological responses that have been recorded in the central areas of the orbital cortex, where cells respond to multimodal food-related stimuli, including the sight, flavor, and ingestion of food items.[18] Furthermore, many of the cells respond to affective qualities of the stimuli as well as to purely sensory qualities.[19,20]

VISCEROMOTOR OUTPUT

It has long been recognized that stimulation of the OMPFC can produce cardiovascular, respiratory, and other visceral reactions, presumably through projections to the hypothalamus and brain stem. In contrast to the sensory character of the orbital network, the medial network appears to be the primary source of such visceromotor outputs from the OMPFC. These have been demonstrated both with anterograde axonal tracers injected into the OMPFC and with retrograde tracers injected into the target regions.[21–23]

Most of the cortical areas within the medial prefrontal network project strongly to the hypothalamus; together these fibers reach all hypothalamic regions[22] (FIG. 1). By contrast the only orbital network connections are weak projections from the agranular insular areas to the posterior lateral hypothalamus. Within the medial network several differences are apparent from different regions. The medial areas 25 and 32 project to all hypothalamic regions, including the medial hypothalamus, whereas the anterior cingulate area 24b projects mainly to the dorsal hypothalamus, and the orbital areas Iai and 12o project mainly to the lateral hypothalamus.[22] This implies that the medial network can be divided into subregions, which differentially affect the endocrine, autonomic, and behavioral functions controlled through the medial, dorsal, and lateral hypothalamus.

In the brain stem, the periaqueductal gray (PAG) is the major target of prefrontal projections in monkeys (FIG. 1). Virtually all of the cortical projections to the PAG arise from the medial network areas or other cortical areas that are closely related to the medial network, such as area 9. As with the hypothalamus, subregions within the medial network project to different columns in the PAG. The medial areas 10m, 25, and 32 project predominantly to the dorsolateral column, whereas the dorsomedial areas 9 and 24b project mainly to the lateral column, and the orbital areas 13a, Iai, and 12o target the ventrolateral column.

The PAG appears to be a center for coordination of visceral and behavioral responses to stress or threatening stimuli. It is organized into rostrocaudal columns that control different responses.[24–26] Microinjections of glutamate into the lateral column evoke an active, "fight or flight" response that would be appropriate for an "escapable" threat. By contrast, excitation of the ventrolateral column elicits a quiescence or "conservation–withdrawal" reaction that resembles the response of an animal to severe injury or defeat in a social encounter, which is not escapable.[26] Both responses also include differential visceral changes and analgesia. For example, activation of the ventrolateral PAG produces hypotension and bradycardia, as well as quiescence, whereas activation of the lateral PAG evokes hypertension and tachycardia along with defensive behavior. Not only does the OMPFC, through the medial network, have a direct role in the control of the stress responses, coordinated through the PAG, but through the differential projections to distinct columns, specific subregions within the network can also affect those responses differentially.

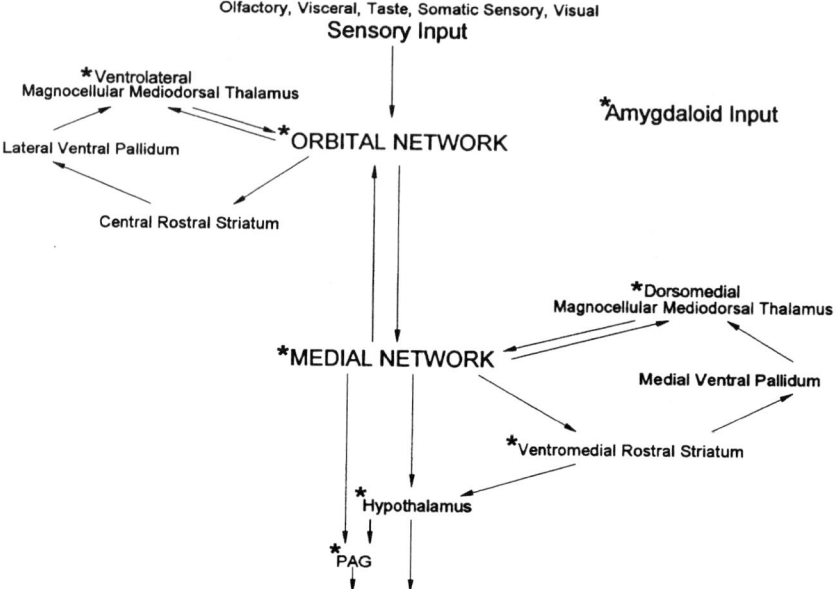

FIGURE 3. Outline of the connectional relations of the orbital and medial prefrontal networks. The orbital network receives sensory inputs from olfactory, visceral, taste, somatic sensory, and visual systems. Cortico-cortical connections, many through areas at the ventromedial edge of the frontal cortex, link the orbital and medial networks. The visceromotor output of the system derives primarily from the medial network. Each network is also linked to largely different circuits through the striatum, ventral pallidum, and mediodorsal thalamic nucleus.

CIRCUIT WITH THALAMUS AND BASAL GANGLIA

The observations summarized above indicate that the OMPFC is divided into two systems or networks, one of which (the orbital network) is related to integration of sensory inputs from several modalities (especially involved in feeding or similar activities), whereas the other (the medial network) is related to visceromotor output to the hypothalamus and brain stem (FIG. 3). Both networks are substantially connected to the amygdala and other limbic structures.

In addition to these connections, the OMPFC and the related limbic structures are involved in a basal ganglia-thalamic circuit that involves the ventral part of the striatum and pallidum, and the medial thalamus. Both the OMPFC and the limbic structures have substantial projections onto the ventromedial part of the striatum, including the nucleus accumbens, the medial caudate nucleus, and the ventrolateral putamen.[21,27,28] Within this system, there are substantial differences between the projections of different cortical regions[21] (FIG. 3). The areas within the medial network of the OMPFC (including the lateral areas Iai and 12o) project primarily to a ventromedial strip of the striatum, including the accumbens nucleus and the medial part of the head, body, and tail of the caudate nucleus. This same striatal region also receives extensive inputs from the amygdala and other limbic structures and projects widely within the hypothalamus, as do the areas in the medial network.[28] By contrast, the areas within the orbital prefrontal network project to an adjacent, more central region of the rostral striatum, immediately dorsal and lateral to the region that receives fibers from the medial network (FIG. 3). Within this region, the agranular insular areas primarily project to the ventral putamen, whereas more rostral orbital areas project to the central putamen and the lateral part of the caudate nucleus.

The projections from these striatal regions to pallidal areas, and from there to the thalamus appear to continue the distinct connections of the orbital and medial prefrontal networks, such that there may be two separate cortico-striato-pallido-thalamic circuits (FIG. 3). The medial part of the accumbens nucleus and the adjacent caudate nucleus (connected to the medial network) project to the rostromedial part of the ventral pallidum, whereas the lateral accumbens nucleus and the adjacent putamen (connected to the orbital network) project to the caudolateral part of the ventral pallidum.[28] These pallidal areas, in turn, project to the dorsomedial and ventrolateral parts of the medial, magnocellular segment of the mediodorsal thalamic nucleus (MDm), respectively.[29,30] Finally, the dorsomedial part of MDm is preferentially interconnected with areas in the medial network, whereas the ventrolateral MDm is preferentially interconnected with the orbital network.[5] To the extent that it is possible to analyze comparable connections from the results of different studies, therefore, the medial and orbital prefrontal networks appear to be involved in distinct circuits in the basal ganglia and thalamus. The precise degree of segregation or interaction between these circuits will need to be defined in further studies.

FUNCTIONAL ASPECTS OF THE OMPFC CORTICO-STRIATO-PALLIDO-THALAMIC CIRCUIT

The anatomical organization of the system described above implies that it may be involved in affective and visceral aspects of feeding. In addition, there are several observations that indicate that several parts of the system are involved in more general guidance of behavior in relation to reward, and in setting of mood.

Neurons in the accumbens nucleus, in particular, have been shown to carry signals related to reward and the anticipation of reward.[31–33] Bilateral lesions of the ventral pallidum or ventral striatum, however, do not prevent rats from learning an odor discrimination task in which one odor is paired with a reward while the other is not. Instead, such lesions prevent rats from correctly performing an odor-reversal task, in which the rewarded odor becomes the unrewarded odor, and vice versa.[34] Lesions of the mediodorsal thalamic nucleus have similar effects,[35,36] as do lesions of the medial or orbital prefrontal cortex (although the deficit following cortical lesions is not as great). By contrast, lesions of the dorsal striatum do not have any significant effect on either the odor-discrimination task or the odor-reversal task (Amon and Price, unpublished observations).

A number of observations have indicated that the dorsal striato-pallido-thalamic system acts to choose between competing motor behaviors by suppressing unwanted or antagonist patterns of motor activity.[37,38] The experiments above suggest that the

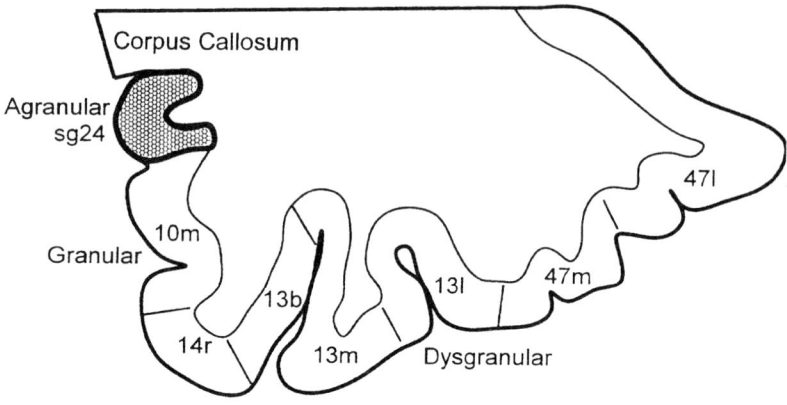

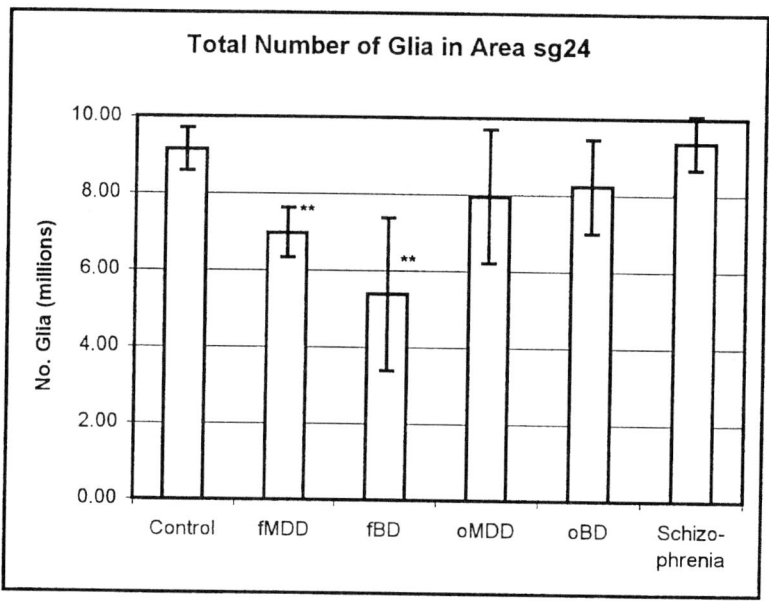

FIGURE 4. The number of glia in the subgenual part of Brodmann's area 24 (sg24) in human subjects that suffered from major depressive disorder (unipolar depression, MDD), bipolar disorder (BD), or schizophrenia, and controls.[45] Significantly lower numbers and density of glia (in relation to controls) were found in mood-disordered subjects with a family history of mood disorders (fMDD and fBD), but little or no change was found in other mood-disordered cases without a clear family history (oMDD and oBD), or in subjects with schizophrenia. There was no difference in the number or density of neurons in area sg24, and no differences were found in either neurons or glia in somatosensory area 3b in the postcentral gyrus.

ventral striato-pallido-thalamic system has a similar role in the realm of stimulus–reward association, acting to inhibit responses to inappropriate or unrewarded stimuli. That is, following lesions of this system, rats are unable to suppress their response to previously rewarded stimuli after the reward has been removed.

Observations on humans with lesions of the OMPFC also indicate that this region is involved in the guidance of behavior in relation to reward (or risk). Such subjects have difficulty in making appropriate judgments and engage in behaviors that are against their own interests.[39] In particular, they appear to be unable to suppress responses to immediate rewards that carry substantial risk of long-term penalties.[4] Because these subjects also have a deficit in visceral responses to affective stimuli, Damasio[41] has suggested that such responses provide a "somatic marker" that tags the stimuli and determines their assessment. Interestingly, an essentially similar mechanism was proposed by Nauta,[42] more than 20 years earlier. He noted that the behavioral effects of frontal-lobe lesions could be due to "interoceptive agnosia," in which the subject is impaired in the ability to integrate information from the internal milieu with information from the environment. Because decisions often appear to be based on analysis of the affective responses evoked by various alternatives, Nauta[42] suggested that this could explain the "loss of foresight" that is seen with large frontal lesions. He further suggested that corollary discharges from the frontal cortex could provide "navigational markers" related to interoceptive information that would influence both the general course and temporal stability of complex goal-directed behavior.

There is also an indication that the OMPFC and related structures are involved in the control of mood. Imaging studies have demonstrated that patients suffering from familial mood disorders have abnormal patterns of activity, and even structural differences in the OMPFC and related areas in the amygdala and medial thalamus, as compared to nondepressed controls. Increases in blood flow and metabolism have been found in the ventrolateral prefrontal cortex, the medial orbital cortex, and the rostral medial cortex, whereas an apparent decrease in blood flow and metabolism was found in the gyrus just ventral to the genu of the corpus callosum (the subgenual part of area 24, or area sg24)[43–45] (see also the chapter by Drevets in this volume). In both unipolar major depressive disorder (MDD) and bipolar disorder (BD), there is also a decrease in the volume of area sg24 on the left side, as measured with MRI.[45]

Finally, examination of tissue from the brains of MDD and BD patients has shown a cellular difference, as compared to either nondepressed controls or schizophrenic patients. In area sg24 and other parts of the PFC, the number of neurons is unchanged in mood-disordered patients, but the number and density of glia is markedly reduced (FIG. 4).[46] This change is seen only in cases with a family history of mood disorders; other MDD and BD brains show no significant glial change. The glial change was also not found in area 3b in the somatic sensory cortex, suggesting that it is specific to the prefrontal cortex. Because of the link to familial cases, it is tempting to suggest that the glial difference might be related to a genetic difference involved in the etiology of depression, but this is unclear at present.

REFERENCES

1. WALKER, A.E. 1940. A cytoarchitectural study of the prefrontal area of the macaque monkey. J. Comp. Neurol. **73:** 59–86.
2. CARMICHAEL, S.T. & J.L. PRICE. 1994. Architectonic subdivision of the orbital and medial prefrontal cortex in the macaque monkey. J. Comp. Neurol. **346:** 366–402.
3. BRODMANN, K. 1909. Vergleichende Lokalisationslehre der Grosshirnrinde in ihren Prinzipien dargestellt auf Grund des Zellenbaues. J. A. Barth. Leipzig.
4. CARMICHAEL, S.T. & J.L. PRICE. 1996. Connectional networks within the orbital and medial prefrontal cortex of macaque monkeys. J. Comp. Neurol. **371:** 179–207.
5. RAY, J.P. & J.L. PRICE. 1993. The organization of projections from the mediodorsal nucleus of the thalamus to orbital and medial prefrontal cortex in macaque monkeys. J. Comp. Neurol. **337:** 1–31.
6. CARMICHAEL, S.T. & J.L. PRICE. 1995. Limbic connections of the orbital and medial prefrontal cortex in macaque monkeys. J. Comp. Neurol. **363:** 615–641.
7. AN, X., D. ÖNGÜR & J.L. PRICE. 1997. Prefrontostriatal projections in relation to cortico-cortical networks in the macaque monkey. Soc. Neurosci. Abstr. **23:** 901.
8. AMARAL, D.G., J.L. PRICE, A. PITKANEN & S.T. CARMICHAEL. 1992. Anatomical organization of the primate amygdaloid complex. In The Amygdala: Neurobiological Aspects of Emotion, Memory and Mental Dysfunction. J. Aggleton, Ed.: 1–66. Wiley-Liss. New York.
9. BARBAS, H. & G.R. BLATT. 1995. Topographically specific hippocampal projections target functionally distinct prefrontal areas in the rhesus monkey. Hippocampus **5:** 511–533.
10. PRICE, J.L., F.T. RUSSCHEN & D.G. AMARAL. 1987. The limbic region. II: The amygdaloid complex. In Handbook of Chemical Neuroanatomy, Vol. 5: Integrated Systems of the CNS, Part I. A. Bjorklund, T. Hokfelt & L.W. Swanson, Eds.: 279–388. Elsevier Science Publishers. Amsterdam.
11. SAUNDERS, R.C., D.L. ROSENE & G.W. VAN HOESEN. 1988. Comparison of the efferents of the amygdala and the hippocampal formation in the rhesus monkey: II. Reciprocal and non-reciprocal connections. J. Comp. Neurol. **271:** 185–207.
12. CARMICHAEL, S.T., M.-C. CLUGNET & J.L. PRICE. 1994. Central olfactory connections in the macaque monkey. J. Comparative Neurol. **346:** 403–434.
13. CARMICHAEL, S.T. & J.L. PRICE. 1995. Sensory and premotor connections of the orbital and medial prefrontal cortex. J. Comp. Neurol. **363:** 642–664.
14. PRITCHARD, T.C., R.B. HAMILTON, J.R. MORSE & R. NORGREN. 1986. Projections of thalamic gustatory and lingual areas in the monkey, *Macaca fascicularis*. J. Comp. Neurol. **244:** 213–228.
15. BECKSTEAD, R.M., J.R. MORSE, R. NORGREN. 1980. The nucleus of the solitary tract in the monkey: projections to the thalamus and brainstem. J. Comp. Neurol. **190:** 259–282.
16. BARBAS, H. 1988. Anatomic organization of basoventral and mediodorsal visual recipient prefrontal regions in the Rhesus monkey. J. Comp. Neurol. **276:** 313–342.
17. WEBSTER, M.J., J. BACHEVALIER & L.G. UNGERLEIDER. 1994. Connections of inferior temporal areas TEO and TE with parietal and frontal cortex in macaque monkeys. Cereb. Cortex **4:** 470–483.
18. ROLLS, E.T. & L.L. BAYLISS. 1994. Gustatory, olfactory and visual convergence within the primate orbitofrontal cortex. J. Neurosci. **14:** 5437–5452.
19. THORPE, S.J., E.T. ROLLS & S. MADDISON. 1983. The orbitofrontal cortex: neuronal activity in the behaving monkey. Exp. Brain Res. **49:** 93–115.
20. ROLLS, E.T., Z.J. SIENCKIEWCZ & S. YAXLEY. 1989. Hunger modulates the responses to gustatory stimuli of single neurons in the caudolateral orbitofrontal cortex of the macaque monkey. Eur. J. Neurosci. **1:** 53–60.
21. AN, X., R. BANDLER, D.ÖNGÜR & J.L. PRICE. 1998. Prefrontal cortical projections to longitudinal columns in the midbrain periaqueductal gray in macaque monkeys. J. Comp. Neurol. **401:** 455–479.

22. ÖNGÜR, D., X. AN & J.L. PRICE. 1998. Prefrontal cortical projections to the hypothalamus in macaque monkeys. J. Comp. Neurol. **401:** 480–505.
23. REMPEL-CLOWER, N.L. & H. BARBAS. 1998. Topographic organization of connections between the hypothalamus and prefrontal cortex in rhesus monkey. J. Comp. Neurol. **398:** 393–419.
24. BANDLER, R. & M.T. SHIPLEY. 1994. Columnar organization in the midbrain periaqueductal gray: modules for emotional expression? Trends Neurosci. **17:** 379–389.
25. BANDLER, R. & K.A. KEAY. 1996. Columnar organization in the midbrain periaqueductal gray and the integration of emotional expression. Prog. Brain Res. **107:** 285–313.
26. BEITZ, A.J. 1995. Periaqueductal gray. *In* The Rat Nervous System. G. Paxinos, Ed.: 173–182. Academic Press. San Diego, CA.
27. RUSSCHEN, F.T., I. BAKST, D.G. AMARAL & J.L. PRICE. 1985. The amygdalostriatal projections in the monkey. An anterograde tracing study. Brain Res. **329:** 241–257.
28. HABER, S.N., E. LYND, C. KLEIN & H.J. GROENEWEGEN. 1990. Topographic organization of the ventral striatal efferent projections in the rhesus monkey: an anterograde tracing study. J. Comp. Neurol. **293:** 282–298.
29. RUSSCHEN, F.T., D.G. AMARAL & J.L. PRICE. 1987. The afferent input to the magnocellular division of the mediodorsal thalamic nucleus in the monkey, *Macaca fascicularis*. J. Comp. Neurol. **256:** 175–210.
30. HREIB, K.K., D.L. ROSENE & M.B. MOSS. 1988. Basal forebrain efferents to the medial dorsal thalamic nucleus in the rhesus monkey. J. Comp. Neurol. **277:** 365–390.
31. SCHULTZ, W., P. APICELLA, E. SCARNATI & T. LJUNGBERG. 1992. Neuronal activity in monkey ventral striatum related to the expectation of reward. J. Neurosci. **12:** 4595–4610.
32. HOLLERMAN, J.R., L. TREMBLAY & W. SCHULTZ. 1998. Influence of reward expectation on behavior-related neuronal activity in primate striatum. J. Neurophysiol. **80:** 947–963.
33. SHIDARA, M., T.G. AIGNER & B.J. RICHMOND. 1998. Neuronal signals in the monkey ventral striatum related to progress through a predictable series of trials. J. Neurosci. **18:** 2613–2625.
34. LU, X.-C. M. & J.L. PRICE. 1994. Lesions of the ventral pallidum interfere with reversal of odor discrimination in rats. Soc. Neurosci. Abstr. **20:** 1017.
35. SLOTNICK, B.M. & J.M. RISSER. 1990. Odor memory and odor learning in rats with lesions of the lateral olfactory tract and mediodorsal thalamic nucleus. Brain Res. **529:** 23–29.
36. MCBRIDE, S.A. & B. SLOTNICK. 1997. The olfactory thalamocortical system and odor reversal learning examined using an asymmetrical lesion paradigm in rats. Behav. Neurosci. **111:**1273–1284.
37. MINK, J.W. & W.T. THACH. 1991. Basal ganglia motor control. III. Pallidal ablation: normal reaction time, muscle cocontraction, and slow movement. J. Neurophysiol. **65:** 330–351.
38. MINK, J.W. 1996. The basal ganglia: focused selection and inhibition of competing motor programs. Prog. Neurobiol. **50:** 381–425.
39. DAMASIO, A.R., D. TRANEL & H. DAMASIO. 1990. Individuals with sociopathic behavior caused by frontal damage fail to respond autonomically to social stimuli. Behav. Brain Res. **41:** 81–94.
40. BECHARA, A., H. DAMASIO, D. TRANEL & A.R. DAMASIO. 1997. Deciding advantageously before knowing the advantageous strategy. Science **275:** 1293–1295.
41. DAMASIO, A.R. 1994. Descartes' Error. Avon Science Publishing. New York.
42. NAUTA, W.J.H. 1971. The problem of the frontal lobe: A reinterpretation. J. Psychiatr. Res. **8:** 167–187.
43. DREVETS, W.C., T.O. VIDEEN, S.H. PRESKORN, J.L. PRICE, S.T. CARMICHAEL & M.E. RAICHLE. 1992. A functional anatomical study of unipolar depression. J. Neurosci. **12:** 3628–3641.

44. DREVETS, W.C. & M.E. RAICHLE. 1994. PET imaging studies of human emotional disorders. *In* The Cognitive Neurosciences. M.S. Gazzaniga Ed.: 1153–1164. MIT Press. Cambridge, MA.
45. DREVETS, W.C., J.L. PRICE, J. SIMPSON, R. TODD, T. REICH, M. VANNIER & M. RAICHLE. 1997. Subgenual prefrontal cortex abnormalities in mood disorders. Nature **386:** 824–827.
46. ÖNGÜR, D., W.D. DREVETS & J.L. PRICE. 1998. Glial reduction in the subgenual prefrontal cortex in mood disorders. Proc. Natl. Acad. Sci. USA **95:** 13290–13295.

Functions of the Amygdala and Related Forebrain Areas in Attention and Cognition

MICHELA GALLAGHER[a] AND GEOFFREY SCHOENBAUM[b]

Department of Psychology, Ames Hall, Johns Hopkins University, 3400 North Charles Street, Baltimore, Maryland 21218-2686, USA

ABSTRACT: This paper will concentrate on two features of the systems described by Alheid and Heimer[1] that have influenced research in our laboratory in recent years. In the first part, we describe our findings on a representational function of the amygdaloid basolateral complex that appears to depend on its interconnections with the prefrontal cortex. In the second part, we describe progress assessing the function of magnocellular corticopetal neurons within the basal forebrain and the strong input to this system from the central amygdaloid group. These lines of behavioral research have revealed that subsystems in the basal forebrain and amygdala serve adaptive functions beyond the domains of motivation and emotion to include attention and cognition.

Behavioral studies, informed by the neuroanatomy of the basal forebrain and amygdaloid complex, have provided links between functions long attributed to these regions, such as motivation and emotion, and more cognitive domains, including attention and representational processes. In describing this recent research a distinction can be made between circuitry that includes the central amygdaloid region and the amygdala basolateral complex. Neuroanatomical considerations led Alheid and Heimer[1] to regard these groupings as components of somewhat separate systems, a view supported by the findings described in this paper.

THE BASOLATERAL COMPLEX

In associative learning, responding to cues that have been paired with an unconditioned stimulus (US), such as a food item, can be used to illustrate the activation of US representations. As demonstrated by an experiment conducted in our laboratory, this type of association is critically dependent on the integrity of the amygdala basolateral complex.

In our study,[2] rats first received pairings of a conditioned stimulus (CS that consisted of a 10 s tone) and food US. FIGURE 1 illustrates the conditioned response that develops using this simple pavlovian appetitive procedure; during the tone that predicts food delivery, rats learn to approach the food cup where pellets are dispensed at the termination of the CS. After establishing this form of conditioning, rats in one

---

[a]Voice: 410-516-0167; fax: 410-516-6205; michela@jhu.edu
[b]Voice: 410-516-0327; schoenbg@jhu.edu

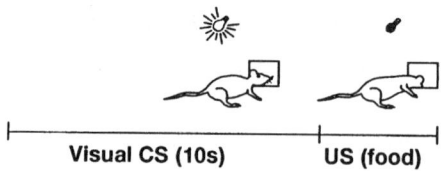

FIGURE 1. Conditioned response elicited in a simple pavlovian appetitive procedure in which delivery of a food US is preceded by a 10 second CS. During the CS, the rats learn to approach the food cup where the reinforcer is delivered.

treatment condition were allowed to freely consume food pellets in another environment, an experience that was followed by administration of LiCl, which produces a conditioned taste aversion for the food. FIGURE 2 shows the behavioral results for this phase of the experiment in which both control and ABL-lesioned rats that received paired food/LiCl suppressed subsequent consumption of the food compared to groups that received unpaired food and administration of LiCl. After the food was "devalued" in this manner, rats were returned to the chamber where they had been previously trained in the pavlovian conditioning task.

Upon initial presentation of the tone CS in the absence of food, FIGURE 2 (right) shows that control rats that had undergone the devaluation procedure were less likely to approach the food cup during the CS than control rats that had received unpaired food and LiCl. The suppression of conditioned responding in these rats demonstrates that the CS has the ability to activate a representation of the US whose value has been altered by the intervening aversive learning episode. In contrast to the control groups, rats with basolateral amygdala (ABL) lesions fail to show any effect of US devaluation, in spite of the fact that they acquired the intervening conditioned taste aversion normally. Also note that the amount of conditioned responding during the devaluation test was comparable for control and ABL groups that received unpaired

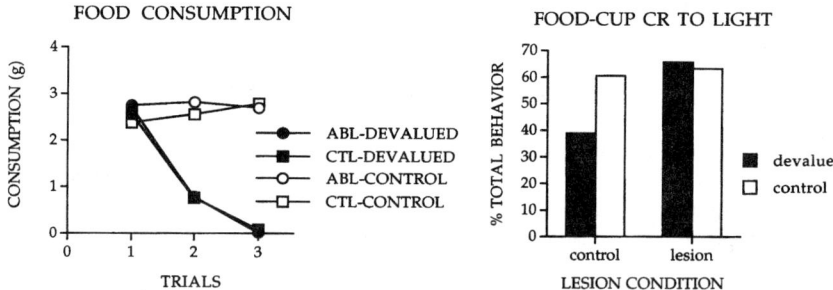

FIGURE 2. In a taste-aversion procedure, a food that previously served as the US in simple appetitive pavlovian conditioning was paired with administration of LiCl; an unpaired treatment was also included for each condition (control and ABL lesion). *Left:* Development of the conditioned taste aversion, which was unaffected by ABL neurotoxic lesions. *Right:* Conditioned responding on re-exposure to the original appetitive conditioning task after the conditioned taste aversion had been acquired. Rats with ABL lesions failed to exhibit a decrease in conditioned responses on re-exposure to the CS (a light) that had been paired with the food.[2]

food and LiCl. Thus, ABL lesions only interfered with the rats' ability to modify their behavior to the CS based on the intervening change in the value of the US. This outcome would be predicted if the representation of the US is unavailable to these rats through an association formed with the CS.

Other studies have confirmed that the amygdala, and specifically the ABL, plays an essential role in the ability of stimuli to gain access to US representations reflecting the current value of those stimuli. Two reports have employed variations of the devaluation procedure used above to test rats with neurotoxic lesions of ABL. In one report,[3] rats were trained to perform an instrumental task that involved pulling a chain or pressing a lever. One action was paired with delivery of a food pellet and the other with delivery of a polycose solution. After acquisition, one of the reinforcers was devalued by allowing the rats to freely consume it for a period of one hour. This specific-satiety procedure was followed by an extinction test in which lever presses and chain pulls were recorded. Although control subjects decreased the response associated with the devalued reinforcer, rats with ABL lesions failed to show this effect. A similar finding was reported using an autoshaping procedure,[4] in which rats were presented with one of two levers just before delivery of either a food pellet or a sucrose solution. The resultant approach behaviors (lever pressing and magazine entry) were unaffected by quinolinic acid lesions of ABL. However, when the rats underwent extinction testing, again following a specific-satiety procedure, in which they were allowed free access to one of the reinforcers, the lesioned rats continued to exhibit approach behaviors to the lever paired with the devalued reinforcer, whereas the controls did not. In addition to these studies using rats, neurotoxic lesions of the amygdala have revealed a similar deficit in nonhuman primates.[5] Rhesus monkeys with excitotoxic lesions of the amygdala fail to decrease responding for a reinforcer that has been devalued through a specific-satiety procedure.

The interpretation that ABL plays a critical role in associations that access US representations is consistent with recent electrophysiological recording data obtained in our laboratory (adapted from refs. 6 and 38). In that study, neurons in ABL developed selective neural activity that was correlated with the impending US. For the majority of those neurons, that encoding was dissociable from neural activity that developed to the discriminative cues that signaled the particular outcome on a trial. In this research, rats were trained on a series of discrimination problems, in which the identity of an odor was informative about the consequence of making a response at a fluid well. The rats were motivated in the task by being maintained on a restricted schedule of water consumption. At the initiation of a trial, rats sampled an odor delivered at an odor port (see FIG. 3A for schematic illustrating the task). Following odor sampling, the rats could respond at a fluid well located just below the odor port. Odors presented at the odor port were either positive, indicating that response at the fluid well would result in delivery of an appetitive sucrose solution, or negative, indicating that response at the fluid well would result in delivery of an aversive quinine solution.

To examine the effect of learning on neural activity, we used novel odors each day; thus rats had to learn the outcomes associated with a new set of odors in every session. In the process of solving each new discrimination, rats typically began by executing a response at the fluid well on every trial (FIG. 3B: positive go and negative go trials) but then gradually learned to withhold this response after sampling an odor that signaled an aversive outcome (FIG. 3B: negative no-go trial). It is important

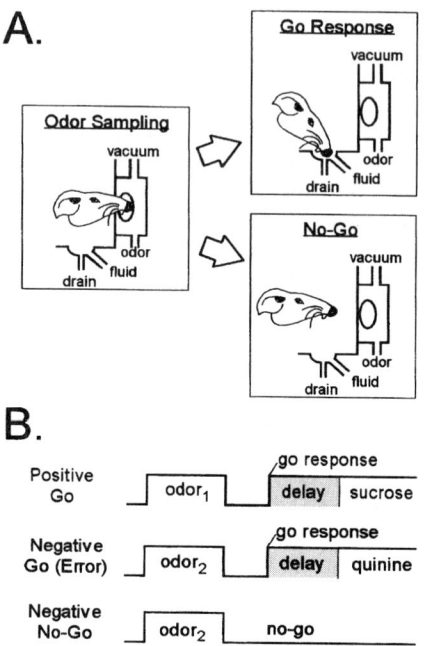

FIGURE 3. Schematic of the odor discrimination task. **A:** At the initiation of a trial, the rat sampled an odor delivered at an odor port (odor sampling), after which the rat could either respond at a nearby fluid well (go response) or withhold that response and wait for the next trial (no-go). One odor signaled a positive outcome, that is, delivery of a preferred sucrose solution at the fluid port, whereas another odor signaled a negative outcome, delivery of a nonpreferred quinine solution. **B:** At the beginning of a session using novel odors, rats typically made responses at the fluid port after sampling either odor. This resulted in positive-go (correct) responses reinforced by sucrose and negative-go (incorrect) responses punished by quinine. Note that a brief variable delay (shaded grey region) was instituted between the response and reinforcer delivery. During the session, rats learned the response contingencies of each odor and adopted the behavioral strategy of responding after sampling a positive odor and withholding responses at the fluid port after sampling a negative odor (negative no-go).[6,38]

to note that a go response at the fluid well was not immediately followed by delivery of reinforcement but rather resulted in a short variable delay period (300–800 ms) before fluid was delivered. During this short delay, the rat was required to remain in the fluid well.

As rats acquired the discrimination appropriate for the odors presented during a session, neurons in ABL developed differential activity during the odor sampling interval that encoded the significance of those cues. Two features of this type of neuronal response were noteworthy. First, the development of differential activity occurred very early during a training session, well before the rat achieved a reliable go, no-go performance. Second, a large proportion of these neurons rapidly reversed differential activity when the task contingencies were reversed. In other words, a

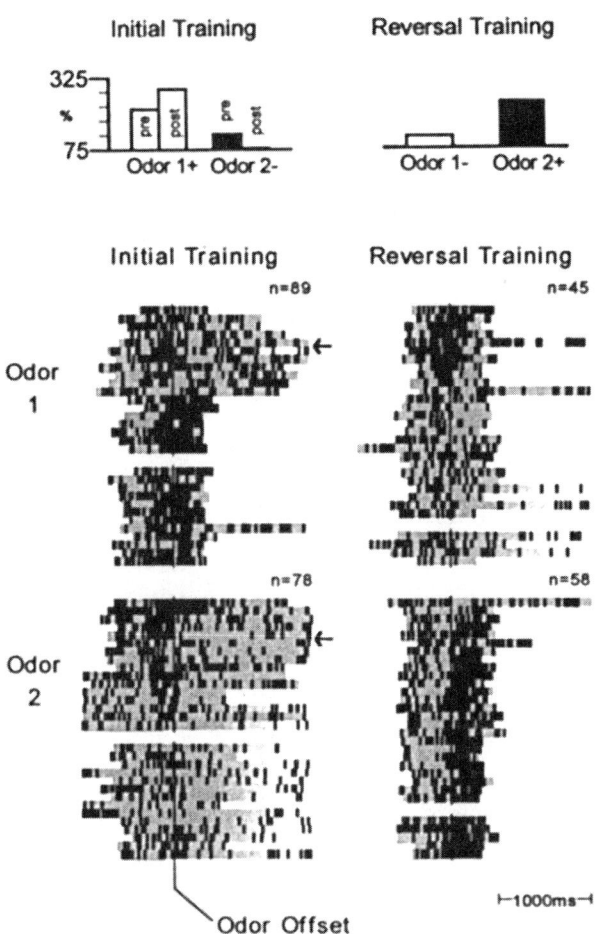

FIGURE 4. Differential activity during odor sampling in a neuron recorded in ABL. The bar graphs show the average activity of this neuron during sampling of positive (odor 1) and negative (odor 2) odors pre- and postcriterion (left graph), and after reversal of the reinforcement contingencies (right graph), represented as a percentage of the pretrial baseline (baseline rate = 24 s/s). Each raster display below illustrates activity on a representative sample of trials of the type noted. The rasters begin with odor onset, are synchronized on odor offset, and end when either a go response was made or after 1000 ms when no response was made. Acquisition of the behavioral criterion is indicated by a space between the rasters in each panel, and the arrows indicate the break point between the early and late segment of precriterion training. This neuron initially showed no selectivity in the precriterion phase but began to fire more strongly during sampling of the positive odor later in precriterion training after several no-go responses had been made (see arrow on rasters) [$F(1, 23) = 23.9$, $p < 0.01$]. Selectivity continued postcriterion [$F(1, 83) = 5.31$, $p < 0.05$] and then reversed after reversal of the response contingencies [$F(1,101) = 22.52$, $p < 0.01$]. Note the rapid change in this neuron's differential firing after reversal.[38]

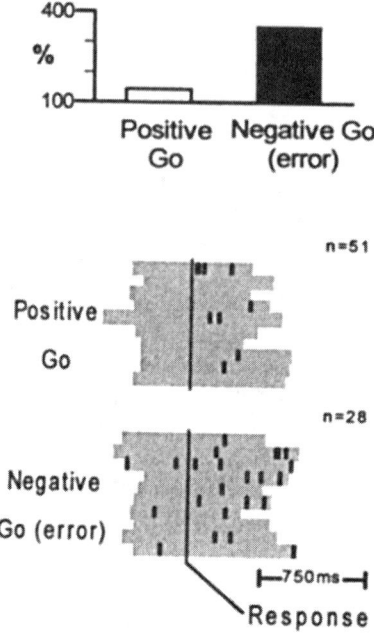

FIGURE 5. Differential activity during the delay after response during precriterion training in a neuron recorded in ABL. The bar graph shows the average activity of this neuron during the delay on positive trials and negative trials, represented as a percentage of the pretrial baseline (baseline rate = 0.78 s/s). Each raster display below illustrates activity on a representative sample of trials of the type noted. The rasters begin with odor offset, are synchronized on the response, and end at reinforcer delivery. This neuron fired more strongly during the delay on negative-go trials, when quinine was about to be delivered, than on positive-go trials, when sucrose was about to be delivered [$F(1, 77) = 21.87, p < 0.001$].[6]

neuron that developed greater activity to the odor cue that signaled sucrose during the initial training phase switched its selectivity during the phase of reversal training when the formerly negative odor cue now became the signal for sucrose availability. A neuron that illustrates these features is shown in FIGURE 4.

The population of neurons that developed selective activity during odor sampling was largely separate from another set of neurons that developed selective activity during the delay that preceded delivery of sucrose or quinine. The response features of these neurons may be of particular importance for the role of ABL in encoding US representations. During the delay period, a large proportion of the neurons recorded in ABL developed selective activity in anticipation of the expected outcome of a trial. Fully 44 (36%) of the 121 neurons recorded in ABL had this type of correlate. These cells exhibited differential activity at the fluid port after a response was made while the rat awaited the delivery of sucrose or quinine. In addition to the fact that this subset of neurons in ABL was largely distinct from the subset that had differential activity during odor sampling, two features of this type of activity were particularly noteworthy. First, similar to the selective activity that developed during odor sampling, selective activity during the delay was evident early in each training session, before the rats had begun to reliably withhold responses to the negative odor. Second, a substantial proportion of these cells had a pattern of selectivity during the delay prior to delivery of sucrose or quinine that was similar to the activity displayed to the reinforcers themselves. In other words, if a neuron had a greater firing rate during the delay prior to quinine delivery (negative-go trials), that neuron also displayed greater activity during the reinforcement interval when contact with quinine was made. FIGURE 5 shows a typical example of an ABL neuron with differential activity during the delay. Activity is shown from early in the training session before the rat had met the behavioral criterion when significant numbers of negative-go responses were made. The bar graphs display the average activity in this neuron during the delay on positive-go and negative-go trials during this "precriterion" phase, and the raster display below depicts the firing activity on a representative selection of those trials. It is evident that the neuron fires more strongly in anticipation of the negative outcome than in anticipation of the positive outcome.

When the activity of the entire population of selective neurons of this type in ABL was examined, the dependence of selectivity on the training experience was clearly evident. FIGURE 6 shows the results of that analysis. An activity contrast was calculated for each cell to reflect the difference in the activity of the neuron during the delay on positive-go and negative-go trials. This activity contrast was determined for the trials in an early segment of training, when few correct no-go responses had occurred, and also for the remaining trials (late segment) prior to acquisition of the behavioral criterion for the discrimination. The activity contrast increased significantly between the early and late segments of precriterion training in ABL, indicating the effect of learning on this type of response.

The information represented by neurons such as those recorded in ABL may provide a basis for behaviors that depend on the representation of the USs evoked by other cues. However, this associative function is likely to be mediated in concert with

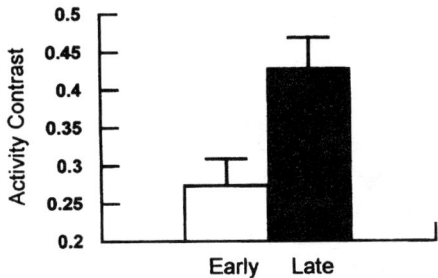

FIGURE 6. Contrast in activity on positive- and negative-go trials during the early (open bars) and late (closed bars) segments of precriterion training for a population of neurons selective during the delay in ABL. The activity contrast was calculated as the absolute difference in the rates on positive- and negative-go trials divided by the sum of those rates, yielding values that ranged from 0 to 1. The activity contrast increased significantly in ABL between the early and late segments of training [t (33) = 3.77, p = 0.00065], reflecting the development of selectivity in the individual neurons over training.[6]

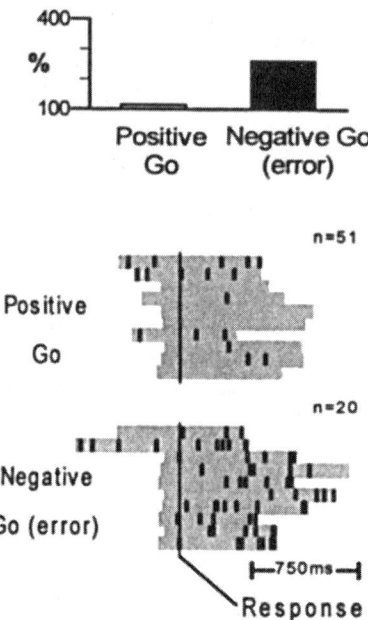

FIGURE 7. Differential activity during the delay after response during precriterion training in a neuron recorded in OFC. The bar graph shows the average activity of this neuron during the delay on positive trials and negative trials, represented as a percentage of the pretrial baseline (baseline rate = 2.33 s/s). Each raster display below illustrates activity on a representative sample of trials of the type noted. The rasters begin with odor offset, are synchronized on the response, and end at reinforcer delivery. This neuron fired more strongly during the delay on negative-go trials, when quinine was about to be delivered, than on positive-go trials, when sucrose was about to be delivered [$F (1, 69) = 37.4, p < 0.001$].[6]

other regions. In describing the quasicortical features of ABL, Alheid and Heimer[1] noted that this region of the amygdaloid complex is distinguished by the large number of cortical circuits in which it participates. Among those, perhaps most notable in the present context are the reciprocal connections between ABL and the orbitofrontal cortex (OFC). Not only are ABL and OFC reciprocally connected,[7–10] but they also receive input from many common sources, such as the mediodorsal thamamic nucleus[11,12] and olfactory-related structures,[9,13] and provide output to common targets.[10,14] Moreover, damage to each of these regions results in somewhat similar syndromes, in which patients have difficulty in recognizing and using appropriately the current motivational value of cues.[15,16] Indeed, studies of animal models have shown that damage to or disconnection of these two structures impairs adaptive goal-directed behavior.[17–20]

For a direct comparison with ABL, we recorded from cells in OFC in the same odor-guided task presented earlier. In the context of the observation that amygdaloid neurons develop correlates for the impending outcome (US), a comparable population of cells was found in the OFC. Of 328 neurons recorded in the OFC, 74 (22%)

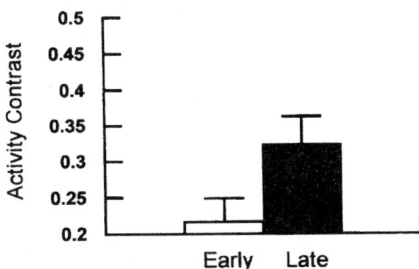

FIGURE 8. Contrast in activity on positive- and negative-go trials during the early (open bars) and late (closed bars) segments of precriterion training for a population of neurons selective during the delay in OFC. The activity contrast was calculated as described in FIG. 6. As in ABL, the activity contrast of the selective neurons in OFC increased significantly between the early and late segments of training [t (34) = 2.32, p = 0.026], reflecting the development of selectivity in the individual neurons over training.[6]

developed selective activity during the delay after a response was made. As had been the case in ABL, this selective activity developed early in training, increasing substantially between the early and late segments of precriterion training. FIGURE 7 shows an example of a neuron recorded in the OFC that fired selectively in anticipation of quinine, similar to the example from ABL in FIGURE 3, and FIGURE 8 shows the increase in relative selectivity during precriterion training for the OFC neurons of this type. Interestingly, in contrast to ABL, only a small number of these neurons exhibited parallel selectivity during the subsequent reinforcement.

The activity of neurons in the OFC during the delay may encode the incentive value of the upcoming US in working memory. The results of a recent experiment examining the effects of selective OFC lesions on devaluation are consistent with this interpretation. Neurotoxic lesions of the OFC, including the region targeted by afferents from ABL and excluding gustatory regions in posterior agranular insular cortex, caused an impairment in devaluation training nearly identical to those seen after lesions of ABL described earlier. Lesioned animals acquired the conditioned response (food-cup approach) and the subsequent conditioned taste aversion normally but failed to decrease the conditioned response relative to controls during testing after devaluation of the reinforcer (unpublished observations, 1998).

By analogy with other component-working memory systems that engage prefrontal neurons, the OFC may depend on its interconnections with ABL to bring into working memory the associative information that is relevant to such tasks. By the same token, the delay activity exhibited by neurons in ABL may depend on the working memory function of the OFC prefrontal system. Thus, in the absence of the OFC, it might be predicted that neural activity during the delay would be eliminated in ABL. In any event, the results of these lines of research serve to further reinforce the concept that ABL is closely allied to cortical circuitry and representational processes.

Pathways for the expression of behaviors based on the associative functions of ABL are available via direct projections from ABL to the striatum and indirect pathways to the striatum via the prefrontal cortex.[7,10,21] In support of the use of such circuitry for the functions described in this section, some other output pathways, such as the central amygdaloid region do not appear to be involved. Notably, neurotoxic lesions of CN do not alter the ability of rats to adjust their behavior in devaluation paradigms.[2] Selective CN lesions also do not affect other associative functions that depend on the reinforcing properties of uncondtioned stimuli in appetitive-conditioning procedures. For example, such damage does not interfere with second-order conditioning, whereas ABL damage produces deficits in both pavlovian second-order conditioning and in the acquisition of new instrumental behavior supported by secondary reinforcers.[2,22] Instead, the CN plays a critical role in controlling the attention that is allocated to cues (conditioned stimuli) in associative learning,[23] a function that makes contact with earlier observations that the amygdala is involved in orienting behavior.

CENTRAL AMYGDALOID REGION

Electrical stimulation of the amygdala and, in particular, stimulation of CN elicits both somatomotor and autonomic components of orienting behavior.[24–26] Damage to the amygdaloid CN does not affect spontaneous orienting to novel cues; however, such damage severely impairs orienting responses that normally develop during conditioning.[27] In addition to its contribution to this type of conditioned response, other studies have shown that CN is critical for more covert changes in the processing of cues in a manner that can promote new learning (for review, see refs. 23 and 28). A theoretical framework for this function is described by Pearce and Hall.[29] Briefly, they specify that "controlled attention" is allocated to a cue when its significance is uncertain. This type of attention is reduced when experience indicates that a cue is not predictive of any behaviorally significant event or if the organism has learned through prior experience that such a cue is an entirely reliable predictor of another event. In either of these cases, little new information is likely to be gained by further processing of a type (i.e., controlled attention) that might lead to new learning. On the other hand, controlled attention is best allocated to a cue when its outcome is uncertain, and such attention can be restored if any stimulus's relation to other events is made uncertain. This account has provided a framework for understanding a number of empirical findings that otherwise would be difficult to explain. Some of those empirical settings have also proven to be informative in the study of amygdaloid CN function.

As specified above, attention that can promote new learning is engaged when a cue's predictive outcome is uncertain or changed from prior expectations. The design of an experiment shown in TABLE 1 has been used to demonstrate this phenomenon and has also proven to be sensitive to the integrity of the amygdaloid CN.

The conditioning procedure includes three phases. Control (CTL) and lesioned (LES) rats are assigned randomly to one of two behavioral treatments, shift and consistent, resulting in four groups: CTL-consistent (CTL-C), CTL-shift (CTL-S), LES-consistent (LES-C), and LES-shift (LES-S). In phase 1, rats in all four groups receive presentations of a light CS, followed by a tone CS. The tone is followed by food reinforcement (the US) in 50% of the trials. This partial reinforcement procedure results in the rapid development of conditioned responding to the tone (due to the temporal contiguity of this CS with the food US). The light, by contrast, does not

TABLE 1. Procedures used to increment attention by altering the predictable relation between two cues

Training Condition (Groups)	Phase 1 Consistent light (L)–tone (T) relationship	Phase 2 Experimental change in light (L)–tone (T) relationship	Phase 3 Test of learning to light (L)
Consistent (CTL-C, LES-C)	L → T → food; L → T	L → T → food; L → T	L → food
Shifted (CTL-S, LES-S)	L → T → food; L → T	L → T → food; L	L → food

NOTE: CTL, control; LES, lesion; L, light-conditioned stimulus (CS); T, tone CS; fd, food; unconditioned stimulus (US); →, signifies serial relation.

develop significant conditioned responding, due to its poor temporal relationship with the US and the presence of a better temporal predictor of the US (the tone). More importantly, because the light consistently predicts the tone during phase 1, attention to the light is gradually reduced, according to the Pearce and Hall[29] model.

During phase 2, the consistent groups continue to receive light→tone→food and light→tone→nothing trials. The shift groups also received light→tone→food trials, but the light→tone→nothing trials are replaced by light-alone trials. Although this procedure maintains the light-food relationship established in phase 1, it makes the light an inconsistent predictor of the tone. According to the Pearce and Hall model, this shift in the light's predictive value increases attention to the light.

Attention to the light is assessed in phase 3 by pairing the light directly with food. Increased attention to the light would be reflected in more rapid acquisition of conditioned responding to the light by rats in the shift groups as compared to rats in the consistent groups. We (and others) have repeatedly obtained this outcome with normal rats.[30–34]

In this paradigm, neurotoxic lesions of the amygdala CN eliminate the increased processing of the light so that learning does not occur more readily to that stimulus. This result is shown in FIGURE 9a, along with the results of two additional studies showing a similar effect after other brain lesions (FIG. 9, b and c). Note that in each study (control groups in FIG. 9, a and c), learning is normally increased in the shift group relative to the consistent group. The sites where lesions were made in these three experiments appear to form a circuit needed for this modulation of attentional processing. The circuit includes CN and its innervation of basal forebrain cholinergic neurons that project to a posterior region of the parietal cortex. Figure 9a shows the impairment in rats with bilateral CN lesions.[33] FIGURE 9b shows the effect of selective removal of the cholinergic neurons in the caudal basal forebrain component of the magnocellular system. These bilateral lesions were made with 192 IgG-saporin, an immunotoxin that selectively targets cholinergic neurons in the basal forebrain that bear low-affinity receptors for nerve growth factor.[35] Similar to the effects of selective removal of CN neurons, this lesion also prevents increases in the processing of the light after its previously established relationship to another stimulus was made uncertain.[31] Those cholinergic neurons innervate widespread regions of neocortex, including an area recently defined in the rat as possessing homology with the primate posterior parietal cortex.[36] The data in FIGURE 9c show the results obtained in the

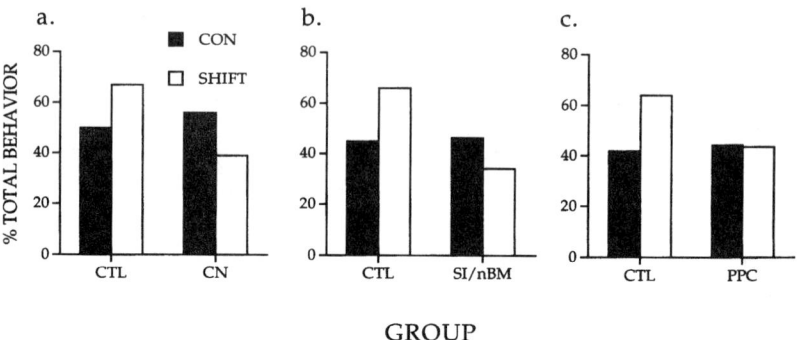

FIGURE 9. Summary data from three experiments.[31,33,37] In each graph the control (CTL) groups show increased conditioning after a shift in the predictive relationship between two cues. Bilateral neurotoxic lesions of CN (**a**), immunotoxic lesions of the cholinergic neurons in the SI/nBM (**b**), and removal of the cholinergic innervation of posterior parietal cortex (**c**) each eliminate this effect.

same attentional processing task after selective removal of the cholinergic innervation of PPC.[37] This lesion was made by microinjection of the cholinergic immunotoxin into the target cortical field. I

As noted by Alheid and Heimer,[1] innervation of the magnocellular corticopetal system in the basal forebrain provides a pathway for amygdala influences on cortical processing systems. Although the behavioral implications of this anatomy remain largely unexplored at that time, the advent of new tools for targeting particular cells in the corticopetal system has greatly aided in understanding the function of this circuitry. Moreover, it has revealed a regulation of the cholinergic component of the magnocellular system by the amygdala. Specifically, a component of the extended amygdaloid system that includes the central amygdaloid region appears to gain regulation of the parietal cortex via this route.

CONCLUSION

Neuroanatomy is an essential guide to understanding the central nervous system. How aggregates of neurons are clustered and share connectivity with other systems serves as a basis for identifying circuitry used for specialized functions. The behavioral neuroscientist relies on such information for targeting manipulations, such as lesions and neuropharmacological interventions and studies of neural activity, to determine the role of specific neural circuitry in a diverse range of psychological functions. The anatomy of the basal forebrain, so elegantly described by Alheid and Heimer,[1] has presented a particular challenge for the behavioral neuroscientist because in this region of the brain multiple systems are not strictly compartmentalized. Instead several systems intermingle and interleave, making it difficult to selectively manipulate one component apart from the others. Two organizing features of the basal forebrain systems and amygdaloid complex highlighted in their report have provided a useful framework for recent behavioral investigations, as highlighted in this paper. Such research supports the existence of subsystems within the basal forebrain and amygdala that serve distinctive functions in adaptive behavior that include not only motivation and emotion, but also attention and cognition.

ACKNOWLEDGMENT

This work was supported by RO1-MH53667 and KO5-MH01149 to M.G.

REFERENCES

1. ALHEID, G.F. & L. HEIMER. 1988. New perspectives in basal forebrain organization of special relevance for neuropsychiatric disorders: the striatopallidal, amygdaloid, and corticopetal components of substantia innominata. Neuroscience 1: 1–39.
2. HATFIELD, T., J.-S. HAN, M. CONLEY, M. GALLAGHER & P. HOLLAND. 1996. Neurotoxic lesions of basolateral, but not central, amygdala interfere with pavlovian second-order conditioning and reinforcer devaluation effects. J. Neurosci. 16: 5256–5265.
3. BALLEINE, B.W., J.C. LIEBESKIND & A. DICKINSON. 1997. Effect of cell body lesions of the basolateral amygdala on instrumental conditioning [abstract]. Soc. Neurosci. Abstr. 34: 786.
4. WILLOUGHBY, P.J. & A.S. KILLCROSS. 1998. The role of the basolateral amygdala in appetitive conditioning [abstract]. X Congreso de la Sociedad Espanola de Psicologia Comparada. Almeria. September, p. 167.
5. MALKOVA, L., D. GAFFAN & E.A. MURRAY. 1997. Excitotoxic lesions of the amygdala fail to produce impairment in visual learning for auditory secondary reinforcement but interfere with reinforcer devaluation effects in rhesus monkeys. J. Neurosci. 17: 6011–6020.
6. SCHOENBAUM, G., A.A. CHIBA & M. GALLAGHER. 1998. Orbitofrontal cortex and basolateral amygdala encode expected outcomes during learning. Nature: Neuroscience 1: 155–159.
7. KRETTEK, J.E. & J.L. PRICE. 1977. Projections from the amygdaloid complex to the cerebral cortex and thalamus in the rat and cat. J. Comp. Neurol. 172: 687–722.
8. KOLB, B. 1984. Functions of the frontal cortex of the rat: a comparative review. Brain Res. Rev. 8: 65–98.
9. PRICE, J.L., F.T. RUSSCHEN & D.G. AMARAL. 1987. The limbic region. II. The amygdaloid complex. In Integrated Systems of the CNS, Part I. Handbook of Chemical Neuroanatomy, vol. 5. A. Bjorklund, T. Hokfelt & L. W. Swanson, Eds.: 279–388. Amsterdam. Elsevier.
10. MCDONALD, A.J. 1991. Organization of amygdaloid projections to the prefrontal cortex and associated striatum in the rat. Neuroscience 44: 1–14.
11. KRETTEK, J.E. & J.L. PRICE. 1977. The cortical projections of the mediodorsal nucleus and adjacent thalamic nuclei in the rat. J. Comp. Neurol. 171: 157–192.
12. GROENEWEGEN, H.J. 1988. Organization of the afferent connections of the mediodorsal thalamic nucleus in the rat, related to the mediodorsal-prefrontal topography. Neuroscience 24: 379–431.
13. PRICE, J.L., S.T. CARMICHAEL, K.M. CARNES, M.-C. CLUGNET, M. KURODA & J.P. RAY. 1991. Olfactory input to the prefrontal cortex. In Olfaction: A Model System for Computational Neuroscience. J. Davis & H. Eichenbaum, Eds.: 101–120. MIT Press. Cambridge, MA.
14. GROENEWEGEN, H.J., H.W. BERENDSE, J.G. WOLTERS & A.H.M. LOHMAN. 1990. The anatomical relationship of the prefrontal cortex with the striatopallidal system, the thalamus, and the amygdala: evidence for a parallel organization. Prog. Brain Res. 85: 95–118.

15. AGGLETON, J.P. 1992. The functional effects of amygdala lesions in humans: a comparison with findings from monkeys. In The Amygdala: Neurological Aspects of Emotion, Memory, and Mental Dysfunction. J. Aggleton, Ed.: 485–503. Wiley. Chichester.
16. BECHARA, A., H. DAMASIO, D. TRANEL & A.R. DAMASIO. 1997. Deciding advantageously before knowing the advantageous strategy. Science **275:** 1293–1294.
17. JONES, B. & M. MISHKIN. 1972. Limbic lesions and the problem of stimulus-reinforcement associations. Exp. Neurol. **36:** 362–377.
18. GAFFAN, D., E.A. MURRAY & M. FABRE-THORPE. 1993. Interaction of the amygdala with the frontal lobe in reward memory. Eur. J. Neurosci. **5:** 968–975.
19. EICHENBAUM, H., R.A. CLEGG & A. FEELEY. 1983. Reexamination of the functional subdivisions of the rodent prefrontal cortex. Exp. Neurol. **79:** 434–451.
20. KILLCROSS, S., T.W. ROBBINS & B.J. EVERITT. 1997. Different types of fear conditioned behavior mediated by separate nuclei within amygdala. Nature **388:** 377–380.
21. KELLEY, A.E., V.B. DOMESICK & W.J.H. NAUTA. 1982. The amygdalostriatal projection in the rat—an anatomical study by anterograde and retrograde tracing methods. Neuroscience **7:** 615–630.
22. EVERITT, B.J., M. CADOR & T.W. ROBBINS. 1989. Interactions between the amygdala and ventral striatum in stimulus-reward associations: studies using a second-order schedule of sexual reinforcement. Neuroscience **30:** 63–75.
23. GALLAGHER, M. & P.C. HOLLAND. 1994. The amygdala complex: multiple roles in associative learning and attention. Proc. Natl. Acad. Sci. USA **91:** 11771–11776.
24. KAADA, B.R. 1951. Somato-motor, autonomic, and electroencephalographic responses to electrical stimulation of rhinencephalic and other structures in primates, cat, and dog. A study of responses from the limbic, subcallosal, orbito-insular, piriform and temporal cortex, hippocampus-fornix and amygdala. Acta Physiol. Scand. **23** (Suppl. 83) 1–285.
25. KAPP, B.S., J.P. PASCOE & M.A. BIXLER. 1984. The amygdala: a neuroanatomical systems approach to its contribution to aversive conditioning. In The Neuropsychology of Memory. L. Squire & N. Butters, Eds.: 473–428. The Guilford Press. New York.
26. KAPP, B.S., W.F. SUPPLE JR. & P.J. WHALEN. 1994. The effects of electrical stimulation of the amygdaloid central nucleus on neocortical arousal in the rabbit. Behav. Neurosci. **108:** 81–93.
27. GALLAGHER, M., P.W. GRAHAM & P.C. HOLLAND. 1990. The amygdala central nucleus and appetitive Pavlovian conditioning: Lesions impair one class of conditioned performance. J. Neurosci. **10:** 1906–1911.
28. HOLLAND, P.C. 1997. Brain mechanisms for changes in processing of conditioned stimuli in Pavlovian conditioning: Implications for behavior theory. Anim. Learn. Behav. **25:** 373–399.
29. PEARCE, J.M. & G. HALL. 1980. A model for Pavlovian learning: variations in the effectiveness of conditioned but not of unconditioned stimuli. Psychol. Rev. **106:** 532–552.
30. BAXTER, M.G., M. GALLAGHER & P.C. HOLLAND. 1997. Disruption of decremental processing of conditioned stimuli by selective removal of hippocampal cholinergic input. J. Neurosci. **17:** 5230–5236.
31. CHIBA, A.A., D.J. BUCCI, P.C. HOLLAND & M. GALLAGHER. 1995. Basal forebrain cholinergic lesions disrupt increments but not decrements in conditioned stimulus processing. J. Neurosci. **15:** 7315–7322.
32. HAN, J-S., P.C. HOLLAND & M. GALLAGHER. 1999. Disconnection of amygdala central nucleus and substantia innominata/nucleus basalis disrupts increments in conditioned stimulus processing in rats. Behav. Neurosci. **113:** 143–151.
33. HOLLAND, P.C., & M. GALLAGHER. 1993. Amygdala central nucleus lesions disrupt increments, but not decrements, in CS processing. Behav. Neurosci. **107:** 246–253.
34. WILSON, P.N., P. BOUMPHREY & J.M. PEARCE. 1992. Restoration of the orienting response to a light by a change in its predictive accuracy. Q. J. Exp. Psychol. **44B:** 17–36.

35. WILEY, R.G., T.N. OELTMANN & D.A. LAPPI. 1991. Immunolesioning: Selective destruction of neurons using immunotoxin to rat NGF receptor. Brain Res. **562:** 149–153.
36. REEP, R.L., H.C. CHANDLER, V. KING & J.V. CORWIN. 1994. Rat posterior parietal cortex: topography of corticocortical and thalamic connections. Exp. Brain Res. **100:** 67–84.
37. BUCCI, D.J., P.C. HOLLAND & M. GALLAGHER. 1998. Removal of cholinergic input to rat posterior parietal cortex disrupts incremental processing of conditioned stimuli. J. Neurosci. **18:** 8038–8046.
38. SCHOENBAUM, G., A.A. CHIBA & M. GALLAGHER. 1999. Neural encoding in orbitofrontal cortex and basolateral amygdala during olfactory discrimination learning. J. Neurosci. 19: 1876–1884.

Associative Processes in Addiction and Reward
The Role of Amygdala-Ventral Striatal Subsystems

BARRY J. EVERITT,[a,d] JOHN A. PARKINSON,[a] MARY C. OLMSTEAD,[b]
MERCEDES ARROYO,[a] PATRICIA ROBLEDO,[c] AND TREVOR W. ROBBINS[a]

[a]*Department of Experimental Psychology, University of Cambridge, Downing Street, Cambridge, United Kingdom, CB2 3EB*
[b]*Department of Psychology, Queens University, Kingston, Ontario, Canada, K7L 3N6*
[c]*Laboratorio de Neuropsicofarmacologia, Hospital de la Santa Creu i Sant Pau, Avgda. Sant Antoni Maria Claret, 167, 08025 Barcelona, Spain*

ABSTRACT: Only recently have the functional implications of the organization of the ventral striatum, amygdala, and related limbic-cortical structures, and their neuroanatomical interactions begun to be clarified. Processes of activation and reward have long been associated with the NAcc and its dopamine innervation, but the precise relationships between these constructs have remained elusive. We have sought to enrich our understanding of the special role of the ventral striatum in coordinating the contribution of different functional subsystems to confer flexibility, as well as coherence and vigor, to goal-directed behavior, through different forms of associative learning. Such appetitive behavior comprises many subcomponents, some of which we have isolated in these experiments to reveal that, not surprisingly, the mechanisms by which an animal sequences responding to reach a goal are complex. The data reveal how the different components, pavlovian approach (or sign-tracking), conditioned reinforcement (whereby pavlovian stimuli control goal-directed action), and also more general response-invigorating processes (often called "activation," "stress," or "drive") may be integrated within the ventral striatum through convergent interactions of the amygdala, other limbic cortical structures, and the mesolimbic dopamine system to produce coherent behavior. The position is probably not far different when considering aversively motivated behavior. Although it may be necessary to employ simplified, even abstract, paradigms for isolating these mechanisms, their concerted action can readily be appreciated in an adaptive, functional setting, such as the responding by rats for intravenous cocaine under a second-order schedule of reinforcement. Here, the interactions of primary reinforcement, psychomotor activation, pavlovian conditioning, and the control that drug cues exert over the integrated drug-seeking response can be seen to operate both serially and concurrently. The power of our analytic techniques for understanding complex motivated behavior has been evident for some time. However, the crucial point is that we are now able to map these components with increasing certainty onto discrete amygdaloid, and other limbic cortical-ventral striatal subsystems. The neural dissection of these mechanisms also serves an important theoretical purpose in helping to validate the various hypothetical constructs and further developing theory. Major challenges remain, not the least of which is an understanding of the operation of the ventral striatum together with its dopaminergic innervation and its interactions with the basolateral amygdala, hippocampal formation, and prefrontal cortex at a more mechanistic, neuronal level.

[d]Voice: +44-1223-333583; fax +44-1223-333548; bje10@cus.cam.ac.uk

INTRODUCTION

Neuroanatomical Considerations

Lennart Heimer and his colleagues, through their innovative neuroanatomical investigations over many years, have radically altered the ways in which the amygdaloid nuclear complex and the nucleus accumbens (NAcc) are viewed. In a quite remarkable series of observations, it was demonstrated that the NAcc is part of a larger structure, the ventral striatum, thereby assimilating the NAcc within the broader context of the striatum and drawing it away from the septal nuclei and more intimate associations with the limbic forebrain.[1,2] One consequence of defining this striatal affinity of the NAcc was an appreciation that, like the rest of the striatum, its major afferents originate from the cortical mantle.[1] However, whereas the dorsal striatum received primarily neocortical afferents, those reaching the ventral striatum, including the NAcc, originated in allocortical and periallocortical areas, such as the hippocampal formation, entorhinal area, and olfactory cortex, as well as from the medial and lateral proisocortical areas, such as the anterior cingulate, prelimbic, and agranular insular cortex.[1,3,4] Moreover, Carlsen and Heimer[5] emphasized that the basolateral amygdala, although not on the surface of the brain and without an obvious laminar structure, is nonetheless a quasicortical structure that also projects richly to the nucleus accumbens. Such observations led directly to a new conceptualization of the NAcc as a "limbic-motor interface"[6] —a rather strange anatomical notation that was meant to convey a functional mechanism by which affective or emotional information gained access to behavioral output, yet which has transformed approaches to the anatomical and functional analysis of the limbic system and emotional behavior.

Having integrated the NAcc within the striatum, it became progressively clear that it is nevertheless a remarkably heterogeneous structure, both histochemically and in terms of its connections, being separable into a core (which has marked striatal characteristics and merges imperceptibly with the overlying caudate-putamen) and a more medial and ventral shell.[2,7–15] The shell, in addition to having a dopaminergic innervation from the ventral tegmental area (VTA), that has different characteristics from that innervating the core,[16] is also distinguished by having efferent projections that not only reach the ventral pallidum (as do efferents from the core), but also the lateral hypothalamus and bed nucleus of the stria terminalis (BNST).[2,13,17,18] Thus, the NAcc shell is apparently not a simple striatal structure but has additional features that indicate a "transitional" organization—but transitional with what?

The latest, and in many ways, most provocative contribution in this revisionist neuroanatomical story concerns the concept of the "extended amygdala."[19] As is discussed elsewhere in this volume, this is an extension of the central and medial nuclei of the amygdala, not only into the bed nucleus of the stria terminalis, which had long been appreciated, but—more controversially—through the basal forebrain (the subcommissural extended amygdala), incorporating the interstitial nucleus of the posterior limb of the anterior commissure (IPAC) and encroaching on the NAcc shell itself.[2,19,20] Thus the shell may be viewed as a complex admixture of striatal neurons and neurons of the extended central amygdala, sharing with it a variety of histochemical features and connections.[2] Notable among the commonalities in the afferent connections of the central nucleus of the amygdala (in the temporal lobe) and the NAcc shell are a rich dopaminergic innervation arising from the VTA and a dense innervation from the basolateral complex of the amygdala.[2,19] These central amygdaloid characteristics of parts of the NAcc shell must also be considered in the context of the striatal characteristics of the central nucleus of the amygdala, Swanson and Petrovich[21] suggesting that the central nucleus is, in fact, a specialized autonomic-projecting region of the striatum.

Functional Implications

These neuroanatomical observations have driven a fundamental reassessment of the functions of the amygdaloid nuclear complex and the ventral striatum in two major ways. First, because a significant projection to the nucleus accumbens core and shell arises from the basolateral parts of the amygdala, it appears logical to investigate possible commonalities in their functions, as suggested by Mogenson[6] and also by Alexander *et al.*,[22] who speculated about this "affective loop" in their general scheme of cortico-striato-pallido-thalamo-cortical circuitry. As we have discussed previously,[23] investigations of the functions of the ventral striatum (especially the NAcc) and of the amygdala have come from somewhat different traditions. Thus, research on the NAcc has primarily sought to identify the neural substrates of reinforcement or incentive, and this endeavour has only marginally implicated the amygdala or, indeed, other limbic structures. This research goal was fueled initially by the phenomenon of intracranial self-stimulation from medial forebrain sites but now is generally focused on the role of dopamine-dependent processes of the ventral striatum.[23,24] As discussed elsewhere in this volume, advances in understanding the neural and neurochemical mode of action of drugs of abuse, such as the psychomotor stimulants and opiates, has strengthened the view that the NAcc is a critical substrate for the rewarding effects of many drugs of abuse and perhaps those of natural reinforcers, such as food and sex.[23,25-28]

By contrast, experimental investigations of the functions of the amygdala have proceeded rather in parallel with the evolution of the concept that the amygdala is implicated in the processes by which environmental stimuli are invested with affective value.[29] Despite many studies demonstrating the importance of the amygdala in the formation of stimulus-reward associations,[23,30,31] there is a widely held view that the amygdala is especially concerned with aversive learning, forming the central component of the brain's fear system.[32-35] However, there are strong grounds for integrating these different strands of research into a more general scheme of the neural basis of emotion.

Second, the proposition that the NAcc shell and centrolateral amygdala are components of a common system, the extended amygdala, raises the question of its possible functions. Does the extended amygdala function as an entity, or do the temporal lobe and basal forebrain components function in a coordinated way to subserve common processes through their shared connectivities? These are difficult questions to approach experimentally, because the neuroanatomical position and extent of the extended amygdala prevent discrete manipulations of its entirety using either psychopharmacological, *in vivo* neurochemical, or lesioning approaches. However, another approach is to manipulate the temporal lobe (amygdala) and basal forebrain (NAcc, BNST) components of the extended amygdala separately within the same behavioral paradigms in order to assess the degree to which there are commonalities in functional effects. This approach is being adopted with success in the context of drug abuse and anxiety research (see Koob and Davis, this volume) to reveal some commonalities of function within temporal and basal forebrain components of the extended amygdala.

Experimental Approach

In the studies summarized here, we have adopted a similar strategy within our investigation of the neural basis of associative mechanisms that are of fundamental importance in the control of incentive motivation, in general, but which also have specific importance for understanding the ways in which drug-associated cues can induce drug craving and control drug-seeking behavior. Thus we have compared the effects of manipulations of the NAcc core and shell, central (CeA) and basolateral (BLA) nuclei of the amygdala, as well as related limbic cortical structures that contribute to the associative processes through which otherwise neutral environmental stimuli acquire motivational salience and thereby control appetitive goal-directed, or instrumental, behavior via ventral striatopallidal circuitry. The pattern of results is summarized in TABLE 1.

APPETITIVE PAVLOVIAN CONDITIONING

The ability of an animal to associate significant biological and motivational events in the environment with cues that may predict those events is clearly adaptive and will aid survival. Such mechanisms may be subserved by relatively simple pavlovian-associative learning rules. Whereas the amygdala has long been known to be involved in pavlovian-conditioning mechanisms, mostly through studies of conditioned fear[33,36–38] but also in appetitive settings,[23,29,39,40] much less is known about the role of the nucleus accumbens in this form of learning, although it has been shown that dopamine release is increased in the nucleus accumbens during aversive conditioning.[41–44] The anterior cingulate cortex and hippocampal formation, both major sources of afferents to the NAcc, have also been implicated in different forms of aversive conditioning,[38,45–47] suggesting that limbic cortical and ventral striatal structures may be differentially involved in associative, information processing that underlies motivational influences on behavior.

Whereas in aversive-conditioning experiments, pavlovian-conditioned responses are readily elicited and quantified (e.g., freezing and startle), this is not so straightforward in appetitive tasks. In the present experiments, we have focused on an "autoshaping" task, in order to provide a relatively easily measurable appetitive pavlovian-conditioned response (approach behavior) and to minimize the contributions of other learning mechanisms in the process by which environmental stimuli are associated with primary reward and thereby gain motivational salience. The apparatus, procedure, and theoretical basis of this task have been discussed in more detail elsewhere.[48] Briefly, a visual stimulus is presented on a VDU, which is then followed by the delivery of food in a different spatial location noncontingently with respect to the animal's behavior. Over training, animals develop a conditioned response of approaching the CS predictive of food before returning to the food hopper to retrieve

TABLE 1. Summary of main results[a]

	Acc DA	CeN	BLA	NAcc core	NAcc shell	Ant Cing	VSub
Autoshaping	↓	↓	NE	↓	NE	↓	NE
Conditioned reinforcement	NE	NE	↓	↓	NE	ND	NE
Amphetamine-potentiation of CRf	↓	↓	NE	NE	↓	ND	↓

[a]Summary of the effects of selective lesions of amygdaloid nuclei and nucleus accumbens regions on pavlovian-approach behavior (autoshaping), conditioned reinforcement, and its potentiation by intra-accumbens D-amphetamine. Downward arrows, impaired; NE, no effect; ND, no data; Acc DA, NAcc dopamine depletion; CeN, central amygdala; BLA, basolateral amygdala; NAcc core/shell, nucleus accumbens core/shell; Ant Cing, anterior cingulate cortex; VSub, ventral subiculum.

the primary reward. This preparatory approach behavior is deemed to be under the control of pavlovian mechanisms, as it lacks the behavioral flexibility of instrumental, goal-directed actions[49] and has been described as a form of sign tracking.[50]

Bilateral, excitotoxic lesions of the BLA had no effect on the acquisition of autoshaping (FIG. 1). By contrast, bilateral lesions of the CeA greatly impaired autoshaping, such that lesioned animals did not increase their approaches to the CS+ (FIG. 1). This dissociation of the effects of lesions of the central and basolateral amygdala on appetitive pavlovian conditioning parallels our earlier data in an aversive task, in which CeA lesions impaired conditioned suppression, while BLA lesions did not.[37]

The effects of CeA lesions on autoshaping were not mirrored by selective excitotoxic lesions of the NAcc shell, which were without effect on autoshaping (FIG. 1), but had other behavioral effects (see below). Thus, this is one instance in which lesions of the temporal and putative NAcc shell components of the extended amygdala do not have a common effect. By contrast, specific lesions of the NAcc core profoundly disrupted autoshaping (FIG. 1).

Clearly, manipulations of both the amygdala and ventral striatum impaired the acquisition of discriminated approach behavior, but these results are difficult to understand within a clear neuroanatomical framework; there is no direct connection between the CeA and NAcc core. To understand what the relationship between these structures might be, it is necessary to look more widely at the neural mechanisms underlying this form of pavlovian conditioning. It is now well established that the anterior, but not posterior, cingulate cortex is critically important for the formation of stimulus-reward associations.[48] We have shown previously that lesions of the anterior cingulate cortex profoundly impair the acquisition of autoshaping[48,51] (see FIG. 1). Moreover, in elegant electrophysiological experiments, Gabriel and colleagues have demonstrated the involvement of the same area of cortex early in aversive-pavlovian conditioning.[52,53] Because our neuroanatomical investigations confirmed that the anterior cingulate cortex is a major source of projections to the NAcc core, we investigated the possible relationship between the two structures in the context of appetitive-pavlovian conditioning by making a "disconnection lesion,"[54] which consists of a unilateral lesion of the anterior cingulate cortex and a contralateral, unilateral lesion of the NAcc core. If these two structures are part of a functional, corticostriatal circuit subserving this form of learning, then the disconnection lesion should disrupt autoshaping in the same way as did bilateral lesions of

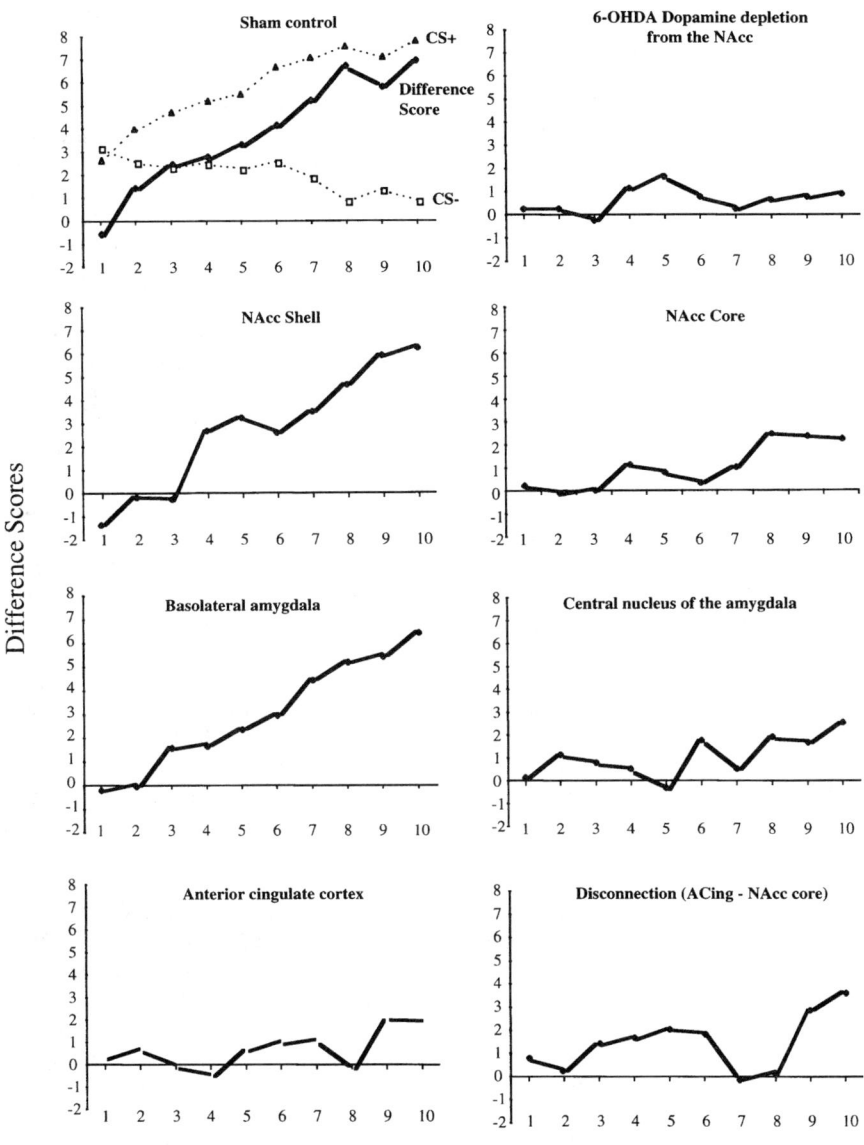

FIGURE 1. The effects of amygdala, nucleus accumbens and cingulate cortex manipulations on pavlovian-approach behavior measured in an autoshaping task. The top left panel shows the acquisition of autoshaping in control subjects, and it can be seen that, over 10 blocks of 10 trials, rats come selectively to approach the CS+ (which is paired with food reward) and to withhold approaches to the CS–. This is also expressed as the difference between CS+ vs. CS– approaches (difference score). This measure alone is then shown in all other panels, which show the effects of a variety of highly specific, excitotoxic lesions to

either structure alone. In fact, as FIGURE 1 shows, this is exactly what happened: the disconnection lesions greatly impaired autoshaping in a way that reflected the specific effects of each lesion. This provides strong evidence for a functional interconnectedness between the anterior cingulate cortex and ventral striatum. But how does the CeA fit into this picture? This is an important question, inasmuch as these studies together indicate that each of these structures is necessary, but not sufficient, for autoshaping to develop.

The answer may involve regulation of the dopaminergic innervation of the NAcc by the CeA. There are clear projections from the CeA to the VTA and substantia nigra. Dopaminergic lesions of the CeA,[55,56] or infusions of dopamine receptor antagonists into the amygdala, have marked effects upon extracellular dopamine levels in the Nacc and cocaine self-administration.[57,58] Moreover, a disconnection lesion of the CeA and the dopaminergic innervation of the dorsolateral striatum has been shown to impair the acquisition of a conditioned-orienting response.[59] In unpublished studies (Parkinson, Bamford, Fehnert, Dalley, Robbins, and Evcritt, 1998), we have also shown that dopamine depletion from the NAcc (by intra-accumbens injection of 6-hydroxydopamine) abolishes the acquisition of autoshaping (FIG. 1).

These results suggest a distributed neural network underlying pavlovian-approach behavior that involves the anterior cingulate cortex, NAcc core, CeA, and mesolimbic dopamine system (FIG. 2). The anterior cingulate cortex may be of prime importance in this network, as it projects not only to the NAcc core, but also to the CeA, which has been suggested to be the route via which this cortical area influences autonomic responses (see also ref. 21). It might be hypothesized that the anterior cingulate cortex–NAcc core system mediates associative processes and gives direction to the behavioral response (somewhat consistent with Mogenson's notion), but that information about appetitive stimuli also impinges on the CeA, which may orchestrate not only autonomic and endocrine responses,[60] but also arousal processes, resulting in behavioral activation through the mesolimbic dopamine system[23] that will influence the coupling of the cingulate cortex with accumbens medium spiny neurons. In addition—and perhaps early in conditioning—the CeA will engage attentional mechanisms through interactions with the basal forebrain cholinergic system, inasmuch as this has also been shown to be an important aspect of the function of this component of the amygdaloid complex (see Holland,[61] for review). Further understanding of these processes requires additional experimentation, most especially to understand the specificity of the effects of manipulations of each of the components of this network on the development of the pavlovian-approach response. For example, it is uncertain whether impairments in autoshaping reflect disruption of the associative process per se or the orchestration and coupling of response mechanisms. Prevailing data would implicate the anterior cingulate cortex in the former[48,53,62] and the NAcc core with its dopaminergic innervation in the latter.[63–65]

---

limbic cortical–ventral striatal structures, as well as 6-hydroxydopamine-induced dopaminergic lesions of the NAcc. It can be seen that BLA and NAcc shell lesions are without effect on autoshaping. By contrast, dopamine depletion from the NAcc, lesions of the CeA, NAcc core, and anterior cingulate cortex all significantly impair autoshaping. The bottom right panel shows that a unilateral lesion of the anterior cingulate cortex coupled with a contralateral lesion of the NAcc core ("disconnection") has the same effect of impairing pavlovian approach as bilateral lesions of either structure alone.

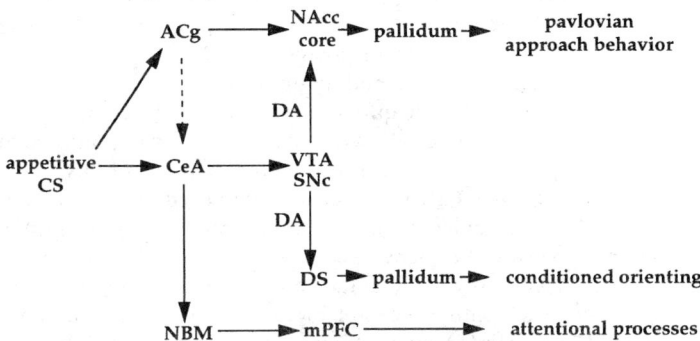

FIGURE 2. A schematic diagram of the neural network underlying aspects of pavlovian-approach behavior based upon the data presented in FIG. 1 and also the data from Gallagher, Holland, and coworkers (see ref. 67). The anterior cingulate cortex (ACg), NAcc core, CeA, and also the dopaminergic innervation of the NAcc are all necessary, but not sufficient, to support the development of pavlovian-approach behavior. We hypothesize that the anterior cingulate cortex and NAcc core are part of a cortico-striatal loop that subserves conditioning per se, that is, subserves informational processes that give direction to approach behavior. We also hypothesize that there is a relationship between the CeA and ventral tegmental area (VTA) dopamine neurons innervating the NAcc, which is also engaged by appetitive conditioned stimuli to activate, or "energize" pavlovian-approach response tendencies (see text for details). In separate, but related experiments, Gallagher, Holland, and colleagues have shown that the CeA is involved in conditioned-orienting responses that depend on corrections via the substantia nigra (SNC) to the dorsal striatum (DS) and in an attentional mechanism and that has been shown to depend upon projections to the cholinergic nucleus basalis magnocellularis (NBM) and thus to the neocortex, especially the medial prefrontal cortex (mPFC).

The CeA, however, may have many more complex functions that transcend associative,[37,66] response selection,[60] attentional,[67] and arousal[68,69] processes. There is little, however, to suggest that any of these processes occur within the NAcc shell, with which the CeA has neuroanatomical and connectional affinity.

CONDITIONED REINFORCEMENT

Appetitive pavlovian-conditioned stimuli not only elicit behavioral arousal and approach responses, but by acquiring some of the properties of a goal they gain motivational salience and thereby control over instrumental behavior as conditioned reinforcers.[70–72] We have studied this pavlovian-to-instrumental transfer of control using a procedure that isolates the conditioned reinforcement process, namely the acquisition of a new instrumental response with conditioned reinforcement.[70,72] Briefly, there are two phases to the procedure. First, rather as in the autoshaping procedure, a neutral stimulus (light, sound, or a compound of both) is paired with primary reward (we have used water in thirsty subjects, sucrose in hungry subjects, or intravenous cocaine), and the development of pavlovian conditioning is assessed by measuring discriminated approach to the CS+. In the second phase, which is carried out in extinction (thereby removing any influence of primary reinforcement), two novel levers enter the testing chamber; responding on one of them (CRf lever) results in presentation of the light CS+. Responding on the second lever (NCRf lever) has no programmed consequence. The acquired motivational valence of the CS to serve as a conditioned reinforcer is therefore assessed by its ability to reinforce the acquisition of this novel and arbitrary response. An important aspect of this process is that the control over behavior by a CRf is powerfully amplified by psychomotor stimulants;[71,73] indeed, this is a fundamentally important property of such drugs,[23,64,74] and this effect has been shown to depend critically upon the dopaminergic innervation of the NAcc.[75] However, even in the face of extensive dopamine depletion from the NAcc,[75] or general dopamine receptor blockade,[76] rats still acquire a new response with conditioned reinforcement, that is, the mesolimbic dopamine system does not mediate conditioned reinforcement but only its potentiation by stimulant drugs. Thus, information about conditioned reinforcers must be derived from another source, presumably one transferring such information to the NAcc, where its impact can be gain amplified by increases in dopamine transmission.[77]

Encouraged by the neuroanatomical data of Heimer, Nauta and Kelley, and Groenewegen,[1,3,4] we investigated the effects on the acquisition of a new response procedure of manipulations of the limbic cortical structures that are the likely sources of information about environmental stimuli, namely the BLA, hippocampal formation, and medial prefrontal cortex.[78–80] Although prelimbic cortex lesions were without effect on responding with conditioned reinforcement, BLA lesions and also lesions of the ventral subiculum, had marked and differential effects (FIGURES 3, A and B). Rats with selective BLA lesions were impaired in their acquisition of a new response, failing to respond selectively upon the CRf lever (FIG. 3B); thus although BLA lesions were without effect on pavlovian conditioning (see also **APPETITIVE PAVLOVIAN CONDTIONING**, above), the pavlovian-to-instrumental transfer of control over behavior by the CS was blocked and, as a consequence, gain amplifying effects on conditioned reinforcement of intra-NAcc infusions of D-amphetamine were greatly attenuated (FIG. 3B). These results are consistent with a burgeoning literature that shows marked effects of BLA lesions on the control over instrumental behavior by pavlovian-conditioned stimuli using a variety of behavioral procedures, including so-called conditioned-place preference, a superficially simple task that, in fact, embodies both pavlovian approach behavior and instrumental response contingencies.[23,37,81–83] By contrast, lesions of the ventral subiculum did not affect the conditioned-reinforcement effect (lesioned subjects still responded selectively on the CRf lever), but the potentiative effects of intra-accumbens amphetamine on the control over behavior by the conditioned reinforcer were abolished (FIG. 3A), in parallel with the locomotor stimulant effects of amphetamine.[78]

Thus, whereas the BLA and ventral subiculum sources of afferents to the ventral striatum are both essential for pavlovian-to-instrumental transfer and its potentiation by increased activity in the mesolimbic dopamine system, their roles are clearly dissociable: (1) the BLA is part of the mechanism whereby pavlovian-conditioned stimuli control instrumental behavior as conditioned reinforcers and the integrity of this process is fundamental to the potentiative effects of stimulant drugs on conditioned reinforcement; (2) the ventral subicular outflow from the hippocampal formation to the NAcc is essential for the potentiation of locomotor activity and conditioned re-

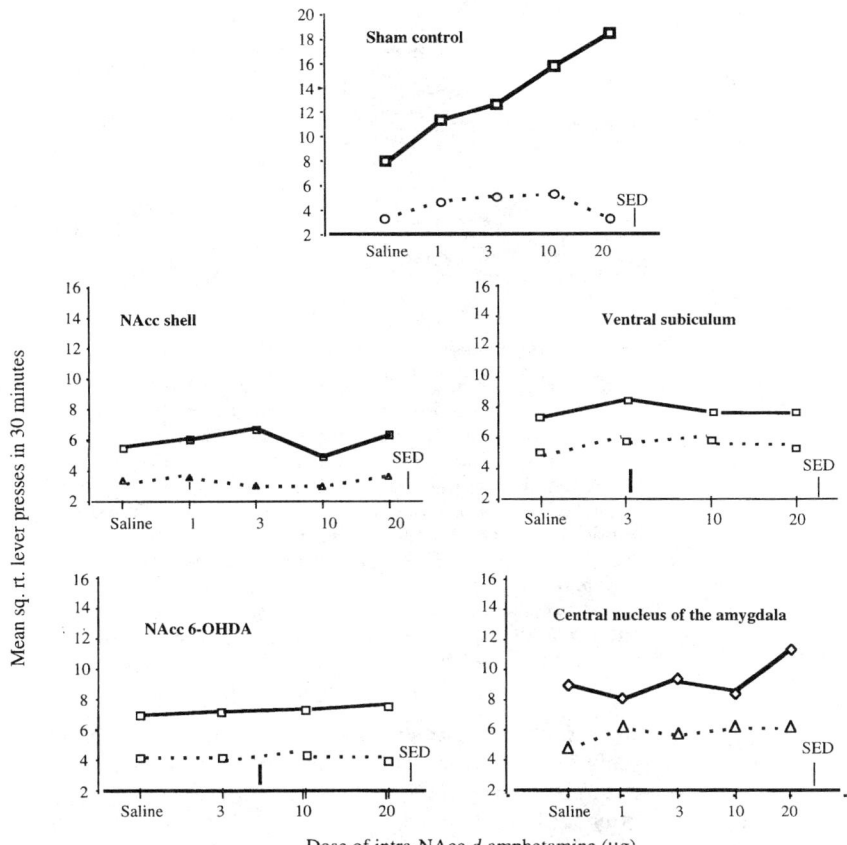

FIGURE 3A. The effects of NAcc dopamine depletion (NAcc 6-OHDA) or selective, excitotoxic lesions of the NAcc shell, ventral subiculum, or central nucleus of the amygdala on the acquisition of instrumental responding with conditioned reinforcement (CRf). The top panel shows the acquisition of a new response with CRf in control subjects. The continuous line represents responding on the lever that results in presentation of the CS+ (CRf lever); the dotted line represents responding on the control lever (NCRf lever). As can be seen, rats respond selectively on the CRf lever under control conditions (infusion of saline into the NAcc), and this responding is dose-dependently potentiated by D-amphetamine infused into the nucleus accumbens. By comparing with the top panel, it can be seen that each of the manipulations in the remaining four panels have a common effect: (1) to abolish the potential effects of intra-Acc D-amphetamine but (2) not to affect the choice behavior controlled by conditioned reinforcement itself. Thus, these lesions do not impair the acquisition of a new response with CRf per se, only its potentiation by stimulant drugs that act by increasing dopamine transmission in the NAcc. SED, standard error of the difference of the means; sq. rt., square root.[75,78,79,84,94]

inforcement by stimulant drugs, but does not mediate informational aspects of the conditioned reinforcement process itself. We have hypothesized that the contribution

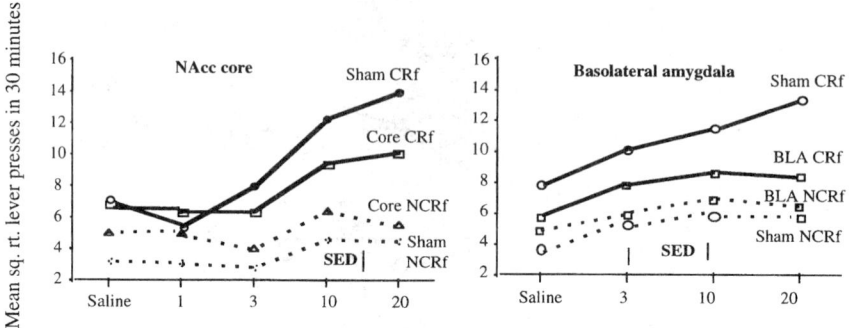

FIGURE 3B. The effects of selective excitotoxic lesions of the NAcc core or basolateral amygdala (BLA) on the acquisition of responding with conditioned reinforcement and its potentiation by intra-accumbens infusions of D-amphetamine. The data are presented as in FIG. 3A, except that control data are shown along with lesion data in each panel. The main effect of both core and BLA lesions is to impair the selectivity of responding and its potentiation of the CRf lever, that is, impair the acquisition of a new response. This is seen especially under saline conditions in BLA-lesioned rats, that is, there is no difference between responses on the CRf and NCRf levers (responding is lower on the CRf lever and higher on the NCRf lever), and the potential effects of intra-NAcc D-amphetamine are correspondingly impaired. In core-lesioned rats, the lack of selectivity in responding is seen somewhat under saline conditions, but also at the two lower doses of intra-Acc D-amphetamine, and is due primarily to increased responses on the NCRf lever.[78,79,84]

of ventral subicular processes to this potentiation may be to provide the contextual background upon which the potentiation of locomotor activity and conditioned reinforcement depend (see FIG. 4); we return to this further, below.

We have recently extended our investigation of the neural basis of conditioned reinforcement and its potentiation by psychomotor stimulants in the light of the neuroanatomical data showing differentiation of the NAcc into a core and shell, the affinities between shell and CeA (extended amygdala), and the functional dissociations within the amygdala of pavlovian and instrumental conditioning.[37,61] First, we have been able to demonstrate that the potentiative effects of amphetamine on conditioned reinforcement depend upon the NAcc shell, but not the core.[84] Thus, selective excitotoxic lesions of the shell abolished the effects of intra-accumbens amphetamine (and significantly attenuated the locomotor stimulant effects of systemic amphetamine) but did not interfere with the control over instrumental behavior by the conditioned reinforcer (FIG. 3A). These effects of shell lesions are remarkably similar to those of ventral subiculum lesions (see FIG. 3A), an observation that is of interest in the context of the strong preferential glutamatergic projection from the ventral subiculum to that part of the NAcc shell (septal pole) which was lesioned in these experiments. Thus, information reaching the NAcc concerned with the nature and direction of behavior, which depends upon the integrity of the BLA,[78,79] presumably via its projections to both the NAcc core and shell,[85,86] may be "gain amplified" by dopamine transmission in the shell in a way that is critically dependent on the integrity of its glutamatergic inputs arising from the ventral subiculum.[78,87–89]

The effects of excitotoxic NAcc core lesions were more complex. First, unlike shell lesions, core lesions retarded reattainment of criterion levels of the pavlovian discriminated approach that preceded the acquisition of a new response, as expected from the autoshaping data summarized above. Second, although NAcc core lesions did not significantly affect the acquisition of responding with conditioned reinforcement under saline conditions (FIG. 3B), the interaction between intra-NAcc D-amphetamine and responding with conditioned reinforcement was affected by lesions of the NAcc core, in that there was a loss of selectivity in the potentiation of responding (FIG. 3B). In FIGURE 3B it can also be seen that animals with lesions of the BLA showed similar impairments,[78, 79] including a loss of control over responding for the CRf under control conditions. We have reported previously similar effects of manipulations of the NAcc and BLA,[23, 80, 90] and this has led us to suggest that the integrity of the BLA is critical for stimulus-reward information to gain influence over voluntary behavior.[23, 24, 78] Thus limbic cortico-striatal circuits involving the BLA and NAcc core may be essential for the influence of associative stimulus-reward information on goal-directed action. The effects of NAcc shell lesions to abolish the potential effects of intra-NAcc D-amphetamine, whereas NAcc core lesions disrupt discriminative control following intra-NAcc infusions of D-amphetamine, bear some similarity to earlier models of striatal function based on separate striatal domains being responsible for "choice" and "vigor."[91–93] However, in animals with NAcc shell lesions and an intact NAcc core, intra-NAcc infusions of D-amphetamine dose-dependently increased magazine approach during the acquisition of a new response with conditioned reinforcement, suggesting that the dopaminergic innervation of the NAcc core may not only modulate the direction of behavioral responses, but also the vigor of pavlovian responses.

One final piece of data completes our current picture of the neural network that underlies conditioned reinforcement and its dopaminergic amplification; this concerns the CeA. Excitotoxic lesions of the CeA did not impair responding with conditioned reinforcement but, like lesions of the NAcc shell and ventral subiculum, completely abolished the effects of intra-NAcc infusions of D-amphetamine[94] (FIG. 3A). This demonstrates an intimate relationship between the CeA and the mesolimbic dopaminergic innervation of the nucleus accumbens—and specifically the shell, so far as the potentiation by stimulants of responding with conditioned reinforcement is concerned.

Therefore, the extended amygdala (CeA and NAcc shell) appears to mediate important effects of psychostimulant drugs. However, the basis of the interaction between the CeA and NAcc shell remains decidedly uncertain. Most likely the CeA, via its projections to the midbrain dopamine neurons, regulates the dopaminergic system innervating the NAcc shell, mediating stimulant drug effects, and core, modulating pavlovian-approach behavior. It is difficult to postulate another mechanism by which damage to the CeA can so effectively prevent the conditioned reinforcement potentiation that follows intra-accumbens infusions of D-amphetamine. Intra-amygdala infusions of D1 dopamine receptor antagonists result in marked changes in extracellular dopamine levels in the NAcc.[58] Moreover, infusions of the D3 receptor agonist 7-OHDPAT into the CeA, but not BLA, significantly enhance stimulus-reward learning.[95, 96] Thus, the evidence to date appears to support an intimate functional relationship between the CeA and NAcc shell, though not in terms of its

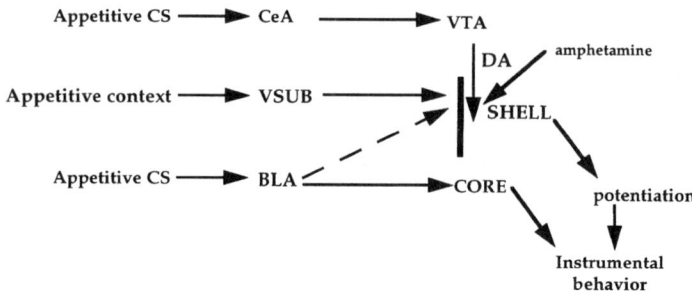

FIGURE 4. A schematic diagram of the neural network underlying conditioned reinforcement and its potentiation by intra-accumbens D-amphetamine, based upon the data presented in Figures 3A and 3B. The pavlovian-to-instrumental transfer of control over behavior, whereby a pavlovian CS+ supports the acquisition of a new response as a conditioned reinforcer, depends upon the integrity of the BLA and NAcc core (CORE); there are rich projections from the BLA to this area of the NAcc. Lesions of either BLA or NAcc core do not directly affect the potentiative effects of D-amphetamine, other than by reducing the conditioned reinforcement effect itself. By contrast, the NAcc shell (SHELL) and CeA appear to be critical substrates for the potentiative effect of D-amphetamine on CRf, but not the pavlovian-to-instrumental transfer of control of behavior by the CS, ultimately acting as a conditioned reinforcer. As in FIG. 2, we hypothesize that the commonality in effects of NAcc shell and CeA lesions, supportive of the "extended amygdala" concept, depends upon regulatory influences of the CeA on the dopaminergic innervation of the NAcc shell via projections to the VTA dopamine cell bodies. The ventral subiculum is also critical for the effects of intra-Acc D-amphetamine on conditioned reinforcement. We hypothesize that this influence of the ventral subiculum depends upon known projections to the caudomedial NAcc shell. Although the BLA and CeA appear to be especially concerned with discrete CS processing, we further hypothesize, based on neuropsychological data, that the ventral subiculum provides contextual information upon which the CRf potentiation effect is based. Clearly, then, there is an interaction between the BLA and ventral subiculum in determining the control over behavior by a conditioned reinforcer and its potentiation by increasing dopaminergic activity in the NAcc shell, and this interaction may be subserved by convergent projections onto NAcc shell neurons.

functioning as an integrated continuum across the basal forebrain. FIGURE 4 represents an attempt to summarize the complex relationships between the basolateral and central amygdala, NAcc core and shell, and also the hippocampal formation in the control over voluntary, goal-directed behavior by pavlovian-conditioned stimuli and its potentiation by psychomotor stimulant drugs acting on the mesolimbic dopamine system.

DRUG CUES, THE AMYGDALA, AND DRUG-SEEKING BEHAVIOR

Cues associated with drugs abused by humans, especially stimulants such as cocaine, acquire powerful motivational effects.[97,98] These drug-associated cues can induce strong cravings for the drug and are considered to be major factors in precipitating drug-seeking behavior and relapse to a drug-taking habit.[99,100] The strength of this conditioned influence on addictive behavior may lie in the fact that,

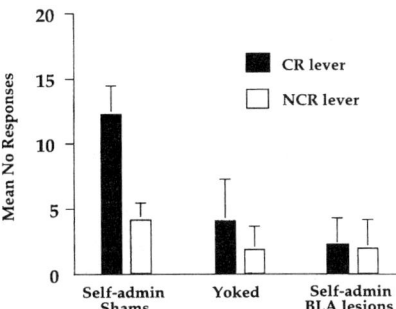

FIGURE 5. The acquisition of responding with conditioned reinforcement in which the CS+ was a cue paired with iv cocaine. In one group of rats, cocaine was self-administered by a nose-poke response (Self-admin Shams), that is, cocaine was contingently administered and each infusion paired with a light CS+. The Yoked group received exactly the same number and pattern of cocaine infusions but without any response contingency (being yoked to a "master" self-administering rat). The data show that only in the case of the master rats did the cocaine cue serve as a conditioned reinforcer to support the acquisition of a new response. This result suggests strongly that having control over the administration of iv cocaine is an important determinant of its rewarding effects. An additional group of rats self-administering cocaine had BLA lesions, which prevented the acquisition of responding reinforced by presentations of the cocaine-paired CS+ (cf. FIG. 3B, right panel).

having precipitated relapse to drug seeking, the renewed self-administration of drugs like cocaine will not only serve to strengthen the conditioned properties of the drug cue but also amplify its impact on behavior, as illustrated in our experiments on the potentiation of conditioned reinforcement by stimulants acting on dopamine transmission in the NAcc.

In a preliminary experiment, we have demonstrated that a light paired with intravenous (iv) cocaine can acquire conditioned reinforcing properties using basically the same acquisition of a new instrumental response procedure described above. However, in this experiment an additional variable was manipulated; that of the contingency of the drug administration. In one group of subjects, a nose-poke response resulted in the iv self-administration of cocaine that was paired with the illumination of a light (the CS+). Thus, in this group the pavlovian pairing of light with the drug effect followed the iv self-administration of cocaine. A second group of rats was yoked to this group, such that they received identical numbers of iv cocaine-light CS pairings, but without any response contingency. A third group also self-administered cocaine but had sustained bilateral excitotoxic lesions of the BLA. The results are summarized in FIGURE 5. It is clear that in the group self-administering cocaine the CS paired with the drug was able to support the learning of a new instrumental response, that is, had acquired conditioned reinforcing properties. Lesions of the BLA completely prevented this, as we had predicted from our earlier work.[78,79] However, at first sight, a surprising result was that, in the yoked subjects, who had no control over their iv infusions of cocaine, the CS did not acquire conditioned-reinforcing properties. This observation emphasizes the importance of contingency as a determinant of the rewarding effects of cocaine, which is known to have mixed rewarding and aversive properties.[101] Thus, under the conditions of this experiment, the aversive (anxiogenic) effects of cocaine may have predominated in the situation in which the subjects had no control over the iv infusion of cocaine. Rats in the yoked group tended to display more arousal and more aggression on being removed from the test chambers at the end of conditioning sessions, and it may have been that the light CS had, in fact, acquired aversive properties, although this has yet to be studied directly.

How might such drug-associated cues be shown to control drug-seeking behavior in experimental animals? It has been demonstrated previously that monkeys will work for prolonged periods of time for cocaine, heroin, or food under second-order schedules of reinforcement in which primary reward-associated cues maintain instrumental behavior prior to the presentation of the primary reward itself.[102,103] We have successfully employed a second-order schedule of reinforcement to study sexual motivation in rats[104] and have recently adapted the procedure to investigate cocaine- and heroin-seeking behavior in rats.[83,105–107] An important principle in using second-order schedules of reinforcement is that it is possible to investigate the rewarding effects of drugs, and the role of drug-associated cues in maintaining drug seeking, in a way that is independent of the pharmacological effects of the drug. This is because the rats are never "primed" with noncontingent infusions of the drug and must work to complete the schedule-response requirements (e.g., respond for 15 min) in order to obtain a single infusion of the drug. During that time, responses are reinforced not only by the eventual infusion of the drug, but also by contingent presentations of the drug-associated cue. A typical cumulative record illustrates this in FIGURE 6.

There are some particularly interesting features of this drug-seeking behavior. Its dependence upon the contingent presentation of the cocaine-associated cue is affirmed by the observation that responding decreases to about 40% of the control level following the omission of the CS+ during each of three daily sessions (despite the fact that iv cocaine is still self-administered at the end of each of five daily fixed intervals of responding). Responding is promptly reestablished at baseline levels following reintroduction of the CS+.[105] Self-administered cocaine increases responding for the drug (see FIG. 6), but under conditions of CS omission, this increase in responding is significantly less than when the drug-associated CS is also presented.[105] This observation illustrates the importance of the interaction between drug cues and self-administered drug in controlling drug-seeking behavior, as discussed above (**CONDITIONED REINFORCEMENT**).

Rats with bilateral, excitotoxic lesions of the BLA could not acquire responding under a second-order schedule of cocaine reinforcement[83] (see FIG. 6); thus, the acquisition of drug-seeking behavior that depends upon presentation of drug-associated cues requires the integrity of this part of the amygdaloid complex, as does the acquisition of a new response with conditioned reinforcement.[78,79] However, BLA lesions did not impair the acquisition of iv cocaine self-administration itself; thus, these lesions did not directly impair the primary rewarding effects of cocaine so that drug-taking behavior was unaffected (or even facilitated).[83] It is apparently only when the behavior depends upon a drug CS that the impact of BLA lesions is revealed. Cocaine self-administration can readily be reinstated following extinction by the presentation of a CS associated with the drug, and this is used increasingly as a model of cue-mediated relapse.[105,108,109] Meil and See[109] have demonstrated that

A. Cumulative record of responding

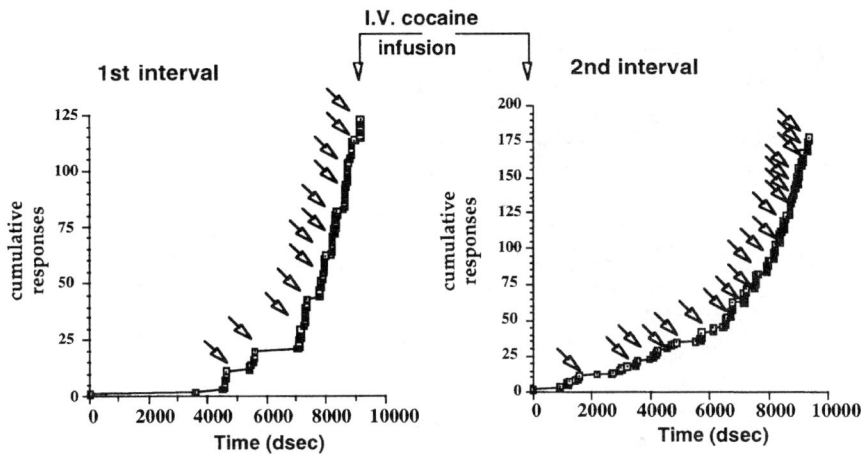

B. Effects of BLA lesions on acquisition

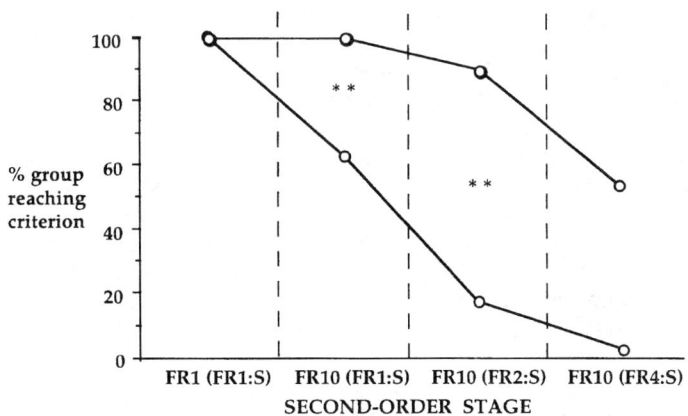

FIGURE 6. The self-administration of cocaine under a second-order schedule of reinforcement. **A:** The upper left panel cumulative record shows a rat responding over a period of 15 min (9000 deciseconds) for a single iv infusion of cocaine, during which time such behavior is maintained by contingent presentations of a cocaine cue (arrows). The iv infusion of cocaine markedly increases this cue-controlled drug-seeking behavior in the subsequent 15-min interval (upper right panel). **B:** Bilateral excitotoxic lesions of the BLA prevent the acquisition of the second-order schedule of cocaine-seeking behavior. The graph

cocaine-associated cues are ineffective in reinstating cocaine self-administration in rats with bilateral BLA lesions, further emphasizing the importance of this region of the amygdala in mediating such conditioned effects on drug-taking behavior. Taken together, these data strongly suggest that the BLA is part of the neural mechanism through which drug-associated conditioned stimuli can control instrumental behavior, presumably by interacting, directly or indirectly, with the ventral striatum, a primary site for the mediation of the rewarding effects of cocaine and other stimulants. We have also shown that rats will acquire responding under a second-order schedule of heroin self-administration, but in a way that is much less obviously dependent upon the contingent presentation of a heroin-associated CS.[107] Under these circumstances, BLA lesions had no effect on the acquisition of heroin-seeking behavior,[107] indicating that only when discrete drug cues support drug-seeking behavior is the BLA a critical structure. Moreover, these results suggest that the psychological processes and neural mechanisms underlying drug-seeking behavior may be different for addictive drugs of different pharmacological classes.

SYNTHESIS

The concept of the extended amygdala has provided a special challenge in terms of specifying what its functions might be and whether the entire continuum, from the temporal lobe through the basal forebrain to the BNST and caudo-medial shell, indeed functions in a unitary way. The data summarized here (see TABLE 1) suggest that the picture for natural behavior is not a simple one, but one consequence of the organization of these structures is that they mediate some of the effects of psychomotor stimulants. Thus, specific lesions of the caudo-medial shell of the NAcc or the CeA both were able to prevent completely the potentiative effects of D-amphetamine on responding with conditioned reinforcement. These results are compatible with several reports suggesting commonalities in the effects of stimulant drugs within the amygdala, presumably the CeA (which receives the majority of the dopaminergic afferents) and the NAcc, presumably the shell.[57,58,110] As discussed elsewhere in this volume, Koob and coworkers have hypothesized that the extended amygdala is a critical structure in which neuroadaptations underlie both the positive effects of many drugs of abuse and the opponent processes that are set in train following abstinence or withdrawal.[111-113] However, the precise mechanisms by which manipulations of the CeA influence drug reinforcement and conditioned reinforcement, whether directly or by virtue of the relationship of the CeA with the NAcc within the extended amygdala, remain unclear. As discussed above, interactions between the CeA and

---

shows the proportion of BLA-lesioned and control rats reaching each stage of training of the second-order schedule, during which the dependence upon presentation of the cocaine cue is progressively increased. For example, at FR1(FR1:S), each response results in an iv cocaine infusion and presentation of the light CS. At FR10(FR2:S), every second response results in presentation of the cocaine cue (CS+), and the rat must earn 10 such CS+ presentations before cocaine is self-administered. Very few BLA-lesioned rats progress beyond this stage, which is considerably less stringent than that shown in the upper panels, in which the CS+ is presented after every 10 responses and rats must continue responding for 15 minutes in order to obtain cocaine.[83,105]

the midbrain dopamine neurons projecting to the striatum seem to be the most likely explanation for many observations, but this has generally not been demonstrated directly except in the case of the disconnection effects revealed by Han et al.[59] Further neurobiological and behavioral studies should address this important issue. But it should also be emphasized that in several instances manipulations of the CeA and NAcc shell do not have common effects, for example, on pavlovian approach[114] or on instrumental behavior.[63] Lesions of the NAcc shell also do not affect aversive pavlovian conditioning,[115] whereas CeA lesions clearly do.[37,60] Similarly, manipulations of the BNST and CeA also have been suggested to have different, but related, effects on fear and anxiety (see Davis, this volume). Although it is important to consider the commonalities in structure and connections of the CeA and NAcc (and BNST), the differences should not be minimized, inasmuch as this will detract from a greater understanding of the functions of these heterogenous areas of the forebrain.

The experiments on appetitive pavlovian conditioning and on the pavlovian-to-instrumental transfer of control (conditioned reinforcement) procedure clearly illustrate the functional importance of "limbic" cortical-ventral striatal mechanisms. Using the disconnection paradigm, we have provided strong evidence for an anterior cingulate cortex-NAcc core system (or "loop") underlying appetitive pavlovian conditioning.[51] Our previous work has also established the comparable importance of interactions between the BLA and ventral striatum in the control over instrumental behavior by pavlovian-conditioned stimuli,[23] including the use of a disconnection procedure to reveal the importance of a BLA-NAcc system in the acquisition of a conditioned place preference.[54]

The data summarized above (**CONDITIONED REINFORCEMENT**; see also TABLE 1) also emphasize the importance of convergent interactions between parallel limbic cortical-ventral striatal systems, the neuroanatomical basis of which is only just becoming clear. For example, the potentiative effects of intra-NAcc D-amphetamine on responding with conditioned reinforcement depends critically upon associative information transferred from the BLA to the NAcc core, because this provides the means by which conditioned environmental stimuli control, or give direction to, instrumental behavior. However, the integrity of the ventral subiculum, which projects preferentially to the NAcc shell, is also critical for the potentiative effects of increased mesolimbic dopaminergic activity. Thus, the whole complexity of the process by which pavlovian-conditioned stimuli control goal-directed actions in a way that can be amplified by dopaminergic activation clearly depends upon interactions, perhaps within the ventral striatum, between these two limbic cortical structures, which are both sources of glutamatergic afferents to the core and shell. There is a clear neuroanatomical basis for such an interaction, because neurons in the ventral subiculum and basolateral amygdala, while having preferential patterns of termination in the NAcc core and shell, also show convergence onto the same medium spiny NAcc neurons.[116,117] Electrical stimulation of one of these projections can markedly affect the striatal neuronal response to coincident stimulation of the other in a way that seems to suggest the existence of neuronal ensembles in the NAcc that are addressed by afferents arising in both the BLA and hippocampal formation.[117] Moreover, these cortical interactions within the NAcc are themselves affected by changes in dopaminergic activity.[87–89,118] There are important theoretical, as well as functional, implications of these data, inasmuch as they suggest that limbic cortical-ventral striatopallidal loops are not simply parallel and segregated, as is generally agreed to be the case for neocortical-dorsal striatopallidal loops, but also show convergence within the ventral striatum. Interactions between the BLA and ventral subiculum within the NAcc core and shell that are also subject to modulation by the mesolimbic dopamine system are well illustrated in the pavlovian-to-instrumental transfer of control over behavior by conditioned stimuli and its potentiation by stimulants (see FIG. 4). These observations also have significant implications for understanding the ways in which drug-associated cues interact with stimulant drugs to control drug-seeking behavior and its reinstatement following drug-cue exposure.

An issue that arises out of the data summarized here is the evidence they provide in favor of amygdala subsystems with dissociable associative/behavioral functions. Thus, lesions of the BLA, but not CeA, markedly disrupted the acquisition of a new response with conditioned reinforcement; by contrast lesions of the CeA, but not BLA, severely impaired appetitive pavlovian conditioning. Thus, simple appetitive pavlovian conditioning and the pavlovian-to-instrumental transfer of control of behavior by a CS+ are doubly dissociable within the amygdala. This argues against the prevailing notion that the CeA does not itself subserve associative processes but relies upon such information relayed to it by the BLA. Indeed, consistent with the dissociations we have shown here, Gallagher, Holland, and colleagues have reported that CeA, but not BLA, lesions disrupt pavlovian-conditioned orienting, whereas BLA, but not CeA, lesions disrupt second-order conditioning,[66,119] which again strongly suggests the involvement of the CeA in pavlovian associations independently of antecedent processing of the CS and US in the lateral and basal nuclei of the amygdala.

We have reported similar dissociations in aversive pavlovian and instrumental conditioning. Thus, in a task that measures the acquisition of pavlovian-conditioned suppression and conditioned avoidance (an instrumental response) simultaneously, we have demonstrated that excitotoxic lesions of the CeA abolished pavlovian-conditioned suppression but were without effect on conditioned punishment (the performance of an action that results in the avoidance of a CS paired with mild foot shock).[37] By contrast, rats with BLA lesions were severely impaired in instrumental-avoidance behavior, but conditioned suppression was unaffected, again emphasizing that the integrity of the lateral and basal amygdala is not essential for the development of the pavlovian-conditioned responses. These data stand in contrast to those of LeDoux and colleagues, which clearly demonstrate the importance of the lateral amygdala in aversive-pavlovian conditioning, including the demonstration of LTP there.[120,121] We have discussed elsewhere[37] that part of the explanation of these apparently discrepant results may depend upon the number of CS–US pairings, which are traditionally very few (3–5) in conventional-conditioned freezing procedures, but that were substantially more in the experiments by Killcross et al.[37] and in the majority of appetitive-conditioning tasks.[48,66,114] These considerations are relevant to the debate concerning the relative importance of the BLA in the formation, as opposed to the storage, of emotional memories.[122,123]

Another aspect to this discussion of dissociable functions of amygdala subsystems based upon CeA or BLA circuitry concerns the affective valence of the conditioned response. It seems highly likely that simple aversive pavlovian-conditioned responses, such as freezing, depend upon well-established caudal projections from the CeA to brain stem motor nuclei, including the periaqueductal grey.[60,124] Indeed, influences of the CeA on appetitive pavlovian-conditioned responses, such as orienting and approach, may also depend upon projections to the brain stem, but perhaps more likely to the ventral tegmental dopaminergic neurons that activate or potentiate response mechanisms within the dorsal and ventral striatum.[59,84,114] However, instrumental behavior is more complex than the more automatic pavlovian responses, enabling an animal voluntarily to act on its environment so as to bring it into contact with a goal, or to avoid danger and predation. Perhaps forebrain projections from the BLA are more relevant in this regard, especially those to the striatum and orbitofrontal cortex, which would appear to provide the basis for voluntary emotional responses. Indeed, in appetitive settings, several experiments, including those summarized here, suggest the importance of such BLA–ventral striatal interactions.[23,78,79,81,90] However, this is a much less clear issue when considering instrumental responses in aversive situations. Although we have shown that amphetamine is able to enhance conditioned punishment, that is, enhance the control over instrumental behavior by aversive-conditioned stimuli,[125] there is no direct evidence that this effect depends upon actions of the drug within the NAcc or upon interactions between the BLA (lesions of which abolish the conditioned-punishment effect) and NAcc, thereby mirroring the conditioned-reinforcement effect and its potentiation. We have established that extracellular dopamine is increased in the ventral striatum during aversive conditioning,[42] but there have been few demonstrations that manipulations of the NAcc core (or shell) affect instrumental avoidance responses (but see ref. 126), although selective NAcc core lesions do impair aversive conditioning to discrete, but not contextual, cues when the behavioral measure is suppression of drinking.[115]

ACKNOWLEDGMENTS

This work was supported by an MRC Programme Grant (G9537855) to B.J.E., T.W.R., and A. Dickinson. J.A.P. was supported by a BBSRC research studentship and an Oon Khye Beng Ch'hia Tsio Scholarship. M.C.O. was supported by an HFSP Long-term Fellowship. P.R. was supported by the Hitchings-Elion Fellowship under the auspices of the Wellcome Trust. This research was conducted within the MRC Co-operative for Brain, Behavior and Neuropsychiatry.

REFERENCES

1. HEIMER, L. & R.D. WILSON. 1975. The subcortical projections of the allocortex: similarities in the neural associations of the hippocampus, the pyriform cortex and the neocortex. *In* Golgi Centennial Symposium. M. Santini, Ed.: 177–192. Raven Press. New York.
2. HEIMER, L. *et al.* 1997. The accumbens: beyond the core-shell dichotomy. J. Neuropsychiatry & Clin. Neurosci. **9:** 354–381.
3. KELLEY, A.E. *et al.* 1982. The amygdalostriatal projection in the rat—an anatomical study by anterogrde and retrograde tracing methods. Neuroscience **7:** 615–630.
4. GROENEWEGEN, H.J. *et al.* 1990. The anatomical relationship of the prefrontal cortex with the striatopallidal system, the thalamus and the amygdala: evidence for a parallel organization. Prog. Brain Res. **85:** 95–118.

5. CARLSEN, J. & L. HEIMER. 1986. The basolateral amygdaloid complex as a cortical-like structure. Brain Res. **441:** 377–380.
6. MOGENSON, G. *et al.* 1984. From motivation to action: functional interface between the limbic system and the motor system. Prog. Neurobiol. **14:** 69–97.
7. GROENEWEGEN, H.J. *et al.* 1989. The compartmental organization of the ventral striatum in the rat. *In* Neural Mechanisms in Disorders of Movement: Current Problems in Neurology, Vol. 19. A.R. Crossman & M.A. Sambrook, Eds.: 45–54. Libbey & Co. London.
8. JONGEN-RELO, A.L. *et al.* 1993. Evidence for a multicompartmental histochemical organization of the nucleus-accumbens in the rat. J. Comp. Neurol. **337:** 267–276.
9. JONGEN-RELO, A.L. *et al.* 1994. Immunohistochemical characterization of the shell and core territories of the nucleus-accumbens in the rat. Eur. J. Neurosci. **6:** 1255–1264.
10. MEREDITH, G.E. *et al.* 1996. Shell and core in monkey and human nucleus accumbens identified with antibodies to calbindin-D-28k. J. Comp. Neurol. **365:** 628–639.
11. VOORN, P. *et al.* 1989. Compartmental organization of the ventral striatum of the rat—Immunohistochemical distribution of enkephalin, substance-P, dopamine, and calcium-binding protein. J. Comp. Neurol. **289:** 189–201.
12. ZABORSZKY, L. *et al.* 1985. Cholecystokinin innervation of the ventral striatum—a morphological and radioimmunological study. Neuroscience **14:** 427.
13. ZAHM, D.S. & L. HEIMER. 1990. Two transpallidal pathways originating in the rat nucleus accumbens. J. Comp. Neurol. **302:** 437–446.
14. ZAHM, D.S. 1991. Compartments in rat dorsal and ventral striatum revealed following injection of 6-hydroxydopamine into the ventral mesencephalon. Brain Res. **552:** 164–169.
15. ZAHM, D.S. & J.S. BROG. 1992. On the significance of subterritories in the "accumbens" part of the rat ventral striatum. Neuroscience **50:** 751–767.
16. DEUTCH, A.Y. & D.S. CAMERON. 1992. Pharmacological characterization of dopamine systems in the nucleus accumbens core and shell. Neuroscience **46:** 49–56.
17. GROENEWEGEN, H.J. & F.T. RUSSCHEN. 1984. Organization of the efferent projections of the nucleus accumbens to pallidal, hypothalamic and mesencephalic structures. A tracing and immunohistochemical study in the cat. J. Comp. Neurol. **223:** 347–367.
18. HEIMER, L. *et al.* 1987. The ventral striatopallidal thalamic projection. I. The striatopallidal link originating in parts of the olfactory tubercle. J. Comp. Neurol. **255:** 571–591.
19. ALHEID, G.F. & L. HEIMER. 1988. New perspectives in basal forebrain organization of special relevance for neuropsychiatric disorders: the striatopallidal, amygdaloid and corticopetal components of the substantia innominata. Neuroscience **27:** 1–39.
20. DE OLMOS, J. 1990. Amygdala. *In* The Human Nervous System. G. Paxinos, Ed.: 583–755. Academic Press. New York.
21. SWANSON, L.W. & G.D. PETROVICH. 1998. What is the amygdala? Trends Neurosci. **21:** 323–331.
22. ALEXANDER, G.E. *et al.* 1986. Parallel organization of functionally segregated circuits linking basal ganglia and cortex. Annu. Rev. Neurosci. **9:** 357–381.
23. EVERITT, B.J. & T.W. ROBBINS. 1992. Amygdala-ventral striatal interactions and reward-related processes. *In* The Amygdala. J.P. Aggleton, Ed.: 401–430. John Wiley & Sons Inc. New York.
24. ROBBINS, T.W. & B.J. EVERITT. 1996. Neurobehavioral mechanisms of reward and motivation. Curr. Opin. Neurobiol. **6:** 228–236.
25. ALTMAN, J. *et al.* 1996. The biological, social and clinical bases of drug addiction: commentary and debate. Psychopharmacology **125:** 285–345.

26. BLACKBURN, J.R. et al. 1992. Dopamine functions in appetitive and defensive behaviors. Prog. Neurobiol. **39:** 247–279.
27. PHILLIPS, A.G. et al. 1991. Dopamine and motivated behavior: insights provided by *in vivo* analyses. *In* The Mesolimbic Dopamine System: From Motivation to Action. P. Willner & J. Scheel-Kruger, Eds.: 473–495. John Wiley & Sons. New York.
28. WISE, R.A. & M.A. BOZARTH. 1987. A psychomotor stimulant theory of addiction. Psychol. Rev. **94:** 469–492.
29. WEISKRANTZ, L. 1956. Behavioral changes associated with ablation of the amygdaloid complex in monkeys. J. Comp. Physiol. Psychol. **49:** 381–391.
30. GAFFAN, D.S. 1992. Amygdala and the memory of reward. *In* The Amygdala. J.P. Aggleton, Ed.: 471–484. Wiley and Sons. Chicester.
31. JONES, B. & M. MISHKIN. 1972. Limbic lesions and the problem of stimulus-reinforcement associations. Exp. Neurol. **36:** 362–377.
32. DAVIS, M. 1992. The role of the amygdala in conditioned fear. *In* The Amygdala. J. P. Aggleton, Ed.: 255–306. Wiley-Liss Inc. New York.
33. PHILLIPS, R.G. & J.E. LEDOUX. 1992. Differential contribution of amygdala and hippocampus to cued and contextual fear conditioning. Behav. Neurosci. **106:** 1–8.
34. LEDOUX, J.E. 1991. Emotion and the limbic system concept. Concepts Neurosci. **2:** 169–199.
35. LEDOUX, J.E. 1993. Emotional memory: in search of systems and synapses. Ann. N. Y. Acad. Sci. **702:** 149–157.
36. HITCHCOCK, J. & M. DAVIS. 1986. Lesions of the amygdala, but not of the cerebellum or red nucleus, block conditioned fear as measured with the potentiated startle paradigm. Behav. Neurosci. **100:** 11–22.
37. KILLCROSS, S., T.W. ROBBINS & B.J. EVERITT. 1997. Different types of fear-conditioned behaviour mediated by separate nuclei within amygdala. Nature **388:** 377–380.
38. SELDEN, N.R.W. et al. 1991. Complementary roles for the amygdala and hippocampus in aversive conditioning to explicit and contextual cues. Neuroscience **42:** 335–350.
39. GAFFAN, D. & S. HARRISON. 1987. Amygdalectomy and disconnection in visual learning for auditory secondary reinforcement in monkeys. J. Neurosci. **7:** 2285–2280.
40. GALLAGHER, M. & A.A. CHIBA. 1996. The amygdala and emotion. Curr. Opin. Neurobiol. **6:** 221–227.
41. SAULSKAYA, N. & C.A. MARSDEN. 1995. Conditioned dopamine release: dependence on *N*-methyl-D-aspartate receptors. Neuroscience **67:** 57–63.
42. WILKINSON, L.S. et al. 1998. Dissociations in dopamine release in medial prefrontal cortex and ventral striatum during the acquisition and extinction of classical aversive conditioning in the rat [Full text delivery]. Eur. J. Neurosci. **10:** 1019–1026.
43. YOUNG, A.M. et al. 1993. Latent inhibition of conditioned dopamine release in rat nucleus-accumbens. Neuroscience **54:** 5–9.
44. YOUNG, A.M. et al. 1998. Increased extracellular dopamine in the nucleus accumbens of the rat during associative learning of neutral stimuli. Neuroscience **83:** 1175–1183.
45. GABRIEL, M. 1990. Functions of anterior and posterior cingulate cortex during avoidance-learning in rabbits. Prog. Brain Res. **85:** 467–483.
46. GABRIEL, M. et al. 1991. Effects of cingulate cortical lesions on avoidance learning and training-induced unit activity in rabbits. Exp. Brain Res. **86:** 585.
47. MAREN, S. et al. 1997. Neurotoxic lesions of the dorsal hippocampus and Pavlovian fear conditioning in rats. Behav. Brain Res. **88:** 261–274.

48. BUSSEY, T.J. *et al.* 1997. Dissociable effects of cingulate and medial frontal cortex lesions on stimulus-reward learning using a novel pavlovian autoshaping procedure for the rat: implications for the neurobiology of emotion. Behav. Neurosci. **111:** 908–919.
49. WILLIAMS, D.R. & H. WILLIAMS. 1969. Auto-maintenance in the pigeon: sustained pecking despite contingent non-reinforcement. J. Exp. Anal. Behav. **12:** 511–520.
50. TOMIE, A. 1996. Locating reward cue at response manipulandum (CAM) induces symptoms of drug abuse. Neurosci. Biobehav. Rev. **20:** 505–535.
51. PARKINSON, J.A. *et al.* 1997. Cortico-striatal circuitry: evidence for a functional connection between anterior cingulate cortex and nucleus accumbens core in pavlovian conditioning. Soc. Neurosci. Abstr. **23:** 779.
52. FREEMAN, J.H. *et al.* 1996. Limbic thalamic, cingulate cortical and hippocampal neuronal correlates of discriminative approach learning in rabbits. Behav. Brain Res. **80:** 123–136.
53. GABRIEL, M. *et al.* 1991. Effects of cingulate cortical-lesions on avoidance-learning and training-induced unit-activity in rabbits. Exp. Brain Res. **86:** 585–600.
54. EVERITT, B.J. *et al.* 1991. The basolateral amygdala-ventral striatal system and conditioned place preference: further evidence of limbic-striatal interactions underlying reward-related processes. Neuroscience **42:** 1–18.
55. LOUILOT, A. *et al.* 1985. Modulation of dopaminergic activity in the nucleus accumbens following facilitation or blockade of the dopaminergic transmission in the amygdala: a study by *in vivo* differential pulse voltammetry. Brain Res. **346:** 141–145.
56. SIMON, H. *et al.* 1988. Lesion of dopaminergic terminals in the amygdala produces enhanced locomotor response to D-amphetamine and opposite changes in dopaminergic activity in prefrontal cortex and nucleus accumbens. Brain Res. **447:** 335–340.
57. CAINE, S.B. *et al.* 1995. Effects of the dopamine D-1 antagonist SCH-23390 microinjected into the accumbens, amygdala or striatum on cocaine self-administration in the rat. Brain Res. **692:** 47–56.
58. HURD, Y.L. *et al.* 1997. *In vivo* amygdala dopamine levels modulate cocaine self-administration behavior in the rat: D1 dopamine receptor involvement. Eur. J. Neurosci. **9:** 2541–2548.
59. HAN, J.S. *et al.* 1997. The role of an amygdalo-nigrostriatal pathway in associative learning. J. Neurosci. **17:** 3913–3919.
60. DAVIS, M. *et al.* 1987. Anxiety and the amygdala: pharmacological and anatomical analysis of the fear-potentiated startle paradigm. *In* The Psychology of Learning and Motivation: Advances in Research and Theory. G. H. Bower, Ed.: 263–305. Academic Press. New York.
61. HOLLAND, P.C. 1997. Brain mechanisms for changes in processing of conditioned stimuli in Pavlovian conditioning: implications for behavior theory. Anim. Learn. Behav. **25:** 373–399.
62. BUSSEY, T.J. *et al.* 1997. Triple dissociation of anterior cingulate, posterior cingulate, and medial frontal cortices on visual discrimination tasks using a touchscreen testing procedure for the rat. Behav. Neurosci. **111:** 920–936.
63. KELLEY, A.E. *et al.* 1997. Response-reinforcement learning is dependent on *N*-methyl-D-aspartate receptor activation in the nucleus accumbens core. Proc. Natl. Acad. Sci. USA **94:** 12174–12179.
64. ROBBINS, T.W. & B.J. EVERITT. 1992. Functions of dopamine in the dorsal and ventral striatum. Sem. Neurosci. **4:** 119–128.
65. SOKOLOWSKI, J.D. & J.D. SALAMONE. 1998. The role of accumbens dopamine in lever pressing and response allocation: effects of 6-OHDA injected into core and

dorsomedial shell. Pharmacol. Biochem. Behav. **59:** 557–566.
66. GALLAGHER, M. *et al.* 1990. The amygdala central nucleus and appetitive Pavlovian conditioning: lesions impair one class of conditioned behavior. J. Neurosci. **10:** 1906–1911.
67. GALLAGHER, M. & P.C. HOLLAND. 1994. The amygdala complex: multiple roles in associative learning and attention. Proc. Natl. Acad. Acad. Sci. USA **91:** 11771–11776.
68. KAPP, B.S. *et al.* 1994. Effects of electrical-stimulation of the amygdaloid central nucleus on neocortical arousal in the rabbit. Behav. Neurosci. **108:** 81–93.
69. SILVESTRI, A.J. & B.S. KAPP. 1998. Amygdaloid modulation of mesopontine peribrachial neuronal activity: implications for arousal. Behav. Neurosci. **112:** 571–588.
70. MACKINTOSH, N.J. 1974. The Psychology of Animal Learning. Academic Press. London.
71. ROBBINS, T.W. 1978. The acquisition of responding with conditioned reinforcement: Effects of pipradrol, methylphenidate, D-amphetamine and nomifensine. Psychopharmacology **58:** 79–87.
72. TAYLOR, J.R. & T.W. ROBBINS. 1984. Enhanced behavioral control by conditioned reinforcers following microinjections of D-amphetamine into the nucleus accumbens. Psychopharmacology **84:** 405–412.
73. ROBBINS, T.W. *et al.* 1983. Contrasting interactions of pipradrol, D-amphetamine, cocaine, cocaine analogues, apomorphine and other drugs with conditioned reinforcement. Psychopharmacology **80:** 113–119.
74. FIBIGER, H.C. *et al.* 1992. The neurobiology of cocaine-induced reinforcement. CIBA Found. Symp. **166:** 96–111.
75. TAYLOR, J.R. & T.W. ROBBINS. 1986. 6-Hydroxydopamine lesions of the nucleus accumbens, but not of the caudate nucleus, attenuate enhanced responding with reward-related stimuli produced by intra-accumbens D-amphetamine. Psychopharmacology **90:** 390–397.
76. WOLTERINK, G. *et al.* 1993. Relative roles of ventral striatal D1 and D2 dopamine receptors in responding with conditioned reinforcement. Psychopharmacology **110:** 355–364.
77. ROBBINS, T.W. *et al.* 1989. Limbic-striatal interactions in reward-related processes. Neurosci. Biobehav. Rev. **13:** 155–162.
78. BURNS, L.H. *et al.* 1993. Differential effects of excitotoxic lesions of the basolateral amygdala, ventral subiculum and medial prefrontal cortex on responding with conditioned reinforcement and locomotor activity potentiated by intra-accumbens infusions of D-amphetamine. Behav. Brain Res. **55:** 167–183.
79. CADOR, M. *et al.* 1989. Involvement of the amygdala in stimulus-reward associations: interaction with the ventral striatum. Neuroscience **30:** 77–86.
80. EVERITT, B.J. *et al.* 1989. Interactions between the amygdala and ventral striatum in stimulus-reward associations: studies using a second-order schedule of sexual reinforcement. Neuroscience **30:** 63–75.
81. Everitt, B.J. *et al.* 1989. The effects of basolateral amygdala and ventral striatal lesions on conditioned place preference in rats. Soc. Neurosci. **15:** 490.11.
82. HIROI, N. & N.M. WHITE. 1991. The lateral nucleus of the amygdala mediates expression of the amphetamine conditioned place preference. J. Neurosci. **11:** 2107–2116.
83. WHITELAW, R.B. *et al.* 1996. Excitotoxic lesions of the basolateral amygdala impair the acquisition of cocaine-seeking behavior under a second-order schedule of reincememt. Psychopharmacology **127:** 213–224.
84. PARKINSON, J.A. *et al.* 1999. Dissociation in effects of lesions of the nucleus accumbens core and shell in appetitive pavlovian approach behavior and the potentiation

of conditioned reinforcement and locomotor activity by D-amphetamine. J. Neurosci. **11:** 1265–1274.
85. GROENEWEGEN, H.J. *et al.* 1991. Functional anatomy of the ventral, limbic system-innervated striatum. *In* The Mesolimbic Dopamine System: From Motivation to Action. P. Willner & J. Scheel-Kruger, Eds.: 19–60. John Wiley and Sons Ltd. Chichester.
86. WRIGHT, C.I. *et al.* 1996. Basal amygdaloid complex afferents to the rat nucleus accumbens are compartmentally organized. J. Neurosci. **16:** 1877–1893.
87. BLAHA, C.D. *et al.* 1997. Gating of hippocampal and amygdalar inputs to the nucleus accumbens by dopamine: a combined *in vivo* extracellular electrophysiological and electrochemical recording study. Soc. Neurosci. Abstr. **23:** 505.6.
88. BRUDZYNSKI, S.M. & C.J. GIBSON. 1997. Release of dopamine in the nucleus accumbens caused by stimulation of the subiculum in freely moving rats. Brain Res. Bull. **42:** 303–308.
89. FLORESCO, S.B. *et al.* 1998. Basolateral amygdala stimulation evokes glutamate receptor-dependent dopamine efflux in the nucleus accumbens of the anaesthetized rat. Eur. J. Neurosci. **10:** 1241–1251.
90. EVERITT, B.J. *et al.* 1989. Interactions between the amygdala and ventral striatum in stimulus-reward associations: studies using a second-order schedule of sexual reinforcement. Neuroscience **30:** 63–75.
91. KELLY, P.H. & K.E. MOORE. 1976. Mesolimbic dopaminergic neurones in the rotational model of nigrostriatal function. Nature **263:** 695–696.
92. KOSHIKAWA, N. *et al.* 1996. Contralateral turning elicited by unilateral stimulation of dopamine D-1 and D-2 receptors in the nucleus accumbens of rats is due to stimulation of these receptors in the shell, but not the core, of this nucleus. Psychopharmacology **126:** 185–190.
93. ROBBINS, T.W. & B.J. EVERITT. 1982. Functional studies of the central catecholamines. Int. Rev. Neurobiol. **23:** 303–365.
94. ROBLEDO, P. *et al.* 1996. Effects of excitotoxic lesions of the central amygdaloid nucleus on the potentiation of reward-related stimuli by intra-accumbens amphetamine. Behav. Neurosci. **110:** 981–990.
95. HITCHCOTT, P.K. *et al.* 1997. Enhanced acquisition of discriminative approach following intra- amygdala D-amphetamine. Psychopharmacology **132:** 237–246.
96. HITCHCOTT, P.K. *et al.* 1997. Enhanced stimulus-reward learning by intra-amygdala administration of a D-3 dopamine receptor agonist. Psychopharmacology **133:** 240–248.
97. CHILDRESS, A. *et al.* 1988. Conditioned craving and arousal in cocaine addiction: a preliminary report. NIDA Res. Monogr. **81:** 74–80.
98. CHILDRESS, A.R. *et al.* 1992. Classically conditioned factors in drug dependence. *In* Substance Abuse: A Comprehensive Text Book. W. Lowinson, P. Luiz, R. B. Millman & J. G. Langard, Ed.: 56–69. Williams and Wilkins. Baltimore.
99. GAWIN, F.H. 1991. Cocaine addiction: psychology and neurophysiology. Science **251:** 1580–1586.
100. O'BRIEN, C.P. & A.T. MCLELLAN. 1996. Myths about the treatment of addiction. Lancet **347:** 237–240.
101. ETTENBERG, A. & T.D. GEIST. 1991. Animal model for investigating the anxiogenic effects of self-administered cocaine. Psychopharmacology (Berl.) **103:** 455–461.
102. GOLDBERG, S.R. *et al.* 1981. Fixed-ratio responding under second-order schedules of food presentation or cocaine injection. J. Pharmacol. Exp. Ther. **218:** 271–281.
103. KATZ, J. 1979. A comparison of responding maintained under second-order schedules of intramuscular cocaine injection or food presentation in squirrel monkeys. J. Exp. Anal. Behav. **32:** 419–431.
104. EVERITT, B.J. *et al.* 1987. Studies of instrumental behavior with sexual reinforcement in male rats (*Rattus norvegicus*): I. Control by brief visual stimuli paired with a receptive female. J. Comp. Psychol. **101:** 395–406.
105. ARROYO, M. *et al.* 1998. Acquisition, maintenance and reinstatement of intravenous

cocaine self-administration under a second-order schedule of reinforcement in rats: effects of conditioned cues and continuous access to cocaine. Psychopharmacology **140:** 331–344.
106. WEISSENBORN, R., T.W. ROBBINS & B.J EVERITT. 1997. Effects of medial prefrontal or anterior cingulate cortex lesions on responding for cocaine under fixed-ratio and second-order schedules of reinforcement in rats. Psychopharmacology **134:** 242–257.
107. ALDERSON, H.L. *et al.* 1997. Establishment of intravenous self-administration of heroin in the rat under a second-order schedule of reinforcement. Soc. Neurosci. Abstr. **23:** 938.7.
108. MALDANADO-IRIZZARY, C.S. *et al.* 1995. Pharmacological and behavioral studies of craving and relapse in rat models of cocaine-seeking behavior. Am. College Neuropsychopharmacol. **34:** 264.
109. MEIL, W.M. & R.E. SEE. 1997. Lesions of the basolateral amygdala abolish the ability of drug associated cues to reinstate responding during withdrawal from self-administered cocaine. Behav. Brain Res. **1997:** 139–148.
110. MCGREGOR, A. & D.C.S. ROBERTS. 1993. Dopaminergic antagonism within the nucleus accumbens or the amygdala produces differential effects on intravenous cocaine self-administration under fixed and progressive ratio schedules of reinforcement. Brain Res. **624:** 245–252.
111. KOOB, G.F. *et al.* 1993. Opponent process and drug dependence: neurobiological mechanisms. Sem. Neurosci. **5:** 351–358.
112. KOOB, G.F. & E.J. NESTLER. 1997. The neurobiology of drug addiction. J. Neuropsychiatry Clin. Neurosci. **9:** 482–497.
113. KOOB, G.F. & M. LEMOAL. 1997. Drug abuse: hedonic homeostatic dysregulation. Science **278:** 52–58.
114. PARKINSON, J.A. *et al.* 1996. Lesions of the nucleus accumbens core, but not basolateral amygdala or subiculum, disrupt stimulus-reward learning in a novel autoshaping procedure. Soc. Neurosci. Abstr. **22:** 111.8.
115. PARKINSON, J.P. *et al.* 1998. Selective excitotoxic lesions of the nucleus accumbens core shell differentially affect aversive pavlovian conditioning to discrete and contextual cues. Psychobiology. In press.
116. WRIGHT, C.I. & H.J. GROENEWEGEN. 1995. Patterns of convergence and segregation in the medial nucleus-accumbens of the rat—relationships of prefrontal cortical, midline thalamic, and basal amygdaloid afferents. J. Comp. Neurol. **361:** 383–403.
117. PENNARTZ, C., M.A. *et al.* 1994. The nucleus accumbens as a complex of functionally distinct neuronal ensembles: an integration of behavioral, electrophysiological and anatomical data. Prog. Neurobiol. **42:** 719–761.
118. BLAHA, C.D. *et al.* 1997. Stimulation of the ventral subiculum of the hippocampus evokes glutamate receptor-mediated changes in dopamine efflux in the rat nucleus accumbens. Eur. J. Neurosci. **9:** 902–911.
119. HATFIELD, T. *et al.* 1996. Neurotoxic lesions of basolateral, but not central, amygdala interfere with pavlovian second-order conditioning and reinforcer devaluation effects. J. Neurosci. **16:** 5256–5265.
120. CLUGNET, M.-C. & J.E. LEDOUX. 1990. Synaptic plasticity in fear conditioning circuits: induction of LTP in the lateral nucleus of the amygdala by stimulation of the medial geniculate body. J. Neurosci. **10:** 2818–2824.
121. LEDOUX, J.E. *et al.* 1990. The lateral amygdaloid nucleus: sensory interface of the amygdala in fear conditioning. J. Neurosci. **10:** 1062–1069.
122. CAHILL, L. & J.L. MCGAUGH. 1998. Mechanisms of emotional arousal and lasting declarative memory. Trends Neurosci. **21:** 294–299.
123. LEDOUX, J.E. & J. MULLER. 1997. Emotional memory and psychopathology. Philos.

Trans. R. Soc. Lond. B Biol. Sci. **352:** 1719–1726.
124. LEDOUX, J.E. *et al.* 1988. Different projections of the central amygdaloid nucleus mediate autonomic and behavioral correlates of conditioned fear. J. Neurosci. **8:** 2517–2529.
125. KILLCROSS, A.S., B.J EVERITT & T.W. ROBBINS. 1997. Symmetrical effects of amphetamine and alpha-flupenthixal on conditioned punishment and conditioned reinforcement: contrasts with midazolam. Psychopharmacology **129:** 141–152.
126. MCCULLOUGH, L.D. *et al.* 1993. A neurochemical and behavioral investigation of the involvement of nucleus-accumbens dopamine in instrumental avoidance. Neuroscience **52:** 919–925.

Functional and Anatomical Relationships among the Amygdala, Basal Forebrain, Ventral Striatum, and Cortex
An Integrative Discussion

THACKERY S. GRAY[a]

Department of Cell Biology, Neurobiology, and Anatomy, Loyola Medical Center, 2160 South First Avenue, Maywood, Illinois 60153, USA

The work of Lennart Heimer and his associates has been an inspiration for many neuroscientists to study the detailed anatomical connections of basal forebrain structures and relate the circuitry to a framework that is tied strongly to function. Consequently, many new and exciting hypotheses have been generated, and old hypotheses have been or are in the process of being discarded. The resulting new scientific data has lead to a substantially increased understanding of the interrelatedness of the amygdala, magnocellular basal forebrain, striatum, and associated cortical regions.

This chapter will attempt to bring together the data and ideas presented in the previous six chapters and the closely related scientific literature into an integrative discussion. The text contains a minimum of scientific citations, because most of the references and ideas presented here are taken from previous highly referenced chapters. The reader is encouraged to refer to these chapters for additional and more complete scientific references.

First, a definition of the anatomical regions that have been discussed in the previous six chapters is presented. For the purposes of brevity, a "simplified" description of the anatomical structures and connections is provided. More detail is conferred later in the chapter, and extensive reviews of the anatomical circuitry are provided in several chapters in this volume.[1–5]

FIGURE 1 is a schematic drawing depicting the regions, reviewed (shaded boxes) in the previous chapters, in the framework of the brain. The cortical regions discussed are predominantly areas connected directly with the amygdala and ventral striatum. For the most part, the cortical regions are allocortical or periallocortical. By contrast, neocortical areas have very limited direct projections into the amygdala and ventral striatum. Cortical connections include prefrontal, insular, entorhinal, perirhinal, piriform cortical areas, and the hippocampus. The magnocellular basal forebrain comprises a seemingly diffuse network of neurons that are distributed within the ventral pallidum, globus pallidus, substantia innominata, septum, and diagonal band of Broca. Basal forebrain neurons have been mainly characterized by large neurons that contain the neurotransmitter, acetylcholine. The basal forebrain has widespread projections to the cerebral cortex and some important subcortical

---

[a]Voice:708-216-3345; fax: 708-216-3913; tgray@bsd.meddean.luc.edu

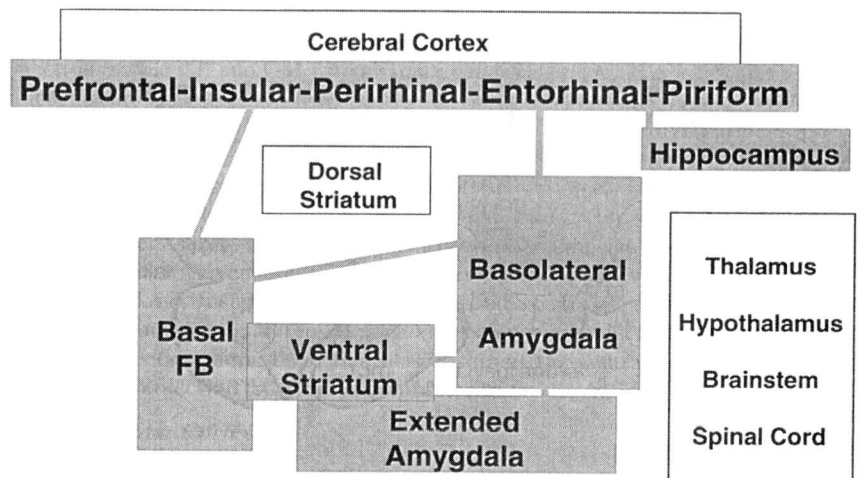

FIGURE 1. Basal forebrain-ventral striatum-amygdala-cortical anatomy.

connections. The magnocellular basal forebrain is reciprocally connected to the amygdala and ventral striatum.

The extended amygdala includes parts of the central and medial amygdaloid nuclei that continue through the substantia innominata into similarly characterized regions of the bed nucleus of the stria terminalis. The extended amygdala has reciprocal connections with the hypothalamus, thalamus, midbrain, and brain stem. The basolateral amygdala refers to the regions of the amygdala that are lateral to the extended amygdala and consist of the basolateral, lateral, and basal amygdaloid nuclei. The basolateral amygdala has reciprocal connections with the aforementioned cortical regions and projections into the extended amygdala, basal forebrain, and ventral striatum. The ventral striatum refers to a continuum of neural tissue that extends through the striatum into and including the nucleus accumbens. The accumbens nucleus is divided into "striatal" core and "transitional" shell regions. The ventral striatum differs from the dorsal striatum in that it receives its cortical input from allocortical regions as opposed to neocortical areas. The ventral striatum, like the extended amygdala, has connections with thalamic and brain stem regions.

In the following discussion, the work of the six chapters will be grouped together for integrative purposes according to their common anatomical and functional features.

CORTICAL CIRCUITRY OF THE BASOLATERAL AND THE EXTENDED AMYGDALA[2,3]

The work of Price and McDonald *et al.* as well as others (e.g., see refs. 6 and 7, and Cassell *et al.*,[1] this volume) demonstrated that there is a high degree of modality specific topography in the connections between various cortical areas that, in turn, are transmitted to cortical areas that innervate the amygdala. The direct cortical input to the amygdala is also segregated and selectively targeted to various amygdaloid subregions. Projections into the amygdala arise from the orbital and medial prefrontal cortex (e.g., limbic and anterior cingulate regions), lateral prefrontal cortex (containing a rostral tip of insular cortex), insular cortex (gustatory, visceral, and somatosensory), perirhinal cortex, lateral entorhinal cortex, piriform cortex, and hippocampus (e.g., subiculum and CA1).

The recipients of these projections are the lateral, basolateral, basal, and extended amygdaloid regions, although the bulk of the incoming cortical projections terminate within the basolateral amygdaloid nuclei. The basolateral and basal amygdaloid nuclei in turn project back upon the cerebral cortex in a highly reciprocally organized topographical manner. The extended amygdala has no direct cortical projections, but, rather, has extensive intrinsic connections and extrinsic pathways that innervate the hypothalamus and lower brain stem regions. In addition, the extended amygdala receives direct visceral and sensory input from the regions in the brain stem (e.g., nucleus of the solitary tract and parabrachial nucleus) and the thalamus.

There are at least several possible functions proposed for these pathways. First, context-specific processed sensory information is provided to the amygdala. This information is probably related to memory consolidation (integration of new information, i.e., learning) and recall (comparing of current information with the past). Further sensory neuronal processing in the amygdala probably results in the attachment of affect or emotion to newly acquired experiences and linking multisensory associations to the consequences of behavior. Inputs from insular cortex could help convey unique auditory, somatosensory, visual, and nociceptive properties of various stimuli. The entorhinal cortex and subiculum provide the amygdala with access to the well-defined trisynaptic circuitry of the hippocampus. The likely function of these connections is spatial and contextual processing of sensory information, and further memory incorporation and recall. Complex sensory properties are also probably linked in time with the rewarding consequences of behavior. The prefrontal cortex is thought to participate in integration of stimulus-reward associations, reward-guided behaviors (especially food seeking), and determination of mood. Deficits associated with damage to this region in humans and animals include disruption of decision making and perseverative behaviors. Consistent with these observations is data from functional imaging studies in humans that demonstrate abnormal prefrontal lobe activity in unipolar and bipolar depressed patients.

MAGNOCELLULAR BASAL FOREBRAIN CIRCUITRY[4,8]

The magnocellular basal forebrain consists of a mixed population of cells distributed loosely through the medial septum, diagonal band of Broca, ventral pallidum, substantia innominata, globus pallidus, and the so-called peripallidal areas. The presence of large cholinergic cells in these regions has been the main criteria for characterization of the magnocellular basal forebrain. However, the work of Zaborszki *et al.*[4] has emphasized the importance of noncholinergic cells that also participate in cortical projections of the basal forebrain. Some of the noncholinergic cells contain GABA and/or peptides. GABAergic neurons project to cortex and subcortically to the diencephalon and brain stem. The GABAergic neurons may also contain calcium-binding proteins. These cells receive convergent inputs from dopaminergic cells of the ventral tegmental area in the brain stem and glutaminergic input from the frontal cortex. The peptidergic neurons are mainly interneurons and contain neuropeptide Y and somatostatin. The cortically projecting cells and interneurons that are located in this region are characterized by somewhat diffuse connections. This diffuse circuitry and other anatomical features have prompted some investigators[9] to propose that the basal forebrain network is a rostral extension of the reticular activating system. Functionally, this hypothesis is consistent with the magnocellular basal forebrain's proposed role in mediating cortical arousal and attention.

The magnocellular basal forebrain system participates in cognition-linked sensory processing necessary for memory recall and consolidation. Cortical acetylcholine seems to be essential for "sustained, selective and divided attention" (Sarter et al.,[8] this volume), which is necessary for integration of sensory perceptions and associations. GABAergic neurons located in either the nucleus accumbens or near basal forebrain neurons are thought to directly modulate cortically projecting cholinergic basal forebrain neurons. The GABAergic neuron activity can be altered by dopamine receptors that are activated by dopamine cells in the brain stem. Thus, dopamine- and glutamate-modulated GABAergic and peptidergic circuitry can, in turn, influence the level of cortical acetycholine released by basal forebrain cholinergic neurons. Cortical acetycholine is critical for the ability to attend to and selectively process incoming sensory stimuli. Cortical-sensory processing is a necessary prerequisite for adaptive responses to changes in the environment that require memory recall and incorporation of new sensory-motor events into memory.

AMYGDALA-VENTRAL STRIATAL CIRCUTRY[10,11]

Probably the greatest contribution of Heimer and his colleagues has been to significantly change our concept of the anatomical relationships among the amygdala, ventral striatum-nucleus/accumbens, and the basal forebrain. The ventral striatum and nucleus accumbens are now generally recognized as being part of the same anatomical system. The nucleus accumbens has been divided into a core that merges with the ventral striatum and a shell, which is located more medially and ventrally. The shell has additional somewhat "nonstriatal" features. For example, it has connections to the hypothalamus and bed nucleus of the stria terminalis. The extended amygdala, an even more recent and controversial, hypothesized region, includes the central and medial amygdala and intervening neural tissue that continues through the substantia innominata into the medial and lateral parts of the bed nucleus of the stria terminalis. The interstitial nucleus of the posterior limb of the anterior commissure and a "packet of cells" that are located along the course of the stria terminalis are also included as part of the extended amygdala. The extended amygdala borders the ventral striatum as it protrudes through the basal forebrain and intermingles with parts of the magnocellular basal forebrain.

Recent studies have demonstrated some significant similarities between the anatomy, neurochemistry, and functions of subregions of the extended amygdala and the ventral striatum-accumbens areas. Both the extended amygdala and ventral striatum receive a dense input from the basolateral amygdaloid nucleus. Both of these regions contain medium, spiny GABAergic neurons and receive a dense dopaminergic input from the brain stem. They also contain a dense innervation of enkephalin. Also, lesion studies have indicated a number of functional similarities between the central extended amygdala and the shell/core parts of the nucleus accumbens, although, it should be noted that there are some distinct difference between the effects of lesions in the extended amygdala and ventral striatum on some behavioral tasks.[10] Regardless, the hypothesis that the central extended amygdala and the nucleus accumbens are part of a common functional and anatomical continuum is worth further exploration. If this hypothesis is further supported, then it represents an even more aggressive addition to Heimer's notion of the extended amygdala's close relationship to the nucleus accumbens-ventral striatum. Regardless, studies of these two regions are beginning to reveal some common organizational features that will contribute to a substantially increased understanding of how these regions operate. These issues have been further explored in detail by other chapters in this volume (e.g., refs. 1 and 10).

The ventral striatum, extended amygdala, and basolateral amygdala circuitry has an important function in associating previously neutral stimuli with positive and negative reward. These include the association of multiple stimuli with the rewarding properties of drugs, food, sex, and other pleasurable stimulus events. These regions are also important for associating sensory stimuli with aversive properties of negative events and sensations, including pain, anxiety, and fear, and other unpleasant experiences. The basolateral amygydala, in concert with prefrontal cortical circuitry, is important for learning and memory, associated with assessing the magnitude and value reward or reinforcement. The basolateral amygdala is also required for making stimulus-stimulus associations to rewarding stimuli. The extended amygdala seems to be more critical for mediating responses associated with engaging and interacting with rewarding stimuli during learning and mediating learning during aversive conditioning. The ventral striatum-nucleus accumbens regions seem to be more responsible for positive reinforcing associations, whereas the central extended amygdala may mediate associations with more negative reinforcing ones. However, exceptions have been noted, especially with regard to the central extended amygdala and some positive reinforcing associations (e.g., opioid addiction, Koob[12]this volume).

Thus, there are important interrelationships among the basolateral amygdala, the extended amygdala, and the ventral striatum. These interactions are reflected in the anatomical circuitry and the neurotransmitters used in these pathways as well as their specialized functions. These regions seem to be essential for single and multiple stimulus associations to rewarding consequences of behaviors and for assessing the value of the reinforcing stimuli. This explains how initially meaningless sensory stimuli acquire potent and complex motivational or emotion-evoking properties.

SUMMARY

Two recent papers[13,14] have questioned the concept of the amygdala as a functional and anatomically separate entity. Swanson and Petrovich[14] go so far as to state that "the amygdala is neither a structural nor a functional unit." This novel concept is derived from the fact that the amygdala is a structure whose anatomical connections and neurochemical features are more strongly interrelated to adjacent parts of the temporal lobe and basal forebrain than to unique characteristics of its own. This is an emerging hypothetical concept of the "amygdala" that seems to repeat itself in many parts of this volume and merits further examination in the future. The basal forebrain and cortical circuitry described here seem to be critical for a set of behaviors/processes that could be collectively described as cognitive–emotive. For example, this would include arousal, attention, sensory processing, reinforcement, and finally associative learning, decision making, and memory. Collectively this circuitry influences the emotional, motivational, and cognitive state of an organism. More and more studies are demonstrating that small and localized manipulations of the brain can result in equally subtle and specific deficits that are associated with definable parts of the anatomical circuitry, neurotransmitters, and receptors of basal forebrain structures. These studies have been guided and influenced by the refined neuroanatomical and neurochemical investigations of Lennart Heimer and his colleagues. Interpretations of these studies are beginning to uncover distinct deficits that suggest explanations and potential treatments for many psychiatric and pathological degenerative disorders.

REFERENCES

1. CASSELL, M.D. et al. 1999. The intrinsic organization of the central extended amygdala. Ann. N. Y. Acad. Sci. This volume.
2. MCDONALD, A.J. et al. 1999. Cortical afferents to the extended amygdala. Ann. N. Y. Acad. Sci. This volume.
3. PRICE, J.L. 1999. Prefrontal cortical networks related to visceral function and mood. Ann. N. Y. Acad. Sci. This volume.
4. ZABORSZKI, L. et al. 1999. The basal forebrain corticopetal system revisited. Ann. N. Y. Acad. Sci. This volume.
5. ZAHM, D.S. 1999. Functional-anatomical implications of the nucleus accumbens core and shell subterritories. Ann. N.Y. Acad. Sci. This volume.
6. TURNER, B.H. 1981. The cortical sequence and terminal distribution of sensory related afferents to the amygdaloid complex of the rat and monkey. In The Amygdaloid Complex. Y. Ben-Ari, Ed.: 51–62. Elsevier/North-Holland Biomedical Press. Amsterdam.
7. VEENING, J.G. 1978. Cortical afferents of the amgydaloid complex in the rat. Neurosci. Lett. **8:** 191–195.
8. SARTER, M. et al. 1999. Basal forebrain afferent projections modulating cortical acetycholine, attention, and implications for neuropsychiatric disorders. Ann. N. Y. Acad. Sci. This volume.
9. LEONTOVICH, T.A. & G.P. ZHUKOVA. 1963. The specificity of the neuronal structure and topography of the reticular formation in the brain and spinal cord of Carnivora. J. Comp. Neurol. **121:** 347–381.
10. EVERITT, B.J. et al. 1999. Associative processes in addiction and reward: the role of amygdala-ventral striatal subsystems. Ann. N. Y. Acad. Sci. This volume.
11. GALLAGHER, M. & G. SCHOENBAUM. 1999. Functions of the amygdala and related forebrain areas in attention and cognition. Ann. N. Y. Acad. Sci. This volume.
12. KOOB, G.F. 1999. The role of the striatopallidal and extended amygdala systems in drug addiction. Ann. N. Y. Acad. Sci. This volume.
13. CASSELL, M.D. 1998. The amygdala: myth or monolith. Trends Neurosci. **21:** 200–201.
14. SWANSON, L. & G.D. PETROVICH. 1998. What is the amygdala? Trends Neurosci. **21:** 323–331.

The Role of the Striatopallidal and Extended Amygdala Systems in Drug Addiction

GEORGE F. KOOB[a]

Department of Neuropharmacology, CVN-7, The Scripps Research Institute, 10550 North Torrey Pines Road, La Jolla, California 92037, USA

ABSTRACT: Evidence suggests that the acute reinforcing actions of drugs of abuse may be mediated by specific elements of the striatopallidal and extended amygdala systems. These include the shell of the nucleus accumbens, the central nucleus of the amygdala, and the sublenticular extended amygdala. Chronic administration of drugs of abuse, including cocaine, amphetamines, nicotine, alcohol, and tetrahydrocannabinol leads to an increasing dysregulation of brain reward systems that is characterized by decreases in reward function. Withdrawal from chronic administration of cocaine, amphetamine, nicotine, alcohol, and tetrahydrocannabinol raises thresholds for brain stimulation reward. Neurochemical elements in the extended amygdala may mediate these changes, including decreases in dopamine and serotonin neurotransmission in the nucleus accumbens and increases in the brain-stress neurotransmitter, corticotropin-releasing factor, in the central nucleus of the amygdala. The combination of decreases in function of neurotransmitters involved in the positive-reinforcing properties of drugs of abuse with recruitment of brain-stress systems within the extended amygdala provides a powerful mechanism for allostatic changes in hedonic set point that can lead to the compulsive drug-seeking and drug-taking behavior characteristic of addiction.

DRUG ADDICTION AND ANIMAL MODELS

Drug addiction can be defined as a compulsion to take a drug with loss of control over drug intake and is characterized by chronic relapses. The term *substance dependence* is used to describe a syndrome basically equivalent to addiction, and the diagnostic criteria used describe symptoms that to a large extent define compulsion and loss of control in drug intake.[1] However, not all substance use leads to substance abuse and substance dependence (addiction),[1] and an important challenge for neurobiological research is to understand how the transition occurs between controlled substance or drug use and the loss of control that defines addiction or substance dependence, and what molecular, cellular, and system processes contribute to the development of substance dependence.

Progress in the neurobiology of drug dependence has depended not only on the development of molecular, neurobiological, and neuropharmacological tools for understanding the neuropharmacological mechanisms of action and neuroanatomical circuits associated with the action of drugs of abuse, but also on the development of

---

[a]Voice: 619-784-7062; fax: 619-784-7405; gkoob@scripps.edu

TABLE 1. Relationship of addiction components and behavioral constructs

Addictive Component	Operational Construct
Pleasure	Positive reinforcement
Self-medication	Negative reinforcement
Habit	Conditioned positive reinforcement
Habit	Conditioned negative reinforcement

animal models of drug dependence that allow interpretation of neuropharmacological advances in the context of the disorder under study. Animal models exist for many elements of the syndrome of drug addiction, and these elements can be constructed according to conceptual frameworks, such as different sources of reinforcement or by symptoms or diagnostic criteria for addiction.[1,2]

MOTIVATIONAL VIEW OF DRUG DEPENDENCE

The motivating factors for the development, maintenance, and persistence of drug addiction can be broken down into four major sources of reinforcement in drug dependence: positive reinforcement, negative reinforcement, conditioned positive reinforcement, and conditioned negative reinforcement[3] (TABLE 1). The striatopallidal/extended amygdala system may be an integral part of the circuitry involved in all four sources of reinforcement. Positive-reinforcing effects of drugs are critical for establishing self-administration behavior and continue to have an important role in all aspects of drug dependence. Indeed, some have argued that positive reinforcement is the key to drug dependence.[4] However, a compelling case can be made for compromises in hedonic processing associated with drug abstinence as a driving force of addiction, even if alleviation of withdrawal symptoms (negative reinforcement) may not be a major motivating factor in the initiation of compulsive drug use.[5,6] Also, the construct of negative reinforcement plays an important role in the maintenance of drug use after the development of dependence. Thus, whereas initial drug use may be motivated by the positive affective state produced by the drug, continued use leads to neuroadaptation to the presence of a drug and reinforcement of another source of reinforcement, the negative reinforcement associated with relieving negative affective consequences of drug termination. Indeed, one can argue that the defining feature of drug dependence is the establishment of a negative affective state.[7]

Perhaps an even more compelling motivational force is that there are neurobiological events that contribute to the reinforcement associated with drug taking by changing the "set point" for hedonic processing.[6] Much progress has been made in identifying the role of subparts of the extended amygdala in the acute positive reinforcing effects of drugs of abuse. A more recent focus has been on the role of the extended amygdala in the negative reinforcement associated with drug dependence and the conditioned reinforcing effects that contribute to relapse.

THE ROLE OF THE EXTENDED AMYGDALA IN THE POSITIVE REINFORCING EFFECTS OF DRUGS

The medial forebrain bundle long has been hypothesized to be the neuronal circuitry forming the neural substrates of reward. The medial forebrain bundle contains both ascending and descending pathways that include most of the brain's monoamine systems,[8–10] and the structures involved include those that support intracranial self-stimulation at low current levels: the ventral tegmental area, the basal forebrain, and the medial forebrain bundle which connects these two areas.[8,9,11,12] Significant insights into the neurochemical and neuroanatomical components of the medial forebrain bundle have provided the key not only to drug reward but also to natural rewards. Perhaps more importantly for the present discussion, the output of the extended amygdala is a massive projection to the medial forebrain bundle and may be the source of much of the descending circuitry hypothesized to be part of the brain reward system.

The principle focus of research on the neurobiology of drug addiction has been the origins and terminal areas of the mesocorticolimbic dopamine system, and there is now compelling evidence for the importance of this system in drug reward. The major components of this drug-reward circuit are the ventral tegmental area (the site of dopaminergic cell bodies), the basal forebrain (the nucleus accumbens, olfactory tubercle, frontal cortex, and amygdala), and the dopaminergic connection between the ventral tegmental area and the basal forebrain. Other components are the opioid peptide, GABA, glutamate, serotonin, and presumably many other neural inputs that interact with the ventral tegmental area and the basal forebrain.[13]

Recent neuroanatomical data and new functional observations have provided support for the hypothesis that a common neural circuitry forms a separate entity within the basal forebrain, termed the *extended amygdala*.[14] Originally described by Johnston,[15] the term extended amygdala represents a macrostructure that is composed of several basal forebrain structures: the bed nucleus of the stria terminalis, the central medial amygdala, the medial part of the nucleus accumbens (e.g., shell),[16] and the area termed the sublenticular substantia innominata. There are similarities in morphology, immunohistochemistry and connectivity in these structures.[14] They receive afferent connections from limbic cortices, the hippocampus, basolateral amygdala, midbrain, and lateral hypothalamus. The efferent connections from this complex include the posterior medial (sublenticular) ventral pallidum, medial ventral tegmental area, various brain stem projections, and perhaps most intriguing from a functional point of view, a considerable projection to the lateral hypothalamus.[17]

The neuronal components of this circuitry for different types of drug reward will be discussed in the following sections with a focus on psychomotor stimulants, and related to the construct of the extended amygdala. This specific neuronal circuitry not only will provide important insights into the relationship of drug reward to natural reward systems but also may be the key to the changes in hedonic set point associated with the development of drug dependence.

Psychomotor stimulants of high-abuse potential interact initially with monamine transporter proteins, which have been cloned and characterized,[18–20] are located on monoaminergic nerve terminals, and terminate a monoamine signal by transporting

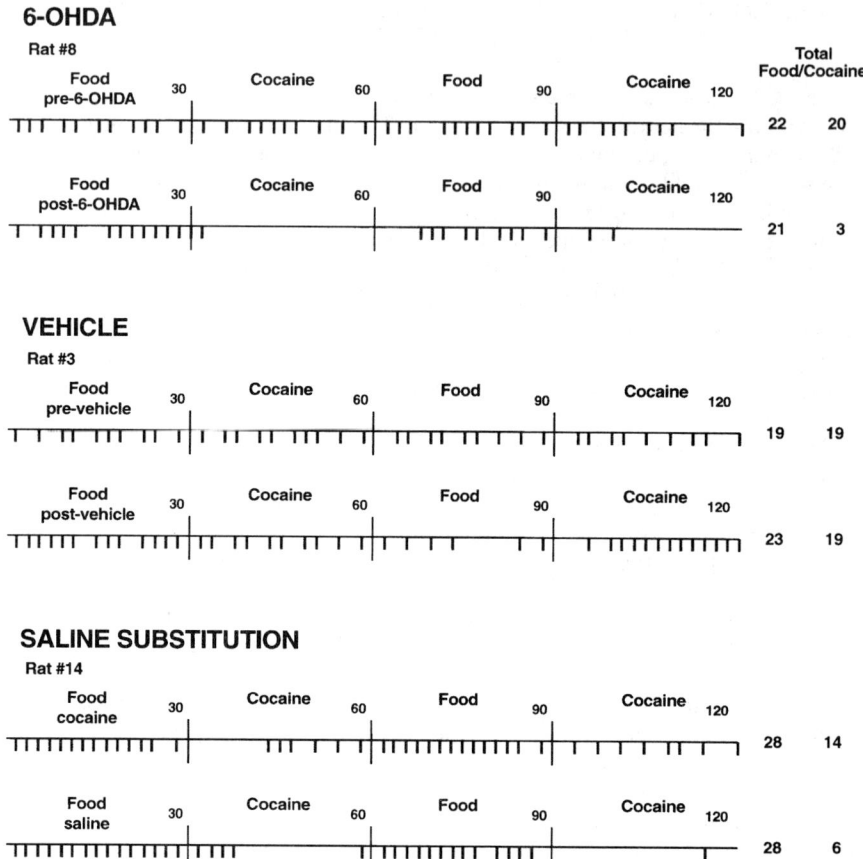

FIGURE 1. The effects of 6-OHDA (top panel) or vehicle (middle panel) infusion into the nucleus accumbens and olfactory tubercle, or substitution of saline for cocaine (bottom panel), on the number of reinforcers earned in the multiple schedule on the last session prior to treatment and on the seventh session posttreatment for three individual animals. Each mark on the time line indicates delivery of a reinforcer (45-mg food pellet or 0.25 mg cocaine iv injection). (Caine and Koob.[41] With permission from *Journal of the Experimental Analysis of Behavior*.)

the monoamine from the synaptic cleft back into the terminals. Cocaine inhibits all three monoamine transporters—dopamine, serotonin, and norepinephrine—thereby potentiating monoaminergic transmission. Amphetamine and its derivatives also potentiate monoaminergic transmission, but by increasing monoamine release. The amphetamine itself is transported into monoaminergic nerve terminals by all three transporters, where it disrupts the storage of the monoamine transmitters. This leads to an increase in extravascular levels of the monoamines and to the reverse transport of the monoamine into the synaptic cleft via the monoamine transporters.[21] Amphetamine and cocaine are psychomotor stimulants and, as such, have many behavioral

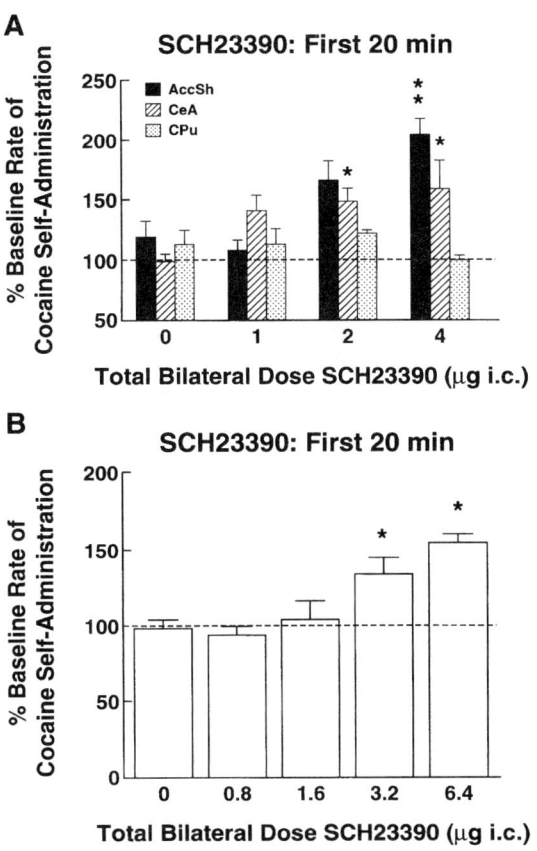

FIGURE 2. A: Effects of SCH23390 (0, 0.5, 1.0, 2.0 µg/0.33µL/side = 0, 1.0, 2.0, 4.0 total bilateral dose) microinjected into the accumbens shell (AccSh), central amygdala (CeA), or dorsal striatum (CPu) on cocaine self-administration (0.25 mg/inj iv; FR5TO 20 s) in separate groups of rats during the first 20 minutes of the self-administration session (values are group means and standard errors; $n = 6$/brain region). Asterisks indicate statistically significant differences from vehicle (saline) injection ($* p < 0.05$; $** p < 0.01$) by Neuman Keuls *a posteori* test following significant main effect of dose by analysis of variance. (Caine *et al.*[47] With permission from *Brain Research*.) **B:** Effects of SCH23390 (0, 0.4, 0.8, 1.6, 3.2 µg/ 0.33 µL/side = 0, 0.8, 1.6, 3.2, 6.4 µg total bilateral dose) microinjected into the dorsal lateral bed nucleus of the stria terminalis (dlBNST) on cocaine self-administration (0.25 mg/inj iv; FR5TO 20 s) within the first 20 minutes of the self-administration session. Values are group means and standard errors ($n = 7$). Asterisks indicate statistically significant differences from vehicle (saline) injection ($p < 0.05$) by post hoc comparisons (using Bonferroni correction) following the observation of a significant main effect of drug using a within-subjects analysis of variance. (Epping-Jordan *et al.*[48] With permission from *Brain Research*.)

effects associated with psychomotor activation. These drugs also have positive reinforcing effects, as shown by their effects to enhance conditioned responding,[22]

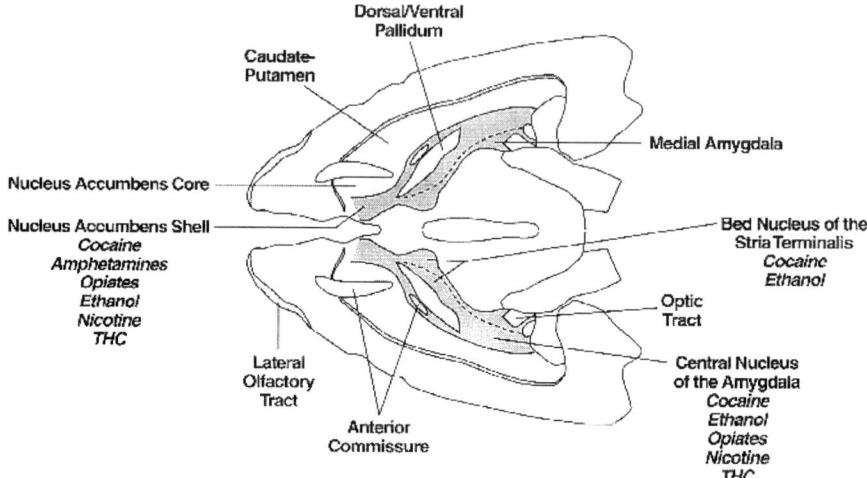

FIGURE 3. Horizontal section of a rat brain depicting the principal structures of the extended amygdala. These structures include the central nucleus of the amygdala, the shell part of the nucleus accumbens, and the bed nucleus of the stria terminalis. The drugs listed below each structure refer to potential sites of action of drug reinforcement during the addiction cycle, either positive or negative. THC, tetrahydrocannabinol. (Koob et al.[85] With permission from *Neuron*.)

decrease thresholds for reinforcing brain stimulation,[23,24] produce preferences for environments where they have been previously experienced (place preferences),[25,26] and readily act as reinforcers for drug self-administration.[27]

The mesocorticolimbic dopamine system, which projects heavily to the extended amygdala, appears to be the critical substrate for both the psychomotor stimulant effects of amphetamine and cocaine[28–30] and their reinforcing actions.[31,32] The most direct evidence implicating dopamine in the reinforcing actions of cocaine comes from studies of intravenous self-administration and studies of conditioned place preference. Dopamine receptor antagonists, when injected systemically, reliably decrease the reinforcing effects of cocaine and amphetamine self-administration in rats and block conditioned place preferences for these drugs.[31–36]

Dopamine antagonists actually shift the cocaine dose-effect function for cocaine self-administration to the right.[37,38] Neurotoxin-induced lesions of the mesocorticolimbic dopamine system with 6-hydroxydopamine (6-OHDA) of the nucleus accumbens or ventral tegmental area produce extinction-like responding and significant, long-lasting decreases in self-administration of cocaine and amphetamine over days.[39,40] These decreases in cocaine self-administration following dopamine-selective lesions of the nucleus accumbens now have been observed in a variety of different tests and conditions, including situations where animals show a decrease in the amount of work they will perform for cocaine[27] and situations where other reinforcers, such as food, were unaffected but cocaine self-administration was abolished[41] (FIG. 1).

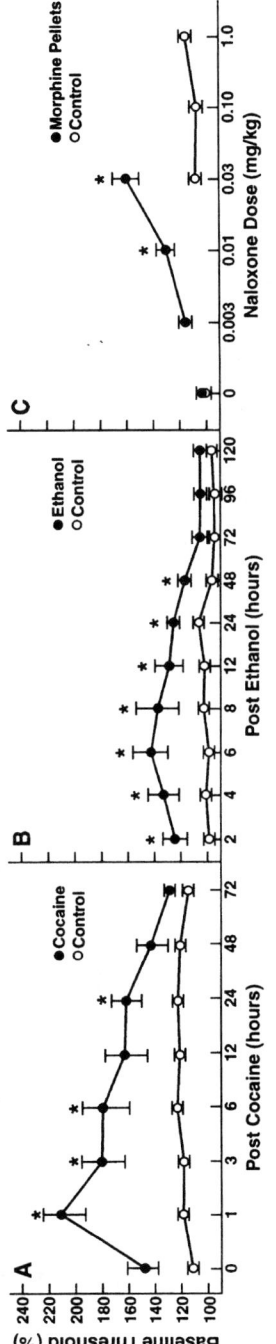

FIGURE 4. Changes in reward threshold associated with chronic administration of three major drugs of abuse. Reward thresholds were determined by a rate-independent discrete trials threshold procedure for intracranial self-stimulation (ICSS) of the medial forebrain bundle. **A:** Rats equipped with intravenous catheters were allowed to self-administer cocaine for 12 hours before withdrawal and reward threshold determinations. Elevations in threshold were dose dependent, with longer bouts of cocaine self-administration yielding larger and longer-lasting elevations in reward thresholds. Asterisks refer to significant differences between treatment and control values. Values are mean ± SEM. **B:** Elevations in reward thresholds with the same ICSS technique after chronic exposure to ethanol of about 200 mg% in ethanol vapor chambers. **C:** Elevations in reward thresholds measured with the same ICSS technique after administration of very low doses (in milligrams per kilogram of body weight) of the opiate antagonist naloxone to animals made dependent on morphine with two, 75-mg morphine (base) pellets implanted subcutaneously. (Koob & Le Moal.[6] With permission from *Science*.)

All three dopamine receptor subtypes have been implicated in the reinforcing actions of cocaine, as measured by intravenous self-administration, including the D1,[42] D2,[38,43] and D3 dopamine receptors.[44] Dopamine D1 and D2 antagonists also block the place conditioning produced by amphetamine.[45,46] However, the evidence for roles of dopamine D1 and D3 receptors directly or indirectly implicates elements of the extended amygdala in psychomotor stimulant reward. D1 dopamine antagonists are particularly effective in blocking cocaine self-administration when the antagonist is administered directly into the shell of the nucleus accumbens, the central nucleus of the amygdala,[47] and the bed nucleus of the stria terminalis[48] (FIG. 2). Dopamine D3 receptors are almost exclusively located in the shell of the nucleus accumbens in the rat,[49] and D3 agonists have powerful agonist effects in suppressing cocaine self-administration.[50]

Previous work has shown that lesions of the sublenticular extended amygdala (substantia innominata) were particularly effective in disrupting cocaine self-administration.[51] This brain region is medial to the subcomissural ventral pallidum and is a major projection area of the shell of the nucleus accumbens.[52]

Additional evidence implicating the extended amygdala in drug reward comes from studies on ethanol. Both GABAergic and opioidergic antagonists when microinjected into the central nucleus of the amygdala are particularly effective in decreasing the acute reinforcing effects of ethanol.[53,54] Finally, selective activation of dopaminergic transmission occurs in the shell of the nucleus accumbens in response to acute administration of virtually all major drugs of abuse[55–57] (FIG. 3).

THE ROLE OF THE EXTENDED AMYGDALA IN NEGATIVE REINFORCEMENT ASSOCIATED WITH DRUG ADDICTION

Acute withdrawal from drugs of abuse is associated with a negative affective state, including various negative emotions, such as dysphoria, depression, irritability, and anxiety that presumably reflects counteradaptive changes in the reward system. For example, cocaine withdrawal in humans in the outpatient setting is characterized by severe depressive symptoms combined with irritability, anxiety, and anhedonia lasting several hours to several days (i.e., the "crash") and may be one of the motivating factors in the maintenance of the cocaine-dependence cycle.[58] Inpatient studies have shown similar changes in mood and anxiety states, but they generally are much less severe.[59] Opiate withdrawal is characterized by severe dysphoria, and ethanol withdrawal produces dysphoria and anxiety.

The neural substrates and neuropharmacological mechanisms of the aversive effects of drug withdrawal, effects that may contribute to the negative reinforcement associated with drug dependence, involve the same neural systems implicated in the positive-reinforcing effects of drugs of abuse. In addition, other nonreward stress systems also involving the extended amygdala appear to be recruited during drug abstinence. Using the technique of intracranial self-stimulation to measure reward thresholds throughout the course of drug dependence, recent studies have shown that reward thresholds are increased (reflecting a decrease in reward) following chronic administration of all major drugs of abuse, including opiates, psychostimulants, ethanol, and nicotine, and can last up to 72 hours, depending on the drug and dose administered[60–65] (FIG. 4).

TABLE 2. Neurotransmitters implicated in the motivational effects of withdrawal from drugs of abuse

↓ Dopamine
↓ Opioid peptides
↓ Serotonin
↓ GABA
↑ Corticotropin-releasing factor

Counteradaptive neurochemical events within the extended amygdala that could contribute to these brain reward changes include decreases in dopaminergic and serotonergic transmission in the nucleus accumbens during drug withdrawal, as measured by *in vivo* microdialysis,[63,66] increased sensitivity of opioid receptor transduction mechanisms in the nucleus accumbens during opiate withdrawal,[67] and decreased GABAergic transmission in the central nucleus of the amygdala during ethanol withdrawal.[68–70] (TABLE 2).

Recruitment of other neurotransmitter systems in the extended amygdala in the adaptive responses to drugs of abuse include neurotransmitter systems not linked to the acute reinforcing effects of the drug, such as brain-stress systems (TABLE 2). Corticotropin-releasing factor (CRF) function, in the central nucleus of the amygdala, also appears to be activated during acute withdrawal from cocaine, ethanol, opiates, and tetrahydrocannabinol and thus may mediate behavioral aspects of stress associated with abstinence.[71–74] Also, rats treated repeatedly with cocaine, nicotine, and ethanol show significant anxiogenic-like responses following cessation of chronic drug administration, which are reversed with intracerebroventricular administration of a CRF antagonist.[75,76] Microinjections into the central nucleus of the amygdala of lower doses of the CRF antagonist also reversed the anxiogenic-like effects of ethanol withdrawal,[75] and similar doses of the CRF antagonist injected into the amygdala were active in reversing the aversive effects of opiate withdrawal.[72]

ANIMAL MODELS FOR CRAVING AND THE EXTENDED AMYGDALA

Substance dependence or addiction not only involves acquisition of drug taking and maintenance of drug taking, but also manifests as a chronic relapsing disorder with reinstatement of drug taking after detoxification and abstinence. Animal models of craving suffer from the validation that comes from clinical studies because clinicians have had major problems defining and measuring drug craving. Nevertheless, one can construct a simple definition and attempt to develop animal models of craving (TABLE 3). An operational definition of craving is "the desire for the previously experienced effects of a psychoactive substance."[77,78] Two particularly important areas for animal model development that potentially use the extended amygdala and its connections are the constructs of conditioned reinforcement and drug set point.

Both the positive and negative affective states can become associated with stimuli in the drug-taking environment or even internal cues through classical conditioning processes.[3] Reexposure to these conditioned stimuli can provide the motivation for continued drug use and relapse after abstention. There is evidence in humans that the

TABLE 3. Animal models of craving for ethanol

- Excessive drinking
    - Resistance to extinction of self-administration
    - Alcohol deprivation effect
    - Self-administration during withdrawal
    - Self-administration during protracted abstinence
- Conditioned reinforcement
    - Cue-elicited prolongation of extinction
    - Cue-elicited reinstatement of self-administration
    - Ethanol reinstatement of self-administration
- Negative affective states
    - Intracranial self-stimulation
    - Conditioned place aversion

positive reinforcing effects of drugs, such as heroin and cocaine, as measured by subjective reports of euphoria or "high," can become conditioned to previously neutral stimuli. Patients being treated for heroin addiction and allowed to self-administer either saline or heroin reported that both saline and heroin injections were pleasurable, particularly in the patient's usual injection environment.[79] Alternatively, patients—even detoxified subjects—can report negative affective symptoms, like those associated with drug abstinence, when returning to environments similar to those associated with drug dependence.[80] Preliminary evidence for a role of the extended amygdala in conditioned drug effects are studies showing that conditioned reinforcement associated with drug self-administration and drug withdrawal depend on the basolateral amygdala.[81,82] Evidence for changes in drug hedonic set point associated with a history of drug use can be found in animal models of chronic drug administration. Animals trained to self-administer ethanol, using a two-lever choice operant test for oral intake of 10% ethanol, show reliable and stable intake of ethanol in daily 30-minute sessions. However, when identically trained rats were subjected to two weeks of dependence induction using the ethanol vapor chambers and then allowed two weeks of detoxification, they showed a dramatic first-day increase in ethanol self-administration (alcohol deprivation effect) and a sustained increase in ethanol self-administration on subsequent testing days. The increase in ethanol on the first day and subsequent days was significantly above that of control animals that experienced identical treatment except with no exposure to ethanol vapors.[83] These results suggested that there was a potential change in "set point" for ethanol intake in animals with a history of sufficient ethanol exposure to produce physical dependence.

With cocaine, recent evidence shows that although limited access to cocaine (1 hour per day) produces stable drug intake from day to day, more prolonged access to cocaine (6 hours) produces an escalation in cocaine intake from day to day. This escalation is associated with a shift of the dose-effect function upward rather than a shift to the right or left[84] (FIG. 5). These data have been interpreted as a change in drug hedonic set point, where a new level of intake is required to maintain the same hedonic effect of the drug.

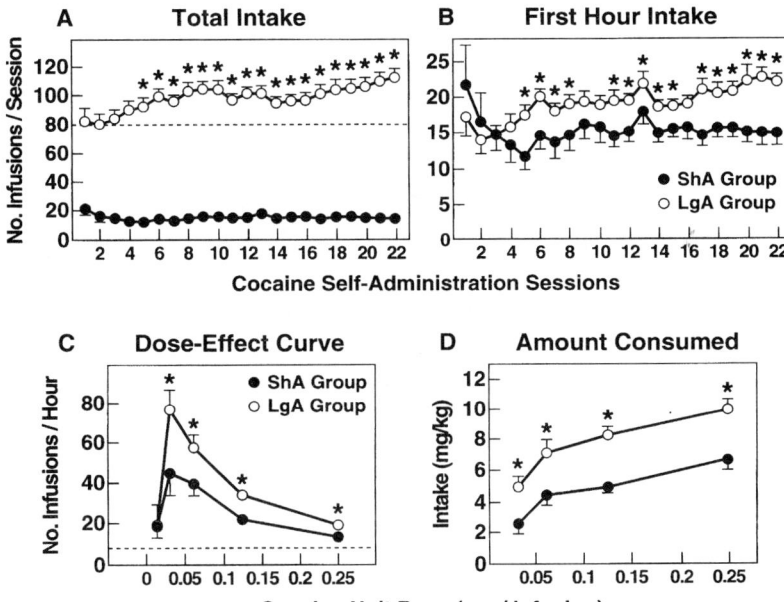

FIGURE 5. Reproduction of escalated cocaine use. **A:** In long-access (LgA) rats ($n = 12$) but not in short-access (ShA) rats ($n = 12$), mean total cocaine intake ($\pm$ SEM) started to increase significantly from session 5 ($p < 0.05$; sessions 5 to 22 compared to session 1) and continued to increase thereafter ($p < 0.05$; session 5 compared to sessions 8 to 10, 12, 13, and 17 to 22). **B:** During the first hour, LgA rats self-administered more infusions than ShA rats during sessions 5 to 8, 11, 12, 14, 15, and 17 to 22 ($p < 0.05$). **C:** Mean infusion ($\pm$ SEM) per cocaine dose tested. LgA rats took significantly more infusions than ShA rats at doses of 31.25, 62.5, 125, and 250 μg per infusion ($p < 0.05$). **D:** After escalation, LgA rats took more cocaine than ShA rats regardless of the dose ($p < 0.05$). Asterisks represent $p < 0.05$ (Student's t-test after appropriate one-way and two-way analysis of variance). (Ahmed & Koob.[84] With permission from *Science*.)

One interpretation of the increases in drug intake associated with a history of dependence (ethanol) or prolonged daily access to drug (cocaine) is that of an allostatic change where the organism has marshaled significant resources to maintain stability in the hedonic domain. The neurobiological bases for the allostasis of protracted abstinence may involve subtle molecular and cellular changes in the circuitry associated with the extended amygdala. Elucidation of these changes will be the challenge of future research on the neurobiology of addiction.

ACKNOWLEDGMENTS

This is publication number 12231-NP from The Scripps Research Institute. Work was supported by National Institutes of Health Grants DA04043 and DA04398 from the National Institute on Drug Abuse, and AA06420 and AA08459 from the

National Institute on Alcohol Abuse and Alcoholism. The author would like to thank Mike Arends for his assistance with manuscript preparation.

REFERENCES

1. AMERICAN PSYCHIATRIC ASSOCIATION. 1994. Diagnostic and Statistical Manual of Mental Disorders, 4th Edition. American Psychiatric Press. Washington, D.C.
2. WORLD HEALTH ORGANIZATION. 1992. International Statistical Classification of Diseases and Related Problems, 10th Revision. World Health Organization. Geneva.
3. WIKLER, A. 1973. Dynamics of drug dependence: implications of a conditioning theory for research and treatment. Arch. Gen. Psychiatry **28:** 611–616.
4. WISE, R.A. 1988. The neurobiology of craving: implications for the understanding and treatment of addiction. J. Abnorm. Psychol. **97:** 118–132.
5. SOLOMON, R.L. 1977. The opponent-process theory of acquired motivation: the affective dynamics of addiction. *In* Psychopathology: Experimental Models. J.D. Maser & M. E. P. Seligman, Eds.: 124–145. W.H. Freeman and Co. San Francisco.
6. KOOB, G.F. & M. LE MOAL. 1997. Drug abuse: hedonic homeostatic dysregulation. Science **278:** 52–58.
7. RUSSELL, M.A.H. 1976. What is dependence? *In* Drugs and Drug Dependence. G. Edwards, M. A. H. Russell, D. Hawks & M. MacCafferty, Eds.: 182–187. Lexington Books. Lexington, MA.
8. OLDS, J. & P. MILNER. 1954. Positive reinforcement produced by electrical stimulation of septal area and other regions of rat brain. J. Comp. Physiol. Psychol. **47:** 419–427.
9. STEIN, L. 1968. Chemistry of reward and punishment. *In* Psychopharmacology, A Review of Progress (1957–1967). D.H. Efron, Ed.: 105–123. U.S. Government Printing Office. Washington, D.C.
10. NAUTA, J.H. & W. HAYMAKER. 1969. Hypothalamic nuclei and fiber connections. *In* The Hypothalamus. W. Haymaker, E. Anderson & W. J. H. Nauta, Eds.: 136–209. Charles C. Thomas. Springfield, IL.
11. LIEBMAN, J.M. & S.J. COOPER. 1989. The Neuropharmacological Basis of Reward. Clarendon Press. Oxford.
12. VALENSTEIN, E.S. & J.F. CAMPBELL. 1966. Medial forebrain bundle-lateral hypothalamic area and reinforcing brain stimulation. Am. J. Physiol. **210:** 270–274.
13. KOOB, G.F. 1992. Drugs of abuse: anatomy, pharmacology, and function of reward pathways. Trends Pharmacol. Sci. **13:** 177–184.
14. ALHEID, G.F. & L. HEIMER. 1988. New perspectives in basal forebrain organization of special relevance for neuropsychiatric disorders: the striatopallidal, amygdaloid, and corticopetal components of substantia innominata. Neuroscience **27:** 1–39.
15. JOHNSTON, J.B. 1923. Further contributions to the study of the evolution of the forebrain. J. Comp. Neurol. **35:** 337–481.
16. HEIMER, L. & G. ALHEID. 1991. Piecing together the puzzle of basal forebrain anatomy. *In* The Basal Forebrain: Anatomy to Function. Advances in Experimental Medicine and Biology. T.C. Napier, P. W. Kalivas & I. Hanin, Eds.: **295.** 1–42. Plenum Press. New York.
17. HEIMER, L., D.S. ZAHM, L. CHURCHILL, P.W. KALIVAS & C. WOHLTMANN. 1991. Specificity in the projection patterns of accumbal core and shell in the rat. Neuroscience **41:** 89–125.
18. KILTY, J.E., D. LORANG & S.G. AMARA. 1991. Cloning and expression of a cocaine-sensitive rat dopamine transporter. Science **254:** 578–579.
19. BLAKELY, R.D., H.E. BERSON, R.T. FREMEAU, JR., M.G. CARON, M.M. PEEK, H.K. PRINCE & C.C. BRADLEY. 1991. Cloning and expression of a functional serotonin transporter from rat brain. Nature **354:** 66–70.
20. GIROS, B., S. EL MESTIKAWY, L. BERTRAND & M.G. CARON. 1991. Cloning and functional characterization of a cocaine-sensitive dopamine transporter. FEBS Lett. **295:** 149–154.

21. RUDNICK, G. & J. CLARK. 1993. From synapse to vesicle: the reuptake and storage of biogenic amine neurotransmitters. Biochim. Biophys. Acta **1144:** 249–263.
22. SPEALMAN, R.D., S.R. GOLDBERG, R.T. KELLEHER, D.M. GOLDBERG & J.P. CHARLTON. 1977. Some effects of cocaine and two cocaine analogs on schedule-controlled behavior of squirrel monkeys. J. Pharmacol. Exp. Ther. **202:** 500–509.
23. KORNETSKY, C. & R.U. ESPOSITO. 1981. Reward and detection thresholds for brain stimulation: dissociative effects of cocaine. Brain Res. **209:** 496–500.
24. KORNETSKY, C. & R.U. ESPOSITO. 1979. Euphorigenic drugs: effects on the reward pathways of the brain. Federation Proc. **38:** 2473–2476.
25. MUCHA, R.F., D. VAN DER KOOY, M. O'SHAUGHNESSY & P. BUCENIEKS. 1982. Drug reinforcement studied by the use of place conditioning in rat. Brain Res. **243:** 91–105.
26. CARR, G.D., H.C. FIBIGER & A.G. PHILLIPS. 1989. Conditioned place preference as a measure of drug reward. *In* The Neuropharmacological Basis of Reward. J.M. Liebman & S. J. Cooper, Eds.: 264–319. Oxford University Press. New York.
27. KOOB, G.F., F.J. VACCARINO, M. AMALRIC & F.E. BLOOM. 1987. Positive reinforcement properties of drugs: search for neural substrates. *In* Brain Reward Systems and Abuse. J. Engel & L. Oreland, Eds.: 35–50. Raven Press. New York.
28. KELLY, P.H., P.W. SEVIOUR & S.D. IVERSEN. 1975. Amphetamine and apomorphine responses in the rat following 6-OHDA lesions of the nucleus accumbens septi and corpus striatum. Brain Res. **94:** 507–522.
29. KELLY, P.H. & S.D. IVERSEN. 1976. Selective 6-OHDA-induced destruction of mesolimbic dopamine neurons: abolition of psychostimulant-induced locomotor activity in rats. Eur. J. Pharmacol. **40:** 45–56.
30. PIJNENBURG, A.J.J., W.M.M. HONIG & J.M. VAN ROSSUM. 1975. Inhibition of D-amphetamine-induced locomotor activity by injection of haloperidol into the nucleus accumbens of the rat. Psychopharmacologia **41:** 87–95.
31. YOKEL, R.A. & R.A. WISE. 1975. Increased lever pressing for amphetamine after pimozide in rats: implications for a dopamine theory of reward. Science **187:** 547–549.
32. ETTENBERG, A., H.O. PETTIT, F.E. BLOOM & G.F. KOOB. 1982. Heroin and cocaine intravenous self-administration in rats: mediation by separate neural systems. Psychopharmacology **78:** 204–209.
33. PHILLIPS, A.G. & H.C. FIBIGER. 1987. Anatomical and neurochemical substrates of drug reward determined by the conditioned place preference technique. *In* Methods of Assessing the Reinforcing Properties of Abused Drugs. M.A. Bozarth, Ed.: 275–290. Springer-Verlag. New York.
34. BENINGER, R.J. & B.L. HAHN. 1983. Pimozide blocks establishment but not expression of amphetamine-produced environment-specific conditioning. Science **220:** 1304–1306.
35. BENINGER, R.J. & R.S. HERZ. 1986. Pimozide blocks establishment but not expression of cocaine-produced environment-specific conditioning. Life Sci. **38:** 1425–1431.
36. MORENCY, M.A. & R.J. BENINGER. 1986. Dopaminergic substrates of cocaine-induced placed conditioning. Brain Res. **399:** 33–41.
37. CAINE, S.B. & G.F. KOOB. 1995. Pretreatment with the dopamine agonist 7-OH-DPAT shifts the cocaine self-administration dose-effect function to the left under different schedules in the rat. Behav. Pharmacol. **6:** 333–347.
38. BERGMAN, J., J.B. KAMIEN & R.D. SPEALMAN. 1990. Antagonism of cocaine self-administration by selective dopamine D1 and D2 antagonists. Behav. Pharmacol. **1:** 355–363.
39. ROBERTS, D.C.S., G.F. KOOB, P. KLONOFF & H.C. FIBIGER. 1980. Extinction and recovery of cocaine self-administration following 6-hydroxydopamine lesions of the nucleus accumbens. Pharmacol. Biochem. Behav. **12:** 781–787.
40. LYNESS, W.H., N.M. FRIEDLE & K.E. MOORE. 1979. Destruction of dopaminergic nerve terminals in nucleus accumbens: effect on D-amphetamine self-administration. Pharmacol. Biochem. Behav. **11:** 553–556.

41. CAINE, S.B. & G.F. KOOB. 1994. Effects of mesolimbic dopamine depletion on responding maintained by cocaine and food. J. Exp. Anal. Behav. **61:** 213–221.
42. KOOB, G.F., H.T. LE & I. CREESE. 1987. The D-1 dopamine receptor antagonist SCH 23390 increases cocaine self-administration in the rat. Neurosci. Lett. **79:** 315–320.
43. WOOLVERTON, W.L. & R.M. VIRUS. 1989. The effects of a D1 and D2 dopamine antagonist on behavior maintained by cocaine or food. Pharmacol. Biochem. Behav. **32:** 691–697.
44. CAINE, S.B. & G.F. KOOB. 1993. Modulation of cocaine self-administration in the rat through D-3 dopamine receptors. Science **260:** 1814–1816.
45. LEONE, P. & G. DI CHIARA. 1987. Blockade of D_1 receptors by SCH 23390 antagonists morphine- and amphetamine-induced place preference conditioning. Eur. J. Pharmacol. **135:** 251–254.
46. BENINGER, R.J., D.C. HOFFMAN & E.J. MAZURSKI. 1989. Receptor subtype-specific dopaminergic agents and conditioned behavior. Neurosci. Biobehav. Rev. **13:** 113–122.
47. CAINE, S.B., S.C. HEINRICHS, V.L. COFFIN & G.F. KOOB. 1995. Effects of the dopamine D1 antagonist SCH 23390 microinjected into the accumbens, amygdala or striatum on cocaine self-administration in the rat. Brain Res. **692:** 47–56.
48. EPPING-JORDAN, M.P., A. MARKOU & G.F. KOOB. 1998. The dopamine D-1 receptor antagonist SCH 23390 injected into the dorsolateral bed nucleus of the stria terminalis decreased cocaine reinforcement in the rat. Brain Res. **784:** 105–115.
49. SOKOLOFF, P., B. GIROS, M.-P. MARTRES, M.L. BOUTHENET & J.-C. SCHWARTZ. 1990. Molecular cloning and characterization of a novel dopamine receptor (D3) as a target for neuroleptics. Nature **347:** 146–151.
50. CAINE, S.B., G.F. KOOB, L.H. PARSONS, B.J. EVERITT, J.-C. SCHWARTZ & P. SOKOLOFF. 1997. D3 receptor test *in vitro* predicts decreased cocaine self-administration in rats. NeuroReport **8:** 2373–2377.
51. ROBLEDO, P. & G.F. KOOB. 1993. Two discrete nucleus accumbens projection areas differentially mediate cocaine self-administration in the rat. Behav. Brain Res. **55:** 159–166.
52. ZAHM, D.S. & L. HEIMER. 1990. Two transpallidal pathways originating in the rat nucleus accumbens. J. Comp. Neurol. **302:** 437–446.
53. HYYTIA, P. & G.F. KOOB. 1995. $GABA_A$ receptor antagonism in the extended amygdala decreases ethanol self-administration in rats. Eur. J. Pharmacol. **283:** 151–159.
54. HEYSER, C.J., A.J. ROBERTS, G. SCHULTEIS, P. HYYTIA & G.F. KOOB. 1995. Central administration of an opiate antagonist decreases oral ethanol self-administration in rats. Soc. Neurosci. Abstr. **21:** 1698.
55. PONTIERI, F.E., G. TANDA & G. DI CHIARA. 1995. Intravenous cocaine, morphine, and amphetamine preferentially increase extracellular dopamine in the "shell" as compared with the "core" of the rat nucleus accumbens. Proc. Natl. Acad. Sci. USA **92:** 12304–12308.
56. TANDA, G., F.E. PONTIERI & G. DI CHIARA. 1997. Cannabinoid and heroin activation of mesolimbic dopamine transmission by a common mu1 opioid receptor mechanism. Science **276:** 2048–2050.
57. PONTIERI, F.E., G. TANDA, F. ORZI & G. DI CHIARA. 1996. Effects of nicotine on the nucleus accumbens and similarity to those of addictive drugs. Nature **382:** 255–257.
58. GAWIN, F.H. & H.D. KLEBER. 1986. Abstinence symptomatology and psychiatric diagnosis in cocaine abusers: clinical observations. Arch. Gen. Psychiatry **43:** 107–113.
59. WEDDINGTON, W.W., JR., B.S. BROWN, C.A. HAERTZEN, J.M. HESS, J.R. MAHAFFEY, A.F. KOLAR & J.H. JAFFE. 1991. Comparison of amantadine and desipramine combined with psychotherapy for treatment of cocaine dependence. Am. J. Drug Alcohol Abuse **17:** 137–152.
60. MARKOU, A. & G.F. KOOB. 1991. Postcocaine anhedonia: an animal model of cocaine withdrawal. Neuropsychopharmacology **4:** 17–26.

61. SCHULTEIS, G., A. MARKOU, L.H. GOLD, L. STINUS & G.F. KOOB. 1994. Relative sensitivity to naloxone of multiple indices of opiate withdrawal: a quantitative dose-response analysis. J. Pharmacol. Exp. Ther. **271:** 1391–1398.
62. LEITH, N.J. & R.J. BARRETT. 1976. Amphetamine and the reward system: evidence for tolerance and post-drug depression. Psychopharmacologia **46:** 19–25.
63. PARSONS, L.H., G.F. KOOB & F. WEISS. 1995. Serotonin dysfunction in the nucleus accumbens of rats during withdrawal after unlimited access to intravenous cocaine. J. Pharmacol. Exp. Ther. **274:** 1182–1191.
64. MARKOU, A. & G.F. KOOB. 1992. Construct validity of a self-stimulation threshold paradigm: effects of reward and performance manipulations. Physiol. Behav. **51:** 111–119.
65. LEGAULT, M. & R.A. WISE. 1994. Effects of withdrawal from nicotine on intracranial self-stimulation. Soc. Neurosci. Abstr. **20:** 1032.
66. WEISS, F., A. MARKOU, M.T. LORANG & G.F. KOOB. 1992. Basal extracellular dopamine levels in the nucleus accumbens are decreased during cocaine withdrawal after unlimited-access self-administration. Brain Res. **593:** 314–318.
67. STINUS, L., M. LE MOAL & G.F. KOOB. 1990. Nucleus accumbens and amygdala are possible substrates for the aversive stimulus effects of opiate withdrawal. Neuroscience **37:** 767–773.
68. ROBERTS, A.J., M. COLE & G.F. KOOB. 1996. Intra-amygdala muscimol decreases operant ethanol self-administration in dependent rats. Alcohol. Clin. Exp. Res. **20:** 1289–1298.
69. WEISS, F., L.H. PARSONS, G. SCHULTEIS, P. HYYTIA, M.T. LORANG, F.E. BLOOM & G.F. KOOB. 1996. Ethanol self-administration restores withdrawal-associated deficiencies in accumbal dopamine and 5-hydroxytryptamine release in dependent rats. J. Neurosci. **16:** 3474–3485.
70. FITZGERALD, L.W. & E.J. NESTLER. 1995. Molecular and cellular adaptations in signal transduction pathways following ethanol exposure. Clin. Neurosci. **3:** 165–173.
71. KOOB, G.F., S.C. HEINRICHS, F. MENZAGHI, E. MERLO-PICH & K.T. BRITTON. 1994. Corticotropin-releasing factor, stress and behavior. Semin. Neurosciences **6:** 221–229.
72. HEINRICHS, S.C., F. MENZAGHI, G. SCHULTEIS, G.F. KOOB & L. STINUS. 1995. Suppression of corticotropin-releasing factor in the amygdala attenuates aversive consequences of morphine withdrawal. Behav. Pharmacol. **6:** 74–80.
73. RODRIGUEZ DE FONSECA, F., M.R.A. CARRERA, M. NAVARRO, G.F. KOOB & F. WEISS. 1997. Activation of corticotropin-releasing factor in the limbic system during cannabinoid withdrawal. Science **276:** 2050–2054.
74. RICHTER, R.M. & F. WEISS. 1998. *In vivo* CRF release in rat amygdala is increased during cocaine withdrawal in self-administering rats. Synapse. In press.
75. RASSNICK, S., S.C. HEINRICHS, K.T. BRITTON & G.F. KOOB. 1993. Microinjection of a corticotropin-releasing factor antagonist into the central nucleus of the amygdala reverses anxiogenic-like effects of ethanol withdrawal. Brain Res. **605:** 25–32.
76. SARNYAI, Z., E. BIRO, J. GARDI, M. VECSERNYES, J. JULESZ & G. TELEGDY. 1995. Brain corticotropin-releasing factor mediates "anxiety-like" behavior induced by cocaine withdrawal in rats. Brain Res. **675:** 89–97.
77. INFORMAL EXPERT GROUP MEETING ON THE CRAVING MECHANISM (Report no. V.92-54439T). 1992. Geneva, Switzerland, United Nations International Drug Control Programme and World Health Organization.
78. MARKOU, A., F. WEISS, L.H. GOLD, S.B. CAINE, G. SCHULTEIS & G.F. KOOB. 1993. Animal models of drug craving. Psychopharmacology **112:** 163–182.
79. MIRIN, R.E. & S.M. MEYER. 1979. The Heroin Stimulus: Implications for a Theory of Addiction. Plenum Press. New York.
80. O'BRIEN, C.P. 1975. Experimental analysis of conditioning factors in human narcotic addiction. Pharmacol. Rev. **27:** 533–543.
81. EVERITT, B.J., K.A. MORRIS, A. O'BRIEN & T.W. ROBBINS. 1991. The basolateral amygdala-ventral striatal system and conditioned place preference: further evidence of limbic-striatal interactions underlying reward-related processes. Neuroscience **42:** 1–18.

82. EVERITT, B.J., G. SCHULTEIS & G.F. KOOB. 1993. Attenuation of conditioned opiate withdrawal following excitotoxic lesions of the basolateral amygdala. Soc. Neurosci. Abstr. **19:** 1246.
83. ROBERTS, A.J., C.J. HEYSER, M. COLE, P. GRIFFIN & G.F. KOOB. 1999. Excessive ethanol drinking following a history of dependence: animal models of allostasis. Submitted.
84. AHMED, S.H. & G.F. KOOB. 1998. Transition from moderate to excessive drug intake: change in hedonic set point. Science **282:** 298–300.
85. KOOB, G.F., P.P. SANNA & F.E. BLOOM. 1998. Neuroscience of addiction. Neuron **21:** 467–476.

Drug Addiction as a Disorder of Associative Learning

Role of Nucleus Accumbens Shell/Extended Amygdala Dopamine

G. DI CHIARA,[a] G. TANDA, V. BASSAREO, F. PONTIERI, E. ACQUAS, S. FENU, C. CADONI, AND E. CARBONI

Department of Toxicology and CNR Center for Neuropharmacology, University of Cagliari, Viale A. Diaz 182, 09126 Cagliari, Italy

ABSTRACT: Conventional reinforcers phasically stimulate dopamine transmission in the nucleus accumbens shell. This property undergoes one-trial habituation consistent with a role of nucleus accumbens shell dopamine in associative learning. Experimental studies with place- and taste-conditioning paradigms confirm this role. Addictive drugs share with conventional reinforcers the property of stimulating dopamine transmission in the nucleus accumbens shell. This response, however, undergoes one-trial habituation in the case of conventional reinforcers but not of drugs. Resistance to habituation allows drugs to repetitively activate dopamine transmission in the shell upon repeated self-administration. This process abnormally facilitates associative learning, leading to the attribution of excessive motivational value to discrete stimuli or contexts predictive of drug availability. Addiction is therefore the expression of the excessive control over behavior acquired by drug-related stimuli as a result of abnormal strenghtening of stimulus-drug contingencies by nondecremental drug-induced stimulation of dopamine transmission in the nucleus accumbens shell.

INTRODUCTION

The heuristic power of the notion of a ventral striatum as part of the striato-pallidal system[1] and of a nucleus accumbens shell as a transition area between the striato-pallidal system and the extended amygdala[2] is best exemplified by the influence these ideas have exerted on the evolution of studies in the field of drug addiction. Drug addiction[3] can be conceptualized as a disorder of motivation characterized by the excessive control over behavior acquired by drugs and drug-related stimuli that act as powerful incentives of drug-seeking and drug-taking behavior.[4–9] Although traditionally viewed in the perspective of reinforcement,[10] drug addiction is not simply a case of drug reinforcement. Caffeine, for example, the active component of coffee beverages, is not listed among addictive drugs,[3] in spite of its reinforcing and psychostimulant properties testifyed by the choice of millions of people.

The positive-reinforcing properties of drugs, although not sufficient, are nonetheless necessary for their addictive properties for at least two reasons: reinforcing

---

[a]Voice: 39.70.303819; fax:39.70.300740; diptoss@tin.it

properties of drugs, by promoting self-administration, are instrumental for repeated drug exposure, which is essential for addiction to develop; and reinforcing properties of drugs are necessary for the associative learning mechanism that confers motivational value to stimuli that predict drug availability and act as powerful incentives of drug-seeking behavior.[4-9]

It is a basic tenet of our hypothesis[9] that the addictive properties of drugs are related to their property of stimulating dopamine (DA) transmission in the shell of the nucleus accumbens (NAc) and in the extended amygdala. Drugs share this property with conventional reinforcers, but this effect is not subjected to habituation upon repeated drug exposure, as instead is the case of conventional reinforcers. The repetitive, nondecremental stimulation of DA transmission induced by drugs in the shell/extended amygdala abnormally facilitates the acquisition of motivational properties by drug-related stimuli, which thus acquire the ability of controlling behavior in that dominant and exclusive manner typical of addiction.

This hypothesis should not be confused with the incentive-sensitization theory of drug addiction,[8] as this theory specifically excludes an involvement of DA in associative learning. Thus, the incentive-sensitization theory posits that drug-related stimuli, having acquired motivational value as a result of a DA-independent associative process, induce the abnormal incentive state of addiction (craving) by eliciting a sensitized release of DA in mesocorticolimbic neurons.[8]

The following is an account of the associative learning hypothesis of drug addiction.

ADDICTIVE DRUGS PREFERENTIALLY STIMULATE *IN VIVO* DA TRANSMISSION IN THE VENTRAL AS COMPARED TO THE DORSAL STRIATUM

In the 1970s three important developments had taken place: first, it was realized that DA is not confined to motor extrapyramidal areas but extends to limbic and cortical areas; second, it was proposed that the nucleus accumbens (NAc) mediates the locomotor effects of psychostimulants and DA agonists; third, the role of DA in brain self-stimulation and in the motivational effects of psychostimulants was fully appreciated.

Until the early 1980s, however, the role of DA in the mechanism of action of non-psychostimulant drugs was debated or simply unknown. The availability of the brain microdialysis technique for estimating *in vivo* DA transmission in specific brain areas[11,12] allowed a systematic study of the effects of drugs of abuse on DA transmission in the dorsal caudate putamen (CPu) and in the NAc, as representatives of the dorsal and of the ventral striatum, respectively.[13] It was found that not only psychostimulants like cocaine and amphetamine[14] but also narcotic analgetics,[15] nicotine,[16] ethanol,[17] and phencyclidine,[14] increase dialysate DA preferentially in the NAc, as compared to the dorsal CPu.[13]

These observations were later confirmed by other laboratories for cocaine,[18] nicotin,[19] and morphine.[29] In the case of amphetamine, however, other studies did not confirm its preferential effect in the NAc versus the dorsal CPu.[18,20] As both these studies used vertical concentric probes rather than transcerebral ones, it was suggest-

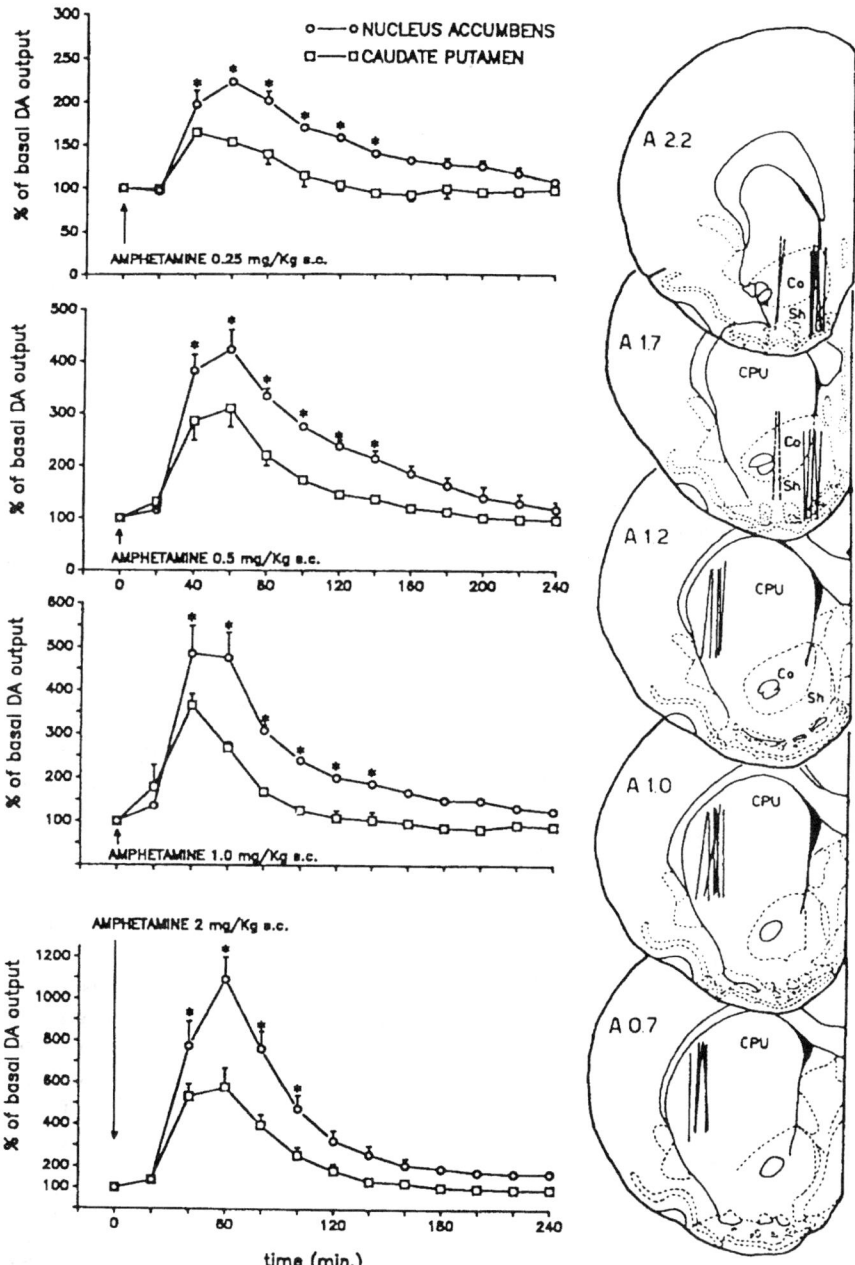

FIGURE 1. Comparison of the effect of different doses of amphetamine on DA output in dialysates from the nucleus accumbens (Acc) (antero-medial site) and from the dorsal caudate-putamen (CPu). Data are means ± SEM of the results expressed as percent of basal

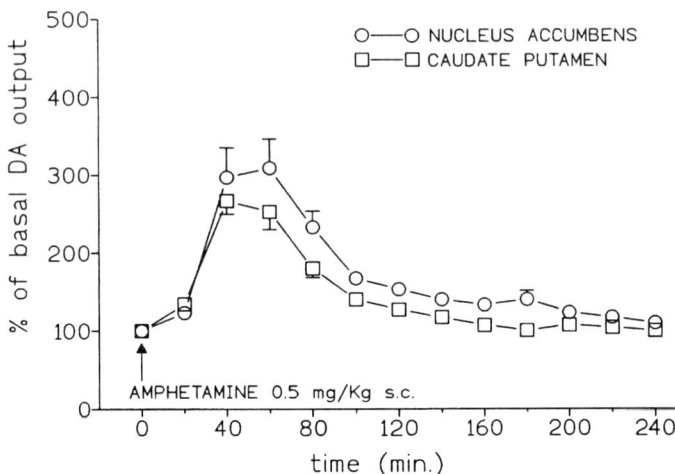

FIGURE 2. Effect of amphetamine (0.5 mg/kg sc) on DA output in dialysates from the nucleus accumbens (antero-central) and the dorsal caudate-putamen. Basal output of DA in pmol/sample (mean ± SEM of 4 rats) was the following: Acc, 0.165 ± 0.018: CPu, 0.278 ± 50. Data are means ± SEM of 4 rats and are expressed as percent of basal values. The location of these probes is shown in FIG. 1. See legend to FIG. 1 for other explanations. (Di Chiara et al.[22] With permission from *Psychopharmacology*.)

ed that topographic differences in the relative location of the probes in the striatum could account for the discrepancies.[21] In agreement with this suggestion, it was showed by vertical concentric probes that, in order to resolve the differences between the NAc and the dorsal CPu in the response to amphetamine, specific topographic conditions had to be satisfied, such as a dorso-lateral placement of microdialysis probes in the CPu and a ventro-medial and anterior placement in the NAc (FIG. 1).[22] Thus, when comparisons were made between the dorsal CPu and the central-lateral part of the NAc, no differences were obtained[22] (FIG. 2).

At the time when these studies were performed the concept of a shell/core dicotomy in the NAc had just been proposed,[1,23] and it appeared perfectly tailored to account for the topographic heterogeneity of the response of striatal DA transmission to addictive drugs. Therefore, the hypothesis was made that the preferential effect of amphetamine and of other drugs of abuse in the NAc was specifically related to differences in DA responsiveness between the dorsal CPu and the NAc shell and that failure to reproduce these differences was due to placement of microdialysis probes

---

uncorrected output of DA. On the right is shown the location of the probes reconstructed on the basis of serial coronal sections. The dialyzing part of the probe was considered to correspond to the 2.2-mm ventralmost portion of the probe track after leaving a 0.3-mm length to account for the sharpened probe tip. Continuous lines refer to the location of the probes in the series of rats whose results are shown in the FIGURE (medial site). Dashed lines correspond to the lateral site (see FIG. 2). On the left of each section, starting from cranial, is indicated the distance from bregma in mm. Co, core; Sh, shell of the nucleus accumbens. (Di Chiara et al.[22] With permission from *Psychopharmacology*.)

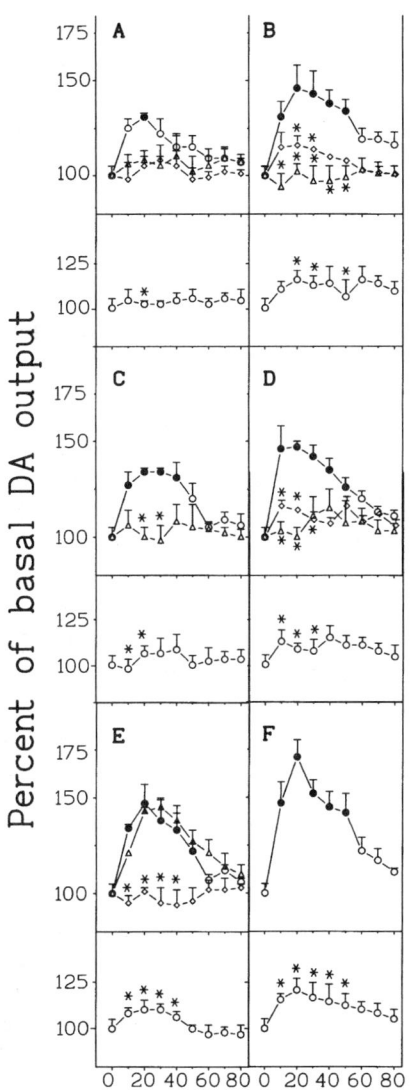

FIGURE 3. Effect of intravenous Δ^9-THC, WIN55212-2, and heroin on dialysate DA in the shell (upper panels) and core (lower panels) of the NAc. **A** and **B**: Δ^9-THC doses of 0.15 and 0.30 mg/kg iv; **C** and **D:** WIN55212-2 doses of 0.15 and 0.30 mg/kg iv; **E** and **F**: heroin doses of 0.018 and 0.030 mg/kg iv. Rats were pretreated with saline (circles), SR141716-A (triangles) (1 mg/kg sc), or with naloxone (diamonds) (0.1 mg/kg ip). Results are means ± SEM of the amount of DA in 10-min dialysate samples, expressed as percent of basal values. Solid symbols: $p < 0.05$, compared with basal values. *$p < 0.05$, compared with the corresponding value obtained in the shell of saline-pretreated controls. (Tanda et al.[26] With permission from *Science*.)

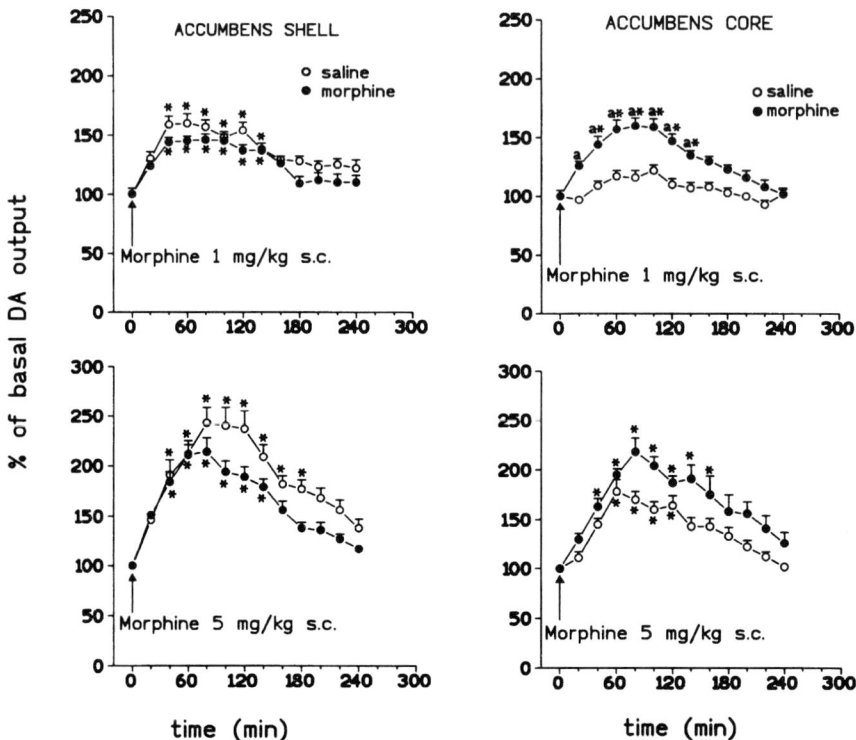

FIGURE 4. Effect of challenge with 1 and 5 mg/kg morphine on basal DA output in dialysates from the NAc shell of control (open circles) and sensitized rats (filled circles). The results (means ± SEM) are expressed as percentage of basal values. *$p < 0.05$, versus respective basal values by two-way ANOVA followed by Tukey's test. (Cadoni & Di Chiara.[27] With permission from *Neuroscience*.)

in the NAc core, the homologous of the dorsal CPu as part of the striato-pallidal system.[23] In order to verify this hypothesis the effect of a variety of drugs of abuse on *in vivo* DA transmission in the NAc shell and core was systematically compared.[24–26] Rats were implanted with concentric probes aimed at the core of one side and at the shell of the other side and with intravenous catheters in order to administer the drugs at unitary doses known from the literature to maintain iv self-administration behavior in the rat. Calbindin immunohistochemistry was used to distinguish shell from core in the histological verification of probe location.[24–26]

ADDICTIVE DRUGS PREFERENTIALLY ACTIVATE DA TRANSMISSION AND ENERGY METABOLISM IN THE NAC SHELL AS COMPARED TO THE CORE

Nonpsychostimulant drugs (including morphine, heroin (FIG. 3), nicotine and (Δ^9THC (FIG. 3) at each of the two doses tested increased dialysate DA selectively

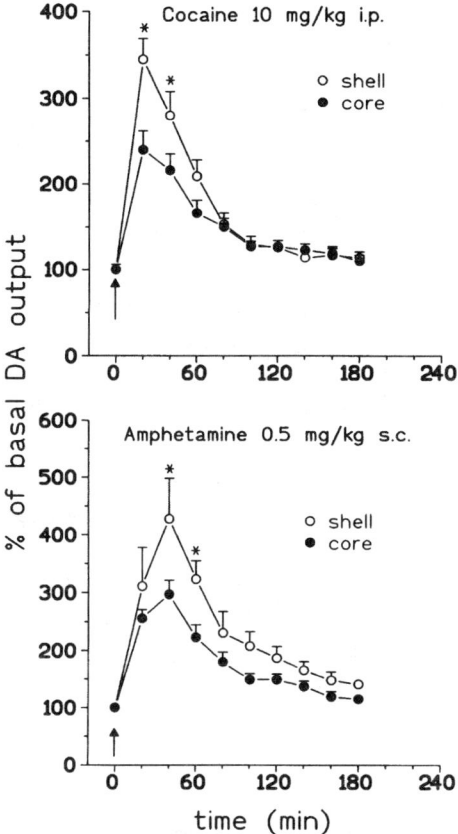

FIGURE 5. Effect of challenge with 10 mg/kg of cocaine ip and of 0.5 mg/kg sc amphetamine on basal DA output in dialysates from the NAc shell and core. The results (means ± SEM) are expressed as percentage of basal values. *$p < 0.05$ versus respective basal values by two-way ANOVA followed by Tukey's test. (Cadoni & Di Chiara.[27] With permission from *Neuroscience*.)

in the NAc shell;[24–26] cocaine showed a selective effect in the shell at the lower dose and a preferential one at the higher dose.[24] Amphetamine had a preferential effect at the lower dose but at the higher one was similarly effective in the shell and in the core.[24] Similar observations were made for morphine (FIG. 4) and amphetamine (FIG. 5) given subcutaneously,[27] and for cocaine (FIG. 5) given intraperitoneally.[27] More recently a preferential effect of amphetamine in the anterior shell has been reported after local intracerebral infusion.[28] Moreover, Barrot *et al.* have recently confirmed the preferential effect of morphine and cocaine on DA of the NAc shell.[29] It is notable that in the case of morphine[27] and cocaine[29] a preferential effect in the NAc, as compared to the dorsal striatum, is obtained also when comparisons are made with the NAc core. This is probably not the case of amphetamine, which dif-

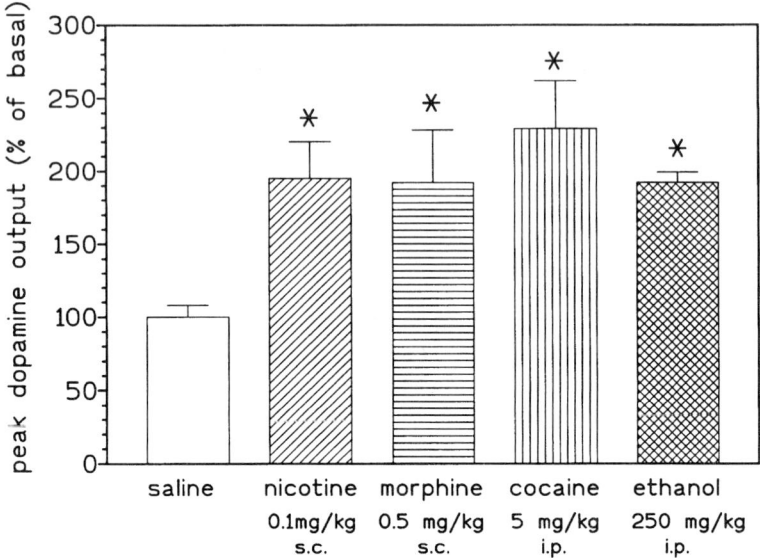

FIGURE 6. Effect of drugs of abuse on extracellular concentration of dopamine in the bed nucleus of the stria terminalis. Results are expressed as maximal percent change from basal and are means ± SEM of at least 4 rats. The probe was implanted with coordinates. Anterior, − 0.1; lateral, 1.1; vertical, 8.1, from the dura, according to the *Atlas* by Paxinos and Watson (1987). Basal extracellular DA concentration was 14.03 ± 1.3 fmoles/20 μL (mean ± SEM; $n = 40$).

ferentially affects NAc shell versus core and dorsal striatum, but not NAc core versus dorsal striatum.

In parallel studies with 2-deoxyglucose autoradiography it was also shown that nicotine,[25] morphine,[30] cocaine, and amphetamine[31] activate, at low doses, energy metabolism selectively in the NAc shell, indicating that stimulation of DA transmission in this area by drugs of abuse increases the activity of intrinsic and afferent neural input.

ADDICTIVE DRUGS ACTIVATE DA TRANSMISSION IN THE BED NUCLEUS OF STRIA TERMINALIS

In view of the proposal by Heimer and colleagues[2,23] that the NAc shell is a transition area between the striatum and the extended amygdala, the observation that addictive drugs activate DA transmission in the shell, coupled to the notion that DA densely innervates a number of areas that belong to the lateral subdivision of the extended amygdala (bed nucleus of stria terminalis, BSTM, and central amygdala)[32] prompted us to investigate the effect of addictive drugs on DA transmission in the BSTM. An alternative area of study, the central amygdala, was discarded because of the possibility of contamination of dialysate DA by DA arising from the adjacent caudate tail.

Nicotine, morphine, cocaine, amphetamine, and ethanol increase dialysate DA in the BSTM (FIG. 6). It is notable that the magnitude of the effect and the sensitivity to the drug is higher in this area as compared to the NAc shell. Therefore, addictive drugs have in common the property of activating DA transmission not only in the NAc shell but also in a major area of the extended amygdala, such as the BSTM.

RELATIONSHIP BETWEEN DA STIMULATION IN THE NAC SHELL AND ADDICTIVE DRUG LIABILITY

In addition to addictive drugs, another class of drugs that increases dialysate DA in the NAc shell is that of neuroleptics. Neuroleptics produce this effect as a result of blockade of DA receptors, mostly D_2/D_3 autoreceptors and postsynaptic D_2-like receptors, and probably also D_1 receptors.[33] Therefore the stimulation of DA release in the NAc shell by neuroleptics, being secondary to DA receptor blockade, has a

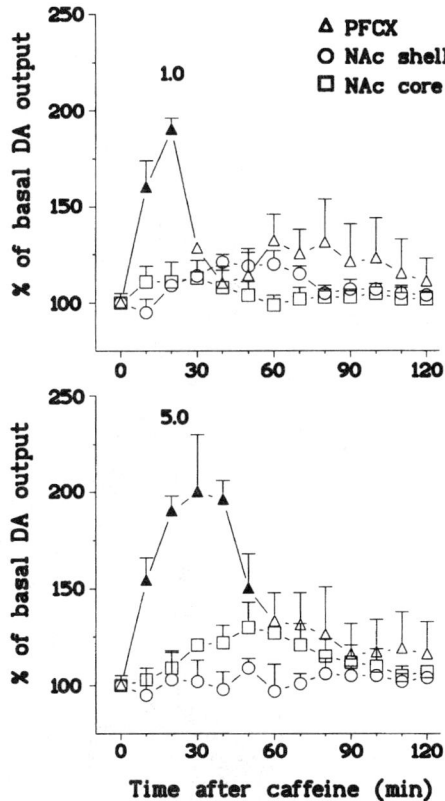

FIGURE 7. Effect of 1.0 and 5.0 mg/kg of caffeine given iv on DA output in dialysates from prefrontal cortex (PFCX) and nucleus accumbens (NAc), shell and core. Results are means ± SEM of 4 rats. Filled symbols: $p < 0.05$ from basal.

significance just opposite to that of the effect of addictive drugs, which primarily activate DA transmission.

Caffeine, a drug with psychostimulant and rewarding properties but devoid of addictive properties,[3] provides an example of the other side of the coin. Thus, caffeine dose-dependently increases dialysate DA in the prefrontal cortex (PFCX) but is ineffective on DA transmission in the NAc shell or core (FIG. 7). The effect of caffeine on DA in the PFCX might be secondary to its psychostimulant properties, which, in turn, might be the result of blockade of A_2 and A_1 adenosine receptors in limbic areas.[34] However, an increase of DA transmission in the PFCX seems unrelated to addictive drug liability (see below). Given the lack of addictive properties of caffeine,[3] its failure to stimulate DA transmission in the NAc shell is consistent with a role of NAc shell DA in the addictive properties of drugs.

MESOLIMBIC SPECIFICITY OF THE DA STIMULANT EFFECT OF ADDICTIVE DRUGS

Nonpsychostimulant drugs, including morphine, ethanol, and nicotine, at doses that fully stimulate DA transmission in the NAc shell, do not increase DA transmission in the medial PFCX where mesocortical DA neurons terminate.[35] Cocaine and amphetamine, however, increase dialysate DA in the PFCX even more effectively than in the NAc shell.[36] The increase in extracellular DA in the PFCX induced by cocaine and amphetamine, however, is not due to an action on the DA carrier (as in the NAc) but to blockade of the noradrenaline (NA) carrier, as shown *in vivo* by the concurrent increase of NA in the PFCX.[36] GBR 12909, a blocker of the DA carrier, devoid of action on the NA carrier, while fully increasing DA in the NAc, is ineffective in raising extracellular DA in the PFCX.[36] Moreover, under selective blockade of the NA carrier by desipramine through reverse dialysis, cocaine fails to increase DA in the PFCX.[36] These observations are explained by the 1000 times difference in the ratio of NA terminals to DA terminals in the PFCX, as compared to the NAc[37] and by the high efficiency (four times more than NA itself) of the NA carrier as a transporter of DA.[38] Therefore, in the PFCX, NA terminals provide the most efficient means for the clearance of DA from the extracellular space so that blockade of the NA carrier provides, in turn, an efficient means for increasing DA in extrastriatal areas where the NA/DA ratio is high.[39,40]

The role of the increase of DA in the PFCX in the addictive properties of cocaine and amphetamine is obscure but is unlikely to be a major one in view of the lack of addictive liability or psychostimulant properties of antidepressants, in spite of the fact that these drugs increase DA in the PFCX but not in the NAc.[40]

MECHANISMS OF DRUG-INDUCED STIMULATION OF MESOLIMBIC DOPAMINE

Addictive drugs stimulate DA transmission by different mechanisms, depending on the drug class they belong to. Psychostimulant (cocaine and amphetamine) and nonpsychostimulant drugs (narcotics, nicotine, ethanol, and Δ^9 THC) differ for the fact that although the first indirectly inhibit the firing activity of DA neurons through DA accumulated extracellularly following inhibition of DA reuptake (e.g., cocaine) or carrier-mediated release of DA (e.g., amphetamine,)[14,41] nonpsychostimulants increase the firing activity of DA neurons,[42–44] and this effect is preferential on VTA as compared to pars compacta neurons, which explains their preferential effect on DA of the NAc.[42–44] A lower efficiency of DA reuptake in the NAc as compared to the dorsal striatum has been suggested to be the basis for the preferential effect of cocaine in the NAc.[45]

A differential property of nonpsychostimulant as compared to psychostimulant drugs is their differential dependence on μ opioid and $5HT_3$ receptors. Thus, systemic administration of naloxonazine, an irreversible μ–opioid antagonist, prevents the *in vivo* stimulation of mesolimbic DA transmission by opiates, ethanol, Δ^9 THC, and nicotine.[26,46] $5HT_3$ antagonists exert a similar effect on morphine, ethanol, and nicotine.[47] Although the μ-dependent effects of narcotics are likely to be due to a direct action of the drug on μ_1 receptors, the effects of ethanol and nicotine, which do not bind to μ_1 receptors, are necessarily indirect. A similar indirect mechanism would apply to the $5HT_3$-dependent effects of morphine, ethanol, and nicotine, which do not bind to $5HT_3$ receptors.

TOPOGRAPHIC SPECIFICITY OF MOTIVATIONAL RESPONSE PROPERTIES OF DA TRANSMISSION IN THE NUCLEUS ACCUMBENS

DA transmission is responsive to stimuli provided of motivational value. Motivational stimuli are distinguished in positive or negative depending on the nature (beneficial or harmful) of their biological consequences. Positive stimuli, in turn, are divided into appetitive and consummatory, depending on the type of behavior they elicit: flexible patterns of search and approach to the reward (appetitive stimuli) or fixed patterns of consumption of the reward for the use of its biological resources (consummatory stimuli).[48]

Feeding of an unfamiliar palatable food stimulates DA transmission in the PFCX, in the NAc shell, and, to a lesser extent, in the NAc core.[49] Repeated predictive association of food smell or extrinsic visual-tactile stimuli with food taste (feeding) results in acquisition by the same stimuli of the property of eliciting conditioned (appetitive) responses (CRs), which consist of orienting towards, approach to the object stimulus (plastic box), and even licking and biting at it.[49] These appetitive effects are associated to an increase of dialysate DA in the PFCX[49] and in the NAc core[50] but not in the shell[49,50] (FIG. 8). Therefore the NAc shell DA responds to primary consummatory but not to secondary appetitive (conditional) olfactory or nonolfactory food stimuli. On the other hand, exposure to conditional olfactory food stimuli for 10–40 min before being reinforced by feeding reduces the responsiveness of the DA transmission shell to subsequent feeding but potentiates that in the NAc core[50] (FIG. 8).

Another aspect of the properties of the responsiveness of DA transmission to motivational stimuli are the adaptive changes it undergoes upon a single exposure to consummatory food stimuli. These changes are quite different in the NAc shell and, respectively, in the NAc core and PFCX. Thus, a single feeding trial of palatable

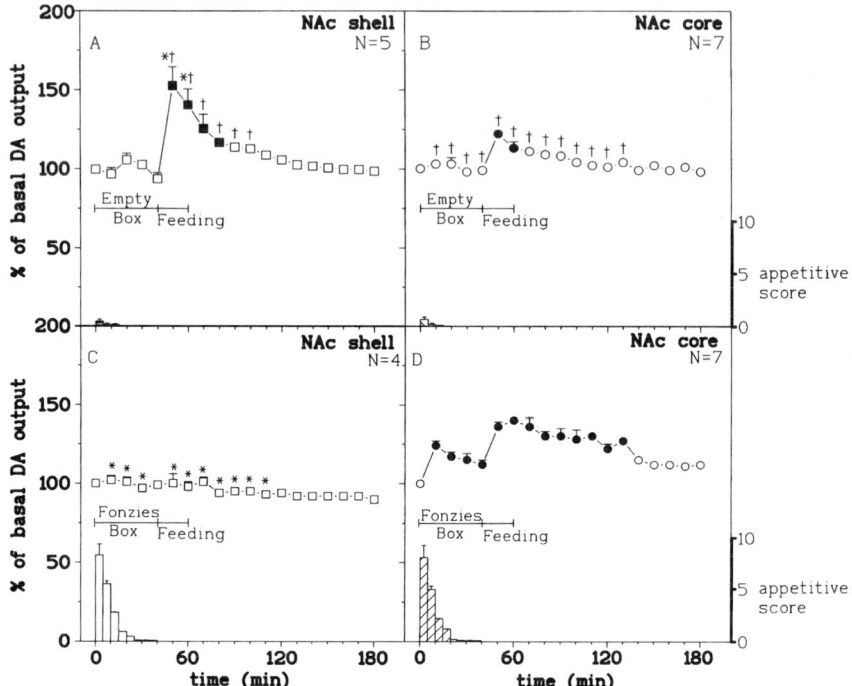

FIGURE 8. Effect of neutral (empty box) or conditional food stimuli (Fonzies, filled box) and of Fonzies feeding on dialysate DA in the NAc shell and core, and on appetitive score. Results are means ± SEM expressed as percent of basal values. Basal values in fmoles DA/sample were NAc shell: 64 ± 6 (means ± SEM of 9 rats); NAc core: 60 ± 6 (means ± SEM of 14 rats). Filled symbols: $p < 0.05$, with respect to basal values; *, $p < 0.05$, with respect to the corresponding value of the group implanted in the NAc core (**A** versus **B**, and **C** versus **D**); †, $p < 0.05$ with respect to the corresponding value of the group preexposed to Fonzies, filled box (**A** versus **C**, and **B** versus **D**). Fonzies (KP Snack foods, Germany) is a snack food made of corn flour, hydrogenated vegetable fat, cheese powder, salt, and monosodium glutamate as a taste enhancer. Rats were fed ad libitum. Rats do not show appetitive responses to the smell of Fonzies placed inside a perforated opaque plastic box, unless they learn the relationship between the smell and taste of Fonzies.[49] Therefore, rats were fed Fonzies 5 days before the experiment by placing 2 g in the home cage. Perforated cylindrical boxes were made of sky-blue plastic and were 8 cm in height and 6 cm in diameter. They were used either empty (**A** and **B**) or filled up with 8 g of Fonzies (**C** and **D**). In order to adapt the rats to the empty plastic box, this was placed in their home cage for the whole day before probe implants. Appetitive behavior in response to perforated cylindrical boxes filled with Fonzies was scored, according to ref. 49. (Bassareo and Di Chiara.[50] With permission from *Neuroscience*.)

food (Fonzies), although inducing habituation of DA responsiveness in the NAc shell,[49] actually sensitizes the response in the NAc core. In the PFCX, a nonsignificant tendency towards potentiation of the response is observed.[49]

These observations indicate that DA transmission is provided with different response properties and is affected by different adaptive mechanisms, depending on the specific subsystem that is taken into consideration. DA of the NAc shell responds to unfamiliar, unpredicted consummatory stimuli, whereas DA in the NAc core and in the PFCX responds to generic motivational stimuli, either appetitive or consummatory, predicted or unpredicted, familiar or unfamiliar.

These response properties are suggestive of a different role of the DA input to the different NAc compartments and to the PFCX in behavior. We suggest that DA of the NAc shell plays a role in associative learning, whereas DA of the NAc core and of the PFCX is involved in the motor expression of motivated behavior.

ROLE OF NAC SHELL DA IN ASSOCIATIVE LEARNING

On the basis of studies with neuroleptics, DA is traditionally considered to be uninvolved in associative learning.[51] However, as neuroleptics act more or less specifically on D_2 receptors, the evidence obtained with these drugs does not exclude that other receptors (e.g., D_1) are involved.

About 10 years ago we reported that blockade of D_1 receptors by SCH 23390 impairs the acquisition but not the expression of place conditioning to a variety of drugs, including rewarding ones like amphetamine, morphine, and diazepam, as well as aversive ones like naloxone, PCP, and lithium[52,53] (FIG. 9). To the mechanism of these, effect is likely to contribute (as in the case of amphetamine) a blockade of the primary rewarding properties of the drug;[53] this mechanism, however, is unlikely for drugs like naloxone, lithium, and diazepam, which do not release DA, and for PCP, which releases DA but is aversive to rats by a non-DA mechanism (NMDA-receptor blockade).[52,53] These observations lead us to postulate that DA plays a role in acquisition of appetitive as well as aversive motivation related to an associative learning mechanism.[52]

More recently a conditioned taste aversion paradigm has been used to investigate the role of D_1 receptors in associative learning. In a CTA paradigm, a novel taste (saccharin) is followed by an intraperitoneal injection of lithium, which induces a state of visceral malaise. As a result of this association, saccharin becomes aversive. According to Caulliez *et al.*[54] postsaccharin infusion of the D_1 antagonist SCH 23390 (25–250 ng) in the lateral hypothalamus impairs CTA learning. We have observed that infusion of the D_1 antagonist SCH 39166 (25–50 ng) in the NAc shell 5 min after saccharin drinking impairs the acquisition of CTA induced by lithium given 1 h later. Infusion of SCH 39166 in the NAc core or in the BSTM does not affect CTA. Administration of SCH 39166 45 min instead of 5 min after saccharin drinking fails to impair the acquisition of CTA. Thus, there appears to be a critical period shortly after perception of the gustatory stimulus when blockade of D_1 receptors disrupts learning of CTA. This period corresponds to the formation and storage of a short-term memory trace of the gustatory stimulus to be later associated with the negative (lithium) state. Therefore, DA acting on D_1 receptors in the NAc shell seems to play a critical role in learning the intrinsic (primary) motivational value of gustatory as well as contextual stimuli.

Indirect evidence for a role of the NAc shell DA in associative learning also arises from the observation that blockade of DA D_2 receptors in the lateral hypothalamus by sulpiride infusion enhances DA transmission in the NAc[55] and consolidation of associative learning.[56] Indeed the role of DA transmission in associative learning

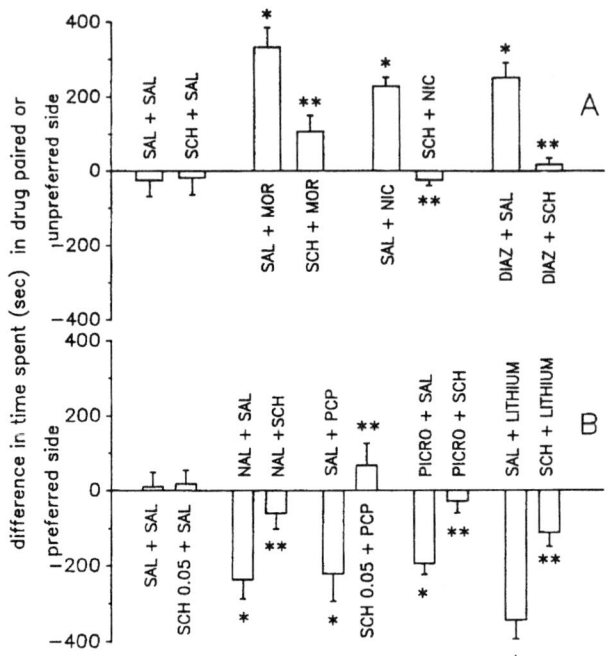

FIGURE 9. Effect of SCH 23390 (0.05 mg/kg sc) on side-preference shift induced by morphine (MOR) (1.0 mg/kg sc), nicotine (NIC) (0.6 mg/kg sc), and diazepam (DIAZ) (1.0 mg/kg ip), paired with the unpreferred compartment (**A**), and by naloxone (NAL) (0.8 mg/kg sc), phencyclidine (PCP) (2.5 mg/kg sc), picrotoxin (PICRO) (2.0 mg/kg ip), and lithium chloride (LITHIUM) (40 mg/kg sc), paired with the preferred compartment (**B**). Results are the mean (± SEM) side-preference shift (expressed in seconds). * $p < 0.05$, for shift in side-preference (Newman-Keuls); ** $p < 0.05$, for differences in the shift in side-preference (Newman-Keuls). SAL, saline. Acquas et al.[52] With permission from *Psychopharmacology*.).

may not be restricted to the NAc shell. Thus, Hitchcott and Phillips[57] have recently provided evidence that postsession infusion of a D_3/D_2 agonist (7 OHDPAT) in the central, but not in the basolateral, amygdala enhances acquisition of a conditioned approach response. If these results are coupled to our observations that drugs of abuse increase DA transmission in the BSTM (see above), which in turn is a cranial extension of the central amygdala as well as an integral part of the extended amygdala, one might hypothesize that drugs of abuse facilitate associative learning by stimulating DA transmission not only in the NAc shell but also in the extended amygdala.

DIFFERENTIAL ROLE OF NAC SHELL AND CORE IN MOTIVATION

The observations on the response properties of motivational stimuli obtained with brain microdialysis, as well the results obtained by intracerebral drug infusion, suggest that, depending on the compartment of the NAc, DA is involved in different aspects of motivation: acquisition in the NAc shell, expression in the NAc core. The role of the NAc shell in acquisition of motivation derives from its role in learning, which has been discussed in the preceding section. Here we will discuss the role of the NAc core in the expression of motivation.

In our view, the role of the NAc core in the expression of motivation coincides with that attributed to by Mogenson to the NAc of an interface between motivation and action.[58] The reason for such coincidence might be indeed a trivial one: previous studies have not distinguished between NAc shell and core and, due to the central location of the core within the NAc, have involved, more often, the core than the shell. This applies not only to lesions and local drug infusion studies but also to brain microdialysis studies. For the same reason, the activational,[59] gain-amplifying,[60] sensory-motor,[61] incentive-motivational[8,62] roles, traditionally attributed to NAc DA, and homologous of Mogenson's view,[58] might refer specifically to DA of the NAc core.

Recent studies indicate that the postulated role of the NAc core in response expression applies in particular to instrumental behavior and might include instrumental learning. This process involves learning of the contingency between the reinforcing stimulus and the response that acquires predictive value for the presentation of the reinforcing stimulus.[63] This type of learning is specifically impaired by infusion of an NMDA antagonist (AP_5) in the NAc core but not in the shell.[64] It is notable that infusion of AP_5 in the NAc core does not impair learning of pavlovian stimulus–reward associations.[64] We speculate that instrumental learning involves an incentive, activational component that is disrupted by manipulation of NMDA transmission in the NAc core. A role of the NAc core in instrumental learning is compatible also with the effect of excitotoxic lesions of the core on the expression of conditioned approach, which is known to involve an instrumental component,[65] and on secondary reinforcement (see Everitt et al., this volume).

DYSADAPTIVE PROPERTIES OF DRUGS AS COMPARED TO CONVENTIONAL REINFORCERS

A comparison between drug and nondrug reinforcers is justified by their behavioral and neurochemical similarities. From the above evidence drug and nondrug reinforcers seem to share the property of activating DA transmission preferentially in the NAc shell. Nonpsychostimulant drugs also share with a conventional reinforcer, like palatable food, a μ-opioid component located in the VTA. Therefore, drugs reproduce certain central neurochemical effects of conventional reinforcers that are the substrate of their motivational effects.[66,67]

Addictive drugs, however, differ from conventional reinforcers for the resistance of their stimulant effects on NAc shell DA transmission to adaptive modulation. Thus, in contrast to palatable food, drug-induced stimulation of DA transmission in the NAc shell does not undergo one-trial habituation.[49] Lack of habituation means that addictive drugs can activate DA transmission in the NAc shell in a manner that is not limited by previous drug history but only by drug availability. Lack of the constraint of adaptive modulation is likely to be per se a major abnormality for a fine mechanism like phasic activation of DA transmission in the NAc shell, which is meant to subserve a learning function. One might hypothesize that, as a result of the repetitive stimulation of DA transmission by the drug, stimuli associated with drug-reward acquire excessive motivational value and become capable of controlling behavior in that exclusive and dominant manner that is typical of addiction.

The above one, however, is not the only abnormality of drugs as compared to conventional reinforcers. Another aspect, which falls under the general property of resistance to negative modulation, is the nondecremental character of drug reward due to lack of satiation. This property ensures that the rewarding effect of the drug is maintained in spite of its continous availability, thus contributing to facilitation of associative learning.

One might object that the rewarding properties of drugs undergo a decremental change as a result of tolerance. It is likely, however, that tolerance to the rewarding effects of the drug is not the result of a reduction in drug efficacy but of a shift in basal affective tone towards a lower, negative level that actually corresponds to the state of abstinence (see below). As a result of this the drug maintains its positive reinforcing properties during abstinence, and a new factor is introduced, abstinence-induced dysphoria, which might contribute to maintaining, by a negative-reinforcing mechanism, drug self-administration (see below).

The property of drugs that allows these adaptive differences with conventional reinforcers is a basic one: drugs do not depend as conventional reinforcers from activation of a neural chain spanning from peripheral sensory receptors to CNS, areas where emotions and associations between emotions and stimuli are formed; drugs enter the brain and directly activate the critical central mechanism that is indirectly activated by conventional reinforcers. As a result of this short-circuit mechanism, drugs escape adaptive modulation, which instead constrains the action of conventional reinforcers. Adaptive constraint, however, is essential for normal learning. Lack of this property leads to defective learning, which, in the case of drugs, corresponds to addiction.

TOLERANCE AND DEPENDENCE

Early and present theories of drug addiction have put a great emphasis on the role of tolerance and dependence mechanisms. According to these theories, addiction is the result of changes induced by the chronic exposure to the drug, which makes the organism dependent for its normal functions and homeostasis on the presence of the drug. Early theories, by referring to opiate addiction as a model, placed major emphasis on physical dependence as a factor of drug addiction.[68] More recent formulations, apart from providing a theory for the mechanism of tolerance and dependence (opponent-process theory),[69] have moved the emphasis from physical dependence to emotional dependence as a motivational factor of drug addiction.[70] The advantage of this modern version over early dependence theories is that emotional dependence has the properties of a factor common to different classes of drugs, whereas physical dependence widely differs, as judged from the phenomenology of physical abstinence from one drug class to the other. Emotional dependence is expressed by a state of anhedonia and dysphoria; this state, by a negative-reinforcing mechanism, would contribute to maintaining drug self-administration (see Koob *et al.*, this volume).

A neurochemical correlate of the aversive state of abstinence might be a reduction of *in vivo* DA transmission in the NAc estimated by microdialysis. These changes have been observed following abstinence from morphine, amphetamine, ethanol, and Δ^9 THC and appear dissociated from the physical signs of abstinence.[71-77] Therefore, reduction of DA transmission in the NAc, like impairement of self-stimulation, appears to be a more sensitive, longer-lasting, and more general sign of dependence than physical signs of abstinence.

Reduction of DA transmission in the NAc following chronic drug exposure can be interpreted in at least two different ways: as the result of an adaptive turning off of endogenous excitatory input on DA neurons secondary to the chronic exposure to the DA stimulant effect of drugs,[72] or as the result of the aversive state induced by abstinence. According to the first interpretation, reduction of DA release in the NAc would be the cause of the negative state of abstinence, whereas in the second case would be a consequence of it. Consistent with the second possibility is the evidence that an aversive state that generalizes to a pentylenetetrazole stimulus is generated during abstinence.[78] A correlate of such an aversive state might be the increase of DA release in the PFCX that is observed during precipitated abstinence from morphine.[79] It is notable that a pattern of increased DA release in the PFCX and reduction in the NAc shell is also observed following exposure to a mild aversive stimulus, like a tail pinch, or to a strong one, like a forced swim (Di Chiara, unpublished). These observations are consistent with the possibility that also the reduction of DA release in the NAc, as the increase in the PFCX, is a response of the DA system to the inescapable aversive state of abstinence.

SENSITIZATION

Repeated drug exposure has been reported to induce sensitization of drug-induced presynaptic stimulation of DA transmission in the ventral and in the dorsal striatum. Existing studies, however, have not distinguished between the NAc shell and core; we have now studied, by brain microdialysis, the responsiveness of DA transmission in the NAc shell and core in rats behaviorally sensitized by three different drugs: morphine,[27] amphetamine, and cocaine. In all three instances no sensitization of DA responsiveness to drug challenge was observed in the NAc shell;[27] in the case of morphine, a small but significant reduction of the DA response was actually obtained[27] (FIG. 4). On the other hand in the NAc core, sensitization of DA responsiveness to drug challenge was observed with morphine at 1.0 and 5.0 mg/kg sc[27] (FIG. 4) and with amphetamine at 0.25 and 0.5 mg/kg sc, but not with cocaine at any of the doses tested (5.0 and 10.0 mg/kg ip).

These results indicate that behavioral sensitization is not associated to changes in the drug-induced stimulation of presynaptic DA transmission in the NAc shell. As to the NAc core, there seems to be no consistent relationship among different drugs, even of the same class (e.g., cocaine and amphetamine), between presynaptic sensitization of DA transmission and behavioral sensitization; this conclusion is in aggreement with the results of various studies that failed to show a relationship between behavioral and presynaptic sensitization of DA responsiveness in the NAc.[80-84] By contrast, there appears to be a striking consistency of changes in functional markers of striato-nigral neurons across different models of sensitization, including a denervated one. Thus, for example, in a unilaterally 6-OHDA denervated model of sensitization (priming), a single administration of a direct DA agonist induces behavioral sensitization to D_1-dependent contralateral turning and increases the striatal expression of glutamic acid decarboxylase,[85] preprotakykinin, and preprodynorphin[86] in striatal neurons that are likely to project to the substantia nigra pars reticulata and express D_1 receptors. Similarly, intermittent amphetamine, cocaine, and morphine administration increases the expression of preprodynorphin, particularly in dorsolateral aspects of the striatum, which are likely to be involved in motor behavior.[87–92] These observations indicate that postsynaptic rather than presynaptic changes play a major role in behavioral sensitization. The observation that these changes take place in the dorsal striatum (dorsal caudate-putamen) rather than in the NAc, is consistent with the motor nature of behavioral sensitization.

These observations bring us to a number of conclusions: (1) sensitization is a generic term that collectively indicates behavioral syndromes, induced by repeated drug exposure, having in common the characteristic of an increased motor response to drug challenge but differing as to their induction mechanism; (2) in spite of differences among different drugs in the mechanism of induction of behavioral sensitization, these conditions might have in common a sensitization of the postsynaptic responsiveness of DA-ceptive elements; and (3) presynaptic sensitization of DA transmission in the NAc might be a consequence rather than the cause of behavioral sensitization being secondary to the postsynaptic changes in DA-ceptive elements that take place in the dorsal striatum.

Robinson and Berridge,[8] on the basis of studies on psychostimulants, have proposed an incentive sensitization theory of drug addiction, which assumes that repeated drug exposure induces a state of sensitization of DA neurons, such that drug-related stimuli elicit a sensitized increase of DA in mesocorticolimbic areas that results in the incentive state of craving. One would argue that if DA neurons are sensitized they should respond in a sensitized fashion not only to drug-related but also to drug-unrelated stimuli. This, however, is clearly incompatible with the stimulus-specificity requirements of drug addiction and with a main characteristic of this condition: that motivated behavior is focused on drug to the exclusion of nondrug stimuli. Therefore a sensitization process like the one hypothesized by Robinson and Berridge[8] is unlikely to provide an interpretative framework of drug addiction.

According to the incentive-sensitization theory, drug-conditional stimuli and drug cues release DA or potentiate drug-induced stimulation of DA transmission in the NAc.[8] Contrary to this prediction, however, operant presentation of a light cue, predictive of cocaine iv infusion, failed to release DA in the NAc from the first extinction test.[93] Moreover, a single noncontingent iv infusion of cocaine, which acts as a powerful incentive of lever pressing in cocaine-trained but not in saline-yoked rats, increases dialysate DA in the NAc to a lesser extent in the cocaine-trained than in the saline-yoked group.[93] Therefore, in contrast with the incentive-sensitization theory, drug-conditioned stimuli as well as drug cues do not stimulate or potentiate *in vivo* DA transmission in the NAc. This conclusion, in turn, is consistent with the hypothesis that conditional appetitive stimuli, in general, do not release DA in the NAc shell.[49]

Rather than for the mechanism of addiction, however, sensitization might be important for the mechanism of psychostimulant psychosis.[94–96] Clinical evidence indicates that this condition is the result of the direct action of the drug as modified by the adaptive changes induced by an escalating binge pattern of drug exposure.[94,95] This pattern of self-administration, in turn, might be the expression of a coping strategy to compensate for the rapid induction of tolerance to the hedonic, orgasm-like effects (rush) of the psychostimulant. Within this framework, sensitization and its expression (psychosis) appear to be side effects of drug taking, a toll to be payed by the subject in its compulsive search for pleasure.

AN ASSOCIATIVE LEARNING HYPOTHESIS OF DRUG ADDICTION

Addictive drugs share with conventional reinforcers two properties that are necessary but not sufficient for their addictive liability: the properties of being rewarding and of facilitating associative learning. Rewarding properties of drugs do not necessarily consist of sheer sensations of pleasure, like the "high" or the "rush" typical of iv amphetamine or heroin, but can take the milder form of, for example, tension relief, reduction of fatigue, improvement of performance, and arousal. To this variety of forms corresponds a variety of neurochemical mechanisms that can account for drug reward. Thus, drug reward, like conventional reward, can be due to final stimulation of GABA, opioid, DA, nicotine, or cannabinoid receptors. This variety of neurochemical mechanisms contrasts with the commonality of the mechanism that determines, across different drug classes, the property of facilitating associative learning, related as it is to the property of stimulating DA transmission in the NAc shell.

Drugs and conventional rewards, although homologous for the property of being rewarding and releasing DA in the NAc shell, differ for the adaptive changes these properties undergo upon repeated exposure. Thus, repeated exposure to conventional reinforcers results in a devaluation of their rewarding properties by satiation and in a reduction of their associative learning properties by habituation of the stimulus responsiveness of DA transmission in the NAc shell. Drug effects, rather than satiation or habituation, undergo tolerance upon repeated exposure. This change, however, may not involve a reduction in the positive-reinforcing efficacy of the drug (see below). Some effects of addictive drugs, such as their motor-activating properties, actually undergo an increase (sensitization) upon repeated administration; it is unlikely, however, that this involves an increase in the rewarding and/or associative learning properties of drugs.

We view drug addiction as the result of the action of four factors: (1) the rewarding properties of drugs; (2) their ability to activate DA transmission in the NAc shell; (3) the resistance of the above properties to negative adaptive modulation (satiation and habituation) after repeated drug exposure; and (4) the adaptive changes induced by repeated drug exposure, resulting in the negative emotional state of abstinence. As the action of these factors is time dependent, drug addiction undergoes different phases or stages.

In the first stage, which we call "controlled drug use" (honeymoon), as a result of, for example, stressful life events, curiosity, peer pressure, social factors, and personality traits, the subject comes into contract with a drug with addictive liability. The reinforcing properties of the drug (first factor) facilitate further exposure to the drug, while its associative learning properties, related to release of DA in the NAc shell (second factor), promote the acquisition of incentive stimuli predictive of drug availability. In this stage the subject responds to the drug and to drug-related stimuli in a controlled manner not dissimilar from normal motivated responding.

With repeated drug exposure the subject progressively enters the second stage, that of drug abuse. In this stage the repeated association of drug reward and drug-related stimuli in the presence of a nonhabituating stimulation of DA transmission in the NAc shell (third factor) results in the attribution of excessive motivational value to drug-associated stimuli. In this stage the subject can still control drug intake in the absence of drug-related stimuli. Their presence, however, elicits compulsive drug seeking, eventually associated with strong urges (craving).

The third stage (addiction) is characterized by the conditions of the preceding stage, to which is added that of tolerance and dependence. In this stage, abstinence results in a negative emotional state (fourth factor), which maintains the motivational relationship between the subject and the drug in the intervals when drug-conditioned incentives are not available. Moreover, the need state of abstinence amplifies the incentive properties of drug-related stimuli. It should be noted here that, even in the presence of the negative motivational state of abstinence, the drug remains the positive reinforcer that maintains responding in spite of the fact that the hedonic properties of the drug (rush) have been reduced by tolerance. This condition, although providing an instructive example of dissociation between positive reinforcing and rewarding properties of a stimulus, might constitute the basis for the escalating dose/binge pattern of drug-taking behavior typical of psychostimulant addiction.

ACKNOWLEDGMENTS

The studies from the authors' laboratory reported in the present article have been supported by funds from MURST (40% and 60%), from CNR, from EC (Biomed Project), and from the Foundation for the Study of Coffee.

REFERENCES

1. HEIMER, L. & R.D. WILSON. 1975. The subcortical projections of allocortex: similarities in the neuronal associations of the hippocampus, the piriform cortex and the neocortex. *In* Golgi Centennial Symposium Proceedings. M. Santini, Ed.: 173–193. Raven Press. New York.
2. HEIMER, L., J. DE OLMOS, G.F. ALHEID & L. ZABORSZKY. 1991. "Perestroika" in the basal forebrain: opening the border between neurology and psychiatry. Prog. Brain Res. **87:** 109–165.
3. AMERICAN PSYCHIATRIC ASSOCIATION. 1994. Diagnostic and Statistical Manual of Mental Disorders. 4th ed. (DSM IV). Washington, D.C.
4. WIKLER, A. 1973. Dynamics of drug dependence: implications of a conditioning theory for research and treatment. Arch. Gen. Psychiatry **28:** 611–616.
5. O'BRIEN, C.P., A.R. CHILDRESS, A.T. MCLELLAN & R. EHRMAN. 1992. Classical conditioning in drug-dependent humans. Ann. N.Y. Acad. Sci. **654:** 400–415.
6. STEWART, J., H. DE WIT & R. EIKELBOOM. 1984. Role of unconditioned and conditioned drug effects in the self-administration of opiates and stimulants. Psychol. Rev. **91:** 251–268.

7. GOLDBERG, S.R. 1976. Stimuli associated with drug injections as events that control behavior. Pharmacol. Rev. 27: 325–340.
8. ROBINSON, T.E. & K.C. BERRIDGE. 1993. The neural basis of drug craving: an incentive-sensitization theory of addiction. Brain Res. Rev. 18: 247–291.
9. DI CHIARA, G. 1998. A motivational learning hypothesis of the role of dopamine in compulsive drug use. J. Psychopharmacol. 12: 54–67.
10. JOHANSON, C.E. 1978. Drugs as reinforcers. In Contemporary Research in Behavioral Pharmacology. Blackman D.E. & D.J. Sanger, Eds.: 325–390. Plenum Press. New York.
11. UNGERSTEDT, U. 1984. Measurements of neurotransmitter release by intracranial dialysis. In Measurement of Neurotransmitter Release in Vivo. C.A. Marsen, Ed.: 81–105. John Wiley. Chichester.
12. DI CHIARA, G. 1990. In vivo brain dialysis of neurotransmitters. Trends Pharmacol. Sci. 11: 116–121.
13. DI CHIARA, G. & A. IMPERATO. 1988. Drugs abused by humans preferentially increase synaptic dopamine concentrations in the mesolimbic system of freely moving rats. Proc. Natl. Acad. Sci. USA 85: 5274–5278.
14. CARBONI, E., A. IMPERATO, L. PEREZZANI & G. DI CHIARA. 1989. Amphetamine, cocaine, phencyclidine and nomifensine increase extracellular dopamine concentrations preferentially in the nucleus accumbens of freely moving rats. Neuroscience 28: 653–661.
15. DI CHIARA, G. & A. IMPERATO. 1988. Opposite effects of mu and kappa opiate agonists on dopamine release in the nucleus accumbens and in the dorsal caudate of freely moving rats. J. Pharmacol. Exp. Ther. 244: 1067–1080.
16. IMPERATO, A., A. MULAS & G. DI CHIARA. 1986. Nicotine preferentially stimulates dopamine released in the limbic system of freely moving rats. Eur. J. Pharmacol. 132: 337–338.
17. IMPERATO, A. & G. DI CHIARA. 1986. Preferential stimulation of dopamine release in the nucleus accumbens of freely moving rats by ethanol. J. Pharmacol. Exp. Ther. 239: 219–228.
18. KUCZENSKI, R. & D.S. SEGAL. 1992. Differential effects of amphetamine and dopamine uptake blockers (cocaine, nomifensine) on caudate and accumbens dialysate dopamine and 3-methoxytyramine. J. Pharmacol. Exp. Ther. 262: 1085–1094.
19. BRAZELL, M.P., S.N. MITCHELL, M.H. JOSEPH & J.A. GRAY. 1990. Acute administration of nicotine increases the in vivo extracellular levels of dopamine, 3,4-dihydroxyphenylacetic acid and ascorbic acid preferentially in the nucleus accumbens of the rat: comparison with caudate-putamen. Neuropharmacology 29: 1177–1185.
20. ROBINSON, T.E. & D.M. CAMP. 1990. Does amphetamine preferentially increase the extracellular concentration of dopamine in the mesolimbic system of freely moving rats? Neuropsychopharmacology 3: 163–173.
21. DI CHIARA, G. 1991. On the preferential release of mesolimbic dopamine by ampheamine. Neuropsychopharmacology 5: 243–244.
22. DI CHIARA, G., G. TANDA, R. FRAU & E. CARBONI. 1993. On the preferential release of dopamine in the nucleus accumbens by amphetamine: further evidence obtained by vertically implanted concentric dialysis probes. Psychopharmacology 112: 398–402.
23. ALHEID, G.F. & L. HEIMER. 1988. New perspectives in basal forebrain organization of special relevance for neuropsychiatric disorders: the striatopallidal, amygdaloid and corticopetal components of substantia innominata. Neuroscience 27: 1–39.
24. PONTIERI, F.E., G. TANDA & G. DI CHIARA. 1995. Intravenous cocaine, morphine and amphetamine preferentially increase extracellular dopamine in the "shell" as compared with the "core" of the rat nucleus accumbens. Proc. Natl. Acad. Sci. USA. 92: 12304–12308.
25. PONTIERI, F.E., G. TANDA, F. ORZI & G. DI CHIARA. 1996. Effects of nicotine on the nucleus accumbens and similarity to those of addictive drugs. Nature 382: 255–257.
26. TANDA, G., F.E. PONTIERI & G. DI CHIARA. 1997. Cannabinoid and heroin activation of mesolimbic dopamine transmission by a common μ_1 opioid receptor mechanism. Science 276: 2048–2050.

27. CADONI, C. & G. DI CHIARA. 1999. Reciprocal changes in dopamine responsiveness in the nucleus accumbens shell and core and in the dorsal caudate-putamen in rats sensitized to morphine. Neuroscience **90:** 447–455.
28. HEIDBREDER, C. & J. FELDON. 1998. Amphetamine-induced neurochemical and locomotor responses are expressed differentially across the anteroposterior axis of the core and shell subterritories of the nucleus accumbens. Synapse **29:** 310–322.
29. BARROT, M., M. MARINELLI, D.N. ABROUS, F. ROUGÉ-PONT, M. LE MOAL & P.V. PIAZZA. 1998. Functional heterogeneity in dopamine release and in the expression of Fos-like proteins within the rat striatal complex. Eur. J. Neurosci. In press.
30. ORZI, F., F. PASSARELLI, M. LA RICCIA, R. DI GREZIA & F.E. PONTIERI. 1996. Intravenous morphine increases glucose utilization in the shell of the rat nucleus accumbens. Eur. J. Pharmacol. **302:** 49–51.
31. PONTIERI, F.E., V. COLANGELO, M. LA RICCIA, C. POZZILLI, F. PASSARELLI & F. ORZI. 1994. Psychostimulant drugs increase glucose utilization in the shell of the rat nucleus accumbens. NeuroReport **5:** 2561–2564.
32. BJÖRKLUND, A. & O. LINDVALL. 1984. Dopamine containing systems in the CNS. In Handbook of Chemical Neuroanatomy. A. Biörklund & T. Hökfelt, Eds.: **2:** 55–122. Classical transmitters in the CNS, part I. Elsevier. Amsterdam.
33. ARNT, J. & T. SKARSFELDT. 1998. Do novel antipsychotics have similar pharmacological charactcristics? A review of the evidence. Neuropsychopharmacology **18:** 63–101.
34. ONGINI, E. & B.B. FREDHOLM. 1996. Pharmacology of adenosine A2 receptors. Trends Pharmacol. Sci. **17:** 364–372.
35. BASSAREO, V., G. TANDA, P. PETROMILLI, C. GIUA & G. DI CHIARA. 1996. Non-psychostimulant drugs of abuse and anxiogenic drugs activate with differential selectivity dopamine transmission in the nucleus accumbens and in the medial prefrontal cortex. Psychopharmacology **124:** 293–299.
36. TANDA, G., F.E. PONTIERI, R. FRAU & G. DI CHIARA. 1997. Contribution of blockade of the noradrenaline carrier to the increase of extracellular dopamine in the rat prefrontal cortex by amphetamine and cocaine. Eur. J. Neurosci. **9:** 2077–2085.
37. PALKOVITS, M. 1979. Dopamine levels of individual brain regions: biochemical aspects of DA distribution in the central nervous system. In The Neurobiology of Dopamine. A.S. Horn, J. Korf & B.H.C. Westerink, Eds.: 343–356. Academic Press. London.
38. RAITERI, M., R. DEL CARMINE, A. BERTOLLINI & G. LEVI. 1977. Effects of sympathomimetic amines on the synaptosomal transport of noradrenaline, dopamine and 5-hydroxytryptamine. Eur. J. Pharmacol. **41:** 133–143.
39. CARBONI, E., G. TANDA, R. FRAU & G. DI CHIARA. 1990. Blockade of the noradrenaline carrier increases extracellular dopamine concentrations in the prefrontal cortex: evidence that dopamine is taken up in vivo by noradrenergic terminals. J. Neurochem. **55:** 1067–1070.
40. TANDA, G., E. CARBONI, R. FRAU & G. DI CHIARA. 1994. Increase of extracellular dopamine in the prefrontal cortex: a trait of drugs with antidepressant potential? Psychopharmacology **115:** 285–288.
41. CADONI, C., A. PINNA, G. RUSSI, S. CONSOLO & G. DI CHIARA. 1995. Role of vesicular dopamine in the in vivo stimulation of striatal dopamine transmission by amphetamine: evidence from microdialysis and Fos immunohistochemistry. Neuroscience **65:** 1027–1039.
42. MATTHEWS, R.T. & D.C. GERMAN. 1984. Electrophysiological evidence for excitation of rat ventral tegmental area dopamine neurons by morphine. Neuroscience **11:** 617–628.
43. GESSA, G.L., F. MUNTONI, M. COLLU, L. VARGIU & G.P. MEREU. 1985. Low doses of ethanol activate dopaminergic neurons in the ventral tegmental area. Brain Res. **348:** 201–203.
44. MEREU, G., K.-W.P. YOON, V. BOI, G.L. GESSA, L. NAES & T.C. WESTFALL. 1987. Preferential stimulation of ventral tegmental area dopaminergic neurons by nicotine. Eur. J. Pharmacol. **141:** 395–399.
45. CASS, W.A., G.A. GERHARDT, R.D. MAYFIELD, P. CURELLA & N.R. ZAHNISER. 1992.

Differences in dopamine clearance and diffusion in rat striatum and nucleus accumbens following systemic cocaine administration. J. Neurochem. **59:** 259–266.
46. TANDA, G. & G. DI CHIARA. 1998. A dopamine-μ_1 opioid link in the rat ventral tegmentum shared by palatable food (Fonzies) and non-psychostimulant drugs of abuse. Eur. J. Neurosci. **10:** 1179–1187.
47. CARBONI, E., E. ACQUAS, R. FRAU & G. DI CHIARA. 1989. Differential inhibitory effects of a $5HT_3$ antagonist on drug-induced stimulation of dopamine release. Eur. J. Pharmacol. **164:** 515–519.
48. KONORSKI, J. 1967. Integrative Activity of the Brain. University of Chicago Press. Chicago.
49. BASSAREO, V. & G. DI CHIARA. 1997. Differential influence of associative and non-associative learning mechanisms on the responsiveness of prefrontal and accumbal dopamine transmission to food stimuli in rats fed ad libitum. J. Neurosci. **17:** 851–861.
50. BASSAREO, V. & G. DI CHIARA. 1999. Differential responsiveness of dopamine transmission to food-stimuli in nucleus accumbens shell/core compartments. Neuroscience. **89(3):** 637–641.
51. BENINGER, R.J. 1983. The role of dopamine in locomotor activity and learning. Brain Res. **6:** 173–196.
52. ACQUAS, E., E. CARBONI, P. LEONE & G. DI CHIARA. 1989. SCH 23390 blocks drug-conditioned place-preference and place-aversion: anhedonia (lack of reward) or apathy (lack of motivation) after dopamine receptor blockade? Psychopharmacology **99:** 151–155.
53. ACQUAS, E. & G. DI CHIARA. 1994. D_1 receptors blockade stereospecifically impairs the acquisition of drug-conditioned place-preference and place-aversion. Behav. Pharmacol. **5:** 555–569.
54. CAULLIEZ, R., M.-J. MEILE & S. NICOLAIDIS. 1996. A lateral hypothalamic D1 dopaminergic mechanism in conditioned taste aversion. Brain Res. **729:** 234–245.
55. PARADA, M.A., M.P. DEPARADA & B.G. HOEBEL. 1995. Rats self-inject a dopamine antagonist in the lateral hypothalamus where it acts to increase extracellular dopamine in the nucleus accumbens. Pharmacol. Biochem. Behav. **52:** 179–187.
56. PHILLIPS, G. & S.L. MORUTTO. 1998. Post-session sulpiride infusions within the perifornical region of the lateral hypothalamus enhance consolidation of associative learning. Psychopharmacology. In press.
57. HITCHCOTT, P.K. & G.D. PHILLIPS. 1998. Double dissociation of the behavioural effects of R(+) 7-OH-DPAT infusions in the central and basolateral amygdala nuclei upon Pavlovian and instrumental conditioned appetitive behaviours. Psychopharmacology. **140(4):** 458–469.
58. MOGENSON, G.J., D.L. JONES & C.Y. YIM. 1980. From motivation to action: functional interface between the limbic system and the motor system. Prog. Neurobiol. **14:** 69–97.
59. SALAMONE, J.D. 1988. Dopaminergic involvement in activational aspects of motivation: effects of haloperidol on schedule-induced activity, feeding and foraging in rats. Psychobiology **16:** 196–206.
60. ROBBINS, T.W., M. CADOR, J.R. TAYLOR & B.J. EVERITT. 1989. Limbic striatal interactions in reward-related processes. Neurosci. Behav. Rev. **13:** 155–162.
61. SALAMONE, J.D. 1992. Complex motor and sensorimotor functions of striatal and accumbens dopamine: involvement in instrumental behavior processes. Psychopharmacology **107:** 160–174.
62. WISE, R.A. 1982. Neuroleptics and operant behavior: the anhedonia hypothesis. Behav. Brain Sci. **5:** 39–87.
63. RESCORLA, R.A. & R.L. SOLOMON. 1967. Two-process learning theory: relationship between Pavlovian conditioning and instrumental learning. Psychol. Rev. **74:** 151–182.
64. KELLY, A.E., S.L. SMITH-ROE & A.R. HOLAHAN. 1997. Response reinforcement learning is dependent on N-methyl-D-aspartate receptor activation in the nucleus accumbens core. Proc. Natl. Acad. Sci. USA **94:** 12174–12179.

65. HOLLAND, P.C. & J.J. STRAUB. 1979. Differential effects of two ways of devaluing the unconditioned stimulus after Pavlovian appetitive conditioning. J. Exp. Psychol. Anim. Behav. **5:** 65–78.
66. DI CHIARA, G., E. ACQUAS, G. TANDA & C. CADONI. 1993. Drugs of abuse: biochemical surrogates of specific aspects of natural reward? Biochem. Soc. Symp. **59:** 65–81.
67. DI CHIARA, G. 1995. The role of dopamine in drug abuse viewed from the perspective of its role in motivation. Drug Alcohol Depend. **38:** 95–137.
68. HIMMELSBACH, C.K. 1943. Morphine, with reference to physical dependence. Fed. Proc. Fed. Am. Soc. Exp. Biol. **2:** 201–203.
69. SOLOMON, R.L. 1977. An opponent-process theory of motivation: IV. The affective dynamics of addiction. *In* Psychopathology: Experimental Models. J.D. Maser & M.E.P. Seligman, Eds.: 66–103. Freeman. San Francisco.
70. KOOB, G.F., L. STINUS, M. LE MOAL & F.E. BLOOM. 1989. Opponent process theory of motivation: neurobiological evidence from studies of opiate dependence. Neurosci. Biobehav. Rev. **13:** 135–140.
71. ACQUAS, E., E. CARBONI & G. DI CHIARA. 1991. Profound depression of mesolimbic dopamine release after morphine withdrawal in dependent rats. Eur. J. Pharmacol. **193:** 133–134.
72. ACQUAS, E. & G. DI CHIARA. 1992. Depression of mesolimbic dopamine transmission and sensitization to morphine during opiate abstinence. J. Neurochem. **58:** 1620–1625.
73. ROSSETTI, Z.L., Y. HMAIDAN & G.L. GESSA. 1992. Marked inhibition of mesolimbic dopamine release: a common feature of ethanol, morphine, cocaine and amphetamine abstinence in rats. Eur. J. Pharmacol. **221:** 227–234.
74. DIANA, M., M. PISTIS, S. CARBONI, G.L. GESSA & Z.L. ROSSETTI. 1993. Profound decrement of mesolimbic dopaminergic neuronal activity during ethanol withdrawal syndrome in rats: elctrophysiological and biochemical evidence. Proc. Natl. Acad. Sci. USA **90:** 7966–7969.
75. POTHOS, E., P. RADA, G.P. MARK & B.G. HOEBEL. 1991. Dopamine microdialysis in the nucleus accumbens during acute and chronic morphine, naloxone-precipitated withdrawal and clonidine treatment. Brain Res. **566:** 348–350.
76. WEISS, F., A. MARKOU, M.T. LORANG & G.F. KOOB. 1992. Basal dopamine levels in the nucleus accumbens are decreased during cocaine withdrawal after unlimited-access self-administration. Brain Res. **593:** 314–318.
77. DIANA, M., M. PISTIS, A. MUNTONI & G. GESSA. 1995. Profound decrease of mesolimbic dopaminergic neuronal activity in morphine withdrawn rats. J. Pharmacol. Exp. Ther. **272:** 781–785.
78. EMMETT-OGLESBY, M.W., D.A. MATHIS, R.T.Y. MOON & H. LAL. 1990. Animal models of drug withdrawal symptoms. Psychopharmacology **101:** 292–309.
79. BASSAREO, V., G. TANDA & G. DI CHIARA. 1995. Increase of extracellular dopamine in the medial prefrontal cortex during spontaneous and naloxone-precipitated opiate abstinence. Psychopharmacology **122:** 202–205.
80. KOLTA, M.G., P. SHREVE, V. DE SOUZA & N.J. URETSKY. 1985. Time course of the development of the enhanced behavioral and biochemical responses to amphetamine after pretreatment with amphetamine. Neuropharmacology **24:** 823–829.
81. SEGAL, D.S. & R. KUCZENSKI. 1992. Repeated cocaine administration induces behavioral sensitization and corresponding decreased extracellular dopamine responses in caudate and accumbens. Brain Res. **577:** 351–355.
82. SEGAL, D.S. & R. KUCZENSKI. 1992. *In vivo* microdialysis reveals a diminished amphetamine-induced DA response corresponding to behavioral sensitization produced by repeated amphetamine pretreatment. Brain Res. **571:** 330–337.
83. KALIVAS, P.W. & P. DUFFY. 1993. Time course of extracellular dopamine and behavioral sensitization to cocaine. I. Dopamine axon terminals. J. Neurosci. **13:** 266–275.
84. WOLF, M.E., F.J. WHITE, R. NASSAR, R.J. BROODERSON & M.R. KHANSA. 1993. Differential development of autoreceptor subsensitivity and enhanced dopamine release during amphetamine sensitization. J. Pharmacol. Exp. Ther. **264:** 249–255.

85. CONSOLO, S., M. MORELLI, M. RIMOLDI, S. GIORGI & G. DI CHIARA. 1999. Increased striatal expression of glutamate decarboxylase 67 after priming of 6-hydroxydopamine-lesioned rats. Neuroscience. **89**(4): 1183–1187.
86. VAN DE WITTE, S.V., H.J. GROENEWEGEN & P. VOORN. 1998. Augmentation of D1-agonist induced upregulation of preprodynorphin mRNA by L-DOPA priming is blocked by MK-801 in the 6-OHDA lesioned striatum. Collected Abstracts of Advancing from the Ventral Striatum to the Extended Amygdala: Implications for Neuropsychiatry and Drug Abuse. Charlottesville, VA. No. P59. New York Academy of Sciences. New York.
87. HURD, Y.L., E.E. BROWN, J.M. FINLAY, H.C. FIBIGER & C.R. GERFEN. 1992. Cocaine self-administration differentially alters mRNA expression of striatal peptides. Mol. Brain Res. **13**: 165–170.
88. STEINER, H. & C.R. GERFEN. 1993. Cocaine-induced c-fos messenger RNA is inversely related to dynorphin expression in striatum. J. Neurosci. **13**: 5066–5081.
89. SPANGLER, R., E.M. UNTERWALD & M.J. KREEK. 1993. "Binge" cocaine administration induces a sustained increase of prodynorphin mRNA in rat caudate-putamen. Mol. BrainRes. **19**: 323–327.
90. DAUNAIS, J.B. & J.F. MCGINTY. 1994. Acute and chronic cocaine administration differentially alters striatal opioid and nuclear transcription factor mRNAs. Synapse **18**: 35–45.
91. WANG, J.Q. & J.F. MCGINTY. 1995. Alterations in striatal zif/268, preprodynorphin and preproenkephalin mRNA expression induced by repeated amphetamine administration in rats. Brain Res. **673**: 262–274.
92. TJON, G.H.K., P. VOORN, L.J.M.J. VANDERSCHUREN, T.J. DE VRIES, N.H.L.M. MICHIELS, A.J. JONKER, H. KLOP, P. NESTBY, A.H. MULDER & A.N.M. SCHOFFELMEER. 1997. Delayed occurrence of enhanced striatal preprodynorphin gene expression in behaviorally sensitized rats: differential long-term effects of intermittent and chronic morphine administration. Neuroscience **76**: 167–176.
93. NEISEWANDER, J.L., L.E. O'DELL, M.A. LY, T.L. TRAN-NGUYEN, M.A. EDWARD CASTAÑEDA & R.A. FUCHS. 1996. Dopamine overflow in the nucleus accumbens during extinction and reinstatement of cocaine. Neuropsychopharmacology **15**: 506–514.
94. ANGRIST, B. 1994. Psychosis-inducing effects of cocaine may show sensitization more than other effects. Neuropsychopharmacology **10**: 197S.
95. GAWIN, F.H. & M.E. KHALSA. 1996. Sensitization and "street" stimulant addiction. *In* Neurotoxicity and Neuropathology Associated with Stimulant Abuse. M.D. Majewska, Ed.: 224–250. NIDA Research Monograph Series, U.S. Government Printing Office, Washington, DC.
96. SEGAL, D.S. & R. KUCZENSKI. 1997. An escalating dose "binge" model of amphetamine psychosis: behavioral and neurochemical characteristics. J. Neurosci. **17**: 2551–2566.

The Bed Nucleus of the Stria Terminalis
A Target Site for Noradrenergic Actions in Opiate Withdrawal

GARY ASTON-JONES,[a] JILL M. DELFS, JONATHAN DRUHAN, AND YAN ZHU

University of Pennsylvania, Department of Psychiatry, VA Medical Center (151), University and Woodland Avenues, Philadelphia, Pennsylvania 19104, USA

ABSTRACT: Hyperactivity of brain norepinephrine (NE) systems has long been implicated in mechanisms of opiate withdrawal (OW). However, little is known about where elevated NE may act to promote OW. Here we report that the bed nucleus of the stria terminalis (BNST), the densest NE target in the brain, is critical for NE actions in OW. (1) Many BNST neurons become Fos+ after OW. Pretreatment with the β antagonist, propranolol, markedly reduces OW symptoms and the number of Fos+ cells in the BNST. (2) Numerous neurons in the nucleus tractus solitarius (A2 neurons) and the A1 cell group are triple labeled for tyrosine hydroxylase, a retrograde tracer from the BNST, and Fos after OW, revealing numerous NE neurons that project to the BNST from the medulla that are stimulated by OW. Fewer such triple-labeled neurons were found in the locus caeruleus. (3) Behavioral studies reveal that local microinjections of selective β-adrenergic antagonists into the BNST attenuate OW symptoms. In particular, withdrawal-induced place aversion is abolished by bilateral microinjection of a cocktail of selective beta 1 (betaxolol) plus the beta 2 (ICI 181,555) antagonists (1.0 nmol each/0.5 μL per side) into the BNST. Similar results were obtained with neurochemically selective lesions of the ventral ascending NE bundle, the pathway for A1 and A2 projections to the BNST. Similar lesions of the dorsal NE bundle of projections from the locus caeruleus had no effect on either aversive or somatic withdrawal symptoms. Together, these results indicate that β-receptor activation in the BNST is critical for aversive withdrawal symptoms, and that A1 and A2 neurons in the medulla are the source of this critical NE.

INTRODUCTION

Hyperactivity of brain norepinephrine (NE) has long been implicated in mechanisms of opiate withdrawal.[1] However, despite significant advances in understanding the neural basis of hyperactivity of NE neurons during opiate withdrawal,[2] it has not been determined where or how heightened NE release acts to contribute to opiate withdrawal–induced behaviors. In this report, we provide anatomical and behavioral evidence that the bed nucleus of the stria terminalis (BNST), a structure with dense NE innervation,[3,4] is an important site where increased NE may act to promote opiate withdrawal.

The BNST is strongly and reciprocally connected with the amygdala. It is a key component of the "extended amygdala," a group of anatomically and functionally

---

[a]Voice: 215-573-5200; fax: 215-573-5202; gaj@mail.med.upenn.edu

related structures that extends rostrocaudally from the BNST to the centromedial nuclei of the amygdala.[5,6] The BNST also projects to the shell of the NAcc as well as to the ventral tegmental area, the main source of dopamine input to the NAcc shell.[5,7] Past studies have demonstrated that structures with the extended amygdala, particularly the NAcc, are critical for the reinforcing and behavioral-activating effects of such opiate drugs as heroin and morphine.[8-11] The NAcc and amygdala have also received considerable attention for their role in the expression of behaviors elicited by opiate withdrawal.[12-16] Curiously, despite the density of NE in the BNST and its relationship to the NAcc and amygdala, the structure has been largely overlooked with respect to its potential role in opiate abuse or opiate withdrawal.

The BNST is an anatomically and functionally heterogeneous brain region. The medial aspect of the BNST connects with the lateral preoptic area, posterior pituitary, and associated nuclei and is thought to be involved in stress and neuroendocrine-related functions.[17-19] The lateral BNST, on the other hand, is strongly connected with the periaqueductal gray, parabrachial area, and dorsal vagal complex, as well as the paraventricular nucleus of the hypothalamus.[17,20,21] Consistent with these projections, the lateral BNST is importantly involved in such autonomic processes as cardiovascular and respiratory function.[22-25] Withdrawal from opiate drugs is associated with profound changes in neuroendocrine, autonomic, aversive and stress-related systems; therefore it seems quite possible that alterations in BNST activity contribute to opiate-withdrawal behaviors. Moreover, the BNST receives one of the densest NE fiber inputs in the brain.[3,4,26,27] Thus, this is a logical site where hyperactivity in NE neurons could influence withdrawal responses.

The NE innervation of the BNST is particularly prominent in its ventral and medial subdivisions. Much of the NE innervation of the BNST presumably arises from the A1 and A2 medullary NE cell groups,[3,28] although to date there have been few systematic studies that have examined the origins of NE innervation of the BNST. One aim of the present study was to determine the source(s) of the NE innervation of the BNST using anatomical tract-tracing techniques and chemical lesions of the dorsal and ventral noradrenergic pathways.

As mentioned previously, NE cells become hyperactive during opiate withdrawal, which results in enhanced NE release at target sites. Previous work from this laboratory demonstrated that systemic administration of the β-adrenergic receptor antagonist, propranolol, attenuated both somatic and aversive signs of naloxone-precipitated opiate withdrawal.[29] A second goal of our study was to determine if such effects of β antagonists are mediated within the BNST. For this, we examined the expression of the immediate early gene, Fos, in the BNST following precipitated opiate withdrawal in rats that were pretreated with propranolol, and we determined the effects of locally administered β antagonists directly into the BNST on the expression of opiate-withdrawal behaviors.

METHODS

Fos Immunohistochemistry: Effects of Propranolol

Rats were made dependent on morphine by subcutaneous implantation of 2 morphine pellets (75 mg morphine sulfate each, NIDA). On the fifth day after pellet implantation, rats were injected with either the β-adrenergic antagonist propranolol (10 mg/kg, ip) or saline. All rats were then given an injection of naltrexone (1 mg/kg, ip) 30 min later, and somatic withdrawal signs were scored over a 30-min period, as described below. Two hours after the naltrexone injection, rats were perfused with fixative and brains were prepared for immunohistochemistry for the Fos protein (and related antigens) using standard procedures. In brief, 40-μm-thick sections were cut on a cryostat and stored in 0.1 M PB with 0.9% saline and 0.3% triton X-100. Sections were incubated with rabbit anti-Fos antiserum (1:50,000, Oncogene Science) for 3 days at 4°C followed by incubations in a biotinylated donkey anti-rabbit secondary antibody (1:1000; Jackson) and finally incubation in avidin-biotin complex (ABC, 1:1000; Vector) for 2 hours at room temperature (RT). Immunodetection was performed with 3,3′-diaminobenzidine (DAB; Sigma) plus nickel ammonium sulfate.

Retrograde Tract Tracing

For triple labeling with retrograde tract tracing plus immunohistochemistry for Fos and tyrosine hydroxylase (TH), microinjections of WGA-apoHRP-gold (WGA-gold) were made into the BNST (400–600 nL over 10 min). These rats were then made dependent on morphine by implantation of pellets, and withdrawal was precipitated 5 days later with naltrexone, as described above. Rats were perfused 2 h after the naltrexone injection, and their brains were processed for visualization of WGA-gold, Fos, and TH in the same tissue sections. Sections were incubated in IntenseM BL silver enhancement kit (Amersham) for 30 min to visualize WGA-gold, followed by incubation in 1° and 2° antibodies and the ABC reaction for Fos (see above). DAB plus nickel ammonium sulfate was used to visualize Fos (purple-black product). To identify TH-containing cells, the sections were subsequently incubated in mouse anti-TH antiserum (1: 6,000, Incstar) overnight at RT. The following day, sections were reacted with donkey anti-mouse IgG (1: 500, Jackson), mouse PAP (1: 500, Jackson), and DAB to yield a brown reaction product. Thus, WGA-gold appeared as small black particles (located in the cytoplasm), Fos was dark purple-black (nucleus), and TH was diffuse brown (cytoplasm).

6-Hydroxydopamine (6-OHDA) Lesions

Male Sprague Dawley rats (Taconic, 250–300 g) were anesthetized with Nembutal (50 mg/kg) and placed in a stereotaxic frame. Bilateral infusion cannulae (28 gauge) were directed toward the dorsal or ventral NE bundles (DNAB, VNAB) in separate groups of animals using the following coordinates: DNAB, AP: −6.0 mm, ML: ±0.8 mm, DV: −6.3 mm from skull, incisor −2.4 mm; VNAB, AP: −6.6 mm, ML: ±2.0 mm, DV: −8.2 and −9.2 mm from skull, incisor + 5.0 mm. Infusions of 2 μL of 6-OHDA (DNAB 2 μg/μL; VNAB 3 μg/μL in 0.1% ascorbic acid/0.9% saline) were made over 8 min (0.25 μL/min) using a Hamilton syringe and a Harvard Apparatus infusion pump. The cannulae were kept in place an additional 5 min to allow tissue to absorb the infusion and limit diffusion upwards along the cannula tract. Ten days after surgery, animals were implanted subcutaneously with 2 pellets of morphine or placebo (as described above). Behavioral testing began 4 days later.

Cannulae Implantation and Intracerebral Microinjections in Behaving Rats

For local microinjection studies, male Sprague-Dawley rats (Taconic, 250–300 g) were anesthetized, and bilateral indwelling guide cannulae (22 gauge) were implanted stereotaxically into the BNST, using the following coordinates: AP: −0.4 mm, ML: ±3.5 mm, DV: −6.2 mm from skull surface, incisor −3.0, 15° angle. Cannulae were affixed to the skull using acrylic cement, and obturators were placed in the guide cannulae to prevent blockage. Approximately 1 week after surgery, 2 morphine pellets were implanted subcutaneously in each rat, and behavioral testing began 4 days later. For intracerebral microinjections, the obturators were removed and 28 gauge injector cannulae were lowered to the final site (1 mm past the guide). Infusions of 0.5 µL per side were made over 1 min using a Hamilton syringe, and the cannulae were left in place an additional 1 minute.

Conditioned Place Aversion and Opiate Withdrawal Behavioral Scoring

A balanced place-conditioning procedure was used to measure aversive effects of opiate withdrawal.[29] On the first day of testing (preconditioning day), animals were placed in the testing chamber with free access to both compartments of a place-conditioning apparatus for 15 minutes. One side of the chamber had black walls and a wire grid floor; the other side had black and white striped walls and a steel bar floor. On each of the next 2 days (pairing days), the animals were given an ip injection of saline (1 mL/kg) or naltrexone (1 mg/kg) and were confined to one compartment or the other for 30 minutes. In this balanced design, if naloxone was injected in one compartment on the first paring day, saline was injected in the other compartment on the second pairing day, and vice versa. Thus, animals had equal exposure to both compartments. For intracerebral microinjection studies, the locally administered drugs were infused just prior to the ip saline and naltrexone injections on both pairing days. During these 2 pairing sessions, the human observer scored opiate withdrawal behaviors. Each occurrence of wet dog shakes, teeth chattering, eye twitching, jumping, penile grooming, and paw tremors was recorded continuously throughout each 30-min pairing session, and the presence of ptosis, rhinorrhea, lachrymation, vocalization on touch, and diarrhea were noted every 5 minutes. On the final day (test day), animals were given no drug injections and were returned to the test apparatus with free access to both compartments for 15 minutes. One day after the experiments, animals were sacrificed by decapitation. For intracerebral microinjection studies, 0.3 µL of Pontamine Sky Blue was injected prior to sacrifice to verify the cannulae placements.

RESULTS

Fos Expression in BNST

Naltrexone-precipitated opiate withdrawal resulted in an prominent increase in Fos+ neurons in the BNST, particularly in the ventral and dorsolateral regions of the nucleus (FIG. 1A) This increase in Fos expression was not observed in the adjacent caudate-putamen, which was virtually devoid of Fos+ neurons (not shown). Systemic pretreatment with 10 mg/kg propranolol, ip, a dose previously shown to significantly reduce opiate withdrawal signs,[29] markedly reduced the number of Fos+

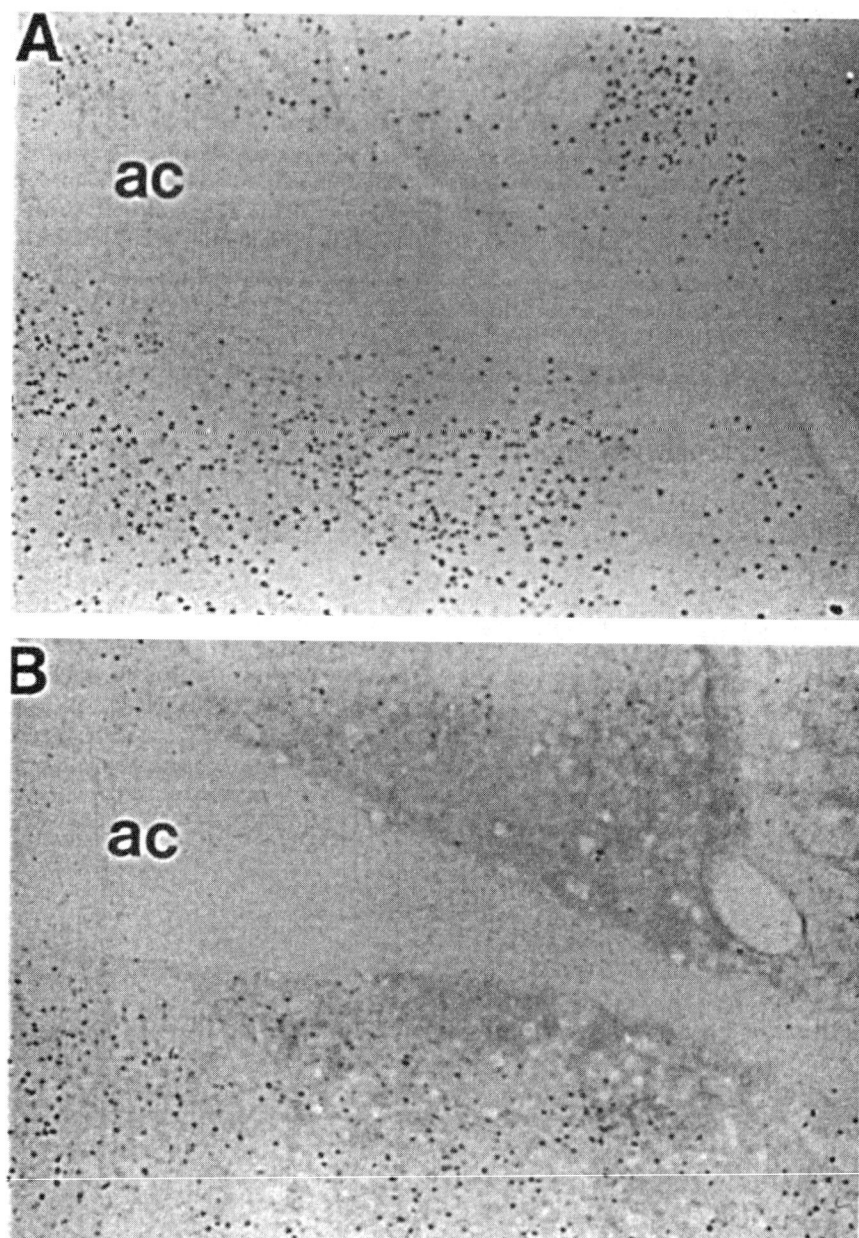

FIGURE 1. Withdrawal-induced increases in Fos expression in the BNST are significantly attenuated by pretreatment with the β antagonist, propranolol. Brightfield photomicrographs of coronal sections through the BNST, illustrating immunohistochemistry for Fos. Each black dot represents a Fos-positive neuron. **A:** A representative section from a

neurons in both the ventral and dorsolateral BNST (FIG. 1B). These same propranolol treatments also substantially reduced the somatic opiate withdrawal behaviors, as previously reported.[29]

Retrograde Tract Tracing: Triple Labeling

Retrograde tract tracing with WGA-gold was used to determine the noradrenergic afferents to the BNST. When combined with Fos and TH immunoreactivity, it was possible to determine which populations of BNST-projecting, NE-containing afferents were activated during opiate withdrawal. Retrogradely labeled neurons were observed in noradrenergic cell groups of the LC, A2 region of the NTS and the A1 region of the caudal ventrolateral medulla following injections of WGA-gold into the BNST. Of these regions, the majority of retrogradely labeled neurons were observed in the NTS. In morphine-dependent rats, which underwent naltrexone-precipitated opiate withdrawal, many retrogradely labeled, TH+ and Fos+ (triple-labeled) neurons were found in the A2 region of the NTS (data not shown). Fewer triple-labeled neurons were observed in the A1 or LC cell groups. This laboratory and others have previously shown an increase in Fos expression in most catecholaminergic neurons of the brain stem following opiate withdrawal.[32,33] The present results indicate that many NE cells, most prominently in the A2 cell group, that project to the BNST are stimulated by opiate withdrawal.

Dorsal and Ventral NE Bundle Lesions: Effects on Opiate Withdrawal-induced Behaviors

We and others had previously demonstrated that chemical lesions of the LC or the dorsal NE bundle (DNAB), which arises from the LC, had no effect on the physical and/or aversive component of opiate withdrawal.[34–37] Our anatomical studies (above) demonstrated that the majority of the NE input to the BNST arises from caudal brain stem NE cell groups (A1 and A2), which give rise to the ventral NE bundle (VNAB). To determine the relative contributions of each of these NE projections to the BNST on the expression of opiate-withdrawal behaviors, 6-OHDA lesions of DNAB or VNAB were made in morphine-dependent and nondependent rats. Lesions of the VNAB significantly attenuated opiate withdrawal-induced place aversion in morphine-dependent animals when compared to sham-operated, morphine-dependent control animals (FIG. 2B). VNAB lesions did not significantly alter the side preference in nondependent (placebo-pelleted) rats. Consistent with previous results, lesions of the DNAB had no significant effect on opiate withdrawal-induced place aversion in morphine-dependent animals compared to sham controls (FIG. 2A). Lesions in placebo-pelleted animals did not significantly affect place conditioning, and these animals did not develop a significant aversion to either side. Notably, neither the DNAB nor VNAB lesions had a significant effect on the expression of so-

---

morphine-dependent animal that underwent naltrexone-induced opiate withdrawal. Note the numerous Fos-positive neurons in the dorsal and ventral BNST. **B:** A section from a morphine-dependent animal that was pretreated with propranolol (10 mg/kg, ip) 30 min prior to precipitation of withdrawal. There were markedly fewer Fos-positive neurons in the dorsal and ventral BNST compared to panel **A.** ac, anterior commissure.

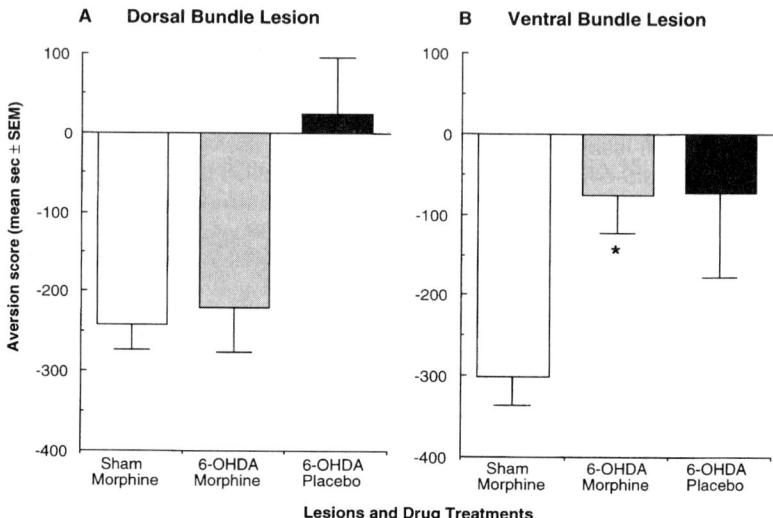

FIGURE 2. Effect of dorsal and ventral noradrenergic bundle lesions on the expression of opiate withdrawal-induced conditioned-place aversion. Aversion score indicates the time spent on the naltrexone-paired side on the test day minus the preconditioning day (a negative number indicates aversion of the naltrexone-paired chamber). **A:** 6-OHDA lesions of the dorsal bundle (DNAB) do not alter the expression of conditioned-place aversion in morphine-dependent rats when compared to sham-lesioned animals. **B:** 6-OHDA lesions of the ventral bundle (VNAB) significantly attenuate withdrawal-induced place aversion when compared to sham-lesioned controls. In **A:** $n = 7$ sham/morphine; $n = 12$ 6-OHDA/morphine; $n = 11$ 6-OHDA/placebo. In **B:** $n = 10$ sham/morphine; $n = 12$ 6-OHDA/morphine; $n = 8$ 6-OHDA/placebo. * $p < 0.05$, compared to sham, ANOVA.

matic signs of opiate withdrawal (data not shown). The VNAB lesion tended to decrease teeth chatters and eye twitches in morphine-dependent rats, although this failed to reach statistical significance.

To rule out the possibility that VNAB-lesioned animals have nonspecific learning deficits, a separate group of rats received VNAB lesions and underwent shock-induced conditioned place aversion. This test was similar, except rats (nondependent) were shocked on one side of the box during the pairing days. VNAB- and sham-lesioned animals had very similar aversion scores (sham control: -376.3 ± 56; VNAB lesion: -371.5 ± 36 s), indicating that VNAB-lesioned animals had no deficit in learning another aversive task.

Intra-BNST Injections of β-receptor Antagonists

This laboratory has previously shown that systemic administration of the β-adrenergic antagonist, propranolol, attenuates somatic and aversive opiate-withdrawal behaviors.[29] Based on the above finding that propranolol could reduce Fos expression in the BNST, we hypothesized that the effects of antagonizing β adrenoceptors on opiate withdrawal were mediated within the BNST. To test this hypothesis, microinjections of a cocktail of the selective β1 (betaxolol) and β2 (ICI 118,555)

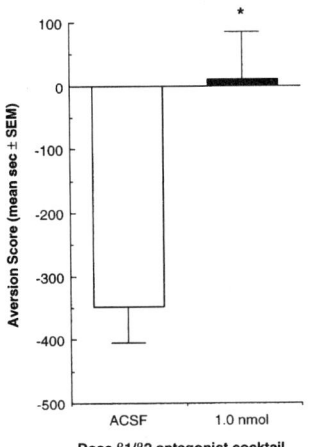

FIGURE 3. Intra-BNST injections of a cocktail of the selective β antagonists, betaxolol and ICI 118,555 significantly attenuated opiate withdrawal-induced conditioned-place aversion. Animals received injections of the β-antagonist cocktail on each of the pairing days (1.0 nmol/0.5 μL per side). Aversion score indicates the time spent on the naltrexone-paired side on the test day minus the preconditioning day (a negative number indicates aversion of the naltrexone-paired chamber). $n = 8$ rats per group. * $p < 0.05$, compared to ACSF, unpaired t-test.

adrenoceptor antagonists were made bilaterally into the BNST just prior to precipitating opiate withdrawal with naltrexone. Microinjection of this cocktail into the BNST markedly reduced conditioned-place aversion in a dose-dependent manner (FIG. 3). At the highest dose (1.0 nmol), the withdrawal aversion was completely abolished. Intra-BNST injections of the β antagonists also caused significant dose-dependent decreases in teeth chatter and eye twitches, as well as a nonsignificant decrease in wet dog shakes (not shown). To test for site specificity, injections of the β antagonist cocktail 3 mm dorsal to the BNST site did not alter the somatic or aversive signs of opiate withdrawal, compared to ACSF-injected rats (data not shown).

Beta antagonists have been shown to act as local anesthetics.[38] Therefore, to rule out the possibility that the observed effects were due to a local anesthetic effect, another group of rats received injections of optical isomers of the nonselective β-antagonist, propranolol (5 nmol/0.5 μL). Both the R- and S-isomers of propranolol possess local anesthetic properties, although only the S isomer blocks the β-adrenoceptor. Intra-BNST injection of the S-isomer of propranolol significantly reduced opiate withdrawal-induced place aversion, whereas the R-isomer did not alter withdrawal-induced aversion (ACSF: −276.2 ± 87; R-Prop: −246.3 ± 71; S-Prop: −11.7 ± 37 s). Similar to the above results, microinjection of the S-, but not R-isomer of propranolol caused significant reductions in TC and ET (data not shown).

DISCUSSION

The present studies are the first to indicate that the BNST is an important target for NE actions during opiate withdrawal. The BNST is stimulated during opiate withdrawal, as indicated by increased Fos expression. This increase in Fos expression was significantly reduced by pretreatment with the β antagonist, propranolol. Using retrograde-labeling techniques we demonstrated that neurons of the A2 (NTS), A1, and A6 (LC) cell groups project to the BNST. These projections were most numerous from the A2 group. We also found that many NE neurons of the A2 and A1 cell groups that project to the BNST were stimulated as revealed by Fos immunoreactivity following naltrexone-precipitated opiate withdrawal. This stimulation of catecholaminergic neurons has been observed previously by our laboratory and others.[32,33] Consistent with these anatomical findings, the results of our behavioral experiments showed that the VNAB, which originates in the A2 and A1 NE cell groups, is critical for the expression of opiate-withdrawal conditioned-place aversion. Local microinjection of β antagonists into the BNST also markedly decreased opiate-withdrawal place aversion, showing that β adrenoceptors in the BNST are a target for elevated NE activity, which drives opiate withdrawal behaviors.

It is noteworthy that a similar pattern of retrograde labeling in NE cell groups was observed following WGA-gold injections in the caudal shell of the NAcc.[30] Future experiments are necessary to test the possible involvement of NE projections to the NAcc in withdrawal-induced aversion. The density of NE innervation in the NAcc is much less than in the BNST.[30] However, previous studies found that local injections of methylnaloxone into the NAcc induced place aversion in morphine-dependent rats.[13]

The finding that the expression of Fos in BNST following naltrexone-induced opiate withdrawal was reduced by the β adrenoceptor antagonist, propranolol, indicates that elevated NE activation of β adrenoceptors may stimulate Fos production in BNST neurons. This possibility is consistent with prior findings that NE inputs potently induce Fos protein in brain neurons.[39,40] It is also consistent with the present result that many of the NE neurons of the A2, A1, and LC, which project directly to the BNST, are stimulated by opiate withdrawal (as revealed by Fos induction).

The majority of the retrogradely labeled neurons observed following injection of tracers into the BNST were found in the A2 NE cell group. The axons of these cell groups course rostrally and ventrally via the VNAB to innervate structures of the ventral forebrain, including the BNST. We hypothesized that the VNAB pathway may be importantly involved in the expression of opiate-withdrawal behaviors, in view of recent evidence for little or no role of the DNAB or the LC in opiate withdrawal behaviors,[34–37] and based upon the current finding of a critical role of NE in the BNST in withdrawal-induced aversion. Consistent with this hypothesis, we found that VNAB lesions (but not DNAB lesions) were very effective at reducing withdrawal-induced conditioned-place aversion. To our knowledge, this is the first demonstration of the involvement of the VNAB system in aversive properties of opiate withdrawal.

The ability of local microinjections of β adrenoceptor antagonists into the BNST to attenuate withdrawal-induced aversion provides further support for the importance of NE in this structure in the manifestation of opiate-withdrawal behaviors. These results also indicate that β receptors in the BNST may be particularly involved. The detailed distribution of β-adrenergic receptors within the BNST is not known, but β1 and β2 receptors have been reported in this nucleus at moderate lev-

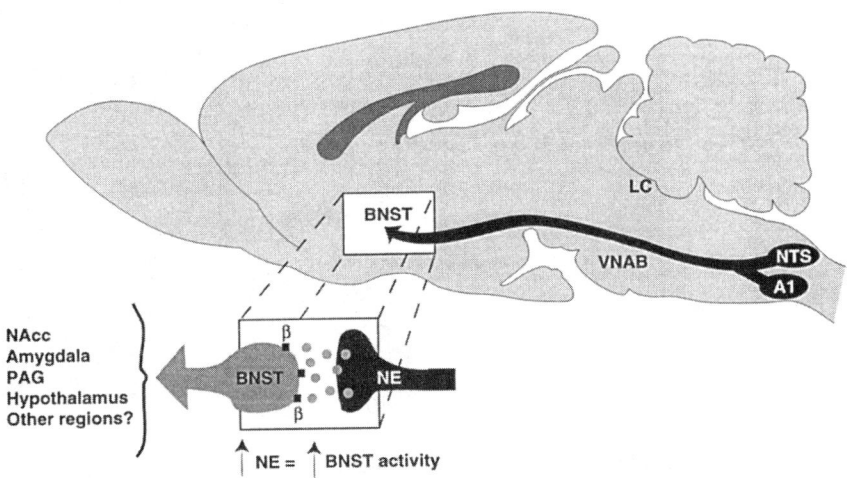

FIGURE 4. Schematic illustrating the effects of opiate withdrawal on the activity of the BNST. Withdrawal-induced activation of NE neurons in the NTS and A1 cell groups (which contribute to the VNAB) would cause enhanced NE release in the BNST. NE acting at β-NE receptors in the BNST would result in activation of BNST neurons projecting to various regions, such as the nucleus accumbens (NAcc), amygdala, periaqueductal gray (PAG), hypothalamus, and perhaps other regions. Blockade of NE release (i.e., lesions of the pathway) or direct blockade of β receptors in the BNST reduce withdrawal-induced conditioned-place aversion, indicating the important role of NE transmission in the BNST in the expression of this behavior. Brain schematic modified from *Brain Maps*.[44]

els.[41] Interestingly, systemic administration of atenolol, a β1 antagonist, which does not cross the blood–brain behavior, was much less effective than propranolol at reducing withdrawal-induced place aversion, providing further support for the central site of action of β antagonists on this behavior.[29]

With regard to the somatic signs of opiate withdrawal, local injections of β antagonists into the BNST significantly reduced teeth chatters, eye twitches, and nonsignificantly decreased wet dog shakes. A recent report by Funada *et al.*[42] showed that icv administration of a β1 or β2 antagonist reduced several signs of opiate withdrawal in mice, including jumping and wet dog shakes. Similar, albeit nonsignificant, reductions in teeth chatters and eye twitches were observed in VNAB-lesioned rats. Although these changes were not as robust as those observed following local administration of β antagonists, these results suggest that these particular somatic signs may be the result of increased NE released from VNAB fibers acting at β receptors in the BNST.

From these anatomical and behavioral results we hypothesize that during opiate withdrawal, hyperactive NE neurons of the caudal brain stem release NE in the BNST (via the VNAB), which in turn stimulates BNST neurons via β-adrenergic receptors (FIG. 4). Activation of BNST neurons by NE acting on β-adrenergic receptors would have downstream effects on a variety of limbic and autonomic areas, such as the NAcc, amygdala, PAG, and hypothalamus. It is reasonable to hypothesize that many of these projections, perhaps especially those to the amygdala and NAcc, are importantly involved in the expression of conditioned-place aversion.[43] Future studies are needed to delineate BNST targets involved in withdrawal-induced aversion. Regardless of the downstream circuit involved, the present study shows that the BNST is an important target of NE actions, subserving the expression of aversive signs of opiate withdrawal.

ACKNOWLEDGMENTS

We thank Carrie Walters for technical assistance. This work was supported by NIH Grants DA06214, DA10088, and DA05810.

REFERENCES

1. MALDONADO, R. 1997. Participation of noradrenergic pathways in the expression of opiate withdrawal: biochemical and pharmacological evidence. Neurosci. Biobehav. Rev. 21: 91–104.
2. ASTON-JONES, G., R. SHIEKHATTAR, J. RAJKOWSKI, P. KUBIAK & H. AKAOKA. 1993. Opiates influence noradrenergic locus coeruleus neurons by potent indirect as well as direct effects. In The Neurobiology of Opiates. R. Hammer, Ed.: 175–202. CRC Press. New York.
3. MOORE, R.Y. 1978. Catecholamine innervation of the basal forebrain: I. The septal area. J. Comp. Neurol. 177: 665–684.
4. PHELIX, C.F., Z. LIPOSITS & W.K. PAULL. 1992. Monoamine innervation of bed nucleus of stria terminalis: an electron microscopic investigation. Brain Res. Bull. 28: 949–965.
5. ALHEID, G.F., J.S. DE OLMOS & C.A. BELTRAMINO. 1995. Amygdala and extended amygdala. In The Rat Nervous System. G. Paxinos, Ed.: 495–578. Academic Press. New York.
6. ALHEID, G.F. & L. HEIMER. 1988. New perspectives in basal forebrain organization of special relevance for neuropsychiatric disorders: the striatopallidal, amygdaloid, and corticopetal components of the substantia inominata. Neuroscience 27: 1–39.
7. BROG, J.S., A. SALYAPONGSE, A.Y. DEUTCH & D.S. ZAHM. 1993. The patterns of afferent innervation of the core and shell in the "accumbens" part of the rat ventral striatum: immunohistochemical detection of retrogradely transported fluoro-gold. J. Comp. Neurol. 338: 255–278.
8. KOOB, G.F., P. ROBELEDO, A. MARKOU & S.B. CAINE. 1993. The mesocorticolimbic circuit in drug dependence and reward—a role for the extended amygdala? In Limbic Motor Circuits and Neuropsychiatry. P. W. Kalivas & C.D. Barnes, Eds.: 289–309. CRC Press, Inc. Boca Raton, FL.
9. KOOB, G.F., F.J. VACCARINO, M. AMALRIC & F.E. BLOOM. 1986. Neurochemical substrates for opiate reinforcement. NIDA Res. Monogr. 71: 146–164.
10. VACCARINO, F.J., F.E. BLOOM & G.F. KOOB. 1985. Blockade of nucleus accumbens opiate receptors attenuates intravenous heroin reward in the rat. Psychopharmacology 86: 37–42.
11. KELSEY, J.E., W.A. CARLEZON, JR. & W.A. FALLS. 1989. Lesions of the nucleus accumbens in rats reduce opiate reward but do not alter context-specific opiate tolerance. Behav. Neurosci. 103: 1327–1334.
12. HARRIS, G. & G. ASTON-JONES. 1994. Involvement of D2 dopamine receptors in the nucleus accumbens in the opiate withdrawal syndrome. Nature 371: 155–157.
13. KOOB, G.F., T.L. WALL & F.E. BLOOM. 1989. Nucleus accumbens as a substrate for the aversive stimulus effects of opiate withdrawal. Psychopharmacology 98: 530–534.

14. POTHOS, E., P. RADA, G.P. MARK & B.G. HOEBEL. 1991. Dopamine microdialysis in the nucleus accumbens during acute and chronic morphine, naloxone-precipitated withdrawal and clonidine treatment. Brain Res. **566:** 348–350.
15. ROSSETTI, Z.L., Y. HMAIDAN & G.L. GESSA. 1992. Marked inhibition of mesolimbic dopamine release: a common feature of ethanol, morphine, cocaine and amphetamine abstinence in rats. Eur. J. Pharmacol. **221:** 227–234.
16. KELSEY, J.E. & S.R. ARNOLD. 1994. Lesions of the dorsomedial amygdala, but not the nucleus accumbens, reduce the aversiveness of morphine withdrawal in rats. Behav. Neurosci. **108:** 1119–1127.
17. DE OLMOS, J., G.F. ALHEID & C.A. BELTRAMINO. 1985. Amygdala. *In* The Rat Nervous System, Vol. 1: Forebrain and Midbrain. G. Paxinos, Ed.: 223–334. Academic Press. New York.
18. GRAY, T.S., R.A. PIECHOWSKI, J.M. YRACHETA, P.A. RITTENHOUSE, C.L. BETHEA & L.D. VAN DE KAR. 1993. Ibotenic acid lesions in the bed nucleus of the stria terminalis attenuate conditioned stress-induced increases in prolactin, ACTH and corticosterone. Neuroendocrinology **57:** 517–24.
19. CASADA, J.H. & N. DAFNY. 1992. Evidence for two different afferent pathways carrying stress-related information (noxious and amygdala stimulation) to the bed nucleus of the stria terminalis. Brain Res. **579:** 93–98.
20. SWANSON, L.W. & P.E. SAWCHENKO. 1980. Paraventricular nucleus: a site for the integration of neuroendocrine and autonomic mechanisms. Neuroendocrinology **31:** 410–417.
21. LOEWY, A.D. 1991. Forebrain nuclei involved in autonomic control. Prog. Brain Res. **87:** 253–268.
22. TERREBERRY, R.R., M. OGURI & R.M. HARPER. 1995. State-dependent respiratory and cardiac relationships with neuronal discharge in the bed nucleus of the stria terminalis. Sleep **18:** 139–144.
23. WILKINSON, M.F. & Q.J. PITTMAN. 1995. Changes in arterial blood pressure alter activity of electrophysiologically identified single units of the bed nucleus of the stria terminalis. Neuroscience **64:** 835–844.
24. CIRIELLO, J. & S.A. JANSSEN. 1993. Effect of glutamate stimulation of bed nucleus of the stria terminalis on arterial pressure and heart rate. Am. J. Physiol. **265:** H1516–1522.
25. RODER, S. & J. CIRIELLO. 1993. Contribution of bed nucleus of the stria terminalis to the cardiovascular responses elicited by stimulation of the amygdala. J. Auton. Nerv. Syst. **45:** 61–75.
26. SWANSON, L.W. & B.K. HARTMAN. 1975. The central adrenergic system. An immunofluorescence study of the location of cell bodies and their efferent connections in the rat utilizing dopamine-beta-hydroxylase as a marker. J. Comp. Neurol. **163:** 467–505.
27. BROWNSTEIN, M.J. & M. PALKOVITS. 1984. Catecholamines, serotonin, acetylcholine, and gamma-aminobutyric acid in the rat brain: biochemical studies. *In* Handbook of Chemical Neuroanatomy, Vol. 2: Classical Transmitters in the CNS, Part 1. A. Björklund & T. Hokfelt, Eds.: 23–54. Elsevier Science Publishers B.V. Amsterdam.
28. UNGERSTEDT, U. 1971. Stereotaxic mapping of monoamine pathways in the rat brain. Acta Physiol. Scand. Suppl. **367:** 1–48.
29. HARRIS, G. & G. ASTON-JONES. 1993. Beta-adrenergic antagonists attenuate somatic and aversive signs of opiate withdrawal. Neuropsychopharmacology **9:** 303–311.
30. DELFS, J.M., Y. ZHU, J.P. DRUHAN & G. ASTON-JONES. 1998. Origin of noradrenergic afferents to the shell subregion of the nucleus accumbens: anterograde and retrograde tract tracing studies in the rat. Brain Res. **806:** 127–140.
31. ASTON-JONES, G., M. ENNIS, V.A. PIERIBONE, W.T. NICKELL & M.T. SHIPLEY. 1986. The brain nucleus locus coeruleus: restricted afferent control of a broad efferent network. Science **234:** 734–737.
32. AKAOKA, H., Y. ZHU, M.T. SHIPLEY & G. ASTON-JONES. 1992. Expression of fos protein in central catecholamine neurons during opiate withdrawal. Soc. Neurosci. Abstr. **18.**

33. STORNETTA, R.L., F.E. NORTON & P.G. GUYENET. 1993. Autonomic areas of rat brain exhibit increased Fos-like immunoreactivity during opiate withdrawal in rats. Brain Res. **624:** 19–28.
34. BRITTON, K., T. SVENSSON, J. SCHWARTZ, F. BLOOM & G. KOOB. 1984. Dorsal noradrenergic bundle lesions fail to alter opiate withdrawal or suppression of opiate withdrawal by clonidine. Life Sci. **34:** 133–139.
35. CHIENG, B. & M.J. CHRISTIE. 1995. Lesions to terminals of noradrenergic locus coeruleus neurones do not inhibit opiate withdrawal behaviour in rats. Neurosci. Lett. **186:** 37–40.
36. DELFS, J.M., J.P. DRUHAN & G. ASTON-JONES. 1997. Involvement of non-locus coeruleus (LC) projections to forebrain in the expression of opiate withdrawal-induced conditioned place aversion (CPA). Soc. Neurosci. Abstr. **23:** 1108.
37. STINUS, L., A. PERON, J.P. RENERIC, M. CADOR & G.F. KOOB. 1997. In morphine dependent rats, the total lesion of locus coeruleus neurons does not impair naloxone-induced withdrawal syndrome and conditioned place aversion, or the protective effects of clonidine upon opiate withdrawal. Soc. Neurosci. Abstr. **23:** 1108.
38. GILMAN, A.G., L.S. GOODMAN, T.W. RALL & F. MURAD. 1985. Goodman and Gilman's The Pharmacological Basis of Therapeutics. Macmillan. New York.
39. BING, G., S. CHEN, Y. ZHANG, D. HILLMAN & E.A. STONE. 1992. Noradrenergic-induced expression of c-fos in rat cortex: neuronal localization. Neurosci. Lett. **140:** 260–264.
40. STONE, E.A., Y. ZHANG, S. JOHN, D. FILER & G. BING. 1993. Effect of locus coeruleus lesion on c-fos expression in the cerebral cortex caused by yohimbine injection or stress. Brain Res. **603:** 181–185.
41. RAINBOW, T.C., B. PARSONS & B.B. WOLFE. 1984. Quantitative autoradiography of $\beta1$- and $\beta2$-adrenergic receptors in rat brain. Proc. Natl. Acad. Sci. USA **81:** 1585–1589.
42. FUNADA, M., T. SUZUKI, Y. SUGANO, M. TSUBAI, M. MISAWA, H. UEDA & Y. MISU. 1994. Role of β-adrenoreceptors in the expression of morphine withdrawal signs. Life Sci. **54:** 113–118.
43. STINUS, L., M. LE MOAL & G.F. KOOB. 1990. Nucleus accumbens and amygdala are possible substrates for the aversive stimulus effects of opiate withdrawal. Neuroscience **37:** 767–73.
44. SWANSON, L.W. 1992. Brain Maps: Structure of the Rat Brain. Elsevier Sciences Publ. Amsterdam.

The Role of Dopamine, Dynorphin, and CART Systems in the Ventral Striatum and Amygdala in Cocaine Abuse

YASMIN L. HURD,[a] PERNILLA SVENSSON, AND MARJAN PONTÉN

Karolinska Institute, Department of Clinical Neuroscience, Psychiatry Section, S-171 76 Stockholm, Sweden

ABSTRACT: Disturbance of the mesolimbic dopamine system has long been hypothesized for the underlying neurobiology of cocaine addiction. Recently, increased attention has been directed towards the opioid neuropeptide system, in particular dynorphin; inasmuch as opioid peptide-containing neurons are regulated by dopamine, these peptides have potent effects on mood and reward, and cocaine consistently modulates dynorphin activity. Our experiments have been directed towards characterizing the specific alterations of dopamine and dynorphin systems during different stages following cocaine administration, as well as assessing the contribution of nucleus accumbens and amygdala dopamine levels to cocaine-intake behavior. We have used the techniques of *in vivo* microdialysis to measure and manipulate extracellular concentrations of dopamine in animals that self-administer cocaine, and *in situ* hybridization to study mRNA expression levels of prodynorphin and dopamine receptors. It is clear from these studies that different stages of the cocaine use cycle are characterized by distinct patterns of prodynorphin and dopamine D_1 mRNA expression levels. Moreover, cocaine-intake behavior is sensitive to very specific concentrations of dopamine in the nucleus accumbens as well as in the amygdala. Recently, the CART (cocaine and amphetamine-regulated transcript) peptide was proposed as a novel target for the actions of psychostimulant drugs. We have noted differences between male and female rats in the mesolimbic mRNA expression of CART that might be relevant for gender differences apparent in drug abuse.

Disturbances of the mesolimbic dopamine (DA) system have long been hypothesized for the underlying neurobiology of cocaine addiction. Of the mesolimbic brain areas, the ventral striatum (nucleus accumbens, NAC) has been extensively studied as to its contribution to cocaine self-administration behavior and drug-reinforcement mechanisms.[1–5] Only recently have a significant number of investigations been undertaken into the potential role of other limbic-related brain areas in drug-taking behavior and how they might interact at the level of the NAC to influence and coordinate drug self-administration. One brain area that presents itself as a potential site for investigation is the amygdala (AMY). The amygdaloid complex has been

---

[a]Voice: 46-8-5177 2379; fax: 46-8-34 65 63; yasmin.hurd@neuro.ks.se

shown to be involved in stimulus-reward associations[6,7] with important contribution to cocaine-taking and cocaine-seeking behavior.[8,9]

Similar to the NAC, the AMY receives a significant innervation from the ventral tegmental area (A10), the origin of DA pathways critical for cocaine self-administration, in addition to receiving some input from the substantia nigra pars compacta (A9) and A8 midbrain cell groups.[10,11] In the AMY, the most dense DA innervation is present in the central nucleus, basal nuclei, and cell clusters at the border of the lateral nuclei.[12] The amygdaloid complex provides discrete inputs to the NAC, with projections arising predominantly from the basal and accessory basal nuclear groups innervating the shell (cell cluster patches) and core (patch and matrix) subregions of the NAC.[13–15] Based on anatomical and behavioral data, the NAC and AMY regions may be key neural sites for the neuroadaptations that underlie cocaine addiction.

DA CONCENTRATIONS IN THE NUCLEUS ACCUMBENS AND AMYGDALA DURING COCAINE SELF-ADMINISTRATION

To determine whether AMY DA levels were affected by cocaine intake and to assess the relationship between DA levels maintained in the NAC to those maintained in the AMY, extracellular levels of DA were monitored in the NAC and AMY of rats (Sprague-Dawley; 300 g) self-administering cocaine by use of the *in vivo* microdialysis technique.[3] The animals had been trained to self-administer cocaine (1.5 mg/kg/injection) under a fixed-ratio reinforcement schedule in 3-h limited sessions. After 5 to 7 days of stable self-administration behavior, a guide cannula was surgically implanted above the NAC and the ipsilateral AMY. A microdialysis probe was subsequently inserted via the guide cannula targeted to either the shell NAC region or the basolateral (i.e., basal nucleus and medial areas of the lateral nucleus) AMY nucleus on the evening prior to the test day. Basal extracellular levels of DA in the

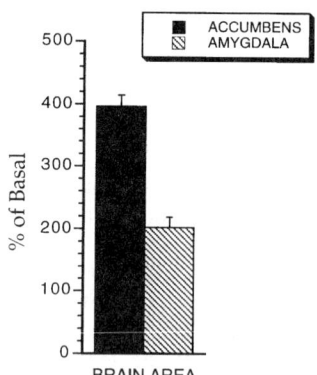

FIGURE 1. Effect of cocaine self-administration on extracellular dopamine levels maintained in the nucleus accumbens ($n = 14$) and amygdala ($n = 6$) of rats. The data (mean ± SEM) are expressed as a percentage of baseline (average of three values obtained prior to initiation of the cocaine self-administration session) of dopamine levels measured during stable cocaine intake.

NAC and AMY were approximately 2.18 ± 0.07 nM and 1.37 ± 0.15 nM in these groups of animals, respectively. DA levels were potentiated twofold higher in the NACC than in the AMY during cocaine self-administration (FIG. 1).[3] Although DA levels in the AMY were significantly lower than those maintained in the NAC, the AMY DA contributed significantly to the cocaine-intake behavior maintained by the animals. Infusion of a D1 antagonist, SCH 23390, into the basolateral AMY caused a concentration-dependent increase of cocaine self-administration behavior. Intra-AMY 0.5 mg and 1.5 mg SCH 23390 induced a 200% and 400% increase of cocaine intake, respectively. Increased rates of cocaine intake are generally interpreted as a compensatory mechanism taken by the animal to overcome a decrease in the reinforcing properties of cocaine. The intra-AMY SCH 23390 effects on cocaine intake behavior were associated with a complementary increase of NAC DA levels.[3] Increased cocaine intake following the intra-AMY SCH 23390 infusion, and thus antagonism of AMY D1-mediated transmission, has been previously reported.[9,16,17] Our results showed that this behavior leads to a subsequent increase in NAC DA levels and suggests that *in vivo* AMY DA also plays a pivotal role in neural processes mediating cocaine self-administration.

An important consideration in the attempt to understand drug self-administration is the question of what maintains cocaine intake behavior: the rate of cocaine intake, and thus rate of DA elevation, or whether there is a "rewarding" DA level that subjects try to achieve.[2,18] It is clear from behavioral studies that animals generally maintain stable cocaine intake during limited-access cocaine self-administration sessions, and *in vivo* studies have shown that stable DA levels are maintained in both the NAC and AMY during these time periods.[3] In order to address whether there are indeed rewarding concentrations of DA maintained in mesolimbic areas associated with the intake of cocaine, DA levels were directly manipulated in the NAC and AMY in rats self-administering cocaine. After animals had maintained a stable level of cocaine intake, which in this study was associated with stable DA levels maintained in the NAC (8.5 nM) and AMY (4.7 nM), different DA concentrations were included in the Ringer's solution perfusing through the microdialysis probe in the respective brain areas. Perfusion of a 90 nM DA concentration resulted in an attenuation or complete inhibition of cocaine intake. A fivefold increase of the perfusing DA concentration doubled the rate of cocaine intake (FIG. 2). Perfusion of the NAC with DA concentrations between the 90 and 450 nM range had no effect on cocaine intake behavior. In the AMY, perfusion of a 45 nM DA concentration during cocaine self-administration attenuated cocaine intake (FIG. 2). Doubling this DA concentration resulted in a twofold increase in the rate of cocaine intake. However, AMY perfusions of DA concentrations in a range up to eight times the normal DA levels failed to alter cocaine intake behavior. These results show that specific concentrations of DA in the NAC and AMY have differential effects on cocaine-intake behavior. Clearly, there appears to be distinct rewarding concentrations of DA in the NAC and AMY. The increased rate of cocaine intake by some concentrations of DA, higher than those maintained by the animal self-administering cocaine, and the inability of a large range of DA concentrations to affect cocaine intake behavior is intriguing. It has to be determined whether certain concentrations of DA might be aversive, thus causing the animal to increase cocaine-intake behavior to block these negative experiences. In addition, these concentrations of DA might activate or block other neural

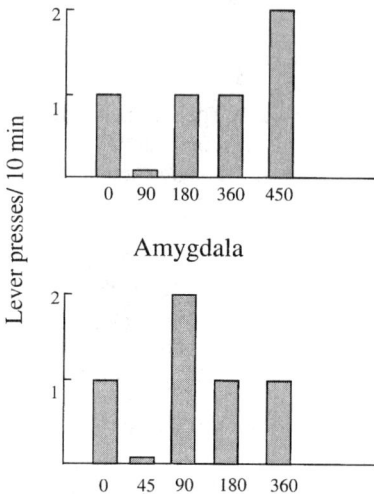

FIGURE 2. General cocaine intake behavior during manipulation of dopamine concentrations perfused through the microdialysis probe situated in either the nucleus accumbens or amygdala of rats with a stable cocaine self-administration behavior. Each lever press results in a 1.5 mg/kg/injection of cocaine.

systems (regulated by DA transmission) that are a critical part of the rewarding effects of the drug. Interestingly, manipulation of a wide range of serotonin (5HT) concentrations in the NAC had no effect on cocaine-intake behavior, whereas specific concentrations of 5HT in the AMY inhibited or increased cocaine-intake behavior. The 5HT system has long been hypothesized to contribute to the effects of cocaine (for a review, see ref. 19). Our results currently point to a larger contribution of the AMY than the NAC 5HT system to cocaine-intake behavior.

THE INFLUENCE OF COCAINE ON DYNORPHIN SYSTEMS

The effects of DA in the NAC are mediated by DA receptors situated on medium spiny neurons located postsynaptic to DAergic terminals. In addition to the inhibitory amino acid, GABA, these medium spiny neurons are abundant in the opioid peptides, dynorphin and enkephalin, and the tachykinin peptide, substance P, and make up the major efferent projection pathways (see ref. 20). A DA-dynorphin interaction has been proposed for the striatal actions of cocaine.[21,22] A large number of studies have now shown that acute and repeated cocaine use consistently increases dynorphin mRNA expression[23–26] and peptide levels[27] in the rat striatum. These dynorphin changes are not only apparent in animals but also in human cocaine users.[28] One aspect, however, of all these results is the fact that the dynorphin alterations are primarily found within the dorsal striatum, rarely within the ventral striatal area. The only conditions under which we have observed significant alterations of the prodynorphin mRNA expression in the ventral striatum is in animals with perinatal exposure to cocaine. Rats exposed to cocaine (50 mg/kg) during postnatal days 11–20, comparable to the third semester of human development, show reduced prodynorphin mRNA expression localized to the shell region of the NAC when studied as adults.[29] These results indicate long-lasting effects of cocaine on the dynorphin system in the most limbic-related area of the NAC, namely the shell, interconnected with the extended AMY.

The reduction of prodynorphin observed in animals with perinatal cocaine exposure most likely reflects neural changes associated with the withdrawal from the drug. This is suggested because whereas increased prodynorphin mRNA expression is apparent following acute and repeated cocaine administration when given to the adult rat,[23–26,30,31] prodynorphin mRNA is reduced following a 10-day drug-free period, subsequent to 10 days of repeated cocaine (30 mg/kg, ip) administration, in the adult animal.[25] Withdrawal from cocaine in humans is often associated with dysphoria, depression, and anxiety, which can contribute to drug craving and the subsequent relapse and self-administration of the drug. The long-term alterations of dynorphin, which is the opioid neuropeptide system mediating dysphoria,[32] might relate to the persistent impaired mood apparent in subjects abstinent from cocaine. Studies are currently ongoing to assess the contribution of the AMY dynorphin system to the effects of cocaine. In the human brain, the prodynorphin mRNA is preferentially expressed in limbic-related areas, including the AMY, hippocampus, patch compartment of the dorsal striatum, and NAC.[33] This discrete limbic expression pattern of the prodynorphin gene suggests a strong involvement of the dynorphin system in emotional behavior.

COCAINE AND AMPHETAMINE-REGULATED TRANSCRIPT (CART) PEPTIDE mRNA EXPRESSION AND COCAINE USE

Recently, another peptide was discovered in the brain that suggests important involvement in drug addiction. Douglas and colleagues,[34] using differential display PCR, localized a gene that was specifically altered in the striatum following administration of cocaine or amphetamine. In situ hybridization showed the distribution pattern of the mRNA expression to be restricted to discrete brain regions important for limbic function, including the NAC, AMY, hippocampus, and hypothalamus.[34,35] Various lines of evidence have now been accumulated showing that the CART peptide is a possible neurotransmitter: the mRNA expression has a similar anatomical distribution as the CART peptide immunoreactivity,[36] the peptide is localized to large dense core vesicles in nerve terminals,[37] the peptide contains a hydrophobic leader sequence that indicates secretion,[34] and the propeptide has several basic amino acids that can be sites for proteolytic cleavage into smaller fragments.[34] In more detailed mapping of the CART mRNA in the forebrain, we have found the expression to be highly localized in islands of the shell and core NAC (no signal in the dorsal caudate putamen), throughout the sublenticular extended AMY and the central AMY (primarily in the lateral and intermediate nucleus) (FIG. 3).[38]

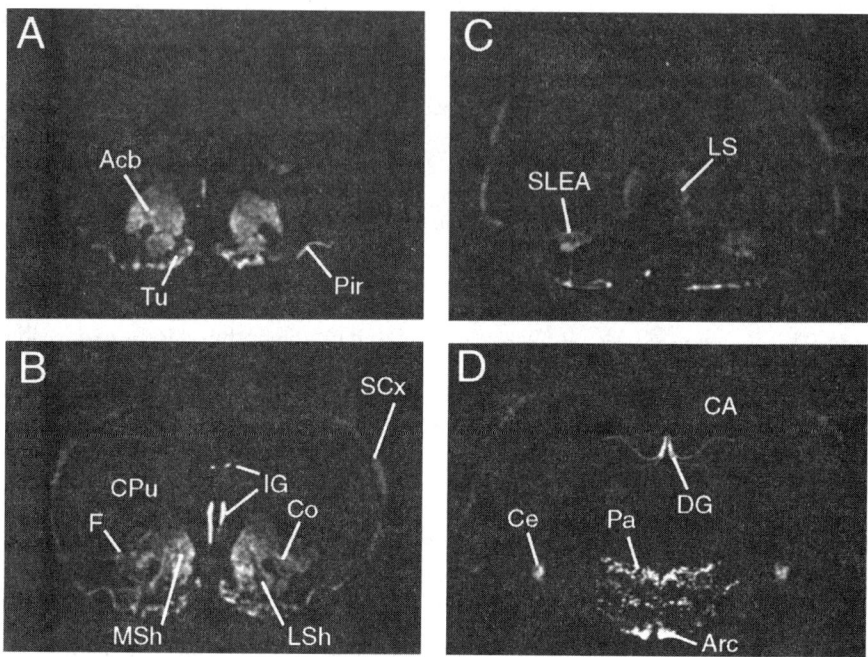

FIGURE 3. CART mRNA expression in the rat brain. Acb, nucleus accumbens; Arc, arcuate nucleus; CA, cornu ammonis hippocampus; Ce, central amygdala; Co, nucleus accumbens core; CPu, caudate-putamen; DG, dentate gyrus; F, fundus striatum; IG, indusium griseum; LS, lateral septum; LSh, lateral nucleus accumbens shell; MSh, medial nucleus accumbens shell; Pa, paraventricular hypothalamic nucleus; Pir, piriform cortex; SLEA, sublenticular extended amygdala; SCx, sensory cortex; Tu, olfactory tubercle.

Our initial studies of the CART mRNA revealed significant basal differences of the expression in the shell NAC between males and females.[38] Administration of cocaine did not alter CART mRNA expression in the NAC of either gender, but there was a significant elevation within the central AMY in males. The physiological actions of CART are still being determined; thus it is preliminary to relate the significance of these CART mRNA alterations to specific behaviors. Further studies are essential to assess its role in drug addiction, but based on the discrete expression to the limbic-related brain areas, it is clear that the CART peptide must have important relevance for the regulation of behaviors associated with emotions.

ACKNOWLEDGMENTS

This work was supported by Grants from the National Institute of Health (DA08912), the Swedish Medical Research Council (11252), and the Karolinska Institute. We thank Mrs. Barbro Berthelsson for her technical assistance.

REFERENCES

1. ROBERTS, D.C., F. KOOB, P. KLONOFF & H.C. FIBIGER. 1980. Extinction and recovery of cocaine self-administration following 6-hydroxydopamine lesions of the nucleus accumbens. Pharmacol. Biochem. Behav. **12:** 781–787.
2. PETTIT, H.O. & J.B. JUSTICE. 1989. Dopamine in the nucleus accumbens during cocaine self-administration as studied by *in vivo* microdialysis. Pharm. Biochem. Behav. **34:** 899–904.
3. HURD, Y.L., A. MCGREGOR & M. PONTÉN. 1997. *In vivo* amygdala dopamine levels modulate cocaine self-administration and modulates cocaine intake behavior in the rat: D1 dopamine receptor involvement. Eur. J. Neurosci. **9:** 2541–2548.
4. KIYATKIIN, E.A. & E.A. STEIN. 1995. Fluctuations in nucleus accumbens dopamine during cocaine self-administration behavior: an *in vivo* electrochemical study. Neuroscience **64:** 599–617.
5. WEISS, F., M.P. PAULUS, M.T. LORANG & G.F. KOOB. 1992. Increases in extracellular dopmaine in the nucleus accumbens by cocaine are inversely related to basal levels: effects of acute and repeated administration. J. Neurosci. **12:** 4372–4380.
6. CADOR, M., T. ROBBINS & B. EVERITT. 1989. Involvement of the amygdala in stimulus-reward associations: interaction with the ventral striatum. Neuroscience **30:** 77–86.
7. EVERITT, B. & T. ROBBINS. 1992. Amygdala-ventral striatal interactions and reward-related processes. *In* The Amygdala. J. P. Aggleton, Eds.: 401–429. Wiley-Liss. New York.
8. WHITELAW, R.B., A. MARKOU, T. ROBBINS & B. EVERITT. 1996. Excitotoxic lesions of the basolateral amygdala impair the acquisition of cocaine-seeking behavior under a second-order schedule of reinforcement. Psychopharmacology **127:** 213–224.
9. MCGREGOR, A. & D.C.S. ROBERTS. 1993. Dopaminergic antagonism within the nucleus accumbens or the amygdala produces differential effects on intravenous cocaine self-administration under fixed and progressive ratio schedules of reinforcement. Brain Res. **624:** 245–252.
10. DAHLSTRŠM, A. & K. FUXE. 1964. Evidence for the existence of monoamine-containing neurons in the central nervous system. I. Demonstration of monoamines in the cell bodies of brain stem neurons. Acta Physiol. Scand. Suppl. **232:** 1–55.
11. LOUGHLIN, S.E. & J.H. FALLON. 1983. Dopaminergic and non-dopaminergic projections to amygdala from substantia nigra and ventral tegmental area. Brain Res. **262:** 334–338.
12. FALLON, J.H. & P. CIOFI. 1992. Distribution of monoamines within the amygdala. *In* The Amygdala. J. P. Aggleton, Eds.: 97–114. Wiley-Liss. New York.
13. WRIGHT, C.I., A.V.J. BEIJER & H.J. GROENEWEGEN. 1996. Basal amygdaloid complex afferents to the rat nucleus accumbens are compartmentally organized. J. Neurosci. **16:** 1877–1893.
14. MCDONALD, A.J. 1991. Topographic organization of amygdaloid projections to the caudate putamen, nucleus accumbens, and related striatal-like areas of the rat brain. Neuroscience **44:** 15–33.
15. BROG, J.S., A. SALYAPONGSE, A.Y. DEUTCH & D.S. ZAHM. 1993. The patterns of afferent innervation of the core and shell of the "accumbens" part of the rat ventral striatum: immunohistochemical detection of retrogradely transported fluoro-gold. J. Comp. Neurol. **338:** 255–278.
16. CALLAHAN, P.M., S.K. BRYAN & K.A. CUNNINGHAM. 1995. Discriminative stimulus effects of cocaine: antagonism by dopamine D1 receptor blockade in the amygdala. Pharmacol. Biochem. Behav. **51:** 759–766.
17. CAINE, S.B. & G.F. KOOB. 1995. Effects of the dopamine D-1 antagonist SCH 23390 microinjected into the accumbens, amygdala or striatum on cocaine self-administration in the rat. Brain Res. **692:** 47–56.
18. WISE, R.A., P. NEWTON, K. LEEB, B. BURNETTE, D. POCOCK & J.B. JUSTICE JR. 1995. Fluctuations in nucleus accumbens dopamine concentrations during intravenous cocaine self-administration in rats. Psychopharmacology **120:** 10–20.

19. WALSH, S.L. & K.A. CUNNINGHAM. 1997. Serotonergic mechanisms invovled in the discriminative stimulus, reinforcing and subjective effects of cocaine. Psychopharmacology **130:** 41–58.
20. GROENEWEGEN, H.J., H.W. BERENDSE, G.E. MEREDITH, S.N. HABER, P. VOORN, J.G. WOLTERS & A.H.M. LOHMAN. 1991. Functional anatomy of the ventral, limbic system–innervated striatum. *In* The Mesolimbic Dopamine System: From Motivation to Action. O. Willner & J. Sheel-Kruger, Eds.: 19–59. John Wiley & Sons. Chichester and New York.
21. HURD, Y.L. 1996. Cocaine effects on dopamine and opioid peptide neural system: implications for human cocaine abuse. *In* Neurotoxicity and Neuropatholology Associated with Cocaine/Stimulants Abuse. M. D. Majewska, Eds.: 94–116. Supt. of Docs., U.S. Govt. Print. Off. Washington, D.C.
22. KREEK, M.J. 1992. Effects of opiates, opioid antagonists and cocaine on the endogenous opioid system: clinical and laboratory studies. NIDA Res. Monogr. Ser. **119:** 44–48.
23. DAUNAIS, J.B., D.C.S. ROBERTS & J.F. MCGINTY. 1993. Cocaine self-administration increases prodynorphin, but not c-fos, mRNA in rat striatum. NeuroReport **4:** 543–546.
24. HURD, Y.L., E. BROWN, J. FINLAY, H.C. FIBIGER & C. GERFEN. 1992. Cocaine self-administration differentially alters mRNA expression of striatal peptides. Mol. Brain Res. **13:** 165–170.
25. SVENSSON, P.S. & Y.L. HURD. 1998. Specific reductions of sriatal prodynorphin and D1 dopamine receptor messenger RNAs during cocaine abstinence. Mol. Brain Res. **56:** 162–168.
26. SPANGLER, R., E.M. UNTERWALD & M.J. KREEK. 1993. "Binge" cocaine administration induces a sustained increase of prodynorphin mRNA in rat caudate-putamen. Mol. Brain Res. **19:** 323–327.
27. SIVAM, S.P. 1989. Cocaine selectively increases striatonigral dynorphin levels by a dopaminergic mechanism. J. Pharmacol. Exp. Ther. **250:** 818–824.
28. HURD, Y.L. & M. HERKENHAM. 1993. Molecular alterations in the neostriatum of human cocaine addicts. Synapse **13:** 357–369.
29. DOW-EDWARDS, D.L. & Y.L. HURD. 1998. Perinatal cocaine decreased the expression of prodynorphin mRNA in nucleus accumbens shell in the adult rat. Mol. Brain Res. **62:** 82–85.
30. DAUNAIS, J.B. & J.F. MCGINTY. 1994. Acute and chronic cocaine administration differentially alters striatal opioid and nuclear transcription factor mRNAs. Synapse **18:** 35–45.
31. STEINER, H. & C. GERFEN. 1993. Cocaine-induced c-fos messenger RNA is inversely related to dynorphin expression in the striatum. J. Neurosci. **13:** 5066–5081.
32. PFEIFFER, A., V. BRANDT & A. HERZ. 1986. Psychotomimesis mediated by kappa opiate receptors. Science **233:** 774–776.
33. HURD, Y.L. 1996. Differential messenger RNA expression of prodynorphin and proenkephalin in the human brain. Neuroscience **72:** 767–783.
34. DOUGLASS, J., A.A. MCKINZIE & P. COUCEYRO. 1995. PCR differential display identifies a rat brain mRNA that is transcriptionally regulated by cocaine and amphetamine. J. Neurosci. **15:** 2471–2481.
35. COUCEYRO, P.R., E.O. KOYLU & M.J. KUHAR. 1997. Further studies on the anatomical distribution of CART by *in situ* hybridization. J. Chem. Neuroanat. **12:** 229–241.
36. KOYLU, E.O., P.R. COUCEYRO, P.D. LAMBERT & M.J. KUHAR. 1998. Cocaine- and amphetamine-regulated transcript peptide immunohistochemical localization in the rat brain. J. Comp. Neurol. **391:** 115–132.
37. SMITH, Y., E.O. KOYLU, P. COUCEYRO & M.J. KUHAR. 1997. Ultrastructural localization of CART (cocaine- and amphetamine-regulated transcript) peptides in the nucleus accumbens of monkeys. Synapse **27:** 90–94.
38. SVENSSON, P.S. & Y.L. HURD. Expression of peptide CART mRNA following acute "binge" cocaine in the male and female rat brain. Submitted.

D_3 Dopamine and Kappa Opioid Receptor Alterations in Human Brain of Cocaine-overdose Victims

DEBORAH C. MASH[a] AND JULIE K. STALEY

Departments of Neurology, and Molecular and Cellular Pharmacology, University of Miami School of Medicine, Miami, Florida 33136, USA

ABSTRACT: Cocaine is thought to be addictive because chronic use leads to molecular adaptations within the mesolimbic dopamine (DA) circuitry, which affects motivated behavior and emotion. Although the reinforcing effects of cocaine are mediated primarily by blockade of DA uptake, reciprocal signaling between DA and endogenous opioids has important implications for understanding cocaine dependence. We have used *in vitro* autoradiography and ligand binding to map D_3 DA and kappa opioid receptors in the human brains of cocaine-overdose victims. The number of D_3 binding sites was increased one- to threefold over the nucleus accumbens and ventromedial sectors of the caudate and putamen from cocaine-overdose victims, as compared to age-matched and drug-free control subjects. D_3 receptor/cyclophilin mRNA ratios in the nucleus accumbens were increased sixfold in cocaine-overdose victims over control values, suggesting that cocaine exposure also affects the expression of D_3 receptor mRNA. The number of kappa opioid receptors in the nucleus accumbens and other corticolimbic areas from cocaine fatalities was increased twofold as compared to control values. Cocaine-overdose victims exhibiting preterminal excited delirium had a selective upregulation of kappa receptors measured also in the amygdala. Understanding the complex regulatory profiles of DA and opioid synaptic markers that occur with chronic misuse of cocaine may suggest multitarget strategies for treating cocaine dependence.

INTRODUCTION

Cocaine dependence is a complex disorder that results from a dysregulation of a number of distinct yet interacting neurochemical systems.[1] Cocaine augments dopamine (DA) neurotransmission by interacting with the DA transporter and inhibiting the clearance of extracellular DA.[2–4] Increased intrasynaptic DA acts on pre- and postsynaptic DA receptors to initiate a sequence of neurochemical events that mediate cocaine's reinforcing effects. Which of the five cloned dopamine receptor subtypes mediates the reinforcing effects of cocaine remains unclear. However, rodent cocaine self-administration studies by Caine and Koob have suggested that the D_3 receptor may be the primary mediator of the reinforcing effects of cocaine.[5,6] D_3 receptor mRNA and protein are expressed almost exclusively in limbic brain re-

---

[a]Address correspondence to Deborah C. Mash, Ph.D., Department of Neurology (D4-5), University of Miami School of Medicine, P.O. Box 016960, Miami, Florida 33101. Voice: 305-243-5888; fax: 305-243-4678; dmash@mednet.med.miami.edu

gions, including the islands of Calleja, nucleus accumbens, and mammillary nuclei in both the rat and human brain.[7-11] Putative D_3-selective agonists enhance or substitute for the effects of cocaine.[6,12] Monkeys trained to self-administer cocaine will self-administer D_3 receptor-selective agonists, whereas cocaine-naive monkeys do not.[13] This observation suggests that continued exposure to cocaine may change the nature of the rewarding experience, perhaps by regulating the number or function of a particular dopamine receptor subtype.

Mesolimbic DA neurotransmission is modulated by endogenous opioids that act at mu and kappa opioid receptors to regulate DA release in striatal reward centers.[14-16] Recent studies in animals have provided evidence for a role of the kappa opioidergic system in the behavioral effects of cocaine.[17] Kappa agonists inhibit cocaine self-administration,[18,19] cocaine-induced place preference,[20,21] and the development of sensitization to the behavioral effects of cocaine.[22,23] The mixed partial mu-agonist/kappa-antagonist buprenorphine reduces cocaine self-administration by rhesus monkeys[24] and prevents the reinstatement of cocaine-reinforced responding in rats.[25] Neuroadaptive changes in the kappa opioidergic system may underlie, in part, the motivational state that triggers binge cocaine abuse.

These observations demonstrate that cocaine affects a number of different neurochemical substrates in the brain and suggest that chronic exposure may lead to complex neuroadaptations within discrete brain loci. Continued exposure to high doses of cocaine may change the nature of the CNS-stimulant experience, leading to psychiatric disorders, as well as toxic physiological reactions. Mortality data have indicated that deaths involving psychostimulant drugs stem not only from overdose, but also from drug-induced mental states that may lead to serious injuries. The arrival of inexpensive smokable "crack" cocaine has radically changed the nature of the epidemic and revealed the serious addictive potential of cocaine. Cocaine, particularly smoked crack cocaine, is known to be one of the most widely abused psychoactive substances. We have used ligand binding and autoradiography to map and quantify the distribution of D_3 DA and $kappa_2$ opioid receptors in the human brain postmortem from cocaine overdose victims who had histories of chronic cocaine abuse. The regulation of these DA and kappa opioid receptor sites was examined also in cocaine-overdose victims, who experienced paranoia and marked agitation prior to death.

MATERIAL AND METHODS

Neuropathological Tissue Specimens

Postmortem neuropathological specimens were obtained during routine autopsy from age-matched and drug-free control subjects. Medicolegal investigations of the deaths were conducted by forensic pathologists. The circumstances of death and toxicology data were reviewed carefully before classifying a death as a cocaine overdose (CO) with or without preterminal excited delirium (ED). Fatal ED victims exhibited an acute onset of bizarre and violent behavior, which was characterized by one or more of the following: aggression, combativeness, hyperactivity, extreme paranoia, demonstration of unexpected strength, or incoherent shouting.[26,27] The syndrome of fatal ED is defined as accidental cocaine toxicity in subjects who exhibited bizarre and violent behavior (as described above) followed by sudden death.[28] Cases were assigned to the ED subgroup if at least two of the behavioral signs and hyperthermia were present prior to death. All cases were evaluated for common drugs of abuse and alcohol, and positive urine screens were confirmed by quantitative analysis of blood. Polydrug abusers identified from the urine toxicology screens were excluded from the study. Blood cocaine was quantified using gas-liquid chromatography with a nitrogen detector. Frozen brain regions were sampled for quantitation of cocaine and benzoylecgonine using gas chromatography/mass spectroscopy techniques.[29] Drug-free and age-matched control subjects were selected from accidental deaths with no cocaine or metabolites detected in toxicology screens of blood or brain tissue.

In Vitro *Ligand Binding and Autoradiography*

Ligand binding and autoradiographic conditions for D_3 receptors have been described previously.[30] For D_3 receptor autoradiography, half-hemisphere slide-mounted tissue sections were incubated with 1 nM [^{3}H]-(+)-7-OH-DPAT in the presence of 300 µM GTP for 2 hours at 25°C. Nonspecific binding was determined in the presence of 10 µM (+) butaclamol. At the end of the incubation, brain tissue sections were washed in two changes of ice-cold assay buffer followed by a quick rinse in ice-cold distilled water to dissociate nonspecifically bound ligand. Tissue sections were apposed with tritium standards to Hyperfilm for 7–8 weeks at 4°C. For [^{125}I]IOXY autoradiography, tissue sections were equilibrated in 10 mM potassium phosphate, pH 7.4, at 4°C prior to treating tissue sections with the site-directed acylating agents, BIT (1 µM) and FIT (1 µM), in 50 mM potassium phosphate, pH 7.4, 100 mM NaCl, to occlude binding to the mu and delta receptors, respectively.[31] Slide-mounted brain tissue sections were incubated with [^{125}I]IOXY (30 pM) in assay buffer containing protease inhibitors at 4°C for 2–3 hours. Nonspecific binding was determined in the presence of 10 µM naloxone. Autoradiograms were prepared by apposing the slide-mounted tissue sections along with coplaced iodine standards to Hyperfilm for 40–48 hours at −80°C.

Measuring Levels of D_3 and Cyclophilin mRNA

Dissected brain regions taken from cryopreserved neuropathological specimens were sampled for analysis of the levels of D_3 and cyclophilin mRNA, using the method of Segal *et al.*[32] Briefly, total RNA (5 µg) prepared by guanadinium-phenol extraction was reverse transcribed (Superscript II RT; GIBCO/BRL) with a $(dT)_{15}$ primer and amplified in a 100 µL polymerase chain reaction (94°C for 30 s, 60°C for 1 min, 72°C for 2 min) with 2.5 U recombinant *Taq* polymerase (BRL) and specific primers for human cyclophilin and D_3 receptor cDNAs. Primers were based on nucleotides 759–783 and 1197–1178 (complementary strand) of human D_3 receptor cDNA sequences. The primer pair directs amplification of putative transmembrane-spanning domains 6 and 7, which includes the third cytoplasmic loop implicated in G-protein coupling. For measurement of cyclophilin mRNA, the primer pair directs amplification of nucleotides 280 to 445 of the human cyclophilin cDNA sequence. cDNAs were amplified for 25 and 30 cycles for cyclophilin and D_3 receptor, respectively, in the presence of [^{32}P]dCTP.

Data Analysis

The competition binding data were analyzed using DRUG, LIGAND for estimates of Ki values. The best fit to a one- or two-site model was based on the partial F-test. For quantitative analysis of receptor autoradiograms, films were scanned using a Howtek Scanmaster 3 at 400 dots per inch using a transparency illuminator. The resulting TIFF (tagged image file format for RGB color) files were converted to grey scale format in specific activity units using the IMAGE (version 1.44; NIH Shareware) and BRAIN (version 1.6; Drexel University) programs. After background subtraction, two-dimensional grey scale maps were created to allow radioactivity levels in fmol/mg to be superimposed on the sections for region-of-interest quantitative analysis. PCR products in denaturing 5% polyacrylamide gels were imaged by chemiluminescent detection on a Molecular Dynamics phosphorimager. The intensity of the signal (pixels) was determined using the Molecular Dynamics IMAGEQUANT (software version 3.0). Statistical significance was determined using the Dunnet's t-test.

RESULTS

Tracking the Epidemic of Cocaine Overdose Deaths in Dade County, Florida

The jurisdiction of the Metropolitan Dade County Medical Examiner's Department (MDCMED) encompasses all of Dade County and includes the city of Miami and other municipalities. The MDCMED routinely performs medicolegal investigations of all deaths from causes other than natural ones. Forensic pathologists identify the victim, evaluate the scene environment and circumstances of death, and autopsy the victim in order to determine the cause and manner of death. The annual incidence of CO deaths in Dade County rose from 8 in 1978 to 50 in 1995 (FIG. 1). The results demonstrate the rise in cases of cocaine lethality, with the increased purity of the street drug and the emergence of crack cocaine abuse in 1986. Fatal ED is a cocaine reaction consisting of an acute onset of a clouded sensorium accompanied by ex-

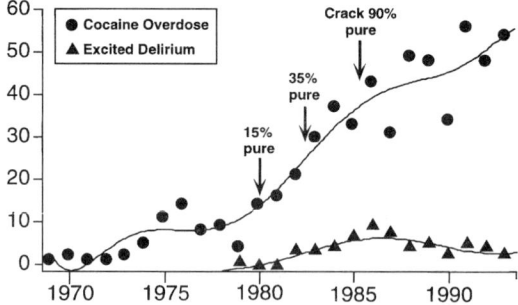

FIGURE 1. Tracking the epidemic of cocaine fatalities in Miami-Dade County, Florida. Closed circles illustrate the annual number of cocaine overdose deaths. Closed triangles illustrate the incidence of excited delirium cases that came to post-mortem evaluation. The increasing street purity of cocaine in Dade County, Florida is noted.

treme hyperactivity or bizarre behavior.[27,28] The annual incidence of fatal ED has a peak that occurs with the rise in crack cocaine abuse (FIG. 1). Compared to a control group (CO deaths *without* evidence of a preterminal ED), the cases of cocaine ED were more likely to be male, to be black, to die in police custody, and to survive longer than one hour after the onset of the overdose symptoms.[29] Controlling for the survival time, the ED cases were more likely to be hyperthermic, to have fewer seizures, and to have a lower blood cocaine concentration, consistent with the extended survival times.[29] Guided by these epidemiologic and toxicologic analyses, a cohort of well-characterized postmortem neuropathological specimens was available for the study of the neurochemical consequences of cocaine abuse in the human brain.

Cocaine Regulates D_3 Receptor Numbers and mRNA in Limbic Sectors of the Striatum

Pharmacological studies with [^{3}H]-(+)-7-OH-DPAT demonstrate that it has 100-fold higher affinity for binding to the cloned D_3 receptor as compared to the cloned D_2 receptor expressed in transfected cell lines. However, binding studies conducted in the brain in regions enriched in the native D_2 receptors have indicated that [^{3}H]-(+)-7-OH-DPAT demonstrates selectivity for the D_3 subtype only when D_2 receptors are uncoupled from their G proteins.[33] This selectivity profile ($D_3 > D_2$) is not seen in the absence of guanine nucleotides, because the high-affinity G-protein coupled state of the D_2 receptor is left shifted, and the binding affinity overlaps with that of the D_3 receptor. Because guanine nucleotides have a minimal effect on agonist binding to the D_3 receptor (2-fold right shift), but markedly decreased agonist binding to the D_2 receptor (100-fold right shift), it is possible to achieve selective labeling of

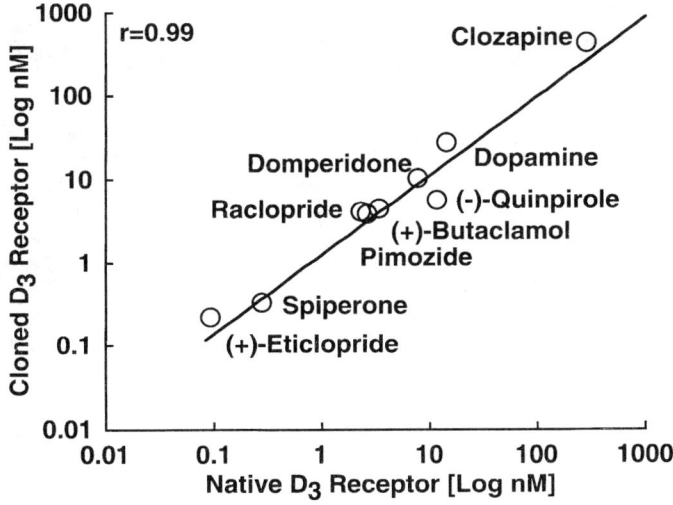

FIGURE 2. Pharmacological profile of [^{3}H]-(+)-7-OH-DPAT binding to cloned and native D_3 receptors. The rank order of inhibition for a series of dopaminergic drugs observed in the human nucleus accumbens correlated significantly with Ki values reported previously for the cloned D_3 receptor.[30]

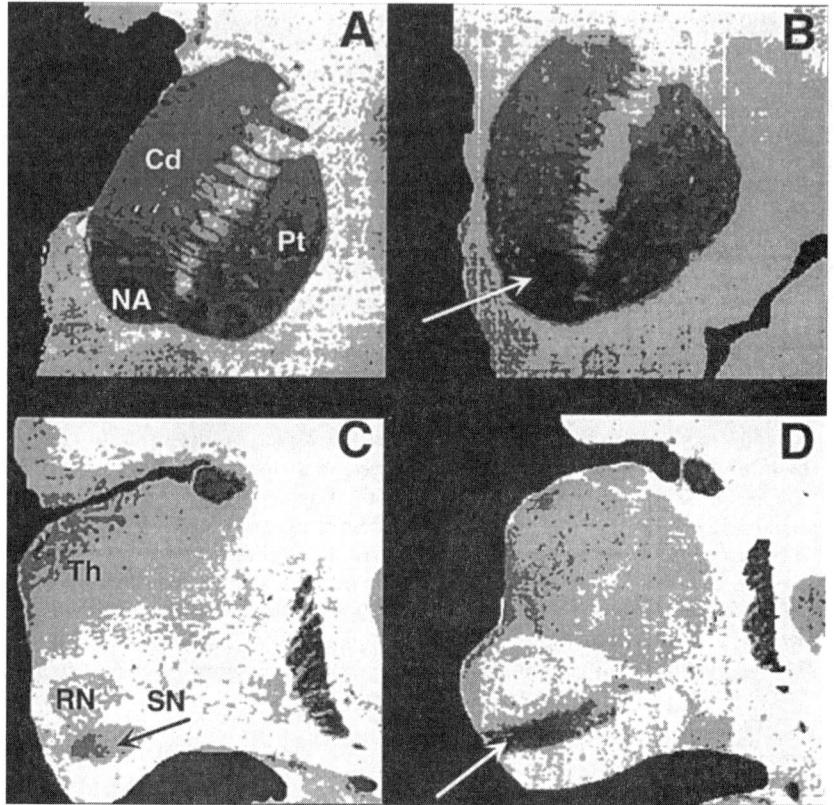

FIGURE 3. Greyscale maps of [^{3}H]-(+)-7-OH-DPAT binding to the D_3 receptor in the anterior striatum of **(A)** a representative drug-free control subject and **(B)** a representative CO victim. Note the significant increase in the density of the D_3 receptors throughout the nucleus accumbens and ventral sectors of the striatum. Cd, caudate; NA, nucleus accubmens; Pt, putamen; RN, red nucleus; Th, thalamus; SN, substantia nigra.

the D_3 receptor in the presence of GTP.[30,34] The specificity of [^{3}H]-(+)-7-OH-DPAT binding to the D_3 receptor in the human nucleus accumbens is demonstrated by the results shown in FIGURE 2. The putative D_3 agonists, (+)-7-OH-DPAT and PD128907, demonstrated the highest potencies for inhibition of [^{3}H]-(+)-7-OH-DPAT binding. The rank order of potency observed for this series of dopaminergic drugs was comparable to those previously reported for the cloned D_3 receptor (FIG. 2).

Quantitative *in vitro* autoradiography was used with D_3-selective assay conditions to map and quantify D_3 receptor densities in human CO victims. The results demonstrate that the binding of [^{3}H]-(+)-7-OH-DPAT was elevated approximately 2-fold in the nucleus accumbens of the CO victims as compared to drug-free and age-matched control subjects (FIGS. 3 and 4A). The intensity of [^{3}H]-(+)-7-OH-DPAT la-

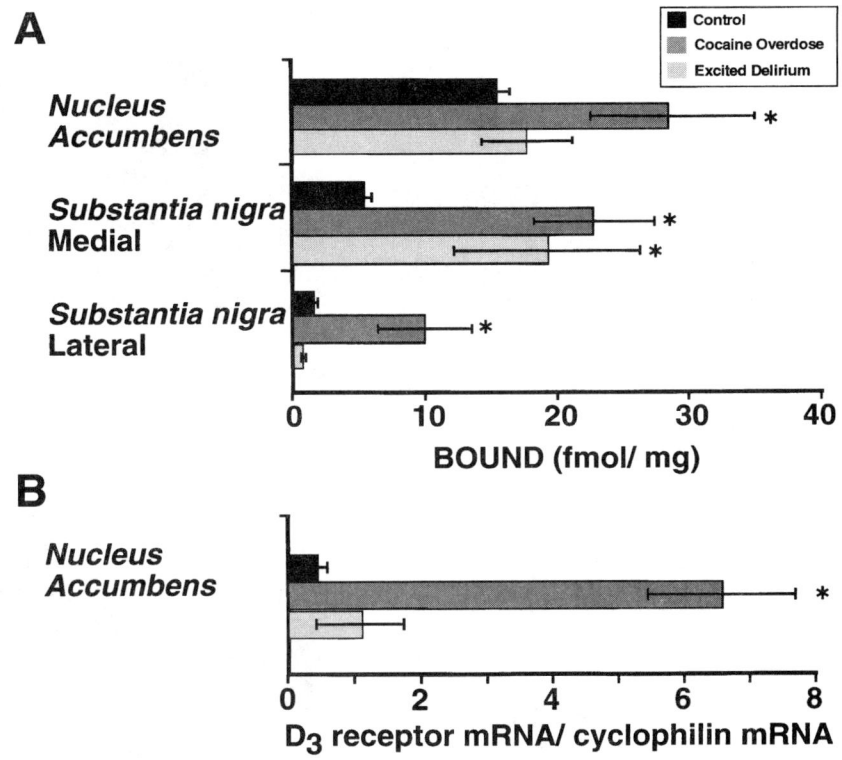

FIGURE 4. A: Summary of the region-of-interest densitometric measurements of [^{3}H]-(+)-7-OH-DPAT binding in the nucleus accumbens and over the cell body fields from control subjects ($n = 9$), CO deaths ($n = 6$), and excited delirium (ED) victims ($n = 6$). **B:** D_3 receptor mRNA/cyclophilin mRNA group ratios (mean + SE). Significant differences from control values, *$p < 0.05$.[30,32]

beling was increased also in the lateral and medial divisions of the substantia nigra in the CO victims. Quantitative densitometric measurements of [^{3}H]-(+)-7-OH-DPAT binding revealed significant elevations in the CO victims, as compared to the drug-free and age-matched control subjects (FIG. 4A; Dunnets t-test, $p < 0.05$). Binding of [^{3}H]-(+)-7-OH-DPAT was not elevated significantly in the nucleus accumbens of the ED subgroup. However, a 2- to 3-fold elevation in D_3 receptor densities was measured over the cell body fields of the medial division of the substantia nigra.

The levels of D_3 receptor mRNA were determined in parallel with ligand-binding assays in the nucleus accumbens, using the reverse transcriptase-polymerase chain reaction technique. D_3 receptor/cyclophilin mRNA ratios in the nucleus accumbens were increased sixfold in CO victims, as compared to age-matched and drug-free control subjects (FIG. 4B). By contrast, the ratios determined for the ED group were not significantly changed from control values (FIG. 4B).

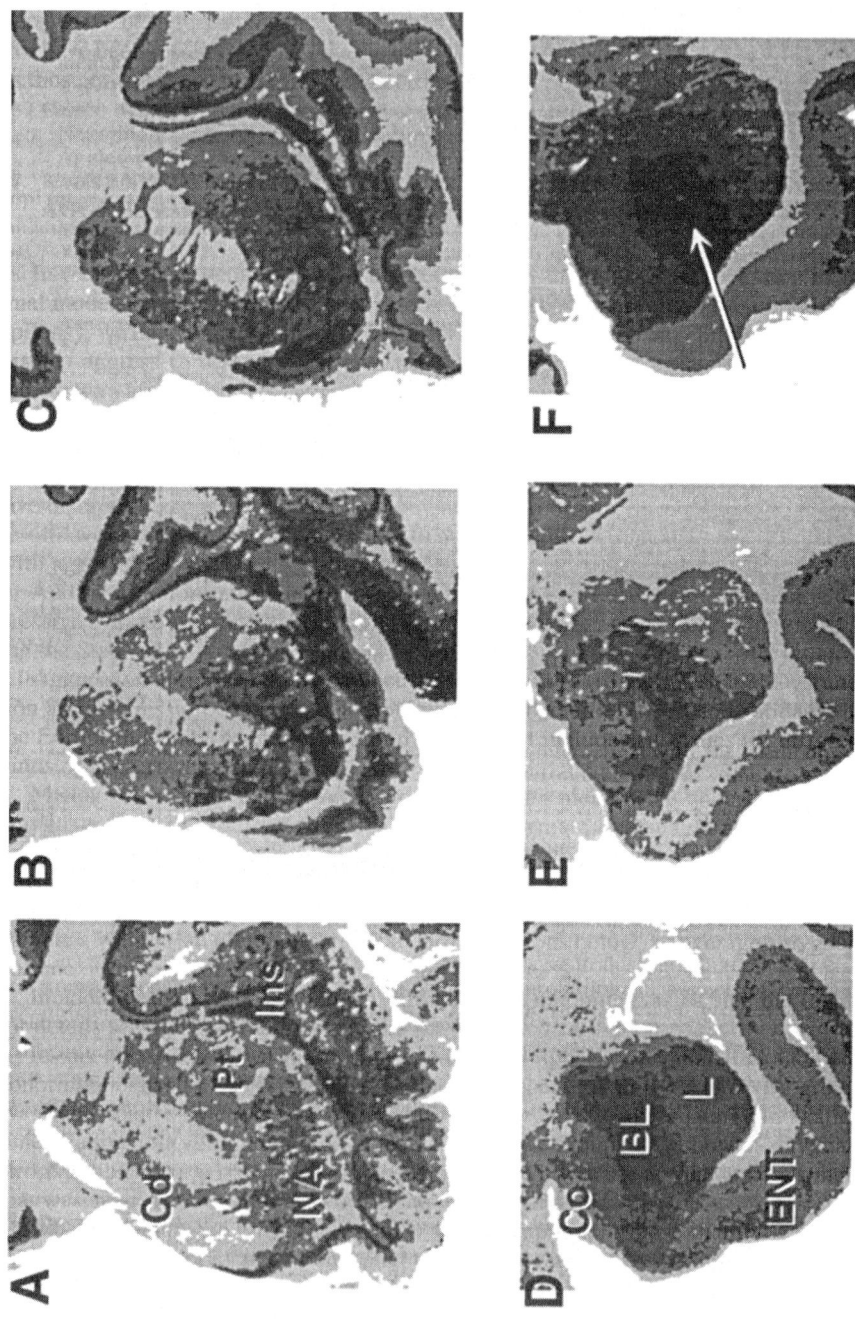

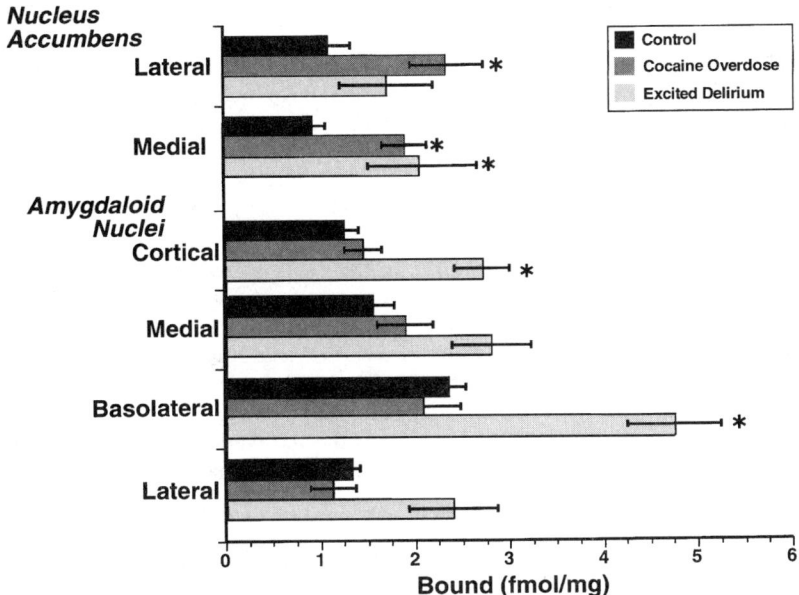

FIGURE 6. Quantitative region-of-interest measurements from the nucleus accumbens and amygdaloid nuclei illustrate the densities of [^{125}I]IOXY binding in the drug-free control subjects ($n = 9$), and CO ($n = 6$) and ED victims ($n = 8$). Dunnet's t-test, *$p < 0.05$.

Regulatory Effects of Cocaine on Kappa Receptors

Quantitative region-of-interest densitometric measurements of [^{125}I]IOXY binding were made to assess the regulatory effects of cocaine on the kappa$_2$ receptor in the human brain. Densitometric measurements of [^{125}I]IOXY binding demonstrated a twofold elevation ($p < 0.05$) in the anterior and ventral sectors of the caudate and putamen and in the nucleus accumbens of the CO and ED victims, as compared to drug-free and age-matched control subjects (FIGS. 5 and 6). The elevation of striatal labeling was confined to the more anterior and ventral sectors of the human striatum. Rosenthal analysis of IOXY-binding data indicated that there was no change in the affinity for [^{125}I]IOXY binding to the high-affinity site assayed in the striatum of the CO and ED victims, as compared to drug-free and age-matched control subjects (data not shown). This observation confirmed that the elevated densities of [^{125}I]IOXY

FIGURE 5. Density maps of [^{125}I]IOXY labeling of kappa$_2$ receptors in the anterior striatum of representative **(A)** drug-free control, **(B)** CO, and **(C)** ED victims. There was a marked increase in the density of the kappa$_2$ receptors in the ventral sectors of the anterior striatum in the CO and ED victims as compared to the drug-free and age-matched control subjects. The bottom panels illustrate [^{125}I]IOXY binding in the amygdala from representative **(D)** control, **(E)** CO, and **(F)** ED victims. BL, basolateral nucleus of the amygdala; Co, cortical nucleus of the amygdala; Cd, caudate nucleus; Ins, insular cortex; L, lateral nucleus of the amygdala; NA, nucleus accumbens; Pt, putamen.

binding in the striatal-reward centers of the CO victims reflected a true increase in binding-site densities and not an altered affinity of receptor for the radioligand. [^{125}I]IOXY binding sites were significantly increased in the cortical and basolateral nuclei of the amygdala in the ED victims ($p < 0.001$), but not in the CO victims, as compared to drug-free and age-matched control subjects.

DISCUSSION

We have investigated the effects of cocaine exposure on the numbers of DA D_3 and kappa opioid receptors within limbic brain regions that are implicated in mediating cocaine reinforcement. The findings suggest that cocaine abuse leads to an adaptive elevation in striatal D_3 receptor densities and mRNA levels in the human brain in response to elevated synaptic DA levels. The upregulation of kappa opioid receptors in the nucleus accumbens and other limbic brain regions from cocaine fatalities suggests that they may play a role in the motivational incentive associated with episodes of binge cocaine use and in the dysphoria that follows abrupt cocaine withdrawal.

Compensatory Changes in DA D_3 Receptors with Chronic Cocaine Abuse

Animal studies have not yet determined an unambiguous role for the D_3 receptor in mediating cocaine's rewarding effects, because most of the purported D_3-selective agonists can produce effects at multiple D_2-like receptors *in vivo*.[35] The recently cloned D_3 receptor is related to the D_2 dopamine receptor sharing considerable sequence homology.[36] Pharmacological studies with [^{3}H]-(+)-7-OH-DPAT demonstrate that it has 100-fold higher affinity for binding to the cloned D_3 receptor, as compared to the cloned D_2 receptor expressed in transfected cell lines.[30] Whereas these observations suggested that 7-OH DPAT is a selective D_3 agonist, binding studies conducted in brain regions enriched in the native D_2 and D_3 receptors have demonstrated overlapping ligand-binding affinities at these receptor subtypes, unless the D_2 receptors are uncoupled from their G proteins and stabilized in a confirmation that has low affinity for agonists.[30]

The D_3 receptor has a neuroanatomical distribution in the human brain, which is distinct from the D_2 receptor, with high densities visualized over the nucleus accumbens and the limbic sectors of the caudate and putamen. This neuroanatomical distribution is relevant, inasmuch as the nucleus accumbens is known to be an anatomical substrate for cocaine's reinforcing effects.[37] Ligand-binding assays conducted in nucleus accumbens membranes demonstrated an overall rank order of inhibition of [^{3}H]-(+)-7-OH-DPAT binding that correlated significantly with its affinity values reported previously for the cloned D_3 receptor. Cocaine-exposure elevated D_3 receptor densities over limbic sectors of the striatum in cases of accidental CO. Thus, cocaine abuse leads to a neuroadaptive elevation in D_3 receptor density in response to increased levels of synaptic DA. This finding provides additional support for a role of the D_3 receptor in the modulation of addictive behaviors, including cocaine dependence.

By contrast, the density for [^{3}H]-(+)-7-OH-DPAT binding to the nucleus accumbens in cocaine ED victims was not significantly different from control values. The

ED victims are marked by intense paranoia, increased body strength, bizarre and violent behavior, and hyperthermia, similar to neuroleptic malignant syndrome.[27,28] Whereas a marked elevation in D_3-receptor density was observed in all CO victims, the number of binding sites was not increased in every fatal ED subject. The reason for heterogeneity within this subgroup of cocaine fatalities is not fully understood, although it may be related to psychiatric comborbidity (trait marker) or a recent pattern of "binge" cocaine use (state marker). Alternatively, differences in the molecular processing of D_3 receptors due to defects in alternatively spliced transcripts might explain the lack of an increase in the D_3-binding sites in the certain ED victims. It is interesting to point out that a different mRNA species has been found in cerebral cortices of chronic schizophrenic patients,[38] suggesting the possibility that similar alterations in D_3-receptor expression may be involved in the psychopathology of the ED syndrome.

The neuroadaptive increase in human D_3 receptor densities by cocaine exposure links this DA receptor subtype to the reinforcing effects of cocaine and its high abuse potential. Medication development for cocaine addiction has focused primarily on drugs that target DAergic synapses. Traditional DA agonists and antagonists have failed to demonstrate significant therapeutic efficacy in clinical trials. Although DA agonists reduce craving, they may be reinforcing and have their own abuse liability. Although DA antagonists are known to attenuate cocaine reinforcement, compliance is hindered by dysphoria and possible extrapyramidal side effects that develop with chronic treatment regimens. Thus, D_3-selective drugs may offer a better lead for the development of pharmacologic interventions for breaking the intractable cycle of cocaine dependence.

Cocaine-induced Adaptations in the Kappa Opioidergic System

Previous studies of the effects of cocaine on kappa receptors in rodent models have used radioligands that do not discriminate among the putative kappa receptor subtypes. For example, binge cocaine administration[39] and chronic continuous exposure[40] in rats caused elevations in [^{3}H]bremazocine and [^{3}H]naloxone binding in the nucleus accumbens. Because these radioligands label both kappa$_1$ and kappa$_2$ receptors, the observed elevations may reflect regulatory increases in either the kappa$_1$ or kappa$_2$ receptor subtype. Hurd and Herkenham previously demonstrated elevated numbers of kappa binding sites in brains from human cocaine abusers.[41] However, in contrast to the present findings, which demonstrated elevated IOXY binding-site densities that were restricted to the ventromedial (limbic) sectors of the striatum, the increased number of kappa receptors labeled with [^{125}I]Tyr^1-D-Pro^{10}-dynorphin A was elevated within the dorsolateral (motor) sectors of the striatum. Kappa receptors are localized on both pre- and postsynaptic elements in the striatum,[42,43] with the ventral striatal regions having higher levels of postsynaptic kappa receptors.[44] One possible explanation for the regional heterogeneity seen in the previous results of Hurd and Herkenham[41] and those of the present study is that the agonist [^{125}I]Tyr^1-D-Pro^{10}-dynorphin A may preferentially label presynaptic sites, whereas the antagonist [^{125}I]IOXY may be a more selective marker of the postsynaptic kappa receptor subtype.

Immunoreactive dynorphin peptides[45–47] and prodynorphin mRNA are elevated by chronic cocaine exposure.[41,47] Direct or indirect DA agonists given chronically to rats also increase prodynorphin mRNA and dynorphin peptides in the striatum.[46,47] Cocaine-induced increases in dynorphin peptides are prevented by the administration of DA receptor antagonists.[45,46] In keeping with this finding, the D_1 receptor knockout mouse had significantly decreased striatal levels of dynorphin, indicating that stimulation of the D_1 receptor by DA affects the level of dynorphin expression.[48] Previous studies have indicated that dynorphin acts in the striatum to blunt the response of striatonigral neurons to dopamine input.[49] Taken together, these observations suggest that a marked upregulation in kappa opioidergic tone occurs as a compensatory response to chronic cocaine exposure.

Role of Kappa Opioidergic System in Cocaine Dependence

Although kappa agonists do not generalize to the cocaine cue in drug discrimination paradigms,[50,51] they suppress the stimulus effects of cocaine in monkeys.[52] Thus, it is unlikely that kappa receptors play a direct role in mediating the reinforcing or euphoric effects of cocaine. Shippenberg and colleagues have suggested that the conditioned-aversive effects related to the hyperactivity of kappa opioidergic neurons in the ventral striatum may underlie the motivational incentive to use cocaine.[17] Cocaine dependence is associated with a withdrawal syndrome characterized by dysphoria, anxiety, depression, and intense craving that begins within thirty minutes after the end of a binge episode and may last for one to ten weeks. Interestingly, in humans the subjective effects of kappa agonists are known to mimic, in part, certain symptoms of cocaine withdrawal. Administration of the nonselective kappa agonists, ketocyclazocine and cyclazocine, to humans caused unpleasant mood and feeling states, distortion of sensory experiences, paranoia, self-reported deficiencies in cognition, and feelings of detachment that may be reversed by administration of naloxone.[53,54] The similarity in the subjective effects of kappa agonists to the symptoms of cocaine withdrawal suggest that increased activity of the kappa opioidergic system may contribute to the dysphoric mood associated with abrupt withdrawal from cocaine.

Cocaine abuse is associated with neuropsychiatric disorders, including acute psychotic episodes, paranoid states, and intoxication delirium. The regionally selective elevation in $kappa_2$ receptor densities in the amygdala may play a role in the neuropsychiatric sequelae of the fatal ED syndrome. The amygdaloid complex has long been seen to have a role in the integration and control of emotional and autonomic behaviors.[55] We have observed an elevation of $kappa_2$ receptors within certain amygdaloid nuclei in the ED cases, as compared to control subjects. By contrast, the regional pattern and local densities of $kappa_2$ receptors were unchanged in the amygdala in accidental CO deaths. The amygdala is the essential component for the association of the appropriate emotional response with extrapersonal objects and aggressive encounters.[56] For example, stimulation of the amygdala in patients with temporal lobe epilepsy elicits discharges from those structures simultaneously with hallucinations or changes in affective behavior.[57] Stereotactic lesions of the amygdala have been done to treat symptoms associated with a hyperresponsive-aggressive syndrome, which includes abnormal behavioral manifestations of aggression (compulsive, combative), vocal expression (screaming, anger), hyperkinesia (running, hyperactive, wild), and emotional status (agitated, hostile). These abnormal behavioral manifestations are reminiscent of the bizarre behaviors reported for cocaine ED. Thus, the selective upregulated kappa opioid numbers within the amygdala may link the dysregulation of the kappa opioidergic system to the resultant clinical display of aberrant complex emotional behaviors in ED victims.

In summary, studies conducted in postmortem human brain from cocaine fatalities demonstrate that cocaine exposure leads to neuroadaptive increases in DA D_3 and kappa$_2$ receptor densities in specific brain loci. Because self-administration of the DA D_3 agonist 7-OH-DPAT in rhesus monkeys is modified by prior cocaine exposure,[13] it is possible that the neuroadaptive increase in human D_3 receptor densities in the nucleus accumbens links the stimulation of this DA receptor subtype to the intractable pattern of chronic cocaine abuse. The downstream dysregulation of kappa$_2$ opioid receptors may underlie, in part, the dysphoric mood and psychological distress associated with the cocaine withdrawal syndrome. Understanding the complex regulatory profiles of subtypes of DA and opioid receptors that occur with chronic misuse of cocaine may suggest combination therapy or multitarget strategy for treating cocaine dependence.

REFERENCES

1. NESTLER, E.J., B.T. HOPE & K.L. WIDNELL. 1993. Drug addiction: a model for the molecular basis of neural plasticity. Neuron **11:** 995–1006.
2. RITZ, M.C., S.R. LAMB, S.R. GOLDBERG & M.J. KUHAR. 1987. Cocaine receptors on dopamine transporters are related to self-administration of cocaine. Science **237:** 1219–1223.
3. REITH, M.E.A., H.K. KRAMER, H. SERSHEN & A. LAJTHA. 1989. Cocaine competitively inhibits catecholamine uptake into brain synaptic vesicles. Res. Commun. Substances Abuse **10:** 205–208.
4. KUHAR, M.J., M.C. RITZ & J.W. BOJA. 1991. The dopamine hypothesis of the reinforcing properties of cocaine. Trends Neurosci. **14:** 299–302.
5. CAINE, S.B. & G.F. KOOB. 1993. Modulation of cocaine self-administration in the rat through D_3 dopamine receptors. Science **260:** 1814–1815.
6. CAINE, S.B. & G.F. KOOB. 1995. Pretreatment with the dopamine agonist 7-OH-DPAT shifts the cocaine self-administration dose-effect function to the left under different schedules in the rat. Behav. Pharmacol. **6:** 333–347.
7. BOUTHENET, M.L., E. SOUIL, M.P. MARTRES, P. SOKOLOFF, B. GIROS & J.C. SCHWARTZ. 1991. Localization of dopamine D3 receptor mRNA in the rat brain using *in situ* hybridization histochemistry: comparison with dopamine D2 receptor mRNA, Brain Res. **564:** 203–219.
8. MENGOD, G., M.T. VILLARO, G.B. LANDWEHRMEYER *et al.* 1992. Visualization of dopamine D1, D2, and D3 receptor mRNAs in human and rat brain, Neurochem. Int. Suppl. **20:** 33S–43S.
9. LEVESQUE, D., J. DIAZ, C. PILON, M.-P. MARTRES, B. GIROS, E. SOUIL, D. SCHOTT, J.L. MORGAT, J.-C. SCHWARTZ & P. SOKOLOFF. 1992. Identification, characterization and localization of the dopamine D3 receptor in rat brain using 7-[^{3}H]hydroxy-*N*,*N*-di-*n*-propyl-2-aminotetralin. Proc. Natl. Acad. Sci. USA **89:** 8155–8159.
10. LANDWEHRMEYER, B., G. MENGOD & J.M. PALACIOS. 1993b. Dopamine D3 receptor mRNA and binding sites in human brain. Mol. Brain Res. **18:** 187–192.
11. MURRAY, A.M., H.L. RYOO, E. GUREVICH & J.N. JOYCE. 1994. Localization of dopamine D3 receptors to mesolimbic and D2 receptors to mesostriatal regions of human forebrain. Proc. Natl. Acad. Sci. USA **91:** 11271–11275.
12. ROBERTS, D.C.S. & R. RANALDI. 1995. Effect of dopaminergic drugs on cocaine reinforcement. Clin. Neuropharmacol. **18:** S84–S95.

13. NADER, M.A. & R.H. MACH. 1996. Self-administration of the dopamine D3 agonist 7-OH-DPAT in rhesus monkeys is modified by prior cocaine exposure. Psychopharmacology. In press.
14. DICHIARA, G. & A. IMPERATO. 1988. Opposite effects of mu and kappa opiate agonists on dopamine release in the nucleus accumbens and in the dorsal caudate of freely moving rats. J. Pharmacol. Exp. Ther. **244:** 1067–1080.
15. SPANAGEL, R., A. HERZ & T. SHIPPENBERG. 1990. The effects of opioid peptides on dopamine release in the nucleus accumbens: an *in vivo* microdialysis study. J Neurochem. **55:** 1734–1740.
16. SPANAGEL, R., A. HERZ & T.S. SHIPPENBERG. 1992. Opposing tonically active endogenous opioid systems modulate the mesolimbic dopaminergic pathway. Proc. Natl. Acad. Sci. USA **89:** 2046–2050.
17. SHIPPENBERG, T.S., A. LEFEVOUR & C. HEIDBREDER. 1996. Kappa opioid receptor agonists prevent sensitization to the conditioned rewarding effects of cocaine. J. Pharmacol. Exp. Ther. **276:** 545–554.
18. SHIPPENBERG, T.S., A. HERZ, R. SPANAGEL, R. BALS-KUBIK & C. STEIN. 1992. Conditioning of opioid reinforcement: neuroanatomical and neurochemical substrates. Ann. N.Y. Acad. Sci. **654:** 347–356.
19. GLICK, S.D., I.M. MAISONNEUVE, J. RAUCCI & S. ARCHER. 1995. Kappa opioid inhibition of morphine and cocaine self-administration in rats. Brain Res. **681:**147–152.
20. SUZUKI, T., Y. SHIOZAKI, Y. MASUKAWA, M. MISAWA & H. NAGASE. 1992. The role of mu- and kappa-opioid receptors in cocaine-induced conditioned place preference. Jpn. J. Pharmacol. **58:** 435–442.
21. HEIDBREDER, C.A., S.R. GOLDBERG & T.S. SHIPPENBERG. 1993. The kappa-opioid receptor agonist U-69593 attenuates cocaine-induced behavioral sensitization in the rat. Brain Res. **616:** 335–338.
22. HEIDBREDER, C.A., D. BABOVIC-VUKSANOVIC, M. SHOAIB & T.S. SHIPPENBERG. 1995. Development of behavioral sensitization to cocaine: Influence of kappa opioid receptor agonists. J. Pharmacol. Exp. Ther. **275:** 150–163.
23. SHIPPENBERG, T.S. & C.H. HEIDBREDER. 1994. Kappa opioid receptor agonists prevent sensitization to the rewarding effects of cocaine. NIDA Res. Monograph **153:** 456.
24. MELLO, N.K., J.B. KAMIEN, S.E. LUKAS, J.H. MENDELSON, DRIEZE J.M. & J.W. SHOLAR. 1993. Effects of intermittent buprenorphine administration on cocaine self-administration by rhesus monkeys. J. Pharmacol. Exp. Ther. **264:** 530–541.
25. COMER, S.D., S.T. LAC, L.K. CURTIS & M.E. CARROLL. 1993. Effects of buprenorphine and naltrexone on reinstatement of cocaine-reinforced responding in rats. J. Pharmacol. Exp. Ther. **267:** 1470–1477.
26. WETLI, C.V. & D.A. FISHBAIN. 1985. Cocaine-induced psychosis and sudden death in recreational cocaine users. J. Forensic Sci. **30:** 873–880.
27. WETLI, C.V., D.C. MASH & S.B. KARCH. 1996. Cocaine-associated agitated delirium and the neuroleptic malignant syndrome. Am. J. Emerg. Med. **14:** 425–428.
28. RUTTENBER, A.J., J. LAWLER-HEAVNER, M. YIN, C.V. WETLI, W.L. HEARN & D.C. MASH. 1997. Fatal excited delirium following cocaine use: epidemiologic findings provide new evidence for mechanisms of cocaine toxicity. J. Anal. Toxicol. **42:** 25–31.
29. HERNANDEZ, A., W. ANDOLLO & W.L. HEARN. 1994. Analysis of cocaine and metabolites in brain using solid phase extraction and full-scanning and GC/ion trap mass spectrometry. Forensic Sci. Int. **65:** 149–156.
30. STALEY, J.K. & D.C. MASH. 1996. Adaptive increase in D_3 dopamine receptors in the brain reward circuits of human cocaine fatalities. J. Neurosci. **16:** 6100–6106.
31. STALEY, J.K. R.B. ROTHMAN, K.C. RICE, J. PARTILLA & D.C. MASH. 1997. Kappa2 opioid receptors in limbic areas of the human brain are upregulated by cocaine in fatal overdose victims. J. Neurosci. 17 (21): 8225–33.
32. SEGAL, D.M., C.T. MOREAS & D.C. MASH. 1997. Upregulation of D3 dopamine receptor mRNA in the nucleus accumbens from human cocaine overdose victims. Mol. Brain Res. 45(2): 335–339.

33. LARGE, C.H. & C.M. STUBBS. 1994. The dopamine D_3 receptor: Chinese hamsters or chinese whispers. Trends Pharmacol. Sci. **15:** 46–47.
34. BURRIS, K.D., T.M. FILTZ, S. CHUMPRADIT, M-P. KUNG, C. FOULON, J.G. HENSLER, H.F. KUNG & P.B. MOLINOFF. 1994. Characterization of $[^{125}I](R)$-*trans*-7-hydroxy-2-[*N*-propyl-*N*-(3'-iodo-2'-propenyl)amino]tetralin binding to dopamine D_3 receptors in rat olfactory tubercle. J. Pharmacol. Exp. Ther. **268:** 935–942.
35. SELF, D.W., W.J. BARNHART, D.A. LEHMAN & E.J. NESTLER. 1996. Opposite modulation of cocaine-seeking behavior by D1-like and D2-like dopamine receptor agonists. Science **271:** 1586–1589.
36. SOKOLOFF, P., B. GIROS, M.P. MARTRES, M.L. BOUTHENET & J.C. SCHWARTZ. 1990. Molecular cloning and characterization of a novel dopamine receptor (D_3) as a target for neuroleptics. Nature **347:** 146–151.
37. KOOB, G.F. & F.E. BLOOM. 1988. Molecular and cellular mechanisms of drug dependence. Science **242:** 715–723.
38. SCHMAUS, C., V. HAROUTUNIAN, K.L. DAVIS & M. DAVIDSON. 1993. Selective loss of dopamine D-3 type receptor mRNA expression in parietal and motor cortices of patients with chronic schizophrenia. Proc. Natl. Acad. Sci. **90:** 8942–8946.
39. UNTERWALD, E.M., J.M. RUBENFELD & M.J. KREEK. 1994. Repeated cocaine administration upregulates kappa and mu but not delta opioid receptors. Neuroreport **5:** 1613–1616.
40. HAMMER, R.P. 1989. Cocaine alters opiate receptor binding in critical brain reward regions. Synapse **3:** 55–60.
41. HURD, Y.L. & M. HERKENHAM. 1993. Molecular alterations in the neostriatum of human cocaine addicts. Synapse **13:** 357–369.
42. WERLING, L.L., A. FRATTALI, P.S. PORTOGHESE, A.E. TAKEMORI & B.M. COX. 1988. Kappa-receptor regulation of dopamine release from striatum and cortex of rats and guinea pigs. . Pharmacol. Exp. Ther. **246:** 282–286.
43. MANSOUR, A., C.A. FOX, H. MENG, H. AKIL & S. WATSON. 1994. k_1 receptor mRNA distribution in the rat CNS: comparison to κ receptor binding and prodynorphin mRNA. Mol. Cell. Neurosci. **5:** 124–144.
44. HURD, Y.L., E.E. BROWN, J.M. FINLAY, H.C. FIBIGER & C.R. GERFEN. 1992. Cocaine self-administration differentially alters mRNA expression of striatal peptides. Mol. Brain Res. **13:** 165–170.
45. SIVAM, S.P. 1989. Cocaine selectively increases striatonigral dynorphin levels by dopaminergic mechanism. J. Pharmacol. Exp. Therap. **250:** 818–824.
46. SMILEY, P.L., M. JOHNSON, L. BUSH, J.W. GIBB & G.R. HANSON. 1990. Effects of cocaine on extrapyramidal and limbic dynorphin systems. J. Pharmacol. Exp. Ther. **253:** 938–943.
47. SPANGLER, R., E.M. UNTERWALD & M.J. KREEK. 1993. "Binge" cocaine administration induced a sustained increase of prodynorphin mRNA in rat caudate-putamen. Mol. Brain Res. **19:** 323–327.
48. XU, M., R. MORATALLA, L.H. GOLD, N. HIROI, G.F. KOOB, A.M. GRAYBIEL & S. TONEGAWA. 1994. Dopamine D_1 receptor mutant mice are deficient in striatal expression of dynorphin and in dopamine-mediated behavioral responses. Cell **79:** 729–742.
49. STEINER, H. & C.R. GERFEN. 1996. Dynorphin regulates D1 dopamine receptor-mediated responses in the striatum: relative contributions of pre- and postsynaptic mechanisms in dorsal and ventral striatum demonstrated by altered immediate early gene induction. J. Comp. Neurol. **376:** 530–541.
50. BROADBENT, J., T.M. GASPARD & S.I. DWORKIN. 1995. Assessment of the discriminative stimulus effects of cocaine in the rat: lack of interaction with opioids. Pharmacol. Biochem. Behav. **51:** 379–385.
51. UKAI, M., E. MORI & T. KAMEYAMA. 1995. Effects of centrally administered neuropeptides on discriminative stimulus properties of cocaine in the rat. Pharmacol. Biochem. Behav. **51:** 705–708.
52. SPEALMAN, R.D. & J. BERGMAN. 1992. Modulation of the discriminative stimulus effects of cocaine by mu and kappa opioids. J. Pharmacol. Exp. Ther. **261:** 607–615.

53. KUMOR, K.M., C.A. HAERTZEN, R.E. JOHNSON, T. KOCHER & D. JASINSKI. 1986. Human psychopharmacology of ketocyclazocine as compared with cyclazocine, morphine and placebo. J. Pharmacol. Exp. Ther. **238:** 960–968.
54. PFEIFFER, A., V. BRANDT & A. HERZ. 1986. Psychotomimesis mediated by kappa opiate receptors. Science **233:** 774–776.
55. BEN-ARI, Y. 1981. *The Amygdaloid Complex.* Elsevier North-Holland Biomedical Press. Amsterdam.
56. KLING, A, H.D. STEKLIS & S. DEUTSCH. 1979. Radiotelemetered activity from the amygdala during social interactions in the monkey. Exp. Neurol. **66:** 88–96.
57. ANDY, O.J. & M.F. JURKO. 1972. Hyperresponsive syndrome. *In* Psychosurgery. E. Hitchcock, L. Laitinen & K. Vaernet, Eds.: 117–126. Thomas. Springfield, IL.

Functional Magnetic Resonance Imaging of Brain Reward Circuitry in the Human

HANS C. BREITER[a,b,c] AND BRUCE R. ROSEN[a]

[a]*Nuclear Magnetic Resonance Center, Department of Radiology, Massachusetts General Hospital and Harvard Medical School, Boston, Massachusetts 02129, USA*
[b]*Department of Psychiatry, Massachusetts General Hospital and Harvard Medical School, Boston, Massachusetts 02114, USA*

ABSTRACT: To produce behavior, motivational states necessitate at least three fundamental operations, including (1) selection of objectives focused on goal-objects, (2) compilation of goal-object information, and (3) determination of physical plans for securing goal-objects. The second of these general operations has been theorized to involve three subprocesses: (a) feature detection and other perceptual processing of putative goal-object "rewards," (b) valuation of goal-object worth in the context of potential hedonic deficit states, and (c) extraction of incidence and temporal data regarding the goal-object. A number of subcortical brain regions appear to be involved in these three informational subprocesses, in particular, the amygdala, sublenticular extended amygdala (SLEA) of the basal forebrain, and nucleus accumbens/subcallosal cortex (NAc/SCC). Components of the amygdala, SLEA, and NAc/SCC together constitute the larger anatomic structure of the extended amygdala. Functional magnetic resonance imaging (fMRI) studies of humans have recently begun to localize these subcortical regions within the extended amygdala during specific experimental conditions. In this manuscript, two human cocaine-infusion studies and one cognitive psychology experiment are reviewed in relation to their pattern of fMRI activation within regions of the extended amygdala. Activation in the NAc/SCC, in particular, is evaluated in relation to a hypothesis that one function of the NAc/SCC and associated brain regions is the evaluation of goal-object incidence data for the computation of conditional probabilities regarding goal-object availability. Further work is warranted to test hypothesized functions for all regions within the extended amygdala and integrate them toward an understanding of motivated behavior.

INTRODUCTION

In the real world, humans appear to alter their behavior by the consequences of previous actions. Their choices are described as being guided by the systematic evaluation (1) of incoming information from the environment, (2) of remembered consequences of previous behavior, (3) of conditions in their bodies, and (4) of conditions in others. In this context, scientists of human behavior infer *drives* or *motivational states* as the postulated mechanisms that explain the intensity and direc-

---

[c]Address correspondence to Hans C. Breiter, MD, MGH-NMR Center, 2nd Floor, Building #149, Thirteenth Street, Charlestown, MA 02129, USA. Voice: 617-726-5715; fax: 617-726-7422; hansb@nmr.mgh.harvard.edu

tion of behavior. The internal drive or motivational state is an inference. This inference is constructed to explain the variability of behavioral responses, when observable stimuli in the environment are not sufficient to completely predict behavioral outcomes. In the context of evolutionary survival, or selection of fitness, motivational states seek to choose goal-objects and activities that will maximize personal fitness over time.[1] Motivational states thus represent the individual's basis for behavioral choice, which may require planning over time, or planning of multiple choice considerations together.

The variable of time injects some complexity into behavioral choice. Some motivational states can be considered to have a simple relationship to time, such as thermoregulation. By contrast, other drives that control behavior do not appear to have any well-defined temporal relationship to environmental events; drives, such as curiosity or sexual arousal, are referred to as drives or motivational states, because like classical homeostatic drives, they still involve arousal and satiation.

To produce motivated behavior, a drive or motivational state must mediate at least three fundamental operations. These operations include (1) selection of short-term and long-term objectives focused on goal-objects, behaviors, and internal physical states that maximize personal fitness over time, (2) integration of perceptual features, worth, and probability/rate data regarding these objectives, and (3) determination of physical plans involving musculature or organ function to obtain these objectives. Motivated behavior necessitates the function of a number of physiological systems, including those for control of large muscle groups, sensory systems, autonomic functions, and other systems for the attainment of motivational objectives. In this manuscript, we will focus on brain systems necessary for the control of large muscle groups; in particular, we will focus on the informatics necessary for the moment-by-moment modulation of behavior, as via the integration of perceptual, evaluative, and timing/probability data for the attainment of goal-objects.

The idea that a goal-object can incite a behavioral response or reinforce a previous or ongoing action rests on an assumption that a number of informational subprocesses are active whenever an animal encounters a potential "reward." These subprocesses have been theorized[1–4] to involve (1) feature detection and other perceptual processing of putative rewards, (2) valuation of goal-object worth in the context of potential hedonic deficit states, and (3) extraction of incidence and temporal features from the object of worth, to allow computation of a probability function for possible outcomes[5] or a rate function.[6]

The relevance of this focus on the informatics necessary for motivated behavior is evident when considering previous research on reward functions. In experiments focused on behavioral choice driven by theorized motivational states, experimental psychologists have investigated the organizing effects of "rewarding" stimuli associated with goal-objects on behavior. Stimuli or goal-objects that produce repeated approach behaviors or response repetitions are termed "rewards." Thus, reward is an operational concept for the positive value that an animal attributes to an object, a behavior, or an internal physical state. Rewarding stimuli can either *incite* a behavioral response, or *reinforce* a previous or ongoing action. As an *incentive* to behavior, a rewarding stimulus can act either via a memory of a previous reward experience or via salient properties (i.e., the sight and smell of food) of the stimulus that orient the animal to it. By contrast, rewarding stimuli acting as *reinforcement* of previous behavior, as during a drug self-administration paradigm, increase the probability that preceding behavioral responses are repeated. Of these two behavioral concepts, the concept of reward acting as a reinforcement of behavior is the closest to the subjective description of pleasure.

Each of the three operations necessary for motivated behavior is constrained by a complex set of variables. As an example, let us consider the subsystem of evaluation of goal-object worth within the larger operation of the informatics needed for moment-by-moment control of motivated behavior. The evaluation of worth occurs in the context that one or more categories of goal objects are needed to compensate a deficit state; the value of a goal object is derived from the degree to which the animal or person needs it. Thus, a thirsty person is said to consider water a reward. A caveat to this observation is that the presence of a deficit state, which can be satiated, does not appear to be necessary for addictive drugs or brain stimulation reward (BSR), neither of which fulfill a known survival-related need. Other variables influencing the value of a natural reward include (1) the rate at which it reinforces behavior,[7] (2) the delay between a behavior and the delivered reward that reinforces this behavior,[8,9] (3) the category of reward and degree to which various categories of reward can be substituted for each other,[10] (4) the ecological constraints shaping behavioral responses so that they are appropriate to the environment of the subject, (i.e., time and effort needed to search and consume food may limit behavior), and (5) the anticipatory mechanisms that directly regulate homeostatic needs before the onset of actual physiological deficits, (i.e., circadian rhythms turn on some physiological behavioral responses before the occurrence of actual tissue needs).

The perceptual processing, evaluation, and rate plus probability analysis of potential goal-objects appears to be mediated by a linked network of brain regions that have traditionally been referred to as the circuitry of "brain reward."[11-13] Among the key components of this network (see FIG. 1) are (1) dopamine-containing neurons in the ventral tegmental area and medial substantial nigra (together referred to here as the ventral tegmentum, VT), (2) neurons in the nucleus accumbens (referred to as NAc/SCC in this manuscript for the nucleus accumbens plus subcallosal cortex given current fMRI spatial resolution) and neighboring ventral striatal regions (which receive a dopaminergic input from the VT), (3) cells in several nuclei of the amygdala proper, and (4) cells in a neighboring portion of the basal forebrain, which have been referred to as the sublenticular extended amygdala (SLEA).[14] Components of regions (2)–(4) are considered to form an anatomic continuum, namely the extended amygdala.[14,15] How the subcomponents of the extended amygdala, along with the VT, interact to produce the informatics necessary for behavioral modulation is far from apparent. Ideally, the functions of each these regions, in terms of their modular contributions to the distributed system, would be separable and interpretable in information processing terms. Dissection of the informational subprocesses that underlie brain reward, using the tools of cognitive neuroscience, would allow us to significantly facilitate our understanding of the larger process of motivation.

To determine how rewarding stimuli have organizing effects on human behavior, and mediate or fulfill motivational states, one must first demonstrate an ability to observe NAc/SCC, amygdala, SLEA, and VT activity in the living human brain, in conjunction with reward functions. Subsequent experiments could then use cognitive tasks to dissect out specific subprocesses, which together are integrated to produce

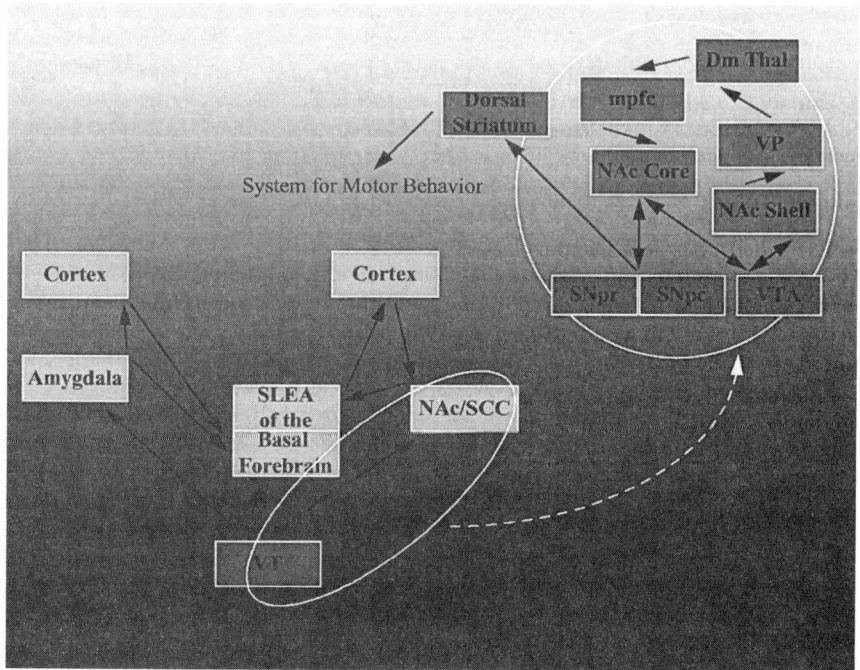

FIGURE 1. Putative reward circuitry. On the left, a cartoon schematizes regions implicated by animal experiments to be involved with brain reward. Abbreviations used for anatomy reflect terminology used for the human fMRI experiments in this manuscript: sublenticular extended amygdala (SLEA), nucleus accumbens/subcallosal cortex (NAc/SCC), and ventral tegmentum of the midbrain (VT). The arrows suggest some of the known connections between these regions. A more detailed construction of the circled connection between VT and NAc/SCC is displayed in the upper right corner. This second cartoon emphasizes some of the complexity of the circuitry between VT and NAc/SCC; a fuller account can be obtained from Heimer and colleagues.[14,15,25] The output arrow from the dorsal striatum symbolizes its contribution to the extended system controlling motor function. Abbreviations include ventral tegmental area (VTA); substantia nigra pars compacta (SNpc); substantia nigra pars reticulata (SNpr); nucleus accumbens (NAc); ventral pallidum (VP); dorsomedial nucleus of the thalamus (Dm Thal); medial prefrontal cortex (mpfc).

reward functions. Over the past four years, we have begun such an endeavor, initially using cocaine infusions in cocaine-dependent subjects to visualize reward circuitry, and then cognitive psychological paradigms to interrogate these regions. In what follows, three separate functional magnetic resonance imaging (fMRI) experiments will be discussed. The first two experiments were double-blind cocaine infusions; the results of these studies[13,16,17] effectively built a bridge between human psychostimulant abuse and animal models of addiction. In these studies, multiple temporal features of NAc/SCC activity were noted, including activation putatively involved with expectancy or anticipation. These data were consistent with, but did not necessitate, an interpretation that the NAc/SCC be involved with processing time and incidence data such as is needed for computation of rate and probability functions describing goal-objects. Amygdala, SLEA, and VT activity were distinct from the activations observed in the NAc/SCC. In contrast to the cocaine-infusion studies, the third project focused on different modes of attentional processing during continuous performance tasks. It observed NAc/SCC activity during the sequential processing of information, unrelated to reward itself, and constrained by the probabilistic incidence of interference in the form of false cues and false targets. This linkage of NAc/SCC activity to a probability function illustrates the use of cognitive paradigms to delineate subsystems that underlie and mediate the functions we define as reinforcement reward and incentive reward. Ultimately, our understanding of motivational state will be based on a reductionistic description of the subprocesses that produce reward and reward-related functions.

STUDY 1

Cocaine is one of the most reinforcing drugs known, both in humans and in animals.[18] This project sought to determine whether regions, such as the VT and NAc/SCC, along with other regions implicated in reinforcement reward, namely the SLEA of the basal forebrain[19] and the amygdala,[20] would show short-term cocaine-induced signal changes, and thus correlate with ratings of euphoria. This project further sought to determine whether or not any regions would show more long-term signal changes and potentially correlate with craving, a monofocused motivational state.

Subjects and Methods

Seventeen subjects were clinically evaluated to have DSM-IV diagnosis of cocaine dependence, without other medical problems. Prior to scanning, they received an unblinded 0.2 mg/kg infusion of cocaine HCl to screen for cocaine-induced arrhythmias, and to practice making behavioral ratings of their rush, high, low, and craving.[13,16]

Prior to scanning, subjects were informed that the identity of one infusion did not imply the identity of the second infusion.[13] Subjects were scanned on a 1.5 T instascan device (General Electric Signa; modified by Advanced NMR Systems, Wilmington, MA) using a head coil (General Electric). Prior to functional scanning, an automated shim procedure was used to improve Bo magnetic field homogeneity. Each subject underwent five functional scans for each infusion (see FIG. 2). The infusion scan lasted 18 minutes, with the cocaine or saline infusion precisely timed to start 5 minutes into the scan. Bracketing the infusion scans were two control experiments to quantify global blood flow changes (scans 2, 4, 7, 9) and to determine that regionally specific activation could still be observed (scans 1, 5, 6, 10). These experiments indicated that despite a global decrease of cerebral blood flow of at least 13-14%, regionally specific brain activation could be observed.[16] Analysis of the infusion scans has been described previously,[13] building upon established techniques.[21,22]

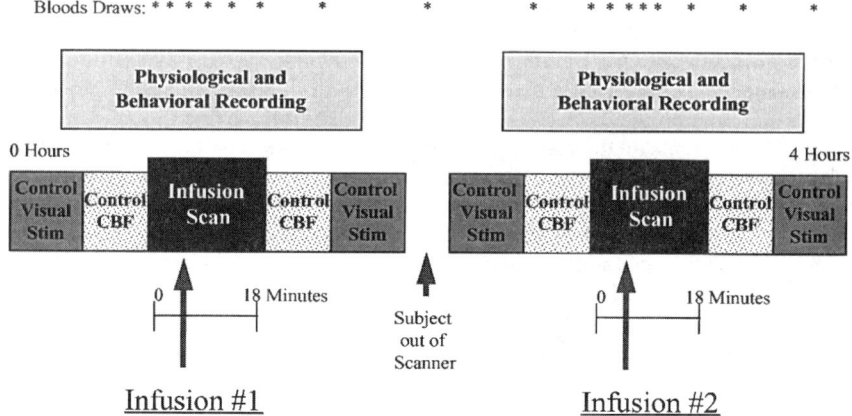

FIGURE 2. Experimental design for the first cocaine infusion study. Over a 4-hour period, subjects participated in 10 experimental scans. The experimental runs were grouped, 5 apiece, around each of the double-blind infusions. Functional scans 1, 3, 5, 6, 8, and 10 used a blood oxygen level-dependent sequence (asymmetric spin echo), whereas scans 2, 4, 7, and 9 used a cerebral blood flow–sensitive sequence (flow-sensitive alternating inversion recovery or FAIR). Physiological recording along with behavioral ratings were initiated prior to the first FAIR scan and continued through the second FAIR scan of each infusion block. After the first infusion, the second double-blind infusion was not initiated until the 120-minute blood sample had been collected. In between the sets of functional scans for each infusion, clinical scans were acquired for neuroradiological assessment. These scans included sagittal T1 images, axial proton density and T2 images, and a 3D time-of-flight angiogram.

Results

Behavioral Measures

No subject reported any rush, high, low, or craving prior to the onset of cocaine or saline infusion. Post hoc, subjects stated they were anticipating receiving cocaine. After cocaine, but not saline, peak rush (2.2 ± 1.1), and peak high (2.1 ± 0.8) occurred ~3 minutes postinfusion. Peak low (primarily reports of dysphoria and paranoia: 0.9 ± 0.8) occurred 11 minutes postinfusion, while peak craving (1.3 ± 0.9) occurred 12 minutes postinfusion.[13,16]

fMRI Results

fMRI signal prior to the onset of both the cocaine and saline infusions was evaluated to determine if it increased in synchrony with drug anticipation. A region of positive signal change meeting the strict Bonferroni significance threshold ($p < 7.1 \times 10^{-6}$) was observed in the ventral region of the NAc/SCC (FIG. 3) prior to both infusions. After its infusion, cocaine induced focal signal increases in NAc/SCC (FIG. 4), basal forebrain, VT, along with signal decreases in the amygdala. Multiple other foci of significant signal change were also noted[13] in the basal ganglia, medial temporal structures, paralimbic cortices, and neocortex. By contrast, saline produced no positive signal change in limbic or paralimbic regions; the limited set of significant

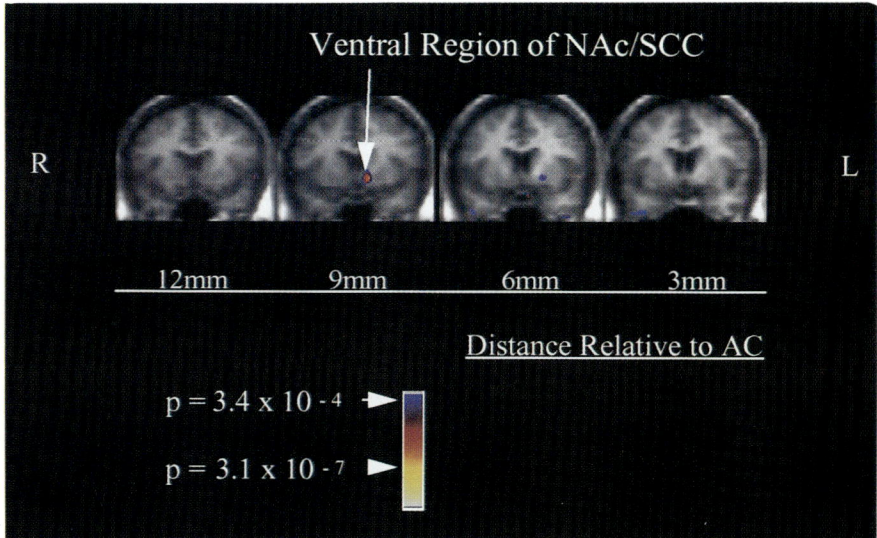

FIGURE 3. Images of subcortical brain regions showing significant fMRI signal changes before both cocaine and saline infusions. These images show Kolmogorov-Smirnov (KS) statistical maps of 4 coronal slices with activation in the NAc/SCC for the average fMRI data from 10 subjects who received cocaine and 10 subjects who received saline. These KS statistical maps are overlaid in pseudocolor on corresponding gray scale average structural maps. Activations with positive signal change are in the ventral region of the NAc/SCC.

activations in frontal and tempero-occipital cortex predominantly matched activations seen in the cocaine maps.

In individuals, the data analysis supported the average results in the NAc/SCC, basal forebrain, and VT, but not the amygdala, which demonstrated response heterogeneity across individuals. This amygdala heterogeneity suggests caution in the interpretation of the negative amygdala activation in the average map. Test/retest in 4 subjects showed good replication for initial activations seen with cocaine and saline; intriguingly, on retest, bilateral NAc/SCC activation was noted for both saline and cocaine infusions.

The majority of brain regions activated by cocaine correlated with rush and high ratings; these regions, including the VT and SLEA of the basal forebrain, showed short duration activation. By contrast, craving ratings correlated with a limited number of brain regions showing sustained signal changes, as was observed with the dorsomedial region of the NAc/SCC and the amygdala.

Summary of Study 1

Cocaine resulted in VT and SLEA signal changes that correlated strongly with rush measures. By contrast, amygdala signal change was noted that correlated more strongly with craving measures, though the heterogeneity of signal change noted in

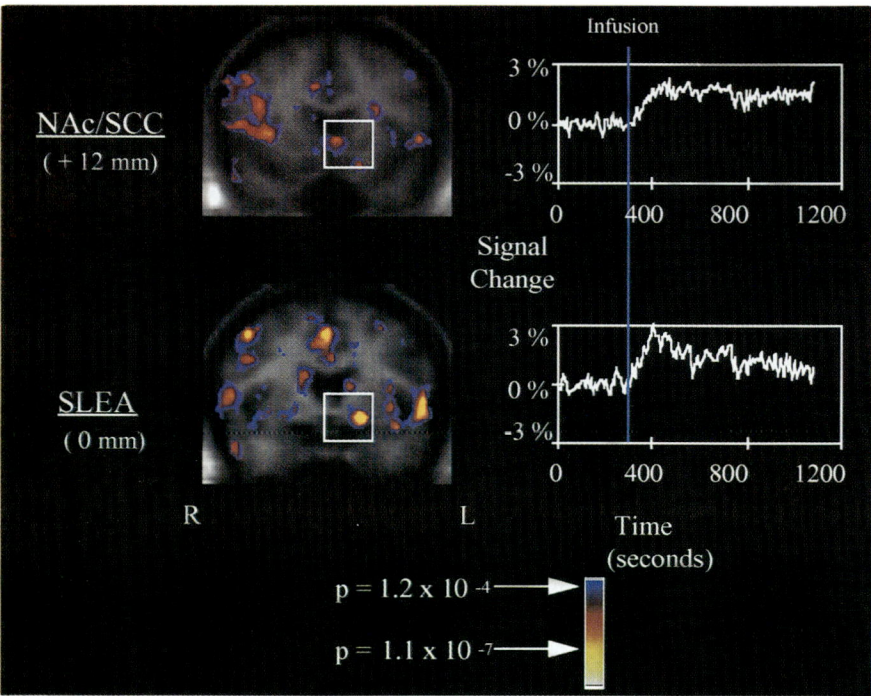

FIGURE 4. Double-blind, investigator-administered cocaine infusion: 0.6 mg/kg in cocaine-dependent volunteers. Images of subcortical brain regions showing significant fMRI signal changes after cocaine, but not after saline, infusions. These Kolmogorov-Smirnov (KS) statistical maps depict 2 coronal levels of pre- versus postinfusion time points for the average fMRI data from 10 subjects who received cocaine. These KS statistical maps are overlaid in pseudocolor on corresponding gray scale average structural maps. Activations with positive signal change include the dorsomedial region of the NAc/SCC and the SLEA. The signal intensity versus time graph for the activations (for all voxels with $p < 10^{-6}$ within the named region) is placed next to each image.

the individual data for this region differentiates it from the other a priori region strongly correlated with craving, namely the NAc/SCC.

This experiment produced activation in the NAc/SCC during the preinfusion period for both saline and cocaine, during which there was a 50% expectancy condition for cocaine. Subsequently, after cocaine infusion alone, NAc/SCC activation had early signal maxima, as seen with subjective measures of rush, which was sustained, leading to its stronger correlation to the incentive-related measure of craving. Analogous to data reported by Carelli and Deadwyler,[23] the preinfusion and postinfusion sustained signal change in the NAc/SCC may reflect the effects of cells that fire before and after cocaine infusions, and that fire to stimuli conditioned to the infusion. Alternately, the preinfusion signal change, given its concordant response before the saline infusion, may reflect an expectancy computation alone, similar to other NAc/SCC cells recorded by Carelli and Deadwyler.[23] In support of this latter interpretation is the nonoverlap of the preinfusion activation in the ventral region of the NAc/SCC and the cocaine postinfusion activation in the dorsomedial region of the NAc/SCC; this nonoverlap is significantly tempered by consideration of altered spatial resolution of this data from signal processing.[13,22,21] Anatomically, the ventral region of the NAc/SCC approximates the shell region of the NAc/SCC,[24,25] to which project medial VT neurons[26] thought to be involved with reward prediction.[12]

Interpretation of the NAc/SCC activations in the context of a temporal function versus a probability function is a significant issue. One might interpret NAc/SCC activation during the phase of putative preinfusion expectancy, along with the phases of postinfusion reinforcement and incentive, as reflecting the processing of specific temporal intervals. These specific temporal intervals would be (1) that before infusion, related to anticipation of onset, (2) that just after infusion, reflecting reinforcement onset plus duration, and (3) that during reinforcement offset/cessation, reflecting incentive function. Alternately, one could interpret the multiple NAc/SCC signal changes in the context of computation of a probabilistic function for reward prediction. In this case, it would be active prior to infusion onset, reflecting the 50% potential incidence of cocaine in the infusate, and following the predictive event of initiating the MRI scan. Postinfusion, the NAc/SCC would further be active, reflecting conditional probability assessment during the wait for subjective drug effects after the predictive event of perceiving cold infusate at the catheter tip. Early NAc/SCC activity after the infusion might also relate to the interaction of probability assessment and reward intensity measurement for the computation of outcome.[5] During the offset/cessation of reinforcement, NAc/SCC activity would potentially relate to probability assessments necessary for incentive functions, such as cocaine-primed craving.

The observation of bilateral NAc/SCC activation on retest cocaine and saline infusion is more consistent with the latter interpretation of probability function computation, because no cocaine euphoria was reported after saline infusion that could be timed (i.e., for this study, no subjective placebo effects were observed). Furthermore, both infusions occurred during a 50% expectancy condition in the novel environment of the magnet, thus defining a partial reinforcement schedule. Conditioned place preference effects are known to occur within one trial, and might have produced the effects seen with these pilot retest experiments. The combination of fMRI test/retest, and subjective data, would support a hypothesis that the NAc/SCC use incidence data to compute a probability function around goal-objects. Such a hypothesis, from limited data, does not displace interpretations of NAc/SCC involvement with temporal information processing, such as marking intertrial intervals,[27] as is necessary for computation of a rate function regarding goal-objects.[6]

STUDY 2

The second cocaine-infusion project[17] sought to confirm the observation of cocaine induced activation in the NAc/SCC, amygdala, SLEA, and VT using a cardiac-gated technique to obviate potential artifacts from cocaine effects on heart rate. It further sought to determine if brain stem regions besides VT, such as the raphe nuclei and locus caeruleus, were concurrently activated with subcortical reward circuitry during cocaine administration. Functional imaging of the brain stem and connected regions is compromised by noise induced by inherent cardiac pulsatility. The next cocaine infusion study thus adapted methods[28] for cardiac-gated fMRI to compensate for brain stem motion. It also used a clustered volume acquisition with sharpened slice profiles[29] to group the acquisition of the brain stem volume and thus reduce effects of imaging noise on cocaine-induced euphoria and craving.

Subjects and Methods

Eleven right-handed, unmedicated men with the DSM-IV diagnosis of cocaine dependence were imaged. All aspects of subject recruitment, characterization, and qualifications were unchanged from our earlier experiment.

Prior to scanning, subjects were informed that the identity of one infusion did not imply the identity of the second infusion. Subsequently, subjects underwent a randomized double-blind infusion of either cocaine HCl (0.6 mg/kg up to maximum dose of 40 mg) or saline 5 minutes into scan acquisition. Behavioral ratings for rush, high, low, and craving were measured via a button-press with ordinal output of 0–3, as in the first study.

Subjects were scanned with the same MRI system as in study 1. A sagittal localizer scan was performed for placement of six experimental slices in the oblique axial plane and covering the brain stem from medulla to inferior colliculus. An automated shim procedure improved Bo magnetic field homogeneity. Functional scans used cardiac gating with an asymmetric spin echo, T2*-weighted clustered volume acquisition.[17,29] Data were analyzed with motion correction, evaluation for residual motion, and statistical mapping with superposition of statistical maps on individual structural scans.[22] Statistical maps were thresholded at the corrected p value for brain regions sampled, $p < 10^{-5}$, and activation localization was performed using previously defined conventions.[13]

Results

As in the first experiment, all subjects produced maximal behavioral ratings for rush and high within 2 minutes of cocaine infusion completion, which returned to baseline within 5–15 minutes. Seven matched sets of cocaine and saline infusion scans were interpretable after motion correction. Compared to the preinfusion baseline, cocaine produced focal positive signal changes (see FIG. 5) in five or more of the subjects in the right NAc/SCC, SLEA, and amygdala, along with bilateral activation in other limbic and paralimbic structures. Bilateral activation in the dorsal raphe and VT was also noted. Following saline infusion, no regions of signal change were observed in five or more subjects for the regions showing activation to cocaine.

Summary of Study 2

Across this study and study 1, double-blind cocaine versus saline infusions produced regionally specific patterns of subcortical and cortical signal change. These two studies represent a bridge between the animal models of addictive processes and human phenomenology of drug effects, in that the same circuitry implicated in animal models of brain reward were observed to be activated in humans after cocaine and not saline. Of these regions, the NAc/SCC, and SLEA of the basal forebrain

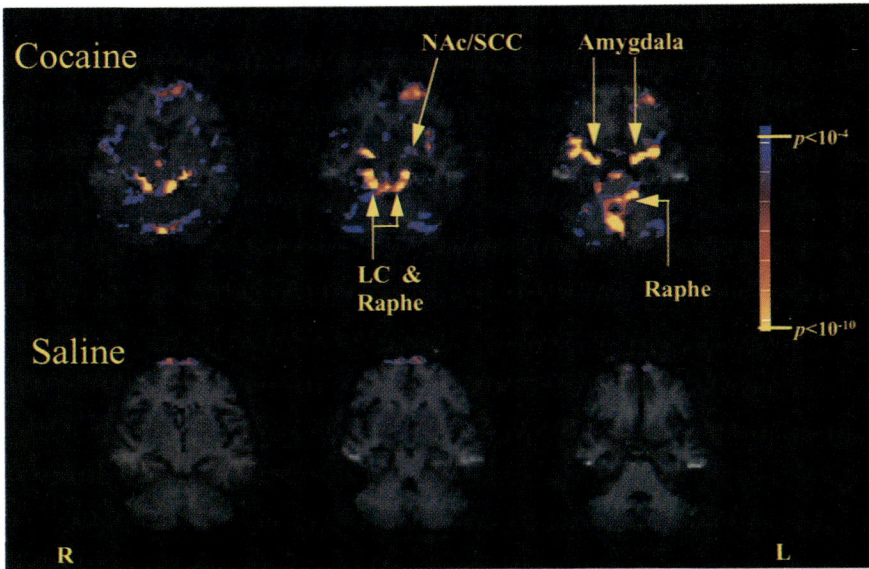

FIGURE 5. Images of subcortical and brain stem activations in one subject after cocaine and saline infusions in the second cocaine infusion experiment. Regions shown include the NAc/SCC, amygdala, and dorsal raphe. Image layout follows the conventions described in FIGURES 3 and 4. The abbreviations signify nucleus accumbens/subcallosal cortex (NAc/SCC), locus caeruleus (LC), and dorsal raphe (raphe). Anatomic definitions for localization have been discussed elsewhere.[17] It is important to note that the nucleus accumbens can be distinguished on this individual's image from the subcallosal cortex, which is adjacent and medial to it. This distinction between nucleus accumbens and subcallosal cortex is not possible on averaged images, and not always possible on individual images. Therefore, we refer to a nucleus accumbens/subcallosal cortex (NAc/SCC) region of interest for both our averaged data and our individual data.

were very consistent findings across studies. Amygdala activation in this second study, in contrast to the first study, was predominantly positive in signal change. Across the two studies, five people had negative amygdala signal changes, eight had positive signal changes, and four had no change; this heterogeneity of amygdala activation across two studies suggests caution in its functional interpretation and distinguishes the data from this region from observations in the NAc/SCC and SLEA. Given the use of cardiac gating, the replicated VT activation from the cocaine infusion indicates that this midbrain activation can be interpreted with greater confidence. The observation of strong dorsal raphe activation further suggests that other monoaminergic systems beyond dopamine, such as serotonin, may be involved with acute cocaine effects.

STUDY 3

The third study involved a cognitive neuroscience experiment that lacked any overt reward associations, yet produced dissociable activation in the NAc/SCC across experimental conditions.[30,31] This study built upon earlier work with a novel continuous performance task (CPT).[32–35] The set of experimental conditions in this study was designed to parse out differences in vigilant attention during a serial processing CPT [CPT-AX(del)], involving a simple probabilistic relationship between a cue and delayed target, versus a dual processing CPT [CPT-AX(int)], with a complex probability relationship between a cue and delayed target. The conditional probability of a subsequent target, given the incidence of a cue, was the same between tasks because the CPT-AX(del) and CPT-AX(int) tasks had the same total number of cue-target pairs and the same total incidence of true cues plus false cues. The tasks were different in that the determination of cue-target pairs was more effortful for the CPT-AX(int) task, due to divided processing and interference suppression needs. The effortful determination of cue-target pairs would impair probability computation and lead to diminished task performance.

Both CPT-AX(del) and CPT-AX(int) were hypothesized to activate an extended set of brain regions for attention, working memory, and interference suppression on the basis of our previous work. Specifically, positive signal change was anticipated in the dorsolateral prefrontal cortex (DLPFC; Brodmann's areas 9/46), supplementary motor area (SMA; Brodmann's area 6), Broca's area (Brodmann's areas 44/45), posterior parietal cortex (PPC; Brodmann's areas 7/40), and thalamus. Negative signal was anticipated in the anterior cingulate/paracingulate (Brodmann's areas 24/32).[32–35] The starting hypotheses of this experiment did not include any component of reward circuitry; thus, NAc/SCC activation was not expected for either the CPT-AX(del) or CPT-AX(int) conditions and had to meet a Bonferroni correction for multiple comparisons to be discussed.

Subjects and Methods

Ten normal right-handed volunteers were studied, five subjects from each gender. The two paradigms involved computer presentation of an auditory letter string, with each letter spoken at a rate of 1 per second. These paradigms had an A-B-A-B design, where the A condition was a simple CPT (referred to as the "QA" sequence), and the B condition was an effortful CPT, with three letters between cue and target pairs (see FIG. 6). The B condition involved either serial processing (CPT-AX(del)) or divided/dual processing (CPT-AX(int)). The CPT-AX(del) was characterized by a lack of false cues or targets between each cue ("q") and target ("a") pair, or by any interdigitated cue-target pairs (i.e., "q"_"q"_"a"_"a"), thus allowing simple probabilistic assessment of cue-to-target pairing with serial association of stimulus and response. The CPT-AX(int) had false cues and/or targets between pairs of cues and targets and had cue-target pairs interdigitate together so that commingled pairs were possible, thus preventing simple counting or rehearsal procedures (i.e., forcing subjects to maintain two or more counts) and increasing the effort needed for probabilistic assessment of cue-to-target pairing. Each A and B epoch lasted 90 seconds. There was a target to distracter ratio of 0.13 for both A and B conditions, and the number of cue-target pairs was the same. Subjects responded with a magnet-compatible button press, so that reaction time and accuracy could be recorded. The order for performing the CPT-AX(del) and the CPT-AX(int) were counterbalanced across subjects.

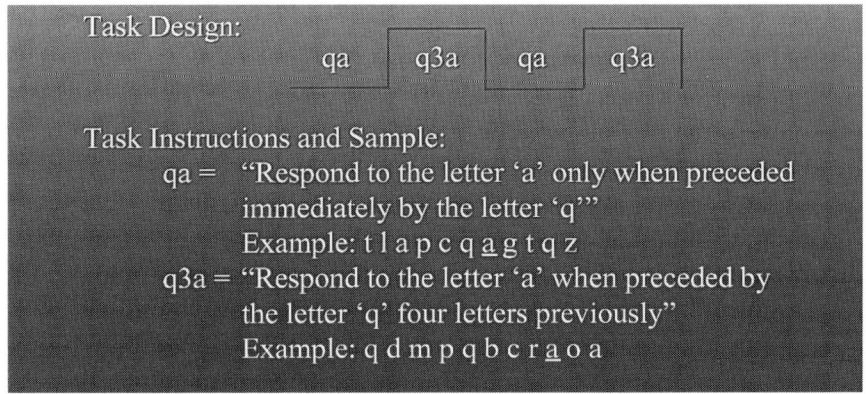

FIGURE 6. Experiment design for the third experiment. This cognitive neuroscience paradigm involved three variants of a continuous performance task, one of which was used as the baseline for the other two. Instructions given for baseline and experimental conditions are shown in quotation marks.

Subjects were scanned on the same 1.5 T device described for the first two studies, with an acquisition of 15 experimental slices in the oblique axial plane and covering much of the brain. Specific experimental procedures and data analysis techniques have been extensively discussed previously.[13,22,21]

Results

On average, reaction times were shorter, and percent accuracy higher, for the CPT-AX(del) condition than for the CPT-AX(int) condition. Both experimental paradigms produced positive signal changes in the DLPFC, SMA, Broca's area, PPC, and thalamus, and negative signal changes in the anterior cingulate/paracingulate, which were consistent with the hypotheses for this study.[35] In both paradigms, at a liberal statistical threshold of $p < 10^{-3}$, voxels associated with activated clusters in the frontal and parietal lobes constituted the majority of observed activation.

Between the CPT-AX(int) condition and the CPT-AX(del) condition, some salient differences were evident. Direct comparison via subtraction of the CPT-AX(del) condition from the CPT-AX(int) condition produced multiple prefrontal foci, and parietal foci. By contrast, the CPT-AX(del) condition produced 2- to 6-fold larger activation volumes than the CPT-AX(int) condition in temporal cortex, occipital cortex, and subcortical structures, such as the basal ganglia. Furthermore, more limbic and paralimbic activation was observed in the CPT-AX(del) condition, including multiple foci in the insula, and bilateral (right ≫ left) activations in NAc/SCC (see FIG. 7). No foci of activation were observed in the amygdala, SLEA of the basal forebrain, or VT for either the CPT-AX(del) or the CPT-AX(int) conditions.[30]

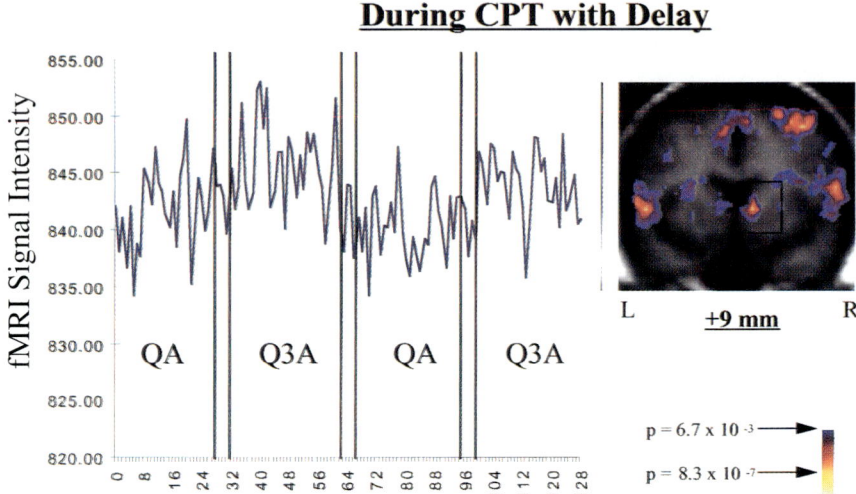

FIGURE 7. Bilateral (right ≫ left) NAc/SCC activation that extends into the ventral striatum. The unsmoothed time course is demonstrated to the left of the statistical map. The three sets of double vertical lines represent five-second intervals between epochs of QA and Q3A conditions for the CPT-AX(del) task, during which recorded instructions were administered to the subject (see FIG. 6 for actual instructions).

Summary of Study 3

The CPT-AX(int) incorporated greater working memory and interference suppression requirements than the CPT-AX(del) and produced more frontal and parietal activation. This is consistent with the implicated function of such regions as the DLPFC and PPC in the active maintenance of task-relevant information, and the maintenance of context information.[35,36] No amygdala, SLEA or the basal forebrain, or VT activation was noted for either task.

Observation of NAc/SCC activation in response to the CPT-AX(del) task, but not the CPT-AX(int) task, raises a number of issues, including a question of whether it is necessarily involved with reward functions. There is salient animal data that suggests that the NAc/SCC is involved with nonreward processes, such as the exploration of novelty,[37] behavioral switching or general behavioral flexibility,[37,38] and the spatial-temporal organization of behavior.[39]

Activation of the NAc/SCC in this experiment with the CPT-AX(del), but not the CPT-AX(int) condition, suggests at least two likely interpretations that can be tested. One possibility is that the NAc/SCC is part of the system for maintaining task-relevant information, which is inhibited or used less when interference suppression needs increase beyond some threshold. Alternately, the NAc/SCC may be part of a system for computation of conditional probabilities for events that may or may not reinforce or incite behavior, and which has a limited processing capacity.[40] For both interpretations, one could imagine that multiple sets of structures are available to perform a particular computational task, and depending on processing demands, one or another set of structures would become active. One might, accordingly, observe NAc/SCC activity during the CPT-AX(del) task, and an absence of NAc/SCC activity, with an increase in frontal and parietal cortex activity during the CPT-AX(int) task.

The possibility that the NAc/SCC is involved with the computation of conditional probabilities will be developed further in the discussion that follows. It is important to note that observation of NAc/SCC signal change in this paradigm with no overt connection to reward indicates that the NAc/SCC can be interrogated and potentially understood in relation to simpler processes that underlie reward function.

DISCUSSION

In the reward literature, there is a long-standing thesis that motivational states, which produce goal-directed behavior, necessitate a complex informatics system composed of multiple subprocesses for the moment-by-moment modulation of behavior.[3,4] These subprocesses can be lumped into three general categories[1,2] for (1) perceptual processing of reward objects, (2) valuation of goal-object worth, and (3) extraction of temporal features and conditional probabilities regarding the object of worth. Feature detection focuses on the identity, placement, and specific hedonic properties of the putative goal-object, whereas valuation of the goal-object determines its motivational salience to the animal. The extraction of temporal information and incidence information regarding the putative goal-object includes extraction of that information necessary to predict when and how often the goal-object is available.[41,42] Such temporal information is necessary for the computation of a rate function[6] and of the conditional probabilities characterizing it in the context of alternate outcomes.[5] Of these subprocesses, those involved with evaluating worth, along with evaluating temporal and incidence features, are sufficient for the determination of payoff/outcome[2] and closely parallel other theories of reward function, such as prospect theory.[5]

The brain circuitry mediating these informational subprocesses includes a central set of regions that has been implicated in brain reward,[13] namely the amygdala, the SLEA of the basal forebrain, and the NAc/SCC. Work focused on attentional processes, and the perception of rewarding versus aversive stimuli, has implicated the amygdala in the modulation of perceptual processing of potential goal-objects.[21,43] Other research suggests that experimental paradigms, such as brain stimulation reward (BSR), are linked to the function of valuation[1,44] and have started to link brain regions, such as the SLEA of the basal forebrain, with this function.[19,45,46] The fMRI data from the three studies synopsized in this manuscript, along with research by others, suggest that the NAc/SCC may be a central component of the subprocess for extracting temporal and incidence data from goal-objects for determining rate and conditional probability functions regarding outcomes. The data presented from studies 1–3 specifically argue that the NAc/SCC in humans may be involved with the processing of conditional probabilities around goal-objects and events; further studies are needed to determine if the human NAc/SCC is also involved with processing rate information for behavioral modulation.

NAC/SCC ACTIVITY AND PROBABILITY ASSESSMENT

There are multiple studies suggesting the NAc/SCC is involved with processing temporal information as would be necessary for computing a rate function regarding potential reward. For instance, Carelli and Deadwyler[23] have reported on multiple sets of cells in the NAc/SCC whose firing patterns are time locked to cocaine self-administration in animals. One set of neurons fires prior to the lever press, suggesting an anticipatory or expectancy response linked to the memory of a contingent relationship between bar-press and potential reward. A second group of neurons changes firing rate after the cocaine infusion, which appears to correspond to the direct effects of reinforcement. A third group of neurons fires both before and after the cocaine infusion, and fires to discrete sensory stimuli that have been paired as conditioned stimuli to the cocaine infusion.[23] This last pattern of NAc/SCC neuron activity is thought to be associated with the cue-induced emotional memory that elicits strong craving in cocaine addicts,[47] and thus to be connected to incentive functions. Other investigators have observed a set of neurons that fires in proportion to the interinfusion interval between consecutive self-administration responses.[27] Other work supports the preinfusion expectancy effect in the primate NAc/SCC for nondrug reward,[48,49] and one pilot study ($n = 4$ subjects) with humans supports this observation with regard to monetary reward.[50] From these studies, it might be generalized that one NAc/SCC function is the extraction of multiple temporal features from reward-related events.

It is important to consider, though, that contingency relationships necessitate not just a rate function for prediction of when goal-objects might be available,[6] but also the construction of a probability function for potential outcomes.[5] Associations between events require some index of event incidence. Indeed, the internal computation of conditional probabilities is an important response by animals to events with variable incidence of reinforcement or punishment. Work implicating the NAc/SCC in the processing and response to conditional probabilities in animals includes experiments that have evaluated the impact of NAc/SCC lesions on partial reinforcement extinction.[51,52] Rodents have specifically been reported to show an increased resistance to extinction with partial reinforcement. When rats with electrolytic lesions of the NAc/SCC and control rats are trained using either a continuous reinforcement or partial reinforcement contingency, both groups of lesioned rats were observed to increase their running speeds in the acquisition phase of the task. During extinction, though, rats with NAc/SCC lesions demonstrated a dissociation in behavioral response, depending on the probability function governing the acquisition phase of the experiment; they showed increased rates of extinction after partial reinforcement, but decreased rates of extinction after continuous reinforcement.[51] A similar response has been reported for NAc/SCC-lesioned primates, in that such lesions result in increased rates of extinction for monkeys trained on a partial reinforcement schedule.[52] These data sets suggest the NAc/SCC may be important for graded responses to probabilistic conditions, so as not to result in all versus nothing responses (i.e., increased versus decreased rates of extinction) during violation of contingencies.

Data implicating such brain regions as the NAc/SCC with the processing of contingency conditions has also been reported in humans.[36] In a study by Berns and colleagues,[36] subjects performed a serial reaction-time task, in which sections of a visually presented sequence of stimuli were predetermined, while others were random. To motivate subjects to maintain a general level of performance, subjects were informed that they would earn monetary bonuses for more accurate performance; subjects accordingly sought monetary reward in return for accurate performance, which was facilitated by implicit learning of predetermined sequences. Ventral striatum (and NAc/SCC) activation was observed at the beginning of the experiment when the initial predetermined sequence was presented; at that time, the predetermined sequence was not novel because there were no prior sequential contingencies for it, in that these stimuli had not yet been probabilistically linked in a sequence and thus not associated with a defined context. Subsequently, when a novel second predetermined sequence was shown that violated the learned contingencies of the first predetermined sequence, an activation was observed in the ventral striatum, including the region of the nucleus accumbens. The data from this experiment suggest that the NAc/SCC may be involved with both (1) the evaluation and learning of new contingencies, and (2) the assessment of the violation of learned contingencies by sequential stimuli, particularly when these contingencies are important for the acquisition of monetary reward.[36]

Such an association between the evaluation of conditional probabilities and NAc/SCC activity is also suggested by the results of the third study of this manuscript. In this study, a continuous performance task with sequential linking of cue and target (CPT-AX(del)) produced focal activation in the NAc/SCC (extending into ventral striatum) which was not seen in a more difficult task (CPT-AX(int)). The CPT-AX(del) task was matched to the CPT-AX(int) task for the total number of false cues and false targets but had none appearing within cue-target pairs. Accordingly, the primary differences between tasks were related to the need for dual processing and the need for interference suppression within potential cue-target pairs of the CPT-AX(int) task. Performance accuracy was less and reaction time longer for the CPT-AX(int) task than the CPT-AX(del) task, suggesting that computation of conditional probabilities regarding cue-target pairing was more effortful with the CPT-AX(int) task. This possibility, in conjunction with the observation that NAc/SCC activation occurred only with the CPT-AX(del) task, suggests that there may be a limit to NAc/SCC function regarding contingency evaluation, beyond which other brain regions may predominate, such as phylogenetically more recent regions like the DLPFC and PPC.[53,54] This interpretation infers that strong demands for interference suppression hampers the evaluation of conditional probabilities. This might seem to contrast with the study by Berns and colleagues,[36] in that a task producing potential error in the computation of a conditional probability function relating cues and targets did not produce activation in the NAc/SCC. Perhaps the most salient observation, though, is that in both the study by Berns and colleagues,[36] and study 3 with the CPT-AX(del) task, successful conditional probability assessment was associated with NAc/SCC activity.

The interaction of dopaminergic neurons from the VT with the NAc/SCC and amygdala raises the question of how to distinguish theorized involvement of VT projections with reward prediction[12] from the current discussion of NAc/SCC involvement with the evaluation of conditional probabilities. Our own initial study with double-blind cocaine versus saline infusions showed signal changes in the VT that correlated strongly with the subjective euphoria, distinguishing the VT from the NAc/SCC and amygdala signal changes, and thus from NAc/SCC plus amygdala function during acute cocaine administration. The function of the mesocorticolimbic dopamine projections remains a topic of intense debate. An early view theorized that mesocorticolimbic dopaminergic neurons were the main circuitry for brain reward, whether from natural rewards, BSR, and drugs of abuse.[55] More recently, arguments have been advanced that dopaminergic neurons set the "incentive salience" of goal objects, and accordingly control such monofocused motivational states as craving.[56] Other theories link dopamine release to anticipatory behaviors,[57] or effortful goal-directed performance.[58] Recent cell physiology and neural modeling work posit that dopaminergic neurons are involved with computing reward prediction on the basis of mismatches between expected rewards and actual outcomes.[12] These ideas regarding VT function may not be inconsistent with each other. Let us consider that the VT receives "feedback" from the regions to which it projects in the amygdala, SLEA of the basal forebrain, and NAc/SCC.[14,25] It is possible that this interaction conveys information regarding goal-object features, goal-object value, and goal-object incidence plus timing to the VT. VT projections from its ventral tier to the dorsal striatum might then reflect this information for the moment-by-moment modulation of behavior,[14,25] in conjunction with output from the extended amygdala through polysynaptic cortical projections to the dorsal striatum. Future work is clearly warranted to determine how the amygdala, SLEA of the basal forebrain, and NAc/SCC interact with the VT, and interact with cortical structures, during the production of motivated behavior.

NAc/SCC ACTIVITY WITH AND WITHOUT CRAVING

The thesis that the NAc/SCC is involved with contingency evaluation would remove an apparent contradiction to its activation appearing postinfusion in conditions without craving (i.e., saline retest infusions) and conditions with craving (i.e., after cocaine infusion). In study 1, bilateral NAc/SCC activation was noted for the saline retest results during which time subjects reported no drug craving. The saline retest NAc/SCC activations closely approximated the same activations seen for the initial cocaine infusion in the total cohort, and the cocaine NAc/SCC activation that correlated more with maximum ratings of craving than with rush. Given observations of altered conditioned responses in animals after only one cocaine dose,[59] it is possible the NAc/SCC activation on saline retest represented one-trial learning to context. The association learned in this case would be between cocaine effects occurring with a 50% incidence and the combined sensory experience of an operating magnet and an infusion that subjects could note as a change in temperature at the catheter site. None of our subjects had ever received cocaine prior to the test/retest experiments in the magnet or any other neuroimaging instrument.

NAc/SCC involvement with the evaluation of conditional probabilities around the contingent relationship of cues to outcomes would also support the presence of its activation during cocaine craving, a monofocused motivational state. There are two main procedures for inducing cocaine craving: one via exposure to conditioned cues, and the other via cocaine infusion. In the first procedure, craving is induced by stimuli that have been conditionally associated with cocaine use and its euphoric effects and that potentially predict its impending consumption and subsequent results. In cue-induced craving, the relationship of craving to contingency evaluation is theoretically apparent in that the craving follows from the perception of cocaine-related cues that have previously been associated with cocaine use, and are presumed to involve classical conditioning with partial reinforcement. In cocaine-induced craving, the relationship of craving to contingency evaluation is less obvious, in that the craving follows some degree of euphoric experience, or occurs in the context of acute withdrawal from cocaine. Cocaine-induced craving may or may not be distinct from cue-induced craving,[60] but arguments for its similarity are suggested (1) by the possibility that a priming dose of cocaine may itself be a cue, and (2) by the process of estimating the value of an event, which involves comparison to prior exemplars. After a cocaine infusion, the experience of cocaine-induced euphoria would involve some retrieval and comparison to its "remembered utility,"[61] or the emotional memory associated with its prior use.

It is noteworthy that only the cocaine infusion work[13] has, to date, shown an association between the NAc/SCC and craving. Indeed, cocaine-induced craving was associated with not just NAc/SCC signal change, but amygdala signal change too. These regions were among the few that demonstrated sustained signal changes, as opposed to the majority of other brain activations with early peaks and shorter duration signal changes. Caveats must be attached to this data, though, in that the amygdala demonstrated considerable heterogeneity of signal change across two sets of cocaine infusion studies,[13,17] with 8 of 17 total subjects showing positive signal change, 5 of 17 showing negative signal change, and 4 of 17 showing no signal change. In contrast to the cocaine-induced craving results, NAc/SCC activation has not been reported for experiments involving cue-induced craving. Most studies of cue-induced craving, which did sample subcortical brain regions, reported signal changes in the amygdala.[62–64] Given the spatial resolution of the PET imaging used in these studies, though, an absence of reported signal change in the NAc/SCC might reflect a false negative result.

An association between the NAc/SCC and amygdala might be expected during conditions of contingency evaluation on the basis of published anatomy and animal behavior data. The NAc/SCC is strongly interlinked to the amygdala, via afferent fibers from it.[65–68] Functionally, the linkage between the amygdala and the NAc/SCC appears to be important for the formation of stimulus-reward associations.[69,70] Aspirative lesions of the amygdala in macaque monkeys prevent the formation of associations between secondary or conditioned reinforcers and the intrinsic properties of primary reward stimuli.[71,72] The connections between amygdala to NAc/SCC further mediate the effects of stimulus-reward associations on behavior, which appears to be dependent on dopamine neurotransmission in the NAc/SCC.[73] Specifically, the amygdala sends information on stimuli previously associated with reward to the same regions where VT dopaminergic input arrives. The level of dopamine transmission in the NAc/SCC is then thought to determine the degree of potentiation of incentive-linked instrumental behavior.[73] These observations suggest that an interaction between the VT, NAc/SCC, and amygdala may be important for producing memories of relative amounts of incentive or reward, as might be hypothesized to be important for cue-induced craving for cocaine.

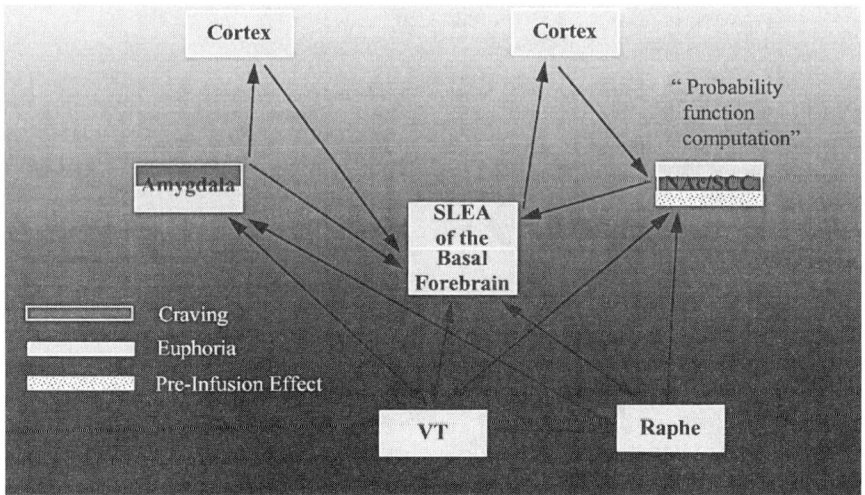

FIGURE 8. Putative human reward circuitry and functional attributions. Summary schematic (for studies 1–3) of brain regions that (1) activate in relation to cocaine-induced euphoria or cocaine-induced craving, (2) activate before either the infusion of cocaine or saline in a 50% expectancy condition, or (3) activate for a serial processing CPT [CPT-AX(del)]. The lines between structures suggest connections between these regions taken from the literature. Anatomic abbreviations follow those used in the text of this manuscript.

SYNOPSIS

In our first cocaine infusion study, NAc/SCC activation was noted in association with drug expectancy, euphoria, and craving. The NAc/SCC also demonstrated activation in a nonreward effortful vigilance task where interference suppression needs were not heavy. When interference suppression needs were increased enough to impair the assessment of the conditional probability for a subsequent target given a cue, as observed with impaired behavioral performance on the CPT-AX(int) task, NAc/SCC activity was significantly diminished. In the context of both animal and human work, which suggest some function in the NAc/SCC with regard to expectancy and detection of contingencies, the two cocaine and one cognitive study reviewed here support the thesis that the NAc/SCC is involved with the computation of conditional probabilities regarding goal-objects. This function is a salient subprocess among those theorized to constitute a motivational state. Other subprocesses of motivational state, such as perceptual processing of goal-object features and evaluation of goal-object worth, have also been tentatively associated with the function of subcortical regions tightly interconnected with the NAc/SCC, namely the amygdala and the SLEA of the basal forebrain.

Functionally, the linkage between the amygdala and the NAc/SCC appears important for the formation of stimulus-reward associations,[69–72] and the effects of these stimulus-reward associations on behavior.[73] Observations such as these, and decades of conditioning research, implicate the amygdala in orienting to and remembering affectively significant stimuli.[20,74,75] Ultimately, these actions may subserve functions such as the attentional modulation of perception,[21,43,76] which is a primary operation of motivational state. The SLEA of the basal forebrain also receives input from the VT and is one of the primary polysynaptic targets of the NAc/SCC and amygdala.[14] Extensive animal research suggests it may be an important component of circuitry involved with the function of goal-object or event valuation.[1,44] The circuitries of the NAc/SCC, amygdala, and SLEA of the basal forebrain appear to be significant components of distributed regions that mediate subprocesses fundamental to the function of motivational state. In the context of their potential functional grouping regarding informatics, it is further intriguing that components of the NAc/SCC, amygdala, and SLEA can also to anatomically linked together as the extended amygdala.[14,15] The interaction of the NAc/SCC and the amygdala with the SLEA of the basal forebrain depends on input from VT and the dorsal raphe (see FIG. 8), along with polysynaptic output through such regions as the thalamus and medial prefrontal cortex. At this time, it appears that these multiple regions in the extended amygdala, and their monoaminergic inputs, are central to the subprocesses that mediate the informatics necessary for motivated behavior. How extensive a set of regions beyond the extended amygdala and its monoaminergic input should be considered as necessary for the complete function of motivation remains to be determined.

ACKNOWLEDGMENTS

This work was supported by Grants to (1) H.C. Breiter and B.R. Rosen from the National Institute of Drug Abuse (Grants #00265 & #09467), and (2) B.R. Rosen from the Heart, Lung and Blood Institute of the NIH (Grant # 39810), Bethesda, MD. This work was also supported by a Young Investigator Award to H.C. Breiter from the National Alliance for Research on Schizophrenia and Depression (NARSAD), and by a Grant to H.C. Breiter from the Scottish Rite Schizophrenia Research Program.

We are deeply indebted to Peter Shizgal, along with Igor Elman and C.J. Malenka, for their critical commentary and support during manuscript preparation.

REFERENCES

1. SHIZGAL, P. 1997. Neural basis of utility estimation. Curr. Opin. Neurobiol. **7:** 198–208.
2. SHIZGAL, P. 1999. On the neural computation of utility: implications from studies of brain stimulation reward. *In* Well-Being: The Foundations of Hedonic Psychology. D. Kahneman, E. Diener & N. Schwarz, Eds.: 502–526. Russell Sage Foundation. New York, NY.
3. PFAFFMANN, C., R. NORGREN & H.J. GRILL. 1977. Sensory affect and motivation. Ann. N. Y. Acad. Sci. **290:** 18–34.
4. ZAJONC, R.B. 1980. Feeling and thinking: preferences need no inference. Am. Psychol. **35(2):** 151–175.
5. KAHNEMAN, D. & A. TVERSKY. 1979. Prospect theory: an analysis of decision under risk. Econometrica **47:** 263–291.
6. GALLISTEL, C.R. 1990. The organization of learning. MIT Press. Cambridge, MA.
7. BAUM, W.M. & H. RACHLIN. 1969. Choice as time allocation. J. Exp. Anal. Behav. **12:** 861–874.

8. MAZUR, J.E. 1986. Choice between single and multiple delayed reinforcers. J. Exp. Anal. Behav. **46:** 67–78.
9. MAZUR, J.E., J.R. STELLAR & M. WARACZYNSKI. 1987. Self-control choice with electrical stimulation of the brain. Behav. Processes **15:** 143–153.
10. GREEN, L. & H. RACHLIN. 1991. Economic substitutability of electrical brain stimulation, food, and water. J. Exp. Anal. Behav. **55:** 133–143.
11. ROBBINS, T.W. & B.J. EVERITT. 1996. Neurobehavioral mechanisms of reward and motivation. Curr. Opin. Neurobiol. **6:** 228–236.
12. SCHULTZ, W., P. DAYAN & P.R. MONTAGUE. 1997. A neural substrate of prediction and reward. Science **275:** 1593–1599.
13. BREITER H.C., R.L. GOLLUB, R.M. WEISSKOFF, D.N. KENNEDY, N. MAKRIS, J.D. BERKE, J.M. GOODMAN, H.L. KANTOR, D.R. GASTFRIEND, J.P. RIORDEN, R.T. MATHEW, B.R. ROSEN & S.E. HYMAN. 1997. Acute effects of cocaine on human brain activity and emotion. Neuron **19:** 591–611.
14. HEIMER, L., R.E. HARLAN, G.F. ALHEID, M.M. GARCIA & J. DE OLMOS. 1997. Substantia innominata: a notion which impedes clinical-anatomical correlations in neuropsychiatric disorders. Neuroscience **76(4):** 957–1006.
15. ALHEID, G.F. & L. HEIMER. 1988. New perspectives in basal forebrain organization of special relevance for neuropsychiatric disorders; the striatopallidal, amygdaloid, and corticopetal components of substantia innominata. Neuroscience **27:** 1–39.
16. GOLLUB, R., H. BREITER, R. WEISSKOFF, W. KENNEDY, H. KANTOR, D. KENNEDY, D. GASTFRIEND, T. MATTHEW, N. MAKRIS, A. GUIMARES, J. RIORDEN, S, HYMAN, B. ROSEN & R. WEISSKOFF. 1998. Cocaine decreases cortical blood flow, but does not obscure regional activation in functional magnetic resonance imaging in human subjects. J. Cereb. Blood Flow Metab. **18(7):** 724–34.
17. BREITER, H.C., R.L. GOLLUB, W. EDMINSTER, T. TALAVAGE, N. MAKRIS, J. MELCHER, D. KENNEDY, H. KANTOR, I. ELMAN, J. RIORDEN, D. GASTFRIEND, T. CAMPBELL, M. FOLEY, R.M. WEISSKOFF & B.R. ROSEN. 1998. Cocaine induced brainstem and subcoartical activity observed through fMRI with cardiac gating. Proc. Int. Soc. Magn. Reson. Med. **1:** 499.
18. JOHANSON, C.E. & M.W. FISCHMAN. 1989. The pharmacology of cocaine related to its abuse. Pharmacol. Rev. **41:** 3–52.
19. ARVANITOGIANNIS, A., M. WARACZYNSKI & P. SHIZGAL. 1996. Effects of excitotoxic lesions of the basal forebrain on MFB self-stimulation. Physiol. & Behav. **59(4/5):** 795–806.
20. EVERITT, B.J., K.A. MORRIS, A. O'BRIEN & T.W. ROBBINS. 1991. The basolateral amygdala-ventral striatal system and conditioned place preference: further evidence of limbic-striatal interactions underlying reward-related processes. J. Neurosci. **42:** 1–18.
21. BREITER, H.C., N.L. ETCOFF, P.J. WHALEN, W.A. KENNEDY, S.L. RAUCH, R.L. BUCKNER, M.M. STRAUSS, S.E. HYMAN & B.R. ROSEN. 1996a. Response and habituation of the human amygdala during visual processing of facial expression. Neuron **17:** 875–887.
22. BREITER, H.C., S.L. RAUCH, K.K. KWONG, J.R. BAKER, R.M. WEISSKOFF, D.N. KENNEDY, A.D. KENDRICK, T.L. DAVIS, A. JIANG, M.S. COHEN, C.E. STERN, J.W. BELLIVEAU, L. BAER, R.L. O'SULLIVAN, C.R. SAVAGE, M.A. JENIKE & B.R. ROSEN. 1996b. Functional magnetic resonance imaging of symptom provocation in obsessive-compulsive disorder. Arch. Gen. Psychiatry **53:** 595–606.
23. CARELLI, R.M. & S.A. DEADWYLER. 1996. Dual factors controlling activity of nucleus accumbens cell-firing during cocaine self-administration. Synapse **24:** 308–311.
24. LYND-BALTA, E. & S.N. HABER. 1994. The organization of midbrain projections to the ventral striatum in the primate. Neuroscience **59:** 609–623.
25. HEIMER, L., G.F. ALHEID, J.S. DE OLMOS, H.J. GROENEWEGEN, S.N. HABER, R.E. HARLAN & D.S. ZAHM. 1997. The accumbens: beyond the core-shell dichotomy. J. Neuropsychiatry Clin. Neurosci. **9(3):** 354–81.

26. SCHULTZ, W., P. APICELLA & T. LJUNGBERG. 1993. Responses of monkey dopamine neurons to reward and conditioned stimuli during successive steps of learning a delayed response task. J. Neurosci. **13**(3): 900–913.
27. PEOPLES, L.L. & M.O. WEST. 1996. Phasic firing of single neurons in the rat nucleus accumbens correlated with the timing of intravenous cocaine self-administration. J. Neurosci. **16**(10): 3459–3473.
28. GUIMARES, A.R., J.R. MELCHER, T.M. TALAVAGE, J.R. BAKER, B.R. ROSEN & R.M. WEISSKOFF. 1996. Detection of inferior colliculus activity during auditory stimulation using cardiac gated functional MRI with T1 correction. NeuroImage **3**(3): S9.
29. EDMINSTER, W.B., T.M. TALAVAGE, P.J. LEDDEN & R.M. WEISSKOFF. 1999. Improved auditory cortex imaging using clustered volume acquisitions. Hum. Brain Map **7**(2): 89–97.
30. SEIDMAN, L.J., H.C. BREITER, J.M. GOLDSTEIN, J.M. GODDMAN, M. WARD, P.W.R. WOODRUFF, S.V. FARAONE, D.N. KENNEDY, R.M. WEISSKOFF, B.R. ROSEN & M.T. TSUANG. 1997. Functional MRI of attention in relatives of schizophrenic patients. Schizophr. Res. **24**: 172.
31. GOLDSTEIN, J.M., L.J. SEIDMAN, R. ANAGNOSON, J.M. GOODMAN, R. WEISSKOFF, M.F. WARD, M.R. PATTI, S.V. FARAONE, M.T. TSUANG, B.R. ROSEN & H. BREITER. 1998. An fMRI study of sex differences in auditory verbal working memory in normals. NeuroImage **7**(4): S854.
32. BREITER, H.C., L.J. SEIDMAN, J.M. GOODMAN, J.M. GOLDSTEIN, K.M. O'CRAVEN, R.M. WEISSKOFF, P.W.R. WOODRUFF, R. SAVOY, A. JIANG, D. KENNEDY, W. KENNEDY, M.T. TSUANG & B.R. ROSEN. 1995a. fMRI of effortful attention using Talairach averaging across subjects. Proc. Soc. Magn. Reson./Eur. Soc. Magn. Reson. Med. Biol. Joint Meeting **3**: 1348.
33. BREITER, H.C., L.J. SEIDMAN, J.M. GOODMAN, J.M. GOLDSTEIN, K.M. O'CRAVEN, R.M. WEISSKOFF, P.W.R. WOODRUFF, R. SAVOY, A. JIANG, D. KENNEDY, W. KENNEDY, M.T. TSUANG & B.R. ROSEN. 1995b. Functional MRI of auditory effortful attention in humans. Proc. Soc. Neurosci. **3**: 1988.
34. SEIDMAN, L.J., H.C. BREITER, J.M. GOODMAN, J.M. GOLDSTEIN, P.W.R., K. O'CRAVEN, R. SAVOY, D. KENNEDY, J. BAKER, K. KWONG, M.T. TSUANG & B.R. ROSEN. 1996. Development of auditory continuous performance tests for functional MRI. Biol. Psychiatry **39**: 636.
35. SEIDMAN, L.J., H.C. BREITER, J.M. GOLDSTEIN, P.W.R. WOODRUFF, K. O'CRAVEN, R. SAVOY, M.T. TSUANG & B.R. ROSEN. 1998. A functional magnetic resonance imagining study of auditory vigilance with low and high information processing demands. Neuropsychology **12**(4): 505–518.
36. BERNS, G.S., J.D. COHEN & M.A. MINTUN. 1997. Brain regions responsive to novelty in the absence of awareness. Science **276**: 1272–1275.
37. TAGHZOUTI, K., A. LOUILOT, J.P. HERMAN, M. LE MOAL & H. SIMON. 1985. Alternative behavioral, spatial discrimination, and 6-hydroxydopamine lesions in the nucleus accumbens of the rat. Behav. Neural Biol. **44**(3): 354–363.
38. MOGENSON, G.J., D.L. JONES & C.Y. YIM. 1980. From motivation to action: functional iterface between the limbic system and the motor system. Prog. Neurobiol. **14**(2–3): 69–97.
39. STERN, C.E. & R.E. PASSINGHAM. 1995. The nucleus accumbens in monkeys (*Macaca fascicularis*): III. Reversal learning. Exp. Brain Res. **106**: 239–247.
40. KAHNEMAN, D. 1973. Attention and effort. Prentice Hall. Englewood Cliffs, NJ.
41. GIBBON, J. 1977. Scalar expectancy theory and Weber's law in animal timing. Psychol. Rev. **84**: 279–325.
42. GIBBON, J., R.M. CHURCH, S. FAIRHURST & A. KACELNIK. 1988. Scalar expectancy theory and choice between delayed rewards. Psychol. Rev. **95**: 102–114.
43. GALLAGHER, M. & A.A. CHIBA. 1996. The amygdala and emotion. Curr. Opin. Neurobiol. **6**: 221–227.
44. SHIZGAL, P. & K. CONOVER. 1996. On the neural computation of utility. Curr. Directions Psychol. Sci. **5**(2): 37–43.

45. ROMPRE, P.P. & P. SHIZGAL. 1986. Electrophysiological characteristics of neurons in forebrain regions implicated in self-stimulation of the medial forebrain bundle in the rat. Brain Res. **364:** 338–349.
46. SHIZGAL, P. & B. MURRAY. 1989. Neuronal basis of intracranial self-stimulation. *In* The neuropharmacological basis of reward. J.M. Lieman & S.J. Coopers, Eds.: 106–163. Oxford University Press. Oxford.
47. KOOB, G.F., P.P. SANA & F.E. BLOOM. 1998. Neuroscience of addiction. Neuron **21:** 1–20.
48. SCHULTZ, W., P. APICELLA, E. SCARNATI & T. LJUNGBERG. 1992. Neuronal activity in monkey ventral striatum related to the expectation of reward. J. Neurosci. **12:** 4595–4610.
49. WILLIAMS, G.V. 1989. Neuronal activity in the primate caudate nucleus and ventral striatum reflects the association between stimuli determining behavior. *In* Neural Mechanisms in Disorders of Movement. A.R. Crossman & M.A. Sambrook, Eds.: 63–73. John Libbey. London.
50. BREITER, H.C., J.D. BERKE, W.A. KENNEDY, B.R. ROSEN & S.E. HYMAN. 1996c. Activation of striatum and amygdala during reward conditioning: an fMRI study. NeuroImage **3(3):** S220.
51. TAI, C.T., A.J.M. CLARK, J. FELDON & J.N.P. RAWLINS. 1991. Electrolytic lesions of the nucleus accumbens in rats which abolish the PREE enhance the locomotor response to amphetamine. Exp. Brain Res. **86:** 333–340.
52. STERN, C.E. & R.E. PASSINGHAM. 1996. The nucleus accumbens in monkeys (*Macaca fascicularis*): II. Emotion and motivation. Behav. Brain Res. **75:** 179–193.
53. ECCLES, J.C. 1989. Evolution of the Brain, Creation of the Self. Routledge. New York.
54. MACLEAN, P.D. 1986. Culminating developments in the evolution of the limbic system: the thalamocingulate division. *In* The Limbic System: Functional Organization and Clinical Disorders. B.K. Doane & K.E. Livingston, Eds. Raven Press. New York.
55. WISE, R.A. 1982. Neuroleptics and operant behavior: the anhedonia hypothesis. Behav. Brain Sci. **5:** 39–87.
56. ROBINSON, T.E. & K.C. BERRIDGE. 1993. The neural basis of drug craving: an incentive-sensitization theory of addiction. Brain Res. Brain Res. Rev. **18:** 247–291.
57. BLACKBURN, J., J. PFAUS & A. PHILLIPS. 1992. Dopamine functions in appetitive and defensive behaviors. Prog. Neurobiol. **3:** 247–279.
58. SALAMONE, J.D., M.S. COUSINS & B.J. SNYDER. 1997. Behavioral functions of nucleus accumbens dopamine empirical and conceptual problems with the anhedonia hypothesis. Neurosci. Biobehav. Rev. **21:** 341–359.
59. WEISS, S.R.B., R.M. POST, A. PERT, R. WOODWARD & D. MURMAN. 1989. Context-dependent cocaine sensitization: differential effect of haloperidol on development versus expression. Pharmacol. Biochem. Behav. **34:** 655.
60. EVERITT, B.J. 1997. Craving cocaine cues: cognitive neuroscience meets drug addiction research. Trends Cogn. Sci. **1(1):** 1–2.
61. KAHNEMAN, D., P.P. WAKKER & R. SARIN. 1997. Back to Bentham? Explorations of experienced utility. Q. J. Economics **112(2):** 375–405.
62. CHILDRESS, A.R. *et al.* 1999. Brain correlates of cue-induced cocaine and opiate craving. Am. J. Psychol. **22:** 933.
63. GRANT, S., E. LONDON, D. NEWLIN, V. VILLEMAGNE, X. LIU, C. CONTOREGGI, R. PHILLIPS & A. MARGOLIN. 1996. Activation of memory circuits during cue-elicited cocaine craving. Proc. Natl. Acad. Sci. USA **93:** 12040–12045.
64. SCHWEITZER, J. *et al.* 1996. The neuroanatomy of drug craving in crack cocaine addiction: a PET analysis. Soc. Neurosci. Abstr. **22:** 933.
65. ITO, N., H. ISHIDA, F. MIYAKAWA & H. NAITO. 1974. Microelectrode study of projections from the amygdaloid complex to the nucleus accumbens in the cat. Brain Res. **67:** 338–341.
66. YIM, C.Y. & G.J. MOGENSON. 1982. Response of nucleus accumbens neurons to amygdala stimulation and its modification by dopamine. Brain Res. **239:** 401–415.

67. RUSSCHEN, F.T., I. BAKST, D.G. AMARAL & J.L. PRICE. 1985. The amygdalostiatal projections in the monkey. An anterograde tracing study. Brain Res. **329:** 241–257.
68. AMARAL, D.G., J.L. PRICE, A. PITKANEN & S.T. CARMICHAEL. 1992. Anatomical organization of the primate amygdala complex. *In* The Amygdala. J.P. Aggleton, Ed. John Wiley-Liss. New York.
69. JONES, B. & M. MISHKIN. 1972. Limbic lesion and the problem of stimulus-reinforcement association. Exp. Neurol. **36:** 362–377.
70. SPIEGLER, B.J. & M. MISHKIN. 1981. Evidence for the sequential participation of inferior temporal cortex and amygdala in the acquisition of stimulus-reward associations. Behav. Brain Res. **3:** 303–317.
71. GAFFAN, D. & S. HARRISON. 1987. Amygdalectomy and disconnection in visual learning for auditory secondary reinforcement by monkeys. J. Neurosci. **7:** 2285–2292.
72. GAFFAN, D. & S. HARRISON. 1988. Disconnection of the amygdala from visual association cortex impairs visual reward-association learning in monkeys. J. Neurosci. **8:** 3144–3150.
73. CADOR, M., T.W. ROBBINS & B.J. EVERITT. 1989. Involvment of the amygdala in stimulus-reward association: interaction with the ventral stratium. Neuroscience **30**(1)**:** 77–86.
74. LEDOUX, J.E. 1992. Emotion and the amygdala. *In* The amygdala: neurobiological aspects of emotion, memory and mental dysfunction. J.P. Aggleton, Ed.: 339–351. Wiley-Liss. New York.
75. HATFIELD, T., J.-S. HAN, M. CONLEY, M. GALLAGHER & P. HOLLAND. 1996. Neurotoxic lesions of basolateral, but not central, amygdala interfere with pavlovian second-order conditioning and reinforcer devaluation effects. J. Neurosci. **16:** 5256–5265.
76. ROLLS, E.T. 1991. The processing of face information in the primate temporal lobe. *In* Processing Images of Faces. V. Bruce & M. Burton, Eds. Ablex. Norwood, NJ.

Epilepsy, Schizophrenia, and the Extended Amygdala

JANICE R. STEVENS[a]

Department of Neurology and Psychiatry, Oregon Health Sciences University, Portland, Oregon 97201, USA

ABSTRACT: Propagation and prolongation of rapid neuronal discharge underlies the epilepsies. However, episodic focal rapid neuronal discharges limited to discrete nuclei and pathways of the amygdala-hippocampal-septal-hypothalamic networks are the language of physiologic message systems for endocrine regulation and reproductive activities vital to the survival of the organism and the species. To prevent prolongation and propagation of physiologic pulsed excitation to areas outside specific networks and resultant epileptic seizures, these discharges must be limited in extent and time by powerful inhibitory processes. The nucleus accumbens, a unit of the extended amygdala, and the monoamines and GABA are components of the inhibitory networks that restrict physiologic rapid discharge in duration and in location. In parallel to the relationship of excessive neuronal excitation to epilepsy, evidence will be presented that excessive inhibition via one or more components of these inhibitory networks or diminished excitation underlies development of some psychoses, including schizophrenia.

INTRODUCTION

Struck by the similarity of the hallucinations of patients with schizophrenia to the auras experienced by some individuals who suffered from temporal lobe epilepsy (TLE), 25 years ago I wrote two papers in which I speculated on the possible common anatomic basis of these two disorders.[1,2] The striking difference between these two afflictions, however, was the fact that the individual with epilepsy always recognizes that his aura is "unreal," that the voices are not really talking to him, but are a warning of an oncoming seizure. By contrast, the schizophrenic patient is generally certain the voices he heard are real, often replies to them, and unfortunately, not too rarely, even acts upon the orders of the voices that could harangue him incessantly and even command him to injure himself or others. Clinically, the difference is that the epileptic aura is brief, rarely lasting more than seconds, whereas the schizophrenic hallucinations and delusions can last for hours, or even days and years. Furthermore, if followed by a motor seizure, the aura of TLE is then always associated with loss of consciousness. Thereafter, activity during the seizure is generally limited to commonplace, stereotyped, or convulsive movements, and there is total amnesia for the motor part of the seizure. Loss of consciousness with TLE indicates that the high frequency discharge of excitatory neurons that is generally initiated in the amygdala,

---

[a]Voice: 503-494-8147; fax: 503-678-3216; stevenja@ohsu.edu

hippocampus, or other temporal lobe structures, propagates to brain centers that maintain consciousness.

By contrast, the schizophrenic patient often suffers cruelly from an incessant barrage of voices or from false sensations or beliefs, does not lose consciousness, and may very rarely, take actions totally against his true inclination. Although the content of hallucinatory or delusory experiences of schizophrenia may resemble some TLE auras, consciousness is not lost but is captured, like victors in a rebellion taking over a radio station and broadcasting their own message while the owner stands by and listens. Where is that radio station and how does it lose focus? Those are the questions that investigators of schizophrenia have been trying to solve for more than a century.

Unfortunately, schizophrenia investigators do not have the lucky clue that Hans Berger offered epileptologists—the electroencephalogram (EEG). The scalp EEG is abnormal in more than 70% of individuals with epilepsy and often points to the region where the seizure is initiated. In schizophrenia, by contrast, the EEG is generally normal, or if abnormal, is nonspecifically so. There is one exception: when depth electrodes were placed in various subcortical loci in schizophrenic patients, by a few intrepid investigators, single intermittent spikes, similar to those recorded over the scalp *between*, but not during, epileptic seizures, and never coalescing into the rapid rhythmic discharges that are characteristic of epileptic seizures, were recorded from the septal-accumbens area.[3] The search for a pathologic substrate for schizophrenia has now, by quite a different route than the EEG, led us to that same area of the brain, the nucleus accumbens septi, part of Heimer's extended amygdala, and a major way station from amygdala nucleus and hippocampus for pathways en route via ventral pallidum to thalamus and cerebral cortex.

A search of Medline for references to the nucleus accumbens will find none prior to 1976, and under septum only 136 references are cited (TABLE 1). Between 1976 and 1980 there were 238 references to nucleus accumbens, and between 1992 and 1997, the number of citations rose to 1161, while septum listed only 203 citations. Much of the interest in the nucleus accumbens springs directly from its possible relationship to schizophrenia, based not on the intracerebral EEG findings, which unfortunately, are not widely known, but derived directly from the work of anatomists, including many of those included in this volume. In this communication, I will try to summarize the neuropathologic studies of schizophrenia, especially as they have progressed since 1985, when I attempted a review of neuropathologic reports up to that time.[4]

The great variety of abnormalities found in subgroups of patients with schizophrenia and the failure to detect any pathology in the brain of substantial numbers of these individuals is reminiscent of neuropathologic studies of epilepsy, in which no specific pathology is detected in more than half the brains examined.[5] Epilepsy is a disorder that represents, physiologically, excessive focal or general neuronal excitation (or decreased inhibition) in some brain region or regions. By contrast, evidence will be presented that schizophrenia appears to be a manifestation of excessive inhibition, that is, a physiologic reciprocal of seizures.[6] This is manifest by abnormal expression of inhibitory transmitters or their receptors in one or more critical brain areas, leading to a loss of focus and of attention allowing intrusion of alien ideas. All neuroleptic drugs, the most successful weapon against the symptoms of schizophrenia, antagonize one or more of these inhibitory mechanisms.

TABLE 1. Nucleus accumbens: Number of citings in Index Medicus, 1966–1997

Year	N. accumbens	Septal nucleus	Ratio
1966–1975 (9 yr)	0	136	0: 136
1976–1980	238	315	0.75: 1
1981–86	650	525	1.2: 1
1987–1992	997	585	1.7: 1
1993–1997	1161	205	5.7: 1

THE NEUROPATHOLOGIES OF SCHIZOPHRENIA

Studies of brain morphology and histopathology have been greatly augmented by the introduction of immunocytochemistry and *in situ* hybridization for specific proteins in post-mortem material and by cerebral imaging with computerized tomography, magnetic resonance imaging, positron emission tomography, functional NMR, and spectroscopy in living patients. Although many differences from normal patients have been reported, no single or constellation of findings appears to be universal or uniquely present in the brains of individuals with schizophrenia .

Usually, only pooled averaged data, with standard deviations and statistical probabilities of differences from controls are presented for schizophrenia. When individual data are available, however, it is evident that each of the abnormalities reported occurs only in some proportion of individuals. This would also be true for brains of individuals with epilepsy if the neuropathologic data from patients with various epilepsies were pooled, averaged, and deviations from normal controls calculated. But no one would pool and average epilepsy data, because it is recognized that epilepsy is a syndrome, a final common path for a number of anatomic and physiologic disturbances. The same may be the case for schizophrenia, demanding similar changes in analytic methods.

In contrast to most neurological disorders, which, with few exceptions exhibit pathologic changes that explain much of the clinical syndrome (e.g., multiple sclerosis, Alzheimer's disease, cerebral palsy, Wernicke's encephalopathy, Parkinson's disease, and Huntington's chorea), no specific neuropathologic lesion, as yet, identifies either epilepsy or schizophrenia. In the case of epilepsy, however, the enormous variety of pathologic and biochemical changes that has been demonstrated led to revision of the old classification of seizures, previously based on a few common phenotypes, to a large number of more narrowly defined syndromes based on specific neurophysiologic, neuropathologic, genetic, and biochemical abnormalities. In this communication, I propose that the neuropathology of schizophrenia might benefit from similar disaggregation, based on the anatomy, histology, genetic markers, and pathophysiology of subgroups of patients. This requires presenting individual pathologic data rather than using only pooled averages as the basis for classification and then seeking which clinical characteristics, including the course of the disorder, characterize individuals with a specific pathology. This could supplement the now common practice of pooling and averaging diverse pathologic data from ever-larger numbers of individuals who meet current criteria for schizophrenia.

TABLE 2. Brain structural deviations of schizophrenics from controls

---
Lateral ventricles: Increased volume of lateral ventricles:[8,15,16]
    12 of 21 imaging studies[9]
    No change: 1st break; [51] Chronic:[52]
III ventricle: Increased volume: 1st break:[51] 7 of 9 studies[9]
Decreased brain weight (fixed specimens):[10,53]
    Not found: (fresh brain)[8,54]
Brain volume decreased: 6/28 MRI meta-analysis ($n = 413$ patients)
    No significant decrease: 22/28 MRI meta-analysis[55]
Intracranial volume: increased 3/19 MRIs and CTs[55]
    No significant change: 16/19 studies[55]
Head circumference: normal or increased[56]
    Normal: 9/10 studies[55]
Thalamus: Decreased volume;[57–59] periventricular grey in 12/13[36]
    No decrease found[7,60]
Amygdala, hippocampus, volume decreased: 7/13 schizphrenic brains[7]
Medial temporal lobe: decreased[14,61]
    Not found: averaged data[62]
Cortical grey matter: Decreased: averaged data,[64]
    No difference: averaged data:[63,54]
Sulcal width increased 4/8 CT studies[9]
Decreased size of superior temporal gyrus[65]
    Not found[66]
Assymetry of planum temporale[67]
    Not found[68]

There are a few changes in *some* schizophrenic brains that are widely accepted, some of which have been noted for nearly a century,[8] and have repeatedly been demonstrated in neuropathologic and cerebral imaging studies. Enlargement of the lateral cerebral ventricles, the most common reported brain abnormality in schizophrenia, is recognized in 20–25% of individuals, and in up to 50% the third ventricle is enlarged (TABLE 2). Seven of 13 schizophrenics have loss of tissue in the amygdala and/or hippocampus in the neuropathologic studies of schizophrenia by Bogerts *et al.*[7] Bilateral decrease in these structures has been reported in pooled, averaged data from several other neuropathologic and neuroimaging studies (TABLE 2). Medial temporal atrophy, usually unilateral, is also characteristic of approximately 50% of individuals with TLE. Widening of cerebral sulci is reported in averaged data from some imaging studies of schizophrenia, but the percentage of individuals affected is seldom given. In contrast to a clear subgroup of individuals with epilepsy and mental retardation in whom cranial size may be reduced, head circumference and intracranial volume are generally normal in schizophrenia (TABLE 2). This suggests that reported tissue loss has occurred after the skull has reached adult size and raises some doubt about currently popular neurodevelopmental theories stressing prenatal etiology. Enlargement of ventricles and cortical sulci are not unique to schizophrenia, nor generally present in the same individual. These findings indicate that there may be at least three kinds of schizophrenia, one in which loss of brain substance is prima-

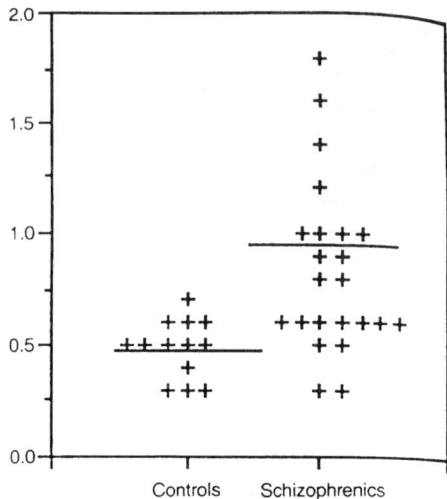

FIGURE 1. Scattergram from MRI of area (cm^2) of the most anterior section of the third ventricle in control (mean 0.480 ± 0.04) and schizophrenic (0.83 ± 0.08) subjects. ($p < 0.05$). Kelsoe et al.[12] (With permission from *Archives of General Psychiatry*.)

rily subcortical, a smaller group in which there is shrinkage or hypoplasia of cortical structures, and a third group in which neither cerebral atrophy nor ventricular enlargement is detected. Fourth and fifth subgroups might be those individuals with medial or lateral temporal lobe pathology.[7,10] As is the case for epilepsy, there are also a number of diverse brain lesions, including neoplasms and anomalies, in which schizophrenia may occur as a secondary phenomenon.[11]

FIGURE 1, which is fairly representative of the few cerebral imaging studies that present individual data, illustrates the distribution of what is perhaps the most common abnormality, increased third ventricular volume. Although the difference in mean area of the third ventricle of 23 schizophrenics is almost twice that of controls ($p < 0.01$), only 12/23 schizophrenic third ventricles in this sample are larger than the largest control.[12] Although it could be argued that in the absence of a bimodal distribution, all the patients have experienced third ventricular enlargement greater than normal, compared to their own baseline, this is not necessarily the case. Instead, the data may indicate that some within the schizophrenia group did not experience an increase in third ventricular volume and have a different pathophysiology. This is even more evident in lateral ventricle studies, in which only 20–25% of schizophrenic brains generally demonstrate enlargement compared to controls.[12]

In an attempt to sort this out, Nair et al.[13] reported that although ventricular volumes in normal patients and schizophrenics are normally distributed, the amount of volume change between scans taken at the first episode of illness and two years later is clearly larger for nearly half of the schizophrenic group than volume change in similarly studied normal patients over the same period. Other investigators, examining patients at both first break and the two-year follow-up have reached similar conclusions.[14] This is the case even though most patients in these studies had been ill

TABLE 3. Histologic and immunohistologic findings reported in schizophrenia: postmortem studies, 1983–1998[a]

Hippocampus: Decreased pyramidal cells[69]
Not found[70]
Abnormal orientation of neurons[71]
Not found[70,72]
Decreased MAP 2, 5, in hippocampal subfields[73]
Decreased synaptophysin mRNA[74]
Decreased Glu R1 Glu R2[75]
Entorhinal cortex: Abnormal architecture in 40% of cases[76,77]
Not found[78]
Thalamus: Decreased neurons in mediodorsal nucleus[79,80]
Prefrontal and cingulate cortex: Upregulation of GABA A receptor binding[81,82]
Decreased small neuron density[83]
Increased neuron density[84]
No change[88]
Increased vertical axons cingulate cortex[86]
Decreased GAD gene expression[85]
Abnormal migration of NADPH cells[87,88]
Association cortex: Increased GAP-43[89]
Gliosis: Periventricular, periaqueductal, subcortical[4,90,91]
No glial increase in cortex, brain stem, thalamus, limbic structures[51,91,92]
None in "purified" sample[53]
Fibrin degradation products increased: possible marker for inflammation[93]

[a]Pooled, averaged data; difference from controls: $p < 0.05$.

for two years or more at the time of the first examination. If the prodromal and early period of the illness had been included, more patients may have shown significant change in ventricular volume, as was reported for subgroups in early pneumoencephalographic studies.[15,16] If, as the neuropathologic data suggest, schizophrenia is, like epilepsy, a heterogeneous syndrome, averaging data from large numbers of patients may obscure the significance of increased ventricular volume (and many other findings) in terms of etiology, clinical course, and response to treatment.

TABLE 2 summarizes some of the gross anatomic data from the very large number of studies reported, and includes, when available, the number or percentage of individuals in whom these measurements are more than one standard deviation from the control mean. As is apparent, there is no unanimity of findings in this representative sample of pathologies, and no single finding is present in all schizophrenic patients. Histology, immunohistochemistry, and *in situ* hybridization studies of various brain areas present an even larger number and more variable galaxy of findings (TABLE 3). Again, actual numbers in subgroups with normal or abnormal values are rarely reported. For this reason, the significance of the data presented in TABLES 2 and 3 is difficult to interpret. When individual values are published, there is nearly always a considerable overlap with control values (FIG. 1).

Inasmuch as it is unlikely that each of the pathologies presented in TABLES 2 and 3 represents a separate cause of schizophrenia, a major question is how many of these individual brains demonstrate significant deviations from the norm in more

TABLE 4. Schizophrenia and epilepsy

	Schizophrenia	Epilepsy
Prevalence	1%	0.5–1%
Concordance MZ twins	45%	40–45%
Enlarged ventricles	20–30%	20-30%
Cortical atrophy	@10%	10%
Cerebral malformations	@1+% ?	@10%
Microneurogenesis	?	5–10%
Atrophic hippocampus	@5–10%	10–20%
Clinical course deterioration	@10%	10–20%
Mental retardation	18.5% (3% after DSM III)	@20%
Obstetrical complications	2–4%	4–5%
Evoked auditory potentials	decreased amplitude	increased amplitude
EEG (scalp) abnormal	20–25%	70%

than one domain. Unfortunately, few laboratories can conduct more than one or two assays in the same areas of the same brains. Thus, the relationship between most of these findings is unknown.

SCHIZOPHRENIA AND EPILEPSY

Over the past 50 years, metabolic and genetic studies, considerably assisted by research in animal models, have disclosed a great variety of causes of epileptic seizures. Although some specific types of epilepsy demonstrate a specific pathology, and are considered "symptomatic," around 65% do not and are hence classified as "idiopathic" or "cryptogenic."[5] More than 100 different genetic abnormalities have been associated with the myoclonic and generalized epilepsies. The most common focal epilepsy, temporal lobe or psychomotor epilepsy, is associated with a specific pathology, hippocampal gliosis, in around 50% of cases. Another 10% of individuals with this diagnosis have neoplasms, scars, or anomalies of temporal lobe structures, whereas the remainder show no gross or histologic pathology.[17] Using special stains, pathologic sprouting of glutamate fibers from the granule cell layer and increase in glutamate AMPA receptors of the hippocampus can be demonstrated in a number of affected individuals whose temporal lobe or hippocampus has been removed for treatment of seizures.[18,19] Other focal epilepsies are associated with a large variety of lesions and anomalies. The most common causes, head injury, obstetric complications, meningitis, encephalitis, and congenital anomalies each contribute 5–10 percent. As in schizophrenia, a family history of epilepsy is present in fewer than half of those affected but is more common in individuals with epilepsy than in those without (TABLE 4). Concordance rates, as for schizophrenia, reach 45% in monozygotic twins.[20] Most commonly, some combination of genetic, maturational, or metabolic disturbances and brain injury or malformation have an additive effect on the expression of the epileptic syndrome.

Epileptic seizures are due to excessive propagation of rapid rhythmic discharges of neurons in focal or diffuse areas of the brain. Such discharges occur secondary to a large variety of neuropathologic, neurochemical, and molecular changes in which the normally carefully regulated control of neuronal excitability is disturbed. Predisposing genetic determinants may define the sites of vulnerability as well as whether and which excitatory or inhibitory systems respond to restore compensation for disequilibria initiated by brain injury, infection, stress, or the physiologic events of maturation and reproduction. In this essay I propose that in schizophrenia the compensatory changes in response to similar events err on the side of excessive inhibition.

EXCESS EXCITATION FOR EPILEPSY; EXCESS INHIBITION FOR SCHIZOPHRENIA

What is the evidence that schizophrenia is related to one or more inhibitory systems or to a pathologic deficit of excitability? The arguments for excess inhibition in schizophrenia are very similar to those for increased excitability as the final cause of epilepsy.

Following his observation that epileptic seizures were uncommon among patients with schizophrenia and that seizures often decreased in epileptics who developed psychotic symptoms, Meduna[21] proposed that there was a biological antagonism between these two disorders. On this basis, he introduced convulsive therapy, which became the first successful remedy for treatment of schizophrenia. The Swiss neurologist Landolt[22] also observed that schizophrenia-like psychoses were prone to occur in some patients with epilepsy when seizures decreased spontaneously or normalization of the EEG followed treatment. Whereas epilepsy is generally associated with a decreased threshold for induced seizures, individuals with schizophrenia have an increased threshold.[23]

All the modern anticonvulsants that are successfully used to treat epilepsy reduce brain excitability, principally via blockade of Ca^+ or Na^+ ion channels or by GABA and monoamine enhancement.[24] By contrast, all of the neuroleptics, the most important pharmacologic agents for treatment of schizophrenia, antagonize inhibitory transmission and are proconvulsive.

One of the most effective of these agents, and one that is often more successful in ameliorating symptoms in otherwise drug-resistant schizophrenia, is clozapine, the most proconvulsive neuroleptic. Clozapine causes epileptiform EEG changes in approximtely 20% of patients, or myoclonic or generalized seizures in 2–10% of those treated with the drug in average doses, and lowers the seizure threshold for myoclonic seizures in animals in a dose-dependent fashion.[25–27] Clozapine opposes the action of a number of inhibitory physiologic transmitters, including dopamine (DA), serotonin, norepinephrine (NE), gamma-amino-butyric acid (GABA), and the action of glutamate antagonists. In addition to reducing the occupation of DA, NE, and serotonin receptors by their respective ligands, clozapine is a potent antagonist of excitatory (NMDA) antagonists,[28–30] opposing their psychotogenic effect and enhancing central excitability. These multiple actions may explain why clozapine is the most proconvulsive (and thus anti-inhibitory) and perhaps why clozapine is the most successful neuroleptic against symptoms of drug-resistant schizophrenia.

Clozapine is more potent than other neuroleptics in causing expression of the early gene product Fos in midline thalamic nuclei, medial frontal lobe paralimbic cortex, and nucleus accumbens shell.[31] "Kindled" myoclonus induced by weekly small doses of clozapine in the rat is associated with expression of cFos mRNA in anterior thalamic and ventral tegmental areas.[32] These findings suggest that the special therapeutic benefit of clozapine may relate to the more effective blockade by this agent of inhibition expressed by specific receptors that normally limit propagation of the physiologic excitatory volleys of the neuroendocrine and attention systems that surround the third ventricle, as well as the striatal projection site for limbic nuclei in the nucleus accumbens.[2,33] Neuroleptics in general, but clozapine in particular, may thus restore more normal excitability to central regions that are damaged or overinhibited in the schizophrenias.

SCHIZOPHRENIA, EPILEPSY, AND REGULATION OF THE NEUROENDOCRINE SYSTEM

The critical balance between excitation and inhibition is manifest everywhere in the nervous system, but nowhere more strikingly than in the neuroendocrine system. The periventricular nuclei of the hypothalamus present a veritable cornucopia of monoamine, glutamate, and GABA axon terminals and receptor types, as well as containing both neurons and receptors of the neuroendocrine system.[34,35] Lesch and Bogerts[36] reported narrowing of the periventricular nuclei in 5 of 13 schizophrenic brains they examined from the Vogt collection. As shown in FIGURE 1, third ventricle enlargement is often the first or only part of the ventricular system that is enlarged, compared to controls in imaging studies of schizophrenia. Neuropathologic studies by a few investigators have shown a decrease in size or number of neurons in specific thalamic nuclei (TABLE 3). Third ventricle enlargement in schizophrenia may or may not relate to a decrease in volume of medial thalamic or hypothalamic nuclei, afferents, efferents, and/or to the reported decrease in size or number of neurons in the amygdala and hippocampal projection sites to these areas, in some cases.

Rapid neuronal discharges, similar in frequency, but shorter in duration and more sharply localized than those that are associated with epileptic seizures, occur in specific subcortical brain nuclei during normal physiologic activity and during sleep.[37,38] These high-frequency circumscribed volleys are part of the normal communication repertoire of many subcortical nuclei of the brain, including hippocampus, amygdala, and other nuclei of the brain stem and limbic system. Under physiologic conditions, hypothalamic excitatory neurons, responsible for regulating the secretion of most hormones, discharge, in brief, high-frequency volleys at regular intervals. Phasic volleys of high-frequency neuronal discharge in specific limbic and hypothalamic nuclei trigger pulsed release of most hormones, including gonadotropic neuron regulatory hormone (GnRH), luteinizing hormone (LH), follicle-stimulating hormone (FSH), and corticotropic-releasing factor (CRF).[38–41] Volleys for the vital hormonal events of the reproductive period commence during puberty and are initially limited to sleep.[41,42] Subsequently, phasic neuronal discharge and hormone release occur in at 60–120 minute intervals throughout the day and night in both men and women.

Glutamate is the principal excitatory transmitter responsible for these vital events. Acetylcholine and estrogen are also excitatory at their appropriate receptors. Given the essential role of these excitatory transmitters in the maintenance of motor, perceptual, memory, and neuroendocrine functions, it is not surprising that nature has been equally generous in providing a wealth of inhibitory safeguards against excessive frequency, prolongation, or propagation of these physiologic excitatory events beyond the discrete times and areas that they are appropriate and necessary, and if unchecked could cause epileptic seizures. GABA and all the monoamines, especially DA, play vital roles in regulating the pulsatile secretion of GnRH, FSH, growth hormone, and prolactin. Some of these rhythms are disturbed in epilepsy and in schizophrenia.[43–45]

Epilepsy results from a number of causes that result in loss of physiologic balance between excitation and inhibition. It is proposed here that schizophrenia may also relate to an imbalance, yielding, however, focal overexpression of inhibition following brain injury or malformation and in limbic and hypothalamic nuclei and their projection sites, or coincident with stress and the events of puberty and the reproductive period. Glutamate axon sprouting and receptor expansion have been demonstrated in experimental epilepsy and in human hippocampi removed for temporal lobe epilepsy.[18,19] In parallel to sprouting of glutamate axons, other injuries or malformations may induce abnormal sprouting or receptor expansion in inhibitory systems in schizophrenia, as has been demonstrated following experimental brain injuries in animals.[47,48]

The normal equilibrium between excitation and inhibition can be permanently altered by repeated focal excitation or kindling, resulting in a permanent state of excessive focal excitability and spontaneous seizures.[49] Similar "kindling" or sensitization may be induced in inhibitory systems in response to focal physiologic pulsed discharges of limbic and hypothalamic neurons.[50] A more or less permanent excess of one or more inhibitory "factors" (transmitters, axons, receptors, or peptides) may then be manifest as a psychosis.

SUMMARY AND CONCLUSIONS

A great variety and number of gross, histologic, and molecular changes have been reported in subgroups of schizophrenic patients. This suggests that either the critical factor has not yet been found, or that there are many routes to schizophrenia. In this respect, schizophrenia resembles epilepsy, in which a wide number of neuropathologies, metabolic abnormalities, and genetic anomalies may lead to a similar final path in susceptible individuals, that is, hyperexcitability expressed in the various forms of the epileptic seizure. In this report, the data presented suggest that schizophrenia may represent a similar compensatory error, which is, however, a physiologic reciprocal of epilepsy, and in which the pathophysiology is excessive inhibition in one or more critical brain areas in response to a variety of factors. To disaggregate these data for schizophrenia, it may be more useful to classify the schizophrenias according to specific brain or cerebrospinal fluid pathologies and then to seek correlations with the clinical phenomenology, course, and epidemiology.

REFERENCES

1. STEVENS, J.R. 1973. Psychomotor epilepsy and schizophrenia: a common anatomy? *In* Epilepsy, Its Phenomena in Man. M.A.B. Brazier, Ed.: 189–214. Academic Press. New York.
2. STEVENS, J.R. 1973. An anatomy of schizophrenia? Arch. Gen. Psychiatry **29:** 177–189.
3. HEATH, R. 1959. Studies in schizophrenia. Harvard University Press. Cambridge, MA.
4. STEVENS, J.R. 1982. Neuropathology of schizophrenia. Arch. Gen. Psychiatry **39:** 1131–1139.
5. HAUSER, W.A. 1997. Incidence and Prevalence *In* Epilepsy: A Comprehensive Textbook. J. Engel Jr. & T.A. Pedley, Eds.: 47–57. Lippincott Raven. Philadelphia.
6. STEVENS, J.R. 1995. Clozapine: The yin and yang of seizures and psychosis. Biol. Psychiatry **37:** 425–426.
7. BOGERTS, B., E. MEERTZ, R. SCHONFELDT-BAUSCH. 1985. Basal ganglia and limbic system pathology in schizophrenia: a morphometric study of brain volume and shrinkage. Arch. Gen. Psychiatry **42:** 784–791.
8. SOUTHARD, E.E. 1915. On the topographical distribution of cortex lesions and anomalies in dementia praecox with some account of their functional significance. Am. J. Insanity **71:** 603–671.
9. LEWIS, S.W. 1990. Computerized tomography in schizophrenia 15 years on. Br. J. Psychiatry **157** (suppl. 9): 16–24.
10. BROWN, R., N. COLTER, J.A.N. CORSELLIS *et al.* 1982. Post-mortem evidence of structural brain change in schizophrenia . Arch. Gen Psychiatry **43:** 46–42.
11. VATAJA, R. & E. ELOMAA. 1988. Midline brain anomalies and schizophrenia in people with CATCH 22 syndrome. Br. J. Psychiatry **172:** 518–520.
12. KELSOE, J.R., J.L. CADET, D. PICKAR *et al.* 1988. Quantitative neuroanatomy in schizophrenia. Arch. Gen. Psychiatry **45:** 533–541.
13. NAIR, T.R., J.D. CHRISTENSEN, S.J. KINGSBURY *et al.* 1997. Progression of cerebroventricular enlargement and the subtyping of schizophrenia. Psychiatr. Res. **74:** 141–150.
14. DE LISI, L.E., M. SAKUMA, W. TEW *et al.* 1997. Schizophrenia as a chronic active brain process: a study of progressive brain structural change subsequent to the onset of schizophrenia. Psychiatr. Res. **74:** 129–140.
15. HUBER, G. 1971. Pneumoencephlographische und psychopathologische Bilder bei endogenen psychoses: Aus dem Gasamtgebiete der neurologie und psychiatrie. Monograph no. 79. Springer Verlag. Berlin.
16. HAUG, O. 1962. Pneumoencephalographic studies of brain atrophy in mental disease. Acta Psychiatr. Scand. **38** (suppl. 165): 57–107.
17. BRUTON, C., J.R. STEVENS & C.D. FRITH. 1994. Epilepsy, psychosis, and schizophrenia. Neurology **44:** 34–42.
18. SUTULA, T.P., G. GOLARAI & J. CAVAZOS. 1992. Assessing the functional significance of mossy fiber sprouting. Epilepsy Res. **57** (suppl.): 251–259.
19. BABB, T.L, G.W. MATHERN, J.P. LEITE *et al.* 1996. Glutamate AMPA receptors in the fascia dentata of human and kainate rat hippocampal epilepsy. Epilepsy Res. **26:** 193–205.
20. TORREY, E.F., A.E. BOWLER, E.H. TAYLOR *et al.* 1994. Schizophrenia and Manic Depressive Disorder. Basic Books. New York.
21. MEDUNA, L.J. 1934. Uber experimentelle Campherepilepsie. Arch. Psychiatr. Nervenkr. **102:** 333–339.
22. LANDOLT, H. 1958. Serial electroencephalographic investigations during psychotic episodes in epileptic patients and during schizophrenic attacks. *In* Lectures on Epilepsy. A.M. Lorentz de Haas, Ed.: 91–133. Elsevier. Amsterdam.
23. SAWA, M. 1969. Epileptoid psychosis: a group of atypical endogenous psychoses. Folia Psychiatr. Neurol. Jpn. **15:** 320–329.
24. MELDRUM, B.S. 1996. Update on the mechanism of action of antiepileptic drugs. Epilepsia **37** (suppl. 6): S4–11.
25. DEVINSKY, O., G. HONIGFELD & J. PATIN. 1991. Clozapine related seizures. Neurology **41:** 369–371.

26. MALOW, B.A, K.B. REESE, S. SATO et al. 1994. Spectrum of EEG abnormalities during clozapine treatment. Clin. Neurophysiol. **91**: 205–211.
27. DENNEY, D. & J.R. STEVENS. 1995. Clozapine and seizures. Biol. Psychiatry **37**: 427–433.
28. ACKENHEIL, M. 1989. Clozapine-pharmocokinetic investigations and biochemical effects in man. Psychopharmacology **99**: S32–37.
29. CORBETT, R., F. CAMACHO, A.T. WOODS et al. 1995. Antipsychotic agents antagonize non-competitive N-methyl-D-aspartate antagonist-induced behaviors. Psychopharmacology **120**: 67–74.
30. MALHOTRA, A.K., C.M. ADLER & S.D. KENNISON. 1997. Clozapine blunts N-methyl-d aspartate antagonist induced psychosis: a study with ketamine. Biol. Psychiatry **42**: 664–668.
31. DEUTCH, A.Y., D. ONGUR & R.S. DUMAN. 1995. Antipsychotic drugs induce fos protein in the thalamic paraventricular nucleus: a novel locus of antipsychotic drug action. Neuroscience **66**: 337–382.
32. STEVENS, J.R., D. DENNEY & P. SZOT. 1997. Sensitization with clozapine: beyond the dopamine hypothesis. Biol Psychiatry **42**: 771–780.
33. GUREVICH, E.V., Y. BORDELON, R.M. SHAPIRO et al. 1997. Mesolimbic dopamine D3 receptors and use of antipsychotics in patients with schizophrenia: a postmortem study. Arch. Gen. Psychiatry **54**: 225–232.
34. SLADEK, J. & C.D. SLADEK. 1995. Morphology of the endocrine brain, hypothalamus and neurohypophysis. In Endocrinology and Metabolism. K.L. Becker, Ed.: 84–90. J.B. Lipincott. Philadelphia.
35. SIMERLY, R.B. 1995. Anatomical substrates of hypothalmic integration. In The Rat Nervous System. G. Paxinos, Ed.: 353–376. Academic Press. New York.
36. LESCH, A. & B. BOGERTS. 1984. The diencephalon in schizophrenia: evidence for reduced thickness of the periventricular grey matter. Eur. Arch. Psychiatry & Neurol. Sci. **234**: 212–219.
37. EVARTS, E.V., E. BENTAL, B. BIHARI et al. 1962. Spontaneous discharge of single neurons during sleep and waking. Science **135**: 726–728.
38. KAWAKAMI, M., T. UEMURA & R. HAYASHI. 1982. Electrophysiological correlates of pulsatile gonadotropin release in rats. Neuroendocrinology **35**: 63–67.
39. KNOBIL, E. 1992. Remembrance: the discovery of the hypothalamic gonadotropin-releasing hormone pulse generator and of its physiological significance. Endocrinology **131**: 1005–1006.
40. KAWAKAMI, M., E. TERASAWA & T. IBUKI. 1970. Changes in multiple unit activity of the brain during the estrous cycle. Neuroendocrinology **6**: 30–48.
41. ORDOG, T., M.D. CHEN, M. NISHIHARA et al. 1997. On the role of gonadotropin-releasing hormone (GnRH) in the operation of the GnRH pulse generator in the rhesus monkey. Neuroenocrinology **65**: 307–313.
42. BOYAR, R.M., R.S. ROSENFELD, J.W. KAPEN et al. 1974. Simultaneous augmented secretion of luteinizing hormone and testosterone during sleep. J. Clin. Invest. **54**: 609–618.
43. HERZOG, A.G., V. RUSSELL, J.L. VAITUKAITIS et al. 1982. Neuroendocrine dysfunction in temporal lobe epilepsy. Arch. Neurol. **39**: 133–135.
44. VAN CAUTER, E., P. LINKOWSKI, M. KERKHOFS et al. 1991. Circadian and sleep related endocrine rhythms in schizophrenia. Arch. Gen. Psychiatry **48**: 348–356.
45. LIEBERMAN, J.A., D. JODY, S. GEISLER et al. 1993. Time course and biological predictors of treatment response in first-episode schizophrenia. Arch. Gen. Psychiatry **50**: 369–376.
46. CSERNANSKY, J.G., C.A. HOLMAN, K.A. BONNET et al. 1983. Dopaminergic supersensitivity at distant sites following induced epileptic foci. Life Sci. **32**: 385–390.
47. GASPAR, P., A. FEBVRET & J. COLOMBO. 1993. Serotonergic sprouting in primate MTP-induced hemiparkinsonism. Exp. Brain Res. **96**: 100–106.
48. STEVENS, J.R. 1991. Kindling of inhibition and psychosis. In Kindling and Synaptic Plasticity. F. Morrell, Ed.: 211–225. Birkhauser. Boston.
49. GODDARD, G.V, G.C. MCINTYRE & C.K. LEECH. 1969. A permanent change in brain function resulting from daily electrical stimulation. Exp. Neurol. **25**: 295–330.

50. STEVENS, J.R. 1992. Abnormal reinnervation as a basis for schizophrenia: a hypothesis. Arch. Gen. Psychiatry **49**: 238–243.
51. IACONO, W.G, G.N. SMITH, M. MOREAU et al. 1988. Ventricular and sulcal size at the onset of psychosis. Am. J. Psychiatry **145**: 820–824.
52. DeMEYER, M.K., R. GILMAR, W.E. DeMEYER et al. 1984. Third ventricular size and ventricular brain ratio in treatment resistant psychiatric patients. J. Operational Psychiatry **15**:2–8.
53. BRUTON, C.J., T.J. CROW, C.D. FRITH et al. 1990. Schizophrenia and the brain: a prospective neuropathological study. Psychol. Med. **20**: 285–304.
54. HECKERS, S., H. HEINSEN, Y.C. HEINSEN et al. 1991. Cortex, white matter, and basal ganglia in schizophrenia: a volumetric postmortem study. Biol. Psychiatry **29**: 556–566.
55. WARD, K.E., L. FRIEDMAN, A. WISE et al. 1996. Meta-analysis of brain and cranial size in schizophrenia. Schizophr. Res. **22**: 197–213.
56. WEINBERGER, D.R, K.F. BERMAN, M. IADAROLA et al. 1987. Hat size in schizophrenia (letter). Arch. Gen. Psychiatry **44**: 672.
57. PAKKENBERG, B. 1992. The volume of the mediodorsal thalamic nucleus in treated and untreated schizophrenics. Schizophr. Res. **7**: 95–100.
58. ANDREASEN, N.C., S. ARNDT, V. SWAYZE et al. 1994. Thalamic abnormalities in schizophrenia visualized through magnetic resonance image averaging. Science **266**: 294–298.
59. BUCHSBAUM, M.S., T. SOMAYA, C.Y. TANG et al. 1996. PET and MRI of the thalamus in never-medicated patients with schizophrenia. Am. J. Psychiatry **153**: 191–199.
60. JERNIGAN, T.L., S. ZISOOK, R.K. HAT et al. 1991. Magnetic resonance imaging abnormalities in lenticular nuclei and cerebral cortex in schizophrenia. Arch. Gen. Psychiatry **48**: 881–890.
61. SUDDATH, R.L., G.W. CHRISTISON, E.F. TORREY et al. 1990. Cerebral anatomical abnormalities in monozygotic twins discordant for schizophrena. N. Engl. J. Med. **322**: 789–794.
62. HECKERS, S. 1990. Limbic structures and lateral ventricle in schizoprenia: a quantitative postmortem study. Arch. Gen. Psychiatry **47**: 1016–1022.
63. PAKKENBERG, B. 1993. Total nerve cell number in neocortex in chronic schizophrenics and controls estimated using optical dissectors. Biol. Psychiatry **34**: 768–772.
64. ZIPURSKY, R.B., K.O. LIM, E.V. SULLIVAN et al. 1992. Widespread cerebral grey matter volume deficits in schizophrenia. Arch Gen Psychiatry **49**: 195–205,
65. SHENTON, M.E., R. KIKINIS, F.A. JOLESZ et al. 1992. Abnormalities of the left temporal lobe and thought disorder in schizophrenia. A quantitative magnetic resonance imaging study. N. Engl. J. Med. **327**: 604–612.
66. KULYNYCH, J.J, K. VLADAR, B.D. FANTIA et al. 1995. Normal asymmetry of the planum temporale in patients with schizophrenia. Three-dimensional cortical morphometry with MRI. Br. J. Psychiatry **166**: 742–749.
67. BARTA, P.E., G.D. PEARLSON, L.B. BRILL et al. 1997. Planum temporale asymmetry reversal in schizophrenia replication and relationship to gray matter abnormalities. Am. J. Psychiatry **154**: 66–67.
68. KULNYCH, J.J., K. VLADA, D.W. JONES et al. 1996. Superior temporal gyrus volume in schizophrenia: a study using MRI morphometry assisted by surface rendering. Am J. Psychiatry **153**: 50–56.
69. FALKAI, P., B. BOGERTS & M. ROZUMEK. 1988. Limbic pathology in schizophrenia: the entorhinal region—a morphometric study. Biol. Psychiatry **24**: 515–521.
70. BENES, F.M., I. SORENSON & E.D. BIRD. 1991. Decreased neuronal size in posterior hippocampus of schizoprenic subjects. Schizophr. Bull. **17**: 597–609.
71. KOVELMAN, J.A. & A.V. SCHEIBEL. 1984. A neurohistological correlate of schizophrenia. Biol. Psychiatry **19**: 1601–1621.
72. ALTSCHULER, L.L., A. CONRAD, J. KOVELMAN et al. 1987. Hippocampal pyramidal cell orientation in schizophrenia. Arch. Gen. Psychiatry **44**: 1094–1098.
73. ARNOLD, S.E., B.T. HYMAN, G.W. VAN HOESEN et al. 1991. Some cytoarchitectual abnormalities of the entorhinal cortex in schizophrenia. Arch. Gen. Psychiatry **48**: 625–632.

74. EASTWOOD, S.L., P.W. BURNET & P.J. HARRISON. 1995. Altered synaptophysin expression as a marker of synaptic pathology in schizophrenia. Neuroscience **66**: 309–319.
75. EASTWOOD, S.L., B. MCDONALD, P.W. BURNET *et al.* 1995. Decreased expression of mRNAs encoding nonNMDA glutamate receptors GluR1 and GR2 in medial temporal lobe neurons in schizophrenia. Brain Res. Mol. Brain Res. **29**: 211–223.
76. JAKOB, H. & H. BECKMANN. 1986. Prenatal developmental disturbances in the limbic allocortex in schizophrenics. J. Neural Transm. **65**: 303–326.
77. ARNOLD, S.E., V.M. LEE, R.E. GUR *et al.* 1991. Abnormal expression of two microtubule associated proteins (MAP 2 and MAP5) in specific subfields of the hippocampal formation in schizophrenia. Proc. Natl. Acad. Sci. USA **88**: 10850–108541.
78. KRIMER, L.S., M.M. HERMAN, R.C. SAUNDERS *et al.* 1997. A qualitative and quantitative analysis of the entorhinal cortex in schizophrenia. Cereb. Cortex **7**: 732–739.
79. PAKKENBERG, B. 1990. Pronounced reduction of total neuron number in mediodorsal thalamic nucleus and nucleus accumbens in schizophrenics. Arch Gen. Psychiatry **47**: 1023–1028.
80. MANAYE, K.F., C-L. LIANG, P.B. HICKS *et al.* 1998. Nerve cell numbers in thalamic anterior and mediodorsal nuclei are selectively reduced in schizophrenia. Soc. Neurosci. Abstr. **24**: 1236.
81. BENES, F.M., S.L.K. VINCENT, B. MARIE *et al.* 1996. Upregulation of GABAa receptor binding on neurons of the prefrontal cortex in schizophrenic subjects. Neuroscience **75**: 1021–1031.
82. BENES, F.M., S.L. VINCENT, G. ALSTERBERG *et al.* 1992. Increased GABA receptor binding in supragranular layers of schizophrenic cingulate cortex. J. Neurosci. **11**: 925–947.
83. BENES, F.M., J. MCSPARREN, E.D. BIRD *et al.* 1991. Deficits in small interneurones in prefrontal and cingulate cortices of schizophrenic and schizoaffective patients. Arch. Gen. Psychiatry **48**: 996–1001.
84. SELEMON, L.D., G. RAJKOWSKA & P.S. GOLDMAN-RAKIC. 1995. Abnormally high neuronal density in the schizophrenic cortex. Arch. Gen. Psychiatry **52**: 805–818.
85. AKBARIAN, S, J.J. KIM, S.G. POTKIN *et al.* 1995. Gene expresssion for glutamic acid decarboxylase is reduced without loss of neurons in prefrontal cortex of schizophrenics. Arch. Gen. Psychiatry **52**: 258–266.
86. BENES, F.M., L. SORENSON, E.D. BIRD *et al.* 1992. Increased density of glutamate immunoreactive vertical processes in superficial laminae in cingulate cortex of schizophrenic brain. Cereb. Cortex **2**: 503–512.
87. AKBARIAN, S., A. VINUUUELA, J.J. KIM *et al.* 1993. Distorted distribution of nicotinamide-adenine dinucleotide phosphate diaphorase neurons in temporal lobe of schizophrenics implies anomalous cortical development. Arch. Gen. Psychiatry **50**:178–187.
88. AKBARIAN, S., W.E BUNNEY, S.G. POTKIN *et al.* 1993. Altered distribution of nicotinamide-adenine dinucleotide phosphate-diaphorase cells in frontal lobe of schizophrenics implies disturbances of cortical development. Arch. Gen. Psychiatry **50**: 169–177.
89. PERRONE-BIZZOZERO, N., A.C. SOWER, E.D. BIRD *et al.* 1996. Levels of the growth-associated protein GAP-43 are selectively increased in association cortices in schizophrenia. Proc. Natl. Acad. Sci. USA **93**: 14182–14187.
90. NIETO, D., A. ESCOBAR. 1972. Major psychoses. *In* Pathology of the Nervous System. J. Mickler, Ed.: 2654–2655. McGraw Hill. New York.
91. WINKELMAN, N.W. & M.H. BOOK. 1949, Observations on the histopathology of schizophrenia. Am. J. Psychiatry **105**: 889–896.
92. HANKOFF, D. & N.S. PERESS. 1981. Neuropathology of the brain stem in psychiatric disorders. Biol. Psychiatry **16**: 945–952.
93. KORSCHENHAUSEN, D.A., H.J. HAMPEL, M. ACKENHEIL *et al.* 1996. Fibrin degradation products in post mortem brain tissue of schizophrenics: a possible marker for underlying inflammatory process. Schizophr. Res. **19**: 103–110.

Mesolimbic Activity Associated with Psychosis in Schizophrenia

Symptom-specific PET Studies

JANE EPSTEIN,[a] EMILY STERN, AND DAVID SILBERSWEIG

Functional Neuroimaging Laboratory, Weill Medical College of Cornell University, New York, New York 10021, USA

> ABSTRACT: Hallucinations and paranoid delusions are prominent among the positive symptoms of schizophrenia. Such psychotic symptoms are notable for their aberrant representations of, and relation to, the external world and for the emotional/motivational valence associated with the representations. As mesolimbic structures, including the amygdala and ventral striatum, are thought to play a significant role in imparting emotional valence to external stimuli, we here examine the mesolimbic findings of $H_2^{15}O$ PET studies designed to probe the functional neuroanatomy of psychosis.
>
> Patients with schizophrenia (including those with active hallucinations, those with active paranoid delusions, and those without active positive symptoms at the time of scanning) and healthy control subjects were studied. An event-related PET paradigm was used to identify the neural correlates of hallucinations, and a modified emotional stroop paradigm (with threat versus neutral words) was used to test the hypothesis that paranoid patients would have increased mesolimbic activity in response to threat, and even in response to neutral stimuli.
>
> The findings suggest that the positive psychotic symptoms of hallucinations and delusions share similar functional neuroanatomical features of increased mesotemporal and ventral striatal activity in the setting of decreased prefrontal activity. The pattern is evident even in a neutral context, unlike the case for normal subjects, who show such features only in response to threat. The implications of these findings for a pathophysiology of psychosis will be discussed in the context of the behavioral neuroanatomical literature in animals and humans.

The expansion of focus in animal studies, from the ventral striatum to the extended amygdala, both facilitates and parallels important developments in the investigation of schizophrenia, in which an early focus on dopaminergic activity has begun to be integrated with evidence of limbic dysfunction.

PATHOPHYSIOLOGY OF SCHIZOPHRENIA

From the early 1960s through the late 1980s, investigations of the pathophysiology of schizophrenia were dominated by the dopamine (DA) hypothesis. Based on

---

[a]Address for correspondence: Functional Neuroimaging Laboratory, Box 171, Weill Medical College of Cornell University, 525 E 68th St., New York, NY 10021. Voice: 212-746-3976; fax: 212-746-8892; jeps@hanazono.med.cornell.edu

the observation that drugs which ameliorate psychotic symptoms decrease DA neurotransmission, the original DA hypothesis posited a general overactivity of DA systems in schizophrenia.[1] Subsequent studies further implicated a relation between DA and psychosis by establishing that dopamine-mimetic drugs can induce psychosis,[2] and that the antipsychotic potency of neuroleptic medications correlates with their affinity for DA D2 receptors.[3,4] Since the majority of these receptors are found in the caudate, putamen, and nucleus accumbens, these anatomical regions became a focus of both animal and human studies of schizophrenia.

The DA hypothesis was refined over the years to incorporate expanding knowledge of dopaminergic pathways,[5] homeostatic mechanisms,[6] interactions with other neurotransmitter systems (serotonergic and glutaminergic currently among the most actively investigated),[7–10] and receptor subtypes.[11,12] During this same period, studies employing postmortem analyses, structural and functional imaging, and neuropsychological paradigms provided mounting evidence of other structural and functional cerebral abnormalities, most prominent in frontal and temporal regions, in patients with schizophrenia.[13–18] These investigations proceeded, for the most part, in parallel with those of the DA system, as the postmortem, imaging and neuropsychological studies were felt to be relevant to deficit, and the neurochemical studies, to psychotic symptoms.[19] Initial efforts to integrate these parallel sets of findings often cited aberrant DA input as the cause of cerebral dysfunction, but were less able to account for structural abnormalities on the basis of a primary DA abnormality (for review, see Weinberger and Lipska[20]). More recent efforts have posited abnormalities of input from limbic structures to the ventral striatum as the source of psychotic symptoms,[20–24] employing a systems-level approach which emphasizes the complex interactions between frontal, temporal and subcortical dopaminergic structures in the production of thought and behavior, possibly leading to both negative and positive symptoms. This approach has emerged, in large part, from advances in functional neuroimaging and cognitive neuroscience, but depends for its integrity on careful studies of cerebral structure, connectivity and function in animals and man.

PHENOMENOLOGY OF PSYCHOSIS

Psychosis, consisting of delusions and hallucinations, represents the most severe part of the psychiatric symptom spectrum. While psychotic symptoms are common in the setting of bipolar affective illness[25] and can occur in a variety of neurologic conditions,[26–32] they are most commonly associated with schizophrenia, occurring in up to 74% of patients with that diagnosis in the course of their illness.[33] The psychotic symptoms that occur in the context of schizophrenia have certain distinguishing features which may provide clues to their pathophysiology and which suggest that, though symptoms found in multiple settings may share common neural substrates,[34] there may also be aspects of the functional neuroanatomy of schizophrenic psychosis particular to that condition. Unlike the hallucinations seen in neurologic disorders, those in schizophrenia, which are most often auditory-verbal, are frequently experienced as real, emotionally relevant, and related to concurrent delusions.[35,36] A factor analysis of schizophrenic symptom-rating scales reveals that hallucinations segregate with delusions, most often paranoid in nature, in a reality distortion/psychosis factor.[16] Hallucinations and delusions in schizophrenic patients tend to respond similarly to neuroleptic treatment,[33] and schizophrenic patients with delusions are more likely to attribute distorted, self-generated speech to an external source.[37] In sum, hallucinations and delusions in the setting of schizophrenia appear to be closely linked, aberrant representations of self-generated and external stimuli, which are imbued with emotional/motivational valence, and endorsed despite conflicting information.

POSITRON EMISSION TOMOGRAPHIC STUDIES OF PSYCHOSIS

We have employed positron emission tomography (PET) to investigate, *in vivo*, the neural correlates of psychotic symptoms in patients with schizophrenia. Our strategy has been to focus on the psychotic state, with studies designed to capture naturally occurring psychotic symptoms, or to probe psychological processes and neuroanatomic circuits that we hypothesize are implicated in symptom formation.

Hallucinations in Schizophrenia

Our initial study of psychosis in schizophrenia, performed with colleagues in London, focused on hallucinations. Subjects were 6 right-handed patients, ranging in age from 23–45, with DSM-IV[38] diagnoses of schizophrenia, paranoid type. Five of the subjects were experiencing frequent, classic auditory verbal hallucinations despite receiving neuroleptic medication; the other, who was analyzed separately, had never received antipsychotic medication, and was experiencing frequent hallucinations in both visual and auditory modalities. For each of 22–25 scans performed in two study sessions, the subjects were instructed to relax, close their eyes, and press a button with their right thumb when they heard voices (which were usually accompanied by visions in the drug-naive patient).

We used PET methods of scanning and analysis that we had previously developed and validated, which can detect and localize brain activity associated with transient, randomly occurring events in single subjects.[39,40] Regional cerebral blood flow (rCBF) distribution was measured, as an index of local neuronal activity, with a Siemens/CPS 953B PET scanner in high-sensitivity three-dimensional mode using a low-dose, slow-bolus $H_2^{15}O$ PET technique.[39] The data were corrected for background activity and attenuation, reconstructed (Hanning filter 0.5, 8.4 mm resolution FWHM), and the images realigned to one another, trimmed to remove scalp artifact, transformed into the stereotactic space of Talairach and Tournoux[41] (for the group) or coregistered[42] with a T1-weighted structural MRI scan of the patient's brain (for the single subject), smoothed with a $15 \times 15 \times 15$ mm Gaussian filter ($15 \times 15 \times 9$ mm for the single subject), and normalized using analysis of covariance to remove the effect of differences in global blood flow across scans or sessions. The timing and duration of each hallucination in relation to the 30 sec of radiotracer delivery was logged by computer. This information was used to derive a weighted score for each scan, reflecting the contribution of radiotracer deposition during hallucinations to the image.[40] An event-related count-rate correlational analysis[40] was then performed on the images within the framework of pixel-by-pixel statistical parametric mapping (SPM).[43] This analysis identifies pixels with intensities covarying with the weighted scores, corresponding to areas of the brain in which activity is specifically associated with hallucinations. The group analysis was performed by determining the significance of the covariate (hallucination scan score) effect, or overall correlation, at each voxel, in a linear model including an effect for global CBF and additive subject effects—the latter adjusted for between-subject differences in mean regional CBF not accounted for by global changes.

This study design should minimize the effect of the patients' medication status, as (1) the symptom, and presumably the associated neural activity, was present despite medication, (2) the analysis was based upon within-subject variance induced by the target events of hallucinations in the setting of constant levels of medication, and (3) medication/dosage differences across subjects were included and controlled for in the analysis of subject effects.

In the group of 5 patients with auditory verbal hallucinations, the pattern of significant activity included bilateral thalamus, bilateral hippocampus/parahippocampal gyri, right anterior cingulate, right ventral striatum, and left orbitofrontal cortex. Areas of activation extended into bilateral amygdalae and the right orbitofrontal cortex, but discrete maxima were absent in these regions. Neocortical activations were absent from the group result, but present (including temporoparietal auditory-linguistic association cortex) in each individual subject. This was probably due to intersubject variability in the precise location of these neocortical activations, perhaps reflecting differences in the exact sensory content and experience of hallucinations from patient to patient. In the patient with the dual sensory modality hallucinations, the pattern of significantly increased brain activity included areas in bilateral visual, auditory and multimodal association cortices (left more extensive than right), left posterior cingulate gyrus, right parahippocampal gyrus and temporal pole, and regions presumably activated during the button press (such as left primary sensorimotor cortices). Of note, decreased activity was found in orbitofrontal cortex.

In sum, these findings suggest that hallucinations in schizophrenia are associated with autonomous activation of bilateral, distributed neural systems including appropriate unimodal association cortices; heteromodal association cortices; paralimbic cortices including cingulate and parahippocampal regions; limbic structures including hippocampus and possibly amygdala; ventral striatum; and thalamic regions.

Paranoid Delusions in Schizophrenia

In a second study of psychosis in schizophrenia, we investigated the other major psychotic symptom, delusions, focusing on a common and defining subtype, paranoid delusions. Subjects were 6 DSM-IV schizophrenic patients with active paranoid delusions, 5 DSM-IV schizophrenic patients without active paranoid delusions, and 6 normal controls. All subjects were right handed, and all schizophrenic subjects were receiving atypical neuroleptics. In order to probe psychological and neurobiological functions which may be involved in the formation of paranoid delusions, we developed a PET activation task based on the emotional Stroop. In particular, we wanted to test the hypothesis that mesolimbic activity in paranoid patients processing neutral stimuli would resemble that seen in control subjects processing threatening stimuli.

The original Stroop task[44] required subjects to name the color in which presented words were written, while ignoring the content of the words. When the content of the words conflicted with the color in which they were written (i.e., denoted a different color), reaction time was lengthened, whereas when the content matched the color in which the words were written (i.e., denoted the same color), reaction time was shortened. This phenomenon suggests that processing of word content and color both occur, with the former interfering with the latter, despite subjects' explicit efforts to focus only on color. In the emotional version of the Stroop task, color naming time is compared for words which are emotionally valenced and those which are neutral in content. Studies using this task with anxiety disordered patients find increased reaction times with words related to the nature of the subjects' anxiety, suggesting a performance bias toward relevant threat-related information at the implicit, preattentive stage of processing.[45,46]

The modified emotional Stroop (MES) developed in our laboratory consists of two word types: neutral (e.g., "rotate," "transfer" and "towel"), and interpersonal-threat (e.g., "whisper," "follow" and "stare"). Word sets are balanced for word length, number of letters and, where possible, part of speech. In a pilot study designed to assess its behavioral validity, the MES was performed outside the scanner by 13 schizophrenic patients, 7 with active paranoid psychosis and 6 without. Analysis of their performance revealed a difference in reaction time based on diagnosis and word type, with paranoid subjects showing significantly increased interference on interpersonal threat-related words (ANOVA, $p < 0.01$).

In the subsequent PET study, subjects were scanned 4 times in each of three conditions: while naming the color of neutral words, naming the color of interpersonal-threat related words, and resting. Conditions were counterbalanced to control for time and order effects. In the two naming conditions, words written in one of five colors appeared every 3 seconds (on screen time 2 seconds) for a total of 60 seconds, beginning with the rise of the whole brain time-activity curve. The high sensitivity slow bolus technique[39] was used for image acquisition, and SPM was used for image processing and analysis,[43] as described above. Predefined contrasts were evaluated for hypothesis testing.

In normal subjects, amygdala activation was noted with semanto-linguistic threat. A similar pattern of increased mesotemporal (periamygdalar/parahippocampal) activity was observed in paranoid patients compared with patient and normal controls, even with neutral stimuli. A double dissociation in right parahippocampal and ventral striatal activity was seen with threat stimuli, with increases noted in paranoid patients, and decreases in patient and normal controls. In paranoid patients, a decrease in dorsal anterior cingulate activity was observed, with failure to modulate with task performance, while ventral frontal activity decreased on task in comparison with controls.

DISCUSSION

Taken together, these studies suggest that both hallucinations and paranoid delusions in schizophrenia are associated with dysfunction or dysmodulation of brain regions in ventral striatal, mesotemporal and medial frontal regions, with a tendency to hyperactivity in the former, and hypoactivity in the latter. These areas of the brain contain interconnected structures which form an integrated network, converging on the ventral striatum, involved in the evaluation of internal and external stimuli in terms of their motivational/emotional significance, and the associated guidance of behavior. This network appears to function according to evolutionary, hierarchic principles of cerebral organization delineated by Hughlings Jackson,[47] with similar functions represented at multiple levels: from the lowest, most organized, and most automatic; to the highest, most flexible, and most voluntary.

The Limbic System and the Ventral Striatum

At the core of the network lies the amygdaloid complex, a heterogeneous collection of nuclei in the medial temporal lobe which serves to evaluate the emotional/motivational significance of internally and externally generated stimuli. The importance of this region for emotional, particularly fear-related, stimulus evaluation was established predominantly through investigations in rats and nonhuman primates,[48–50] but more recent studies suggest that it plays a similar role in humans.[51–57] The amygdaloid complex is reciprocally connected[58–65] with limbic, paralimbic, and sensory association regions which process highly integrated information—including the hippocampus, which mediates contextual aspects of emotional evaluation,[66,67] and anterior insular, anterior cingulate, orbital frontal, and temporal polar cortices. It also has reciprocal connections with several less differentiated structures or systems which serve to translate limbically processed information into motivationally based behaviors: the hypothalamus, ventral tegmentum (via the extended amygdala), and modulatory neurotransmitter systems (including dopaminergic, noradrenergic, and serotonergic). The pathways which transmit exteroceptive information to the amygdala are consistent with its role in shaping behavioral responses to motivationally relevant stimuli. In the auditory system of the rat, sensory input arrives via both direct thalamo-amygdalar, and indirect thalamo-cortico-amygdalar pathways, with the former providing crude but rapid representations of stimuli allowing for rapid response and the latter, more detailed information.[58] In humans, there is evidence that motivational evaluation can occur prior to, or in the absence of, conscious awareness of the stimulus in question,[68,69] and that such nonconscious affective processing involves the amygdala.[70,71]

A more primitive form of motivational evaluation occurs at the level of the hypothalamus,[72] a structure with reciprocal connections to the amygdaloid complex. Ascending input to the hypothalamus comes mainly from visceral organs, circulating hormones, neurotransmitters and osmotic components of the blood stream; its descending output goes to the autonomic nervous system, pituitary gland, and subcortical motor centers that elicit stereotypic movements. This connectivity enables it to coordinate somatic responses to changes in the internal milieu, or to stimuli initially processed at higher levels of the evaluative system, via a system of antagonistic excitatory and inhibitory nuclei which mediate the production of preprogrammed adaptive behaviors, or fixed-action patterns. Whereas input to the amygdala is compared with information largely attained through experience, in the form of stimulus-reinforcement associations, the significance of input to the hypothalamus is determined by comparison with genetically encoded information, and modifiable only by descending inputs from higher levels of the system.

At the highest level of the evaluative hierarchy lie the paralimbic cortices, rings of increasingly differentiated neural tissue which fall between limbic and isocortical levels of structural organization[62] and support a more flexible, voluntary form of emotional evaluation. The paralimbic areas most densely interconnected with the amygdaloid body are the temporal pole, anterior insula, and medial prefrontal cortices (anterior cingulate and caudal orbital frontal).[60–62,65] Like the amygdala, these regions receive exteroceptive and interoceptive input, and participate in the evaluation of emotional significance. In contrast to the amygdala, the medial prefrontal region is able to modulate emotional responsivity and rapidly readjust behavioral responses to stimuli when their reinforcement value is changed, or when a more complex assessment of the current context suggests the need for modification.[50,60,73–75] The paralimbic cortices project to a number of isocortical regions. Output to posterior isocortex may provide a pathway for the emotional modulation of perceptual and conceptual processing. Output to anterior isocortex appears to be involved in realistically planning and sustaining goal-related activity, anticipating the consequences of behavior, and acting in accordance with socially determined norms.[73,76,77]

Efferents from the amygdaloid complex and several of its interconnected structures, including medial frontal cortex, hippocampus, and ventral tegmental area, converge on the ventral striatum, creating yet another opportunity for complex interaction and integration of their functions. There is evidence that both hippocampal and amygdalar input to the nucleus accumbens affect its processing of information from prefrontal efferents through facilitory roles at the level of electrical activity. Hippocampal input provides repetitive, long-duration depolarizing plateaus which enable prefrontal afferents to create action potentials in accumbens cells, while amygdalar input appears to work on an event-related basis, facilitating prefrontal-evoked spiking only if it precedes stimulation from that source by less than 40 ms.[23] Similarly, dopaminergic input from the ventral tegmentum appears to modulate the responsiveness of ventral striatal neurons to stimulation from other afferents, affecting the translation of motivationally relevant information into goal-directed behavior.[78–81] Phasic activity of ventral tegmental neurons in response to motivationally relevant stimuli is itself affected by input from evaluative regions to A10 dopamine neurons,[81] as well as by tonic background dopamine release, which in turn may be regulated by both prefrontal and amygdalar activity.[82,83]

The multiple opportunities for interaction and modulation of evaluative inputs to the ventral striatum is characteristic of limbic processing, in which regions involved in the processing of motivationally relevant information appear to function as a distributed, multiply interconnected system.[60,61,84] Similarly, the basal ganglia-thalamocortical circuits that center on the ventral striatum appear to be more "open" than those associated with the dorsal striatum, with greater interconnections both to non-circuit structures, and to other corticostriatal loops.[61,78,85,86] While differences beween the frontal lobes of rats, non-human primates, and humans make it difficult to establish exact connectivity and function in the latter, it appears that information contained in corticostriatal circuits centered on the ventral striatum flows from regions with predominantly evaluative to those with predominantly behavioral functions.[61,78,86–88] This flow is reflected in the interaction of the ventral striatum with midbrain dopamine neurons, which can be divided into dorsal and ventral tiers: the dorsal tier receives input from limbic structures, and projects to the ventral striatum; the ventral tier, in turn, receives input from the ventral striatum, and projects to dorsal basal ganglia-thalamocortical circuits involved in motor activity.[81,83,84]

Implications

The results of our studies are consistent with a model of psychosis in schizophrenia involving dysmodulated input to the ventral striatum from systems involved in the evaluation of motivational significance, with hyperactivity of lower level, and hypoactivity of higher level evaluative structures. More specifically, both hallucinations and delusions appear to be associated with increased mesotemporal and ventral striatal activity in the setting of decreased prefrontal activity, most notably in the absence of veridically threatening stimuli. While the complexity and heterogeneity of schizophrenia and the circularly dependent nature of limbic structures make it difficult to implicate dysfunction of any one structure or system as a primary etiologic factor in symptom formation, there are several pieces of evidence which support such a model of psychosis in schizophrenia. The first of these is the phenomenology of the symptoms.

As noted above, hallucinations and delusions in the setting of schizophrenia are closely linked, aberrant representations of self-generated and external stimuli, which are imbued with emotional/motivational valence and endorsed despite conflicting information. This constellation of features is consistent with a model of amygdalar overactivity (increased assignment of motivational relevance) improperly integrated with and modulated by hypoactive medial frontal regions (impaired higher level evaluative functions) and hyperactive hippocampal/parahippocampal regions (abnormal processing of contextual and higher sensory information),[23,66,67] with subsequent overactivation of ventral striatal and other amygdalofugal targets (dysregulated translation of evaluative inputs into goal-directed behavior) including ventral tegmental DA neurons (aberrant modulation of ventral striatal neuronal response). In the normally functioning brain, the balance of inputs to the ventral striatum from various evaluative regions is used to prepare, initiate or prevent selected behaviors, and maintain a coherent steam of goal-oriented activity.[89] A disturbance in this balance might lead not only to aberrant representations of input, as manifested in hallucinations and delusions, but to dyscoherence of thought and action, as frequently seen in schizophrenia. It is notable, then, that medications which ameliorate hallucinations, delusions, and thought disorder are associated with modulation of DNA transcription in the shell of the nucleus accumbens, the region of the ventral striatum where inputs from prefrontal and temporolimbic cortices converge.[20,84]

Further evidence of a role for limbic dysfunction in the generation of schizophrenic symptoms is provided by postmortem, neuropsychological, and neuroimaging studies, noted above,[13–16,18] which reveal structural and functional abnormalities of temporofrontal regions in patients with schizophrenia, including both hypofunction of prefrontal regions associated with deficit symptoms, and hyperactivity of temporal regions associated with reality distortion and overall psychopathology. While most studies of prefrontal functions and activity have focused on dorsolateral areas, a substantial number show disturbances in higher level socioemotional evaluation (for review, see Penn et al.[90]) or in medial frontal structure or activity.[91–95] Dysmodulated evaluative input to the ventral striatum is also implicated in the formation of schizophrenic psychosis by studies of latent inhibition. This behavioral phenomenon—a retardation of conditioning seen when the to-be-conditioned stimulus is first presented a number of times without consequences—can be viewed as a modulation of motivational evaluation by information concerning past experience.[96] In rats, latent inhibition has been shown to be dependent on DA release in the nucleus accumbens, and on the integrity of the hippocampal formation and retrohippocampal region. In humans with schizophrenia, it has been shown to be disrupted in the setting of acute psychotic symptoms—a disruption proposed as a model of the cognitive abnormality underlying such symptoms.[97]

Future Directions

The model of schizophrenic psychosis presented above, involving dysmodulated ventral striatal input from limbic evaluative structures, requires further empiric validation, and alternative or more detailed theories will clearly be developed as new data emerge. Nonetheless, the *in vivo*, systems-level approach made possible by functional neuroimaging technologies and cognitive neuroscience, combined with ongoing advances at the level of mapping individual cell populations and pathways, holds great potential for expanding and refining our knowledge of this complex and devastating illness.

REFERENCES

1. CARLSSON, A. & M. LINDQVIST. 1963. Effect of chlorpromazine or haloperidol on formation of 3-methoxytyramine and normetanephrine in mouse brain. Acta Pharmacol. Toxicol. **20:** 140–144.
2. ANGRIST, B., *et al.* 1974. Amphetamine psychosis: behavioral and biochemical aspects. J. Psychiatr. Res. **11:** 13–23.
3. CREESE, I., D.R. BURT & S.H. SNYDER. 1976. Dopamine receptor binding predicts clinical and pharmacological potencies of antischizophrenic drugs. Science **192**(4238): 481–483.
4. SEEMAN, P., *et al.* 1976. Antipsychotic drug doses and neuroleptic/dopamine receptors. Nature **261**(5562): 717–719.
5. STEVENS, J.R. 1973. An anatomy of schizophrenia? Arch. Gen. Psychiatry **29**(2): 177–189.
6. FRIEDHOFF, A.J. & J.C. MILLER. 1983. Clinical implications of receptor sensitivity modification. Annu. Rev. Neurosci. **6:** 121–148.
7. TANDON, R. & J.F. GREDEN. 1989. Cholinergic hyperactivity and negative schizophrenic symptoms. A model of cholinergic/dopaminergic interactions in schizophrenia. Arch. Gen. Psychiatry **46**(8): 745–753.
8. KAPUR, S. & G. REMINGTON. 1996. Serotonin-dopamine interaction and its relevance to schizophrenia. Am. J. Psychiatry **153**(4): . 466–476.
9. CARLSSON, A. 1995. Neurocircuitries and neurotransmitter interactions in schizophrenia. Int. Clin. Psychopharmacol. **3:** 21–28.
10. BENES, F.M. 1997. The role of stress and dopamine-GABA interactions in the vulnerability for schizophrenia. J. Psychiatr. Res. **31**(2): 257–275.
11. SEEMAN, P., H.C. GUAN & H.H. VAN TOL. 1993. Dopamine D4 receptors elevated in schizophrenia. Nature **365**(6445): 441–445.
12. GUREVICH, E.V., *et al.* 1997. Mesolimbic dopamine D3 receptors and use of antipsychotics in patients with schizophrenia. A postmortem study. Arch. Gen. Psychiatry **54**(3): 225–232.
13. BACHUS, S.E. & J.E. KLEINMAN. 1996. The neuropathology of schizophrenia. J. Clin. Psychiatry **11:** 72–83.
14. FRISTON, K.J., *et al.* 1992. The left medial temporal region and schizophrenia. A PET study. Brain **115**(2): 367–382.
15. LAWRIE, S.M. & S.S. ABUKMEIL. 1998. Brain abnormality in schizophrenia. A systematic and quantitative review of volumetric magnetic resonance imaging studies. Br. J. Psychiatry **172:** 110–120.

16. LIDDLE, P.F., et al. 1992. Patterns of cerebral blood flow in schizophrenia. Br. J. Psychiatry **160:** 179–186.
17. TAMMINGA, C.A., et al. 1992. Limbic system abnormalities identified in schizophrenia using positron emission tomography with fluorodeoxyglucose and neocortical alterations with deficit syndrome. Arch. Gen. Psychiatry **49**(7): 522–530.
18. WEINBERGER, D.R., et al. 1994. The frontal lobes and schizophrenia [published erratum appears in J. Neuropsychiatry Clin. Neurosci. 1995. Winter **7(1):**121]. J. Neuropsychiatry Clin. Neurosci. **6**(4): 419–427.
19. CROW, T.J., I.N. FERRIER & E.C. JOHNSTONE. 1986. The two-syndrome concept and neuroendocrinology of schizophrenia. Psychiatr. Clin. North Am. **9**(1): 99–113.
20. WEINBERGER, D.R. & B.K. LIPSKA. 1995. Cortical maldevelopment, anti-psychotic drugs, and schizophrenia: a search for common ground. Schizophrenia Res. **16**(2): 87–110.
21. BOGERTS, B. 1997. The temporolimbic system theory of positive schizophrenic symptoms. Schizophrenia Bull. **23**(3): . 423–435.
22. CSERNANSKY, J.G., G.M. MURPHY & W.O. FAUSTMAN. 1991. Limbic/mesolimbic connections and the pathogenesis of schizophrenia. Biol. Psychiatry **30**(4): 383–400.
23. GRACE, A.A. & H. MOORE. 1998. Regulation of information flow in the nucleus accumbens: a model for the pathophysiology of schizophrenia. *In* Origins and Development of Schizophrenia: Advances in Experimental Psychopathology. M.F. Lenzenweger & R.H. Dworkin, Eds.: 123–157. American Psychological Association. Washington, D.C.
24. GRAY, J.A., et al. 1991. The neuropsychology of schizophrenia. Behavioral & Brain Sci. **14**(1): 1–84.
25. DIEPERINK, M.E. & J.R. SANDS. 1996. Bipolar mania with psychotic features: diagnosis and treatment. Psychiatr. Ann. **26**: 633–637.
26. BENSON, M.T. & I.G. RENNIE. 1989. Formed hallucination in the hemianopic field. Postgrad. Med. J. **65**(768): . 756–757.
27. BERRIOS, G.E. 1985. Hallucinosis. *In* Handbook of Clinical Neurology: Neurobehavioural Disorders. J.A.M. Frederiks, Ed.: 561–572. Elsevier Science Publishers. New York.
28. FERNANDEZ, W., G. STERN & A.J. LEES. 1992. Hallucinations and parkinsonian motor fluctuations. Behav. Neurol. **5**(2): 83–86.
29. MALLOY, P.F. & E.D. RICHARDSON. 1994. The frontal lobes and content-specific delusions. J. Neuropsychiatry Clin. Neurosci. **6**(4): 455–466.
30. NODA, S., M. MIZOGUCHI & A. YAMAMOTO. 1993. Thalamic experiential hallucinosis. J. Neurol. Neurosurg. Psychiatry **56**(11): 1224–1226.
31. SERRA CATAFAU, J., F. RUBIO & J. PERES SERRA. 1992. Peduncular hallucinosis associated with posterior thalamic infarction. J. Neurol. **239**(2): 89–90.
32. TRIMBLE, M.R. 1991. The psychoses of epilepsy. New York. Raven Press.
33. KAPLAN, H.I. & B.J. SADOCK. 1995. Comprehensive Textbook of Psychiatry. Williams & Wilkins. Baltimore, MD.
34. DOLAN, R.J., et al. 1993. Dorsolateral prefrontal cortex dysfunction in the major psychoses; symptom or disease specificity? J. Neurol. Neurosurg. Psychiatry **56**(12): 1290–1294.
35. BENTALL, R.P., Ed. 1990. Reconstructing schizophrenia. Routledge. London, p. 308.
36. SCHNEIDER, K. 1959. Clinical psychopathology, 5th edit., Vol. 173. Grune & Stratton. New York.
37. CAHILL, C., D. SILBERSWEIG & C. FRITH. 1996. Psychotic experiences induced in deluded patients using distorted auditory feedback. Cog. Neuropsychiatry **1**: 201–211.
38. Diagnostic and Statistical Manual of Mental Disorders, 4th edit. 1994. American Psychiatric Association. Washington, D.C.
39. SILBERSWEIG, D.A., et al. 1993. Detection of thirty-second cognitive activations in single subjects with positron emission tomography: a new low-dose $H_2(15)O$ regional cerebral blood flow three-dimensional imaging technique. J. Cereb. Blood Flow Metab. **13**(4): 617–629.

40. SILBERSWEIG, D.A., et al. 1994. Imaging transient, randomly occurring neuropsychological events in single subjects with positron emission tomography: an event-related count rate correlational analysis. J. Cereb. Blood Flow Metab. **14**(5): . 771–782.
41. TALAIRACH, J. & P. TOURNOUX. 1989. Co-Planar Stereotaxic Atlas of the Human Brain. Thieme. Stuttgart.
42. WOODS, R.P., J.C. MAZZIOTTA & S.R. CHERRY. 1993. MRI-PET registration with automated algorithm. J. Comput. Assist. Tomogr. **17**(4): 536–546.
43. FRISTON, K.J., et al. 1995. Statistical parametric maps in functional imaging: a general linear approach. Human Brain Mapping **2**: 189–210.
44. STROOP, J.R. 1935. Studies of interference in serial verbal reactions. J. Exp. Psychol. **18**: 643–662.
45. MOGG, K., et al. 1993. Subliminal processing of emotional information in anxiety and depression. J. Abnormal Psychol. **102**(2): 304–311.
46. WILLIAMS, J.M.G., et al. 1988. Cognitive Psychology and Emotional Disorders. John Wiley & Sons. Chichester, England.
47. TAYLOR, J., Ed. Selected Writings of John Hughlings Jackson. 1958. Basic Books. New York.
48. LEDOUX, J.E. 1992. Emotion and the amygdala. In The Amygdala: Neurobiological Aspects of Emotion, Memory, and Mental Dysfunction. J.P. Aggleton, Ed.: 339–351. Wiley-Liss. New York.
49. ONO, T. & H. NISHIJO. 1992. Neurophysiological basis of the Kluever-Bucy syndrome: responses of monkey amygdaloid neurons to biologically significant objects. In The Amygdala: Neurobiological Aspects of Emotion, Memory, and Mental Dysfunction. J.P. Aggleton, Ed.: 167–190. Wiley-Liss. New York.
50. ROLLS, E.T. 1990. A theory of emotion, and its application to understanding the neural basis of emotion. Cognition & Emotion **4**(3): 161–190.
51. BONDA, E., et al. 1996. Specific involvement of human parietal systems and the amygdala in the perception of biological motion. J. Neurosci. **16**(11): 3737–3744.
52. CAHILL, L., B. ROOZENDAAL & J.L. MCGAUGH. 1997. The neurobiology of memory for aversive emotional events. In Learning, Motivation, and Cognition: The Functional Behaviorism of Robert C. Bolles. M.E. Bouton, Ed.: 369–384. American Psychological Association. Washington, D.C.
53. ADOLPHS, R., et al. 1995. Fear and the human amygdala. J. Neurosci. **15**(9): 5879–5891.
54. ADOLPHS, R., et al. 1997. Impaired declarative memory for emotional material following bilateral amygdala damage in humans. Learning & Memory **4**(3): 291–300.
55. ADOLPHS, R., D. TRANEL & A.R. DAMSIO. 1998. The human amygdala in social judgment. Nature **393**(6684): 470–474.
56. MORRIS, J.S., et al. 1996. A differential neural response in the human amygdala to fearful and happy facial expressions. Nature **383**(6603): 812–815.
57. MORRIS, J.S., et al. 1998. A neuromodulatory role for the human amygdala in processing emotional facial expressions. Brain **121**(1): 47–57.
58. ARMONY, J.L. & J.E. LE DOUX. 1997. How the brain processes emotional information. Ann. N.Y. Acad. Sci. **821**: 259–270.
59. DAVIS, M. 1997. Neurobiology of fear responses: the role of the amygdala. J. Neuropsychiatry & Clin. Neurosci. **9**(3): 382–402.
60. DEVINSKY, O., M.J. MORRELL & B.A. VOGT. 1995. Contributions of anterior cingulate cortex to behaviour. Brain **118**(1): 279–306.
61. MEGA, M.S., et al. 1997. The limbic system: an anatomic, phylogenetic, and clinical perspective. J. Neuropsychiatry Clin. Neurosci. **9**(3): 315–330.
62. MESULAM, M.M. 1985. Patterns in behavioral neuroanatomy: association areas, the limbic system, and hemispheric specialization. In Principles of Behavioral Neurology. M.M. Mesulam, Ed.: 1–70. F. A. Davis. Philadelphia.
63. PRICE, J.L. & D.G. AMARAL. 1981. An autoradiographic study of the projections of the central nucleus of the monkey amygdala. J. Neurosci. **1**(11): 1242–1259.
64. ROSEN, J.B. & J. SCHULKIN. 1998. From normal fear to pathological anxiety. Psychol. Rev. **105**(2): 325–350.

65. ZALD, D.H. & S.W. KIM. 1996. Anatomy and function of the orbital frontal cortex, I: anatomy, neurocircuitry; and obsessive-compulsive disorder. J. Neuropsychiatry Clin. Neurosci. **8**(2): 125–138.
66. PHILLIPS, R.G. & J.E. LE DOUX. 1992. Differential contribution of amygdala and hippocampus to cued and contextual fear conditioning. Behav. Neurosci. **106**(2): 274–285.
67. KIM, J.J. & M.S. FANSELOW. 1992. Modality-specific retrograde amnesia of fear. Science **256**(5057): 675–677.
68. MURPHY, S.T. & R.B. ZAJONC. 1993. Affect, cognition, and awareness: affective priming with optimal and suboptimal stimulus exposures. J. Personality & Soc. Psychol. **64**(5): 723–739.
69. OHMAN, A. & J.J. SOARES. 1993. On the automatic nature of phobic fear: conditioned electrodermal responses to masked fear-relevant stimuli. J. Abnorm. Psychol. **102**(1): 121–132.
70. WHALEN, P.J., et al. 1998. Masked presentations of emotional facial expressions modulate amygdala activity without explicit knowledge. J. Neurosci. **18**(1): 411–418.
71. MORRIS, J.S., A. OHMAN & R.J. DOLAN. 1998. Conscious and unconscious emotional learning in the human amygdala. Nature **393**(6684): 467–470.
72. BEAR, D. 1991. Neurological perspectives on aggressive behavior. J. Neuropsychiatry & Clin. Neurosci. **3**(2): S3–S8.
73. DERRYBERRY, D. & D.M. TUCKER. 1992. Neural mechanisms of emotion. J.Consulting & Clin. Psychol. **60**(3): 329–338.
74. MORGAN, M.A., L.M. ROMANSKI & J.E. LEDOUX. 1993. Extinction of emotional learning: contribution of medial prefrontal cortex. Neurosci. Lett. **163**(1): 109–113.
75. MORGAN, M.A. & J.E. LEDOUX. 1995. Differential contribution of dorsal and ventral medial prefrontal cortex to the acquisition and extinction of conditioned fear in rats. Behav. Neurosci. **109**(4): 681–688.
76. BECHARA, A., et al. 1994. Insensitivity to future consequences following damage to human prefrontal cortex. Cognition **50**(1–3): 7–15.
77. DAMASIO, A.R., D. TRANEL & H. DAMASIO. 1990. Individuals with sociopathic behavior caused by frontal damage fail to respond autonomically to social stimuli. Behav. Brain Res. **41**(2): 81–94.
78. FERRE, S. 1997. Adenosine-dopamine interactions in the ventral striatum. Implications for the treatment of schizophrenia. Psychopharmacology (Berl.) **133**(2): 107–120.
79. MOGENSON, G.J. & C.C. YIM. 1991. Neuromodulatory Functions of the mesolimbic dopamine system: electrophysiologic and behavioural studies. *In* The Mesolimbic Dopamine System: From Motivation to Action. P. Willner & J. Scheel-Kruger, Eds.: 105–130. John Wiley & Sons. New York.
80. ROBBINS, T.W. & B.J. EVERITT. 1992. Functions of dopamine in the dorsal and ventral striatum. Semin. Neurosci. **4**: 119–127.
81. WHITE, F.J. 1991. Neurotransmission in the mesoaccumbens dopamine system. *In* The Mesolimbic Dopamine System: From Motivation to Action. P. Willner & J. Scheel-Kruger, Eds.: 61–103. John Wiley & Sons. New York.
82. GRACE, A.A. 1991. Phasic versus tonic dopamine release and the modulation of dopamine system responsivity: a hypothesis for the etiology of schizophrenia. Neuroscience **41**(1): 1–24.
83. HABER, S.N. & J.L. FUDGE. 1997. The interface between dopamine neurons and the amygdala: implications for schizophrenia. Schizophrenia Bull. **23**(3): 471–482.
84. HEIMER, L., et al. 1997. The accumbens: beyond the core-shell dichotomy. J. Neuropsychiatry & Clin. Neurosci. **9**(3): 354–381.
85. ALEXANDER, G.E., M.D. CRUTCHER & M.R. DE LONG. 1990. Basal ganglia-thalamo-cortical circuits: parallel substrates for motor, oculomotor, "prefrontal" and "limbic" functions. Prog. Brain Res. **85**: 119–146.
86. GROENEWEGEN, H.J. 1997. Cortical-subcortical relationships and the limbic forebrain. *In* Contemporary Behavioral Neurology. Blue Books of Practical Neurology.

M.R. Trimble, Ed.: 29–48. Butterworth-Heinemann. Boston, MA.
87. DEUTCH, A.Y., A.J. BOURDELAIS & D.S. ZAHM. 1993. The nucleus accumbens core and shell: accombal compartments and their functional attributes. *In* Limbic Motor Circuits and Neuropsychiatry. P.W. Kalivas & C.D. Barnes, Eds.: 45–88. CRC Press. Boca Raton, FL.
88. PREUSS, T.M. 1995. Do rats have prefrontal cortex? The Rose-Woolsey-Akert program reconsidered. J. Cog. Neurosci. **7**(1): 1–24.
89. ROLLS, E.T. 1994. Neurophysiology and cognitive functions of the striatum. Rev. Neurol. **150**(8–9): 648–660.
90. PENN, D.L., *et al.* 1997. Social cognition in schizophrenia. Psychol. Bull. **121**(1): 114–132.
91. BARTHA, R., *et al.* 1997. Measurement of glutamate and glutamine in the medial prefrontal cortex of never-treated schizophrenic patients and healthy controls by proton magnetic resonance spectroscopy. Arch. Gen. Psychiatry **54**(10): 959–965.
92. BENES, F.M. 1996. The defects of affect and attention in schizophrenia: a possible neuroanatomical substrate, *In* Psychopathology: The Evolving Science of Mental Disorder. S. Matthysse, Ed.: 127–151. Cambridge University Press. New York.
93. FLETCHER, P.C., *et al.* 1996. Local and distributed effects of apomorphine on frontotemporal function in acute unmedicated schizophrenia. J. Neurosci. **16**(21): 7055–7062.
94. LIDDLE, P.F. 1994. Volition and schizophrenia. *In* The Neuropsychology of Schizophrenia. A.S. David, Ed.: 39–49. Lawrence Erlbaum Associates. Hove, England.
95. SCHROEDER, J., *et al.* 1995. Structural and functional correlates of subsyndromes in chronic schizophrenia. Psychopathology **28**(1): 38–45.
96. HEMSLEY, D.R. 1987. An experimental psychological model for schizophrenia. *In* Search for the Causes of Schizophrenia. H. Hafner, W.F. Gattaz & W. Janzarik, Eds.: 179–188. Springer-Verlag. Berlin.
97. GRAY, J.A., *et al.* 1995. The role of mesolimbic dopaminergic and retrohippocampal afferents to the nucleus accumbens in latent inhibition: implications for schizophrenia. Behav. Brain Res. **71**(1–2): 19–31.

Ventromedial Temporal Lobe Pathology in Dementia, Brain Trauma, and Schizophrenia

GARY W. VAN HOESEN,[a–c] JEAN C. AUGUSTINACK,[a] AND SARAH J. REDMAN[a]

[a]*Department of Anatomy and Cell Biology and the* [b]*Division of Cognitive Neuroscience, Department of Neurology, University of Iowa, Iowa City, Iowa 52242, USA*

ABSTRACT: The ventromedial temporal area contains numerous anatomical structures collectively or selectively involved in a wide range of neurological and psychiatric disorders. Collective involvement is exemplified best by Alzheimer's disease where a host of anatomical structures and a host of cognitive and behavioral changes are manifested. Selective disease of the amygdala can yield deficits in the ability to judge and evaluate emotional expressions. While memory functions are nearly synonymous with the concept of ventromedial temporal area, they overshadow other functions associated with the diverse anatomical structures in this part of the brain. For example, it could be argued that in addition to output directed toward the hippocampal formation, the output of the ventromedial temporal area is equally strong to the ventral striatopallidal system of the basal forebrain. Denervation of these structures could be associated with the behavioral changes that occur in tandem with the memory-related changes of ventromedial temporal lobe pathology. Here we explore the anatomical and pathological correlates associated with ventromedial temporal area pathology and consider how these may impact on ventral striatopallidal conceptualizations. We conclude that ventromedial temporal area pathology deprives the basal forebrain of multimodal association information from the endstages of corticocortical sensory processing. This endstage information carries with it an analysis of real-time sensory awareness, historical-time or past sensory experiences, and decisions from hippocampal output structures regarding relevancy and novelty. In this sense, basal forebrain structures are in a unique position to regulate behavioral responses to a wide range of stimuli and to organize appropriate emotional, motor, autonomic, and endocrine responses to them.

INTRODUCTION

The ventromedial temporal area is a functionally diverse and anatomically complex part of the cerebral hemisphere inserted along the ventral and medial parts of the temporal fossa.[29,83,85] It borders the sphenoid bone and the petrous part of the temporal bone. Portions of the ventromedial temporal area are traversed by the free edge of the tentorium cerebelli prior to its attachment to the petrous apex and the anterior and posterior clinoid processes.[24,51,63] The paired free edges of the tentorium cerebelli form an aperture through which the upper brain stem passes and the ante-

---

[c]Author for correspondence: Department of Anatomy and Cell Biology, University of Iowa, Iowa City, IA 52242, USA. Voice: 319-335-7741; fax: 319-335-7198; gary-vanhoesen@uiowa.edu

rior and medial parts of the ventromedial temporal area protrude into and over the aperture unprotected by dura mater.

The component structures of the ventromedial temporal area include the cortical and subcortical parts of the amygdala, the enfolded allocortical areas rolled into the inferior horn of the lateral ventricle known as the hippocampal formation and the surface allocortical and periallocortical areas that form the pyriform lobe of the parahippocampal gyrus. Anteriorly, the latter is formed largely by the primary olfactory allocortex, whereas posteriorly, the pyriform lobe is formed by the sizable entorhinal periallocortex, or Brodmann's area 28. The latter extends posteriorly in all species where it approximates occipital areas. The lateral border of the ventromedial temporal area is the rhinal sulcus in all mammals. It contains the perirhinal cortex, or Brodmann's area 35, in its fundus and lateral bank.[29,47,71,84] However, in the human brain, the rhinal sulcus is normally short, if present at all, and the perirhinal cortex courses into the collateral sulcus and forms a part of its medial bank. It retains, however, its exact anatomical position sandwiched between the olfactory and entorhinal cortices and the more laterally located temporal isocortices whether the rhinal sulcus is present to any degree or not.[83,85]

In functional terms, the ventromedial temporal area has been linked historically to three major realms of behavior, namely, olfaction, emotion and memory. Olfactory sensation has never been disputed, although great debate over the extent of olfactory bulb projections, and hence, the olfactory brain, occupied many decades. Clearly, several brain areas receive direct olfactory bulb projections and these along with secondary olfactory projections reach many parts of the ventromedial temporal area.[9,22,27,28] A role in emotion for ventromedial temporal areas was championed by Papez and the "emotive process" was assembled or "built up", according to his thinking, in its hippocampal and/or hippocampal-related structures. Although historical interest is still given to Papez's bold proposal,[67] and its anatomical underpinnings, it never received definitive support in the temporal lobe. While it is clear that the amygdala of the ventromedial temporal area plays a role in emotional perception and memory, and governs some of the key autonomic and endocrine responses paired with emotion,[9] core elements of affect and feelings are governed by larger neural systems in which the amygdala is only one player.[25] Ironically, the amygdala was not a part of Papez's circuit.

A definitive role for the ventromedial temporal area in memory is a cornerstone of neuroscience teaching and the first thought that occurs when this geographic area of the cerebral hemisphere is mentioned.[75] Moreover, the case has been steadily strengthened and elaborated as time has passed.[7,66,80,96] While much of the neuroanatomical organization of ventromedial temporal area seems geared to subserving memory-related mechanisms,[84] it is easy to lose sight of the fact that many large hippocampal output neural systems arise here that contribute to other forms of behavior. These systems may not play a definitive role in memory-related behavior per se, but instead contribute critical memory-related information to other behaviors.[86] One of the major non-hippocampal targets of output from the ventromedial temporal areas is the basal forebrain, and particularly, the ventral striatopallidal and magnocellular cell groups that form these areas.[3,5,8,39,42,52,56,87,95] These areas have been linked more strongly to emotional mechanisms than was ever the case for ventromedial temporal areas, and it is likely, that it is via these systems, an integrated emotional behavior is achieved.[41,42] To explore this concept, we will examine several types of temporal lobe pathology that affects neural systems that contribute powerful input to basal forebrain structures. The general theme to be considered is that behavioral changes in these disorders, including schizophrenia, may be understood, at least, in part, by considering the fact that ventromedial temporal area pathology deafferents basal forebrain areas depriving them of real-time, historical-time and memory-related awareness critical for emotional, motor and homeostatic mechanisms.

ALZHEIMER'S DISEASE

Hippocampal Formation

Hippocampal pathological changes in Alzheimer's disease (AD) have been observed for nearly a century, and documenting them is recommended in all neuropathological diagnostic protocols.[11,19–21,44–46] In terms of neurofibrillary tangles (NFTs), this signature feature of AD is observed primarily in the subicular and CA 1 pyramidal neurons, with the CA 3 pyramids negative, or largely spared. In general, there is typically more subicular/CA 1 pathology in patients who have been ill for a long time and less in those with illnesses of shorter duration. NFTs among the various hilar neurons that form the CA 4 zone of the dentate gyrus are not unusual, but seldom total more than 8–10 affected neurons per cross-section, with many cases having none. Curiously, CA 1 and subicular NFT pathology fails to have a differential anterior-posterior distribution.[46] These neurons often have classical NFTs with dense filamentous paired helices extending for long distances in the apical and basal dendrites and more delicate filaments surrounding the nucleus in the region of the soma. Many, in long duration cases, form the so-called "extraneuronal or ghost" NFTs, meaning simply that they are marking the location of a once viable neuron which at death contained no stainable cytoplasm. In shorter duration cases, it is not unusual to see subicular and CA 1 pyramids with conspicuous tangles in their apical dendrites, but retaining stainable cytoplasm and a still concentric well-defined nucleus and nucleolus.[45] One has to assume that these neurons are altered greatly from a functional viewpoint, but the apparent integrity of the soma, and presumably, intact axon hillock might provide an altered abnormal output to areas where they send axons. NFTs are observed occasionally in the granule cell neurons that form the dentate gyrus, but this is the exception rather than the rule, and typically, these cases have a lengthy duration of illness.

Neuritic plaques (NPs) are also observed in the hippocampal formation in AD. Unlike the isocortex, where their distribution is often more random across several cortical laminae, their distribution in the hippocampal formation is more conservative in AD. For example, NPs are often observed in the molecular layer of the dentate gyrus where they form a band between the granule cell somas and the hippocampal fissure. In the subiculum and CA 1 zones they are often seen among the somas that form these fields, but also in the stratum radiatum and stratum laconosum-moleculare areas of their apical dendrites. Both in the dentate gyrus, and for parts of the CA 1/subicular zones, NPs seem to show a preference for the terminal fields of the perforant pathway.[45,46]

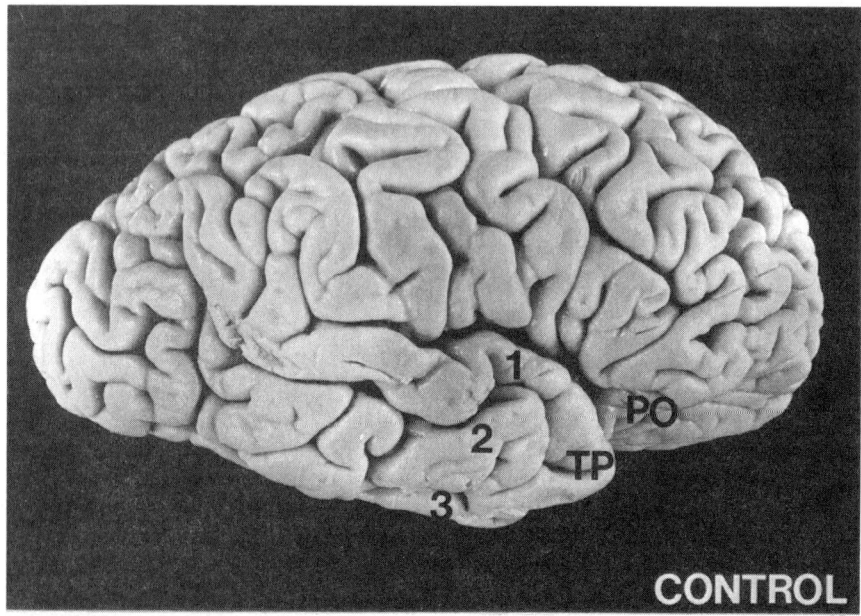
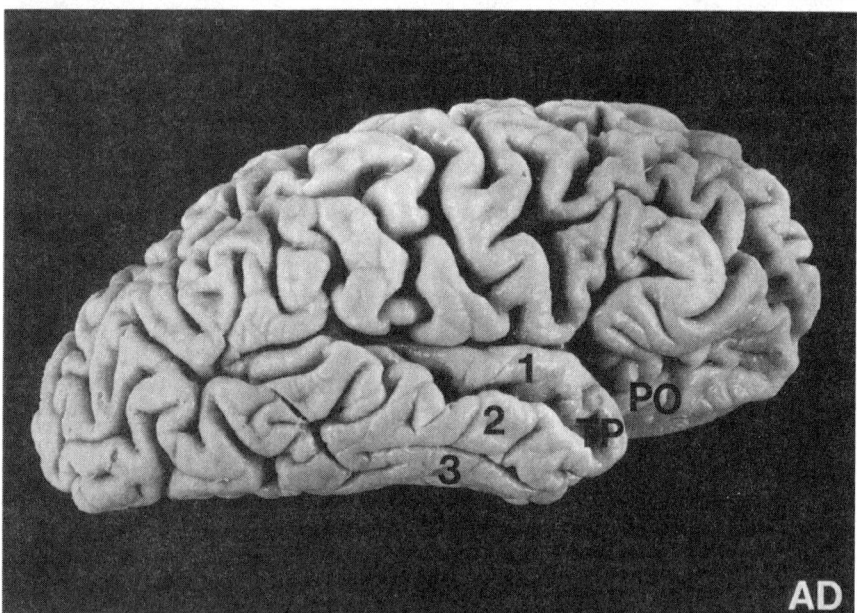

FIGURE 1. The upper panel shows a lateral view of the right hemisphere of a 93-year-old non-demented control donor with no history of neurological or psychiatric illness. Brain weight was 1214 g. The lower panel shows a lateral view of the right hemisphere of a 66-year-old demented donor with clinical and neuropathological evidence of AD. Brain-weight was 940 g. The superior, middle and inferior temporal gyri are labeled 1, 2, and 3, respective-

In summary, hippocampal formation pathology in AD is extensive, affecting pyramidal projection neurons that in other mammals send axons to widespread parts of the telencephalon and diencephalon.[70] This would include hippocampal projections to the entorhinal, posterior parahippocampal, perirhinal and temporal polar parts of the temporal lobe, and to the orbital and medial frontal parts of the frontal lobe (FIG. 1).[39,70,93,94] Additional input to the anterior and posterior cingulate cortices would be expected to be compromised also. Other non-cortical telencephalic projections altered in AD would be CA 1/subicular input to the amygdala, septum, vertical limb of the diagonal band nucleus and nucleus accumbens of the ventral striatum.[70,71] Subcortical diencephalic projections to the anterior thalamus and hypothalamus would no doubt degenerate as well in a severely affected AD case. On the basis of animal research, some of the neurons affected by NFTs would be expected to send axons directly to cortical areas that in turn send axons to the ventral striatum.[40,62,68] The net affect in AD would be a profound disconnection between this part of the ventromedial temporal area and the ventral striatum.

Entorhinal Cortex

There is little doubt that the entorhinal (Brodmann's area 28) and perirhinal (Brodmann's area 35) cortices are the initial focal points for the formation of NFTs in AD and the entorhinal cortex is the most heavily ravaged by the illness at all points in its course (FIG. 2).[21,45] Indeed, the normally conspicuous layer II islands of neurons can disappear entirely in cell stains in endstage AD;[36] however, pathological stains, such as thioflavin-S and Bielschowsky, reveal their continued presence, but in the form of extraneuronal NFTs without stainable rough ER and ribosomes. The superficial parts of layer III in entorhinal cortex also contain NFTs as does layer IV deep to the lamina dissecans. However, the latter is typically a later occurrence in AD after a duration of illness that exceeds three years (FIG. 3). It is not unusual in early onset familial AD and in sporadic AD with a long duration of illness to see nearly all neurons in all layers of the entorhinal cortex affected by NFTs.

In addition to differential laminar changes, a clear lateral to medial gradient of NFT formation also occurs, with the first islands affected lying near the collateral sulcus and the last affected lying more medially nearer the periamygdaloid cortex or parasubiculum depending on the anterior-posterior level examined.

In summary, entorhinal cortex pathology in AD greatly compromises the cells of origin for both the entorhino-dentate and entorhino-hippocampal components of the perforant pathway.[88,90,93,94] In addition, neurofibrillary tangles selectively destroy many of the large modified pyramidal neurons that form layer IV. These neurons receive a strong hippocampal output[70] and project directly to the ventral striatum.[38,78,81,93] Moreover, they project to the temporal and frontal cortices[54] that project strongly to the ventral striatum and the magnocellular parts of the basal forebrain (FIG. 1).[40,62,68,87]

---

ly. In the AD donor, dense NFTs were observed in the subicular/CA 1 zone of the hippocampal formation. The pyramids that occupy this zone in non-human primates project to cortical regions such as the temporal polar (TP) and posterior orbital (PO) cortices. Note in the AD brain that these areas are discolored and atrophic, suggesting that non-direct relayed ventromedial temporal area input to the ventral striatum and magnocellular cell group of the basal forebrain is also compromised in AD along with direct subicular/CA 1 projections.

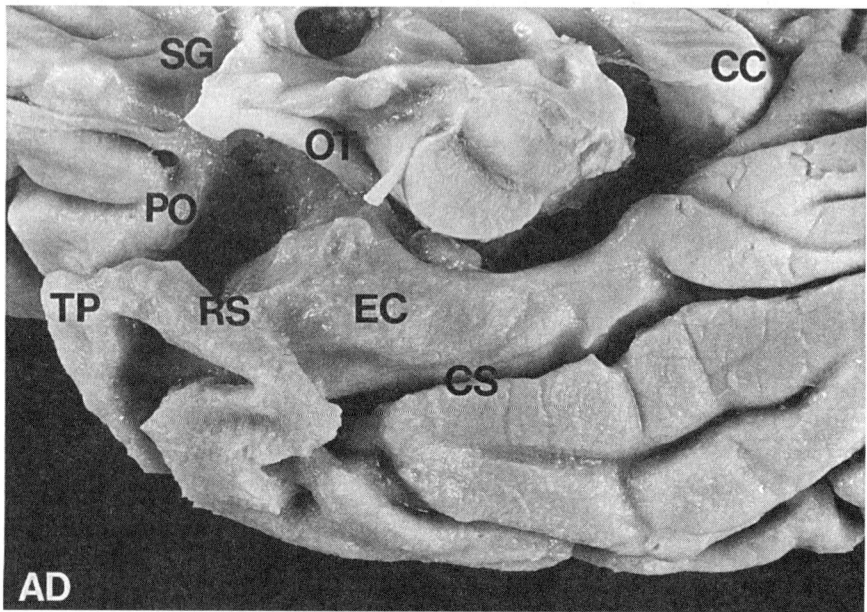

FIGURE 2. This photograph shows a ventromedial temporal view of the right hemisphere in an endstage AD donor. Note the highly atrophic entorhinal cortex (EC), temporal polar cortex (TP), posterior orbital cortex (PO), and subgenual cortex (SG). All of these areas have been shown in non-human primates to project directly to the ventral striatum and magnocellular cell groups of the basal forebrain. (Other abbreviations: CC, corpus callosum; CS, collateral sulcus; OT, optic tract; RS, rhinal sulcus).

Amygdala

Like the hippocampal formation and entorhinal cortex, the amygdala is damaged heavily, but selectively, in AD and a number of recent investigations have brought these changes into sharp focus.[30,53,58,65] In so far as NFTs are concerned, the most heavily damaged amygdaloid nuclei are the accessory basal and cortical nuclei. The cortical transition area of the posterior amygdala is also damaged heavily, but the lateral, laterobasal, mediobasal, central and medial nuclei have a more moderate quantity of neurofibrillary changes. Changes in these nuclei can also be variable in a population of AD victims, such that it is not unusual to find cases with little or no NFT pathology in the lateral, central and medial amygdaloid nuclei.

A somewhat similar picture emerges when one considers the amygdaloid distribution of NPs. For example, these are most dense in the accessory basal nucleus with slightly lesser quantities in the cortical nuclei and the cortical transition area. However, in contrast to the moderate quantity of NFTs, NPs are typically dense in the mediobasal nucleus equaling or exceeding those of the accessory basal nucleus. The lateral, laterobasal, central and medial nuclei frequently contain NPs, but their quantity is often modest or lacking significant numbers altogether.[58]

In summary, it is probably accurate to state that the amygdala as a whole is more variably damaged by the pathology of AD than the hippocampal formation and en-

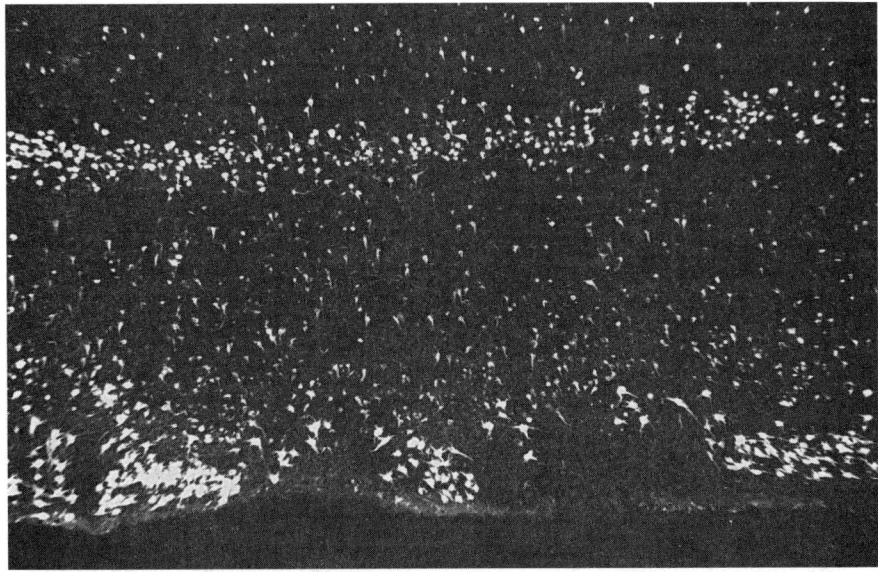

FIGURE 3. This is a photomicrograph of a thioflavin-S stained cross-section through the entorhinal cortex at endstage AD viewed under fluorescent illumination to reveal neurofibrillary tangles. The superficial layer II islands contain dense NFTs as does layer IV near the top of the photomicrograph. The latter receives a powerful hippocampal output and projects directly to the ventral striatum and to temporal and frontal cortices that project to the basal forebrain.

torhinal cortex parts of the ventromedial temporal area. However, selective nuclei such as the accessory basal and cortical nuclei are always damaged by dense NFTs, and the former, plus the mediobasal nucleus, contain large quantities of NPs. As a general rule, the lateral, central and medial nuclei are consistently the least affected. Caution here though is probably recommended since most AD investigators have focused largely on only NFTs and NPs, and not neuron loss. There is a suggestion in the literature preceding these more recent studies that neuron loss may be extensive in amygdaloid nuclei that do not contain classic AD pathology.[43,91] Irrespective of this, it is clear that the basal complex of the amygdala is damaged heavily in AD. As with the hippocampal formation and entorhinal cortex, this pathology affects neurons that are sources of a powerful afferent input to the ventral striatum and magnocellular cell groups of the basal forebrain and to frontal and temporal cortices that in turn project to these same basal forebrain targets (FIGS. 4 and 5).[3,8,9]

TEMPORAL LOBE INJURY

The Tentorial Incisura

Although nearly all components of the ventromedial temporal area are affected severely, but selectively, by pathology in AD, and partially so in Pick's disease, these

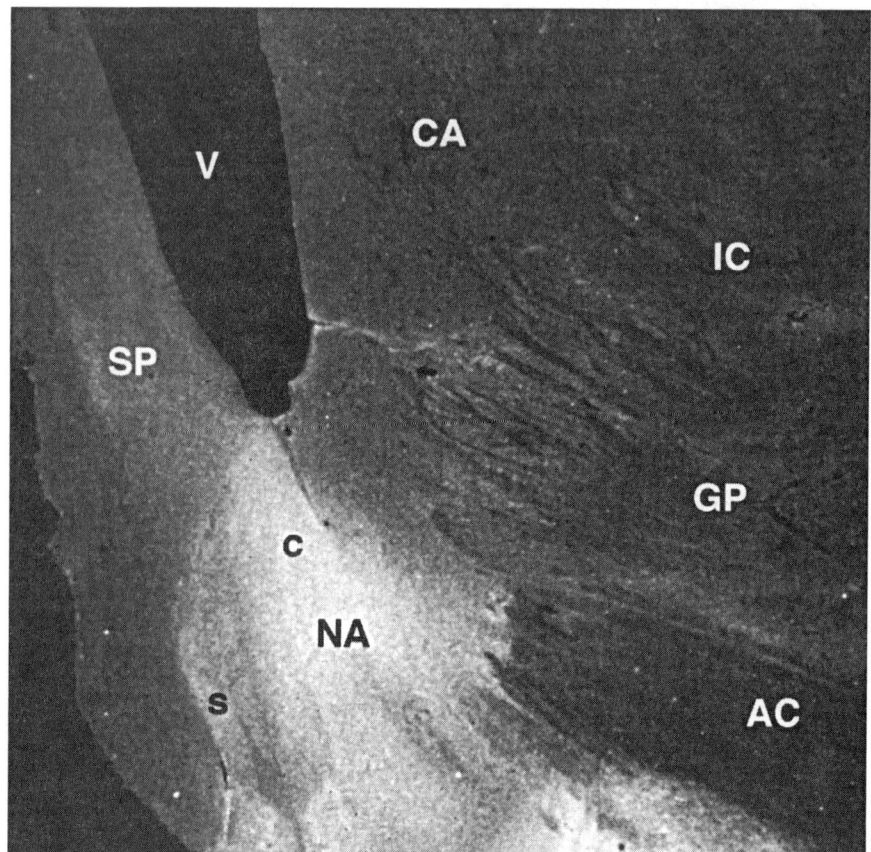

FIGURE 4. This photomicrograph shows a dark field image of terminal axon labeling (*white*) over the core (c) and shell (s) of the nucleus accumbens (NA) of a rhesus monkey following an injection of tritiated amino acids into the dorsal portions of the laterobasal and accessory basal amygdaloid nuclei. (Other abbreviations: AC, anterior commissure; CA, caudate nucleus; GP, globus pallidus; IC, internal capsule; SP, septum; V, anterior horn of lateral ventricle).

conditions form only one class of injury that can affect the temporal lobe. Another large class of injury relates to the tight encasement and insertion of the ventromedial temporal area into the temporal fossa adjacent to the irregular boney structure of this part of the skull. The vulnerability of the temporal lobe from direct forces and forces generated by impact at many points on the skull in head injury is well known.[2,37] Likewise, the proximity of ventromedial temporal areas to the inferior horn of the lateral ventricle is of consequence since injury can occur with increased intracranial pressure in the supratentorial space, no matter what its etiology—tumor, abscess, hematoma, edema, infection or infarction.[1,64]

Central to both head injury and increased intracranial pressure in the supratentorial space is the free edge of the tentorium cerebelli which traverses across the ven-

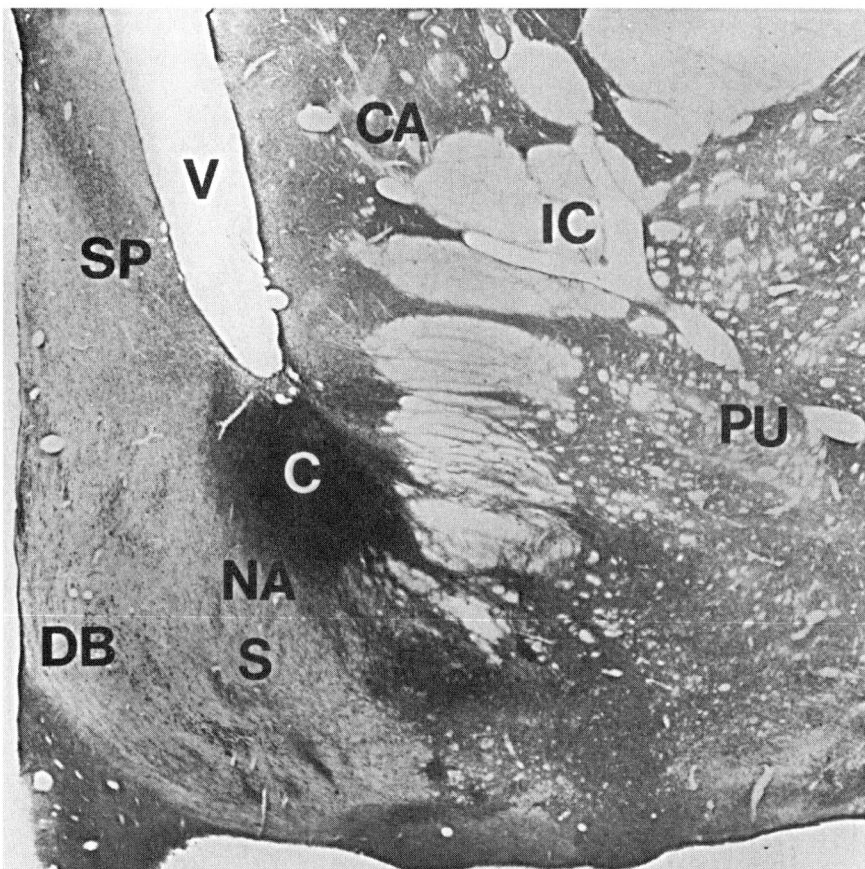

FIGURE 5. This photomicrograph shows a bright field image of dense biotinylated detran amine axon labeling in the core (c) of the nucleus accumbens (NA) following an injection into the ventral part of the laterobasal amygdaloid nucleus in the rhesus monkey. (Other abbreviations: CA, caudate nucleus; DB, vertical limb of diagonal band of Broca; IC, internal capsule; PU, putamen; SP, septum; V, anterior horn of lateral ventricle.)

tromedial temporal area of each hemisphere before its attachment to the petrous apex and anterior and posterior clinoid processes (FIG. 6). This arrangement forms an aperture through which the upper brain stem passes with a sharp dural incisura surrounding the aperture. It is through this aperture that communication between the supratentorial and infratentorial spaces is achieved.[51,63]

The anterior part of the parahippocampal gyrus, the so-called gyrus ambiens, lies directly in the tentorial aperture unprotected by dura mater.[69] The size of the tentorial aperture varies among humans, but it has been estimated that the free edge of the tentorium cerebelli contracts or grooves the parahippocampal gyrus in 70% of the population, that this groove is visible in neonates, and visible in both the unfixed or fixed brain.[24] Retzius[69] labeled this groove the inferior rhinal sulcus, but others have

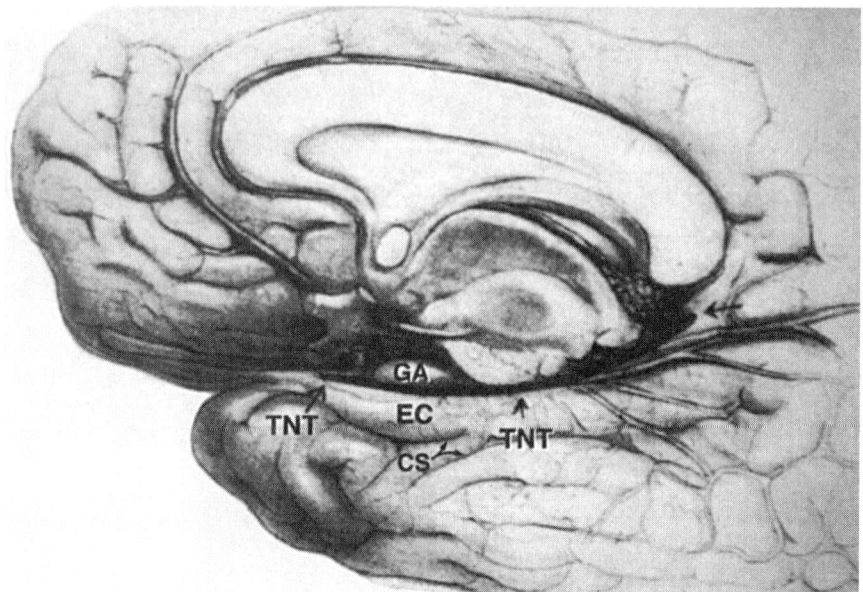

FIGURE 6. A reproduction of FIGURE 1 from Jefferson's classic article "The Tentorial Pressure Cone" showing the course of the free edge of the tentorium cerebelli (TNT) across the parahippocampal gyrus. At the level of the entorhinal cortex (EC) the free edge contacts and notches the cortex. Note that the gyrus ambiens (GA) of the entorhinal cortex bulges over the free edge of the tentorium cerebelli and sits without dural protection in the tentorial aperture. (Other abbreviations: CS, collateral sulcus).

labeled it the tentorial notch or groove reflecting, in their estimation, that it represents an indentation and surface marking consistent with the disposition of the free edge of the tentorium cerebelli.[12,29] It is doubtful that it deserves the label of sulcus since it is merely an indentation and bears no relationship to the rhinal sulcus.

Uncal Herniation with Head Injury and Increased Intracranial Pressure

The location of the tentorial incisura and the complications it can create in neurological disease and diagnosis has long been appreciated.[63] Quite simply, potential space in the supratentorial space is not extensive, and when exhausted, supratentorially located brain structures will herniate across the free edge of the tentorium cerebelli into the space of Bichat and infratentorial space. The consequent compression of the brain stem necessitates emergency efforts to preserve life. The pathological concept of uncal herniation is an appropriate description for extreme herniation and in autopsy specimens where death occurred. Indeed, in such cases the uncal hippocampal formation has herniated, and dominates the pathological picture.[24] However, in technical terms, it is not the uncal hippocampus that lies in the tentorial aperture, but instead the entorhinal cortex of the gyrus ambiens of the ventromedial temporal area, and it leads the herniation. Thus, partial herniation in-

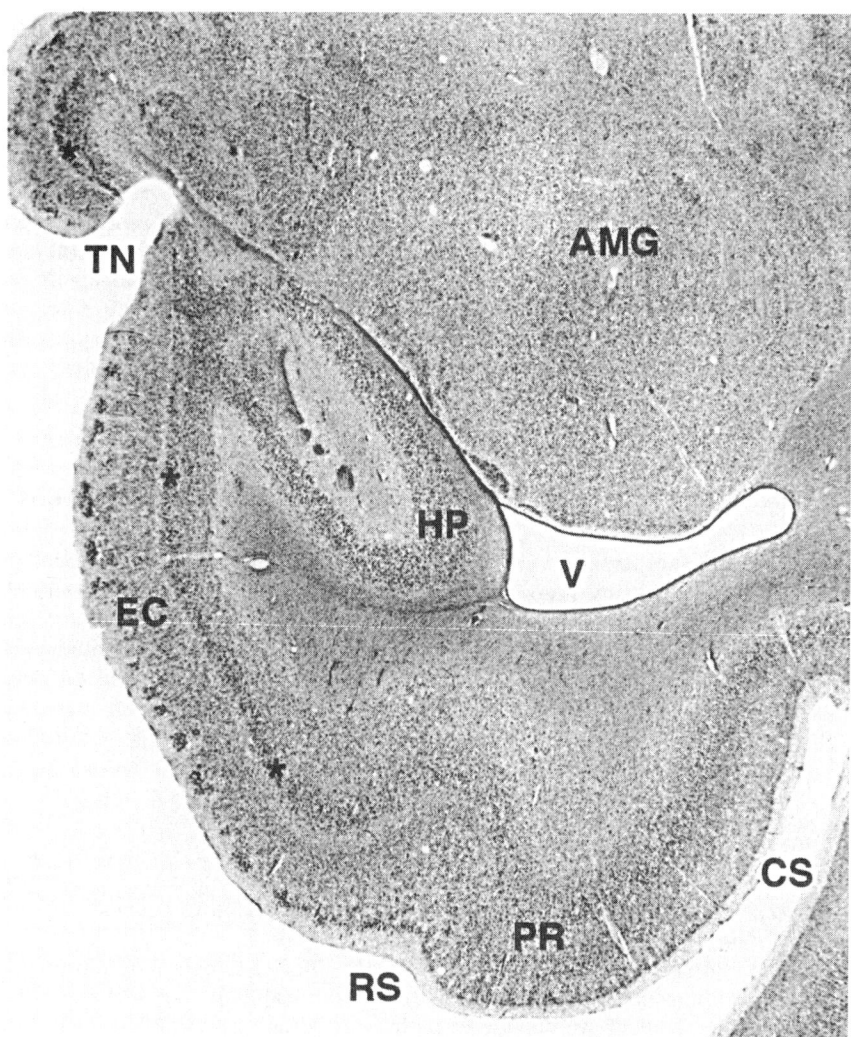

FIGURE 7. A Nissl-stained cross-section of the ventromedial temporal area showing injury at the tentorial notch (TN) by the free edge of the tentorium cerebelli in a 62-year-old donor who suffered from agitated depression and psychoses after head injury at age 43. The asterisks denote layer IV of the entorhinal cortex (EC) which projects to the nucleus accumbens of the ventral striatum. The unusual, more vertical positioning, of the amygdala (AMG) and hippocampal formation (HP) are no doubt due to the ventromedial temporal area being forced onto the fixed free edge of the tentorium cerebelli. Gliosis and vascular hypertrophy can still be seen in the amygdala immediately above the tentorial notch. (Other abbreviations: CS, collateral sulcus; PR, perirhinal cortex; RS, rhinal sulcus).

jures ventromedial temporal areas that provide input to the ventral striatum and to areas that project to it, and behavior changes in such patients could reflect this situation as much as direct entorhinal cortex injury. In this sense, abnormal behavior following temporal lobe injury and entorhinal herniation could represent a false localizing sign in the same manner as cranial nerve signs do, due to brain stem compression, in full uncal herniation.[51,63]

In a related matter, many patients suffering head trauma recuperate from their injuries physically, but are left with post-traumatic behavioral changes. In many of these cases, it is likely that ventromedial temporal area injury occurred around the free edge or incisura of the tentorium cerebelli due to the brain being forced onto it (FIG. 7). Thus, post-traumatic behavioral changes in head injury survivors may reflect distal changes in the basal forebrain equally as much as direct damage to the ventromedial temporal area. We suspect that temporal injury around the free edge of the tentorium cerebelli, whatever its cause, is more widespread than appreciated and a contributor to poorly understood behavioral changes in humans of all ages. Anatomically detailed imaging studies will shed light on such patients.

SCHIZOPHRENIA AND THE VENTROMEDIAL TEMPORAL AREA

The ventromedial temporal area has been of special interest relative to schizophrenia research for many years because of clinical observations of psychotic-like behavior in temporal lobe disease. Some of the disorders discussed above have contributed to this interest. For example, in AD, a memory disorder is the hallmark of the associated behavioral changes throughout the entire illness, but confusion, delusions, aggression, agitation, and hallucinations are not uncommon in many patients.[26,34,59–61] These are also common in Pick's disease and Lewy Body disease, and in fact, may be a more prominent motivator for medical attention than a memory impairment. These latter degenerative dementias, however, are less uniquely associated anatomically with the temporal lobe, but nevertheless, involve it to a significant degree. Pick's disease, for example, often involves the dentate gyrus and the subicular/CA 1 zone of the hippocampal formation (FIG. 8). Other temporal lobe disorders in which psychotic-like behaviors occur include herpes simplex encephalitis[86] and temporal lobe epilepsy.[77]

The neurobiology of schizophrenia relative to medial temporal structures has been included in recent reviews,[13,14,79] and we will not attempt to repeat these very adequate efforts. Instead, we will comment only on certain issues pertaining to ventromedial temporal area cytoarchitecture and neuropathology that have a bearing on the comments of the text above in the two previous sections.

Postmortem studies in schizophrenia have many difficulties well before they reach the microscope. Agonal state before death is often problematic as are long histories of neuroleptic medication. In many instances, death cannot be anticipated and medical examiners frequently have agendas and obligations not compatible with short autolysis times, brain fixation and neuroscience research. Despite this, postmortem studies have become more common in the past two decades and their results point toward ventromedial temporal area changes, particularly in the hippocampal formation and entorhinal cortex.[13,14,79] In the former structure, decreased quantities of microtubule-associated proteins have been observed in the subicular/CA 1 parts of the hippocampal formation and entorhinal cortex in schizophrenics.[12,72] These

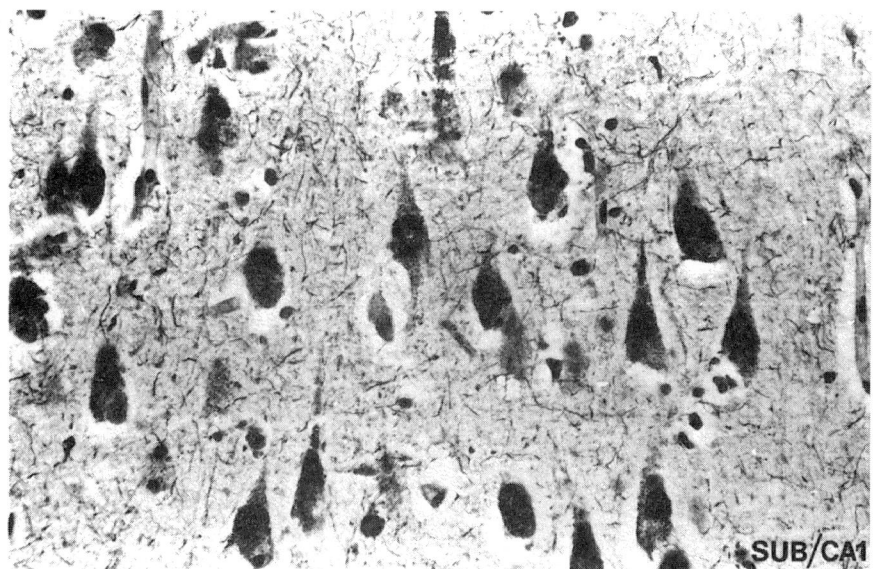

FIGURE 8. This photomicrograph is a Bielschowsky-stained cross-section through the subicular/CA 1 zone of the hippocampal formation in Pick's disease. Note that nearly every pyramidal neuron contains a large darkly stained Pick body that displaces the nucleus and nucleolus to the periphery of the soma away from their normal central position within the cytoplasm. Abnormal neurites can be seen in the neuropil between neurons as well as remnants of organelles and isolated Pick bodies from degenerating neurons. Psychoses and other behavioral disturbances are observed typically in Pick's disease.

molecules are expressed strongly during development and are known to play a role in microtubule cell biology, and particularly, dendritic orientation and elaboration. One might expect on the basis of these results alterations in pyramidal neuron dendritic morphology, but results on this issue are variable in the hippocampal formation,[6,23,55,73,74] but well documented in other limbic cortical areas.[15] Smaller neuron size, however, has been well documented in the subicular/CA 1 zone and entorhinal cortex in schizophrenics, as have volume changes.[10,16,31,32]

Laminar heterotopy in the entorhinal cortex of schizophrenics has been reported in several articles[12,48–50] and diminished density of neurons in key entorhinal layers is a consistent result.[4,32,57] An abnormal spatial arrangement of entorhinal neurons has also been observed.[13] Although the observations of entorhinal laminar heterotopy have been challenged,[4,57] those regarding density and spatial arrangement have not. Clearly, it is too early to judge entorhinal changes in schizophrenia, but variable results across patients seems likely. The affirmative or disaffirmative result in this regard is probably less critical than understanding why some schizophrenics have entorhinal cellular alterations and others do not. Interactions with abnormalities elsewhere in the brain would certainly be suspected to contribute to this variability.

Finally, it is of interest that abnormalities around the tentorial notch of the entorhinal cortex have been reported in some schizophrenics.[4,12,48–50,57] Several

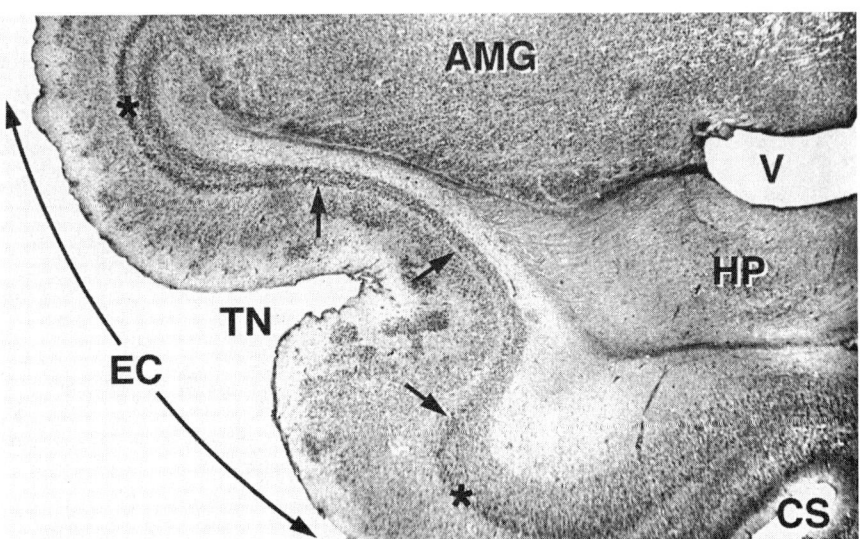

FIGURE 9. This is a photograph of a Nissl-stained cross-section through the entorhinal cortex (EC) of a brain from a schizophrenia patient in the Yakovlev Collection at the Armed Forces Institute of Pathology. Note, the deep tentorial notch (TN) and the laminar heterotopy of layer II cell islands at and around the injury. For many reasons, this is regarded as a developmental abnormality. The absence of gliosis is apparent as is the inappropriate migrational positioning of layer II neurons. Also, note that layer III pyramidal neurons are sparse at the tentorial notch and for several millimeters medial and lateral to it. Layer IV (*arrows*) is greatly depleted also at and around the tentorial notch. Both layers III and IV contain predominantly pyramidal neurons whose apical dendrites reach the molecular layer and pial surface. Injury or compression of the neuropil would compromise dendritic elaboration and may be associated with the paucity of neurons seen in these layers. Finally, the normal positioning of the amygdala (AMG) and hippocampal formation (HP) suggest that trauma due to head injury (see FIG. 8) was probably not a factor in the heterotopy and abnormal tentorial notch. For similar reasons it is unlikely that a previous lobotomy had anything to do with these dramatic cytoarchitectural changes in the entorhinal cortex of this schizophrenic. The patient was an adult, well beyond the age of developmental neural migration.

brains in the Yakovlev Collection have this abnormality (FIG. 9). Those in this collection have been questioned because of a prior prefrontal lobotomy.[57] However, numerous brains in that collection had lobotomies for reasons other than schizophrenia and lacked this abnormality in the ventromedial temporal area. While enthusiasm for abnormalities in the entorhinal cortex caused by the free edge of the tentorium cerebelli in some schizophrenics is dampened by similar changes in occasional normals, the key question may be related to timing of injury. If an injury reflected an intra-uterine infection, or was related to birth trauma, it may yield wholly different long-term outcomes than those occurring with episodic increased intracranial pressure in adulthood. Deep invaginations in the entorhinal cortex around the free edge of the tentorium cerebelli are not a normal anatomic variation in the human brains as some authors suggest. Instead, they speak clearly to previous head trauma or abnormalities in the supratentorial space. Why such changes are over-represented in populations of schizophrenics deserves further study and their presence in occasional normals does not diminish this interest.

In summary, ventromedial temporal changes in schizophrenia are commonplace and the weight of the evidence with all measures employed from molecules[12] to brain and ventricular volumes[17,18] adds to the picture. Understanding the variability within a population of schizophrenics could be key to further isolating the mechanisms that cause the disease. As with the other forms of temporal lobe disease highlighted here, the ventromedial temporal areas that are suspect in schizophrenia are precisely those that project powerfully to basal forebrain structures or to cortical areas that in turn send axons to this part of the brain. This is the key consideration.

CONCLUDING REMARKS

In the sections above, we have highlighted only selective examples of ventromedial temporal area abnormalities that could deafferent the ventral striatopallidal and magnocellular parts of the basal forebrain. Many others could be added to the list, and they also have behavioral sequela as clinical features. While it is partially arbitrary to focus only on basal forebrain targets of the ventromedial temporal area axons, it is also important to recognize that the latter structures do not have widespread frontal lobe projections.[33,35,92] Indeed, ventromedial temporal areas project primarily to only those frontal areas that give rise to ventral striatopallidal and magnocellular nuclei projections. For example, the subicular/CA 1 zone of the hippocampal formation, the deep layers of the entorhinal cortex and the basal nuclei of the amygdala project powerfully to the anterior cingulate, medial frontal and the orbitofrontal cortices, and only modestly so, if at all, to the dorsolateral and frontal polar cortex—the classical prefrontal granular cortices. Temporal input to these areas arise largely from more proximal sensory association cortices in the parietal, occipital and temporal lobes. We are far more impressed with the fact that diseases and injury to the ventromedial temporal area often target exactly those structures and layers of cortex that project powerfully to the basal forebrain and to those frontal areas that also send axons to the ventral striatum and magnocellular cell groups.

A fundamental principle of mamallian neuroanatomy is that ventromedial temporal areas are at the endstation of corticocortical association systems for all modalities[82,89] and process on line sensory events in real time. These same cortical association pathways that converge onto ventromedial temporal areas sequentially pass through both proximal and distal association cortices that are repositories for past learning and memory. Thus, the input to ventromedial temporal areas, that project to the basal forebrain, has both real-time and historical-time elements associated with it. Moreover, hippocampal output is adjoined with this for elements of significance, novelty and relevancy.[84,89] The same cannot be said for proximal association projections to classical dorsolateral and frontal polar prefrontal cortices.

All things considered, we view the basal forebrain in a highly unique position where, by virtue of the digest of its multimodal and hippocampal input, it can organize, or at least predispose, the organism for appropriate emotional, motor, endocrine and autonomic responses exactly in register with real time perception in the context of past history, novelty and its relevance. It is certainly arguable that deficits involving psychoses are reducible to deficiencies in appropriate response selections to the richly textured real-time, historical-time and memory-related information that the basal forebrain receives. As demonstrated recently by Richmond and his collaborators,[76] these are essential elements for a predictable reality, and ventral striatal units are tuned keenly to these contingencies in primates. A major deficit in schizophrenia may lie largely in utilizing real-time, historical-time and memory-related information for predictions about reality. If this is the case, altered ventromedial temporal areas would be expected to have a large voice in the abnormality.

ACKNOWLEDGMENTS

This research was supported by NIH Grants NS 14944 and PO NS 19632. We thank Sherry Lohman for library research and typing the manuscript, Paul Reimann for photography, and Darrell Wilkins for tissue acquisition from the University of Iowa Deeded Body Program.

REFERENCES

1. ADAMS, J.H. 1984. The pathophysiology of raised intracranial pressure. *In* Greenfield's Neuropathology, 4th edit. J.H. Adams, J.A.N. Corsellis & L. W. Dunchen, Eds. John Wiley & Sons. New York.
2. ADAMS, J.H., D.I. GRAHAM, G. SCOTT, L.S. PARKER & D. DOYLE. 1980. Brain damage in non-missile head injury. J. Clin. Pathol. **33:** 1132–1145.
3. AGGLETON, J.P., D.P. FRIEDMAN & M. MISHKIN. 1987. A comparison between the connections of the amygdala and hippocampus with the basal forebrain in the macaque. Exp. Brain Res. **67:** 556–568.
4. AKIL, M. & D.A. LEWIS. 1997. Cytoarchitecture of the entorhinal cortex in schizophrenia. Am. J. Psychiatry **154:** 1010–1012.
5. ALHEID, G.F. & L. HEIMER. 1988. New perspectives in basal forebrain organization of special relevance for neuropsychiatric disorders: the striatopallidal, amygdaloid, and corticopetal components of substantia innominata. Neuroscience **27:** 1–39.
6. ALTSCHULER, L.L., A. CONRAD, J.A. KOVELMAN & A. SCHEIBEL. 1987. Hippocampal pyramidal cell orientation in schizophrenia. Arch. Gen. Psychiatry **44:** 1094–1098.
7. ALVAREZ, P., S. ZOLA-MORGAN & L.R. SQUIRE. 1995. Damage limited to the hippocampal region produces long-lasting memory impairment in monkeys. J. Neurosci. **15(5):** 3796–3807.
8. AMARAL, D.G. & J.L. PRICE. 1984. Amygdalo-cortical projections in the monkey. J. Comp. Neurol. **230:** 465–496.
9. AMARAL, D.G., J.L. PRICE, A. PITKANEN & S.T. CARMICHAEL. 1992. Anatomical organization of the primate amygdaloid complex. *In* The Amygdala. J.P. Aggleton, Ed.: 1–66. Wiley-Liss. New York.
10. ARNOLD, S.E., B.R. FRANZ, R.C. GUR, R.E. GUR, R.M. SHAPIRO, P.J. MOBERG & J.Q. TROJANOWSKI. 1995. Smaller neuron size in schizophrenia in hippocampal subfields that mediate cortical-hippocampal interactions. Am. J. Psychiatry **152:** 738–748.
11. ARNOLD, S.E., B.T. HYMAN, J. FLORY, A.R. DAMASIO & G.W. VAN HOESEN. 1991. The topographical and neuroanatomical distribution of neurofibrillary tangles and neuritic plaques in the cerebral cortex of patients with Alzheimer's disease. Cerebral Cortex **1(Jan/Feb):** 103–116.
12. ARNOLD, S.E., V.M.Y. LEE, R.E. GUR & J.Q. TROJANOWSKI. 1991. Abnormal expression of two microtubule-associated proteins (MAP2 and MAP5) in specific sub-

fields of the hippocampal formation in schizophrenia. Proc. Natl. Acad. Sci. USA **88:** 10850–10854.
13. ARNOLD, S.E., D.D. RUSCHEINSKY & L.-Y. HAN. 1997. Further evidence of abnormal cytoarchitecture of the entorhinal cortex in schizophrenia using spatial point pattern analyses. Biol. Psychiatry 42(8): 639–647.
14. ARNOLD, S.E. & J.Q. TROJANOWSKI. 1996. Recent advances in defining the neuropathology of schizophrenia. Acta Neuropathol. **92:** 217–231.
15. BENES, F.M. 1993. Neurobiological investigations in cingulate cortex of schizophrenic brain. Schizophrenic Bull. **19:** 537–549.
16. BENES, F.M., I. SORENSON & D.E. BIRD. 1991. Reduced neuronal size in posterior hippocampus of schizophrenic patients. Schizophrenic Bull. **17:** 597–608.
17. BOGERTS, B., M. ASHTARI, G. DEGREEF, J.M. ALVIR, R.M. BILDER & J.A. LIEBERMAN. 1990. Reduced temporal limbic structure volumes on magnetic resonance images in first episode schizophrenia. Psychiatry Res. Neuroimaging **35:** 1–13.
18. BOGERTS, B., J.A. LIEBERMAN, M. ASHTARI, R. BILFRT, G. DEGREEF, G. LERNER, C. JOHNS & S. MASIAR. 1993. Hippocampus-amygdala volumes and psychopathology in chronic schizophrenia. Biol. Psychiatry. **33:** 236–246.
19. BRAAK, H. & E. BRAAK. 1992. The human entorhinal cortex: normal morphology and lamina-specific pathology in various diseases. Neurosci. Res. **15:** 6–31.
20. BRAAK, H. & E. BRAAK. 1991. Neuropathological staging of Alzheimer-related changes. Acta Neuropathol. **82:** 239–259.
21. BRAAK, H. & E. BRAAK. 1985. On areas of transition between entorhinal allocortex and temporal isocortex in the human brain. Normal morphology and lamina-specific pathology in Alzheimer's Disease. Acta Neuropathol. **68:** 325–332.
22. CARMICHAEL, S.T., M.-C. CLUGNET & J.L. PRICE. 1994. Central olfactory connections in the macaque monkey. J. Comp. Neurol. **346:** 403–434.
23. CHRISTISON, G.W., M.F. CASANOVA, D.R. WEINBERGER, R. RAWLINGS & J.E. KLEINMAN. 1989. A quantitative investigation of hippocampal pyramidal cell size, shape, and variability of orientation in schizophrenia. Arch. Gen. Psychiatry **46:** 1027–1032.
24. CORSELLIS, J.A.N. 1958. Individual variation in the size of the tentorial opening. J. Neurol. Neurosurg. Psychiatry **21:** 279–283.
25. DAMASIO, A. R. 1994. Descartes' Error: Emotion, Reason, and the Human Brain. Grosset/Putnam. New York.
26. DAVISON, K. 1983. Schizophrenia-like psychoses associated with organic cerebral disorders: a review. Psychiatr. Dev. **1:** 1–34.
27. DE OLMOS, J.S. 1990. Amygdala. *In* The Human Nervous System. G. Paxinos, Ed.: 583–710. Academic Press, Inc. San Diego.
28. DE OLMOS, J.S., G.F. ALHEID & C.A. BELTRAMINO. 1985. Amygdala. *In* The Rat Nervous System. G. Paximos, Ed.: 223–334. Academic Press. Sydney.
29. DUVERNOY, H.M. 1988. The Human Hippocampus: An Atlas of Applied Anatomy. Bergmann. Munich.
30. ESIRI, M. M., R. C. A. PEARSON, J. E. STEELE, D. M. BOWEN & T. P. S. POWELL. 1990. A quantitative study of the neurofibrillary tangles and the choline acetyltransferase activity in the cerebral cortex and the amygdala in Alzheimer's disease. J. Neurol. Neurosurg. Psychiatry **53:** 161–165.
31. FALKAI, P. & B. BOGERTS. 1986. Cell loss in the hippocampus of schizophrenics. Eur. Arch. Psychiatry in Neurol. Sci. **236:** 154–161.
32. FALKAI, P., B. BOGERTS & M. ROZUMEK. 1988. Limbic pathology in schizophrenia: The entorhinal region—a morphometric study. Biol. Psychiatry **24:** 515–521.
33. FLETCHER, P. 1998. The missing link: a failure of fronto-hippocampal integration in schizophrenia. Nature Neurosci. 1(4): 266–267.
34. FÖRSTL, H., A. BURNS, R. LEVY & N. CAIRNS. 1994. Neuropathological correlates of psychotic phenomena in confirmed Alzheimer's disease. Br. J. Psychiatry **165:** 53–59.
35. GOLDMAN-RAKIC, P.S. 1991. Prefrontal cortical dysfunction in schizophrenia: the relevance of working memory. *In* Psychopathology and the Brain. B.J. Carroll & J.E. Barrett, Eds.: 1–23. Raven Press. New York.

36. GÓMEZ-ISLA, T., J.L. PRICE, D.W. MCKEEL, JR., J.C. MORRIS, J.H. GROWDON & B.T. HYMAN. 1996. Profound loss of layer II entorhinal cortex neurons occurs in very mild Alzheimer's disease. J. Neurosci. **16**(14): 4491–5000.
37. GRAHAM, D.I., J.H. ADAMS & T.A. GENNARELLI. 1993. Pathology of brain damage in head injury. *In* Head Injury. P. R. Cooper, Ed.: 91–113. Williams and Wilkins. Baltimore, MD.
38. GROENEWEGEN, H.J., P. ROOM, M.P. WITTER & A.H.M. LOHMAN. 1982. Cortical afferents of the nucleus accumbens in the cat, studied with anterograde and retrograde transport techniques. Neuroscience **7**: 977–996.
39. GROENEWEGEN, H.J., E. VERMEULEN-VAN DER ZEE, A. TE KORTSCHOT & M.P. WITTER. 1987. Organization of the projections from the subiculum to the ventral striatum in the rat. A study using anterograde transport of phaseolus vulgaris leucoagglutinin. Neuroscience **23**(1): 103–120.
40. HABER, S. N., K. KUNISHIO, M. MIZOBUCHI & E. LYND-BALTA. 1995. The orbital and medial prefrontal circuit through the primate basal ganglia. J. Neurosci. **15**: 4851–4867.
41. HEIMER, L., G.F. ALHEID, J.S. DE OLMOS, H.J. GROWENEWEGEN, S.N. HABER, R.E. HARLAN & D.S. ZAHM. 1997. The accumbens: beyond the core-shell dichotomy. J. Neuropsychiatry Clin. Neurosci. **9**: 354–381.
42. HEIMER, L., J. DE OLMOS, G.F. ALHEID & L. ZABORSKY. 1991. "Perestroika" in the basal forebrain: opening the border between neurology and psychiatry. Prog. Brain Res. **87**: 109–165.
43. HERZOG, A. G. & T. L. KEMPER. 1980. Amygdaloid changes in aging and dementia. Arch. Neurol. **37**: 625–629.
44. HYMAN, B.T., L.J. KROMER & G.W. VAN HOESEN. 1988. A direct demonstration of the perforant pathway terminal zone in Alzheimer's disease using the monoclonal antibody Alz-50. Brain Res. **450**: 392–397.
45. HYMAN, B.T., G.W. VAN HOESEN, A.R. DAMASIO & C.L. BARNES. 1984. Alzheimer's disease: cell-specific pathology isolates the hippocampal formation. Science **225**: 1168–1170.
46. HYMAN, B.T., G.W. VAN HOESEN, L.J. KROMER & A.R. DAMASIO. 1986. Perforant pathway changes and the memory impairment of Alzheimer's disease. Ann. Neurol. **20**(4): 472–481.
47. INSAUSTI, R. 1993. Comparative anatomy of the entorhinal cortex and hippocampus in mammals. Hippocampus **3**(Special issue): 19–26.
48. JAKOB, H. & H. BECKMANN. 1994. Circumscribed malformation and nerve cell alterations in the entorhinal cortex of schizophrenics. J. Neural Transmission **98**: 83–106.
49. JAKOB, H. & H. BECKMANN. 1989. Gross and histological criteria for developmental disorders in brains of schizophrenics. J. Royal Soc. Med. **82**: 466–469.
50. JAKOB, H. & H. BECKMANN. 1986. Prenatal developmental disturbances in the limbic allocortex in schizophrenics. J. Neural Transmission **65**: 303–326.
51. JEFFERSON, G. 1938. The tentorial pressure cone. Arch. Neurol. Psychiatry **40**: 857–876.
52. KELLEY, A. E. & V. B. DOMESICK. 1982. The distribution of the projection from the hippocampal formation to the nucleus accumbens in the rat: an anterograde- and retrograde-horseradish peroxidase study. Science **7**(10): 2321–2335.
53. KEMPER, T.L. 1983. Organization of the Neuropathology of the amygdala in Alzheimer's disease. *In* Biological Aspects of Alzheimer's Disease, Banbury Report 15. R. Katzman, Ed.: 31–35. Cold Spring Harbor Laboratory.
54. KOSEL, K.C., G.W. VAN HOESEN & D.L. ROSENE. 1982. Non-hippocampal cortical projections from the entorhinal cortex in the rat and rhesus monkey. Brain Res. **244**: 210–213.
55. KOVELMAN, J. A. & A. B. SCHEIBEL. 1984. A neurohistological correlate of schizophrenia. Biol. Psychiatry **19**: 1601–1621.
56. KRAYNIAK, P. F., R. C. MEIBACH & A. SIEGEL. 1981. A projection from the entorhinal cortex to the nucleus accumbens in the rat. Brain Res. **209**: 427–431.

57. KRIMER, L.S., M.M. HERMAN, R.C. SAUNDERS, J.C. BOYD, T.M. HYDE, J.M. CARTER, J.E. KLEINMAN & D.R. WEINBERGER. 1997. A qualitative and quantitative analysis of the entorhinal cortex in schizophrenia. Cerebral Cortex **7**: 732–739.
58. KROMER VOGT, L.J., B.T. HYMAN, G.W. VAN HOESEN & A.R. DAMASIO. 1990. Pathological alterations in the amygdala in Alzheimer's disease. Neuroscience **37**(2): 377–385.
59. LYKETSOS, C.G., C. STEELE, E. GALIK, A. ROSENBLATT, M. STEINBERG, A. WARREN & J.-M. SHEPPARD. 1999. Physical aggression in dementia patients and its relationship to depression. Am. J. Psychiatry **156**: 66–71.
60. MCSHANE, R., J. KEENE, C. FAIRBURN, R. JACOBY & T. HOPE. 1998. Psychiatric symptoms in patients with dementia predict the later development of behavioral abnormalities. Psychol. Med. **28**: 1119–1127.
61. MEGA, M.S. & J.L. CUMMINGS. 1994. Frontal-subcortical circuits and neuropsychiatric disorders. J. Neuropsychiatry **6**: 358–370.
62. MESULAM, M.M. & E.J. MUFSON. 1984. Neural inputs into the nucleus basalis of the substantia innominata (Ch4) in the rhesus monkey. Brain **107**: 253–274.
63. MEYER, A. 1920. Herniation of the brain. Arch. Neurol. Psychiatry. **4**: 387–400.
64. MILLER, J.D. & J.H. ADAMS. 1984. The pathophysiology of raised intracranial pressure. *In* Greenfield's Neuropathology, 4th edit. J.H. Adams, J.A.N. Corsellis & L.W. Duchen, Eds. John Wiley & Sons. New York.
65. MURPHY, G.M., JR. & W.G. ELLIS. 1991. The amygdala in Down's syndrome and familial Alzheimer disease: four clinicopathological case reports. Biol. Psychiatry **30**: 92–106.
66. MURRAY, E. A., D. GAFFAN & M. MISHKIN. 1993. Neural substrates of visual stimulus-stimulus association in rhesus monkeys. J. Neurosci. **13**: 4549–4561.
67. PAPEZ, J.W. 1937. A proposed mechanism of emotion. Arch. Neurol. Psychiatry **38**: 725–743.
68. PRICE, J.L., S.T. CARMICHAEL & W.C. DREVETS. 1996. Networks related to the orbital and medial prefrontal cortex. *In* The Emotional Motor System. G. Holstege, R. Bandler & D.B. Saper, Eds.: 461–484. Elsevier Science, Ltd.
69. RETZIUS, G. 1896. Das menschenhirn. Studien in der makroskopischen morphologie. Norstedt & Sohne. Stockholm.
70. ROSENE, D.L. & G.W. VAN HOESEN. 1977. Hippocampal efferents reach widepread areas of cerebral cortex and amygdala in the rhesus monkey. Science **198**: 315–317.
71. ROSENE, D. L. & G. W. VAN HOESEN. 1987. The hippocampal formation of the primate brain: a review of some comparative aspects of cytoarchitecture and connections. *In* Cerebral Cortex, vol. 6. Plenum Press. New York.
72. ROSOKLIJA, G., M.A. KAUFMAN & D. LIU. 1995. Subicular MAP-2 immunoreactivity in schizophrenia (abstract). Soc. Neurosci. Abstracts **21**: 2126.
73. SCHEIBEL, A.B. & J.A. KOVELMAN. 1981. Disorientation of the hippocampal pyramidal cells and its processes in the schizophrenic patient. Biol. Psychiatry **16**: 101–102.
74. SCHMAJUK, N.A. & M. TYBERG. 1990. The hippocampal lesion model of schizophrenia. *In* Neuromethods: Animal Models in Psychiatry, vol. 19. A.A. Boulton, G.B. Baker & M.T.P. Martin-Iverson, Eds. Humana Press. Clifton, NJ.
75. SCOVILLE, W.B. & B. MILNER. 1957. Loss of recent memory after bilateral hippocampal lesions. J. Neurol. Neurosurg. Psychiatry **20**: 11.
76. SHIDARA, M., T.G. AIGNER & B.J. RICHMOND. 1998. Neuronal signals in the monkey ventral striatum related to progress through a predictable series of trials. J. Neurosci. **18**(7): 2613–2625.
77. SLATER, E. & A.W. BEARD. 1963. The schizophrenia-like psychoses of epilepsy. Br. J. Psychiatry **109**: 95–150.
78. SORENSEN, K.E. 1985. Projections of the entorhinal area to the striatum, nucleus accumbens, and cerebral cortex in the guinea pig. J. Comp. Neurol. **238**: 308–322.
79. STEVENS, J.R. 1997. Anatomy of schizophrenia revisited. Schizophrenic Bull. **23**: 373–383.

80. SUZUKI, W.A., S. ZOLA-MORGAN, L.R. SQUIRE & D.G. AMARAL. 1993. Lesions of the perirhinal and parahippocampal cortices in the monkey produce long-lasting memory impairment in the visual and tactual modalities. J. Neurosci. **13**(6): 2430–2451.
81. TOTTERDELL, S. & G.E. MEREDITH. 1997. Topographical organization of projections from the entorhinal cortex to the striatum of the rat. Neuroscience **78**(3): 715–729.
82. VAN ESSEN, D.C., D.J. FELLEMAN, E.A. DEYOE, J. OLAVARRIA & J. KNIERIM. 1990. Modular and hierarchical organization of extrastriate visual cortex in the macaque monkey. Cold Spring Harbor Symp. Quant. Biol. **3**: 679–696.
83. VAN HOESEN, G.W. 1995. Anatomy of the medial temporal lobe. Mag. Resonance Imaging **13**(8): 1047–1055.
84. VAN HOESEN, G.W. 1982. The parahippocampal gyrus: new observations regarding its cortical connections in the monkey. Trends Neurosci. **5**: 345–350.
85. VAN HOESEN, G.W. 1997. Ventromedial temporal lobe anatomy, with comments on Alzheimer's disease and temporal injury. J. Neuropsychiatry Clin. Neurosci. **9**: 331–341.
86. VAN HOESEN, G.W. & A.R. DAMASIO. 1987. Neural correlates of the cognitive impairment in Alzheimer's disease. *In* Higher Functions of the Nervous System, the Handbook of Physiology. F. Plum, Ed.: 871–898.
87. VAN HOESEN, G.W., M.-M. MESULAM & R. HAAXMA. 1976. Temporal cortical projections to the olfactory tubercle in the rhesus monkey. Brain Res. **109**: 375–381.
88. VAN HOESEN, G.W. & D.N. PANDYA. 1975. Some connections of the entorhinal (area 28) and perirhinal (area 35) cortices of the rhesus monkey. I. Temporal lobe afferents. Brain Res. **95**: 1–24.
89. VAN HOESEN, G.W., D.N. PANDYA & N. BUTTERS. 1972. Cortical afferents to the entorhinal cortex of the rhesus monkey. Science **175**: 1471–1473.
90. VAN HOESEN, G.W., D.N. PANDYA & N. BUTTERS. 1975. Some connections of the entorhinal (area 28) and perirhinal (area 35) cortices of the rhesus monkey. II. Frontal lobe afferents. Brain Res. **95**: 25–38.
91. VEREECKEN, H.L.G., O.J.M. VOGELS & R. NIEUWENHUYS. 1994. Neuron loss and shrinkage in the amygdala in Alzheimer's disease. Neurobiol. Aging **15**(1): 45–54.
92. WEINBERGER, D.R. 1991. Anteromedial temporal-prefrontal connectivity: a functional neuroanatomical system implicated in schizophrenia. *In* Psychopathology and the Brain. B.J. Carroll & J.E. Barret, Eds.: 25–43. Raven Press. New York.
93. WITTER, M., H.J. GROENEWEGEN, F.H. LOPES DA SILVA & A.H.M. LOHMAN. 1989. Functional organization of the extrinsic and intrinsic circuitry of the parahippocampal region. Prog. Neurobiol. **33**: 161–254.
94. WITTER, M.P. 1993. Organization of the entorhinal-hippocampal system: A review of current anatomical data. Hippocampus **3**: 33–44.
95. WRIGHT, C.I., A.V. BEIJER & H.J. GROENEWEGEN. 1996. Basal amygdaloid complex afferents to the rat nucleus. J. Neurosci. **16**(5): 1877–1893.
96. ZOLA-MORGAN, S., L.R. SQUIRE, R.P. CLOWER & N.L. REMPEL. 1993. Damage to the perirhinal cortex exacerbates memory impairment following lesions to the hippocampal formation. J. Neurosci. **13**(1): 251–265.

D_3 Receptors and the Actions of Neuroleptics in the Ventral Striatopallidal System of Schizophrenics

JEFFREY N. JOYCE[a] AND EUGENIA V. GUREVICH

Christopher Center for Parkinson's Disease Research, Sun Health Research Institute, 10515 W. Santa Fe Drive, Sun City, Arizona 85351, USA

ABSTRACT: The mesolimbic dopamine (DA) system and an important target receptor, the D_3 receptor, have been implicated in schizophrenia. We have identified, using non-radioactive *in situ* hybridization histochemistry, that D_3 mRNA-positive neurons are highly concentrated in the ventral striatum, efferents of the ventral striatum (globus pallidus internal, ventral palladium, substantia nigra pars reticulata), and in regions projecting to the ventral striatum (medial dorsal thalamus, nucleus basalis, extended amygdala). D_3 receptors are also highly enriched in the "limbic" striatal-pallidal-thalamic loop, exhibiting segregation from the D_2 receptor–enriched "motor loop." This supports data developed in rats showing that the D_3 receptor is a target of the mesolimbic DA system that can modulate the limbic striato-palladial-thalamic loop. However, D_2 and D_3 receptors and their mRNAs are co-localized in many sensory regions (lateral and medial geniculate nuclei, basolateral and basomedial amygdala, regions of thalamus), suggesting mechanisms of cross-talk. We have also demonstrated that there are 45% elevations in D_3 receptor number in ventral striatal neurons and their striatopalladial targets in schizophrenics that is reduced by concurrent antipsychotic treatment. Chronic haloperidol treatment to rats for 6 months with a 2-month withdrawal does not result in elevated D_3 receptor number. We hypothesize that antipsychotic treatment via D_3 receptors returns balance to limbic efferents of the ventral striatum. We established that early neonatal damage to the nigrostriatal DA system in rats produces characteristic adaptations in the pre- and post-synaptic components of the mesolimbic DA system that can provide a model to explore regulation by antipsychotics. This includes elevated release of DA from the mesolimbic DA terminals, elevated D_3 receptor mRNA in the Islands of Calleja and nucleus accumbens, and enhanced behavioral response to psychostimulants.

INTRODUCTION

The dopamine (DA) hypotheses of schizophrenia are varied in their hypothesized mechanisms but have been based largely on the evidence that pharmacological manipulations of the DA systems either augment the symptoms or depress the symptoms of schizophrenia. With the identification, in 1976, that antipsychotics (e.g., Haldol, haloperidol) bind to DA D_2 receptors[1,2] it has become widely believed that is the blockade of one or more members of the D_2-family of receptors[3] that alleviates

---

[a]Author to whom correspondence should be addressed. Voice: 623-876-5439; fax: 623-876-5695 (fax); jjoyce@mail.sunhealth.org

schizophrenia and the corollary that alterations in the density of DA receptors is an important component of the pathology of schizophrenia. Direct studies of brains derived at post-mortem from schizophrenics have identified that one more members of the D_2 receptor family are elevated in density in the striatum of schizophrenics as compared to age-matched controls.[4] However, these results remain difficult to interpret for several reasons. First, as is widely acknowledged the increase of striatal D_2 receptors obtained from postmortem studies may not be due to the illness, but rather to long-term adaptations of DA receptors to chronic antipsychotic treatment. In animal studies, both short-term (one to three weeks) and chronic treatment (6 or more months) with haloperidol elevates striatal D_2 receptors, which remain elevated even after drug withdrawal.[5] Accordingly, elevations in D_2 receptors in striatum identified in schizophrenics may be related to the use of the antipsychotics rather than to the illness itself. Secondly, many of these investigations have focused on DA receptors located in the striatum, but it has been difficult to support the hypothesis that it is the actions of antipsychotics at D_2 receptors in the striatum that modulate psychosis. For example, while typical antipsychotics can induce behavioral and neurochemical changes in striatum through actions at D_2 receptors, the atypical class of antipsychotics appear to be much less efficacious at striatal D_2 receptors.[6] By definition, the atypical antipsychotics possess a lower likelihood of inducing extrapyramidal (motor) side effects than the typical antipsychotics (e.g., Haldol). Thus, blockade of D_2 receptors within the striatum is likely the site of induction of the extrapyramidal side effects and not antipsychotic effects. This has raised the issue of whether the beneficial actions of antipsychotics occurs through the mesolimbic DA system and DA receptors mediating the actions of this system.[7]

LIMBIC AND MOTOR REGIONS OF THE BASAL GANGLIA

The midbrain DA neurons of the primate show a complex organization of subgroups of neurons, which can be differentiated, into different populations based on morphology and regions of innervation. Two tiers of TH-immunoreactive (TH-IR) neurons are evident in the human SN:

(1) a dorsal tier of neurons whose dendrites stretch in a mediolateral direction and
(2) a ventral group of clustered cells in the SNpc and in the SNpr with dendrites extending ventrally.[8]

Based on the tracer studies, the mesolimbic DA system of the primate, which includes the A10 region and the dorsal tier of the SNpc, innervates the ventral striatum. The ventral striatum is composed of the nucleus accumbens (NAS) and the ventral putamen. Whereas the origination of the "nigrostriatal" DA system innervating the dorsal caudate and putamen would be more restricted to the ventral tier of the SNpc.[9] As initially postulated by Heimer and Wilson,[10] it has now been convincingly demonstrated that there are parallel dorsal and ventral striatal-pallidal-thalamo circuits.[11] The dorsal putamen receives afferents from the sensory/motor cortex projects to both the globus pallidus external (GPe) and globus pallidus internal (GPi), and integrates information while under the control of the nigrostriatal DA system.[12] The GPi and SNpr project to specific nuclei in the thalamus (ventro posterior), which in turn projects to the premotor cortex and supplementary motor cortex. The ventral striatum has as its target the ventral pallidum (VP), the GPi and the substantia nigra.[13,14] In the primate the predominant efferents of the VP are the STN, substantia nigra (SN) and lateral hypothalamus,[15] whereas that for the GPi include the anteroventral (AV) and mediodorsal (MD) nuclei of the thalamus,[13,14] which in turn influence cortical regions innervating the limbic zones of the basal ganglia.[13,14,16]

The NAS and ventral putamen is known to receive afferents from the prefrontal cortex, thalamus, amygdala, cingulate, superior and inferior temporal cortices,[17-19] and integrate these signals under the modulatory influence of the mesolimbic DA system.[9,20] There is now considerable evidence that these limbic regions of the cortex are directly affected in schizophrenia; changes include smaller size, cytoarchitectonic abnormalities, and signs of disturbances in morphological development.[21] Functional studies involving *in vivo* imaging of local cerebral glucose utilization in schizophrenic subjects also show alterations in several limbic regions, including the medial temporal lobe.[22,23] Presumably this altered neuronal circuitry would result in disturbed processing and output of regions of brain functionally involved in a number of higher order cognitive processes. This would be "gated" through the limbic ventral striatal-pallidal-thalamo circuit under the control of the mesolimbic DA system. With the cloning of the members of the D_2-like receptor family, D_2, D_3 and D_4,[3] it became apparent they exhibited different anatomical patterns of high expression.[24,25] The D_2 receptor is highly expressed in the terminal region of the nigrostriatal DA system and the D_3 receptor in the terminal regions of the mesolimbic DA system, whereas the D_4 receptor resides largely outside the basal ganglia. The differential anatomy of the D_2 and D_3 receptor has reintroduced the hypothesis that is the pharmacological actions of the antipsychotics acting through the mesolimbic DA system that is most directly implicated in the ameliorative effects of these drugs.[26] However, this hypothesis has been based, until recently, on research in the rat. We and others, have provided new information in the human regarding anatomy of the mRNAs and receptor proteins for these receptors, altered expression in schizophrenia and their modulation by antipsychotics that provide new insight into mechanisms of action of antipsychotics.[7,27]

HETEROGENEITY OF DOPAMINE SYSTEMS AND THEIR TARGET RECEPTORS

It has been shown that in the rodent the D_3 receptor is much less abundant than the D_2 receptor, has a restricted distribution, and exhibits a significant degree of segregation from the D_2 receptor in the NAS.[24,28,29] The highest concentration of D_3 receptor and mRNA is in the Islands of Calleja followed by the NAS shell and then the NAS core, with considerably lower levels in the dorsal caudate-putamen. The two major sub-populations of striatal medium spiny neurons that preferentially express the D_1 mRNA or D_2 mRNA[29,30] also differentially express D_3 mRNA. Striatonigral substance P containing neurons preferentially express mRNA encoding the D_1 receptor and striatopallidal neurons that express enkephalin preferentially co-ex-

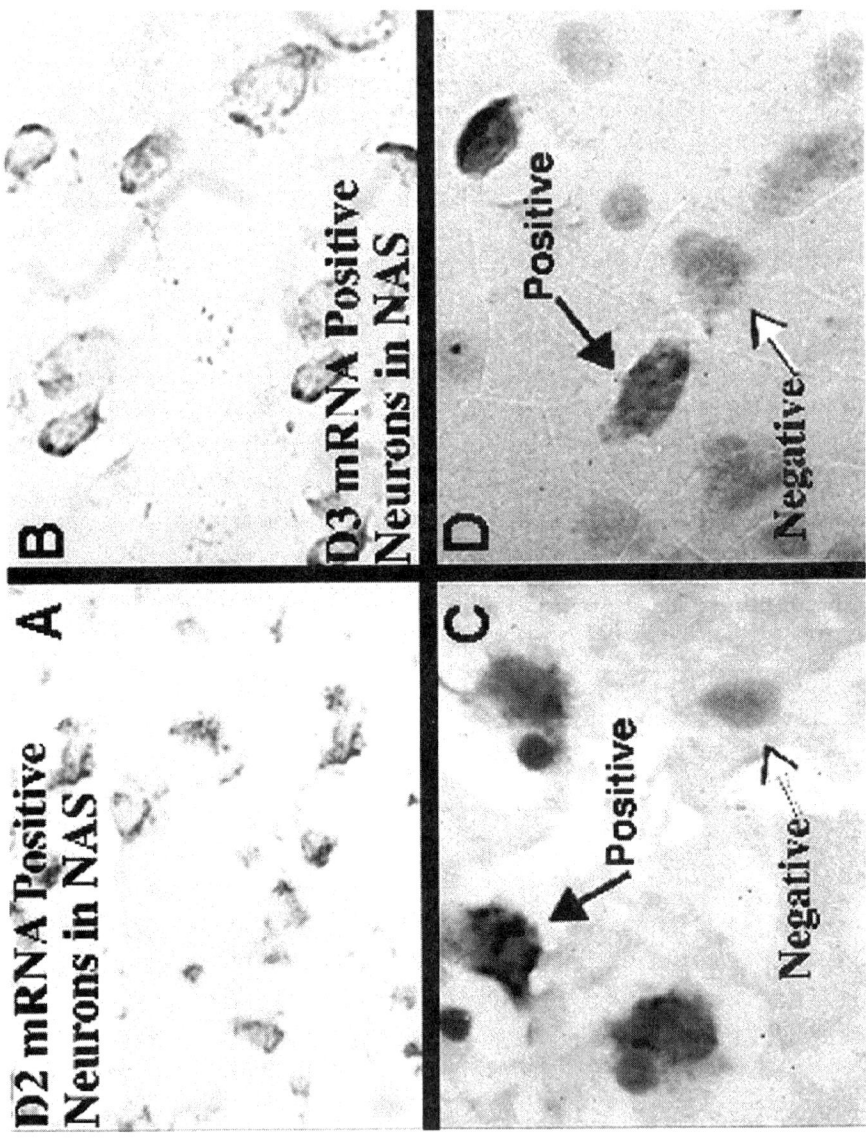

press mRNA encoding the D_2 receptor. There is, however, co-expression of D_1 and D_2 mRNA in a subset of striatal neurons, especially those co-expressing substance P and enkephalin.[31] Several studies have shown that in the NAS the D_3 receptor is likely to be expressed at higher concentrations in neurons expressing the D_1 DA receptor, substance P, and/or neurotensin than in other populations of neurons.[28,29,31]

It is much less evident that there is a similar clear compartmentalization of D_2 and D_3 receptors in human brain.[32–35] Nonetheless, we believe that in the human one can demonstrate cortico-striatal-pallidal-thalamo circuits that segregate the D_2 from D_3 receptor and regions of significant overlap. In fact, we believe that the ventral striatum, its efferents and afferents are highlighted by the degree of D_2/D_3 interactions. This differs from the "motor" cortico-striatal-pallidal-thalamo circuit in which D_3 receptor actions would not play a significant role. Radioligand binding for the D_2 receptor demonstrates that it is enriched in the matrix compartment with a dorsolateral to medioventral gradient.[34,36] In contrast, the D_3 receptor is enriched in the ventral striatum, and within that region highest in the striosomal compartment.[27,32,34] D_2 receptor mRNA is homogeneously distributed in the striatum, whereas the ventral striatum is enriched in D_3 receptor mRNA.[7,33] Using non-radioactive *in situ* hybridization histochemistry to allow for visualization of different populations of neurons expressing D_2 mRNA or D_3 mRNA we can demonstrate neurons expressing D_2 mRNA but not for D_3 mRNA are relatively homogeneously distributed in the striatum.[32] D_2 mRNA-positive neurons were numerous in all regions of the striatum, including the NAS (FIG. 1A). Higher concentrations of D_3 mRNA-positive neurons exist in the ventral striatum than in the dorsal striatum, and within the ventral striatum there are distinct clustering (patches) of D_3 mRNA-positive neurons (FIG. 1B; see also FIG. 5). Interestingly, the high proportion of D2 mRNA positive (75% of total) or D_3 mRNA-positive (30% of total) neurons in the NAS (FIG. 1, C,D) would suggest that there is overlap of D_2 mRNA with D_3 mRNA in a subset of neurons.

The differential organization of the D_2 and D_3 receptors in striatum is maintained in the efferents,[32,34] with high levels of D_2 receptors in the GPe and not the GPi (FIG. 2A). In contrast, the D_3 receptor is enriched in the VP, GPi and SNpr (FIG. 2, C–F). Large neurons stained positively for D_2 mRNA or D_3 mRNA are evident in both the GPe and GPi with higher numbers of D_3 mRNA positive neurons in the GPi (FIG. 3). Many neurons co-expressed D_2 and D_3 mRNA (FIG. 4C). D_2 mRNA is highly expressed in the SNpc (FIG. 2B) and double *in situ* hybridization histochemistry demonstrates its co-localization with TH-containing cells in that region (FIG. 4B). In contrast, D_3 mRNA is expressed in few TH-containing cells in the SNpc (FIG. 4A) and then in neurons co-expressing D_2 mRNA (FIG. 4D). D_3 mRNA is found frequently in small presumably GABAergic projection neurons of the SNpr. These may be the source of the GABAergic nigrothalamic pathway.[37,38] One important difference from the rat is that D_3 receptors were virtually absent in the ventral tegmental area and are

---

FIGURE 1. D_2 and D_3 mRNA positive neurons in the NAS. Tissue sections were labeled for D_2 mRNA with the digoxigenin-labeled riboprobe (**A, C**) and D_3 mRNA with the fluorescein-labeled riboprobe (**B, D**) and counterstained with Nuclear Fast Red (**A**) or Methyl Green (**D**). As the original color images were photographed in grey tones, only the most darkly stained neurons are visible. Neurons that are postive (*black arrow*) and negative (*light arrow*) for double labeling are identified in **C** and **D**.

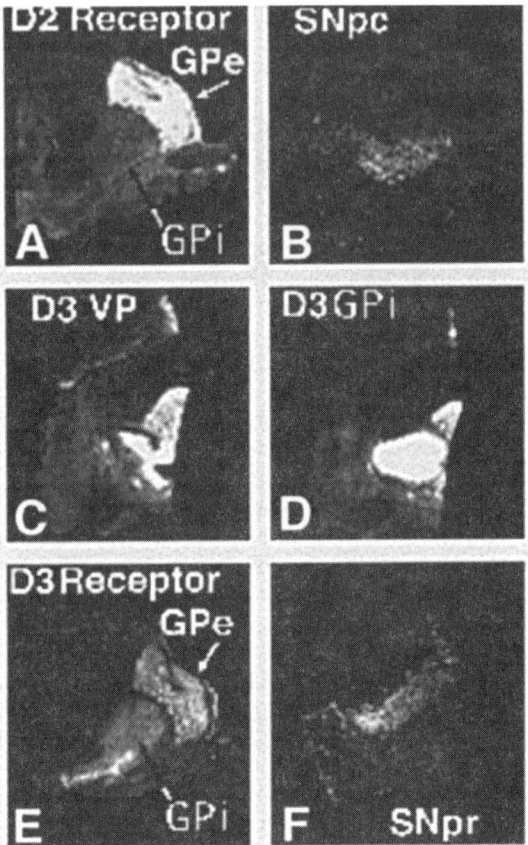

FIGURE 2. Darkfield photomicrographs of [^{125}I]epidepride binding to D$_2$ (**A,B**) or [^{125}I]7-*trans*-hydroxy-PIPAT binding to D$_3$ receptors (**C–F**) in efferents of the pallidum. Abbreviations: GPe, globus pallidus external; GPI, globus pallidus internal; SNpc, substantia nigra pars compacts, SNPr, substantia nigra pars reticulata; VP, ventral pallidum.

unlikely to provide a role as autoreceptor in the mesolimbic DA system. D$_3$ receptors and D$_3$ mRNA positive neurons were also observed in sensory, hormonal, and association regions such as the nucleus basalis, anteroventral, mediodorsal, and geniculate nuclei of the thalamus, mammillary nuclei, the basolateral, basomedial, and cortical nuclei of the amygdala. Many of these regions provide input to the ventral striatum, and within these regions are many neurons that co-express D$_2$ and D$_3$ mRNA.

The regions of relatively higher expression of the D$_3$ receptor and its mRNA appeared linked through functional circuits and segregated from those circuits with highest expression of D$_2$ mRNA, yet the significant co-expression of D$_2$ and D$_3$ mRNA in many neurons suggests a functional interaction in many regions (FIG. 5). Based on studies of the neuronal localization of the D$_2$ receptor mRNA in the rodent,[30] it would be predicted that the enkephalin-containing neurons that give rise to

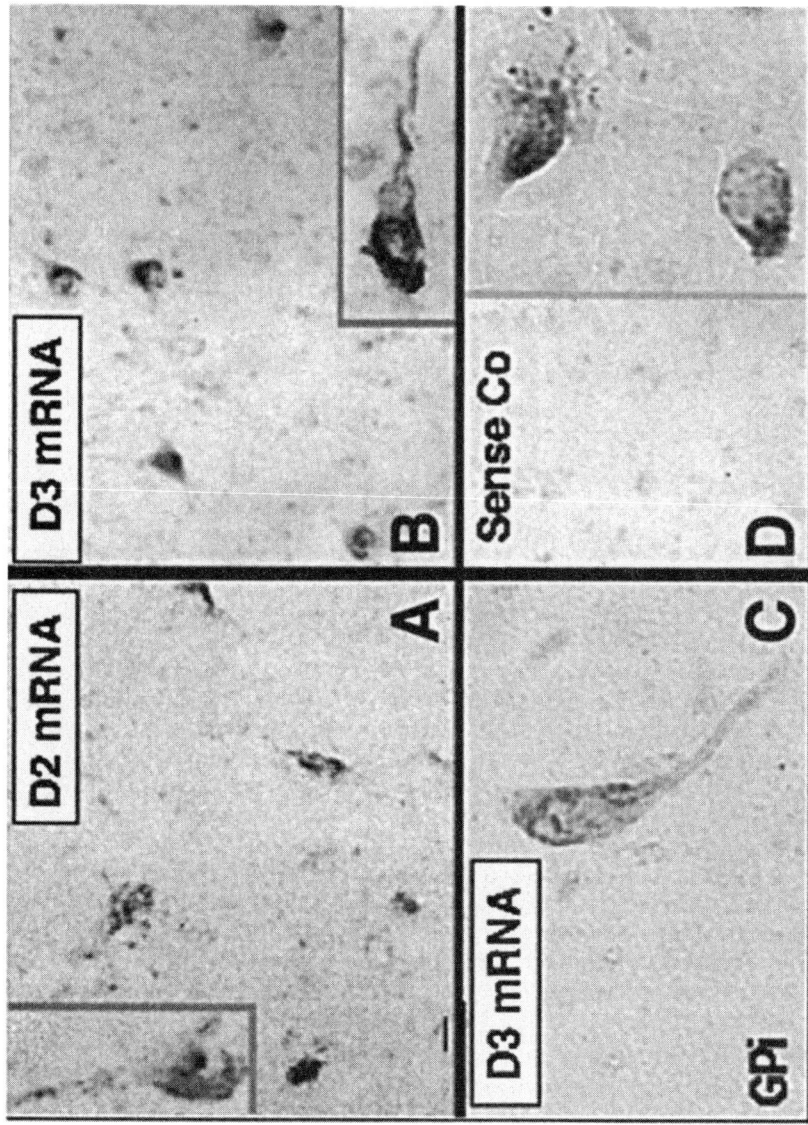

FIGURE 3. Neurons labeled for D_2 (**A**) and D_3 receptor (**B–D**) mRNA in the GPe (**A**), GPi (**B**, **C**); **D** displays absence of labeling with sense probe but intense labeling of neurons with antisense probe in GPi. **A**, **B**–GPi (inserts–enlarged individual pallidal neurons labeled for D_2 and D_3 mRNA, respectively); Bar = 40 μm **A**, **B**; 23 μm in inserts in **A** and **B** and **C**, **D**.

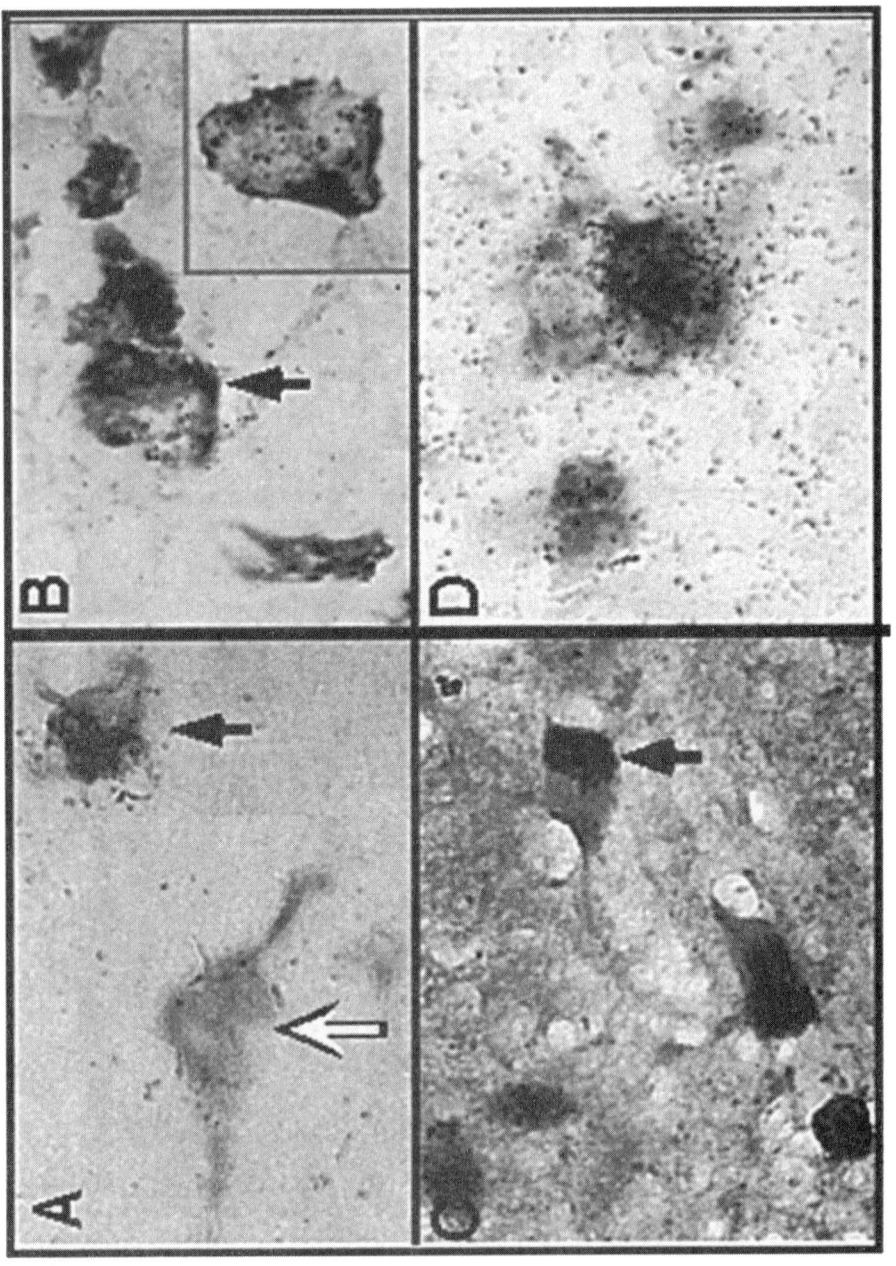

the striatopallidal pathway to the GPe in the primate[14] would be largely segregated with the D_2 receptor (FIG. 5). In contrast, the substance P–positive neurons that project to the GPi and ventral tier of the SNpc would express the D_1 receptor.[14,29] Our results would further suggest that the dynorphin-positive pathway from the ventral striatum to the VP, GPi, VTA and dorsal tier of the SNpc (mesolimbic DA cell bodies) is likely to express the D_3 receptor (FIG. 5). In primates, the VP stains intensely for enkephalin, similar to the GPe and poorly for substance P, whereas the GPi stains intensely for substance P and weakly for enkephalin.[39] Therefore, based on efferents of the VP and its histochemical composition it has been postulated that the VP in primates is an extension of the GPe.[15] It is interesting that in the human D_3 receptor binding is enriched in the VP and the GPi but not the GPe. We hypothesize that in human ventral striatum neurons co-expressing D_2 and D_3 mRNA project to the VP and those co-expressing D_3 and D_1 project to the GPi. Our data using nonradioactive labeling of D_2 and D_3 mRNA also shows that there are neurons within pallidum that express these mRNAs. As the pallidum receive DA input,[40,41] it would suggest there DA could exert local control over efferents of the pallidum. Hence, the different compartments of the striatum, and their striatopallidal, striatonigral, and pallido-thalamic efferents would be influenced by different dopaminergic systems mediated, in part, by different DA receptors.

DOPAMINE RECEPTORS IN SCHIZOPHRENIA

Because the positive symptoms of schizophrenia respond to neuroleptic treatment and the clinical potency of all neuroleptics correlates well with their activity at D_2-like sites,[1,2] changes in D_2 receptor number may be related to the positive symptoms of schizophrenia. However, any interpretation has been complicated by the fact that the majority of cases examined were treated ante mortem with neuroleptics, which by themselves increase D_2-like receptor number. Some investigators have attempted to substantiate a role for the increases in D_2 receptor numbers in schizophrenia based on the argument that amplitude of the effect cannot be accounted for by a drug effect,[4] but this argument is limited by the types of comparisons that are made. Second, most investigators have examined the striatum for changes in D_2 receptor number and it has only been recently that other regions of human brain have been examined. We have been interested in exploring if specific changes in DA receptors that mediate the effects of the mesolimbic DA system are altered in schizophrenia. We also wanted to take approaches that allowed us to directly test if D_2 and D_3 re-

---

FIGURE 4. Neurons labeled for D_2 and D_3 mRNA in the SN and VTA. **A**, D_3 mRNA positive neurons; **B, C, D**, D_2 mRNA positive neurons. A–colocalization of D_3 mRNA (grains) and TH immunoreactivity (dark grey) in the SNc. *Black arrows* indicate double labeled cells; *white arrows*, TH-positive cells that were negative for D_3 receptor mRNA. B–colocalization of D_2 mRNA (grains) and TH immunoreactivity (dark grey) in a melanin-containing cell in SNpc; insert shows a non-melanized TH-positive cell containing D_2 receptor mRNA. C–double labeling for D_2 and D_3 mRNA utilizing nonradioactive probes in the GPi. D_2 mRNA was visualized as black granulated precipitate and D_3 mRNA as brown more homogenously distributed precipitate. **D**–colocalization of D_2 (grains) and D_3 mRNA (dark grey) in neuron in SNpc.

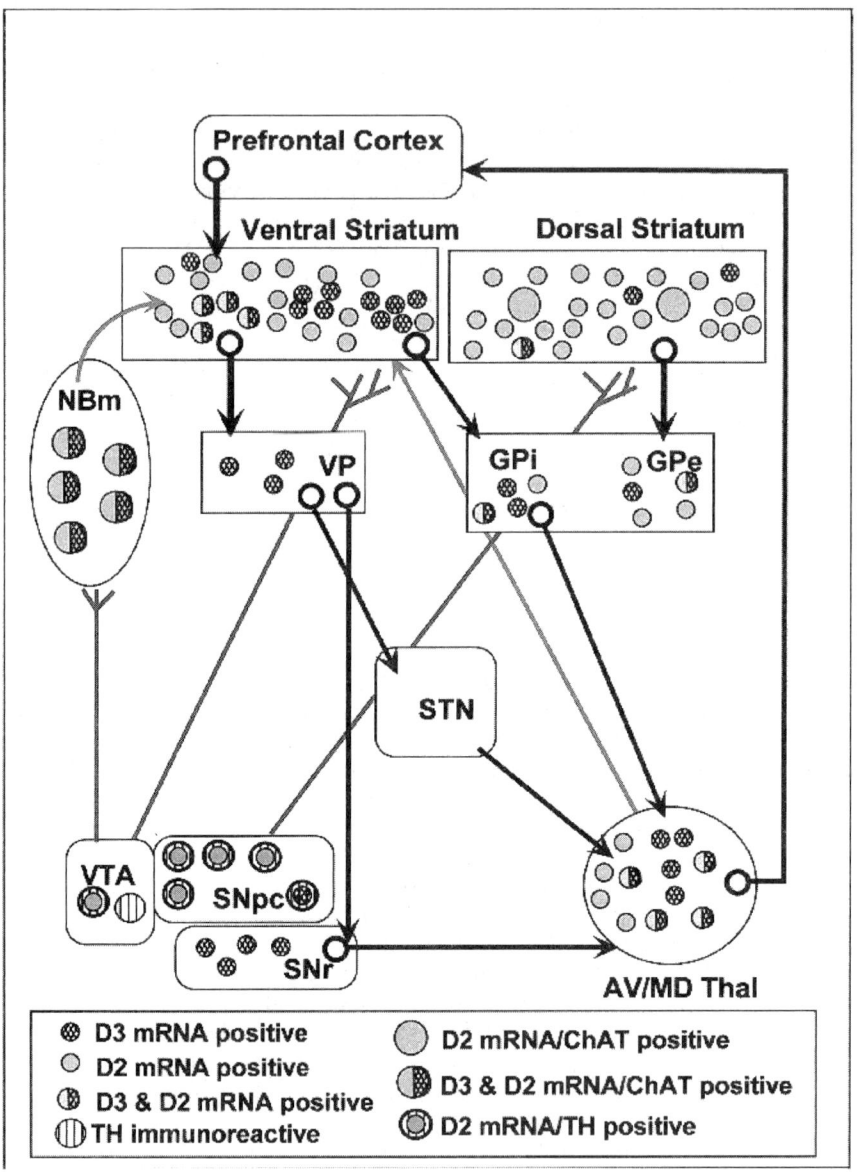

FIGURE 5. Diagram of the connections of the striato-pallidal-thalmic circuits indicating localization of neurons expressing D_2 mRNA, D_3 mRNA or co-expression of both mRNAs in different structures. Connecting arrows indicate efferent connections.

ceptors were modified in dissimilar ways and if the changes could be accounted for by a previous history of medication. In an initial study of a small number of unmedicated schizophrenic patients we determined that [^{3}H]spiroperidol binding to D_2-like

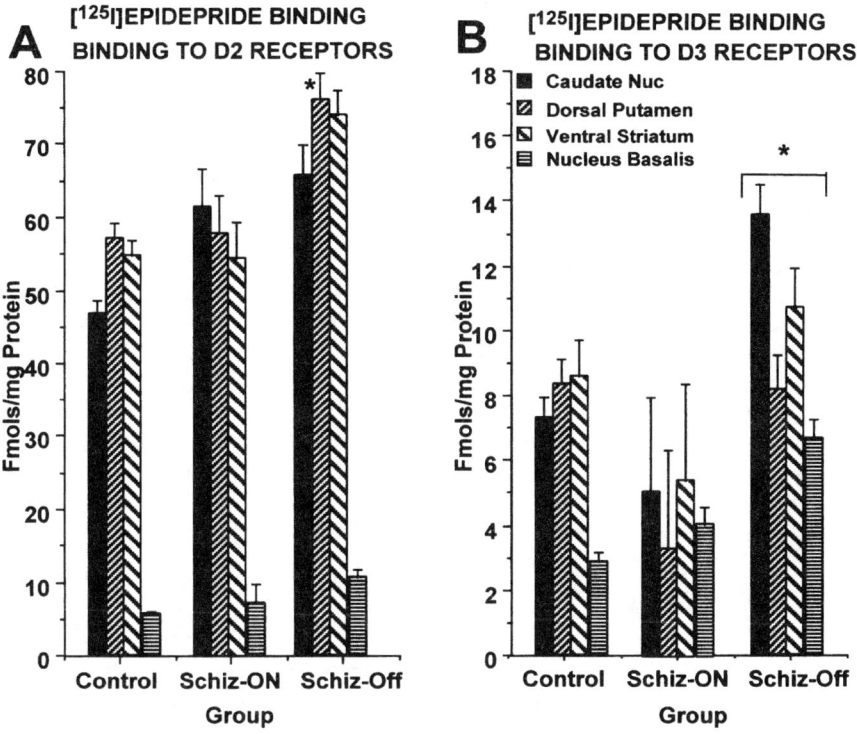

FIGURE 6. [^{125}I]epipride binding to D_2 (**A**) or to D_3 receptors (**B**) in different regions of the striatum and nucleus basalis in three groups of cases. Adjacent sections were labeled with 50 pM [^{125}I]epipride (Kd = 50 pM) in the presence of 100 μM Gpp and either 100 nM 7-OH-DPAT (to block D_3 receptors) to quantify D_2 receptors or 10 μM domperidone (to block D_2 receptors) to quantify D_3 receptors. Mean values ± S.E.M for specific binding in control, schizophrenic on antipsychotic treatment, and schizophrenic off treatment for 1 month or more. Asterisk indicates significant difference from control at $p < 0.05$.

receptors was significantly elevated in the ventral striatum. There was a 200% increase in density of D2 receptors in the NAS and ventral putamen and a smaller increase in the dorsal caudate nucleus and dorsal putamen (dorsal striatum).[42] This suggested to us that D_2-like receptors in these two regions were affected differentially in schizophrenia. This might be accounted for by changes in D_3 receptors, but [^{3}H]spiroperidol does not sufficiently discriminate between D_2 and D_3 receptors so as to specifically label D_2 receptors.[43] We characterized the conditions for selective binding of the radioligand [^{125}I](R)-*trans*-7-hyroxy-2-[*N*-propyl-*N*-(3′-iodo-2′-propenyl)-amino]tetralin ([^{125}I]*trans*-7-OH-PIPAT) to the human D_3 receptor.[27] Using quantitative autoradiography we determined the concentration of D_3 receptors in regions of the rostral and caudate striatum and pallidal structures in postmortem tissue derived from schizophrenics and age-matched controls, but in which one schizophrenic group had been removed from antipsychotics at least a month before death.[27] We found about twofold elevations in the number of D_3 receptors in the ventral striatum, VP, GPe and GPi of chronically hospitalized schizophrenics free of antipsychotics for at least a month before death ($n = 7$), with the majority drug free for a year or more, as compared to matched controls ($n = 15$). Schizophrenics receiving antipsychotics at death ($n = 8$) actually had levels below that of control values. There were no differences in the binding characteristics or affinity of [^{125}I]*trans*-7-OH-PIPAT binding to D_3 receptors between control and schizophrenic cases. Thus, the lower D_3 receptor number in the schizophrenics on medication does not reflect residual drug effects on the kinetics of the binding of the compound but an actual decrease in Bmax values. Similarly, the increase in D_3 receptor number in the schizophrenics off antipsychotic treatment reflects an increase in Bmax.

In order to examine if D_2 receptors were affected in similar ways we examined the binding of [^{125}I]epidepride to D_2 and D_3 receptors in a subset of the same cases (unpublished findings). [^{125}I]epidepride labels D_2 and D_3 receptors with equally high affinity but can be displaced from either the D_3 receptor with 7-OH-DPAT to measure D_2 receptors or from the D_2 receptor with domperidone to quantify D_3 receptor number.[34] Similar to our results with [^{125}I]*trans*-7-OH-PIPAT binding to D_3 receptors we observed decreased binding in the schizophrenics receiving antipsychotics at death ($n = 4$) as compared to the control group (FIG. 6B). Elevated [^{125}I]epidepride binding to D_3 receptors was observed in the schizophrenics free of antipsychotics for at least a month before death ($n = 5$), as compared to matched controls ($n = 8$). D_2 receptor number was also affected with small elevations in the schizophrenics receiving antipsychotics at death and greater elevations in the chronically treated cases withdrawn from antipsychotics for at least a month (FIG. 6A). The D_3 receptor elevation observed in the drug-free schizophrenics was restricted to the ventral striatum, and within that region was elevated most in patches of dense binding likely associated with the striosomal compartment.[34] These regional effects, we blieve are regulated by antipsychotic medication. The elevation of D_2 receptors within the motor subdivision of the striatum is, on the other hand, likely the result of the chronic treatment with antipsychotics. However, the interpretation of the results depends on an interpretation of the effects of chronic antipsychotic treatment of D_2 and D_3 receptor number in the different brain regions.

Regulation of Subtypes of the D_2-Family of Receptors

It is now well recognized that blockade of DA receptors leads to increased D_2 receptor synthesis, which is coupled to mRNA expression in the adult rat striatum.[44-46] It is less clear if chronic antipsychotic treatment modifies the mesolimbic DA D_2-like receptors in the same way as that in the nigrostriatal DA system. Under conditions of continuous, chronic treatment with typical antipsychotics (e.g., Hal-

---

FIGURE 7. Photomicrographs representing [^{125}I]7-*trans*-hydroxy-PIPAT binding to D_3 receptors in different treatment groups. **A**, Vehicle control for acute haloperidol; **B**, acute treatment haloperidol decanoate intramuscular for 48 hours; **C**, vehicle control for 11 month chronic haloperidol; **D**, haloperidol decanoate intramuscular for 11 months plus 48 hour withdrawal; **E**, vehicle control for 9 month chronic haloperidol; **F**, haloperidol decanoate intramuscular for 9 months plus 2 month withdrawal. D_3 receptors are not changed in any haloperidol treatment group.

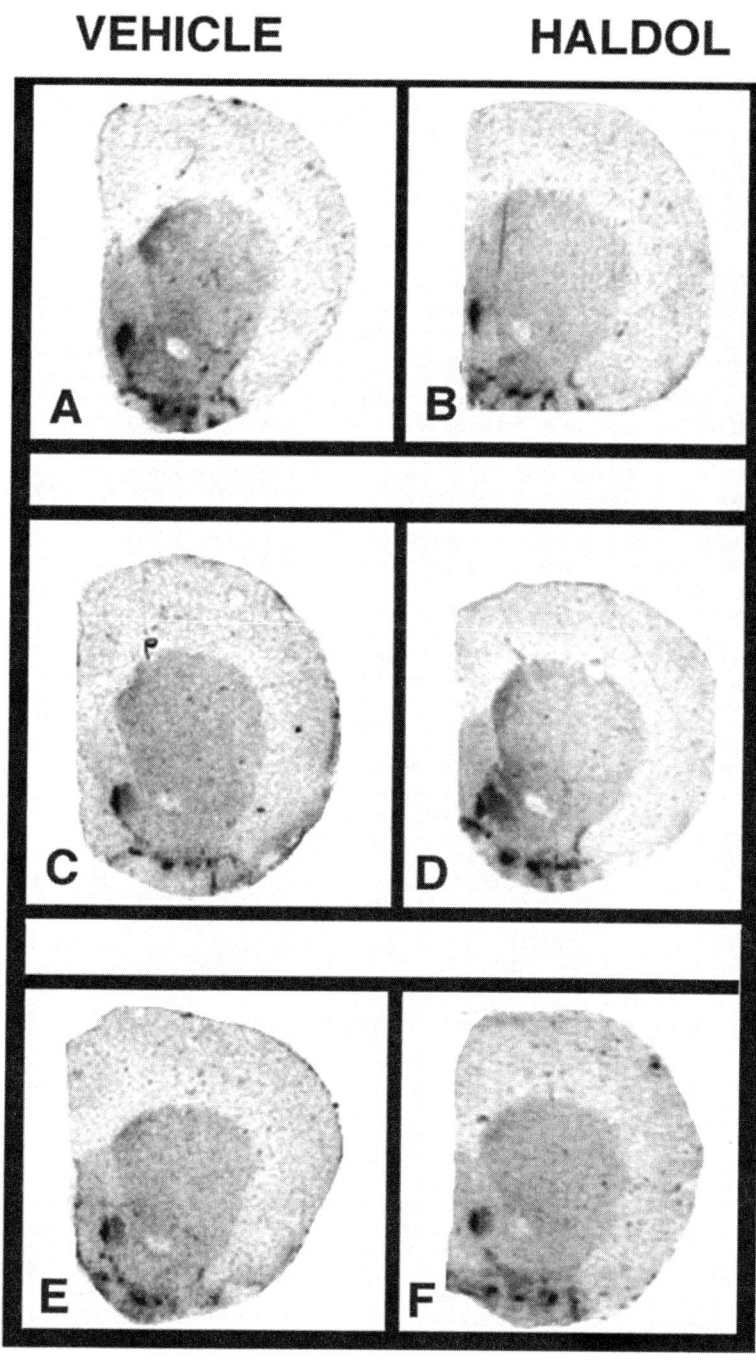

dol, haloperidol) some investigators have reported that [^{3}H]spiroperidol binding to D_2 receptors is either not elevated in mesolimbic regions (e.g., nucleus accumbens) or may not persist with continuous treatment[47–49] in contrast to that in striatum. Furthermore, it has been reported that behavioral responses to DA agonists thought to be mediated by the mesolimbic DA system does not evidence a functional supersensitivity during continuous treatment with antipsychotics.[50] However, other investigators have failed to find a development of the behavioral tolerance to chronic antipsychotic treatment.[5,51] For example, using methods of continuous haloperidol treatment that clearly sustain high plasma levels for long periods of time (8 months) one group has shown it leads to persistent elevations in [^{3}H]spiroperidol binding in both nigrostriatal and mesolimbic regions.[5] However, this same group failed to find elevations in D_2 receptor mRNA in the NAS when elevations were evident in the striatum.[52] This would suggest the possibility that it is changes in D_3 receptors in NAS that account for alterations in [^{3}H]spiroperidol binding there. However, three groups has failed to find elevations in D_3 mRNA in the mouse or rat, either in specific regions (e.g., olfactory tubercle) or whole brain with chronic antipsychotic treatment, when conditions were sufficient to induce elevations in D_2 mRNA in the caudate-putamen.[53–55] Those studies, however, utilized short-term treatment regimens. Of more value would be to utilize treatment regimens more closely approximating conditions associated with treatment of schizophrenia. One group[5,52] has reported that intramuscular injections of haloperidol decanoate, at a dose of 28.5 mg/kg every three weeks (equivalent of 1.5 mg/kg/day), for 36 weeks showed elevated concentrations of D_2 receptors and levels of D_2 mRNA for at least 28 weeks after the last injection. This treatment paradigm also resulted in extrapyramidal side effects in the animals resembling tardive dyskinesias in humans. This suggests that this regimen of chronic antipsychotic treatment more closely resemble the effects of chronic Haldol treatment in humans.

We utilized this same method to examine effects of chronic haloperidol treatment with and without a long-term withdrawal period on D_2 and D_3 receptors in the nigrostriatal and mesolimbic DA system (unpublished findings). Treatment was initiated at 8 weeks of age and rats were administered haloperidol decanoate or the oil vehicle for 9 months plus a 2 month withdrawal (long withdrawal group), 11 months with a 48 hour withdrawal (acute withdrawal), or age-matched rats were administered a single dose of haloperidol and a 48 hour withdrawal (acute treatment). Our results demonstrate that long-term chronic treatment with haloperidol led to elevations in D_2 receptors in the CPu but not the NAS. The effect was more pronounced with the 2 month than the 48 hour withdrawal group. D_3 receptor number was largely unaffected by the long-term chronic treatment with haloperidol except for a nonsignificant increase in D_3 receptor number in the acute withdrawal group in the NAS (FIG. 7). Thus our data support the hypothesis that neither the D_2 or D_3 receptor and mRNA are elevated in the NAS under chronic DA receptor blockade, even with conditions which lead to elevation in D_2 receptor and mRNA in the caudate-putamen. Our results also indicate that in the postmortem studies of schizophrenics in which there was a decrease in D_3 receptor number in the group on antipsychotics (withdrawn for less than 72 h) and an elevation in the group of antipsychotics withdrawn for month is not due to chronic treatment with antipsychotics. Our results for D_2 receptors are remarkably similar to the postmortem studies indicating the elevations in the dorsal striatum in chronically treated schizophrenics are likely to reflect a drug effect.

Hypothesis

Many investigators have proposed that the limbic regions of the striatum, recipient of limbic efferents, play a particularly important role in the gating of disturbed "limbic"-related neuronal processing in schizophrenia (see, e.g., ref. 20). Since this, in turn, is modulated by the mesolimbic DA system, we,[7,27] and others,[26] have proposed that the mesolimbic D_3 receptor mediates this "gate". Our results do support this hypothesis. First, the D_3 receptor mRNA and binding sites are expressed by neurons within the ventral striatum and within the limbic ventral striatal-pallidal-thalamo circuit (FIG. 5).[7,32,33] Second, our own data demonstrate that there is overproduction of D_3 receptors in the ventral striatum of unmedicated schizophrenic patients and those removed from antipsychotics but down-regulated in those on medication.[27,42] In a separate study, we identified that D_2 receptors were elevated in those on or off antipsychotics at time of death. Thus, in contrast to the previously detected elevation of D_2 receptors in schizophrenia, elevation of D_3 receptors in limbic striatum and its efferents observed in schizophrenics may be reduced by antipsychotics. The mechanism for this differential regulation of D_2 and D_3 receptors is not known. It is unlikely to be due to release from chronic antipsychotic treatment as we and others[53–55] have not found that D_3 receptor or mRNA levels are elevated with chronic antipsychotic treatment in rats. The higher expression of D_3 receptors in the ventral striatum and its efferents in schizophrenics and their down-regulation by antipsychotics may reflect direct modification of transcript levels in the striatal neurons. However, one study has indicated that levels of D_3 mRNA are not different in ventral striatum of schizophrenics as compared to controls, regardless of the drug treatment at the time of death.[56] Second, it may reflect co-regulation of non-striatal sources of presynaptic D_3 receptors such as the afferents from the mesolimbic DA system, amygdala or thalamus. Third, it may reflect modifications in the mesolimbic DA system and its regulation of the target D_3 receptor, but results in the adult rat would not indicate this.[55] Another approach, which we have taken, is to identify an animal model with neurochemical changes in the ventral striatum that are characteristic of schizophrenia.

We have identified other characteristics of the mesostriatal DA system in schizophrenia that does suggest there is a model available. We have previously observed a small reduction in D_1 receptors and dopamine transporter (DAT) sites in the caudate nucleus of schizophrenic cases,[42] suggesting a subtotal lesion to the presynaptic DA system. Our data also suggest that elevations in D_2 receptors are a consequence of chronic antipsychotic action and not the pathologic processes involved in schizophrenia. Consequently, the limbic region of the striatum may show significant alterations in DA systems, particularly in the expression of D_3 receptors in ventral striatum and a small reduction in DA fibers in caudate nucleus. These alterations in the DA system may be related to marked alterations in other monoaminergic systems in the ventral striatum, including serotonin hyperinnervation, elevated densities of 5-HT_2 receptors and β-adrenergic receptors.[57,58] We have proposed that this is similar in many respects to what occurs in rats with lesions made to the nigrostriatal DA system in early development that spares the mesolimbic DA system and modifies monoaminergic systems of the striatum, including serotonin hyperinnervation of the striatum.[59] In this model the mesolimbic DA system shows a great deal more plasticity than the nigrostriatal DA system. We have found in such animals with small lesions to the nigrostriatal DA system in early development that in the adult there is loss of TH and DAT sites in the medial caudate but recovery of TH in the NAS and ventral caudate-putamen. Regions of the midbrain subserving the nigrostriatal DA system undergoes loss of TH mRNA while the region subserving the mesolimbic DA system (VTA) show elevations in TH mRNA but reduced DAT following the neonatal lesion. We also have found in such animals with small lesions to the mesostriatal DA system that the striatum does not show modifications in D_2 receptor number or D_2 mRNA levels but evidence small losses of D_1 receptors.

We recently showed that there is a biphasic development-related response of D_3 mRNA-positive neurons to this subtotal loss of DA.[60] There is initially a reduction in the number of D_3 mRNA positive neurons in the ventral striatum of the rat in early development, and this effect is magnified by the loss of DA. However, by adulthood there is an elevation in the proportion of neurons that are D_3 mRNA positive, and elevated levels of D_3 mRNA per neuron. Thus, the early loss of DA appears to modify the normal developmental regulation of expression of D_3 mRNA. These changes are different from what happens following adult lesions of the nigrostriatal DA system in which D_2 receptors and mRNA are up regulated and D_3 receptor/mRNA levels are not modified (see, e.g., refs. 44, 55). If the DA system of the schizophrenics had been damaged subtotally in early development one would expect to observe similar changes in the DA systems, as compared to age-matched controls, that we have observed in the animal studies. If this can be confirmed, then we could examine the effects of antipsychotic treatment on the regulation of D_3 receptors and their mRNAs under conditions of experimental up-regulation in a rodent model. These data also suggest a novel process for the elevation of D_3 receptors in schizophrenics. Presumably the increased number of D_3 receptors in the ventral striatum and efferents observed in unmedicated schizophrenics results in altered neural processing in their output through the striatal-pallidal-thalamic-cortical "limbic loop." The increase in D_3 receptor number, we believe, reflects an increase in the proportion of neurons expressing high levels of D_3 mRNA and not simply elevations in the amount of transcript/neuron. This could occur on a background of reduced cell number that is induced by loss of DA in early development.[61] Under those conditions, antipsychotics could act to down-regulate D_3 mRNA concentrations/neuron and thereby affect protein levels. Antipsychotic down-regulation of the D_3 receptor-mediated limbic loop may provide a means of resolving the imbalance in this loop. Interestingly, atypical antipsychotics should produce this effect without also affecting D_2 receptors of the dorsal striatum.

ACKNOWLEDGMENTS

This research was supported by an award from Scottish Rite Benevolent Foundation's Schizophrenia Research Program, N.M.J., USA, and by US Public Health Service Grants MH 56824, and AG 09215.

REFERENCES

1. CREESE, I., et al. 1976. Dopamine receptor binding predicts clinical and pharmacological potencies of antischizophrenic drugs. Science **192**: 596–598.

2. SEEMAN, P, et al. 1976. Antipsychotic drug doses and neuroleptic/dopamine receptors. Nature **261:** 717–719.
3. SIBLEY, D. & F. MONSMA. 1992. Molecular biology of dopamine receptors. Trends Pharmacol. Sci. **13:** 61–65.
4. SEEMAN, P., et al. 1987. Human brain D1 and D2 dopamine receptors in schizophrenia, Alzheimer's, Parkinson's and Huntington's disease. Neuropsychopharmacology **1:** 5-15.
5. LARUELLE, M., et al. 1992. D1 and D2 receptor modulation in rat striatum and nucleus accumbens after chronic haloperidol treatment, Brain Res. **575:** 47–56.
6. MERCHANT, K.M., et al. 1992. Expression of the proneurotensin gene in the rat brain and its regulation by antipsychotic drugs. Ann. N.Y. Acad. Sci. **668:** 54–69.
7. JOYCE, J.N. & J.H. MEADOR-WOODRUFF. 1997. Linking the family of D2 receptors to neuronal circuits in human brain: insights into schizophrenia. Neuropsychopharmacology **16:** 375–384.
8. GIBB, W.R.G. 1992. Melanin, tyrosine hydroxylase, calbindin and substance P in the human midbrain and substantia nigra in relation to nigrostriatal projections and differential neruonal susceptibility in Parkinson's disease. Brain Res. **581:** 283–291.
9. LYND-BALTA E. & S.N. HABER. 1994. The organization of midbrain projections to the ventral striatum in the primate. Neuroscience **59:** 609–623.
10. HEIMER, L. & R.D. WILSON. 1975. The subcortical projections of the allocortex: similarities in the neural associations of the hippocampus, the priform cortex, and the neocortex. *In* Golgi Centennial Symposium. M. Santini, Ed.: 177–193. Raven Press. New York.
11. ALEXANDER, G.E. & M.D. CRUTCHER. 1990. Functional architecture of basal ganglia circuits: neural substrates of parallel processing. TINS **13:** 266–271.
12. LYND-BALTA, E. & S.N. HABER. 1994. The organization of midbrain projections to the striatum in the primate: sensorimotor-related striatum versus ventral striatum. Neuroscience **59:** 625–640.
13. HABER, S.N. et al. 1985. Efferent connections of the ventral pallidum: evidence of a dual striatopallidofugal pathway. J. Comp. Neurol. **235:** 322–335.
14. HABER, S.N., et al. 1994. Integrative aspects of basal ganglia circuitry. Advances Behav. Biol. **41:** 71–80.
15. HABER, S.N., et al. 1993. The organization of the descending ventral pallidal projections in the monkey. J. Comp. Neurol. **329:** 111–128.
16. GIGUERE, M. & P.S. GOLDMAN-RAKIC. 1988. Mediodorsal nucleus: areal, laminar, and tangential distribution of afferents and efferents in the frontal lobe of rhesus monkeys. J. Comp. Neurol. **277:** 195–213.
17. ROOM, P., et al. 1985. Efferent connections of the prelimbic (area 32) and the infralimbic (area 25) cortices: an anterograde tracing study in the cat. J. Comp. Neurol. **242:** 40–55.
18. SAUNDERS, R.C., et al. 1988. Comparison of the efferents of the amygdala and the hippocampal formation in the rhesus monkey: II. Reciprocal and non-reciprocal connections. J. Comp. Neurol. **271:**185–207.
19. SELEMON, L.D. & P.S. GOLDMAN-RAKIC. 1985. Longitudinal topography and interdigitation of corticostriatal projections in the rhesus monkey. J. Neuroscience **5:** 776–794.
20. MOGENSON, G.J., et al. 1988. Influence of dopamine on limbic inputs to the nucleus accumbens. Ann. NY. Acad. Sci. **537:** 86–100.
21. SHAPIRO, R.M. 1993. Regional neuropathology in schizophrenia: Where are we? Where are we going? Schizophrenia Res. **10:** 187–239.
22. TAMMINGA, C.A., et al. 1988. Dopamine neuronal tracts in schiozphrenia; their pharmacology and in vivo glucose metabolism. Ann. N.Y. Acad. Sci. **537:** 443–450.
23. TAMMINGA, C.A., et al. 1992. Limbic system abnormalities identified in schizophrenia using positron emission tomography with fluorodeoxyglucose and neocortical alterations with deficit syndrome. Arch. Gen. Psychiatry **49:** 522–530.
24. BOUTHENET, M.L., et al. 1991. Localization of dopamine D3 receptor mRNA in the rat brain using in situ hybridization histochemistry: comparison with dopamine D2 receptor mRNA. Brain Res. **564:** 203–219.

25. VAN TOL, H.H.M., et al. 1991. Cloning of the gene for a human dopamine D4 receptor with high affinity for the antipsychotic clozapine, Nature **350:** 610–614.
26. SCHWARTZ, J.-C., et al. 1993. Dopamine D3 receptor: basic and clinical aspects. Clinical Neuropharmacol. **16:** 295–314.
27. GUREVICH, E.V., et al. 1997. Dopamine D3 receptors and use of antipsychotics in patients with schizophrenia: a postmortem study. Arch. Gen. Psychiatry **54:** 225–232.
28. LE MOINE, C. & B. BLOCH. 1996. Expression of the D3 dopamine receptor in peptidergic neurons of the nucleus accumbens: comparison with the D1 and D2 dopamine receptor. Neuroscience **73:** 131–143.
29. LE MOINE, C., et al. 1991. Phenotypical characterization of the rat striatal neurons expressing the D1 dopamine receptor gene. Proc. Natl. Acad. Sci. USA **88:** 4205–4209.
30. LE MOINE, C. & B. BLOCH. 1995. D1 and D2 dopamine receptor gene expression in the rat striatum: sensitive cRNA probes demonstrate prominent segregation of D1 and D2 mRNAs in distinct neuronal populations of the dorsal and ventral striatum. J. Comp. Neurol. **355:** 418–426.
31. SURMEIER, D.J., et al. 1996. Coordinated expression of dopamine receptors in neostriatal medium spiny neurons. J. Neurosci. **16:** 6579–6591.
32. GUREVICH, E.V. & J.N. JOYCE. 1999. Cellular distribution and co-expression of dopamine D2 and D3 receptors in the human brain. Neuropsychopharmacology **20:** 60–80.
33. MEADOR-WOODRUFF, J.H., et al. 1996. Dopamine receptor mRNA expression in human striatum and neocortex. Neuropsychopharmacol. **15:** 17–29.
34. MURRAY, A.M., et al. 1994. Localization of dopamine D3 receptors to mesolimbic and D2 receptors to mesostriatal regions of human forebrain. Proc. Natl. Acad. Sci. USA **91:** 11271–1127.
35. SUZUKI M., et al. 1998. D3 dopamine receptor mRNA is widely expressed in the human brain. Brain Res. **779:** 58–74.
36. JOYCE, J.N., et al. 1986. Human striatal dopamine receptors are organized in compartments. Proc. Natl. Acad. Sci. USA. **83:** 8002-8006.
37. ILINKSY, I.A., et al. 1985. Organization of the nigrothalamocortical system in the rhesus monkey. J. Comp. Neurol. **236:** 315–330.
38. KULTAS-ILINSKY, K. & I.A. ILINSKY. 1990. Fine structure of the magnocellular subdivision of the ventral anterior thalamic nucleus (Vamc) of *Macaca mulatta*: II. Organization of nigrothalamic afferents as revealed with EM autoradiography. J. Comp. Neurol. **294:** 479–489.
39. HABER, S.N. & S.J. WATSON. 1985. The comparative distribution of enkephaline, dynorphine and substance P in the human globus pallidus and basal forebrain. Neuroscience **14:** 1011–1024
40. KLITENICK, M A., et al. 1992. Topography and functional role of dopaminergic projections from the ventral mesencephalic tegmentum to the ventral pallidum. Neuroscience **50:** 371–386.
41. PARENT A., et al. 1990. The dopaminergic nigropallidal projection in primates: distinct cellular origin and relative sparing in MPTP-treated monkeys. Advances Neurol. **53:** 111–116.
42. JOYCE, J.N., et al. 1988. Organization of dopamine D1 and D2 receptors in human striatum: receptor autoradiographic studies in Huntington's disease and schizophrenia. Synapse **2:** 546–557.
43. SOKOLOFF, P., et al. 1990. Molecular cloning and characterisation of a novel dopamine receptor (D3) as a target for neuroleptics. Nature **347:** 146–151.
44. ANGULO, J.A., et al. 1991. Regulation by dopaminergic neurotransmission of dopamine D2 mRNA and receptor levels in the striatum and nucleus accumbens of the rat. Mol. Brain Res. **11:** 161–166.
45. COIRINI, H., et al 1990. Increase in striatal dopamine D2 receptor mRNA after lesions or haloperidol treatment. Eur. J. Pharmacol. **186:** 369–371.

46. QIN, Z.-H. & B. WEISS. 1994. Dopamine receptor blockade increases dopamine D2 receptor and glutamic acid decarboxylase mRNAs in mouse substantia nigra. Eur. J. Pharmacol. **269:** 25–33.
47. MURUGAIAH, K., et al. 1985. Chronic continuous administration of neurolepteic drugs alters cerebral dopamine receptors and increases spontaenous dopaminergic action in striatum. Nature **296:** 570–573.
48. CLOW, A., et al. 1980. A comparison of striatal and mesolimbic dopamine function in the rat during 6-month trifluoperazine administration. Psychopharmacology **69:** 227–233.
49. PROSSER, E.S., et al. 1989. Differences in the time course of dopaminergic supersensitvity following chronic administration of haloperidol, molindone, or sulpiride. Psychopharmacology **99:** 109–116.
50. RUPNIAK, N.M.J., et al. 1985. Mesolimbic dopamine function is not altered during continuous chronic treatment of rats with typical or atypical neuroleptic drugs. J. Neural Transm. **62:** 249–266.
51. WADDINGTON, J.L. & S.J. GAMBLE. 1980. Neuroleptic treatment for a substantial proportion of adult life: behavioural sequelae of 9 months haloperidol administration. Eur. J. Pharmacol. **67:** 363–369.
52. EGAN, M.F., et al. 1994. Alterations in mRNA levels of D2 receptors and neuropeptides in striatonigal neurons of rats with neuroleptic-induced dyskenesias. Synapse **18:** 178–189.
53. DAMASK, S.P., et al. 1996. Differential effects of clozapine and haloperidol on dopamine receptor mRNA expression in rat striatum and cortex. Mol. Brain Res. **41:** 241-249.
54. FISHBURN, C.S., et al. 1994. The effect of haloperidol on D2 dopamine receptor subtype mRNA levels in the brain. FEBS Letters **339:** 63–66.
55. LÉVESQUE D, et al. 1995. A paradoxical regulation of the dopamine D3 receptor expression suggests the involvement of an anterograde factor from dopamine neurons. Proc. Natl. Acad. Sci. USA **92:** 1719–1723.
56. MEADOR-WOODRUFF, J.H., et al. 1997. Dopamine receptor transcript expression in striatum and prefrontal and occipital cortex. Focal abnormalities in orbitofrontal cortex in schizophrenia. Arch. Gen. Psychiatry **54:** 1089–1095.
57. JOYCE, J.N., et al. 1992. Distribution of Beta-adrenergic receptor subtypes in human post-mortem brain: alterations in limbic regions of schizophrenics. Synapse **10:** 228–246.
58. JOYCE, J.N., et al. 1993. Serotonin uptake sites and serotonin receptors are altered in limbic system of schizophrenics. Neuropsychopharmacol. **8:** 315–336.
59. JOYCE, J.N., et al. 1997. Functional and molecular differentiation of the dopamine system induced by neonatal denervation. Neurosci. Biobehav. Rev. **20:** 453–486.
60. GUREVICH, E.V., et al. 1999. Developmental regulation of expression of the D3 dopamine receptor in rat nucleus accumbens and islands of Calleja. J. Pharmacol Exp. Ther. **289:** 587–598.
61. PAKKENBERG, B. 1990. Pronounced reduction of total neuron number in medialdorsal thalamic nucleus and nucleus accumbens in schizophrenics. Arch. Gen. Psychiatry **47:** 1023–1027.

Prefrontal Cortical-Amygdalar Metabolism in Major Depression

WAYNE C. DREVETS[a]

Departments of Psychiatry and Radiology, University of Pittsburgh School of Medicine, Pittsburgh, Pennsylvania 15213, USA

ABSTRACT: Functional neuroimaging studies of the anatomical correlates of familial major depressive disorder (MDD) and bipolar disorder (BD) have identified abnormalities of resting blood flow (BF) and glucose metabolism in depression in the amygdala and the orbital and medial prefrontal cortical (PFC) areas that are extensively connected with the amygdala. The amygdala metabolism in MDD and BD is positively correlated with both depression severity and "stressed" plasma cortisol concentrations measured during scanning. During antidepressant drug treatment, the mean amygdala metabolism decreases in treatment responders, and the persistence of elevated amygdala metabolism during remission is associated with a high risk for the development of depressive relapse. The orbital C metabolism is also abnormally elevated during depression, but is negatively correlated with both depression severity and amygdala metabolism, suggesting that this structure may be activated as a compensatory mechanism to modulate amygdala activity or amygdala-driven emotional responses. The posterior orbital C and anterior cingulate C ventral to the genu of the corpus callosum (subgenual PFC) have more recently been shown in morphometric MRI and/or *post mortem* histopathological studies to have reduced grey matter volume and *reduced* glial cell numbers (with no equivalent loss of neurons) in familial MDD and BD. These data suggest a neural model in which dysfunction of limbic PFC structures impairs the modulation of the amygdala, leading to abnormal processing of emotional stimuli. Antidepressant drugs may compensate for this dysfunction by inhibiting pathological limbic activity.

INTRODUCTION

Pathological interactions between the amygdala and related parts of the ventral striatum and prefrontal cortex (PFC) appear to play a central role in the genesis of major depression. Neuroimaging, lesion analysis, and *post mortem* histopathological studies of clinically depressed subjects suggest that elements of the emotional/stress-response systems are pathologically activated in major depression, and that this activity is associated with abnormalities in the prefrontal cortical and monoamine neurotransmitter systems that normally modulate such responses. This chapter overviews the neurophysiological abnormalities identified in the amygdala and the orbital and medial PFC in depression. These findings are integrated with converging information from electrophysiological, histological, and anatomical studies in hu-

---

[a]Address for correspondence: B 938, Presbyterian University Hospital, University of Pittsburgh Medical Center, 200 Lothrop St., Pittsburgh, PA 15213; Voice: 412-647-1005; fax: 412-647-0700; drevets@pet.upmc.edu

mans and experimental animals to generate hypotheses concerning the neurobiological mechanisms underlying specific clinical manifestations of major depression.

PHENOMENOLOGY OF MAJOR DEPRESSIVE DISORDERS

Depressed mood is to a major depressive episode (MDE) as an immunological response is to an autoimmune disorder. The former condition in these parallel cases, is an adaptive, physiological response to a stressor or threat, while the latter comprises a disease state in which responses occur irrespective of an appropriate stimulus and become severe, persistent, and debilitating. Major depression thus appears, in many cases, to reflect dysfunction of the neural substrates supporting emotional and motivated behavior.

The MDE is characterized by persistent negative emotions and thoughts that coexist with disturbances of sleep, energy, and motivated behavior.[1] Such episodes may arise as primary, idiopathic disorders in the absence of clear medical or psychiatric antecedents [termed "major depressive disorder" (MDD) when only depressive episodes occur, or "bipolar disorder" (BD) when manic as well as depressive episodes occur],[2] or as syndromes that occur secondary to a specific neurological, endocrinological, or psychiatric disorders or pharmacological substances. The most common of these conditions, MDD, rivals hypertension as the most common illness encountered in primary health care.[3]

"Major depression" is a misnomer in the sense that anxiety symptoms, irritability and hypohedonia (diminished ability to find interest or reward in previously motivating activities) are endorsed at least as commonly by subjects meeting criteria for MDD than "depressed mood" itself.[1] Food, sex, hobbies, social behavior and work accomplishments are no longer rewarding, and depressives become inactive because of the inability to motivate themselves to engage in such behaviors. Social activity is also avoided because social contacts become anxiety provoking and minor stressors overwhelming. Panic attacks occur in one-third of cases of MDD and up to one-half of cases of BD. These emotional symptoms are accompanied by prominent fatigue, psychomotor slowing or agitation, and the perception of "psychic pain."[4] The psychological manifestations include preoccupation with death, suicide, guilt, self depreciation and hopelessness. About 15% of patients hospitalized for a MDE eventually die by suicide, and about one-half of completed suicides occur within the context of a MDE.[1] The intrusive and perseverative nature of thoughts of death, suicide, or guilt and their responsiveness to antidepressant drugs or electroconvulsive therapy suggest that abnormal brain processes underlie and maintain such symptoms.[5]

Illness onset can occur throughout the life span, although the first MDE usually occurs after puberty.[1] The usual course of MDD consists of recurrent MDE separated by, early in the illness course, a return to the premorbid level of function. Later, however, returns to the premorbid baseline are often incomplete, and depressive symptoms and functional impairment may become chronic or intermittent. Antidepressant treatment shortens the duration of depressive episodes, reduces the likelihood of chronicity, and, if continued, decreases the risk of recurrence.[5,6] Mortality risks from suicide, accidental death, and cardiovascular disease are elevated in MDD.[1,7–9]

Mania and depression reflect phenomenological antitheses of one another, being characterized by increases and decreases, respectively, in mood, motivation, energy, psychomotor activity, self-esteem, libido, and hedonia.[2,10] In BD (formerly "manic-depressive illness"), a MDE will typically follow a manic episode, although MDE may occur spontaneously as well. The hedonic state of mania often reflects both a tonic euphoria and an increased capacity for deriving pleasure and reward from social, work-related, or creative activities.[10] Patients consequently increase their engagement in such activities. This "hypermotivational" state is fueled by a sense of boundless energy, decreased need for sleep, motor restlessness, and racing thoughts. Moreover, the increased engagement in pleasurable activities and the impairment of judgment may lead to ruinous buying sprees, sexual indiscretions, or substance abuse.[1,10]

The etiology of MDD and BD are unknown. Twin, adoption and family studies indicate that genetic factors contribute substantially to the liability for developing both disorders.[1] Since the symptoms of a MDE resemble those of a severe stress response (e.g., to bereavement), stressful events are expected to constitute "acquired factors" that interact with genetic susceptibility in the development of mood disorders.[1,11] A link between stressors and MDE has been difficult to establish, however, and patients with recurrent episodes often report that their pattern of depressive symptoms is inappropriate to and not explained by stressful life situations. Moreover, when substantial "precipitating events" are reported, a critical evaluation of the chronology often reveals that the MDE onset preceded those events (e.g., job loss and marital separation may be consequences of depression). The life events that are clearly associated with the development of MDE include pregnancy and delivery, with the post-partum period comprising the epoch of greatest risk in females.[1,10]

NEUROPHYSIOLOGICAL CORRELATES OF MAJOR DEPRESSION

Neuroimaging investigations into the functional anatomical correlates of MDD have revealed a complex set of regional cerebral blood flow (CBF) and glucose metabolic abnormalities in multiple limbic and prefrontal cortical structures that have been implicated by other types of evidence in emotional behavior.[12] These abnormalities include both state-dependent physiological changes that appear to comprise nonspecific correlates of emotional or stress responses and trait-like abnormalities that may be disease specific. Consensus within the functional imaging literature regarding the anatomical correlates of depression has not been achieved, partly because of experimental design differences across studies.

Issues salient to subject sample selection are discussed elsewhere,[12] but can be briefly summarized:

(1) Sample sizes employed in most studies are small and the magnitude of CBF and metabolic abnormalities relative to the variability of such measures is also small. Therefore, some failures to replicate previous findings reflect limitations of statistical power.

(2) Most published studies are uninterpretable because of confounding medication effects in the depressed subjects. Regional CBF and metabolism in the PFC are reduced by antidepressant, antipsychotic and antianxiety

drugs.[12–14] Studies including subjects taking these agents may thus report artifactual differences between groups and fail to detect the areas of hypermetabolism identified in unmedicated depressives.

(3) Depressed subjects with illness onset after age 55 to 60 have neuromorphological MRI evidence of cerebrovascular disease, which most commonly involve the left PFC and striatum in such cases.[12] Unless such cases are excluded from functional imaging studies, the CBF and metabolic results cannot be interpreted as describing alterations in local synaptic activity, since the relationship between neuronal activity, blood flow, and metabolism are altered.[12,23]

(4) MDD and BD likely encompass a group of disorders that are heterogenous with respect to etiology and pathophysiology. These conditions are thus likely to be characterized by an assortment of distinct functional imaging abnormalities. The extant literature supports this hypothesis, since subtyping of depressed subjects appears critical to the reproducibility of results.

In the studies described below, the variability of image data in depressed samples was reduced by exclusion of medicated subjects, subjects with depression-onset beyond age 50, and subjects whose depressive syndrome arose temporally after other major medical or psychiatric conditions (who have imaging correlates that generally differ from those of primary MDD).[12] We also selected our benchmark depressed samples using criteria for BD or familial pure depressive disease[15] (FPDD; primary MDD subjects with a first degree relative with MDD, but not mania, alcoholism, or antisocial personality disorder), since these subtypes have been more likely than the depression spectrum disease[15] (DSD; primary MDD subjects with a first degree relative with alcoholism or sociopathy) or sporadic depressive disease[15] subtypes (primary MDD subject with no first degree relatives with MDD, alcoholism or sociopathy) to have abnormal dexamethasone suppression of cortisol,[15,16] premature nadir in cortisol release,[17] blunted hypoglycemic response to insulin,[18,19] reduced platelet [^{3}H]-imipramine binding sites,[20] decreased latency to rapid eye movement (REM) sleep,[21] and greater likelihood of response to somatic antidepressant treatments.[22] BD and FPDD samples thus appear "enriched" for the likelihood having biological abnormalities.

Technical issues regarding image acquisition and analysis also contribute to differences across studies.[12,23] Anatomical localization in functional brain images has been enhanced by improving spatial resolution [now 4 mm for state-of-the-art PET cameras and 0.5 mm for functional MRI (fMRI)], techniques for co-registering PET and MRI images, and statistical mapping methods that delimit inherent physiological differences between depressives and controls. Functional anatomical localization is now limited as much by anatomical variability across individuals as by the inherent spatial resolution of imaging technologies. However, the literature largely consists of data acquired using early generation, relatively low-resolution PET and SPECT scanners or non-tomographic techniques (that provide CBF measures limited to the cortical grey matter near the scalp).[23] Moreover, most PET studies performed with state-of-the-art scanners blurred their images to spatial resolutions of 2 cm or more prior to analysis to reduce the effects of anatomical variability across subjects, eliminating the ability to resolve small structures such as the amygdala and subgenual PFC.[24]

We have employed a combination of low- and relatively high-resolution image analysis strategies to sensitively identify and precisely localize abnormalities in depression. To generate hypotheses regarding regional abnormalities in depression we initially generate composite images of voxel t-values by summing spatially normalized CBF or metabolic images.[25] Regions where such "t-images" showed the greatest differences between depressives and controls are used to define regions-of-interest (ROI) for hypothesis-testing in an independent subject sample.[25] This latter step is currently performed by defining ROI on each subject's MR image and obtaining the corresponding metabolic measure from a co-registered PET image.[26] Although this two-step approach is sensitive for identifying larger cortical areas of abnormal CBF and metabolism in depression, detecting abnormalities in smaller structures such as the amygdala is more sensitively accomplished using MRI-based ROI analysis alone.

Since the first step in this approach involves computations in a few hundred thousand image voxels, the second step is needed to distinguish true from false positive findings. An alternative approach is to correct *p*-values obtained using statistical parametric maps (e.g., SPM) for the number of comparisons.[27] Unfortunately, few other laboratories using omnibus, statistical mapping approaches have applied either approach for protecting against Type I error, and the literature has been diluted with results that cannot be distinguished from multiple comparison artifact. The findings described below review many of the functional imaging abnormalities in MDD and BD which have been found and replicated using rigorous experimental design.

AMYGDALA METABOLISM IN DEPRESSION

Resting CBF and glucose metabolism are abnormally elevated in depressives relative to controls in the amygdala, although limitations in spatial resolution have precluded distinctions among specific amygdala nuclei (FIG. 1).[24,25,28–31] This finding is highly reproducible in unmedicated samples with FPDD or BD, being demonstrable in four consecutive, independent series studied by the author. The magnitude of the abnormal elevation measured by PET is about 6% in FPDD. Because of the low spatial resolution of PET relative to the size of the amygdala and the low recovery coefficient of radioactive counts from the amygdala, measuring an intergroup difference of 6% using PET requires an actual 50 to 70% increase in amygdala CBF and glucose metabolism in the depressed samples.[25,33] This magnitude (50%) approximates that of the CBF increases measured by autoradiography in the rat amygdala during exposure to fear-conditioned stimuli.[34]

The amygdala has been the only structure where regional CBF and glucose metabolism consistently correlate positively with depression severity ratings.[24,25,28] In addition to being elevated in the depressed state, CBF and metabolism in the left amygdala appear abnormally elevated (although to a lesser extent) in asymptomatic (i.e., between MDE), familial depressives who are not taking antidepressant drugs (AD).[25] Conversely, during AD treatment that both induces and maintains symptom remission, amygdala metabolism decreases toward normal,[35] compatible with preclinical evidence that chronic AD administration has inhibitory effects on amygdala function.[36–38,40] Consistent with these observations, AD-medicated, remitted sub-

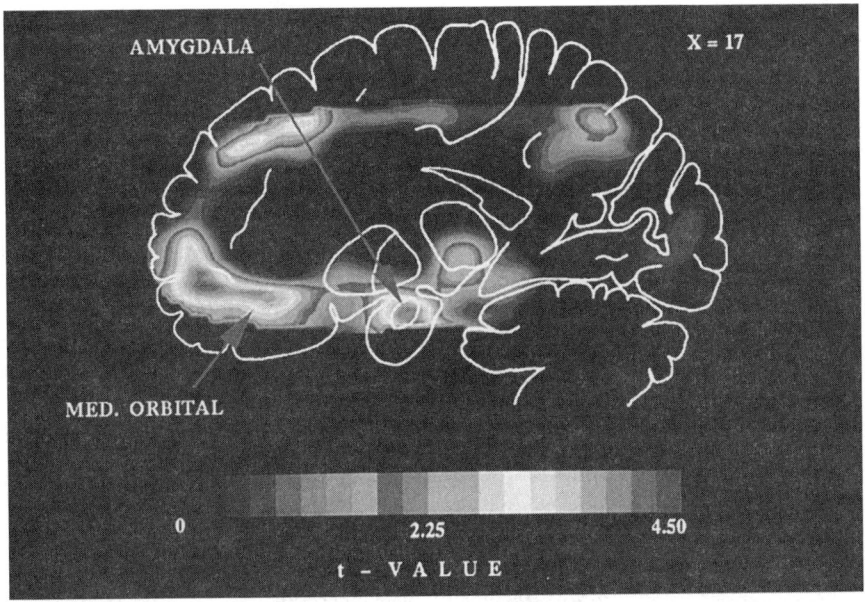

FIGURE 1. Areas of abnormally increased blood flow in familial MDD. The image section shown is from an image of t-values, produced by a voxel-by-voxel computation of the unpaired t-statistic to compare CBF between depressed and control samples.[25] The positive t-values in this sagittal section at 17 mm to the left of midline show areas of increased CBF in the depressives relative to the controls in the amygdala and the medial (MED) orbital cortex. Abnormal activity in these regions in MDD has been confirmed using higher resolution, glucose metabolism measurements in other studies.[24,28,30] Anterior is to the left. Reproduced with permission from Price *et al.*[32]

jects with MDD who relapse when given a tryptophan-free diet (which putatively reduces CNS serotonin levels) have higher baseline amygdala metabolism (i.e., prior to depletion) than similar subjects who do not relapse.[41] These data are compatible with the hypothesis that abnormally elevated amygdala activity confers susceptibility to recurrence of depressive episodes.[11,25] Abnormal *resting* metabolism in the amygdala has generally not been reported in other psychiatric conditions, suggesting that this finding may be specific to primary mood disorders.

The elevated activity in the left amygdala in depression may result from reduced inhibitory tone on amygdala neurons which would increase local synaptic transmission within the amygdaloid complex, or reflect increased synaptic transmission from afferent structures.[23] Increased afferent input could potentially arise from the posterior orbital cortex, the anterior insula and the subgenual and pregenual portions of the anterior cingulate cortex, where metabolic activity is increased in depression (see below) and which extensively project to the basal nucleus of the amygdala.[42,43] Modulatory systems which may function deficiently to disinhibit neuronal activity in these regions include the serotonergic system, which has been implicated in the pathophysiology of MDD by multiple types of evidence.[44–50] For example, recent *post mortem* studies demonstrate reduced numbers of Nissl-staining neurons in the dorsal raphe nucleus in MDD and BD subjects studied *post mortem*,[47] decreased raphe nucleus area 5HT1A somatodendritic autoreceptor density in suicide victims,[48] and abnormally decreased hippocampal 5HT1A receptor mRNA expression in MDD subjects who died by suicide.[49] Using PET and paired ^{18}FDG and [^{11}C]WAY100635 scans, we showed that abnormally elevated amygdala metabolism is associated with reduced 5HT1A receptor binding potential in the mesiotemporal cortex and the raphe in depressives with MDD and BD.[30]

In the amygdala, hippocampus, and PFC, postsynaptic 5HT1A receptors are abundantly expressed on the axon hillock of pyramidal neurons where, when stimulated, they inhibit action potential formation.[50] If the reduction in raphe neurons is associated with deficient 5HT release, or if 5HT1A receptor density is decreased in the amygdala, amygdala activity may conceivably increase.[44] AD drugs may compensate for such effects, since chronic SSRI and MAOI administration desensitizes presynaptic 5HT1A autoreceptors, increasing the amount of 5HT released per action potential,[51] and chronic AD and repeated ECS produce tonic activation of mesiotemporal cortical postsynaptic 5HT1A receptors which inhibits pyramidal neuron firing activity.[44,52]

Implications of Amygdala Hypermetabolism for Clinical Manifestations of Depression

The observation that amygdala metabolism correlates positively with Hamilton Depression Rating Scale (HDRS) score is remarkable because this scale covers a diverse set of clinical signs and symptoms related to mood, sleep, energy, motivation, anxiety, thought content, appetite, weight, libido, and psychomotor activity.[25,28] Electrical stimulation of the amygdala in humans can produce anxiety, fear, and dysphoria, recollection of emotionally provocative events that occurred in the distant past, and increased cortisol release, all of which are associated with MDD.[1,39,53,54] A preliminary PET study of depressives imaged during sleep found that glucose metabolism in the amygdala/periamygdaloid cortex is abnormally increased in MDD at baseline, and during sleep shows a further, incremental increase that is more prominent than that seen in healthy controls.[55] Elevated amygdala activity during sleep may conceivably account for the increased arousal evident in sleep EEG studies of MDD, as manifested clinically by interval insomnia.[21]

Additional depressive features may be explained if elevated amygdala activity stimulates efferent neurons in the hypothalamus and periaqueductal grey (PAG).[56,57] In experimental animals stimulation of the ventrolateral PAG produces social withdrawal, inactivity, and analgesia while stimulation of the lateral PAG produces defensive behaviors, analgesia and autonomic changes resembling those of a defense/flight response or panic attack.[57] Social withdrawal, inactivity, panic attacks, and reduced pain sensitivity are all manifested in MDD.

Evidence of excessive limbic-hypothalamic stimulation is provided by studies showing that severely depressed subjects have increased CSF levels of corticotropin releasing factor (CRF), hypersecretion of cortisol, and pituitary and adrenal gland enlargement.[4,12,58] In addition, depressives show a blunted ACTH response to CRF and suicide victims studied *post mortem* have decreased CRF receptor density in the frontal cortex along with pituitary mRNA levels indicative of chronic HPA axis activation.[58,59] Finally, some depressives show reduced sensitivity to dexamethasone negative feedback and/or to glucocorticoid "fast feedback."[60]

This pathological drive on CRF release may involve dysfunction of brain systems that mediate negative feedback inhibition of cortisol release, such as the hippocampus or the ventromedial PFC,[60,61,62] or excessive stimulation from the amygdala or extended amygdala. The central nucleus of the amygdala stimulates CRF release from the paraventricular nucleus of the hypothalamus via indirect anatomical connections through other hypothalamic nuclei and the bed nucleus of the stria terminalis.[62,63] "Stressed" plasma cortisol levels measured during PET scanning (i.e., following arterial and venous cannulation and > one hour of head restraint within the scanner) correlate positively with concomitant measures of left amygdala metabolism.[64] During successful—but not unsuccessful—treatment, amygdala metabolism decreases, serum cortisol and CSF levels of CRF normalize, and cortisol secretion becomes suppressible by dexamethasone, while subjects who show persistent elevations of amygdala metabolism or LHPA axis activity are at high risk for relapse in spite of treatment.[35,64] These treatment-associated changes may reflect the ability of chronic AD to suppress amygdala activity[36,37,52] and increase hippocampal glucocorticoid receptor binding capacity (augmenting feedback inhibition of CRF release).[64]

Although preliminary neuroimaging evidence that resting CBF is abnormally elevated in the hypothalamus and midbrain in MDD exists, these data have been difficult to interpret because of the low resolution of PET relative to these structures' small size.[32] The functional responsivity of these structures has thus been probed using PET to measure hemodynamic changes during visual stimulation with pictures of human faces exhibiting fearful expressions. Healthy subjects increase regional CBF in the amygdala, the lateral hypothalamus and the PAG when viewing fearful faces as compared with viewing emotionally "neutral" faces.[65] In contrast, depressives show no significant changes in these areas because their CBF values in the amygdala, hypothalamus and PAG remain elevated during exposure to both the neutral and fearful face stimuli.[65]

PREFRONTAL CORTICAL ABNORMALITIES IN MAJOR DEPRESSION

Neuroimaging abnormalities in the PFC in MDD and BD have been located in regions implicated by PET and fMRI studies of healthy subjects imaged during experimentally induced emotional states.[12] An important contribution of these studies in MDD and BD has been to identify areas where abnormalities of both brain structure and function exist in MDD and BD. Such findings have begun to guide *post mortem* studies to identify histopathological abnormalities in these disorders.

The Dorsomedial/Dorsal Anterolateral Prefrontal Cortex

The most widely reported abnormalities in the PFC in MDD have been that CBF and glucose metabolism are abnormally decreased in the dorsal anterolateral and dorsomedial PFC.[41,66–69,71,72,77] These abnormalities have been reversible with effective antidepressant therapy in some[66,74,70] but not all studies.[67,75,76] The specific location of these abnormalities remained unclear partly because early studies used very low resolution PET images (blurred to 2 to 4 cm full-width at half-maximum) or large ROI that precluded restricted localization within the large human PFC.[12] Moreover, because many types of psychotropic medications and the cerebrovascular disease associated with late-life onset depression diffusely decrease CBF and metabolism in the dorsolateral PFC, studies including image data for subjects with these confounding effects have reported reduced physiological activity in widely disparate areas of the dorsal PFC. Other studies localize these areas to the dorsomedial and dorsal anterolateral PFC area corresponding to the cortex lying dorsal and anterior to the dorsal anterior cingulate gyrus (BA 9) and to the dorsal anterior cingulate cortex itself.[66–68] The dorsomedial PFC (BA 9) was also found to have reduced CBF in depressed versus non-depressed patients with Parkinson's Disease, possibly related to the dense DA innervation this region receives from the VTA.[77]

In brain-mapping studies performed in healthy humans, CBF increases in these areas of BA 9 during performance of tasks that elicit emotional responses[78,79] or require emotional evaluations.[80] The relationship between the hemodynamic response and emotion ratings in these studies suggests that this region is activated to modulate emotional responses. For example, during anticipation of a painful electrical shock CBF increases in this region relative to resting or teeth clenching control conditions, but within each condition the change in anxiety ratings and heart rate correlate inversely with ΔCBF.[78]

The dorsomedial PFC (BA 9) receives and sends extensive efferent projections to the PAG, through which it may modulate emotional behavior or cardiovascular responses.[57] Lesions placed in the dorsomedial PFC in experimental animals result in elevated HR responses during exposure to fear-conditioned stimuli,[81] and electrical and chemical stimulation sites in the dorsal mPFC attenuate or inhibit the defensive behavior and associated cardiovascular responses evoked by amygdala stimulation (reviewed in Frysztak and Neafsey[81]). It is thus hypothesized that the dorsomedial mPFC normally acts to decrease HR during stress.[81]

Rajkowska et al.[82] recently reported that the cortical thickness is abnormally reduced in BA 9 of the dorsal anterolateral/dorsomedial PFC in MDD subjects studied *post mortem*. This observation could account for the reduction in CBF and glucose metabolism found in this area in MDD.[83] Moreover, if the dorsomedial PFC participates in modulating behavioral and cardiovascular responses to stress, the reduced grey matter identified by Rajkowska et al.[82] may indicate that impairment of the dorsomedial PFC function underlies the exaggerated stress responses seen in MDD. Dorsomedial PFC dysfunction acquired from other causes may similarly alter stress or emotional responses, as suggested by evidence that reduced CBF in this area distinguishes depressed from non-depressed patients with Parkinson's Disease.[77]

The Subgenual Prefrontal Cortex

In the anterior cingulate cortex ventral to the genu of the corpus callosum (i.e., the subgenual PFC) CBF and metabolism are decreased in unipolar and bipolar depressives relative to healthy controls (FIG. 2).[70,84] This metabolic decrement appears to be explained by a corresponding reduction in cortex, initially demonstrated by MRI-based neuromorphometric measures as a left-lateralized, mean grey matter volume reduction of 39% and 48% in the familial BD and MDD samples, respectively.[84] This volumetric difference persisted during treatment and was present in various mood states. Because of the low resolution of PET, a reduction of grey matter

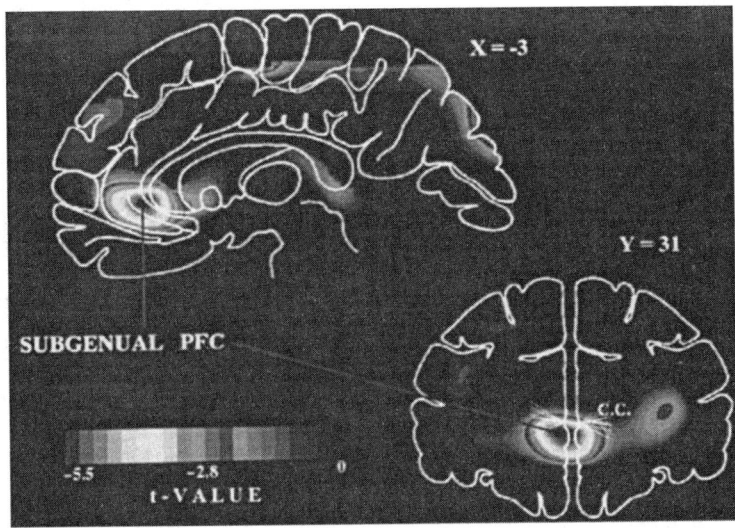

FIGURE 2. Coronal ($y = 31$ mm anterior to the anterior commissure) and sagittal ($x = -3$ mm left of midline) sections showing negative voxel t-values where glucose metabolism is decreased in depressives relative to controls.[84] Although none of these subjects were involved in the study[25] that generated the images in FIGURES 2–5, the mean metabolism in this set of depressives and controls was also abnormally increased in the depressives in the amygdala, orbital cortex, and medial thalamus shown in FIGURES 1, 3, and 5, and decreased in the caudate head as shown in FIGURE 6.[28] Anterior or left is to left. Reproduced with permission from Drevets et al.[84]

would appear as reduced CBF and metabolism due to partial volume averaging effects.[83] These MRI-based findings were replicated and extended by Hirayasu et al.,[86] who confirmed this left lateralized abnormality in familial but not non-familial BD samples, and Botteron et al.,[87] who showed this abnormality is present in both affected and unaffected co-twins from monozygotic twin pairs (ages 18 to 24) discordant for MDD.

Computer simulations performed to correct the PET measures for the effects of a reduction in cortex concluded that glucose metabolism in the remaining subgenual PFC tissue is actually abnormally *increased* in depressives relative to controls. This result is compatible with observations that effective AD treatment results in a further *decrease* in glucose metabolism in the subgenual PFC,[70,88] and that in healthy subjects, CBF increases in the subgenual PFC during sadness induced via contemplation of sad autobiographical material.[89,90] These data converge with evidence that other PFC structures implicated in emotional behavior also have reductions in cortex volume together with elevated physiological activity in the unmedicated-depressed relative to the medicated-remitted state (see below).

Post mortem assessments of subgenual PFC tissue (in humans this cortex comprises area 24b and, to a lesser extent, 24a on the prelimbic anterior cingulate gyrus) from BD or MDD subjects confirmed the abnormal reduction in cortex volume.[88,91] These studies demonstrated that the reduction in grey matter is associated with a reduction in glia without an equivalent loss of neurons in familial MDD and BD cases relative to psychiatrically healthy and schizophrenic controls. Neuronal counts were not decreased and neuronal density trended toward being abnormally increased in the mood-disordered samples.

Given the importance of glia (e.g., astroglia) in providing trophic factors and energy substrates to neurons, maintaining potassium homeostasis, and transporting glutamate and GABA from the extracellular fluid suggests mechanisms by which glial hypofunction could disturb synaptic activity within the subgenual PFC.[92] While it is unclear that this reduction in glial number is associated with glial hypofunction, it is noteworthy that the proportion of high affinity, glycine-displaceable [^{3}H]CGP-39653 binding to NMDA glutamatergic receptors is reduced in the PFC of suicide victims, possibly because impaired glutamate transport increases these receptors' exposure to glutamate.[93] Antidepressant treatments may compensate for impaired glutamate transport, as repeated electroconvulsive shock (ECS) and chronic AD administration desensitizes glutamatergic-NMDA receptors in the frontal cortex of rats.[94,95] In addition, anticonvulsant agents which putatively inhibit glutamate release appear effective in treating depression and preventing abnormal mood episodes in BD.[96]

Clinical Implications of Subgenual PFC Dysfunction

The subgenual PFC has extensive connections with the amygdala, lateral hypothalamus, nucleus accumbens, VTA, substantia nigra, raphe, locus ceruleus, PAG, and brain stem autonomic nuclei in monkeys and other experimental animals.[43,81,97,98,101] Since these structures have been implicated in various aspects of emotional behavior, abnormal synaptic interactions between these areas and the subgenual PFC may conceivably alter emotional processing, monoaminergic neurotransmitter release, neuroendocrine function, or autonomic regulation.[88]

Humans with lesions that include the subgenual PFC demonstrate abnormal autonomic responses to emotional experiences, inability to experience emotion related to concepts that ordinarily evoke emotion, and inability to use information regarding the likelihood of punishment versus reward in guiding social behavior.[99] Partly on the basis of these observations, Damasio *et al.*[99,100] proposed that the ability to evaluate the consequences of social behavior depends upon interactions between the ventromedial PFC, hypothalamic autonomic centers, and brain stem monoamine neurotransmitter systems. If so, disordered interactions between the subgenual PFC and these latter structures may disrupt evaluative processing, conceivably manifested by the heightened sensitivity to failure, pathological guilt, and exaggerated self criticism seen in depression, and the swings toward inappropriate elation, emotional lability, and insensitivity to the negative social consequences of pleasurable or violent behavior in mania.[84,100]

Rats with experimental lesions of prelimbic cortex (an apparent homologue of the primate subgenual PFC) demonstrate altered neuroendocrine responses to stress that resemble changes in these systems in humans with mood disorders.[101] For example, Diorio *et al.*[61] showed that lesions of the prelimbic and infralimbic anterior cingulate cortex increased plasma ACTH and corticosterone (CORT) responses to restraint stress, while implants of crystalline CORT in the same areas decreased these responses. Diorio et al.[61] concluded that the glucocorticoid receptors located in these areas are involved in the negative feedback of glucocorticoids on stress-related LHPA activity. Subgenual PFC dysfunction could thus contribute to the abnormal central drive on cortisol release, glucocorticoid negative feedback, and cortisol responses to stressors seen in MDD.[4,60,61]

Lesions of the medial PFC also alter autonomic and behavioral responses to stressors in rats. Bilateral lesions of the dorsal prelimbic and anterior cingulate cortex increase freezing behavior and heart rate (HR) elevations during exposure to fear-conditioned stimuli, while bilateral lesions of infralimbic and ventral prelimbic cortex reduce HR responses to fear-conditioned stimuli, suggesting that the latter regions play a role in increasing HR during stress.[81,102] The drive on sympathetic autonomic arousal and CORT release during stress were more specifically linked to the *right* ventromedial PFC by evidence that rats with lesions of the *left* infralimbic, prelimbic, and anterior cingulate cortices show heightened sympathetic arousal and exaggerated CORT responses to restraint stress, while right-lesioned animals showed attenuation of the CORT rise and gastric stress pathology associated with restraint stress.[103] Sullivan and Grattan[103] hypothesized that *left* ventromedial PFC lesions disinhibit the *right* ventromedial PFC, yielding heightened sympathetic and HPA-axis arousal. Given the left-lateralization of neuroimaging abnormalities in the subgenual PFC[84,86,87] it might be hypothesized that *left* subgenual PFC dysfunction contributes to the heightened neuroendocrine and sympathetic autonomic arousal seen in depression.[58,60,104]

Prelimbic and infralimbic cortex lesions reduce HR variability at rest and during exposure to fear-conditioned stimuli. HR variability is thought to reflect parasympathetic control of the sinus node via vagal nerve transmission,[81,105] and lesions of these cortical areas may alter parasympathetic tone because the ventral prelimbic and adjacent infralimbic cortex contain neurons that project to the nucleus tractus solitarius (NTS) of the vagus.[81,106] Depressed humans show reduced HR variability and elevated resting HR relative to non-depressed controls, findings that may conceivably relate to subgenual PFC dysfunction.[7,104] The reduced HR variability in MDD has been linked to the elevated risk for developing ventricular tachycardia, myocardial infarction and sudden death in depressed versus non-depressed patients matched for extent of cardiovascular disease.[7-9]

Finally, the subgenual PFC appears to participate in evaluating the behavioral significance of stimuli by modulating monoaminergic neurotransmitter function. The midbrain connections of the subgenual PFC include projections to neurons in the VTA, the substantia nigra, the raphe, and the locus ceruleus,[97,98,107,108] and of the PFC areas that receive dopaminergic inputs, Area 24 of the anterior cingulate gyrus (part of which is subgenual PFC) receives the most dense DA innervation, principally from the VTA.[109] In rats, electrical or glutamatergic stimulation of mPFC areas that would include the subgenual PFC elicits burst firing patterns from DA cells in the VTA and increases DA release in the nucleus accumbens.[110-113] The phasic, burst firing of DA neurons and accompanying rise in DA release appear to participate in encoding information regarding stimuli that predict reward and deviations between such predictions and the actual occurrence of reward.[114] If the subgenual PFC participates in modulating electrophysiological responses of VTA DA neurons in humans, then dysfunction of this region in mood disorders may alter hedonic perceptions and motivated behavior.

The subgenual PFC abnormalities found in MDD and BD may thus relate to evidence that DA function is reduced in depression.[115,116] Unmedicated MDD subjects consistently show reduced CSF concentrations of the DA metabolite, homovanillic acid (HVA),[116] although this abnormality may not relate specifically to mesolimbic DA function. Receptor imaging studies report that the apparent DA D_2/D_3 receptor binding potential is abnormally increased in non-psychotic MDD subjects when measured using the selective D_2/D_3 receptor radioligand ([^{123}I]IBZM), which is sensitive to competition from endogenous DA,[123–125] but not when measured using [^{11}C]-N-methylspiperone (NMSP),[126] which is insensitive to endogenous DA. Together these imaging data suggest that the intrasynaptic DA concentration is abnormally decreased in nonpsychotic depressives. These observations are consistent with evidence that DA depletion associated with reserpine treatment or Parkinson's Disease increases the risk for developing MDE (the risk for MDE in Parkinson's Disease is 2- to 5-fold higher than that in other similarly disabling conditions, and the majority of depressed Parkinson's cases experience depression onset prior to the appearance of motor signs).[117,118] In primary MDD, depressive symptoms may remit during i.v. dextroamphetamine administration, and both direct DA agonists (bromocriptine, piribedil) and DA reuptake inhibitors (nomifensine) are as effective as conventional antidepressant drugs (AD) in double-blind trials.[115,119] Conventional

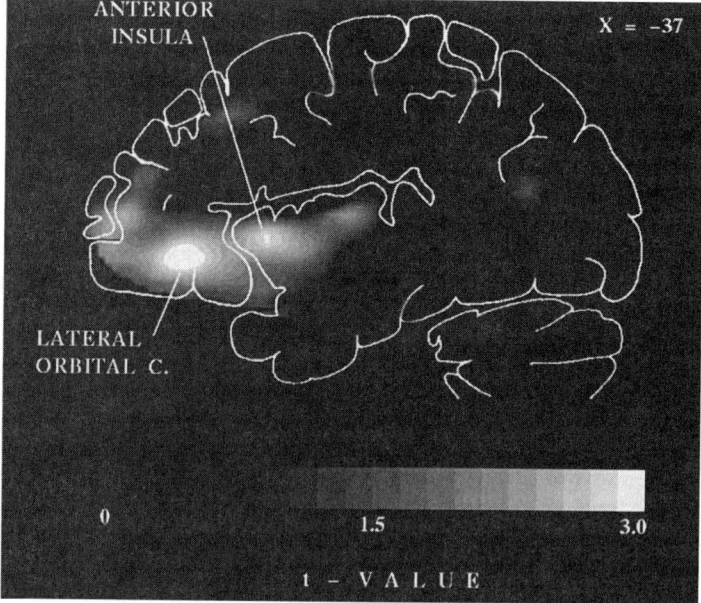

FIGURE 3. Sagittal t-image section 37 mm left of midline ($X = -37$) shows an area of increased CBF in depressed with MDD relative to healthy controls in the left ventrolateral PFC (VLPFC), lateral orbital C (L. Orbital) and anterior insula.[25] Reproduced with permission from Drevets and Botteron.[135]

AD also enhance mesolimbic DA D_2/D_3 receptor function via pharmacodynamic effects, and repeated ECS and chronic administration of AD that inhibit norepinephrine (NE) reuptake increase extracellular DA concentrations in the mPFC and accumbens shell.[120–122]

The Orbital Cortex

In the ventrolateral PFC (VLPFC) and the posterolateral and posteromedial orbital cortex (FIGS. 1 and 3) and in some cases, in the anterior cingulate cortex anterior to the genu of the corpus callosum (i.e., the "pregenual" anterior cingulate) CBF and metabolism are abnormally *increased* in unmedicated subjects with primary MDD.[25,28,69,71,72,139] These findings are not specific to depression, as flow and me-

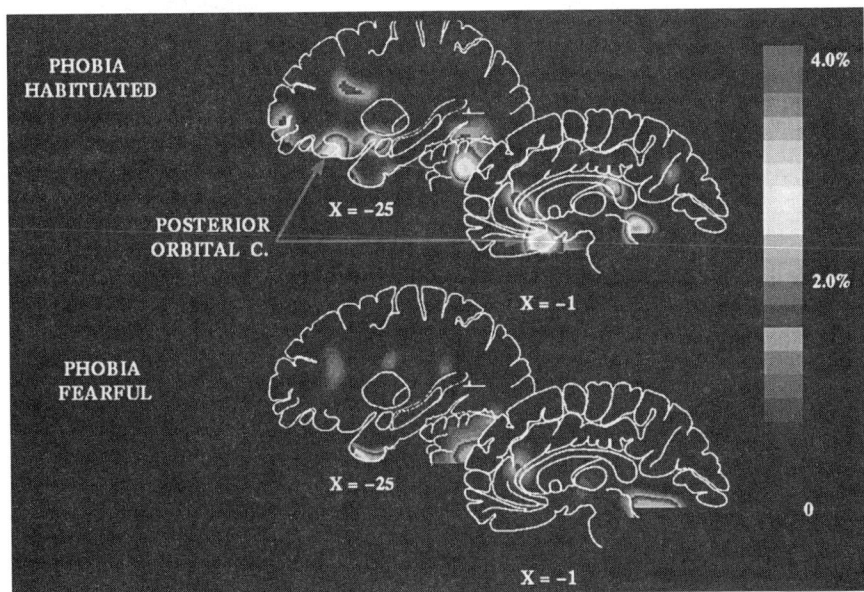

FIGURE 4. Images of CBF changes in subjects with simple animal phobias during exposure to relevant phobic stimuli (live snake or tarantula).[129] Habituation to a phobic stimulus is accompanied by the development of a blood flow response in the posteromedial orbital cortex during repeated exposure to a phobic stimulus (*phobia habituated*). The magnitude of ΔCBF in this region correlated inversely with the accompanying changes in heart rate and anxiety ratings. In contrast, CBF did not change in this area during initial exposures to the same animal (*phobia fearful*). In PET studies involving healthy or obsessive-compulsive subjects exposed to anxiety provoking stimuli, CBF generally increases in the posterior orbital cortex during the initial exposure to anxiogenic stimuli, with the magnitude of ΔCBF correlating inversely with symptom ratings. In contrast, the phobic subjects fail to activate this region until undergoing repeated *in vivo* exposure to the phobic stimulus. Anterior is to the left. The grey-scale bar indicates ΔCBF in percent in the anxious minus control conditions. The *X* coordinate provides the position (in mm) of each sagittal image plane relative to the midline, with negative *X* indicating left. Reproduced by permission from Drevets and Botteron.[135]

TABLE 1. Antidepressant treatment effects on ventral prefrontal cortical CBF and metabolism in depression

Authors	Treatment Modality	Change in CBF or glucose metabolism post- vs. pretreatment scans
Bonne et al.[74]	ECT	↑ anterior cingulate in responders, n.s. in ventral anterolateral PFC
Buchsbaum et al.[70]	Sertraline	↓ dorsal anterior cingulate, ↓ ventromedial (subgenual) PFC
Cohen et al.[71]	Phototherapy	↓ medial orbital C[a]
Drevets & Raichle[38]	Desipramine	↓ left ventrolateral PFC
Drevets et al.[35]	Sertraline	↓ ventrolateral PFC and orbital C
Ebert et al.[72]	Sleep deprivation	↓ orbital C in responders[a]
George et al.[b]	RTMS	↓ orbital C in responders
Goodwin et al.[131]	Various drug treatments	↑ anterior cingulate, n.s. ventral anterolateral
Nobler et al.[75]	ECT	↓ left ventrolateral PFC, responders[c]
Rubin et al.[76]	Nortriptyline or sertraline	↓ left ventrolateral PFC, responders[c]
Wu et al.[31]	Sleep deprivation	↓ anterior cingulate, responders

ABBREVIATIONS: C, cortex; ECT, electroconvulsive therapy; PFC, prefrontal cortex. RTMS, repeated transcranial magnetic stimulation. ↑, ↓, and n.s. indicate increases, decreases, or no significant changes, respectively, in the treated relative to the untreated state. Not all studies examined the same regions, and the absence of a listed result for a specific region indicates that no image data were provided for that region.

[a]The treatment-associated change reported in this study was not shown by paired statistical tests.

[b]Presented at the Annual Meeting of the American College of Neuropsychopharmacology, San Juan, Puerto Rico, 1996.

[c]Studies performed using xenon-133, which only provides CBF measures from cerebral cortex lying near the scalp.

tabolism increase in these areas during experimentally induced sadness or anxiety in healthy subjects and during induced anxiety and/or obsessional states in subjects with obsessive-compulsive disorder, panic disorder, post-traumatic stress disorder, and simple animal phobia (FIG. 4).[90,128–130] The CBF and metabolic increases in these areas are mood-state dependent in MDD,[25] and studies comparing images acquired before and during effective antidepressant treatment show that VLPFC/orbital PFC activity decreases in the remitted relative to the depressed phase of MDD (TABLE 1). Treatment-effects in the pregenual anterior cingulate have been more variable (TABLE 1).

Complex Relationship between Orbital Metabolism and Illness Severity

Although CBF and metabolism are elevated in the VLPFC and orbital cortex in the unmedicated depressed phase relative to the remitted phase of MDD, these measures correlate inversely with ratings of depression severity and depressive ideation.[25,28] Similarly, in subjects with obsessive-compulsive disorder or animal phobias scanned during exposure to phobic stimuli and in healthy subjects imaged during induced sadness, CBF in the posterior orbital cortex increases, yet the magnitude of the CBF change correlates inversely with concomitant changes in obsessive thinking, anxiety, and sadness, respectively.[128–130] These observations are consistent with evidence that the posterior orbital cortex plays a role in modulating defensive autonomic and behavioral responses and redirecting psychological and behavioral response patterns as reward contingencies change.[132,133]

Humans with lesions of the orbital cortex exhibit difficulty shifting intellectual strategies in response to changing demands [i.e., they perseverate in strategies that become inappropriate[132]] Likewise, monkeys with surgical lesions of the lateral orbital/ventrolateral PFC demonstrate "perseverative interference," characterized by difficulty in learning to withhold responses to non-rewarding stimuli.[134] During single unit recordings from orbital cortex, nearly one-half of pyramidal cells demonstrate altered firing rates during the delay period between stimulus and response, and post-trial activity is related to the presence or absence of reward.[132] One type of cells appears to encode the availability of reward, and a second type, deviations from expectancy of reward.[132] Thus, during depressive episodes activation of the posterior orbital cortex may reflect endogenous attempts to break perseverative patterns of self-depreciating and non-rewarding thought and emotion.

The orbital cortex may also play a role in extinguishing responses to stimuli that are not reinforced.[129] Consistent with this hypothesis, we demonstrated that as humans with animal phobias habituate to a phobic stimulus, the magnitude of changes in anxiety ratings and heart rate correlate inversely with changes in posterior orbital cortex CBF (FIG. 4). This effect may be mediated at a level fugal to the amygdala, since defensive behaviors and cardiovascular responses produced by electrical stimulation of the amygdala are attenuated or ablated by concomitant stimulation of sites in the orbital cortex, which when stimulated alone produce no autonomic changes.[133] Given evidence that somatic antidepressant treatments may directly modulate neuronal activity in the amygdala,[36,37,44,52] the reduction in orbital cortex CBF and metabolism following successful treatment may indicate that the orbital cortex can "relax" as such treatments inhibit the pathological limbic activity to which they respond (TABLE 1).

Dysfunction of the orbital cortex may also yield a state in which obsessive ruminations and exaggerated stress responses appear (depressives note that their ability to interrupt perseverative melancholic thoughts and anxious responses to ordinarily non-threatening stimuli seems impaired).[92] Abnormally reduced grey matter wet weight and cortical thickness have been reported in the posterolateral orbital cortex in *post mortem* studies of MDD and BD.[46,82,136] Histological assessment of these areas show that the posterior orbital C has a reduction in glia like that found in the subgenual PFC, which could potentially disturb interactions between the orbital cortex neurons and their projections to the amygdala, striatum, cingulate, hypothalamus or PAG.[57,82,88,91,136]

Partial volume averaging effects associated with this reduction in posterior orbital cortex volume may contribute to the inverse relationship found between metabolism and depression severity.[83] If the magnitude of the grey matter reduction determines how severely depressed one is likely to become during a MDE, then subjects with more severe depression would tend to show the lowest apparent CBF and metabo-

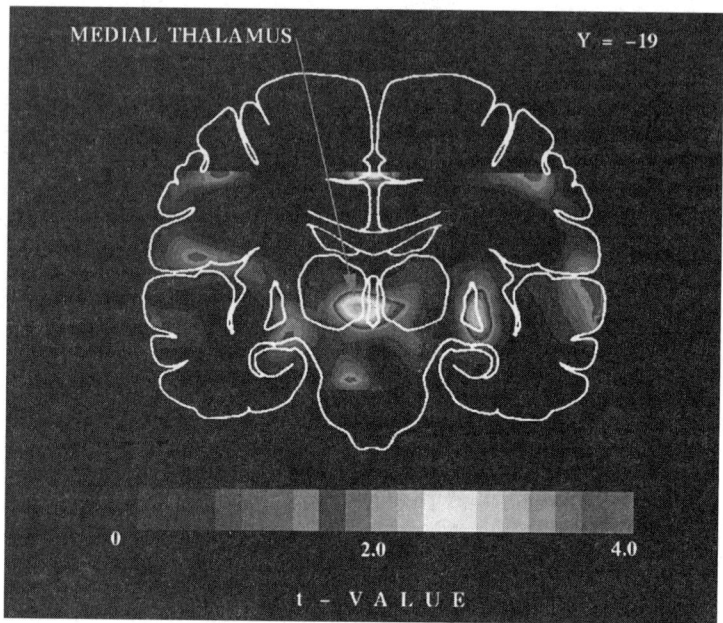

FIGURE 5. Coronal t-image section 19 mm caudal to the anterior commissure (i.e., $y = -19$) showing the area corresponding to increased CBF in the left medial thalamus of depressed subjects relative to controls.[25] Reproduced by permission from Drevets and Todd.[1]

lism in these regions. This effect would also reduce sensitivity for detecting abnormal increases in orbital cortex metabolism in more severely ill MDD samples.

Implications for the Pathogenesis of Secondary Major Depressive Syndromes

Compatible with the hypothesis that orbital cortex plays a modulatory role over depressive symptoms in primary MDD, lesions of this cortex or interruption of neural interactions between the orbital cortex and related parts of the striatum increase the risk for developing major depressive syndromes.[1,137] The neuroimaging findings in the amygdala and PFC coupled with evidence that metabolic activity is abnormal in related parts of the striatum and thalamus in primary MDD implicate a limbic-thalamo-cortical circuit, involving the amygdala, the mediodorsal nucleus (MD) of the thalamus and the orbital and medial PFC, and a limbic-striatal-pallidal-thalamic circuit, involving related parts of the striatum and ventral pallidum as well as the components of the other circuit (FIGS. 5 and 6).[25,28,139,108] Lesions involving the parts of the PFC that participate in the limbic-thalamo-cortical circuit (i.e., left middle cerebral artery stroke involving the frontal cortex and striatum) and diseases of the basal ganglia (e.g. Parkinson's Disease and Huntington's Disease) are associated with higher rates of major depression than other similarly debilitating conditions.[117,118,137,138] Because these conditions affect this system in different ways, imbalances within these circuits, rather than overall increased or decreased synaptic activity within a particular structure, may give rise to the depressive syndrome.[25,138]

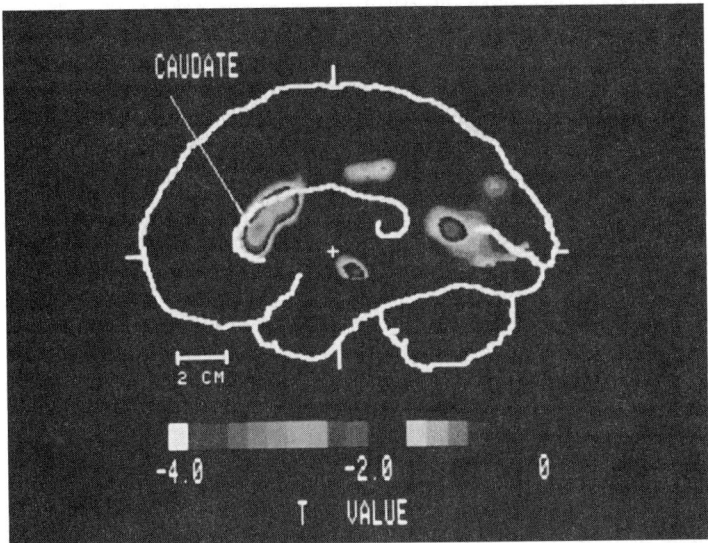

FIGURE 6. The t-image demonstrating areas of decreased activity in the depressed subjects with MDD relative to the controls in the left medial caudate. The image shown is a sagittal projection of the greatest voxel t-values in all planes between the midline and 10 mm left of midline. This observation replicated an earlier finding reported by Baxter et al.[139] Anterior is to the left. Reproduced with permission from Drevets et al.[25]

SUMMARY

Although the neurobiological correlates of mood disorders remain poorly understood, neuroimaging and histopathological studies are beginning to delineate anatomical systems involved in their pathophysiology. Such studies support a neural model in which dysfunction of modulatory systems within the PFC, striatum and brain stem disinhibit emotional and stress responses generated through the amygdala and its projections to the hypothalamus, PAG, and "extended amygdala." Antidepressant therapies may compensate for dysfunction in these modulatory systems by directly inhibiting this pathological limbic activity, augmenting monoamine neurotransmission, and/or altering neuroreceptor sensitivity at various points in the pathways mediating abnormal emotional expression.

REFERENCES

1. DREVETS, W.C. & R.D. TODD. 1997. Depression, Mania and Related Disorders. In Adult Psychiatry. S.B. Guze, Ed. **8:** 99–141. Mosby Press. St.Louis, MO.
2. AMERICAN PSYCHIATRIC ASSOCIATION. 1994. Diagnostic and Statistical Manual of Mental Disorders (DSM-IV). APA Press. Washington, D.C.
3. REGIER, D.A., J.H. BOYD, J.D. BURKE, et al. 1988. One-month prevalence of mental disorders in the United States. Arch. Gen. Psychiatry **45:** 977–986.
4. CARROLL, B.J. 1994. Brain mechanisms in manic depression. Clin. Chem. **40:** 303–308.

5. ELKIN, I., T. SHEA, J.T. WATKINS, et al. 1989. National Institute of Mental Health treatment of depression collaborative research program. Arch. Gen. Psychiatry **46:** 971–982.
6. KUPFER, D.J., E. FRANK, J.M. PEREL, et al. 1992. Five-year outcome for maintenance therapies in recurrent depression. Arch. Gen. Psychiatry **49**(10): 769–773.
7. CARNEY, R.M., M.W. RICH, K.E. FREEDLAND, J. SAINI, A. TEVELDE, C. SIMEONE & K. CLARK. 1988. Major depressive disorder predicts cardiac events in patients with coronary artery disease. Psychosom. Med. **50:** 627–633.
8. CARNEY, R.M., K.E. FREEDLAND, M.W. RICH, L.J. SMITH & A.S. JAFFE. 1993. Ventricular tachycardia and psychiatric depression in patients with coronary artery disease. Am. J. Med. **95:** 23–28.
9. FRASURE-SMITH, N., F. LESPÉANCE & M. TALAJIC. 1995. Depression and 18 month prognosis after myocardial infarction. Circulation **91**(4): 999–1005.
10. GOODWIN, F.K. & K.R. JAMISON. 1990. Manic-Depressive Illness. Oxford. New York.
11. POST, R.M. 1992. Transduction of psychosocial stress into the neurobiology of recurrent affective disorder. Am. J. Psychiatry **149:** 999–1010.
12. DREVETS, W.C., K. GADDE & R. KRISHNAN. Neuroimaging studies of depression. *In* The Neurobiological Foundation of Mental Illness. D.S. Charney, E.J. Nestler & B.J. Bunney, Eds. Oxford University Press. In press.
13. MAES, M., R. DIERCKX, H.Y. MELTZER, et al. 1993. Psychiatry Res. Neuroimaging **50:** 77–88.
14. SILFVERSKIOLD, P. & J. RISBERG. 1989. Arch. Gen. Psychiatry **46:** 253–259.
15. WINOKUR, G. 1982. Pharmacopsychiatry **15:** 142–146.
16. ARANA, G.W., R.J. BALDESSARINI & M. ORNSTEEN. 1985. Arch. Gen. Psychiatry **42:** 1193–1204.
17. WINOKUR, G. & W. CORYELL. 1992. Biol Psychiatry **32:** 1012–1018.
18. LEWIS, D.A., R.G. KATHOL, B.M. SHERMAN, G. WINOKUR & M.A. SCHLESSER. 1984. Arch. Gen. Psychiatry **40:** 167–170.
19. WINOKUR, A., G. MAISLIN, J.L. PHILLIPS & J.D. AMSTERDAM. 1988. Am. J. Psychiatry **145:** 325–330.
20. LEWIS, D.A. & C. MCCHESNEY. 1985. Arch. Gen. Psychiatry **42:** 485–488.
21. KUPFER, D.J., E. TARG & J. STACK. 1992. J. Nerv. Ment. Dis. **170**(8): 494–498.
22. CORYELL, W. & ZIMMERMAN. 1984. Outcome following ECT for primary unipolar depression: a test of newly proposed response predictors. Am. J. Psychiatry. **141**(7): 862–867.
23. RAICHLE, M.E. 1987. Circulatory and metabolic correlates of brain function in normal humans. *In* Handbook of Physiology—The Nervous System V. J.M. Brookhart & V.B. Mountcastle, Eds. Vol. 5, Chap. 16: 643–674. Am. Physiol. Soc.
24. ABERCROMBIE, H.C., C.L. LARSON, R.T. WARD, et al. 1996. Neuroimage **3:** S217.
25. DREVETS, W.C., T.O. VIDEEN, J.L. PRICE, et al. 1992. Functional anatomical study of unipolar depression. J. Neurosci. **12:** 3628–3641.
26. WOODS, R.P., J.C. MAZZIOTTA & S.R. CHERRY. 1993. MRI-PET registration with automated algorithm. J. Comput. Assist. Tomogr. **17:** 536–546.
27. WORSLEY, K.J., S. MARRETT, P. NEELIN, et al. 1995. Brain Mapping **4:** 58–73
28. DREVETS, W.C., E. SPITZNAGEL & M.E. RAICHLE. 1995. Functional anatomical differences between major depressive subtypes. J. Cerebral Blood Flow Metab. **15**(1): S93.
29. DREVETS, W.C., J.L. PRICE, J.R. SIMPSON, et al. 1997. Soc. Neurosci. Abstr. **23**(2): 1407.
30. DREVETS, W.C., J.C. PRICE, D.J. KUPFER, et al. Biol. Psychiatry. In press.
31. WU, J.C., J.C. GILLIN, M.S. BUCHSBAUM, et al. 1992. Am. J. Psychiatry **149:** 538–543.
32. PRICE, J.L., S.T. CARMICHAEL, W.C. DREVETS. 1996. Prog. Brain Res. **107:** 523–536.
33. LINKS, J.M., J.K. ZUBIETA, C.C. MELTZER, M.J. STUMPF & J.J. FROST. 1996. J. Comput. Assist. Tomogr. **20**(4): 680–687
34. LEDOUX, J.E., M.E. THOMPSON, C. IADECOLA, et al. 1983. Science **221:** 576–578.
35. DREVETS, W.C., J.L. PRICE, J.R. SIMPSON, et al. 1996. Soc. Neurosci. Abstr. **22**(1): 66.
36. BROEKKAMP, C.L. & K.G. LLOYD. 1981. The role of the amygdala on the action of psychotropic drugs. *In* The Amygdaloid Complex. Y. Ben-Ari, Ed.: 219–225. Elsevier-North Holland Biomedical. Amsterdam.

37. DUNCAN, G.E., G.R. BREESE, H. CRISWELL, W.E. STUMPF, R.A. MUELLER & J.B. COVEY. 1986. Effects of antidepressant drugs injected into the amygdala on behavioral responses of rats in the forced swim test. J. Pharmacol. Exp. Ther. **238:** 758–762.
38. DREVETS, W.C. & M.E. RAICHLE. 1992. Psychopharm. Bull. **28:** 261–274
39. RUBIN, R.T., A.J. MANDELL & P.H. CRANDALL. 1966. Corticosteroid responses to limbic stimulation in man: localization of stimulus sites. Science **153:** 767–768.
40. ORDWAY, G.A., C. GAMBARANA, S.M. TEJANI-BUTT, P. ARESO, M. HAUPTMANN & M. FRAZER. 1991. Preferential reduction of binding of ^{125}I-iodopindolol to beta-1 adrenoceptors in the amydala of rats after antidepressant treatments. J. Pharmacol. Exp. Ther. **257:** 681–690.
41. BREMNER, J.D, R.B. INNIS, R.M. SALOMON, et al. 1997. Arch. Gen. Psychiat. **54:** 346–374.
42. AMARAL, D., J. PRICE, A. PITKANEN & S. CARMICHAEL. 1992. Anatomical organization of the primate amygdaloid complex. In The Amygdala. J. Aggleton, Ed.: 1–66. Wiley-Liss, Inc. New York.
43. CARMICHAEL, S.T. & J.L. PRICE. 1995. Limbic connections of the orbital and medial prefrontal cortex in Macaque Monkeys. J. Comp. Neurol. **363:** 615–641.
44. HADDJERI, N., P. BLIER & C. DE MONTIGNY. 1998. J. Neurosci. **18(23):** 10150–10156
45. FRANCIS, P.T., A. POYNTON, S.L. LOWE, et al. 1989. Brain amino acid concentrations and Ca^{2+}-dependent release in intractable depression assessed antemortem. Brain Res. **494:** 314–324.
46. BOWEN, D.M., A. NAJLERAHIM, A.W. PROCTER, P.T. FRANCIS & E. MURPHY. 1989. Proc. Natl. Acad. Sci. USA **86:** 9504–9508.
47. BAUMANN, B.G. & B. BOGERTS. 1998. Post mortem studies of bipolar disorder. Presented at the Stanley Bipolar Symposium, Royal Society, London, September 24.
48. KASSIR, S.A., M.D. UNDERWOOD, M.J. BAKALIAN, et al. 1998. Soc. Neurosci. Abstr. **24:** 1274.
49. LÓPEZ, J.F., D.T. CHALMERS, K.Y. LITTLE & S.J. WATSON. 1998. Biol. Psychiatry **43:** 547–573
50. AZMITIA, E.C., P.J. GANNON, N.M. KHECK & P.M. WHITAKER-AZMITIA. 1996. Neuropsychopharmacology **14:** 35–46.
51. CHAPUT, Y., C. DEMONTIGNY & P. BLIER. 1991. Neuropsychopharmacology **5:** 219–229.
52. WANG, R.Y. & G.K. AGHAJANIAN. 1980. Commun. Psychopharmacol. **4:** 83–90.
53. GLOOR, P., A. OLIVIER, L.F. QUESNEY, F. ANDERMANN & S. HOROWITZ. 1982. Ann. Neurol. **12:** 129–144.
54. BROTHERS, L. 1995. In The Cognitive Neurosciences. M.S. Gazzaniga, Ed. Chap. 73: 1107–1116. MIT Press. Cambridge, MA.
55. NOFZINGER, E.F., T.E. NICHOLS, D.J. KUPFER & R.Y. MOORE. 1998. Soc. Neurosci. Abstr. **24:** 1519.
56. LEDOUX, J.E. 1987. Emotion. In Handbook of Physiology—The Nervous System V. J. Mills, V.B. Mountcastle, F. Plum & S.R. Geiger, Eds.: 373–417. Williams & Wilkins. Baltimore.
57. PRICE, J.L. 1999. Networks within the orbital and medial prefrontal cortex. Neurocase **5.** In press.
58. MUSSELMAN, D.L. & C.B. NEMEROFF. 1993. The role of corticotropin-releasing factor in the pathophysiology of psychiatric disorders. Psychiatric Ann. **23:** 676–681.
59. LOPEZ, J.F., M. PALKOVITS, M. ARATO, A. MANSOUR, H. AKIL & S.J. WATSON. 1992. Localization and quantitation of proopiomelanocortin mRNA and glucocorticoid receptor mRNA in pituitary of suicide victims. Neuroendocrinology **56:** 491–501.
60. YOUNG, E.A., J. KOTUN, R.F. HASKETT, L. GRUNHAUS, J.F. GREDEN, S.J. WATSON & H. AKIL. 1993. Dissociation between pituitary and adrenal suppression to dexamethasone in depression. Arch. Gen. Psychiatry **50:** 395–403.
61. DIORO, D., V. VIAU & M.J. MEANEY. 1993. The role of the medial prefrontal cortex (cingulate gyrus) in the regulation of hypothalamic-pituitary-adrenal responses to stress. J. Neurosci. **13(9):** 3839–3847.
62. MCEWEN, B.S. 1995. Stressful experience, brain, and emotions: developmental,

genetic and hormonal influences. *In* The Cognitive Neurosciences. M. Gazzaniga, Ed.: 1117–1135. MIT Press. Cambridge, MA.
63. HERMAN, J.P. & W.E. CULLINAN. 1997. Neurocircuitry of stress: central control of the hypothalamo-pituitary-adrenocortical axis. Trends Neurosci. **20**(2): 78–84.
64. BARDEN, N., J. REUL & F. HOLSBOER. 1995. Trends Neurosci. **18**: 6–11.
65. DREVETS, W.C., S. PROPER, C. GAUTTIER, D.I. PERRETT & D.J. KUPFER. Hemodynamic responses to facial emotion in amygdala, inferotemporal cortex altered in depression. 1998. Presented at a conference entitled Advancing from the Ventral Striatum to the Extended Amygdala: Implications for Neuropsychiatry and Drug Abuse. Charlottesville, VA.
66. BAXTER, L.R., J.M. SCHWARTZ, M.E. PHELPS, *et al.* 1989. Arch. Gen. Psychiatry **46**: 243–250.
67. BELL, K., D.J. KUPFER & W.C. DREVETS. Biol. Psychiatry. In press.
68. BENCH, C.J., K.J. FRISTON, R.G. BROWN, *et al.* 1992. Psychol. Med. **22**: 607–615.
69. BIVER, F., S. GOLDMAN, V. DELVENNE, *et al.* 1994. Biol. Psychiatry **36**: 381–388.
70. BUCHSBAUM, M.S., J. WU, B.V. SIEGEL, E. HACKETT, M. TRENARY, L. ABEL & C. REYNOLDS. 1997. Effect of sertraline on regional metabolic rate in patients with affective disorder. Biol. Psychiatry **41**: 15–22.
71. COHEN, R.M., M. GROSS, T.E. NORDAHL, *et al.* 1992. Arch. Gen. Psychiatry **49**: 545–552.
72. EBERT, D., H. FEISTEL & A. BAROCKA. 1991. Psychiatry Res. Neuroimaging **40**: 247–251.
73. MAYBERG, H.S., S.K. BRANNAN, R.K. MAHURIN, *et al.* 1997. Neuroreport. **8**(4): 1057–1061.
74. BONNE, O., Y. KRAUSZ, B. SHAPIRA, *et al.* 1996. J. Nucl. Med. **37**: 1075–1080.
75. NOBLER, M.S., H.A. SACKEIM, I. PROHOVNIK, *et al.* 1994. Arch. Gen. Psychiatry **51**: 884–897.
76. RUBIN, R.T., A.J. MANDELL & P.H. CRANDALL. 1966. Science **153**: 767–768.
77. RING, H.A., C.J. BENCH, M.R. TRIMBLE, *et al.* 1994. Br. J. Psychiatry **165**: 333–339.
78. DREVETS, W.C., T.O. VIDEEN, A.Z. SNYDER, *et al.* 1994. Soc. Neurosci. Abstr. **20**(1): 368.
79. REIMAN, E.M., R.D. LANE, G.L. AHERN, *et al.* 1997. Am .J. Psychiatry **154**(7): 918–925.
80. DOLAN, R.J., P. FLETCHER, J. MORRIS, *et al.* 1996. Neuroimage. **4**: 194–200.
81. FRYSZTAK, R.J. & E.J. NEAFSEY. 1994. The effect of medial frontal cortex lesions on cardiovascular conditioned emotional responses in the rat. Brain Res. **643**: 181–193.
82. RAJKOWSKA, G., J.J. MIGUEL-HIDALGO, J. WEI *et al.* 1999. Biol. Psychiatry **45**(9): 1085–1098.
83. MAZZIOTTA, J.C., M.E. PHELPS, D. PLUMMER & D.E. KUHL. 1981. J. Comput. Assist. Tomogr. **5**: 734–743.
84. DREVETS, W.C., J.L. PRICE, J.R. SIMPSON, R.D. TODD, T. REICH, M. VANNIER & M.E. RAICHLE. 1997. Nature **386**: 824–827.
85. Baxter, L.R., M.E. Phelps, J.C. Mazziotta, *et al.* 1987. Arch. Gen. Psychiatry **44**: 211–218.
86. HIRAYASU, Y., M.E. SHENTON, D.F. SALISBURY, *et al.* Am. J. Psychiatry. In press.
87. BOTTERON, K.N., M. RAICHLE, A. HEATH & R.D. TODD. 1998. Presented at a conference entitled Advancing from the Ventral Striatum to the Extended Amygdala: Implications for Neuropsychiatry and Drug Abuse. Charlottesville, VA.
88. DREVETS, W.C., D. ÖNGÜR & J.L. PRICE. 1998. Mol. Psychiatry **3**(3): 220–226.
89. DAMASIO, A.R., T.J. GRABOWSKI, A. BECHARA, *et al.* 1998. Soc. Neurosci. Abstr. **24**: 258.
90. GEORGE, M.S., T.A. KETTER, P.I. PAREKH, B. HORWITZ, P. HERSCOVITCH, R.M. POST. 1995. Brain activity during transient sadness and happiness in healthy women. Am. J. Psychiatry **152**: 341–351
91. ÖNGÜR, D., W.C. DREVETS & J.L. PRICE. 1998. Proc. Natl. Acad. Sci. USA **95**: 13290–13295.
92. MAGISTRETTI, P.J., L. PELLERIN & J.L. MARTIN. 1995. Brain energy metabolism: an integrated cellular perspective. *In* Psychopharmacology: The Fourth Generation of

Progress. F.E. Bloom & D.J. Kupfer, Eds.: 921–932. Raven Press. New York.
93. NOWAK, G., G.A. ORDWAY & I.A. PAUL. 1995. Alterations in the N-methyl-D-aspartate (NMDA) receptor complex in the frontal cortex of suicide victims. Brain Res. **675:** 157–164.
94. NOWAK, G., R. TRULLAS, R.T. LAYER, P. SKOLNICK & I.A. PAUL. 1993. Adaptive changes in the N-methyl-D-aspartate receptor complex after chronic treatment with imipramine and 1-aminocyclopropanecarboxylic acid. J. Pharmacol. Exp. Ther. **265:** 1380–1386.
95. PAUL, I.A., G. NOWAK, R.T. LAYER, P. POPIK & P. SKOLNICK. 1994. Adaption of the N-methyl-D-aspartate receptor complex following chronic antidepressant treatments. J. Pharmacol. Exp. Ther. **269**(1): 95–102.
96. SPORN, J. & G. SACHS. 1997. The anticonvulsant lamotrigine in treatment-resistant manic-depressive illness. J. Clin. Psychopharmacol. **17**(3): 185–189.
97. SESACK, S.R., A.Y. DEUTCH, R.H. ROTH & B.S. BUNNEY. 1989. Topographic organization of the efferent projections of the medial prefrontal cortex in the rat: an anterograde tract-tracing study using *Phaseolus vulgaris* leucoagglutinin. J. Comp. Neurol. **290:** 213–242.
98. SESACK, S.R. & V.M. PICKEL. 1992. Prefrontal cortical efferents in the rat synapse on unlabeled neuronal targets of catecholamine terminals in the nucleus accumbens septi and on dopamine neurons in the ventral tegmental area. J. Comp. Neurol. **320:** 145–160.
99. DAMASIO, A.R., D. TRANEL & H. DAMASIO. 1990. Individuals with sociopathic behavior caused by frontal damage fail to respond autonomically to social stimuli. Behav. Brain Res. **41:** 81–94.
100. DAMASIO, A.R. 1994. Descarte's Error: Emotion, Reason, and the Human Brain. Grosset/Putnam. New York. [Picador MacMillan. London (1995).]
101. NEAFSEY, E.J., R.R. TERREBERRY, K.M. HURLEY, K.G. RUIT & R.J. FRYSZTAK. 1993. Anterior cingulate cortex in rodents: connections, visceral control functions, and implications for emotion. *In* Neurobiology of Cingulate Cortex and Limbic Thalamus. B.A. Vogt & M. Gabriel, Eds.: 206–223. Birkhauser. Boston.
102. MORGAN, M.A. & J.E. LEDOUX. 1995. Differential contribution of dorsal and ventral medial prefrontal cortex to the acquisition and extinction of conditioned fear in rats. Behav. Neurosci. **109:** 681–688.
103. SULLIVAN, R.M. & A. GRATTON. 1997. Lateralization of medial prefrontal cortical modulation of autonomic and neuroendocrine stress responses in rats. Soc. Neurosci. Abstr. **23**(2): 1085.
104. VEITH, R.C., N. LEWIS, O.A. LINARES, R.F. BARNES, M.A. RASKIND, E.C. VILLACRES, M.M. MURBURG, E.A. ASHLEIGH, S. CASTILLO, E.R. PESKIND, M. PASCUALY & J.B. HALTER. 1994. Sympathetic nervous system activity in major depression. Arch. Gen. Psychiatry **51:** 411–422.
105. PAGANI, M., F. LOMBARDI, S. GUZZETTI, O. RIMOLDI, R. FURLAN, P. PIZZINELLI, G. SANDRONE, G. MALFATTO, S. DEL'ORTO, E. PICCALUGA, M. TURIEL, G. BASELLI, S. CERUTTI & A. MALLIANI. 1986. Power spectral analysis of heart rate and arterial pressure variabilities as a marker for sympathovagal interaction in man and conscious dog. Circ. Res. **59:** 178–193.
106. NEAFSEY, E.J., K.M. HURLEY-GIUS & D. ARVANITIS. 1986. The topographical organization of neurons in the rat medial frontal, insular and olfactory cortex projecting to the solitary nucleus, olfactory bulb, periaqueductal gray and superior colliculus. Brain Res. **377:** 261–270.
107. LEICHNETZ, G.R. & J. ASTRUC. 1976. The efferent projections of the medial prefrontal cortex in the squirrel monkey (*Saimiri sciureus*). Brain Res. **109:** 455–472.
108. NAUTA, W.J. & V. DOMESICK. 1984. Afferent and efferent relationships of the basal ganglia. *In* Function of the Basal Ganglia. CIBA Foundation Symposium 107: 3–29. Pitman Press. London.
109. CRINO, P.B., J.H. MORRISON & P.R. HOF. 1993. Monoaminergic innervation of cingulate cortex. *In* Neurobiology of Cingulate Cortex and Limbic Thalamus. B.A. Vogt & M. Gabriel, Eds.: 285–312. Birkhauser. Boston.
110. CHERGUI, K., G.G. NOMIKOS, J.M. MATHE, F. GONON & T.H. SVENSSON. 1993.

Tonic activation of NMDA receptors causes spontaneous burst discharge of rat midbrain dopamine neurons in vivo. Eur. J. Neurosci. **5:** 137–144.
111. MURASE, S., J. GRENHOFF, G. CHOUVET, F. GONON & T.H. SVENSSON. 1993. Prefrontal cortex regulates burst firing and transmitter release in rat mesolimbic dopamine neurons. Neurosci. Lett. **157:** 53–56.
112. ROTH, R.H. & J.D. ELSWORTH. 1995. Biochemical pharmacology of midbrain dopamine neurons. *In* Psychopharmacology: The Fourth Generation of Progress. F.E. Bloom & D.J. Kupfer, Eds.: 227–243. Raven Press. New York.
113. TABER, M.T. & H.C. FIBIGER. 1993. Electrical stimulation of the medial prefrontal cortex increases dopamine release in the striatum. Neuropsychopharmacology **9:** 271–275.
114. SCHULTZ, W. 1997. Dopamine neurons and their role in reward mechanisms. Curr. Opin. Neurobiol. **7:** 191–197.
115. FIBIGER, H.C. 1991. The dopamine hypotheses of schizophrenia and mood disorders. *In* The Mesolimbic Dopamine System: From Motivation to Action. P. Willner & J. Scheel-Kruger, Eds.: 615–638. Wiley. New York.
116. WILLNER, P. 1995. Dopaminergic mechanisms in depression and mania. *In* Psychopharmacology: The Fourth Generation of Progress. F.E. Bloom & D.J. Kupfer, Eds.: 921–932. Raven Press. New York.
117. MAYEUX, R. 1982. Depression and dementia in Parkinson's Disease. *In* Movement Disorders. C.O. Marsden & S. Fahn, Eds.: 75–95. Butterworth, London.
118. SANTAMARIA, J., E. TOLOSA & A. VALLES. 1986. Parkinson's disease with depression: a possible subgroup of idiopathic parkinsonism. Neurology **36:** 1130–1133.
119. FAWCETT, J. & V. SIOMOPOULOS. 1971. Arch. Gen. Psychiatry **25:** 247–255.
120. CARBONI, E., G.L. TANDA, R. FRAU & G. DICHIARA. 1990. J. Neurochem. **55:** 1067–1070.
121. NOMIKOS, G.G., A.P. ZIS, G. DAMSMA & H.C. FIBIGER. 1991. Neuropsychopharmacology **4:** 65–69.
122. TANDA, G., E. CARBONI, R. FRAU & G. DICHIARA. 1994. Increase of extracellular dopamine in the prefrontal cortex: a trait of drugs with antidepressant potential? Psychopharmacology **115:** 285–288.
123. D'HAENEN, H.A. & A. BOSSUYT. 1994. Biol. Psychiatry **35:** 128–132.
124. EBERT, D., H. FEISTEL, T. LOEW & A. PIRNER. 1996. Psychopharmacology **126:** 91–94.
125. SHAH, P.J., A.D. OGILVIE, G.M. GOODWIN, K.P. EBMEIER. 1997. Psychol. Med. **27:** 1247–1256.
126. PEARLSON, G.D., D.F. WONG, L.E. TUNE, *et al.* 1995. Arch. Gen. Psych. **52:** 471–477.
127. SEEMAN, P., H. GUAN & C. NIZNIK. 1989. Synapse **3:** 96–97.
128. RAUCH, S.L., M.A. JENIKE, N.M. ALPERT, *et al.* 1994. Arch. Gen. Psychiatry **51:** 62–70.
129. DREVETS, W.C., J.R. SIMPSON & M.E. RAICHLE. 1995. J. Cereb. Blood Flow Metab. **15**(1): S856.
130. SCHNEIDER, F., R.E. GUR, A. ALAVI, *et al.* 1995. Psychiatry Res. Neuroimaging **61:** 265–283.
131. GOODWIN, G.M., M.P. AUSTIN & N. DOUGALL. 1993. J. Affective Disorders **29:** 243–253.
132. ROLLS, E.T. 1995. A theory of emotion and consciousness, and its application to understanding the neural basis of emotion. *In* The Cognitive Neurosciences. M.S. Gazzaniga, Ed.: 1091–1106. MIT Press. Cambridge, MA.
133. TIMMS, R.J. 1977. J. Physiol. Lond. **266:** 98–99.
134. IVERSON, S.D. & M. MISHKIN. 1970. Perserverative interference in monkeys following selective lesions of the inferior prefrontal convexity. Exp. Brain. Res. **11:** 376–386.
135. DREVETS, W.C. & K. BOTTERON. 1997. Neuroimaging in psychiatry. *In* Adult Psychiatry. S.B. Guze, Ed.: 53–82. Mosby. St. Louis, MO.
136. RAJKOWSKA, G., L.D. SELEMON & P.S. GOLDMAN-RAKIC. 1997. Schizophr. Res. **24:** 41.

137. STARKSTEIN, S.E. & R.G. ROBINSON. 1989. Affective disorders and cerebral vascular disease. Br. J. Psychiatry **154:** 170–182.
138. YOUNG, A.B., J.B. PENNEY, S. STAROSTA-RUBINSTEIN, D.S. MARKEL, S. BERENT, B. GIORDANI, R. EHRENKAUFER, D. JEWETT & R. HICHWA. 1986. PET scan investigations of Hunnington's disease: cerebral metabolic correlates of neurological features and functional decline. Ann. Neurol. **20:** 296–303.
139. BAXTER, L.R., M.E. PHELPS, J.C. MAZZIOTTA, *et al.* 1985. Arch. Gen. Psychiatry **42:** 441–447.

On Some Clinical Implications of the Ventral Striatum and the Extended Amygdala

Investigations of Aggression

MICHAEL R. TRIMBLE[a,c] AND LUDGER TEBARTZ VAN ELST[b]

[a]*Institute of Neurology, Queen Square, London, England WC1N3BG*
[b]*Department of Psychiatry, Albert-Ludwig's University Freiburg, Germany*

ABSTRACT: In this paper, we have first reviewed the animal studies which suggest an association between the amygdala and aggressive behavior. This is followed by a review of the literature of aggression in epilepsy, emphasizing the less controversial peri-ictal aggressions, with the more controversial assertion that temporal lobe epilepsy in particular is associated with an increase in interictal aggression. We then go on to describe the results of some investigations using the MRI to examine amygdala pathology in a group of patients presenting with affective aggression in comparison with a control group. The main findings are that the patients with aggression tend to have lower IQs and more psychopathology than the control group. There is no difference in amygdala T2 and volumetric assessments between the groups, but a subgroup of patients are defined with aggression, left-sided amygdala atrophy, and a history of encephalitis.

INTRODUCTION

It is easy to underestimate the importance of neuroanatomy for a full understanding of the regulation of behavior, both in humans and in animals. It seems to be the case that in the last century psychopathologists were also neuropathologists, and vice versa. Both would be fully aware of the neuroanatomy of their time, and many startling advances were made by European neuropsychiatrists in the last century, which gave us a base for an understanding of behavior disorders and their relationship to normal or abnormal brain function.

Those not aquatinted with neuroanatomy, and indeed those who, for their own reasons, were put off this exciting subject in medical school, preferring alternative distractions, are often unfamiliar with the dynamic growth of the subject in the last few decades. One consequence of this has been a clearer understanding of the way the brain may work, but also a clarification of the way disturbed brain structure and function may be reflected in disturbed behavior.

The growth of neuroanatomical concepts has led us far away from the concept that the brain is the static geography that one sees reflected in a brain slice, either macroscopic or microscopic, to an appreciation of the complexity of functional in-

---

[c]Author to whom correspondence should be addressed: Voice: 44-171-837-3611, ext. 4273; fax: 44-171-278-8772; mtrimble@ion.ucl.ac.uk

terrelationships between various brain areas and their dynamic interplay. A number of neuroanatomical concepts, some of which are old, have been revived by a need to interpret neuroimaging studies, in particular with PET technology. A simply example is von Monakov's idea of diaschisis, subtly, but brilliant conceived at the time, a word lost to several generations of neurologists, but which has once again become part of our neuroanatomical language.

With regards to neuropsychiatry, several important advances have occurred in recent years, which help explain behavior and its disturbances. Foremost amongst these would be the development of the concept of the limbic system by authors such as MacLean,[1] which gave psychiatry a firm neurological foundation for the neuroanatomical expression of the emotions. Although still arousing controversy, and open to several obvious criticisms, the limbic system concept is still alive and well. However, it has been developed; for example, Nieuwenhuys[2] refers to the "greater limbic system," breaking down some of the conceptual and anatomical barriers which the original term may have inadvertently erected. A much greater appreciation of the various components of the limbic system in relation to behavior has developed, and in particular the work of Heimer and his colleagues on the ventral striatum and the extended amygdala stand out as milestones for clinical neuropsychiatrists trying to explain behavioral syndromes they see in patients with various disorders of brain structure and function.

AGGRESSION

From the 1939 observations of Kluver and Bucy[3] it seemed clear that the medial temporal lobes, and the limbic system were somehow related to controlling mood and to the expression of aggression. Their clinical syndrome, central to which was loss of fear and aggressive responses, has been seen in the clinical setting, and has formed the basis for attempts to further disentangle the neuroanatomical substrates for aggressive behaviors.

Later work seems to have substantiated, in animal models at least, a relationship of the amygdala to aggression, with a reciprocal link to the hypothalamus and the frontal cortex. Following up on the Kluver-Bucy experiments, Schreiner and Kling,[4] tamed various aggressive feline species with bilateral amygdala lesions, an effect which could be abolished with additional lesions in the ventro-lateral hypothalamus.

Aggression can be provoked by stimulation of the amygdala, hypothalamus and the area around the fornix in the diencephalon, and the hypothalamic-elicited aggression can be inhibited by the stimulation of the ipsilateral frontal cortex (Siegel et al.[5]). Animal experiments by both Delgado[6] and Rosvold et al.,[7] further demonstrated a close link between stimulation or lesions of the amygdala and either aggressive behavior or dominance within a social hierarchy.

More recently, the studies of Adamec[8] using limbic kindling revealed that in cats behavioral changes, particularly aggressiveness or defensiveness, can be kindled and that "limbic permeability," namely the degree and facility of seizure propagation from limbic structures to hypothalamic areas could be related to these behavior changes.

AGGRESSION AND EPILEPSY

Thus, although not wishing to emphasize a purely modular, localizationalist view of cerebral function, the animal literature suggested close links between alteration of limbic system, in particular amygdala and hypothalamic function, and the modulation of aggression. Clearly, many other factors are involved. The expression of any particular behavior must be seen from a connectivist view point, and the role of neurotransmitters in regulating activity in the system are clearly relevant.

The literature of various transmitters potentially involved in aggressive behavior is confusing, and appears at first sight to be species dependent. Generally however, depletion of serotonin and GABA or increasing cholinergic or catcholaminergic drive, facilitate aggressive behavior. Then there is the role of hormones, testosterone in particular being associated with an increased tendency to aggressive displays.[9]

The amygdala, and by implication therefore the extended amygdala, may well be nodal points in circuits which regulate expressive behaviors such as aggression. Since the amygdala is frequently damaged in patients with epilepsy, who display in clinical practice, usually but not always, complex partial seizures occasionally with specific aurae, it may be expected that patients with epilepsy may display more aggression than patients who do not have epilepsy, but have other forms of neurological disease that do not affect these areas of the brain. Further, it might be thought that patients with temporal lobe epilepsy in particular would display more aggression than those with other forms of epilepsy.

This however is an area of considerable clinical controversy. In part this reflects the difficulty of actually measuring aggression in the human setting (and also in the animal setting) where so many different forms of aggression, for example, predatory aggression, etc., have been described. Further it reflects on the difficult of monitoring aggressive behavior in societies where the borderline between the expression of aggression as an accepted human behavior and one that is pathological shifts not only with the culture, but also with the historical time point, and also with the microenvironment of any individual.

Clinicians for well over a hundred and fifty years, writing on the subject of the psychiatry of epilepsy, have identified the clinical fact that patients with epilepsy could have outbursts of aggressive behavior, sometimes, but not always associated with a seizure. Some authors (Samt) considered some behaviors which had an acute onset, were expressed in aggressive, violent and extravagant behavior, but which then appeared to have an acute end, could be classified as an epileptic syndrome, simply on account of the clinical pattern, irrespective of whether or not they were ictally driven. Further, many descriptions were given in which patients with recognized epileptic seizures would have such extravagant behavioral outbursts, which sometimes seemed to substitute for the epileptic seizures themselves.[10]

Behavioral syndromes of epilepsy are usually subdivided into two major categories, those which are peri-ictal, and those which are inter-ictal. Peri-ictal violence is less controversial. Any physician who treats patients with difficult-to-control epilepsy will have seen patients who develop a post-ictal confusion, and during that confusion, perhaps because attempts are made improperly to restrain them, may become aggressive. However, the aggression is usually part of a delirium, the patient is confused, and the aggression is poorly directed. Less well described, but of more interest, are post-ictal aggressions, that form part of a post-ictal psychosis. These commonly occur following a cluster of seizures, when there then occurs the so-called lucid interval, in which the patient appears to be in normal consciousness and not emotionally disturbed, and then perhaps 24 to 48 hours later an acute episode of paranoia with release of aggression erupts. The aggression can be directed towards others or the self, but because the patient is in relatively clear consciousness, the outcome can be very dangerous. These episodes were probably what was referred to as epileptic furore in the 19*th* century.

Ictal violence, namely an episode of aggression directly related to the ictus, is rare but has been clearly described.[11] One problem is that the episode has to be monitored using video telemetry. Video telemetry requires the patient to be in a well-controlled, non-spontaneous environment, and the patient in such a setting is not only less likely to display such behaviors, but also is less likely to have environmental triggers for the release of the behavior.

There is no clear consensus as to the anatomical sites of relevance for the release of these aggressive behaviors, although they most commonly occur in patients who have complex partial seizures, which are difficult to treat, and the latter clinically implies a temporal lobe localization-related focal epilepsy.

Kligman and Goldberg[12] examined studies of inter-ictal aggression. They reviewed the results of eight controlled studies where a relationship between aggression and epilepsy had been investigated, and noted only two that supported the link.

Hermann and Whitman[13] noted the high risk factors for aggression in epilepsy, which included organic cerebral disease, low socio-economic status, and up bringing in a poor environment.

The area of aggression and epilepsy was reviewed thoroughly by Fenwick[14] who noted the evidence from intracranial implanted electrode studies suggesting that the amygdala was involved in the mediation of aggression in man, and further commented that amygdalectomy improves aggressive behavior in the few series where this operation has been tried. In addition, patients with temporal lobe epilepsy who undergo a temporal lobectomy show a reduction of seizures, but also often show an improvement in aggressive behavior. Fenwick's conclusion was that a relationship between seizure discharges and aggressive behavior had been shown, but he went on to suggest that the relationship was more between poor impulse control and brain damage, than anything necessarily to do with the seizure process itself or where in the brain that might be localized.

An additional related topic which should be just noted is that of the episodic dyscontrol syndrome.[14,15] This condition presents as sudden episodes of spontaneously released violence, often in a setting of minimal provocation, which tends to be short lived. The episodes may be provoked by small amounts of alcohol, and after the events patients usually feel considerable remorse. Generally, the condition is associated with non-specific variables which can also be seen in epilepsy, for example evidence of cerebral damage, low socio-economic status, and a disturbed upbringing. Evidence of minimal neurological damage, with soft neurological signs and abnormal EEGs are often found, although there is no evidence that these episodes have the same pathophysiology as epileptic seizures. Their paroxysmal nature has led to the comparison with epilepsy, a carryover from the 19*th* century literature already noted.

However links between episodic dyscontrol, temporal lobe abnormalities, and epilepsy have been readily made.[15] The phenomenological criteria of episodic dyscontrol have been restated by the American Psychiatric Association's DSM IV (1994)[16] as those of Intermittent Explosive Disorder.

AN INVESTIGATION OF THE ROLE OF THE AMYGDALA IN AGGRESSION IN PATIENTS WITH TEMPORAL LOBE EPILEPSY

In view of the potential relationship between the amygdala and aggression in animal models, and the possible associations with epilepsy, particularly temporal lobe epilepsy, we have undertaken an MRI assessment of patients with epilepsy who also display aggressive behavior. Patients with epilepsy and what we had referred to as intermittent affective aggression were the study group. All patients had complex partial seizures and temporal lobe epilepsy, the diagnoses being confirmed by the semiology of the attacks, EEG investigations, and MRI studies.

The aggressive patients ($N = 25$) fulfilled DSM IV criteria for intermittent explosive disorder (except for the fact that they all had an organic brain disease), and the results were compared to 25 control patients who did not appear to have problems with aggression.

Additional information on patients psychopathology was collected including depressive symptoms using the Beck Depression Inventory, and anxiety symptoms using the State–Trait Anxiety Inventory.

Aggression was assessed by carers by asking them to fill out the Social Dysfunction and Aggression Scale, an instrument that had been developed and validated by the European Rating Aggression Group (1992).[17] It includes subscales for different kinds of aggressive behavior.

MRI scans were obtained, and volumetric measurements were undertaken of the amygdala (for full details see Tebartz Van Elst, Worman, Lemeux, and Trimble—in preparation). Amygdala volumes were corrected for total brain size, and interrater reliability assessed and shown to be satisfactory.

We defined a subgroup of patients who were said to have amygdala atrophy, namely a volume smaller than three standard deviations below the average amygdala volume of the control group.

In addition to amygdala volumes, amygdala T2 mapping was carried out (again for details see Tebartz Van Elst *et al.*).

In this investigation we found significantly less right-sided focal EEG and MRI abnormalities, and more bilateral EEG changes in patients in the aggressive group. We found no differences between the groups with regards to amygdala T2 relaxation time or amygdala volumes, although in the aggressive group, 20% showed amygdala atrophy, which was a significant finding. In all cases it was the dominant hemisphere that was affected, although in two patients it was bilateral.

When patients with amygdala atrophy were compared to those that did not have such atrophy, the incidence of encephalitis was increased in the atrophy group.

Finally, patients with aggressive behavior showed significantly lower verbal and performance IQs, and higher rating scores for both depression and state and trait anxiety.

CONCLUSIONS

The suggestion that the amygdala, and by implication the extended amygdala, plays some role in the neuronal circuitry for the expression of aggressive behavior has a long and respectable history. The suggestion that patients with epilepsy, particularly temporal lobe epilepsy, may be more susceptible to the development of these behaviors is considerably more controversial, and appropriate epidemiological studies have not been carried out to allow any conclusions to be reached. However, in clinical practice it is a fact that patients with neurological disease often demonstrate the release of aggression.

We have studied aggressive behavior in a group of patients with temporal lobe epilepsy, specifically examining the role of the amygdala. We have not reliably demonstrated an association between aggression and either amygdala volumes or T2 relaxation times; it may well be in the future neuroimaging studies will allow alternative variables to be measured, that may provide a different perspective on underlying pathological processes.

In our study, patients with aggressive behavior tended to show lower IQs, and higher psychopathology and also suggestions of more defuse, predominantly bilateral neuropathology. However, the dominant hemisphere seems more likely to be involved, and we have identified a sub-group of patients who might suffer from amygdala atrophy, secondary to encephalitis, who may be particularly susceptible to displaying aggressive behavior. There may well be links therefore between early encephalitis (as opposed to mesial temporal sclerosis, which we did not find associated with aggressive behavior), and more diffuse neuropathology. Further, such patients may be more susceptible to affective disorders, increasing the propensity to aggressive outbursts.

We would not wish to conclude that the amygdala is some modular brain area where aggression is somehow represented. However, the investigations reviewed above, and our data do suggest that in some patients at least, the amygdala should be viewed as part of an important cerebral circuitry, often damaged in patients with epilepsy, that is involved in the mediation of aggressive behavior. Other critical sites, such as the periaquaductal grey matter, the hypothalamus, and indeed the frontal lobes have not been evaluated in our study, which has concerned itself with the amygdala. Neither can we comment on any nuclear subdivisions of the amygdala, which of course may be of relevance. However, we believe that further neuropsychiatric investigations of the neurological underpinning of aggressive behavior, based on currently developed and developing neuroanatomical principles, are important areas of future research.

REFERENCES

1. MacLean, P.D. 1989. The Triune Brain in Evolution. Plenum Press. New York.
2. Nieuwenhuys, R. 1996. The greater limibic system, the emotional motor system and the brain. *In* The Emotional Motor System. R. Holstege Bandler & C.B. Saper, Eds.: 551–582. Elsevier. Amsterdam.
3. Kluver, H. & B.C. Bucy. 1939. Preliminary analysis of functions of the temporal lobe in monkeys. Arch. Neurol. Psychol. **42:** 979–1000.
4. Schreiner, L. & A. Kling. 1956. Rhinencephalon and behaviour. Am. J. Psychiatry **184:** 486–490.

5. SIEGEL, A., H. EDINGER & M. DOTTO. 1975. Effects of electrical stimulation of the lateral aspects of the prefrontal cortex upon attack behaviour. Brain **93:** 473–484.
6. DELGADO, J.M.R. 1966. Aggressive behaviour evoked by radiostimulation in monkey colonies. Am. Zool. **6:** 669–681.
7. ROSVOLD, A.G., A.F. MIRSKY & K.H. PRIBRAM. 1954. Influence of amygdalectomy on social behaviour in monkeys. J. Comp. Physiol. Psychol. **47:** 173–180.
8. ADAMEC, R.E. & C. STARK-ADAMEC. 1983. Limbic kindling and animal behaviour. Biol. Psychiatry **18:** 269–293.
9. TRIMBLE, M.R. 1996. Biological Psychiatry, 2nd edit. J. Wiley & Sons. Chichester, England.
10. TRIMBLE, M.R. & B. SCHMITZ, Eds. 1998. Forced Normalisation and Alternative Psychoses of Epilepsy. Wright Biomedical Publications. Petersfield, England.
11. DELGADO-ESCUETA, A., R.H. MATTSON, L. KING, *et al.* 1981. The nature of aggression during epileptic seizures. N. Engl. J. Med. **305:** 711–716.
12. KLIGMAN, D. & D.A. GOLDBERG. 1975. Temporal lobe epilepsy and aggression. J. Nerv. Ment. Dis. **160:** 324–341.
13. HERMANN, B.P. & S. WHITMAN. 1984. Behavioural and personality correlates of epilepsy: a review, methodological critique and conceptual model. Psychol. Bull. **95:** 451–492.
14. FENWICK, P. 1986. Aggression and epilepsy. *In* Aspects of Epilepsy in Psychiatry. M.R. Trimble & T. Bolwig, Eds.: 31–60. J. Wiley & Sons. Chichester, England.
15. MONROE, R. 1970. Episodic Behaviour Disorders. Harvard University Press. Cambridge, MA
16. AMERICAN PSYCHIATRIC ASSOCIATION. 1994. Diagnostic and Statistical Manual of Mental Disorders, IVth edit. APA Press. Washington, D.C.
17. EUROPEAN RATING AGGRESSION GROUP. 1992. Social dysfunction and aggression scale (SDAS-21) in generalised aggression and in aggressive attacks: a validity and reliability study. Int. J. Meth. Psych. Res. **2:** 15–29.

The Interstitial Nucleus of the Posterior Limb of the Anterior Commissure: A Novel Layer of the Central Division of Extended Amygdala

GEORGE F. ALHEID,[a,d] SARA J. SHAMMAH-LAGNADO,[b] AND CARLOS A. BELTRAMINO[c]

[a]*Department of Physiology and Institute for Neuroscience, Northwestern University Medical Center, Chicago, Illinois 60611, USA*

[b]*Department of Physiology and Biophysics, Institute of Biomedical Sciences, University of São Paulo, São Paulo 05508-900, Brazil*

[c]*Department of Psychology, University of Córdoba and Istituto de Investigación Médica, Córdoba, Argentina*

The topic of this volume encompasses two macrostructures within basal forebrain, the *ventral striatopallidal system*[1–4] and the *"extended amygdala."*[4–7] The ventral striatum, encompassing primarily the olfactory tubercle and nucleus accumbens and their main target, the ventral subcommissural extension of the pallidum, is now recognized by virtually every investigator whose work touches on basal forebrain. The ventral pallidum occupies a zone previously described as the anterior (subcommissural) substantia innominata, while the caudal sublenticular portion of the substantia innominata is occupied by sublenticular portions of the extended amygdala. For this reason, we have argued[4,8] that the term "substantia innominata" should be abandoned in favor of specific structural names that reflect the actual functional anatomical associations of these forebrain areas.

THE VENTRAL STRIATOPALLIDAL SYSTEM

The theory of the ventral striatopallidal system has allowed us to plan investigations of the ventral forebrain in comparison with the circuits in the dorsal striatum (i.e., in caudate and putamen). For example, the ventral striatopallidal system includes a prominent output reaching the frontal/cingulate cortex transsynaptically via the mediodorsal thalamus.[2,9–11] This appears to be analogous to the dorsal striatum's transpallidal route via the ventral anterior and ventral lateral thalamus to premotor cortex.[1,2]

ACCUMBENS CORE AND SHELL

In comparing the ventral striatum with its dorsal counterpart, it became clear that the accumbens appears to have at least two major subdivisions, i.e., a "core and

---

[d]Corresponding author: George F. Alheid Ph.D., Department of Physiology and Institute for Neuroscience, Morton, Rm 5-654, Northwestern University, 303 E. Chicago Ave., Chicago, Illinois 60611-3008. Voice: 312-503-0188; fax: 312-503-5101; gfa@nwu.edu

shell."[12] This dual nature of the accumbens was initially suggested by the observation that dense cholecystokinin terminals appeared in the accumbens shell but were not characteristically found in the core or in the dorsally adjacent territories of the striatum.[12,13] The significance of this histochemical variation was subsequently reinforced by the demonstration that "nonstriatal" projections from the accumbens to lateral hypothalamus, amygdala, and midbrain[14] originate preferentially from the accumbens shell,[15,16] while connections originating in the core of the accumbens follow a more typical striatal pattern. The functional significance of this dichotomy has been supported by a growing number of observations which have shown that the shell area of the accumbens seems to be most relevant to behaviors such as rewarding aspects of drugs of abuse[17,18] and modulation of ingestion.[19–21] The shell rather than the core also seems to be a possible site of action for antipsychotic drugs, including typical and atypical neuroleptics,[22–25] and drugs used in treating affective disorders.[26]

CENTRAL AND MEDIAL EXTENDED AMYGDALA

At the same time that the dichotomy of the accumbens core and shell was realized, we also introduced a second anatomical model[5] to describe the anatomical relations in the posterior sublenticular "substantia innominata." This model argued for the continuity of the centromedial amygdala with the bed nucleus of the stria terminalis, suggested by their similar morphology and connections. The similarity between these two forebrain areas is shared by cells accompanying the stria terminalis,[27] as originally observed by Johnston,[28] and by neurons traversing the sublenticular gray areas caudal to the ventral pallidum.[5,29–31] This continuum consists of at least two major columns,[5,32,33] related to the the central or medial amygdaloid nucleus, respectively. We therefore termed these columns, along with their allied nuclei in the amygdala and bed nucleus of the stria terminalis, the central and medial divisions of amygdala's extension into the forebrain,[5] or the central or medial "extended amygdala"[4,7] (for schematic, see FIG. 1). The remaining nuclei of the classically defined amygdala are for the time being grouped as the "cortical-like nuclei."[7,34]

As might be predicted from its constituent nuclei, the medial extended amygdala is generally related to the medial hypothalamus and seems to be most relevant in considering functions related to social behaviors (sex and parental behaviors) and to the neuroendocrine component of these behaviors. The central division of extended amygdala is more closely related to the lateral hypothalamus and to the autonomic and affective motor systems in the brainstem. Since the various cortical-like nuclei of the amygdala (basolateral, lateral, and superficial amygdaloid nuclei) project to the medial and central divisions of extended amygdala, and considering the well established role of the amygdala in emotional behavior, it is natural to assume that the extended amygdala has a significant role to play in the expression of these emotions. Extended amygdala may be able to influence behavior either by its projections directly to the hypothalamus and brainstem, or via afferents that appear to terminate on dopamine cells in substantia nigra.[35] This suggests that extended amygdala can also function as a target of psychotherapeutic drugs, or alternatively as a target for

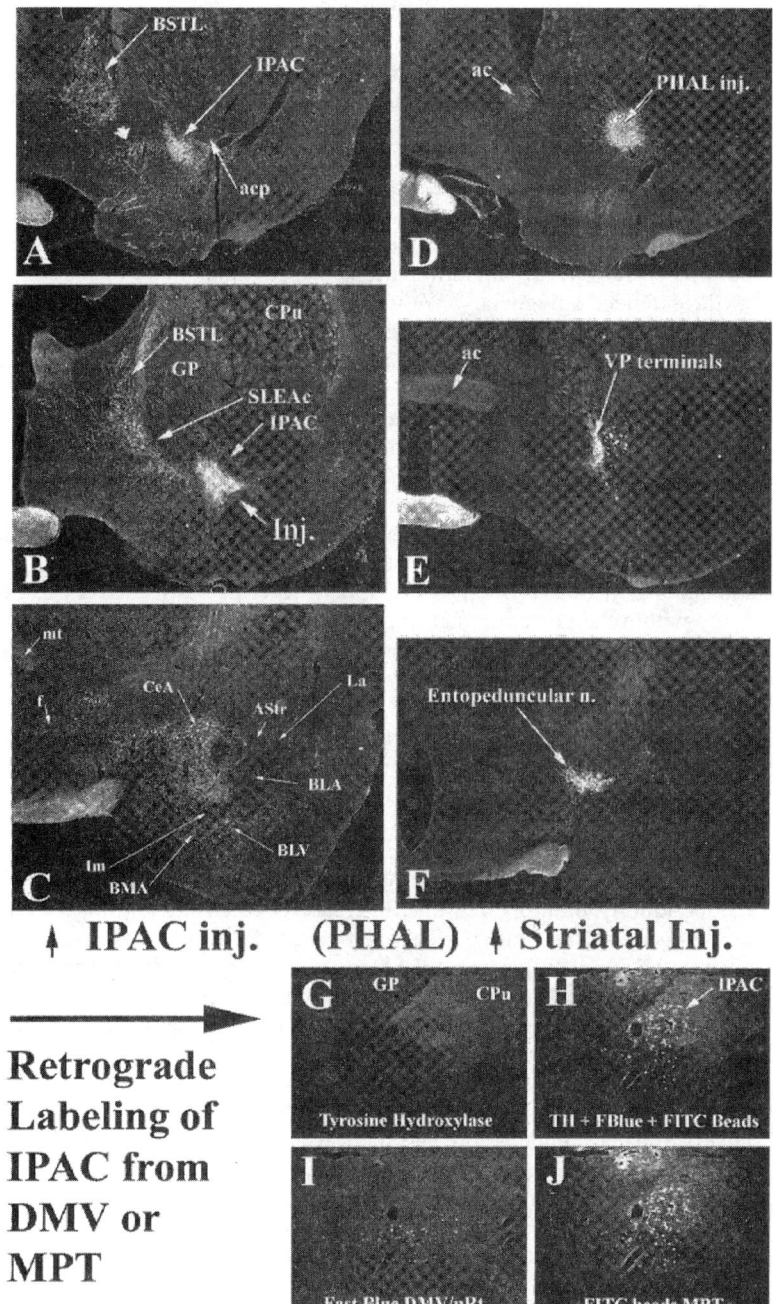

densely within the confines of the central division of extended amygdala, including the lateral bed nucleus of the stria terminalis, central amygdaloid nucleus, and interconnecting sublenticular columns of neurons that we have termed the central division of the sublenticular extended amygdala (FIG. 2). Moreover, we found that the long projections of IPAC in many ways resemble the projections of the central amygdaloid nucleus with terminations in mid-level and posterior lateral hypothalamus, the mesopontine reticular formation and retrorubral area, parabrachial nucleus, vagal-solitary nuclear complex, and the parvocellular reticular formation. A complementary picture is presented by the afferents to IPAC with particularly the medial portion of this corridor receiving terminations that resemble those of the central division of the extended amygdala.[56] We would, therefore, argue that IPAC, and particularly its medial part, can be considered the outermost "dopamine-rich layer" of the central division of extended amygdala.

This realization is important, since it reinforces both the growing perception of the role played by the extended amygdala in central nervous system (CNS) pharmacology and therapeutics and the understanding of the impact of dopamine agonists and antagonists in behaviors ranging from schizophrenia to drug addiction. Within the context of the ventral striatum, it suggests that a column of cells related to the amygdala traverses the caudal accumbens, and predicts that the rostral-to-caudal dimension in accumbens should be functionally differentiated. While differences along this dimension are less often reported, they nevertheless seem to exist. For example, only within the posterior shell region can the dopamine-evoked increase in dye coupling between accumbens neurons be blocked by clozapine,[23] an effect postulated to be relevant to the drug's antipsychotic efficacy. In a similar vein, when injected in the posterior accumbens, CCK-8 preferentially inhibits exploratory activity through a decrease in dopamine turnover that is dependent on functioning D2 receptors.[57] Finally, in rats receiving electroconvulsive shock, dopamine receptor (D1 and D2) messenger RNA is acutely increased, but only in the posterior part of nucleus accumbens.[58] IPAC may be implicated as a relevant site of neuroleptic action by the fact that subcutaneous clozapine has selective effects on IPAC, releasing γ-aminobutyric acid (GABA, as measured by microdialysis), an effect not seen after subcutaneous haloperidol. Both drugs, however, increase GABA release from dorsolateral striatum.[59] In general, the similarity between the caudal accumbens shell and IPAC is reflected in the fact that they react the same when subjected to experimental manipulations that include IPAC as a dependent variable. As a particular example, chronic cocaine administration in the rat preferentially increases neurotensin mRNA not only in the shell of the accumbens, but also in IPAC.[60]

In summary, the model of the ventral striatum has provided a productive perspective for investigation of the functions of the basal forebrain. This was amplified by the discovery of the accumbens core and shell, which provided anatomically distinct compartments which predictably supported distinct behavioral functions. The extended amygdala provides a highly differentiated forebrain structure with many layered compartments as a context for interpreting novel functional anatomical experiments in basal forebrain. IPAC as a novel component of the central division of extended amygdala, lends itself to investigations of the impact of dopamine on the function of this division of the amygdala, and provides a rationale for interpreting data that are already accumulating with respect to rostro-caudal distinctions in accumbens functions.

ACKNOWLEDGMENTS

This work was supported by Grants from the U.S. Public Health Service (NS-17743), the Brazilian Foundation FAPESP (94/0387-0 and 96/7794-5), and Conicet, Argentina.

REFERENCES

1. HEIMER, L. & R.D. WILSON. 1975. The subcortical projections of allocortex: similarities in the neuronal associations of the hippocampus, the piriform cortex and the neocortex. *In* Golgi Centennial Symposium Proceedings. M. Santini, Ed.: 173–193. Raven Press. New York.
2. HEIMER, L. 1978. The olfactory cortex and the ventral striatum [review, 194 refs.]. *In* Limbic Mechanisms. K.E. Livingston & O. Hornykiewicz, Eds.: 95–187. Plenum Press. New York, NY.
3. HEIMER, L., G.F. ALHEID & L. ZÁBORSZKY. 1985. The basal ganglia. *In* The Rat Nervous System. G. Paxinos, Ed.: 37–74. Academic Press. Sydney.
4. ALHEID, G.F. & L. HEIMER. 1988. New perspectives in basal forebrain organization of special relevance for neuropsychiatric disorders: the striatopallidal, amygdaloid, and corticopetal components of substantia innominata [review, 334 refs.]. Neuroscience **27:** 1–39.
5. DE OLMOS, J.S., G.F. ALHEID & C.A. BELTRAMINO. 1985. Amygdala. *In* The Rat Nervous System. G. Paxinos, Ed.: 223–334. Academic Press. Sydney.
6. DE OLMOS, J.S. 1990. Amygdala. *In* The Human Nervous System. G. Paxinos, Ed. 583–710. Academic Press, Inc. San Diego, CA.
7. ALHEID, G.F., J.S. DE OLMOS & C.A. BELTRAMINO. 1995. Amygdala and extended amygdala. *In* The Rat Nervous System, 2nd edit. G. Paxinos, Ed.: 495–578. Academic Press, Inc., San Diego.
8. HEIMER, L., R.E. HARLAN, G.F. ALHEID, M.M. GARCIA & J. DE OLMOS. 1997. Substantia innominata: a notion which impedes clinical-anatomical correlations in neuropsychiatric disorders [review, 562 refs.]. Neuroscience **76:** 957–1006.
9. PRICE, J.L. & B.M. SLOTNICK. 1983. Dual olfactory representation in the rat thalamus: an anatomical and electrophysiological study. J.Comp.Neurol. **215:** 63–77.
10. YOUNG, W.S., G.F. ALHEID & L. HEIMER. 1984. The ventral pallidal projection to the mediodorsal thalamus: a study with fluorescent retrograde tracers and immunohistofluorescence. J. Neurosci. **4:** 1626–1638.
11. GROENEWEGEN, H.J. 1988. Organization of the afferent connections of the mediodorsal thalamic nucleus in the rat, related to the mediodorsal-prefrontal topography. Neuroscience **24:** 379–431.
12. ZÁBORSZKY, L., G.F. ALHEID, M.C. BEINFELD, L.E. EIDEN, L. HEIMER & M. PALKOVITS. 1985. Cholecystokinin innervation of the ventral striatum: a morphological and radioimmunological study. Neuroscience **14:** 427–453.
13. FALLON, J.H., R. HICKS & S.E. LOUGHLIN. 1983. The origin of cholecystokinin terminals in the basal forebrain of the rat: evidence from immunofluorescence and retrograde tracing. Neurosci. Lett. **37:** 29–35.
14. NAUTA, W.J.H., G.P. SMITH, R.L.M. FAULL & V.B. DOMESICK. 1978. Efferent connections and nigral afferents of the nucleus accumbens septi in the rat. Neuroscience **3:** 385–401.
15. ZAHM, D.S. & L. HEIMER. 1990. Two transpallidal pathways originating in the rat nucleus accumbens. J. Comp. Neurol. **302:** 437–446.
16. HEIMER, L., D.S. ZAHM, L. CHURCHILL, P.W. KALIVAS & C. WOHLTMANN. 1991. Specificity in the projection patterns of accumbal core and shell in the rat. Neuroscience **41:** 89–125.
17. KOOB, G.F. & E.J. NESTLER. 1997. The neurobiology of drug addiction [review]. J. Neuropsychiatry Clin. Neurosci. **9:** 482–497.

18. KOOB, G.F. & M. LEMOAL. 1997. Drug abuse: hedonic homeostatic dysregulation. Science **278:** 52–58.
19. MALDONADO-IRIZARRY, C.S., C.J. SWANSON & A.E. KELLEY. 1995. Glutamate receptors in the nucleus accumbens shell control feeding behavior via the lateral hypothalamus. J. Neurosci. **15:** 6779–6788.
20. STRATFORD, T.R. & A.E. KELLEY. 1997. GABA in the nucleus accumbens shell participates in the central regulation of feeding behavior. J. Neurosci. **17:** 4434–4440.
21. STRATFORD, T.R., M.R. HOLAHAN & A.E. KELLEY. 1997. Injections of nociceptin into nucleus accumbens shell or ventromedial hypothalamic nucleus increase food intake. Neuroreport **8:** 423–426.
22. DEUTCH, A.Y., D.A. LEWIS, R.E. WHITEHEAD, J.D. ELSWORTH, M.J. IADAROLA, D.E.J. REDMOND & R.H. ROTH. 1996. Effects of D2 dopamine receptor antagonists on Fos protein expression in the striatal complex & entorhinal cortex of the nonhuman primate. Synapse **23:** 182–191.
23. O'DONNELL, P. & A.A. GRACE. 1993. Dopaminergic modulation of dye coupling between neurons in the core and shell regions of the nucleus accumbens. J. Neurosci. **13:** 3456–3471.
24. O'DONNELL, P. & A.A. GRACE. 1995. Different effects of subchronic clozapine and haloperidol on dye coupling between neurons in the rat striatal complex. Neuroscience **66:** 763–767.
25. ONN, S.P. & A.A. GRACE. 1995. Repeated treatment with haloperidol and clozapine exerts differential effects on dye coupling between neurons in subregions of striatum and nucleus accumbens. J. Neurosci. **15:** 7024–7036.
26. ZACHRISSON, O., A.A. MATHE, C. STENFORS & N. LINDEFORS. 1995. Region-specific effects of chronic lithium administration on neuropeptide Y and somatostatin mRNA expression in the rat brain. Neurosci. Lett. **194:** 89–92.
27. ALHEID, G.F., C.A. BELTRAMINO, J.S. DE OLMOS, M.S. FORBES, D.J. SWANSON & L. HEIMER. 1998. The neuronal organization of the supracapsular part of the stria terminalis in the rat: the dorsal component of extended amygdala. Neuroscience **84:** 967–996.
28. JOHNSTON, J.B. 1923. Further contribution to the study of the evolution of the forebrain. J. Comp. Neurol. **35:** 337–481.
29. DE OLMOS, J.S. 1969. A cupric-silver method for impregnation of terminal axon degeneration and its further use in staining granular argyrophilic neurons. Brain Behav. Evol. **2:** 213–237.
30. DE OLMOS, J.S. 1972. The amygdaloid projection field in the rat as studied with the cupric silver method. *In* The Neurobiology of the Amygdala. B.E. Eleftheriou, Ed.: 145–204. Plenum Press. New York.
31. SCHWABER, J.S., B.S. KAPP, G.A. HIGGINS & P.R. RAPP. 1982. Amygdaloid and basal forebrain direct connections with the nucleus of the solitary tract and the dorsal motor nucleus. J. Neurosci. **2:** 1424–1438.
32. GROVE, E.A. 1988. Neural associations of the substantia innominata in the rat: afferent connections. J. Comp. Neurol. **277:** 315–346.
33. GROVE, E.A. 1988. Efferent connections of the substantia innominata in the rat. J. Comp. Neurol. **277:** 347–364.
34. MCDONALD, A.J. 1992. Cell types and intrinsic connections of the amygdala. *In* The Amygdala: Neurobiological Aspects of Emotion, Memory, and Mental Dysfunction. J.P. Aggleton, Ed.: 67–96. Wiley-Liss, Inc. New York.
35. HABER, S.N. & J.L. FUDGE. 1997. The primate substantia nigra and VTA: integrative circuitry and function [review, 159 refs.]. Crit. Rev. Neurobiol. **11:** 323–342.
36. ALHEID, G.F. & L. HEIMER. 1987. The "extended amygdala" as a receptor area for psychotherapeutic drugs. Behav. Brain Sci. **10:** 208–208.
37. HEIMER, L., J. DE OLMOS, G.F. ALHEID & L. ZABORSZKY. 1991. "Perestroika" in the basal forebrain: opening the border between neurology and psychiatry [review, 404 refs.]. Prog. Brain Res. **87:** 109–165.
38. SHIBATA, K., D.M. HAVERSTICK & M.J. BANNON. 1990. Tachykinin gene expression in rat limbic nuclei: modulation by dopamine antagonists. J. Pharmacol. Exp. Ther. **255:** 388–392.

39. KROESEN, S., J. MARKSTEINER, S.K. MAHATA, M. MAHATA, R. FISCHER-COLBRIE, A. SARIA, I. KAPELLER & H. WINKLER. 1995. Effects of haloperidol, clozapine and citalopram on messenger RNA levels of chromogranins A and B and secretogranin II in various regions of rat brain. Neuroscience **69:** 881–891.
40. REBEC, G.V., K.D. ALLOWAY & T.R. BASHORE. 1981. Differential action for classical and atypical antipsychotic drugs on spontaneous neuronal acitvity in the amygdaloid complex. Pharmacol. Biochem. Behav. **14:** 49–56.
41. WANG, Z. & G.V. REBEC. 1996. Amygdaloid neurons respond to clozapine rather than haloperidol in behaving rats pretreated with intra-amygdaloid amphetamine. Brain Res. **711:** 64–72.
42. O'DONNELL, P., A. LAVIN, L.W. ENQUIST, A.A. GRACE & J.P. CARD. 1997. Interconnected parallel circuits between rat nucleus accumbens and thalamus revealed by retrograde transynaptic transport of pseudorabies virus. J. Neurosci. **17:** 2143–2167.
43. LIND, R.W., L.W. SWANSON & D. GANTEN. 1985. Organization of angiotensin II immunoreactive cells and fibers in the rat central nervous system. Neuroendocrinology **40:** 2–24.
44. SKOFITSCH, G. & D.M. JACOBOWITZ. 1985. Immunohistochemical mapping of galanin-like neurons in the rat central nervous system. Peptides **6:** 509–546.
45. SKOFITSCH, G. & D.M. JACOBOWITZ. 1985. Calcitonin gene-related peptide: detailed immunohistochemical distribution in the central nervous system. Peptides **6:** 721–745.
46. SEXTON, P.M., J.S. MCKENZIE, R.T. MASON, J.M. MOSELEY, T.J. MARTIN & F.A.O. MENDELSOHN. 1986. Localization of binding sites for calcitonin gene-related peptide in rat brain by *in vitro* autoradiography. Neuroscience **19:** 1235–1245.
47. SEXTON, P.M., G. PAXINOS, M.A. KENNEY, P.J. WOOKEY & K. BEAUMONT. 1994. *In vitro* autoradiographic localization of amylin binding sites in rat brain. Neuroscience **62:** 553–567.
48. HILTON, J.M., S.Y. CHAI & P.M. SEXTON. 1995. *In vitro* autoradiographic localization of the calcitonin receptor isoforms, C1a and C1b, in rat brain. Neuroscience **69:** 1223–1237.
49. CHRISTOPOULOS, G., G. PAXINOS, X.F. HUANG, K. BEAUMONT, A.W. TOGA & P.M. SEXTON. 1995. Comparative distribution of receptors for amylin and the related peptides calcitonin gene related peptide and calcitonin in rat and monkey brain. Can. J. Physiol. Pharmacol. **73:** 1037–1041.
50. MELANDER, T., C. KÖHLER, S. NILSSON, G. FISONE, T. BARTFAI & T. HÖKFELT. 1992. ^{125}I-Galanin binding sites in the rat central nervous system. *In* Handbook of Chemical Neuroanatomy. Vol. 11. Neuropeptide Receptors in the CNS. A. Björklund, T. Hökfelt & M.J. Kuhar, Eds.: 187–221. Elsevier. Amsterdam.
51. TRIBOLLET, E. 1992. Vasopressin and oxytocin receptors in the rat brain. *In* Handbook of Chemical Neuroanatomy. Vol. 11. Neuropeptide Receptors in the CNS. A. Björklund, T. Hökfelt & M.J. Kuhar, Eds.: 289–320. Elsevier. Amsterdam.
52. VEINANTE, P. & M.J. FREUND-MERCIER. 1997. Distribution of oxytocin- and vasopressin-binding sites in the rat extended amygdala: a histoautoradiographic study. J. Comp. Neurol. **383:** 305–325.
53. ALHEID, G.F., C.A. BELTRAMINO, A. BRAUN, R.R. MISELIS, C. FRANÇOIS & J.S. DE OLMOS. 1994. Transition areas of the striatopallidal system with the extended amygdala in the rat and primate: observations from histochemistry and experiments with mono- and transsynaptic tracer. *In* The Basal Ganglia IV. Vol. 41. New Ideas and Data on Structure and Function. G. Percheron, J.S. McKenzie & J. Feger, Eds.: 95–107. Plenum Press. New York.
54. ALHEID, G.F., S.J. SHAMMAH-LAGNADO, C.A. BELTRAMINO, M. YANG, R.R. MISELIS, J.S. DE OLMOS & L. HEIMER. 1996. Efferent projections of the "interstitial nucleus of the posterior limb of the anterior commissure." PHA-L transport from a dopamine-rich lateral wing of the extended amygdala. Soc. Neurosci. Abstr. **22:** 806.13.
55. BROCKHAUS, H. 1942. Zur feineren Anatomie des Septum und des Striatum. J. Psychol. Neurol. **51:** 1–56.

56. SHAMMAH-LAGNADO, S.J., G.F. ALHEID & L. HEIMER. 1999. Afferent connections of the interstitial nucleus of the posterior limb of the anterior commissure and adjacent amygdalostriatal transition areas in the rat. Neuroscience. In press.
57. DERRIEN, M., C. DURIEUX, V. DAUGE & B.P. ROQUES. 1993. Involvement of D2 dopaminergic receptors in the emotional and motivational responses induced by injection of CCK-8 in the posterior part of the rat nucleus accumbens. Brain Res. **617:** 181–188.
58. SMITH, S., N. LINDEFORS, Y. HURD & T. SHARP. 1995. Electroconvulsive shock increases dopamine D1 and D2 receptor mRNA in the nucleus accumbens of the rat. Psychopharmacology **120:** 333–340.
59. DREW, K.L., W.T. O'CONNOR, J. KEHR & U. UNGERSTEDT. 1990. Regional specific effects of clozapine and haloperidol on GABA and dopamine release in rat basal ganglia. Eur. J. Pharmacol. **187:** 385–397.
60. BETANCUR, C., W. ROSTENE & A. BEROD. 1997. Chronic cocaine increases neurotensin gene expression in the shell of the nucleus accumbens and in discrete regions of the striatum. Brain Res. Mol. Brain Res. **44:** 334–340.

Projections of the Amygdalopiriform Transition Area (APir)

A PHA-L Study in the Rat

SARA J. SHAMMAH-LAGNADO[a] AND ADRIANA C. SANTIAGO

Department of Physiology and Biophysics, Institute of Biomedical Sciences, University of São Paulo, São Paulo, SP, 05508-900, Brazil

The amygdalopiriform transition area (APir) is a poorly understood region located at the junction of the piriform, periamygdaloid and entorhinal cortices. This transition area, which is characterized by a well developed molecular layer, a poorly laminated organization and distinctive staining features, receives direct projections from the olfactory bulb.[1] In spite of its peculiar cytoarchitecture, APir has often been considered a rostral extent of the ventrolateral entorhinal cortex.[2] However, it is of note that, in contrast to the lateral entorhinal cortex, APir receives only modest projections from midline thalamic nuclei.[3] Moreover, incidental observations indicate that APir and the lateral entorhinal cortex have different amygdalopetal projections.[4,5] Since APir efferent connections have not been thus far examined with anterograde tracing techniques, they were presently investigated in the rat using the sensitive *Phaseolus vulgaris* leukoagglutinin (PHA-L) tracer.

MATERIALS AND METHODS

Unilateral deposits of PHA-L were placed stereotaxically in different APir districts as well as in the adjacent posterior basolateral amygdaloid nucleus and lateral entorhinal cortex. The tracer was delivered via glass micropipettes (internal tip diameter 10–15 μm) filled with a 2.5% solution of PHA-L in 0.1 M sodium phosphate buffer at pH 7.4. Iontophoresis was achieved with a positive-pulsed (7 seconds on, 7 seconds off) current of 5 μA for 15–25 min. After 10–14 days, the animals were deeply anesthetized and perfused transcardially with 50 ml saline followed by 500 ml fixative consisting of ice-cold 4% paraformaldehyde in 0.1 M sodium phosphate buffer (pH 7.4). The brains were postfixed for several hours, cryoprotected by immersion in a 20% sucrose solution in 0.1 M sodium phosphate buffer (pH 7.4) and sectioned coronally on a sliding microtome. Brain sections were processed for PHA-L immunohistochemistry[6] by using the avidin-biotin-peroxidase (ABC) technique. An adjacent series was stained with thionin. The immunostained sections were examined under both bright- and darkfield illumination.

---

[a]Corresponding author: Sara J. Shammah-Lagnado, Department of Physiology and Biophysics, Institute of Biomedical Sciences, University of São Paulo, 05508-900, São Paulo, SP, Brazil. Voice: 55-11 818-7216; fax: 55-11 818-7285; sara@fisio.icb1.usp.br

APir 23

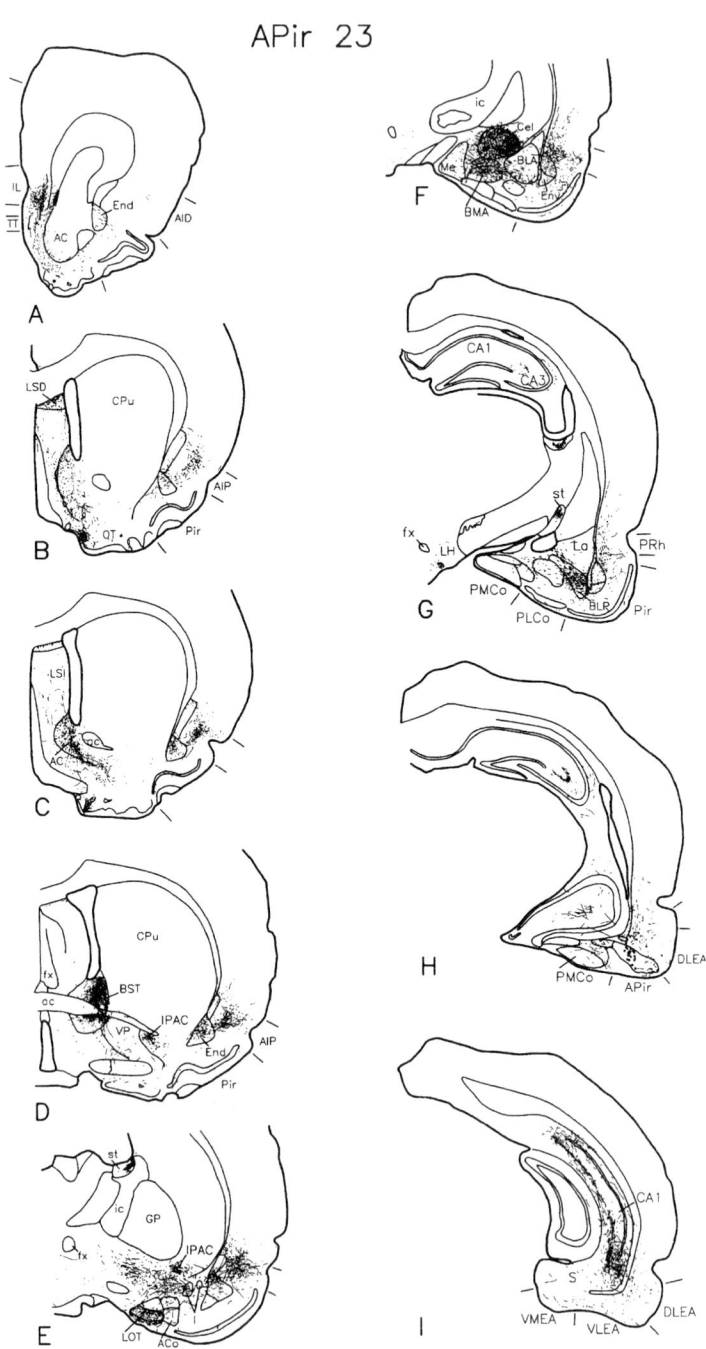

RESULTS

The anterograde labeling observed in case 23, which has a PHA-L deposit in the middle third of APir mediolateral extent, is illustrated in FIGURE 1. Labeled fibers issuing rostromedially from the injection site arborize in the posterior basolateral and anterior basomedial amygdaloid nuclei, central extended amygdala, nucleus of the lateral olfactory tract, ventral striatum, lateral septum, mainly in its dorsal part, infralimbic cortex, tenia tecta and anterior olfactory nucleus. The terminal plexus in the central extended amygdala is particularly dense and encompasses all the divisions of the central nucleus and of the lateral bed nucleus of the stria terminalis, the sublenticular corridor, the interstitial nucleus of the posterior limb of the anterior commissure and the supracapsular bed nucleus of the stria terminalis. In contrast, the medial amygdaloid nucleus and the intraamygdaloid bed nucleus of the stria terminalis appear much less densely labeled. In the ventral striatum, terminal labeling is observed in the caudomedial part of the olfactory tubercle, and in the medial shell of the accumbens including its posterodorsal region, i.e., its septal pole. Issuing laterally from the injection site, labeled fibers course in the external capsule and endopiriform nucleus to distribute to the lateral entorhinal, perirhinal and posterior piriform cortices, and, very prominently, to the posterior division of the agranular insular cortex. In addition, APir efferents, via perforant path, reach the molecular layer of the ventral subiculum and the stratum lacunosum-moleculare of Ammon's horn, but the dentate gyrus, in stark contrast to cases with PHA-L injections into the lateral entorhinal cortex, is free of labeling.

The analysis of cases in which PHA-L deposits were placed in different APir districts or in adjacent structures, i.e., the posterior basolateral amygdaloid nucleus and lateral entorhinal cortex, indicate that projections arising from medial APir districts (case 25) are very similar to those from the posterior basolateral amygdaloid nucle-

---

FIGURE 1. Distribution of PHA-L-labeled fibers in case 23. *Dots* in **(H)** indicate PHA-L immunoreactive cells bodies. The labeling was nearly exclusively found in the ipsilateral side. Abbreviations: AC, accumbens nucleus; ac, anterior commissure; ACo, anterior cortical amygdaloid nucleus; AID, agranular insular cortex, dorsal division; AIP, agranular insular cortex, posterior division; APir, amygdalopiriform transition area; BLA, anterior basolateral amygdaloid nucleus; BLP, posterior basolateral amygdaloid nucleus; BMA, anterior basomedial amygdaloid nucleus; BST, bed nucleus of the stria terminalis; BSTS, supracapsular bed nucleus of the stria terminalis; CA1 and CA3, Ammon's horn, fields CA1 and CA3; Cec, central amygdaloid nucleus, capsular part; Cel, central amygdaloid nucleus, lateral part; Cem, central amygdaloid nucleus, medial part; CPu, caudate-putamen; DLEA, dorsolateral entorhinal area; End, endopiriform nucleus, dorsal part; Env, endopiriform nucleus, ventral part; fx, fornix; GP, globus pallidus; I, intercalated amygdaloid nuclei; ic, internal capsule; IL, infralimbic cortex; IPAC, interstitial nucleus of the posterior limb of the anterior commissure; Ju, juxtacapsular part of the lateral bed nucleus of the stria terminalis; La, lateral amygdaloid nucleus; LH, lateral hypothalamus; LOT, nucleus of the lateral olfactory tract; LSD, lateral septal nucleus, dorsal part; LSI, lateral septal nucleus, intermediate part; LSV, lateral septal nucleus, ventral part; Me, medial amygdaloid nucleus; OT, olfactory tubercle; Pir, piriform cortex; PLCo, posterolateral cortical amygdaloid nucleus; PMCo, posteromedial cortical amygdaloid nucleus; PRh, perirhinal cortex; S, subiculum; st, stria terminalis; TT, tenia tecta; VLEA, ventrolateral entorhinal area; VMEA, ventromedial entorhinal area; VP, ventral pallidum.

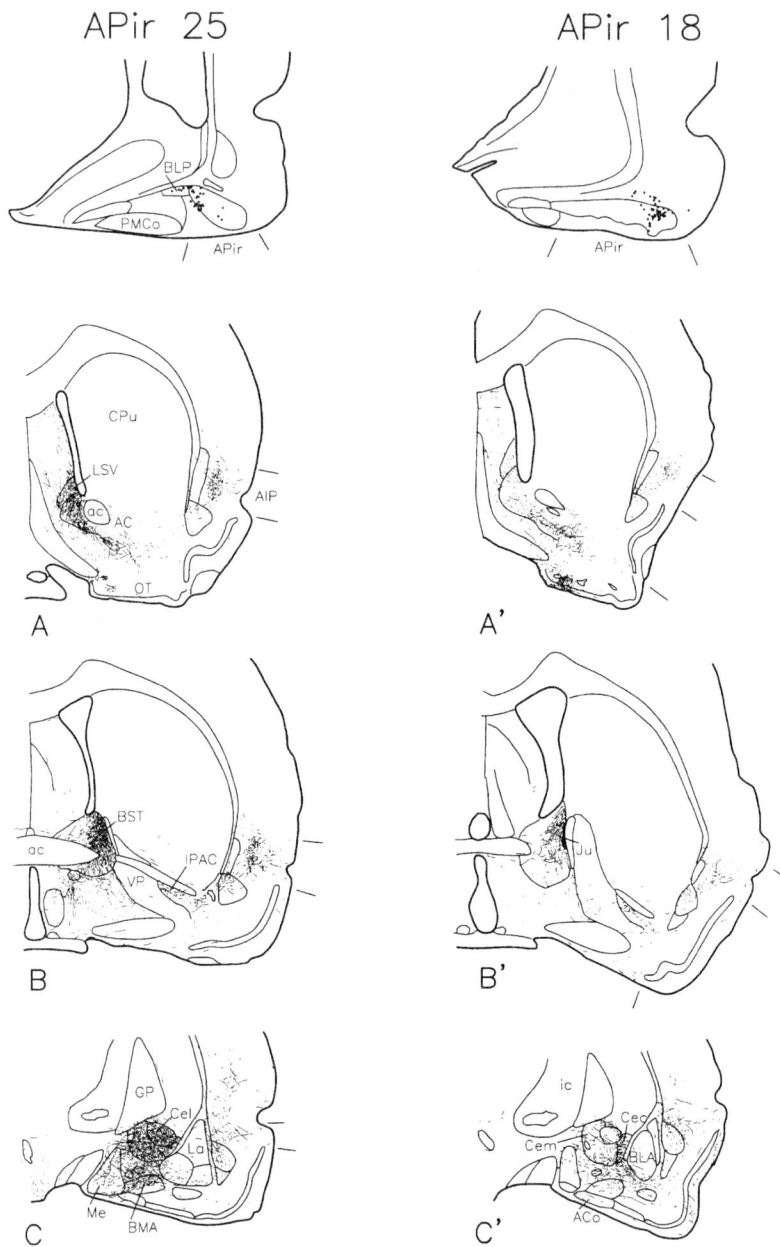

FIGURE 2. Distribution of PHA-L-labeled fibers following PHA-L injection (*shown on top*) in medial (case 25) and lateral (case 18) APir districts showing that APir projections to the ventral striatum and extended amygdala are topographically organized. See FIG. 1 for abbreviations.

us, while projections from lateral APir districts (case 18) resemble those of the laterally contiguous entorhinal cortex. These cases also reveal that APir projections to the ventral striatum, extended amygdala and hippocampal formation are organized according to a mediolateral topographical plan (FIG. 2). Thus, medial APir districts innervate the medial shell of the accumbens including its septal pole and the caudomedial part of the olfactory tubercle (FIG. 2A). Lateral APir districts project heavily to the latter, and, to a lesser degree, to the ventral shell of the accumbens and largely avoid its septal pole (FIG. 2A'). Medial APir districts innervate heavily all the components of the central extended amygdala and provide also moderately dense projections to the medial extended amygdala, particularly to the anterodorsal division of the medial amygdaloid nucleus, the intraamygdaloid bed nucleus of the stria terminalis and the ventral and posterolateral parts of the medial bed nucleus of the stria terminalis (FIG. 2B,C). Lateral APir districts project much less densely to the extended amygdala and terminate nearly exclusively in the central division, arborizing chiefly in the capsular part of the central nucleus and the juxtacapsular part of the lateral bed nucleus of the stria terminalis (FIG. 2B',C'). Medial and intermediolateral APir districts project to the lateral septal nucleus targeting chiefly its ventral and dorsal parts, respectively (FIGS. 1B,C and 2A), while lateral APir districts project only lightly to the septum (FIG. 2A'). Medial APir districts project to the ventral subiculum and the adjoining temporal field CA1. Lateral APir projections to the hippocampal formation have a wider temporo-septal distribution. In the ventral subiculum, the outermost portion of the molecular layer is labeled after lateral APir injections, and the stratum radiatum after medial APir injections. In none of the present APir cases were projections to the dentate gyrus observed.

CONCLUSIONS

Our results suggest that APir projects to the main olfactory system, mesocortical areas, ventral striatum, central extended amygdala, ventral subiculum and temporal field CA1, and as such is expected to play a role in the expression of emotional and motivated behaviors.

Although APir has often been considered a rostral extent of the ventrolateral entorhinal cortex,[2] our observations, in agreement with other studies,[4,5,7] suggest that APir differs from the latter by its dense projections to the central extended amygdala and by the absence of projections to the molecular layer of the dentate gyrus. APir, however, retains certain typical entorhinal organizational features. In particular, lateral APir projections to the hippocampal formation have a wider temporo-septal distribution and they also target more distal portions of the apical dendrite of pyramidal cells than do projections from medial APir districts. In this sense, lateral and medial APir projections to the hippocampal formation resemble those arising from lateral and medial entorhinal cortices, respectively.[8]

ACKNOWLEDGMENTS

We thank Ana Maria Peraçoli for excellent histological assistance. This study was supported by FAPESP Grants 96/7794-5 and 96/11787-4.

REFERENCES

1. ALHEID, G F., J.S. DE OLMOS & C.A. BELTRAMINO. 1995. Amygdala and extended amygdala. *In* The Rat Nervous System. 2nd edit. G. Paxinos, Ed.: 495–578. Academic Press. San Diego.
2. KRETTEK, J.E. & J.L PRICE. 1977. Projections from the amygdaloid complex and adjacent olfactory structures to the entorhinal cortex and to the subiculum in the rat and cat. J. Comp. Neurol. **172:** 723–752.
3. BECKSTEAD, R.M. 1978. Afferent connections of the entorhinal area in the rat as demonstrated by retrograde cell-labeling with horseradish peroxidase. Brain Res. **152:** 249–264.
4. OTTERSEN, O.P. 1982. Connections of the amygdala of the rat. IV. Corticoamygdaloid and intraamygdaloid connections as studied with axonal transport of horseradish peroxidase. J. Comp. Neurol. **205:** 30–48.
5. McDONALD, A.J. & F. MASCAGNI. 1997. Projections of the lateral entorhinal cortex to the amygdala: a *Phaseolus vulgaris* leucoagglutinin study in the rat. Neuroscience **77:** 445–459.
6. GERFEN, C.R. & P.E. SAWCHENKO. 1984. An anterograde neuroanatomical tracing method that shows the detailed morphology of neurons, their axons, and terminals: immunohistochemical localization of an axonally transported plant lectin, *Phaseolus vulgaris* leucoagglutinin (PHA-L). Brain Res. **290:** 219–238.
7. SWANSON, L.W. & G.D. PETROVICH. 1998. What is the amygdala? Trends Neurosci. **21:** 323–331.
8. WYSS, J.M. 1981. An autoradiographic study of the efferent connections of the entorhinal cortex in the rat. J. Comp. Neurol. **199:** 495–512.

The Ventral Striatum of the Syrian Hamster

LUKE R. JOHNSON[a] AND RUTH I. WOOD

Department of Obstetrics and Gynecology, Yale University School of Medicine, New Haven, Connecticut 06520, USA

INTRODUCTION

The Syrian hamster, *Mesocricetus auratus*, was first used in laboratory experiments some fifty years ago in the Middle East, from animals captured in the wild.[1] Since then the Syrian hamster has been domesticated and used extensively in laboratory studies of motivation, incluiding reproduction, feeding, aggression and circadian behaviors.[2] In comparison to the rat, the male Syrian hamster is a solitary animal known for its territorial aggression, photoperiodic mating and hoarding behaviors. Many neural circuits controlling reproductive behaviors are now known.[3] While these motivated behaviors have been demonstrated to be regulated by endocrine status there is increasing evidence that dopamine within the nucleus accumbens conveys the rewarding tone of sexual motivation.[4]

The nucleus accumbens not only regulates appetitive behaviors but its amygdalar afferents allow environmental stimuli to gain predictive association via their interactions with dopamine in the nucleus accumbens[5] and thus regulate sexual motivation.[6] The pattern of limbic afferentation to the ventral striatum correlates with immunocytoarchitectural demarcations in the rat.[7] Winans and Newman have investigated and defined the Syrian hamster nucleus accumbens and olfactory tubercles based on hodological studies.[8,9] While much is known about motivated behaviors in the Syrian hamster and the cytoarchitecture of the rat ventral striatum, in this study we investigate and juxtapose, the cytoarchitecture of the ventral striatum of the Syrian hamster with the rat, using immunocytochemisty for calbindin D28k, calretinin and tyrosine hydroxylase.

METHODS

Standard immunocytochemistry and histology techniques were employed. Four male Syrian hamsters and four male Sprague-Dawley rats were anesthetized and transcardially perfused with 4% paraformaldehyde. Coronal sections were cut at 50 µm and stained with either cresyl violet or immunocytochemistry for calbindin D28k (CaBP, 1:25000, Sigma, MO); calretinin (1:30000, Dr. J. Rogers, Cambridge University); or tyrosine hydroxylase (1:15000, Eugene Tech, OR). Sections were incubated in the appropriate secondary antibody followed by avidin-biotin complex, and the antigens visualized with diaminobenzidine (DAB) or nickel-enhanced diami-

---

[a]Address for correspondence: Luke R. Johnson, PhD, Department of Obstetrics and Gynecology, Yale University School of Medicine, 333 Cedar Street, New Haven, CT 06520. Voice: 203-737-1217; fax: 203-785-9294; Luke.Johnson@yale.edu

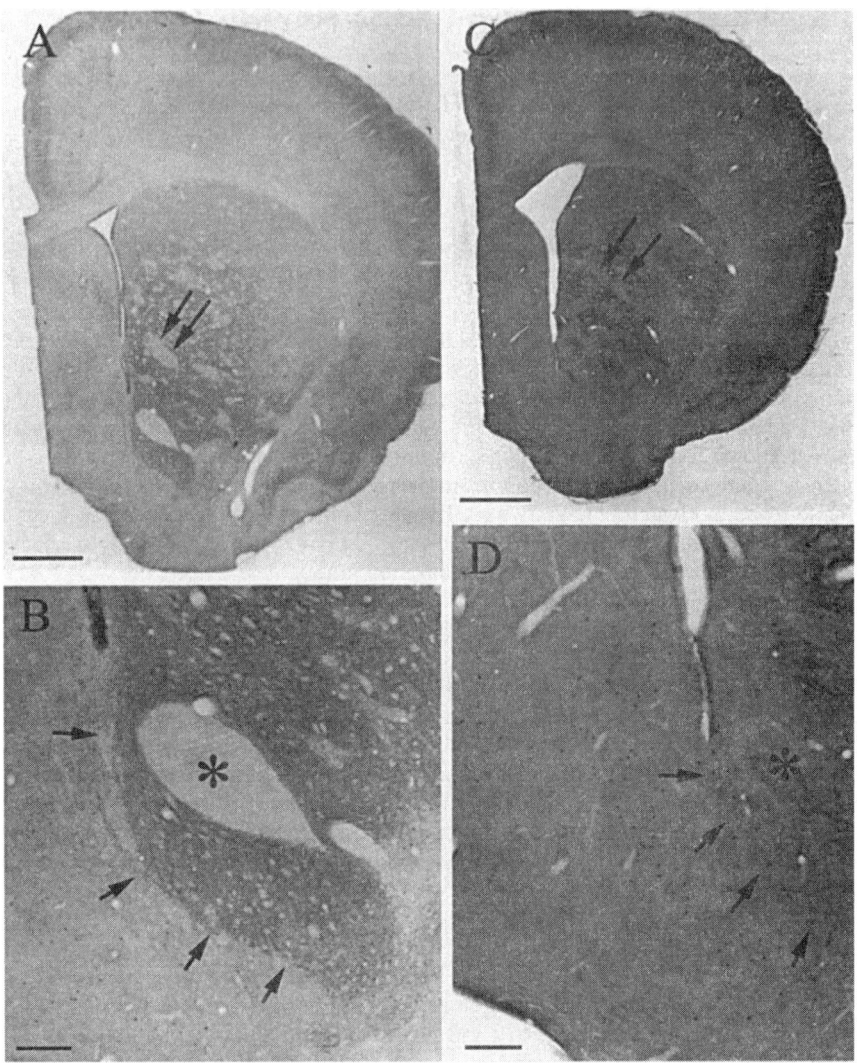

FIGURE 1. Immunoreactivity for calcium binding protein D28k revealed with DAB in the caudal ventral striatum of rat (**A,B**) and the Syrian hamster (**C,D**). A similar pattern of labeling was observed in both species, although the demarcation between dark and light staining was not as clear in the hamster. A patch-matrix labeling was observed throughout the dorsal striatum, except the dorsolateral quadrant, where no staining was observed in either species. The lighter stained patches appeared more elongated in hamster (C, *arrows*), compared to rat (A, *arrows*). The boundary between core and shell on the nucleus accumbens was clearly demarcated by CaBP immunoreactivity in the rat (B, *arrows*), and no immunoreactivity was observed in the anterior commissure (*asterisk*). In contrast, the demarcation between core and shell was less clear in hamster (D, *arrows*); in addition the anterior commissure appeared immunoreactive (*asterisk*). Scale bars = 1 mm (A,C) and 200 μm (B,D).

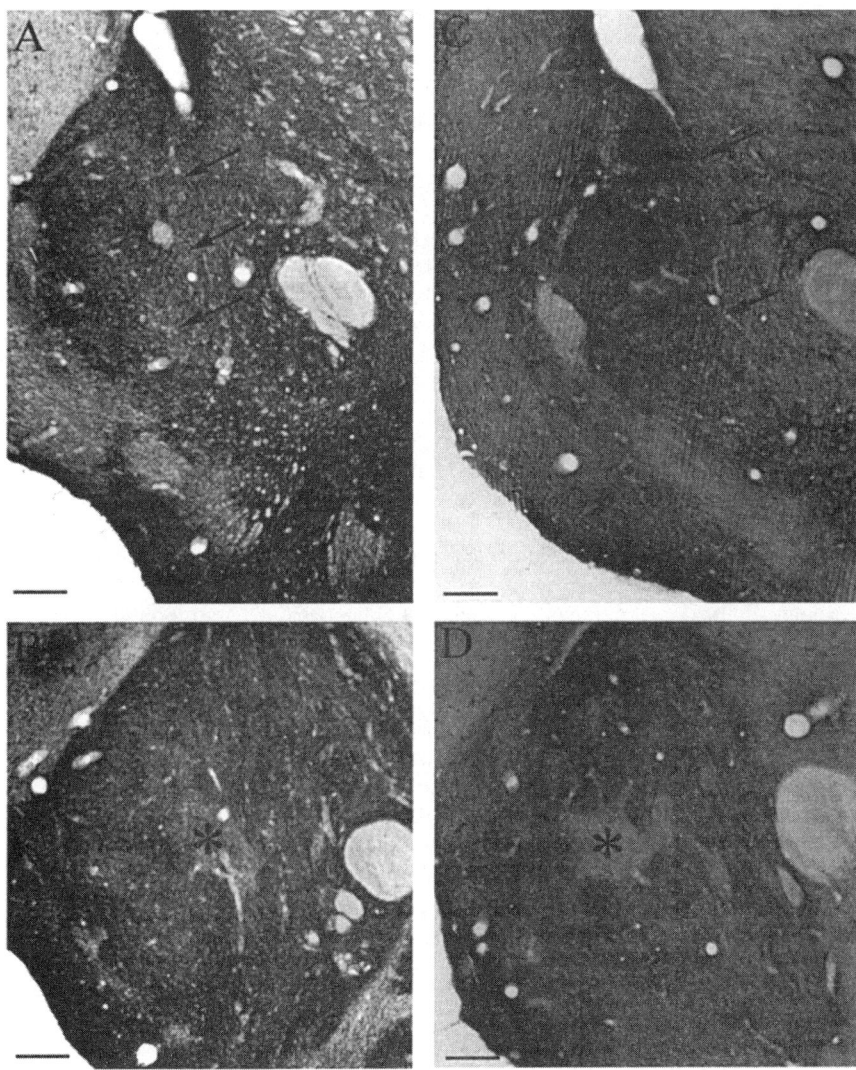

FIGURE 2. Immunoreactivity for tyrosine hydroxylase (**A,B**) and calretinin (**C,D**) revealed with nickel-DAB in the rostral and midventral striatum of the Syrian hamster. With tyrosine hydroxylase immunoreactivity (A,B), note the darker staining in the dorsal nucleus accumbens shell (*arrows*) and olfactory tubercles (A). In the rostral nucleus accumbens, a prominent irregular-shaped zone of light staining was observed (B, *asterisk*). Calretinin immunoreactivity showed similar patterns of staining. Note the darker staining also observed in the dorsal nucleus accumbens shell (C, *arrows*). In the rostral nucleus accumbens an irregular-shaped zone of lighter staining, approximately corresponding to that observed in tyrosine hydroxylase-stained material, was observed (D, *asterisk*). Scale bar = 200 μm.

nobenzidine (Ni-DAB). Negative control sections were included by omitting the primary antibody. All sections for direct comparison were processed in parallel and photomicrographs were taken under the same conditions.

RESULTS

Immunocytochemistry for calbindin D28k, calretinin and tyrosine hydroxylase revealed distinctive compartmental staining in both hamster and rat. Immunostaining in the hamster for CaBP labeled with DAB, revealed a 'patch/matrix' compartmentalization throughout the rostrocaudal extent of the striatum (FIG. 1C) which was similar to that seen in the rat (FIG. 1A). In keeping with the gross morphology of the hamster brain, lightly stained patches appeared elongated in the mediolateral plane. The dorsolateral striatum was devoid of CaBP immunoreactivity in both species. Ventrally in the striatum, a core of the nucleus accumbens could be delineated by the presence of immunoreactivity surrounding the anterior commissure which declined medially and ventrally towards the olfactory tubercles (FIG. 1B,D). The anterior commissure was immunostained in the hamster but not in the rat (FIG. 1B,D). Calbindin-immunoreactive neurons were occasionally identified within the anterior commissure itself.

Immunocytochemistry for calretinin and tyrosine hydroxylase, labeled with Ni-DAB, both revealed complex reactivity in the hamster. Calretinin immunoreactivity was dense in the dorsal nucleus accumbens shell (FIG. 2C). Throughout the core and olfactory tubercles, calretinin immunostaining was moderate. In the rostral nucleus accumbens, calretinin immunoreactivity revealed a distinctive irregular-shaped zone of light staining (FIG. 2D). Tyrosine hydroxylase immunoreactivity defines the entire striatum. The pattern of tyrosine hydroxylase immunoreactivity in the ventral striatum of the hamster was similar to that of calretinin immunoreactivity. Reactivity was especially dense in the ventrolateral striatum, where it coursed through the lateral side of the islands of Calleja and delineated the entire olfactory tubercles. Staining was intense in the dorsal nucleus accumbens shell (FIG. 2A) but also showed patches of lighter staining in the rostral accumbens (FIG. 2B) in a manner similar to calretinin immunoreactivity (FIG. 2).

Nissl-stained sections from the hamster revealed heterogeneously distributed neurons in the ventral striatum. A core of the closely packed neurons was identified around the anterior commissure akin to the rat nucleus accumbens core. Medially and laterally, cell density decreased with the exception of cell clusters which demarcated the core/shell border. Further ventrally, cell bridges connecting the nucleus accumbens with the olfactory tubercles divided the islands of Calleja. Medially a very prominent major island of Calleja was also observed.

DISCUSSION

Our observations define the hamster ventral striatum cytoarchitecturally for the first time. The ventral striatum of the male Syrian hamster shares mostly similar cytoarchitectural heterogeneity as previously identified in other species, as defined with tyrosine hydroxylase, calretinin and calbindin D28k immunoreactivity. The identification of a nucleus accumbens shell region[10] based on a diminished CaBP immunoreactivity and increased calretinin and tyrosine hydroxylase immunoreactivity is in agreement with previous findings in the rat.[7,11–14] Compared to the rat, CaBP immunoreactivity was less effective in demarcating subregions of the striatum due to low contrast staining between patch and matrix and core and shell. Also, unlike the rat, the hamster anterior commissure appeared positively stained and occasionally contained CaBP positive cells. The irregular shaped patches of light calretinin immunostaining in the rostral nucleus accumbens resemble those defined by Hussain and colleagues in the rat.[13] Hiroi observed that this pattern of staining correlates with regions of tightly packed cells that are known to contain mu-opioid receptor patches.[15] The hodological studies of Winans and Newman[8,9] defined the hamster ventral striatum as receiving topographically based afferent connections from limbic structures including the amygdala and hippocampus and the limbic cortex. Efferents of the hamster ventral striatum projected to the substantia nigra and ventral pallidal structures. The seminal work of Groenewegen and colleagues working in the rat has identified the interrelation between ventral striatum circuitry and cytoarchitecture.[7] Whether similar relationships also exist in hamster and how such arrangements may determine differences in motivated behavior between rat and hamster, remains to be determined.

REFERENCES

1. MURPHY, M.R. 1985. History of the capture and domestication of the Syrian hamster (*Mesocricetus auratus*). *In* The Hamster, Reproduction and Behaviour. H.I. Siegel, Ed.: 3–20. Plenum Press. New York.
2. LISK, R. D. 1985. The estrous cycle. *In* The Hamster, Reproduction and Behaviour. H.I. Siegel, Ed.: 23–51. Plenum Press. New York.
3. WOOD, R.I. & S.W. NEWMAN. 1995. Integration of chemosensory and hormonal cues is essential for mating in the male Syrian hamster. J. Neurosci. **15**: 7261–7269.
4. DAMSMA, G., J.G. PFAUS, D. WENKSTERN, A.G. PHILLIPS & H.C. FIBIGER. 1992. Sexual behavior increases dopamine transmission in the nucleus accumbens and striatum of male rats: comparison with novelty and locomotion. Behav. Neurosci. **106**: 181–191.
5. JOHNSON, L.R., R.L. AYLWARD, Z. HUSSAIN & S. TOTTERDELL. 1994. Input from the amygdala to the rat nucleus accumbens: its relationship with tyrosine hydroxylase immunoreactivity and identified neurons. Neuroscience **61**: 851–865.
6. EVERITT, B.J. 1990. Sexual motivation: a neural and behavioural analysis of the mechanisms underlying appetitive and copulatory responses of male rats. Neurosci. Biobehav. Rev. **14**: 217–232.
7. GROENEWEGEN, H.J., H.W. BERENDSE, G.E. MEREDITH *et al.* 1991. Functional anatomy of the ventral, limbic system-innervated striatum. *In* The Mesolimbic Dopamine System: from Motivation to Action. P. Wilner & J. Scheel-Kruger, Eds.: 19–59. John Wiley & Sons. New York.
8. NEWMAN, R. & S.S. WINANS. 1980. An experimental study of the ventral striatum of the golden hamster. I. Neuronal connections of the nucleus accumbens. J. Comp. Neurol. **191**: 167–192.
9. NEWMAN, R. & S.S. WINANS. 1980. An experimental study of the ventral striatum of the golden hamster. II. Neuronal connections of the olfactory tubercle. J. Comp. Neurol. **191**(2): 193–212.
10. ZABORSZKY, L., G.F. ALHEID, M.C. BEINFELD, L.E. EIDEN, L. HEIMER & M. PALKOVITS. 1985. Cholecystokinin innervation of the ventral striatum: a morphological and radioimmunological study. Neuroscience **14**(2): 427–453.

11. VOORN, P., B. JORRISTSMA-BYHAM & C. VAN DIJK. 1986. The dopaminergic innervation of the ventral striatum in the rat: a light and electron microscopical study with antibodies against dopamine. J. Comp. Neurol. **251:** 84–99.
12. MEREDITH, G.E., A. PATTISELANNO, H.J. GROENEWEGEN & S.N. HABER. 1996. Shell and core in monkey and human nucleus accumbens identified with antibodies to calbindin-D28k. J. Comp. Neurol. **365:** 628–639.
13. HUSSAIN, Z., L.R. JOHNSON & S. TOTTERDELL. 1996. A light and electron microscopic study of NADPH-diaphorase-, calretinin- and parvalbumin-containing neurons in the rat nucleus accumbens. J. Chem. Neuroanat. **10:** 19–39.
14. HEIMER, L., G.F. ALHEID, J.S. DE OLMOS, H.J. GROENEWEGEN, S.N. HABER, R.E. HARLAN & D.S. ZAHM. 1997. The accumbens: beyond the core-shell dichotomy. J. Neuropsychiatry Clin. Neurosci. **3:** 354–381.
15. HIROI, N. 1995. Compartmental organization of calretinin in the rat striatum. Neurosci. Lett. **197:** 223–226.

Afferent Connections to the Ventral Striatum from the Medial Prefrontal Cortex (Area 25) and the Thalamic Nuclei in the Macaque Monkey

K. NAKANO,[a,c] T. KAYAHARA,[a] AND T. CHIBA[b]

[a]*Department of Anatomy, Faculty of Medicine, Mie University, Mie 514-8507, Japan*
[b]*Department of Neurobiology, School of Medicine, Chiba University, Chiba 260-8670, Japan*

ABSTRACT: The ventral striatal inputs in the macaque monkey were studied in relation to the connections from the orbitofrontal cortex, focusing on the infralimbic area (IL or area 25), thalamic nuclei and the vagal-solitary nuclear complex (NTS-X). The IL projects to more restricted parts of the ventral striatum (shell and core of nucleus accumbens, Acb; ventricular margin of caudate nucleus, CN), whereas the striatal projections of the prelimbic area (PL) are more extended than those of IL. The dorsal midline nuclei project densely to area 13, agranular insular cortex (Ia), and Acb. The nucleus ventralis anterior pars magnocellularis (VAmc) projects to the IL, perigenual area and to the region of CN between the limbic and association striatum with partial overlapping, and seems to play a role as an interface between the limbic and motor systems. The distribution pattern of retrogradely labeled neurons was similar in the midline-intralaminar thalamic nuclei following injections in the IL and ventral striatum.

INTRODUCTION

The heterogeneous ventral striatum consists of a number of smaller modules, and participates in the mechanisms of the subchannels of limbic basal ganglia-thalamo-cortical system. Although the neural circuits of the striatum were studied in detail in rats and cats,[3] only a limited number of studies have been done in monkeys.[2–4] In this paper we studied inputs to the ventral striatum from the infralimbic area (IL), prelimbic area (PL), thalamic nuclei, and the vagal-solitary nuclear complex (NTS-X) using axonal tracers of biotinylated dextran amine (BDA) and wheat germ agglutinin-conjugated horseradish peroxidase (WGA-HRP).

---

[c]Corresponding author: Dr. Katsuma Nakano, Department of Anatomy, Faculty of Medicine, Mie University, Tsu, Mie 514-8507, Japan. Voice: 81-59-231-5002; fax 81-59-231-5219; nakano@doc.medic.mie-u.ac.jp

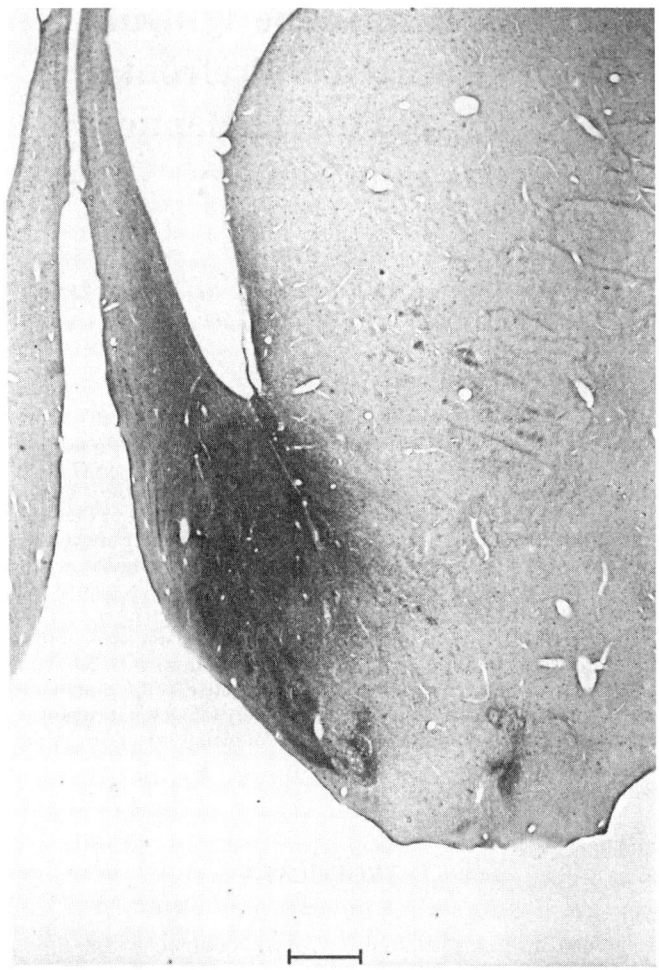

FIGURE 1. Low-power photograph illustrating the projection region in ventral striatum from the infralimbic area (IL) following injections of biotinylated dextran amine (BDA) into the IL. BDA reaction with diaminobenzidine tetrahydrochloride and nickel ammonium sulfate. Bar = 1 mm.

RESULTS AND DISCUSSION

With BDA injections in the IL, labeled terminals were found in more restricted portions of the shell and core of nucleus accumbens (Acb), and the ventricular margin of the rostro-caudal extent of caudate nucleus (CN, FIG. 1), whereas BDA injections in the PL produced terminal labelings more extensively in the ventral striatum. These findings were also confirmed by retrograde labeling with WGA-HRP injections in the various parts of the ventral striatum. Following injections of BDA in the dorsal midline nuclei (paraventricular, Pv; paratenial, Pt; reuniens nuclei, Rh), labeled terminals were found in the Acb, lateral preoptic area, central (Ce) and cortical amygdaloid nuclei and entorhinal cortex as well as the orbitofrontal cortices (IL, areas 14, 13, 12, and Ia). These terminal labelings were densest in Ia, areas 13m, 13l and 13b. WGA-HRP injections in NTS-X resulted in retrograde labeling cells somewhat dense in Acb, bed nucleus of the stria terminalis (BST), substantia innominata and preoptic area, dense in the interstitial nucleus of the posterior limb of anterior commissure, Ce, and most dense in the paraventricular hypothalamic nucleus. Anterogradely HRP-labeled terminals were observed in Acb, BST and preoptic areas. With a WGA-HRP injection in the IL, PL, or in the various parts of the ventral striatum, retrogradely labeled cells were seen in the midline and intralaminar (iLa) thalamic nuclei. Labeled cells in the iLa were noted only in the ventromedial part of the parafascicular nucleus (Pf) and the central medial nucleus (CeM). The distribution pattern of these labeled cells in the thalamus was essentially similar in all cases, but with injections in IL and Acb, labeled cells were denser in Pv, Rh, and Re, and only in these cases were labeled cells detected in Pt. Labeled cells in the Pv, Rh, and Re were more limited in the midline region following a WGA-HRP injection in the perigenual area. With a WGA-HRP injection in the PL, labeled cells were seen only in

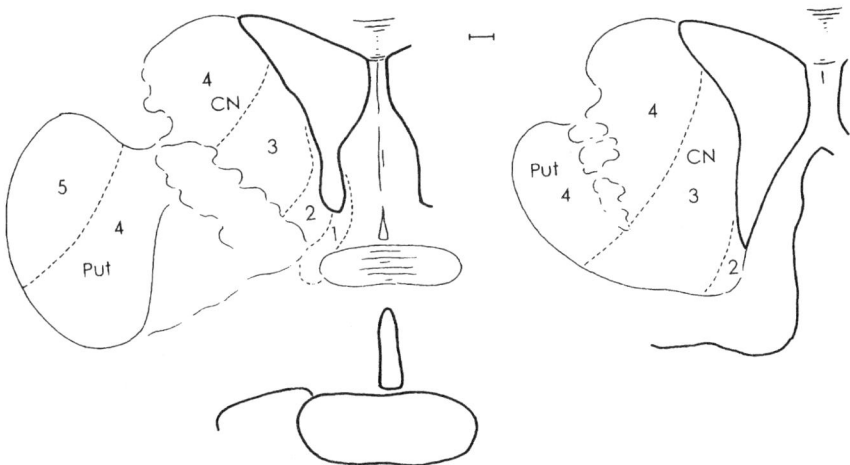

FIGURE 2. Summary diagrams showing topographical projections to the striatum from the motor thalamic nuclei, midline-intralaminar nuclei, IL, prelimbic area (PL), and from the solitary-vagal nuclear complex (NTS-X). The NTS-X territory (1) was located in the most ventromedial part of the striatum; the territory of the midline thalamic nuclei, the ventromedial part of the parafascicular nucleus (Pf) and IL (2) was in the shell and core of Acb; the territory of the nucleus ventralis anterior pars parvicellularis (VApc) and lateral Pf (4) in the dorsolateral part of the caudate nucleus (CN) and in the rostromedial part of the putamen (Put); and the territory of the nucleus ventralis anterior pars magnocellularis (VAmc), medial Pf and PL (3) was in the intermediate part of CN. The territory of the nucleus ventralis lateralis pars oralis (VLo) and the centromedian nucleus (CM) (5) was located in the postcommissural part of Put dorsolateral to the VApc and lateral Pf territories (4). Bar = 1 mm.

the lateral parts of Rh and Re, and in the rostral end of the nucleus ventralis anterior pars parvicellularis (VApc). There were also labeled cells in the VAmc in the cases with injections in IL and perigenual area.

A precise topographic organization of the thalamostriatal projection from the midline and iLa was described in rats.[3] This topography remains largely undetermined in our study due to the difficulty in making an injection within each midline nucleus. According to Royce,[8] the striatum receives some collaterals of thalamocortical fibers arising from the midline-iLa nuclei. Recently, a retrograde double-labeling study in rats revealed branching projections to the medial prefrontal cortex and the Acb from single neurons in the midline thalamic nuclei as well as in the medial part of the Pf.[7] Although double-labeling studies are needed, the present findings in the monkey also suggest these branching projections. Motor thalamic nuclei connecting with the motor-related cortical areas also reportedly project topographically to the striatum.[5] On the basis of these[5] and the present findings, the topographical subdivisions of the striatum are schematically indicated in FIGURE 2. The IL connects with basal and accessory basal amygdaloid nuclei,[1,6] and the ventral striatum and limbic thalamic nuclei connect with amygdaloid nuclei.[3] The amygdaloid complex seems to exert a powerful influence on the orbitoprefrontal cortex, ventral striatum and the limbic thalamic nuclei,[2] a phenomenon corroborated by our present and previous experiments in the monkey.[1,6] It appears that the projections from the orbitofrontal subfields receiving limbic thalamic afferents converge in the ventral striatum with those of limbic thalamo-striatal afferents as well as amygdaloid afferents. The ventral striatum is a key station for the limbic basal ganglia-thalamo-cortical channels, and plays an important role in motivational behavior.

REFERENCES

1. CHIBA, T. & K. NAKANO. 1997. Efferent projection of infralimbic area of the medial prefrontal cortex (area 25) in the monkey, *Macaca fuscata*. J. Auton. Nerv. Syst. **65:** 98.
2. GIMENEZ-AMAYA, J. M. *et al.* 1995. Organization of thalamic projections to the ventral striatum in the primate. J. Comp. Neurol. **354:** 127–149.
3. GROENEWEGEN, H. J. *et al.* 1997. The anatomical relationships of the prefrontal cortex with limbic structures and the basal ganglia. J. Psychopharmacol. **11:** 99–106.
4. HABER, S. *et al.* 1995. The orbital and medial prefrontal circuit through the primate basal ganglia. J. Neurosci. **15:** 4851–4867.
5. NAKANO, K. *et al.* 1990. Topographical projections from the thalamus, subthalamic nucleus and pedunculopontine tegmental nucleus to the striatum in the Japanese monkey, *Macaca fuscata*. Brain Res. **537:** 54–68.
6. NAKANO, K. & T. CHIBA. 1997. Afferent connections of the infralimbic area in the medial prefrontal cortex (area 25) of the monkey, *Macaca fuscata*. J. Auton. Nerv. Syst. **65:** 103.
7. OTAKE, K. & Y. NAKAMURA. 1998. Single midline thalamic neurons projecting to both the ventral striatum and the prefrontal cortex in the rat. Neuroscience **86:** 635–649.
8. ROYCE, G. J. 1983. Single thalamic neurons which project to both the rostral cortex and caudate nucleus studied with the fluorescent double labeling method. Exp. Neurol. **79:** 773–784.

Expression of Enkephalin in Pallido-Striatal Neurons

PIETER VOORN,[a] SERGE VAN DE WITTE, GUNO TJON,
AND ALLERT JAN JONKER

Department of Anatomy, Research Institute of Neurosciences, Vrije University, 1081 BT Amsterdam, The Netherlands

INTRODUCTION

Lesions of the ascending dopaminergic system in the rat or neuroleptic treatment may lead to an upregulation of activity in globus pallidus, which is contrary to what would be expected based on current models of basal ganglia function.[1] It is not known if such a response occurs in all pallidal neurons or whether subpopulations of pallidal neurons react differently. Pallidal neurons reach several different target nuclei.[2] In the present experiments we tried to differentiate between subpopulations of pallidal neurons by determining the presence of prepro-enkephalin mRNA. Next, possible projection targets of the enkephalin-expressing pallidal neurons were identified. Finally, we determined the response of the enkephalin-expressing cells to unilateral dopamine depletion by midbrain 6-hydroxydopamine (6-OHDA) lesion.

METHODS

In situ hybridization was performed with ^{35}S-UTP-labeled cRNA probes for prepro-enkephalin (ENK) on cryostat brain sections. After hybridization sections were exposed to Ilford K5 photographic emulsion. Retrograde neuroanatomical tract-tracing was performed by injecting 0.5 µl of 2% Fluorogold into the caudate-putamen, entopeduncular nucleus, subthalamic nucleus and substantia nigra pars reticulata. Unilateral lesions of the dopamine system were made by injecting 5 µg 6-OHDA in 1 µl 0.9% NaCl + 0.01% ascorbic acid into the medial forebrain bundle. Rats ($n = 7$) survived for 3 weeks before decapitation. Quantification was performed by grain counting in emulsion-coated sections (2 sections per animal) over cresyl-violet-stained or fluorescent pallidal neurons. Cells with number of grains higher than mean + 2 standard deviations of background were considered specifically labeled.

---

[a]Corresponding author: Pieter Voorn, Ph.D., Dept. of Anatomy, Research Institute of Neurosciences, Vrije Universiteit, van der Boechorststraat 7, 1081 BT Amsterdam, The Netherlands. Voice: +31 20 444-8051; fax: +31 20 444-8054; P.Voorn.Anat@med.vu.nl

RESULTS

Quantification of the number of globus pallidus neurons containing hybridized ENK probe showed that approximately 40% of all large-sized pallidal neurons identified in cresyl-violet-counterstained sections were labeled for ENK mRNA. Per section 86 ± 9 (mean ± SEM) neurons were counted of which 33 ± 4 were positive for ENK mRNA. In FIGURE 1 the size of the ENK-positive population can be appreciated at low magnification. It becomes clear from this figure that the intensity of labeling of the pallidal neurons for ENK mRNA is considerably lower than that of the striatal neurons.

FIGURE 2 shows labeling for ENK mRNA in pallidiostriatal projection neurons. None of the tracer injections in the other brain regions resulted in the retrograde filling of ENK mRNA-positive pallidal neurons. In contrast, an average of 54% of fluorescently labeled neurons from injections in the striatum were labeled for ENK mRNA.

Quantification of the amount of hybridized ENK cRNA probe to GP neurons in unilaterally 6-OHDA-lesioned animals, showed a 40% increase in the lesioned side compared to the nonlesioned side, with 52 ± 1 grains per neuron in the nonlesioned side and 37 ± 1 grains per neuron in the lesioned side ($p < 0.05$ in Student t-test).

DISCUSSION

The present study for the first time demonstrates the presence of a sizable population (40%) of pallidal neurons expressing prepro-enkephalin in the rat. The majority of these enkephalinergic pallidal neurons projects to the caudate-putamen. A pallido-striatal connection has been known for some time.[3] There is evidence that pallidal neurons give rise to collaterals reaching several basal ganglia targets.[4] The enkephalinergic pallido-striatal neurons at this point do not appear to have collaterals to the other regions studied, since retrograde tracing from the substantia nigra, subthalamic nucleus and entopeduncular nucleus did not result in any labeling of enkephalinergic cells. However, the possibility of the enkephalinergic neurons collateralizing to other regions cannot be excluded.

The enkephalinergic pallidal neurons were found to respond with an upregulation of ENK mRNA synthesis to dopamine depletion. This may be a direct effect of decreased dopaminergic input to the pallidal neurons, and/or an indirect effect via the striato-pallidal projections. Interestingly, the striato-pallidal connection is also enkephalinergic and responds with higher levels of ENK mRNA to dopamine depletion.[5] This means that the net effect of the midbrain dopamine lesion is an upregulation of both legs of an enkephalinergic striato-pallido-striatal loop. Similar findings, with respect to upregulation of pallidal neurons, have been reported for γ-aminobutyric acid decarboxylase (GAD) mRNA.[1] It will be interesting to see if the enkephalinergic pallidal neurons also contain γ-aminobutyric acid (GABA) and if an upregulation of pallidal activity preferentially affects the pallido-striatal connection.

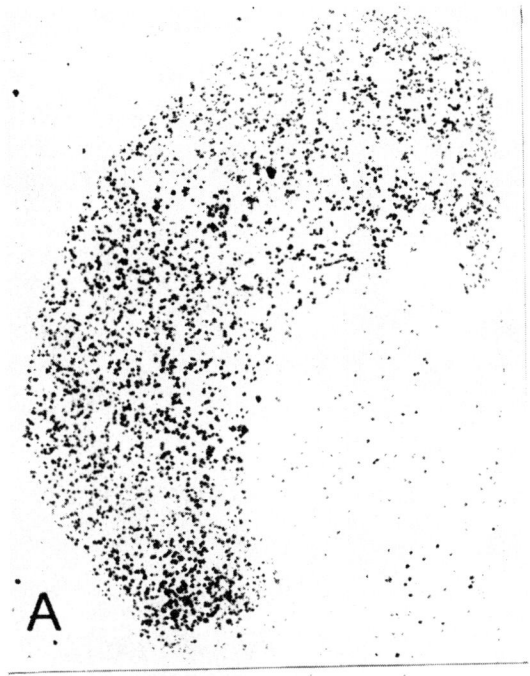
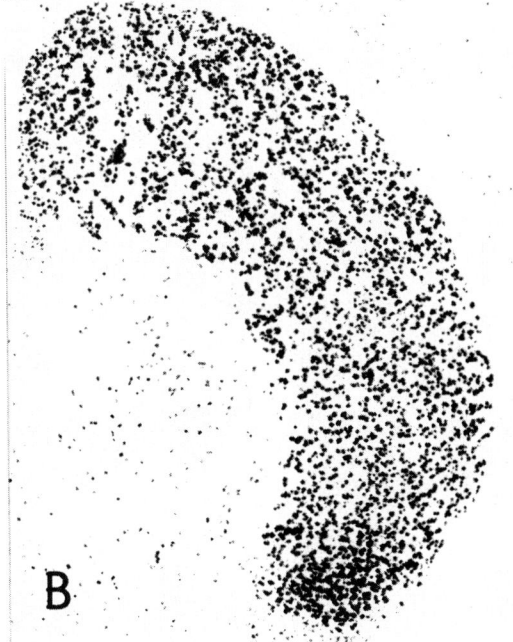

FIGURE 1. Inverted dark-field images of emulsion autoradiogram of transverse section through caudate-putamen (CP) and globus pallidus (GP) hybridized with [^{35}S]-labeled cRNA ENK probe. **(A)** shows the unlesioned hemisphere and **(B)** the lesioned hemisphere.

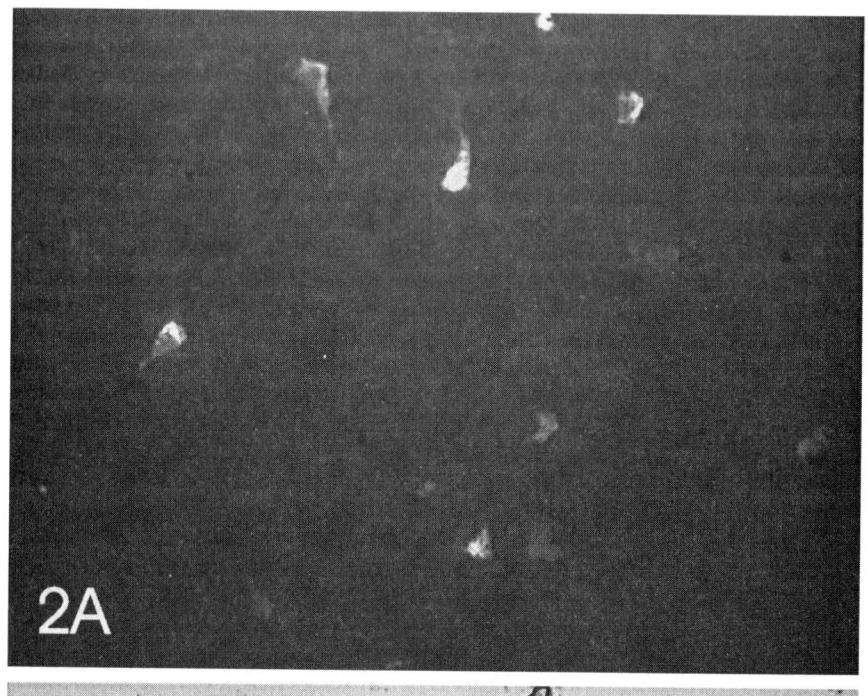
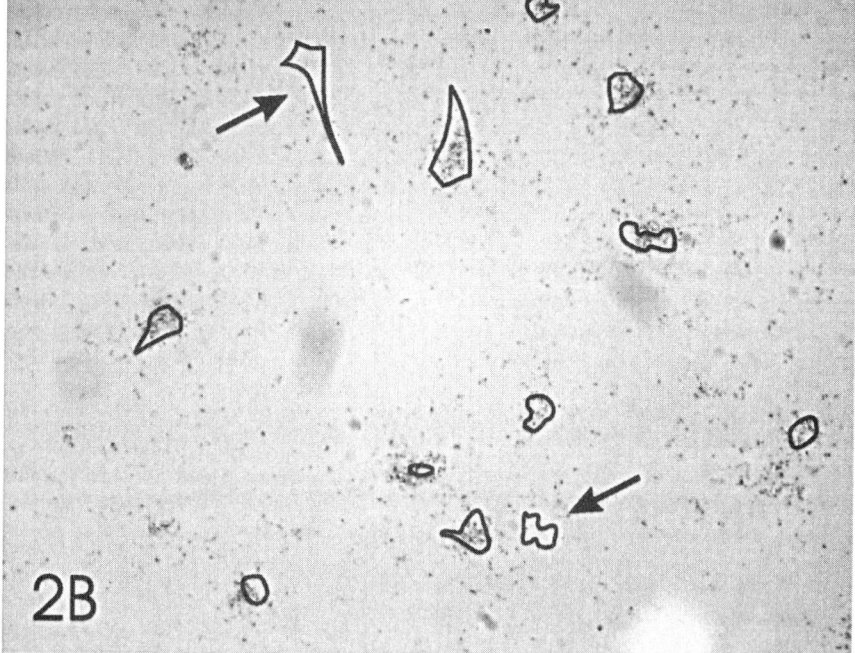

REFERENCES

1. CHESSELET, M.F. & J.M. DELFS. 1996. Basal ganglia and movement disorders: an update. Trends Neurosci. **19:** 417–422.
2. PARENT, A. & L.N. HAZRATI. 1995. Functional anatomy of the basal ganglia. II. The place of subthalamic nucleus and external pallidum in basal ganglia circuitry. Brain Res. Rev. **20:** 128–154.
3. STAINES, W.A., S. ATMADJA & H.C. FIBIGER. 1981. Demonstration of a pallido-striatal pathway by retrograde transport of HRP-labeled lectin. Brain Res. **206:** 446–450.
4. KITA, H. & S.T. KITAI. 1994. The morphology of globus pallidus projection neurons in the rat: an intracellular staining study. Brain Res. **636:** 308–319.
5. YOUNG, W.S., T.I. BONNER & M.R. BRANN. 1986. Mesencephalic dopamine neurons regulate the expression of neuropeptide mRNAs in the rat forebrain. Proc. Natl. Acad. Sci. USA **83:** 9827–9831.

FIGURE 2. Double-labeling for Fluorogold and ENK mRNA in one section through globus pallidus at 10× magnification. Fluorogold injection site was in rostral caudate-putamen. **(A)** With epifluorescent illumination, retrogradely labeled pallido-striatal neurons are visible. **(B)** Outline of fluorescent neurons from (A) is superimposed on image obtained with transmitted light illumination showing aggregates of silver grains indicating the presence of ENK mRNA-containing GP neurons. *Arrows* point to pallido-striatal neurons not labeled for ENK mRNA.

Terminals from the Rat Prefrontal Cortex Synapse on Mesoaccumbens VTA Neurons

DAVID B. CARR AND SUSAN R. SESACK[a]

Departments of Neuroscience and Psychiatry, University of Pittsburgh, Pittsburgh, Pennsylvania 15260, USA

The firing rates and patterns of dopamine (DA) neurons in the ventral tegmental area (VTA) are dependent, at least in part, on glutamatergic input.[1] One of the principal glutamatergic inputs to the VTA arises from the prefrontal cortex (PFC).[2] This PFC input to the VTA regulates the output of ascending DA projections, as PFC stimulation increases levels of extracellular DA in the nucleus accumbens (NAc),[3,4] while inactivation of the PFC produces the opposite effect.[4] These actions may be due to direct monosynaptic inputs from PFC neurons to DA cells in the VTA. For example, stimulation of the PFC increases burst firing of DA neurons,[4,5] while inactivation of the PFC reduces burst firing in these cells.[4] Furthermore, our previous anatomical experiments have demonstrated that afferents from the PFC synapse upon both DA and non-DA neurons within the VTA.[2]

The efferent targets of the VTA neurons that receive direct input from the PFC are not known. PFC afferents may target VTA neurons that project to the NAc, as the distribution of PFC terminals in the VTA is similar to the location of neurons that project to the NAc.[2,6] In addition, increases in DA levels in the NAc produced by PFC stimulation are blocked by the administration of glutamate receptor antagonists within the VTA, but not within the NAc.[3] Based on this evidence, we hypothesize that PFC terminals form direct synaptic connections onto mesoaccumbens DA neurons.

In addition to the well-characterized DA-containing mesolimbic pathway, the VTA also sends a γ-aminobutyric acid (GABA)-containing projection to the NAc.[7] As the majority of PFC terminals within the VTA synapse on non-DA containing neurons,[2] and as PFC stimulation produces excitatory effects in non-DA neurons,[8] we hypothesize that PFC terminals in the VTA may also target GABA-containing mesoaccumbens neurons.

To examine these questions, anterograde labeling of PFC afferents with biotinylated dextran amine (BDA) and retrograde labeling of mesoaccumbens VTA neurons with Fluorogold (FG) was combined with immunohistochemistry for tyrosine hydroxylase (TH) or GABA. A dual-labeling electron microscopic method was used in which mesoaccumbens VTA neurons labeled with FG and PFC afferents labeled by BDA were visualized with immunoperoxidase labeling, and the neurotransmitter phenotype of retrogradely labeled VTA neurons was determined by immunogold-silver labeling for TH or GABA.

---

[a]Corresponding author: Susan R. Sesack, Ph.D. Department of Neuroscience, 446 Crawford Hall, University of Pittsburgh, Pittsburgh, PA 15260. Voice: 412-624-5158; fax: 412-624-9198; Sesack@brain.bns.pitt.edu

Within the VTA, PFC terminals labeled by BDA transport formed asymmetric synaptic contacts primarily onto unlabeled dendrites. PFC terminals also synapsed onto dendrites singly labeled for TH or GABA. In tissue labeled for FG and GABA, PFC terminals occasionally synapsed onto dendrites that contained FG retrogradely transported from the NAc, and typically these dendrites were also labeled for GABA. However, in tissue labeled for FG and TH, the dendrites that both received synaptic input from a PFC terminal and contained FG retrogradely transported from the NAc were typically immunonegative for TH. In one case, a PFC terminal was observed to synapse on a dendrite that contained both retrogradely transported FG and immunoreactivity for TH.

These data provide the first anatomical demonstration that PFC afferents to the VTA synapse directly onto the dendrites of mesoaccumbens projection neurons. As such, our findings are consistent with physiological reports of excitatory effects of PFC stimulation on DA[4,5] and non-DA[8] neurons. Our preliminary investigation of phenotype suggests that PFC terminals preferentially target mesoaccumbens neurons that utilize GABA as a neurotransmitter. However, this preliminary investigation must be substantiated by a more extensive analysis of the tissue generated for this study. Furthermore, technical limitations that may have contributed to early data need to be ruled out. Nevertheless, these data are intriguing, since the majority of mesoaccumbens VTA neurons are dopaminergic,[6] and a random distribution of PFC terminals to TH- versus GABA-containing mesoaccumbens cells should have produced a greater incidence of synaptic input to TH-positive neurons.

The circuitry of the VTA that is being revealed by the present investigation has important implications in understanding the regulation of dopamine transmission in the NAc. In addition, PFC terminals may also contact DA- and GABA-containing VTA neurons that project to other sites. Preliminary data from our laboratory indicate that one target for these neurons is the PFC itself (Carr & Sesack, unpublished observations). Although future investigation will be required to thoroughly address this issue, such an interaction may represent an important regulatory feedback pathway between these two areas.

ACKNOWLEDGMENTS

This work is supported by USPHS Grants MH11368 (DBC) and MH50314 (SRS).

REFERENCES

1. GRACE, A.A. & B.S. BUNNEY. 1995. Electrophysiological properties of midbrain dopamine neurons. *In* Psychopharmacology: The Fourth Generation of Progress. F. E. Bloom & D. J. Kupfer, Eds.: 163–177. Raven Press. New York.
2. SESACK, S.R. & V.M. PICKEL. 1992. Prefrontal cortical efferents in the rat synapse on unlabeled neuronal targets of catecholamine terminals in the nucleus accumbens septi and on dopamine neurons in the ventral tegmental area. J. Comp. Neurol. **320:** 145–160.
3. KARREMAN, M. & B. MOGHADDAM. 1996. The prefrontal cortex regulates the basal release of dopamine in the limbic striatum: an effect mediated by ventral tegmental area. J. Neurochem. **66:** 589–598.

4. MURASE, S. *et al.* 1993. Prefrontal cortex regulates burst firing and transmitter release in rat mesolimbic dopamine neurons studied *in vivo*. Neurosci. Lett. **157:** 53–56.
5. TONG, Z.-Y., P.G. OVERTON & D. CLARK. 1996. Stimulation of the prefrontal cortex in the rat induces patterns of activity in midbrain dopaminergic neurons which resemble natural burst events. Synapse **22:** 195–208.
6. Swanson, L.W. 1982. The projections of the ventral tegmental area and adjacent regions: a combined fluorescent retrograde tracer and immunofluorescence study in the rat. Brain Res. Bull. **9:** 321–353.
7. VAN BOCKSTAELE, E.J. & V.M. PICKEL. 1995. GABA-containing neurons in the ventral tegmental area project to nucleus accumbens in rat brain. Brain Res. **682:** 215–221.
8. TONG, Z.-Y. *et al.* 1998. Do non-dopaminergic neurons in the ventral tegmental area play a role in the responses elicited in A10 dopaminergic neurons by electrical stimulation of the prefrontal cortex? Exp. Brain Res. **118:** 466–476.

Dopamine D_4 Receptors Are Strategically Localized for Primary Involvement in the Presynaptic Effects of Dopamine in the Rat Nucleus Accumbens Shell

ADENA L. SVINGOS,[a] SUNDARI PERIASAMY, AND VIRGINIA M. PICKEL

Department of Neurology and Neuroscience, Division of Neurobiology, Cornell University Medical College, New York, New York 10021, USA

INTRODUCTION

Clozapine, an atypical neuroleptic, ameliorates the symptoms of schizophrenia without causing the motor impairments associated with typical antipsychotic drugs.[4] Clozapine also has a relatively higher affinity for D_4 receptors, as compared to other dopamine receptors.[9] The therapeutic efficacy of clozapine may be associated with D_4 receptor-mediated modulation of dopamine transmission in distinct anatomical areas, including the nucleus accumbens shell (AcbSh).[8] The present study used immunoperoxidase labeling of the D_4 receptor and immunogold-silver labeling of tyrosine hydroxylase (TH) to examine (1) the cellular sites for D_4 receptor activation, and (2) whether D_4 receptors are localized to modulate the presynaptic release of dopamine in this brain region.

MATERIALS AND METHODS

Antisera

A rabbit antipeptide antibody (amino acids 176–185) raised against the D_4 receptor N-terminus[2] (R&D Antibodies, Berkeley, CA), and a monoclonal antiserum raised in mouse against TH (Incstar, Stillwater, MN) were used to immunocytochemically detect the receptor and dopaminergic afferents, respectively.

Tissue Preparation

Briefly, 9 adult male Sprague-Dawley rats were anesthetized and perfused through the aorta with acrolein (3.75%) and paraformaldehyde (2%) in phosphate buffer. Vibratome sections (30–40 μm) were incubated in 1% sodium borohydride, rinsed in Tris-buffered saline (TBS), and incubated in 1% bovine serum albumin (BSA).

---

[a]Corresponding author: Dr. Adena L. Svingos, Department of Neurology and Neuroscience, Division of Neurobiology, Cornell University Medical College, 411 E. 69th Street, New York, NY 10021. Voice: 212-570-2900; fax: 212-988-3672; asvingos@mail.med.cornell.edu

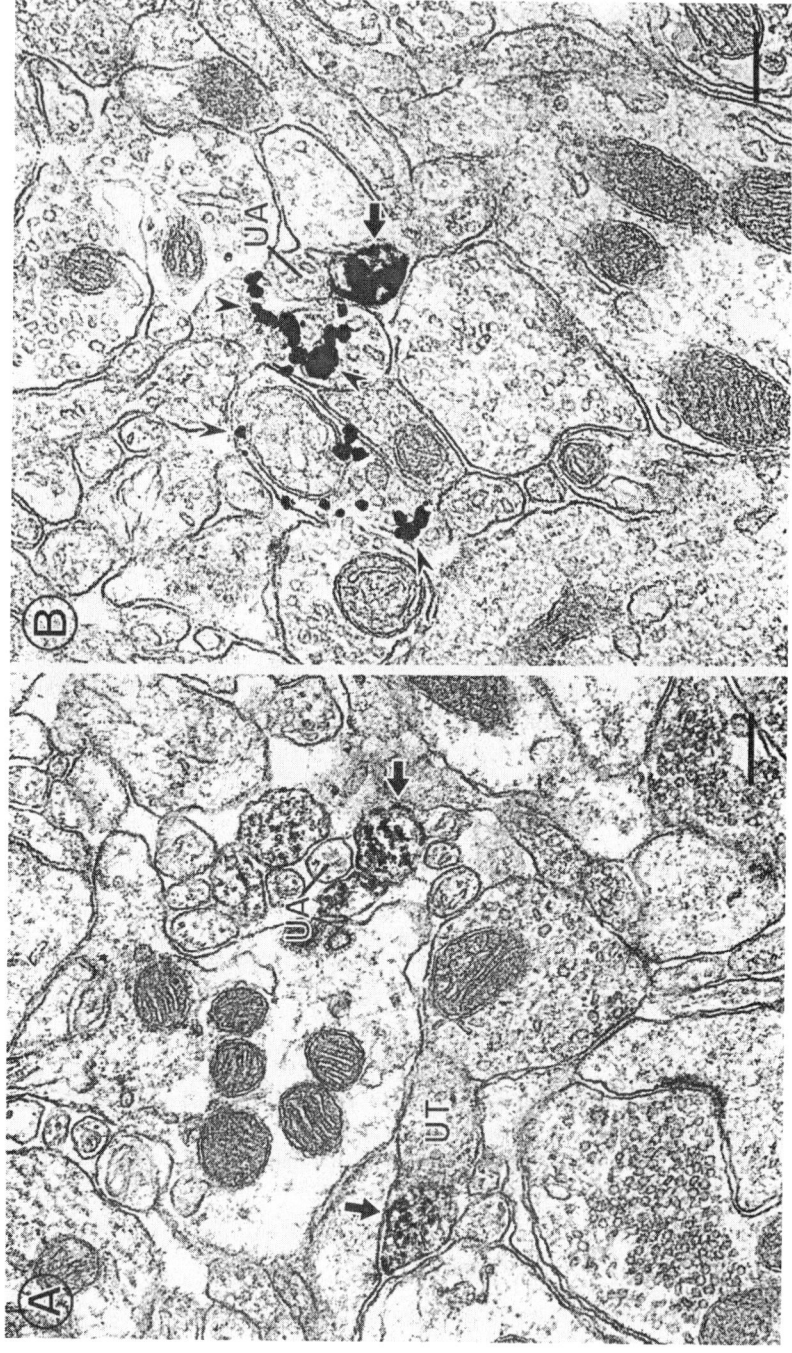

Immunocytochemistry

Tissue sections were incubated for 48 hours at 4°C in a solution containing the D_4 receptor antibody (1:10,000) for single labeling, or antisera for the D_4 receptor (1:8,000) and TH (1:3,000) for dual labeling in 0.1% BSA/TBS. For peroxidase detection of the D_4 receptor, the avidin-biotin complex (ABC) method was used. Tissue sections were incubated for (1) 30 min in rabbit biotinylated immunoglobulin G (IgG, 1:400), (2) 30 min in ABC (1:100), and (3) 6 min in a solution of 3,3'-diaminobenzidine and H_2O_2 in 0.1 M TBS. For immunogold-silver detection of TH, tissue sections were (1) incubated for 2 hr in mouse colloidal gold IgG (1:50), (2) fixed in 2% glutaraldehyde, and (3) reacted with a silver solution. On completion of immunolabeling, sections were processed for electron microscopy.[1]

RESULTS

Axon Terminals and Axons

Of all D_4 receptor-labeled profiles, 65% were axon terminals and axons. D_4 receptor labeling was prominently localized to plasma and vesicular membranes of morphologically heterogenous axon terminals that either formed punctate junctions or lacked synaptic specializations. Of all D_4 receptor-immunoreactive terminals and axons examined in tissue processed for dual labeling, 56% apposed TH-labeled terminals, and 17% also contained TH (FIG. 1).

Dendrites and Dendritic Spines

Twenty-two percent of D_4 receptor-immunoreactive profiles were dendrites and dendritic spines, some of which were contacted by TH-containing terminals. D_4 labeling most often was localized to segments of the plasma membrane, including postsynaptic densities of spines, but also was associated with cytoplasmic organelles, including the smooth endoplasmic reticulum of dendrites.

Astrocytic Processes

Thirteen percent of D_4 receptor labeling was associated with of glial processes, which were interspersed among various unlabeled profiles.

FIGURE 1. Electron micrographs showing D_4 receptor immunoreactivity localized to axons and axon terminals that appose unlabeled and TH-labeled terminals. (**A**) shows peroxidase immunoreactivity for the D_4 receptor associated with plasma and vesicular membranes of small axon terminals and unmyelinated axons (*small arrows*) that are apposed by unlabeled terminals (UT) and axons (UA). (**B**) shows an axon with intense peroxidase reaction product for the D_4 receptor (*small arrow*) apposed to a terminal containing immunogold-silver particles for TH (*arrowheads*) and an unlabeled axon (UA). In the same field, another axon terminal contains gold-silver particles for TH (*arrowheads*). Scale bars = 0.2 µm.

DISCUSSION

The results of the present study are the first to show that in the AcbSh, D_4 receptors primarily are localized to modulate presynaptic nondopaminergic neurotransmission.

D_4 Receptors Primarily Are Localized to Regulate Presynaptic Neurotransmitter Release

D_4 receptor immunoreactivity was prominently localized to plasma and vesicular membranes of morphologically heterogenous terminals. These data suggest that activation of D_4 receptors may modulate the release of various neurotransmitters.[3]

D_4 Receptors Are Localized to Modulate Postsynaptic Responses

D_4 receptor immunoreactivity was associated with synaptic and nonsynaptic sites along plasma membranes of dendrites and dendritic spines, suggesting that D_4 receptors may modulate postsynaptic responses within inhibitory-type neurons.[6]

Sites for D_4 Receptor and Dopamine Interactions

D_4 receptor immunoreactivity was seen in axons that mainly apposed TH-labeled terminals but also was observed in terminals containing TH, suggesting that the D_4 receptor primarily functions as a heteroreceptor but also mediates the release of dopamine.[5] D_4 receptor-labeled dendrites and dendritic spines were apposed to TH-immunoreactive terminals, suggesting that postsynaptic responses to dopamine may be modulated by D_4 receptors.[7]

ACKNOWLEDGMENTS

This work was supported by a grant from the Stanley Foundation to A.L.S. and by NIMH Grants MH 00078 and 40342 to V.M.P.

REFERENCES

1. CHAN, J. et al. 1990. Optimization of differential immunogold-silver and peroxidase labeling with maintenance of ultrastructure in brain sections before plastic embedding. J. Neurosci. Methods **33:** 169–181.
2. HARLAN, R.E. et al. 1996. Characterization of antibodies to dopamine D_4 receptors in the rat brain. Soc. Neurosci. Abstr. **22:** 825.
3. GARDNER, E.L. et al. 1994. Clozapine produces potent antidopaminergic effects anatomically specific to mesolimbic system. J. Clin. Psychiatry **55:** 15–22.
4. MELTZER, H.Y. 1994. An overview of the mechanism of action of clozapine. J. Clin. Psychiatry **55:** 47–52.
5. MOGHADDAM, B. & B.S. BUNNY. 1990. Acute effects of typical and atypical antipsychotic drugs on the release of dopamine from prefrontal cortex, nucleus accumbens, and striatum of the rat: an in vivo microdialysis study. J. Neurochem. **54:** 1755–1760.
6. MRZLJAK, L. et al. 1996. Localization of dopamine D4 receptors in GABAergic neurons of the primate brain. Nature **381:** 245–248.

7. OLNEY, J.W. & N.B. FARBER. 1995. Glutamate receptor dysfunction and schizophrenia. Arch. Gen. Psychiatry **52**: 998–1007.
8. ONN, S.P. & A.A. GRACE. 1995. Repeated treatment with haloperidol and clozapine exerts differential effects on dye coupling between neurons in subregions of striatum and nucleus accumbens. J. Neurosci. **15**: 7024–7036.
9. VAN TOL, H.H.M. *et al.* 1991. Cloning of the gene for a human dopamine D4 receptor with high affinity for the antipsychotic drug clozapine. Nature **350**: 610–614.

Glutamatergic Modulation of Subcortical Motor and Limbic Circuits

DANIEL J. HEALY[a] AND JAMES H. MEADOR-WOODRUFF

Mental Health Research Institute, Department of Psychiatry, University of Michigan, Ann Arbor, Michigan 48109-0720, USA

The ventral striatum is a critical component of parallel circuits associated with motor and limbic functions, termed the corticostriatopallidothalamic circuit (CSPT).[1] The interconnectivity of the regions comprising these circuits is believed to mediate the processing of sensory information that leads to the modulation of both motor and limbic behaviors. This well-defined circuitry allows for the neurochemical anatomical examination of functionally integrated regions. The striatum is one of the critical integrative areas in the CSPT because of the convergence of its glutamatergic and dopaminergic afferents, and the modulatory effects of its efferents.[1]

Corticostriatal glutamate projections synapse on mesostriatal dopaminergic projections, and modulate dopamine release in the dorsal and ventral striatum.[2] Modulators of all four glutamate receptor subtypes—NMDA, AMPA, kainate, and metabotropic—affect dopamine release in dorsal and ventral striatum. We previously reported that systemic treatment with the NMDA receptor antagonist MK-801 alters D_2 receptor mRNA in the ventral tegmental area (VTA) but not the substantia nigra, pars compacta (SNc), or in the dorsal or ventral striatum.[2] These data suggest that NMDA receptors exert a tonic effect on dopamine autoreceptor expression preferentially in limbic regions. We now present data from a follow-up experiment to determine the effects of other glutamate receptor modulators on dopamine receptor expression in caudate-putamen (CPu), nucleus accumbens, core (core), and nucleus accumbens, shell (shell).

Sprague-Dawley male rates (225–275 g) were treated with seven daily injections of CNQX (an antagonist of both AMPA and kainate receptors), GYKI52466 (an AMPA receptor desensitization facilitator), riluzole (a glutamate release inhibitor), or DMSO (vehicle), and rats were sacrificed 24 hours after the last injection.[3] Ten animals were treated per group. *In situ* histochemistry for preprodynorphin and preproenkephalin transcripts, and D_1 and D_2 receptor mRNAs was performed as previously described.[2] Results are shown in FIGURE 1. D_1 and opioid peptide precursor mRNA were not affected by any of the treatments, while D_2 mRNA was significantly decreased by riluzole and GYKI52466 treatments.

Riluzole and GYKI52466 equally decreased the expression of D_2 receptors in both dorsal and ventral striatal regions. This is in contrast to the effects of MK-801,[2] and suggests that our previously reported results after NMDA receptor antagonist

---

[a]Corresponding author: Daniel J. Healy, M.D., Mental Health Research Institute, Dept. of Psychiatry, University of Michigan, 205 Zina Pitcher Place, Ann Arbor, MI 48109-0720. Voice: 734-936-2061; fax: 734-647-4130; drdan@umich.edu

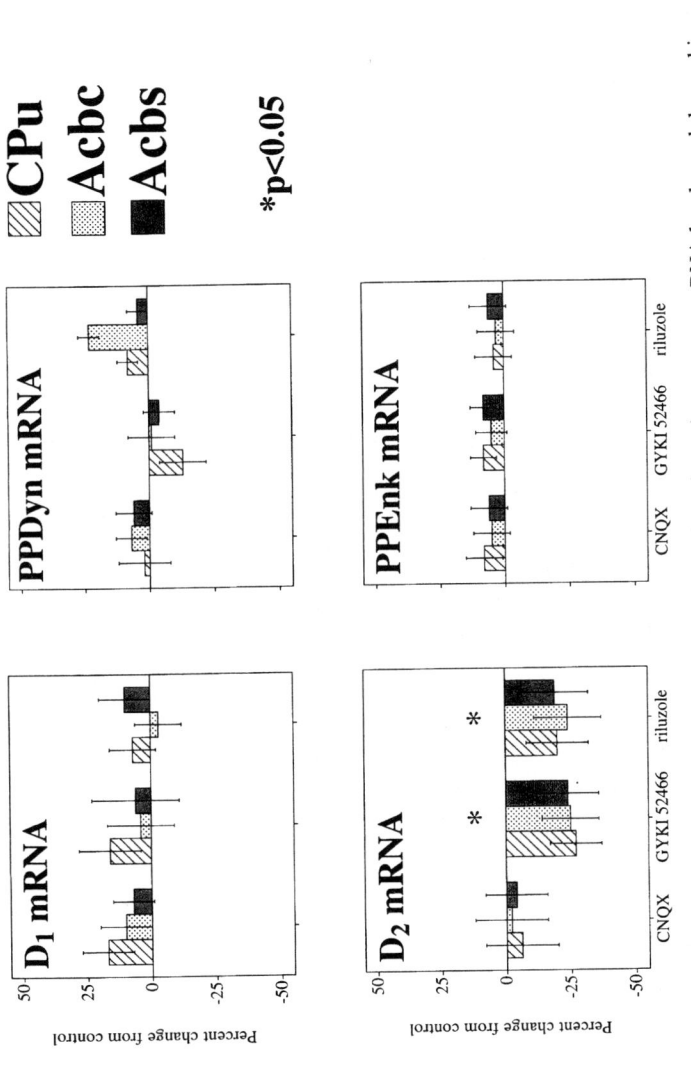

FIGURE 1. Effects of CNQX, GYKI52466, and riluzole on D_1 and D_2 dopamine receptor mRNA levels, and dynorphin and enkephalin peptide precursor mRNA levels in the caudate-putamen (CPu), nucleus accumbens core (Acbc), and nucleus accumbens shell (Acbs). Data are reported as percent change from control.

treatment do not represent a general property of ionotropic glutamate receptor blockade, but may be subtype specific.

D_2 mRNA levels were decreased by GYKI52466 but not CNQX, indicating that the less selective AMPA and kainate receptor antagonist had a different effect than the more selective AMPA receptor antagonist. Perhaps the different synaptic localization of AMPA and kainate receptors is associated with this pattern. Kainate receptors are predominantly presynaptic autoreceptors, while AMPA receptors are predominantly postsynaptic.[3] Modulation of autoreceptors and postsynaptic receptors by CNQX may affect overall glutamatergic activity differently than GYKI52466, which may not induce alterations in striatal dopamine receptor expression. However, riluzole would be expected to have similar effects to CNQX, if this is due to concomitant autoreceptor and postsynaptic effects. The change in presynaptic release of glutamate would be expected to affect activity of postsynaptic glutamate receptors, but riluzole had an effect similar to a relatively selective AMPA receptor antagonist. There appears to be a complicated pattern of regulation that requires further elucidation.

Opioid peptide precursor levels did not change, although we only measured mRNA levels. There are multiple levels of regulation for the expression of fully processed endogenous opioid peptides; it is possible that these drugs affected opioid peptide expression, but we could not detect it with *in situ* histochemistry. Likewise, this study does not address whether the mRNA levels of the D_1 and D_2 dopamine receptors reflect final receptor protein levels. These questions are important because the intrinsic striatal circuitry suggests that D_2 receptor and enkephalin expression should both be affected. There are direct and indirect striatal efferent pathways that participate in the balance of striatal activity.[4] The direct pathway is comprised of dopaminergic projections from SNc and VTA to the CPu, core, and shell, and reciprocal striatal projections directly back to the substantia nigra, pars reticulata (SNr) or VTA.[4] The indirect pathway also serves as a feedback loop, but involves several other regions. CPu neurons project to the globus pallidus, which in turn sends GABAergic projections to the subthalamic nucleus.[4] Glutamatergic neurons in this nucleus project back to the SNr directly, completing the loop.[4] Core and shell neurons both project to the ventral pallidum, and then back to the SNr or VTA. Activation of the direct and indirect pathways appears to have opposite electrophysiological effects on midbrain dopaminergic neurons.[4] Further, the striatal neurons in the direct and indirect pathways differ phenotypically from each other. CPu cells of the direct pathway express the D_1 receptor and prodynorphin, while those that project to the pallidum express D_2 receptors and proenkephalin-derived peptides.[5] The colocalization of dopamine receptor subtype and neuropeptide is more strongly associated with motor than limbic function, as this colocalization appears to break down in the shell.[6] In addition, the identification of a striatal neuron as being part of the indirect or direct circuit based on D_1 versus D_2 expression also seems to breakdown in core and shell.[7] D_1 receptors are expressed in both direct and indirect pathway neurons, though D_2 expression is limited to the indirect pathway.[7] Still, altered expression of these receptors may reflect a differential activation of these two pathways, providing a neurochemical anatomical basis to examine the direct and indirect pathways. Our findings of changes in D_2—but not D_1—receptor expression would be consistent with a preferential effect of AMPA receptor modulation of the indirect striatal efferent pathways.

REFERENCES

1. CARLSSON, M. & A. CARLSSON. 1990. Schizophrenia: a subcortical neurotransmitter imbalance syndrome? Schizophr. Bull. **16:** 425–432.
2. HEALY, D.J. & J.H. MEADOR-WOODRUFF. 1996. Differential regulation, by MK-801, of dopamine receptor gene expression in rat nigrostriatal and mesocorticolimbic systems. Brain Res. **708:** 38–44.
3. WHEAL, H.V. & A.M. THOMSON. 1995. Excitatory Amino Acids and Synaptic Neurotransmission. Academic Press. London.
4. KALIVAS, P.W. & C.D. BARNES. 1993. Limbic Motor Circuits and Neuropsychiatry. CRC Press. Boca Raton, FL.
5. GERFEN, C.R. 1992. The neostriatal mosaic: multiple levels of compartmentalization. Trends Neurosci. **15:** 133–139.
6. CURRAN, E.J. & S.J. WATSON. 1995. Dopamine receptor mRNA expression patterns by opioid peptide cells in the nucleus accumbens of the rat: a double *in situ* hybridization study. J. Comp. Neurol. **361:** 57–76.
7. LU, X.Y., M.B. GHASEMZADEH & P.W. KALIVAS. 1998. Expression of D_1 receptor, D_2 receptor, substance P, and enkephalin messenger RNAs in the neurons projecting from the nucleus accumbens. Neuroscience **82:** 767–780.

Modulation of Ventral Tegmental Area Dopamine Cell Activity by the Ventral Subiculum and Entorhinal Cortex

CHRISTOPHER L. TODD[a,c,d] AND ANTHONY A. GRACE[a,b,c,e]

Departments of [a]Neuroscience and [b]Psychiatry, [c]Center for Neuroscience, University of Pittsburgh, Pittsburgh, Pennsylvania 15260, USA

The nucleus accumbens (NAC) is at the core of a circuit that is in a strategic position to relay information about motivation, drive and affective state to motor systems, thus providing a link "from motivation to action"[7] that is necessary for any animal to display goal-directed behavior. The NAC receives input from several limbic structures, most notably the amygdala, hippocampal formation (via the ventral subiculum; vSub) and medial prefrontal cortex (mPFC), and innervates the ventral pallidum (VP), subpallidal area (SP), and substantia nigra (SN), which provide inputs to motor structures. The ventral tegmental area (VTA) supplies a dopaminergic (DA) input to several nuclei in this circuit, and it has been shown repeatedly that DA in the NAC plays an essential role in the functioning of this circuit. For example, the locomotor response that can be induced by the infusion of amphetamine or DA agonists into the NAC or by the infusion of NMDA into the vSub can be blocked by DA antagonists in the NAC.[7] Furthermore, electrical stimulation of the mPFC,[10] amygdala, or vSub[1,2] increase DA levels in the NAC, but it is not yet clear to what extent this release is mediated at the cell body or at the terminal. Relatively few studies have directly analyzed the influence of this circuit on VTA DA cell activity, which is surprising given the prominent inputs to the VTA from several of these structures, in particular the mPFC, NAC, and VP/SP. Given the complex actions of DA in this circuit, understanding how this circuit modulates VTA DA cell activity may lend further insight into the role played by DA in the modulation of goal-directed behavior.

In this study, single-unit recordings were made from physiologically identified VTA DA neurons[3] in chloral hydrate-anesthetized rats. NMDA (0.75 µg), TTX (1 µM), or vehicle (Dulbecco's buffer) was infused into the vSub or entorhinal cortex (EC) in 0.5 µL aliquots over a period of two minutes. Immediately following infusion, a recording electrode was lowered into the VTA. The relative proportion of DA neurons firing was determined by counting the number of spontaneously firing DA neurons encountered in nine electrode tracks made through the VTA in a predefined stereotaxic pattern, with each electrode track separated by 200 µm. The order in which the tracks were made was psuedo-random. Each neuron was recorded for 2–3 minutes to determine the mean firing rate and mean percentage of spikes fired in

---

[d]Corresponding author: Christopher L. Todd, Dept. of Neuroscience, 446 Crawford Hall, University of Pittsburgh, Pittsburgh, PA 15260. Voice: 412-624-7332; fax: 412-624-9198; Todd@neurosci.bns.pitt.edu

[e]Voice: 412-624-4609; fax: 412-624-9198; Grace@bns.pitt.edu

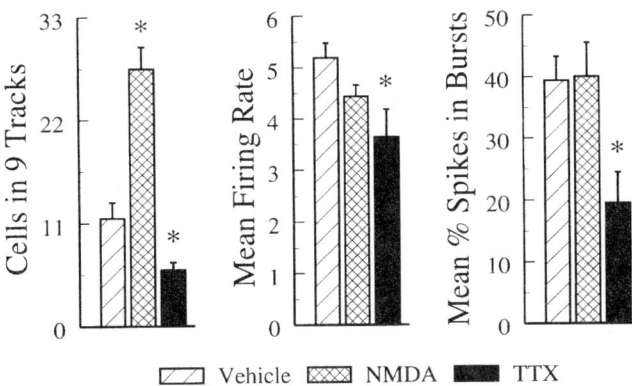

FIGURE 1. The effects of vSub/EC stimulation or inhibition on VTA DA cell activity. Mean firing rate is in spikes/sec. All values are mean ± SEM. *, $p < 0.05$ compared to vehicle group.

bursts (%SIB). In some rats, 10 μg/1.0 μL kynurenic acid (KYN) was infused into the NAC shell a few minutes prior to infusion of 0.75 μg NMDA or vehicle into the vSub.

Chemical stimulation of the vSub or EC by NMDA infusion markedly increased the number of spontaneously firing DA neurons encountered in the VTA (FIG. 1) while having little effect on their baseline firing rate or pattern. In contrast, chemical inhibition of the vSub or EC by infusion of TTX markedly decreased the number of spontaneously firing VTA DA neurons, in addition to causing a substantial decrease in the percentage of spikes these neurons fired in bursts. Our preliminary experiments suggest that these effects are mediated via the NAC, as infusion of the glutamate receptor antagonist kynurenic acid (KYNA) into the NAC blocked the effect of vSub NMDA infusion (15 DA cells/9 tracks, mean firing rate = 5.6 spikes/sec, mean %SIB = 46.4, $n = 1$ rat). In contrast, infusion of KYNA into the NAC alone resulted in 12 cells in 9 tracks with a mean firing rate of 7.7 spikes/sec and 65.8% SIB ($n = 1$ rat). There was no evidence that the number of cells encountered per electrode track changed over the course of sampling the VTA, which typically took 3–4 hours, since these effects were observed to be consistent across all nine electrode tracks (data not shown).

The present study demonstrates that the vSub and EC provide substantial modulatory control over VTA DA neuron activity, and that this effect may be mediated via the vSub/EC projection to the NAC. Furthermore, the increase in VTA DA cell firing rate and burst firing seen when KYNA was infused into the NAC (in the absence of vSub/EC NMDA infusion) is consistent with data showing that this manipulation increases extracellular DA levels in the NAC.[10] Thus, the vSub is in a position to facilitate goal-directed behavior not only by directly gating information flow through NAC neurons,[8] but also by potently modulating DA cell activity and, thus, DA input to the NAC. An increase in DA in the NAC would be expected to suppress excitatory synaptic input to these cells[9] while exerting state-dependent effects on NAC neuron membrane potential.[4] These actions, combined with the actions of DA on NMDA receptor function,[6] may serve to selectively enhance the relative efficacy of less well-established synaptic inputs to influence NAC cell activity. In this manner, DA-induced synaptic plasticity in the NAC would serve to enhance behavioral flexibility. Recent reports that DA neurons recorded in behaving monkeys emit a 'teaching' signal[5] are consistent with this view. Furthermore, dysfunction within this circuit, as may occur in schizophrenia, might be expected to result in an inappropriate selection of behaviors given the context and affective state of the individual.

REFERENCES

1. BLAHA, C.D. *et al.* 1997. Stimulation of the ventral subiculum of the hippocampus evokes glutamate receptor-mediated changes in dopamine efflux in the rat nucleus accumbens. Eur. J. Neurosci. **9:** 902–911.
2. FLORESCO, S.B. *et al.* 1998. Basolateral amygdala stimulation evokes glutamate receptor-dependent dopamine efflux in the nucleus accumbens of the anesthetized rat. Eur. J. Neurosci. **10:** 1241–1251.
3. GRACE, A.A. & B.S. BUNNEY. 1983. Intracellular and extracellular electrophysiology of nigral dopaminergic neurons. 1. Identification and characterization. Neuroscience **10:** 301–315.
4. HERNANDEZ-LOPEZ, S. *et al.* 1997. D1 receptor activation enhances evoked discharge in neostriatal medium spiny neurons by modulating an L-type Ca^{+2} conductance. J. Neurosci. **17(9):** 3334–3342.
5. HOLLERMAN, J.R. & W. SCHULTZ. 1998. Dopamine neurons report an error in the temporal prediction of reward during learning. Nat. Neurosci. **1:** 304–309.
6. LEVINE, M.S. *et al.* 1996. Neuromodulatory actions of dopamine on synaptically-evoked neostriatal responses in slices. Synapse **24:** 65–78.
7. MOGENSON, G.J. *et al.* 1993. From motivation to action: a review of dopaminergic regulation of limbic→nucleus accumbens→ventral pallidum→pedunculopontine nucleus circuitries involved in limbic-motor integration. *In* Limbic Motor Circuits in Neuropsychiatry. P.W. Kalivas & C.D. Barnes, Eds.: 193–236. CRC Press. Boca Raton, FL.
8. O'DONNELL, P. & A.A. GRACE. 1995. Synaptic interactions among excitatory afferents to nucleus accumbens neurons: hippocampal gating of prefrontal cortical input. J. Neurosci. **15(5):** 3622–3639.
9. O'DONNELL, P. & A.A. GRACE. 1994. Tonic D_2-mediated attenuation of cortical excitation in nucleus accumbens neurons recorded *in vitro*. Brain Res. **634:** 105–112.
10. TABER, M.T. & H.C. FIBIGER. 1995. Electrical stimulation of the prefrontal cortex increases dopamine release in the nucleus accumbens of the rat: modulation by metabotropic glutamate receptors. J. Neurosci. **15:** 3896–3904.

Electrophysiological Properties of Anatomically Identified Ventral Pallidal Neurons in Rat Brain Slices

C. PETER BENGTSON AND PEREGRINE B. OSBORNE[a]

Department of Physiology and Pharmacology, The University of Queensland, Brisbane, Qld 4072, Australia

Remarkably little is known about the functional properties of pallidal neurons despite the critical role these cells have in determining the output from the striatopallidal system. For example, the ventral pallidum has been studied extensively using extracellular recording (e.g., Napier, this volume) but the electrophysiological properties of the neurons have been described using higher resolution techniques in only a single *in vivo* intracellular microelectrode recording study.[1]

To address this situation, and as a prelude to *in vitro* pharmacological studies in the future, we have used patch clamp techniques to record from ventral pallidal neurons visualized in brain slices with DIC-IR optics. The slices were prepared using standard methods from rats aged 6–16 days that had been anesthetized with halothane and decapitated. The electrode solutions contained Neurobiotin in order to fill neurons during recordings so that they could subsequently be selectively stained and visualized in fixed slices, and also immunostained for choline acetyltransferase (ChAT).

Viewing brain slices with DIC-IR optics showed that medium neurons with soma diameters around 15 μm were the most abundant neurons in the ventral pallidum, but that significant numbers of much larger and smaller cells were also present. By recording from a range of different sized neurons in voltage-clamp and using a hyperpolarizing voltage step protocol we identified three basic cell types. The medium neurons ($n = 88$) characteristically had a prominent h-current (FIG. 1, top right): an inwardly rectifying current that slowly activated over approximately 1 sec and was blocked by extracellular cesium ions (2 mM, $n = 6$). Large neurons ($n = 32$) showed a pronounced inwardly rectifying potassium current at hyperpolarized potentials (FIG. 1, middle right) that activated instantaneously and was blocked by extracellular barium ions (200 μM, $n = 3$). In contrast a majority of small neurons ($n = 18$) had little or no rectifying currents (FIG. 1, bottom right).

Confocal microscope images representing the major three cell types are also shown in FIGURE 1 (left panels). Medium neurons generally had triangular shaped somata (FIG. 1, top left) with large primary dendrites and had a sparse-to-medium covering of spines. ChAT staining showed that these were noncholinergic (2/16 ChAT positive). Large neurons were multipolar cells (FIG. 1, middle left) that also had spiny dendrites, but were cholinergic (11/12 ChAT positive). Small cells were more diverse in their morphologies (FIG. 1, bottom left), but most commonly had a

---

[a]Corresponding author. Voice: +617-3365-4757; fax: 617-3365-1766; osborne@plpk.uq.edu.au

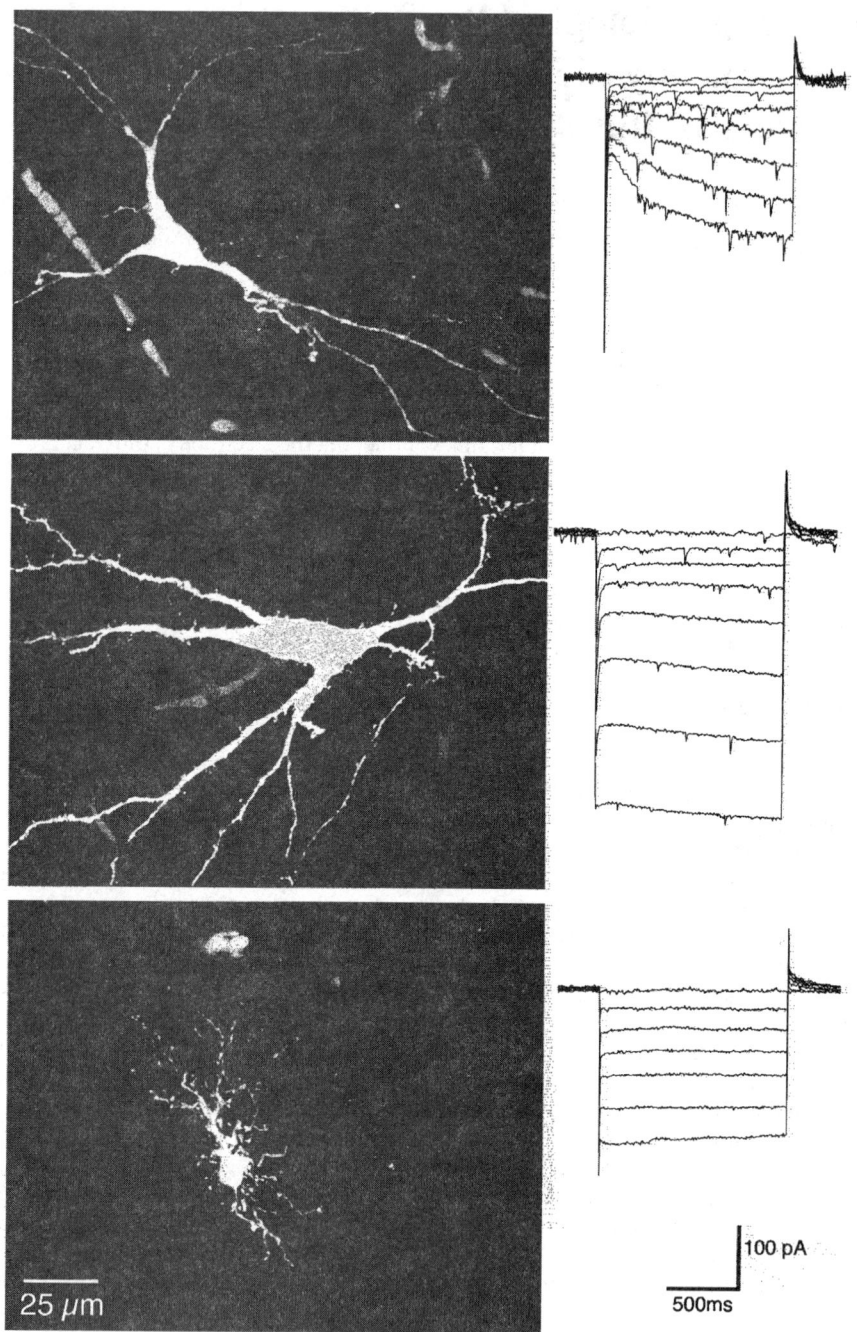

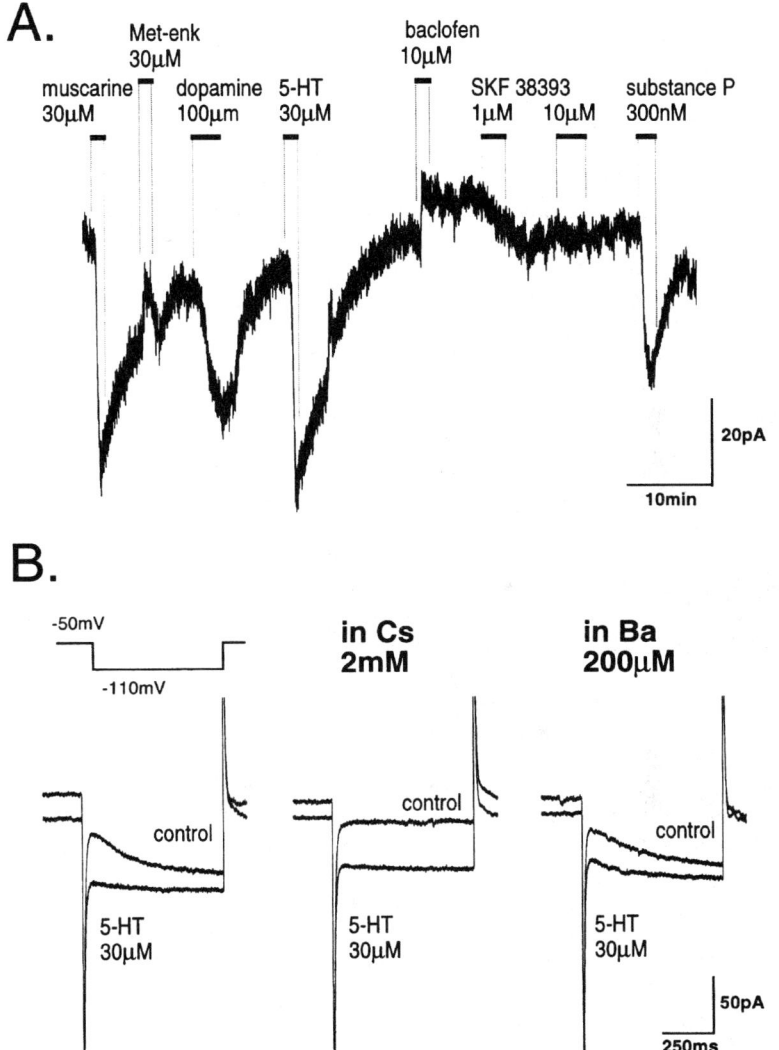

FIGURE 2. In (**A**) is shown various agonist-evoked current responses in a medium (h-current) neuron voltage-clamped to a holding potential of −50 mV. In (**B**) is shown the effect of 5-HT on currents evoked in a medium neuron by single voltage step from −50 to −110 mV. The *left panel* shows how 5-HT causes a current that is inward at both −50 and −110 mV. The *middle panel* shows the lack of effect of cesium on the 5-HT current although this treatment completely blocked the time-dependent h-current. The *right panel* shows the lack of a significant effect of the potassium channel blocker, barium, on the 5-HT current.

FIGURE 1. In the *left three panels* are shown confocal images of Neurobiotin-filled neurons representing the major cell types identified in the ventral pallidum. In the *right panels* are shown the corresponding voltage-clamp recordings made in each neuron of currents evoked by a hyperpolarizing step protocol (V_{hold} −50 mV, −10 mV steps).

multitude of short dendrites that terminated within a few diameters of the soma. These were all noncholinergic (0/7 ChAT positive). The appearance and electrophysiological properties of these small cells, especially our inability to evoke action potentials when recording in current clamp, suggested these could be nonneuronal cells such as oligodendrocytes.

Spontaneous action potentials were observed using on-cell recording (prior to going whole cell) in 38/48 of neurons subsequently shown to be medium cells with h-currents. In contrast, no spontaneous action potential firing was ever seen in large neurons, and recordings in current-clamp showed that these cells were strongly polarized with a resting membrane potential of −73 ± 10 mV.

A number of agonists were tested against receptors for endogenous neurotransmitters known to be present in the ventral pallidum. In FIGURE 2A is shown an example of a medium h-current neuron in which inward currents were caused by muscarine, dopamine, 5-HT and substance P, and small outward currents were caused by the opioid agonist [Met]^5-enkephalin, and the $GABA_B$ receptor agonist baclofen. We have studied the agonist actions of 5-HT in more detail and found that it produced inward currents in 74% of medium neurons. As yet we have not identified the 5-HT-receptor subtype involved but have shown that the inward current is caused neither by an increase in the h-current (which in fact appeared to be inhibited by 5-HT) nor by a decrease in a resting potassium conductance. This is demonstrated by the experiment shown in FIGURE 2B. Firstly, cesium (2 mM) completely blocked the h-current but had no significant effect on the 5-HT current. Secondly, the 5-HT current got bigger at hyperpolarized potentials (i.e., did not reverse at the potassium equilibrium potential, −105 mV) and was not reduced by barium at a concentration (200 µM) which would block potassium channels.

In conclusion, this study is the first in which the electrophysiological properties of morphologically identified ventral pallidal neurons have been described. We have shown that the two major output neurons in the ventral pallidum—medium, spiny GABA neurons and cholinergic neurons—have distinctly different electrophysiological properties that allows them to be easily identified in brain slice preparations. Medium spiny projection neurons are mostly spontaneously active and can be regulated by many of the endogenous neurotransmitters found in the ventral pallidum. These neurons are functional homologues of medium spiny neurons in the globus pallidus.[2] In contrast, cholinergic projection neurons in the ventral pallidum are silent and may depend on excitatory synaptic input in order to be activated. These cholinergic neurons have electrophysiological properties remarkably similar to cholinergic neurons present in the rat medial septum.[3]

REFERENCES

1. LAVIN, A. & A.A. GRACE. 1996. Physiological properties of rat ventral pallidal neurons recorded extracellularly *in vivo*. J. Neurophysiol. **75:** 1433.
2. NAMBU, A. & R. LLINAS. 1994. Electrophysiology of globus pallidus neurons *in vitro*. J. Neurophysiol. **72:** 1127.
3. GORELOVA, N. & P.B. REINER. 1996. Role of the afterhyperpolarization in control of discharge properties of septal cholinergic neurons *in vitro*. J. Neurophysiol. **75:** 695.

Neurons of the Bed Nucleus of the Stria Terminalis (BNST)

Electrophysiological Properties and Their Response to Serotonin

DONALD G. RAINNIE[a]

Harvard Medical School and Department of Psychiatry, Brockton Veterans Affairs Medical Center, Brockton, Massachusetts 02301, USA

INTRODUCTION

A descending pathway from the bed nucleus of the stria terminalis (BNST) to nuclei within the hypothalamus and brainstem has been implicated in the generation of anxiety.[1] Drugs such as the 5-HT$_{1A}$ agonist, buspirone, and specific serotonin reuptake inhibitors (SSRIs), which are used to treat anxiety behaviors, act to modulate serotonin (5-HT) transmission.[2] Hence, 5-HT may act as a neuromodulator in the BNST to regulate anxiety states. The BNST receives serotonergic afferents from the midbrain raphé nuclei,[4] and has high densities of 5-HT1-like receptors.[3] Moreover, infusion of buspirone into the BNST blocks light-enhanced startle.[1] It is, therefore, important to know how excitation is regulated within the BNST, and how 5-HT may affect neuronal excitation and hence signal transduction. The aim of this study was to determine the electrophysiological properties of individual neurons, and to examine the effects of serotonin on these intrinsic properties, using whole-cell patch clamp recording from BNST neurons, *in vitro*.

METHODS

Whole-cell patch clamp records were obtained from neurons of the dorsal subdivisions of the BNST in an *in vitro* slice preparation of the rat using standard techniques. Briefly, 25–35-day-old Long-Evans rats were decapitated, and the brains were rapidly removed and placed in ice-cold, oxygenated, ACSF containing in mM: NaCl, 124; KCl, 2.2; KH$_2$PO$_4$, 3.0; MgCl$_2$, 1.3; CaCl$_2$, 2.5; NaHCO$_3$, 26; and glucose, 10. Slices, 500 µm thick, containing the BNST were prepared and incubated in oxygenated ACSF at room temperature for at least 1 hour prior to experimentation. Patch electrodes (6–8 MΩ) were filled with recording solution containing, in mM: KGluconate, 120; KCl, 10; phosphocreatinine, 10; MgCl$_2$, 3; HEPES, 10; MgATP, 2; NaGTP, 0.2; biocytin 0.40% and titred to pH 7.2 and 280 mOsm. Whole-cell patch clamp records were obtained using an Axopatch-1D preamplifier and pClamp 6.0

---

[a]Address for correspondence: Dr. Donald G. Rainnie, Dept. of Psychiatry, Neuroscience Laboratory 151C, Brockton Veterans Affairs Medical Center, 940 Belmont Street, Brockton, MA 02401. Voice: 508-583-4500, ext. 2589; fax: 508-895-0059; donald_rainnie@hms.harvard.edu

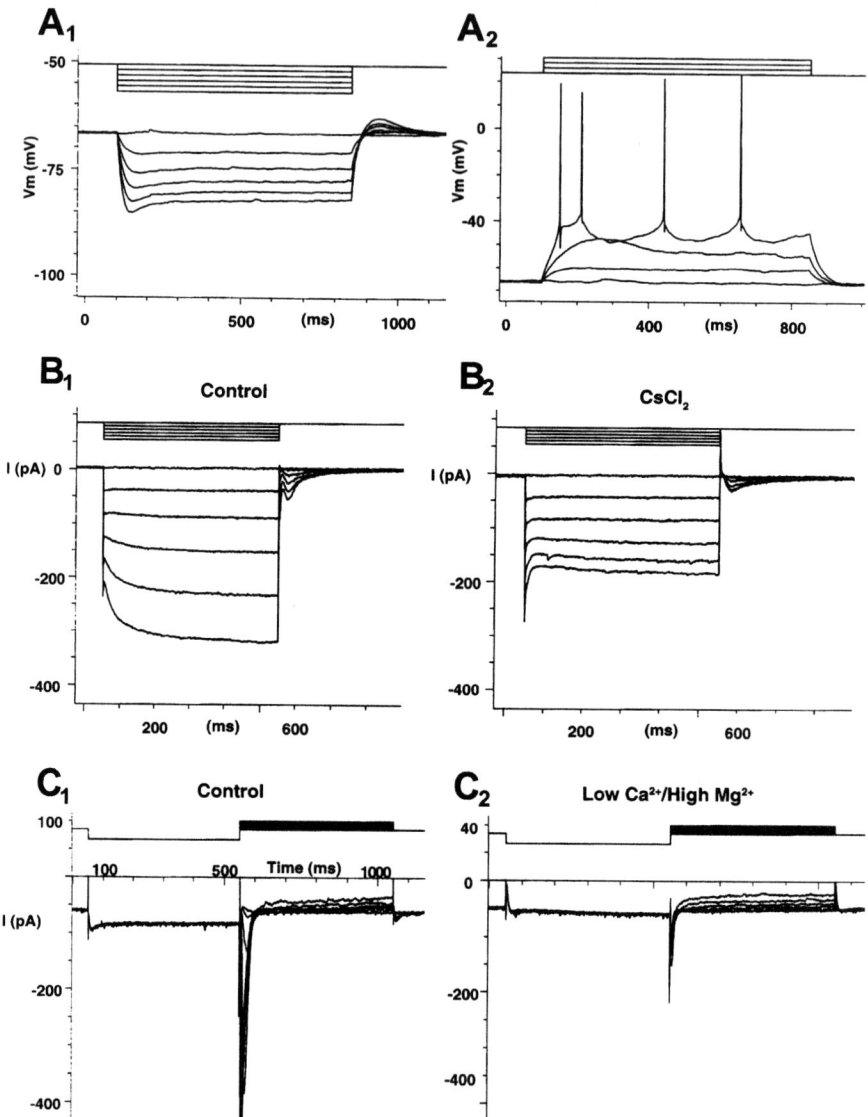

FIGURE 1. Typical whole-cell patch clamp records obtained from a neuron located in the medial-dorsal BNST. (A_1) Voltage excursions of a medial BNST neuron in response to transient hyperpolarizing current injection of increasing amplitude (−10 to −50 pA). (A_2) In the same neuron depolarizing current injection evoked a depolarizing prepotential subthreshold to action potential generation. (B_1) In control ACSF hyperpolarizing voltage commands of increasing amplitude (*upper trace*) activate a time- and voltage-dependent inward current. (B_2) Application of $CsCl_2$ (3 mM) to the ACSF blocked the expression of the inward current and revealed a time-independent rectification. (C_1) In the presence of TTX (0.6 μM), a dual-pulse protocol elicited a voltage-dependent rapidly activating inward current. (C_2) The inward current was blocked by reducing the ACSF calcium concentration from 3 to 0.3 mM.

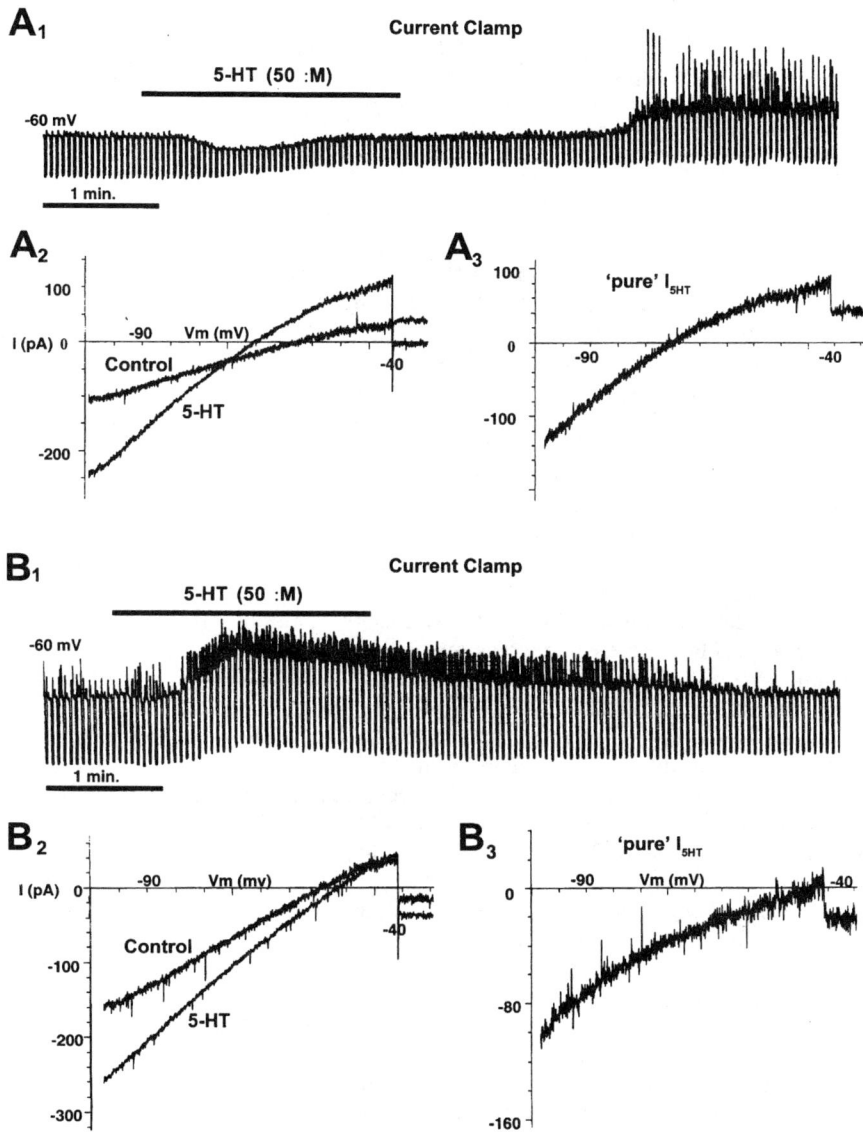

FIGURE 2. Exogenous serotonin activates both an outward and an inward conductance in BNST neurons. In 39% of BNST neurons 5-HT (50 μM) evoked a monophasic membrane hyperpolarization (-4.2 ± 0.34 mV, $n = 15$). (A_1) In 33% of BNST neurons a biphasic hyperpolarization-depolarization was observed in current clamp. The hyperpolarization decayed during the period of 5-HT application and was followed by a period of rebound excitation following washout. (A_2) In voltage clamp, in the presence of TTX, the 5-HT-induced membrane hyperpolarization was associated with an outward current (~50 pA) at -60 mV, and an increased conductance. (A_3) Subtraction of the steady state conductances dem-

software for data acquisition and analysis. Only those cells that showed a stable resting membrane potential (< −55 mV) for at least 5 minutes, and an overshooting action potential were accepted for drug application. Drugs were applied in the ACSF at known concentrations. Serotonin stock solution was made fresh on the day of experimentation and stored on ice until used.

RESULTS

Patch clamp records were obtained from 53 neurons of the BNST, dorsal to the anterior commissure, between 0.0 and −0.6 Bregma. Of the 22 neurons successfully recovered for visualization, 10 were located in the medial subdivision (mBNST), and 12 were located in the lateral subdivision (lBNST). Neurons of the mBNST had a significantly higher R_m (680 ± 120 MΩ) than those of the lBNST (250 ± 26 MΩ; $p = 0.001$, $F = 12.727$). Similarly, τ was significantly greater for mBNST neurons (34 ± 4.8 ms) than that for lBNST (21 ± 1.1 ms, $n = 11$, $p = 0.024$, $F = 5.93$). In contrast, no significant difference was observed in Vm (−63 ± 0.6 mV) for each neuronal population. Seventy percent of all BNST neurons examined expressed a depolarizing sag in the voltage response to transient hyperpolarizing current injection (FIG. 1A$_1$), that was mediated by activation of the time- and voltage-dependent nonspecific cation conductance, I_h (FIG. 1B$_{1-2}$). Upon transient depolarization, these same neurons expressed a depolarizing envelope on which rode two or more action potentials (FIG. 1A$_2$). The depolarizing envelope was mediated by activation of the low threshold calcium current (I_T; FIG. 1C$_{1-2}$). At the resting Vm, electrical stimulation of the stria terminalis evoked an excitatory postsynaptic potential (EPSP), or an EPSP followed by an inhibitory postsynaptic potential (IPSP). The IPSP was abolished by the GABA$_A$ receptor antagonist, bicuculline methiodide (30 µM), whereas the EPSP was almost totally abolished by the AMPA receptor antagonist, DNQX (10 µM).

Serotonin (5-HT; 50–100 µM) was applied to 38 BNST neurons; 15 responded with a membrane hyperpolarization, 13 with a hyperpolarization followed by a depolarization, and 7 with a membrane depolarization. The remaining 3 neurons were unresponsive to 5-HT application. No difference was observed in the response of mBNST or lBNST neurons to 5-HT. The response persisted in the presence of tetrodotoxin (TTX, 1.2 µM) suggesting activation of postsynaptic 5-HT receptors. In current clamp, the hyperpolarization was associated with a reduction of the membrane input resistance (FIG. 2A), and by an increased outward current in voltage clamp mode (FIG. 2B). The outward current reversed polarity at ~ −80 mV, which is close to the potassium reversal potential for this preparation. The depolarization was associated with a small increase in membrane input resistance, and was mediated by an inward current that reversed polarity at ~ −40 mV.

---

onstrated that the "pure" I_{5-HT} was an inwardly rectifying conductance. (**B$_1$**) A typical example of the 18% of BNST neurons that expressed a 5-HT-induced membrane depolarization. (**B$_2$**) In voltage clamp, a comparison of the steady state conductance before and during 5-HT application revealed an inward current at all points on the ramp protocol (−100 to −40 mV). (**D**) The pure I_{5-HT} current was inward at −60 mV (~30 pA) and showed a reversal potential close to −40 mV.

In 7/8 neurons examined, application of 5-HT (50 µM) also reduced the amplitude of evoked EPSPs by 41 ± 8%, irrespective of the postsynaptic response of BNST neurons. In the remaining neuron the EPSP amplitude was increased by 20%. In voltage clamp, the 5-HT-induced reduction of evoked EPSP amplitude was mediated by an equivalent reduction in the amplitude of the EPSC. These data suggest that serotonin also may regulate BNST excitability at a presynaptic locus. Experiments are in progress to determine the 5-HT receptor subtype/s involved in the pre- and postsynaptic response of BNST neurons to 5-HT application.

DISCUSSION

These data demonstrate for the first time that the excitability of neurons of the mBNST and lBNST can be directly, and indirectly, regulated by serotonin. Hence, activation postsynaptic 5-HT receptors can result in either (1) a membrane hyperpolarization mediated by activation of an inwardly rectifying potassium conductance, and/or (2) a membrane depolarization, the mechanism of which has yet to be determined. In addition, 5-HT acts at a presynaptic locus on glutamatergic afferents to reduce the release of glutamate and, hence, indirectly reduce the excitability of the BNST.

Although a continuum was observed in the response of BNST neurons to 5-HT, a correlation has yet to be established between the relative expression of either I_h and/or I_T in any given neuron, and its response to 5-HT. However, these results suggest that the input-output responses of these two BNST subdivisions are regulated by multiple 5-HT receptor subtypes. If activation of these 5-HT receptors has a direct impact on the behavioral expression of anxiety, the duality of response to 5-HT, demonstrated here, may act as a feedback control mechanism. Moreover, Davis and co-workers (1997) have reported that perfusion of the AMPA receptor antagonist, NBQX, into the BNST attenuates light-enhanced startle. Attenuation of the AMPA receptor-mediated EPSC by 5-HT, reported here, may represent an endogenous anxiolytic mechanism. Experiments are in progress to identify the 5-HT receptor subtypes responsible for the responses reported here. It is hoped that identification of these receptors may ultimately lead to the development of more specific treatments for anxiety.

REFERENCES

1. DAVIS, M. *et al.* 1997. Amygdala and bed nucleus of the stria terminalis: differential roles in fear and anxiety measured with the acoustic startle reflex. Phil. Trans. R. Soc. Lond. **352:** 1675–1687.
2. DE VRY, J. 1995. 5-HT$_{1A}$ receptor agonists: recent developments and controversial issues. Psychopharmacology **121:** 1–26.
3. PAZOS, A. & J.M. PALACIOS. 1985. Quantitative autoradiographic mapping of serotonin receptors in the rat brain. I. Serotonin-1 receptors. Brain Res. **346:** 205–230.
4. PHELIX, C.E. *et al.* 1992. Monoamine innervation of bed nucleus of stria terminalis: an electron microscopic investigation. Brain Res. Bull. **28:** 949–965.

Distribution of [³H]Citalopram Binding Sites in the Nonhuman Primate Brain

HILARY R. SMITH, JAMES B. DAUNAIS, MICHAEL A. NADER, AND LINDA J. PORRINO[a]

Department of Physiology and Pharmacology, Wake Forest University School of Medicine, Winston-Salem, North Carolina 27157, USA

The serotonergic system plays a role in mediating the effects of several drugs of abuse.[1,2] In addition, it has been shown to play a major role in the neurobiology of mood disorders.[3–5] Many of these effects can be attributed in part to perturbations in the normal function of the serotonin transporter (5-HTT).[1,2,4,5] The distribution of 5-HTT binding sites has been described extensively in the rodent,[6–8] and there have been several descriptive studies utilizing human postmortem tissue.[8–10] Comparisons of 5-HTT-rich areas in primate and rodent brain point out substantial species differences in a variety of limbic sites that include elements of the extended amygdala.[8] The density of 5-HTTs within components of the extended amygdala such as the bed nucleus of the stria terminalis and the substantia innominata, however, has not been described in detail, particularly in the primate. The goal of this study, therefore, was to describe the normal distribution of serotonin transporters in the nonhuman primate forebrain using the 5-HTT-selective ligand [³H]citalopram.

Three rhesus monkey brains were fresh-frozen and prepared for [³H]citalopram autoradiography. Procedures for labeling serotonin transporters were adapted from those described by D'Amato and colleagues.[6] Slide-mounted tissue sections were preincubated for 15 min at 25°C in buffer (50 mM Tris, 120 mM NaCl, 5 mM KCl, pH 7.4). Slides were then incubated in the same buffer containing 1 nM [³H]citalopram (New England Nuclear, Boston, MA) to assess total binding. Adjacent sections were incubated under identical conditions in the presence of 20 µM paroxetine (SmithKline Beecham, Sussex, UK) to determine nonspecific binding. Sections were washed, dried under a cool stream of air, and apposed to Hyperfilm (Amersham, Arlington Heights, IL) for 4 weeks along with tritium standards (Amersham). Autoradiographic analysis of [³H]citalopram binding to the 5-HTT was conducted by quantitative densitometry with a computerized image processing system (MCID, Imaging Research, St. Catharines, Ontario). Specific binding was determined by subtracting nonspecific binding values from the total binding values, as measured in adjacent sections. Data are expressed as fmol/mg of wet weight tissue.

Binding patterns of [³H]citalopram in the monkey striatum were markedly heterogeneous. In the rostral striatum the binding sites were uniformly distributed throughout the caudate, putamen, and rostral accumbens. All three structures exhibited a low-to-moderate level of binding. The olfactory tracts had the densest degree

---

[a]Corresponding author: Linda J. Porrino, Ph.D., Dept. of Physiology and Pharmacology, Wake Forest University School of Medicine, Medical Center Boulevard, Winston-Salem, NC 27157. Voice: 336-716-8575; fax: 336-716-8501; lporrino@wfubmc.edu

TABLE 1. [^{3}H]Citalopram binding in the rhesus monkey extended amygdala and related structures

Region of interest	fmol/mg wet weight tissue
Anterior Putamen	19.53 ± 0.9
Anterior Accumbens	21.51 ± 2.4
Anterior Dorsal Caudate	20.22 ± 0.2
Anterior Ventral Caudate	20.70 ± 2.2
Dorsal Caudate	16.92 ± 2.5
Ventral Caudate	33.26 ± 2.4
Accumbens Core	21.85 ± 1.1
Accumbens Shell	52.96 ± 12.5
Precommissural Putamen	16.95 ± 2.7
BNST	67.77 ± 8.1
Substantia Innominata	39.44 ± 4.4
VM Hypothalamus	56.55 ± 5.4
Amygdala	
Basal	45.93 ± 9.2
Accessory Basal	40.09 ± 9.7
Medial	38.42 ± 4.8
Central	66.73 ± 12.5
Lateral	41.34 ± 7.3

of binding at this level of the brain, while cortical areas exhibited very low levels of binding sites. At a more caudal level of the striatum, at which there is a clear distinction between the subdivisions of the nucleus accumbens, the pattern of binding was quite different. The caudate exhibited a distinct heterogeneity in binding sites at this level, with a clear ventrodorsal gradient of decreasing density. The shell of the nucleus accumbens also showed a distinct subregional pattern of binding. There appeared to be a cap of extremely dense binding at the dorsomedial tip of the shell, while the remainder of the structure exhibited a dense pattern of binding in the medial portions and more moderate levels laterally. The core of the accumbens, however, again had a homogeneously low to moderate level of binding, as did the putamen. More caudally, the anterior hypothalamic area, substantia innominata, and anterior aspects of the amygdaloid complex exhibited moderate [^{3}H]citalopram binding levels. Most striking at this level was the extremely dense binding in the bed nucleus of the stria terminalis. There was a notable heterogeneity of [^{3}H]citalopram binding sites within nuclei of the central amygdaloid complex in the monkey brain. The central nucleus exhibited the densest binding levels, while the lateral and basal nuclei bound [^{3}H]citalopram moderately to densely, and the medial nucleus exhibited a lower level of binding sites. The accessory basal nucleus showed a dorsoventral gradient, with the magnocellular division binding [^{3}H]citalopram more densely than the parvocellular division. There was moderate-to-dense binding in the hypothalamic area, particularly in the ventromedial nuclei, where binding was very dense. The emerging midline thalamic nuclei also exhibited moderate levels of binding sites.

The densest [^{3}H]citalopram binding in the monkey forebrain occurs in an array of structures which include those associated with the extended amygdala. Highest levels of binding were seen in the ventral striatum, bed nucleus of the stria terminalis, the amygdaloid complex, and the ventromedial hypothalamus. The distribution of 5-HTTs in the rhesus monkey extended amygdala and related structures appears to be similar to that of the human. Binding patterns in the amygdala resemble those seen in human brain, with a greater density of binding sites in the central and less in the basolateral nucleus than has been observed in the rat. The topography of binding sites in both ventral striatum and ventromedial hypothalamus also display similar patterns to those seen in the human. The parallels in the topography of 5-HTTs in the monkey and human forebrain attest to the nonhuman primate's value as a model of human drug abuse and psychopathology.

In summary, these results show that binding of [^{3}H]citalopram in the nonhuman primate forebrain is concentrated largely within the extended amygdala and associated structures. Measurements of neuroadaptation within this system may elucidate the extended amygdala's role in drug abuse and mood disorders.

ACKNOWLEDGMENT

This work was supported by NIDA Grant DA 09085 (LJP).

REFERENCES

1. HEINZ, A. et al. 1998. In vivo association between alcohol intoxication, aggression, and serotonin transporter availability in non-human primates. Am. J. Psychiatry **155:** 1023–1028.
2. LITTLE, K.Y. et al. 1998. Cocaine, ethanol, and genotype effects on human midbrain serotonin transporter binding sites and mRNA levels. Am. J. Psychiatry **155:** 207–213.
3. MELTZER, H.Y. 1990. Role of serotonin in depression. Ann. N.Y. Acad. Sci. **600:** 486–499.
4. COLLIER, D.A. et al. 1996. A novel functional polymorphism within the promoter of the serotonin transporter gene: possible role in susceptibility to affective disorders. Mol. Psychiatry **1:** 453–460.
5. MEADOR-WOODRUFF, J.H. et al. 1997. Serotonin transporter mRNA in schizophrenia. Mol. Psychiatry **2:** 446–447.
6. D'AMATO, R.J. et al. 1987. Selective labelling of serotonin uptake sites in rat brain by [^{3}H]citalopram contrasted to multiple sites by [^{3}H]imipramine. J. Pharmacol. Exp. Ther. **242:** 362–371.
7. DESOUZA, E.B. & B.L. KUYATT. 1987. Autoradiographic localization of [^{3}H]paroxetine-labeled serotonin uptake sites in rat brain. Synapse **1:** 488–496.
8. DUNCAN, G.E. et al. 1992. Autoradiographic characterization of [^{3}H]imipramine and [^{3}H]citalopram binding in rat and human brain: species differences and relationships to to serotonin innervation patterns. Brain Res. **591:** 181–197.
9. CORTES, R, et al. 1988. Autoradiography of antidepressant binding sites in the human brain: localization using [^{3}H]imipramine and [^{3}H]paroxetine. Neuroscience **27:** 473–496.
10. GUREVICH, E.V. & J.N. JOYCE. 1996. Comparison of [^{3}H]paroxetine and [^{3}H]cyanoimipramine for quantitative measurement of serotonin transporter sites in human brain. Neuropsychopharmacology **14:** 309–323.

Antidepressants and Atypical Neuroleptics Induce Fos-like Immunoreactivity in the Central Extended Amygdala

M. MORELLI[a] AND A. PINNA

Department of Toxicology, University of Cagliari, 09126 Cagliari, Italy

On the basis of anatomical connections, it has been suggested that the extended amygdala plays an important role in neuropsychiatric disorders characterized by emotional and affective alterations.[1,4] However, specific data showing the effect of drugs used in the therapy of these disorders are scarce.

Induction of the early-gene c-fos is secondary to neuronal activation and is correlated to an increased function of specific areas in the CNS.[8] Moreover, detection of the c-fos encoded protein Fos through Fos-like immunoreactivity (FLI) allows the study of the influence of drugs in small brain areas like those examined in this study. Using this methodology it was shown that antidepressant drugs increased FLI in specific limbic areas of the rat brain and that classical and atypical antipsychotics induced a different pattern of FLI in the striatum and prefrontal cortex which was predictive of their ability to induce extrapyramidal side effects (striatum) and to be effective on the negative symptoms of schizophrenia (prefrontal cortex).[2,3,5–7,9]

In order to evaluate the potential role of areas belonging to the extended amygdala in the effects of antidepressant and antipsychotic drugs, we have evaluated the induction of FLI in the rat central amygdaloid nucleus, sublenticular extended amygdala (SLEA), interstitial nucleus of posterior limb of the anterior commissure (IPAC) and the bed nucleus of stria terminalis (BST). As antidepressants, we utilized citalopram, which belongs to the class of serotonin reuptake inhibitors, and the tricyclic imipramine, which blocks the reuptake of both serotonin and noradrenaline. As antipsychotics, we used clozapine, which reduces the negative symptoms of schizophrenia, and haloperidol, which belongs to classical antipsychotics and which, differently from clozapine, induces extrapyramidal side effects.

Two hr after treatments male Sprague-Dawley rats were anesthetized and then perfused transcardially with paraformaldehyde. Coronal brain sections, cut with a vibratome, were incubated for 48 hr with a Fos primary antibody (OA-11-824, CRB), at a dilution of 1:1,400. The reaction was visualized using biotinylated secondary antisera and by standard avidin-biotin horseradish-peroxidase technique.[6]

---

[a]Corresponding author: Micaela Morelli, Dept. of Toxicology, University of Cagliari, Viale A. Diaz 182, 09126 Cagliari, Italy. Voice: +39-070-303819; fax: +39-070-300740; micmor@tin.it

TABLE 1. Number of Fos-like positive neurons after clozapine and haloperidol

		Fos-like Positive Nuclei (0.5 mm² grid)			
		clozapine		haloperidol	
	vehicle	(10 mg/kg)	(20 mg/kg)	(0.1 mg/kg)	(1 mg/kg)
PFCx	20 ± 9	50 ± 4*	56 ± 5**	14 ± 2	16 ± 2
Acb shell	7 ± 2	51 ± 7**	55 ± 6**	66 ± 5**	68 ± 14**
Acb core	1 ± 0.5	10 ± 2*	9 ± 3	18 ± 2**	20 ± 1**
ICPu	0.2 ± 0.1	5 ± 1*	10 ± 2*	39 ± 5**	44 ± 4**
BSTL	8 ± 3	25 ± 2**	26 ± 3**	16 ± 4	5 ± 2
IPAC	0.5 ± 0.2	13 ± 2**	14 ± 2**	43 ± 3**	71 ± 8**
SLEA	0.2 ± 0.1	14 ± 1**	17 ± 2**	4 ± 2	3 ± 2
Amyg Ce	6 ± 3	30 ± 3**	33 ± 3**	19 ± 3*	8 ± 2

Number ± SEM of Fos-like positive neurons in the prefrontal cortex (PFCx), nucleus accumbens shell (Acb shell), core (Acb core), dorso-lateral striatum (1CPu), bed nucleus of stria terminalis lateral division (BSTL), interstitial nucleus of posterior limb of the anterior commissure (IPAC), sublenticular extended amygdala (SLEA), central amygdaloid nucleus (Amyg Ce). The values are the means of 4–7 rats. When not receiving the drugs, rats were treated with the vehicle. Clozapine and haloperidol were injected i.p. and s.c., respectively. Statistically different from vehicle treated rats, *$p < 0.05$, **$p < 0.005$.

FOS-LIKE IMMUNOREACTIVITY AFTER ANTIDEPRESSANTS

Administration of imipramine (IM) (20 mg/kg i.p.) or a high dose of citalopram (CI) (20 mg/kg i.p.) increased FLI, in respect to control (CT), in the central amygdaloid nucleus (CT = 10 ± 4, IM = 57 ± 13*, CI = 34 ± 9*), BST lateral division (BSTL) (CT = 11 ± 2, IM = 80 ± 19*, CI = 45 ± 12*) and IPAC (CT = 3 ± 0.5, IM = 7 ± 1*, CI = 6 ± 1*) while they did not affect FLI in SLEA (CT = 0 ± 0, IM = 0 ± 0, CI = 0 ± 0) and decreased FLI in the nucleus accumbens (Acb) shell (CT = 26 ± 4, IM = 10 ± 2*, CI = 6 ± 1*). At a low dose, citalopram (5 mg/kg i.p.) did not induce FLI in the IPAC.[6] Doses of citalopram and imipramine were selected on the basis of studies in rats and considering that clinically equivalent doses of the two drugs have fourfold difference.

FOS-LIKE IMMUNOREACTIVITY AFTER ANTIPSYCHOTICS

Acute administration of clozapine at either 10 or 20 mg/kg i.p. induced a marked increase in FLI in the prefrontal cortex, Acb shell, BSTL and central amygdaloid nucleus (TABLE 1 and FIG. 1). A lower increase in FLI was observed in the Acb core, dorso-medial striatum, IPAC and SLEA (TABLE 1 and FIG. 1). FLI was already maximal after 10 mg/kg of clozapine in all areas examined. Acute administration of haloperidol (0.1 and 1 mg/kg s.c.) induced an increase in FLI in the Acb shell, dorso-lateral striatum and IPAC, while a lower increase in FLI was observed in the Acb core (TABLE 1). In the prefrontal cortex, BSTL and SLEA, haloperidol did not in-

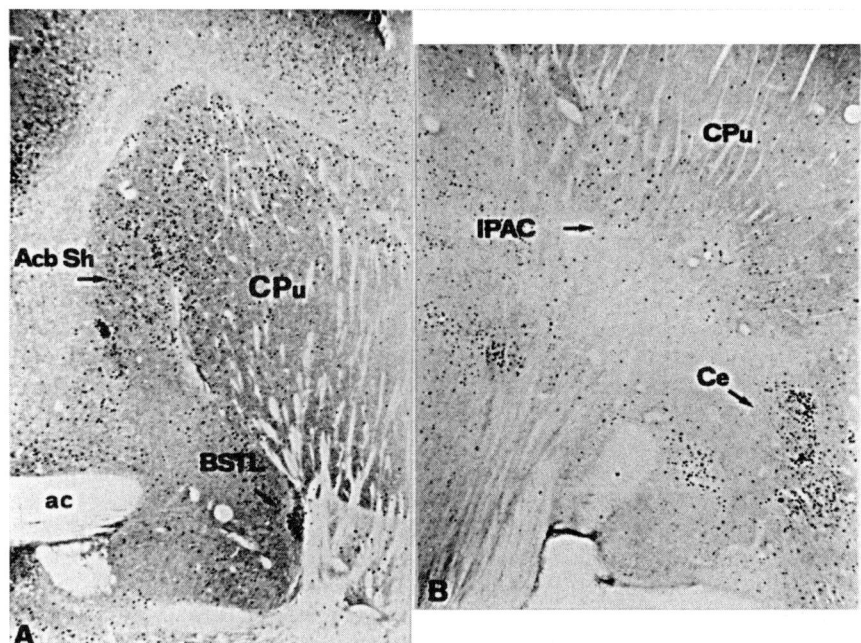

FIGURE 1. Photomicrographs of an horizontal section showing Fos-like positive nuclei in (A) nucleus accumbens shell (Acb Sh) and bed nucleus of stria terminalis lateral division (BSTL) and (B) interstitial nucleus of posterior limb of the anterior commissure (IPAC) and central amygdaloid nucleus (Ce) after 20 mg/kg i.p. of clozapine. Ac = anterior commissure, CPu = striatum.

crease FLI at any dose. In the central amygdaloid nucleus a small increase in FLI was observed after 0.1 mg/kg, whereas 1 mg/kg did not modify FLI (TABLE 1). In both the central amygdaloid nucleus and BSTL, FLI was less pronounced after 1 mg/kg than 0.1 mg/kg. The doses of drugs used were selected on the basis of studies in rats and considering that clinically equivalent doses of the two drugs have approximately a 70-fold difference.

The present results, by showing that acute administration of citalopram and imipramine activated FLI in areas belonging to the central extended amygdala, indicate a new important target for the action of antidepressants and suggest that the extended amygdala might play an important role in the mediation of disorders characterized by alterations of motivational behaviors and cognitive processes. Similarly to antidepressants, clozapine but not haloperidol induced FLI in central amygdaloid nucleus, IPAC, BSTL, and also SLEA. The only area of the extended amygdala in which haloperidol strongly increased FLI was the IPAC. This result, however, is probably due to the large rise in FLI induced by haloperidol in the striatum from which IPAC, otherwise called fundus striati, is not distinguished. Therefore, this result might not indicate a specific action of haloperidol in the extended amygdala. The only effect of haloperidol that could be regarded as specifically due to an effect on the extended amygdala was the increase of FLI observed in the central amygdaloid nucleus after the low dose. The increase observed, however, was of low intensity suggesting a limited effect of haloperidol in this area. The central amygdaloid nucleus and BSTL receive projections from the prefrontal cortex. In this area, as already reported,[5,7] clozapine but not haloperidol increased FLI. Therefore, induction of FLI in the central extended amygdala, as in the prefrontal cortex, might be a way to differentiate atypical from typical antipsychotics. The central amygdaloid nucleus elaborates components of the integrated emotional behavior, therefore, a prominent activation of FLI by antidepressants and clozapine but not haloperidol in the central extended amygdala, as that reported by this study, might explain the efficacy of these drugs on symptoms such as blunted affect and social withdrawal and in general in diseases characterized by alteration of emotional and motivational behavior. The central amygdaloid nucleus and BSTL receive large serotoninergic and noradrenergic innervation which might mediate the effects of antidepressants and clozapine on FLI. Moreover, the BSTL and the central amygdaloid nucleus, both directly and through the Acb shell and the IPAC, which belong to the most densely dopamine-innervated areas of the forebrain, are strongly affected by dopaminergic inputs. Each of these neurotransmitters might be responsible for the effects observed. However, the specific mechanism and the receptor types responsible for the increase in FLI cannot be determined from the present study. In conclusion, the elevation of FLI in the central extended amygdala after antidepressants and also after clozapine which, differently from haloperidol, ameliorate the negative symptoms of schizophrenia, provides evidence of the importance of the extended amygdala in neuropsychiatric disorders characterized by affective alterations.

REFERENCES

1. ALHEID, G.F. & L. HEIMER. 1996. Theories of basal forebrain organization and the "emotional motor system." Prog. Brain Res. **107:** 461–484.
2. BECK, C.H.M. 1994. Acute treatment with antidepressant drugs selectively increases the expression of c-fos in the rat brain. J. Psychiatry Neurosci. **20:** 25–32.
3. DUNCAN, G.E. *et al.* 1996. Functional classification of antidepressants based on antagonism of swim stress-induced fos-like immunoreactivity. J. Pharmacol. Exp. Ther. **277:** 1076–1080.
4. HEIMER, L. *et al.* 1997. Substantia innominata: a notion which impedes clinical-anatomical correlations in neuropsychiatric disorders. Neuroscience **76:** 957–1006.
5. MACGIBBON, G.A. *et al.* 1994. Clozapine and haloperidol produce a differential pattern of immediate early gene expression in rat caudate-putamen, nucleus accumbens, lateral septum and islands of Calleja. Mol. Brain Res. **23:** 21–32.
6. MORELLI, M. *et al.* 1999. Induction of Fos-like-immunoreactivity in the central extended amygdala by antidepressant drugs. Synapse **31:** 1–5.
7. ROBERTSON, G.S. *et al.* 1994. Induction patterns of fos-like immunoreactivity in the forebrain as predictors of atypical antipsychotic activity. J. Pharmacol. Exp. Ther. **271:** 1058–1066.
8. SAGAR, S.M. *et al.* 1988. Expression of c-fos protein in brain: metabolic mapping at the cellular level. Science **240:** 1328–1331.
9. SEBENS, J.B. *et al.* 1995. Differential Fos-protein induction in rat forebrain regions after acute and long-term haloperidol and clozapine treatment. Eur. J. Pharmacol. **273:** 175–182.

Stimulation of Dopamine Release in the Bed Nucleus of Stria Terminalis

A Trait of Atypical Antipsychotics?

EZIO CARBONI,[a] ALESSANDRA SILVAGNI, MARIA T. P. ROLANDO, AND GAETANO DI CHIARA

Department of Toxicology, University of Cagliari, 09126 Cagliari, Italy

It has been hypothesized that schizophrenia involves an alteration of dopamine (DA) transmission in specific brain areas. This hypothesis is based in part on the observation that the therapeutic potency of neuroleptics correlates with their affinity for DA D_2 receptor. Atypical neuroleptics (e.g., clozapine) differ from classical neuroleptics through having fewer side extrapyramidal effects and higher efficacy on negative symptoms of schizophrenia.[1] Atypical neuroleptics enhance DA output in dialysates preferentially in the prefrontal cortex rather than in the striatum or in the n. accumbens, which is the case with classical neuroleptics.[2] Some of the areas densely innervated by DA neurons such as the bed nucleus of stria terminalis (BNST) and the central amygdala have been assigned to the so-called extended amygdala. As no information exists on the effect of neuroleptics on DA transmission in these areas, we investigated the effect of typical and atypical neuroleptics on DA transmission in the BNST with concentric microdialysis probes in freely moving rats.[3]

MATERIALS AND METHODS

Animals

Male Sprague-Dawley rats (Charles River, Calco, Italy) 230–250 g were used.

Probe Preparation

Concentric probes were prepared with a 7-mm piece of AN 69 (sodium methallyl sulfate copolymer) dialysis fiber (310 µm o.d., 220 µm i.d., Hospal, Dasco, Italy).

Surgery

Rats were anesthetized with ketamine (Ketalar, Park-Davis, Milan, Italy). The probe was implanted vertically in the BNST (anterior: −0.1, lateral: 1.1, vertical: 8.1, from the dura), according to the atlas of Paxinos and Watson,[5] and then fixed on the skull with dental cement. Experiments were performed on freely moving rats 24 hr after implant.

---

[a]Corresponding author: Dr. Ezio Carboni, Dept. of Toxicology, Viale A. Diaz 182, 09126 Cagliari, Italy. Voice: +39-070-303819; fax: +39-070-300740; ecarboni@unica.it

Experiments

Ringer's solution (147 mM NaCl; 2.2 mM $CaCl_2$; 4 mM KCl) was pumped through the dialysis probe at a constant rate of 1 µl/min. Samples were analyzed every 20 min.

Analytical Procedure

Dialysate samples (20 µl), were injected without any purification into an HPLC apparatus equipped with reverse-phase column (LC-18 DB Supelco) and a coulometric detector (ESA Coulochem II, Bedford, MA) to quantitate DA. The composition of the mobile phase was: 50 mM $Na\ H_2\ PO_4$; 5 mM Na_2HPO_4; 0.1 mM Na_2EDTA; 0.5 mM octyl sodium sulfate; 15% (vol/vol) methanol, pH 5.5. The assay sensitivity allowed detecting 5 fmol DA.

Histology

At the end of the experiment, rat brains were cut on a vibratome in serial coronal slices, in order to locate the position of fiber.

Statistics

One-way or two-way analysis of variance (ANOVA) for repeated measures was applied to the data obtained. Post-hoc Tukey test with significance for $p < 0.05$ was applied. Basal values were the means of three consecutive samples differing less than 10%.

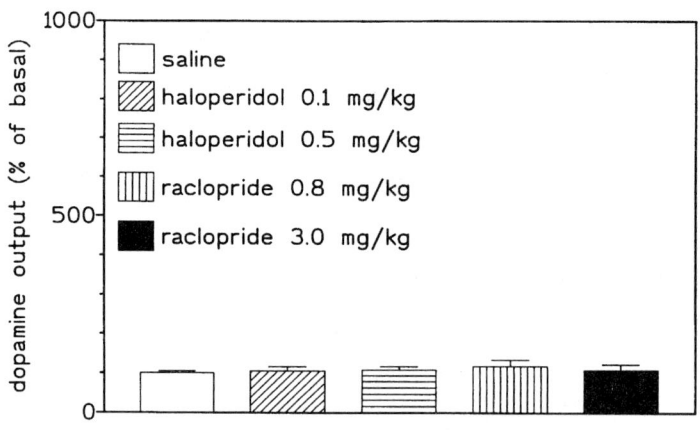

FIGURE 1. Effect of saline (0.1 ml/100 g, s.c.), haloperidol (0.1 and 0.5 mg/kg s.c.) and raclopride (0.8 and 3.0 mg/kg s.c.) on extracellular dopamine concentration at 40 min after treatment. Results (expressed as change of basal values in %) are mean of at least 4 rats.

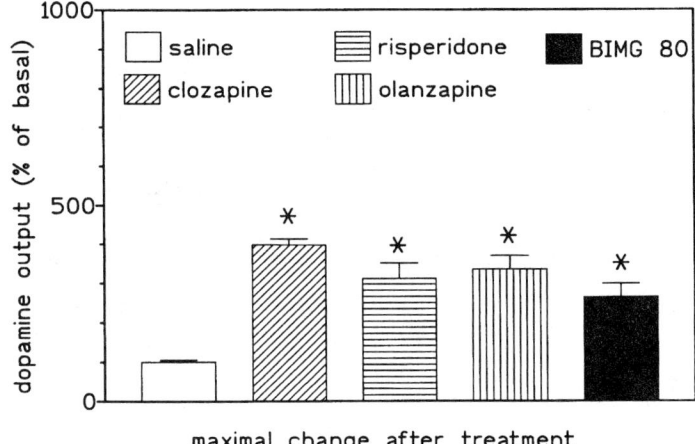

FIGURE 2. Effect of saline (0.3 ml/100 g, i.p.), clozapine (10 mg/kg i.p.), risperidone (3 mg/kg i.p.), olanzapine (6 mg/kg i.p.) and BIMG 80 (5 mg/kg i.p.) on extracellular dopamine concentration at 40 min after treatment. Results (expressed as change of basal values in %) are mean of at least 4 rats. *, $p < 0.05$ compared to saline treatment.

RESULTS

Basal extracellular DA concentration in the BNST was 14.03 ± 1.3 fmol/20 µl (mean ± SEM, $n = 40$). The typical neuroleptics haloperidol (0.1 and 0.5 mg/kg s.c.) and raclopride (0.8 and 3.0 mg/kg s.c.), as shown in FIGURE 1, did not modify significantly basal extracellular DA concentration (ANOVA, $F_{4,19} = 0.194$; $p = 0.93$). The atypical neuroleptics clozapine (10 mg/kg i.p.), risperidone (3 mg/kg i.p.), olanzapine (6 mg/kg i.p.) and BIMG 80[4] (5 mg/kg i.p.) but not saline (0.3 ml/100 g, i.p.), as shown in FIGURE 1, significantly increased DA extracellular concentration in the BNST (ANOVA/Tukey, $F_{4,16} = 9.7$; $p < 0.001$); maximal increases (297, 211, 235, and 164% above basal values, respectively) were observed at 40 min after treatment.

CONCLUSIONS

Dopamine transmission can be evaluated by microdialysis in the BNST. Atypical neuroleptics like clozapine, olanzapine, risperidone and BIMG 80 have in common the ability to stimulate, dose dependently, DA transmission in the BNST.

Typical neuroleptics like haloperidol and raclopride do not stimulate DA transmission in the BNST but stimulate it in the n. accumbens.[2] The receptor affinity profile of the atypical neuroleptics tested indicate that all have high affinity for DA D_4 and D_2, serotonin 5-HT_{2A}, and α_1 adrenoceptors and suggests that these receptors might play a relevant role in their effect on DA transmission in the BNST. These results suggest that BNST plays a role in the atypical properties of neuroleptics.

REFERENCES

1. ARNT, J. & M. SKARSFELDT. 1998. Do novel antipsychotics have similar pharmacological characteristics? A review of the evidence. Neuropsychopharmacology **18:** 63–101.
2. MOGHADDAM, B. & B.S. BUNNEY. 1990. Acute effects of typical and atypical antipsychotics drugs on the release of dopamine from prefrontal cortex, n. accumbens and striatum of the rat: an *in vivo* microdialysis study. J. Neurochem. **54:** 1755–1760.
3. DI CHIARA, G. 1990. "*In vivo*" brain dialysis of neurotransmitters. Trends Pharmacol. Sci. **11:** 116–121.
4. VOLONTÈ, M. *et al*. 1997. BIMG 80, a novel potential antipsychotic drug: evidence for multireceptor actions and preferential release of dopamine in prefrontal cortex. J. Neurochem. **69:** 182–190.
5. PAXINOS, G. & C. WATSON. 1987. The Rat Brain Stereotaxic Coordinates. 2nd edit. Academic Press. New York.

Involvement of the Ventral Pallidum in Working Memory Tasks With or Without a Delay

STAN B. FLORESCO,[a] DEANNA N. BRAAKSMA, AND ANTHONY G. PHILLIPS[b]

Department of Psychology, University of British Columbia, Vancouver, British Columbia, V6T 1Z4, Canada

The ventral pallidum (VP) forms an integral part of the extended amygdala.[1] The VP shares dense reciprocal connections with the nucleus accumbens[2] and also sends projections to both the medial-dorsal thalamus and motor effector sites in the hindbrain.[3] The reciprocal connectivity between the VP and the ventral striatum has led to the speculation that this pallidal region is the major target for nucleus accumbens outflow.[3] As such, the VP may contribute to goal-directed behaviors dependent on the activity of the nucleus accumbens. Previous studies have shown that lesions of the VP disrupt learning of stimulus-reward associations,[4] as do lesions of the nucleus accumbens, or disconnections between the amygdala and the nucleus accumbens.[5] However, it remains to be determined whether the VP is also involved in tasks that require working memory to guide goal-directed behavior. We have shown previously that spatially mediated foraging behavior on different variants of the radial arm maze task is dependent on specific neural circuits that link the hippocampus and the prefrontal cortex to the nucleus accumbens.[6–8] Therefore, the present study was conducted to assess the role of the VP in search behavior on a radial arm maze that is guided by working memory, subserved by limbic-cortical-striatal circuits.

METHOD

Male Long Evans rats weighing between 300–450 g prior to surgery were implanted with bilateral guide cannulae into the VP (mouth bar –3.3 mm; AP = 0.0 mm from bregma, ML = ±2.4 mm from midline, and DV = –8.0 mm from dura) using standard stereotaxic techniques. Each rat was given at least 7 days to recover from surgery prior to testing. Rats were trained on either the delayed spatial win-shift (SWSh) radial arm maze task (FIG. 1A) or the random foraging (RF) radial-maze task without a delay period (FIG. 1B). The day after criterion performance was reached, rats received bilateral infusions of either lidocaine (20 µg in 0.5 µL of saline at a rate of 0.5 µL/1.2 min) or vehicle into the VP. Each rat remained in its home cage for an additional 3 min prior to being placed on the maze. Following the first

[a]Voice: 604-822-6789; fax: 604-822-6923; stanbf@unixg.ubc.ca
[b]Voice: 604-822-3245; fax: 604-822-6923; aphillips@cortex.psych.ubc.ca

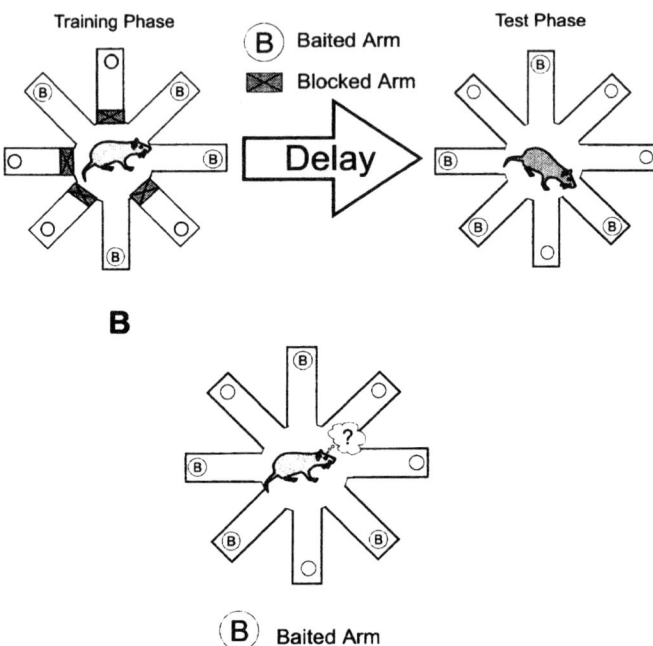

FIGURE 1. A: The delayed spatial win-shift (SWSh) task consisted of a training phase and a test phase, separated by a delay. Prior to the training phase, a set of four arms was chosen randomly and blocked, and food pellets were placed in the food cups of the four remaining open arms. Each rat was allowed to retrieve the pellets from the four open arms and then return to its home cage for the delay period. During the test phase of each daily trial, all arms were open, but only the arms that were previously blocked contained food. Errors were scored as entries into unbaited arms. Rats were trained to a criterion of one error or less during the test phase, for two consecutive days. The following day, rats were given an infusion of lidocaine or saline into the VP. **B:** The random foraging (RF) task required rats to forage for pellets placed at random in food cups of 4 of the 8 arms. A different set of arms was baited each day. Rats were trained to a criterion of one reentry error or less per daily trial for four consecutive days. The following day, rats were administered an infusion of lidocaine or saline into the VP.

injection test day, rats were retrained to criterion performance on the respective task and then given a counterbalanced infusion of either saline or lidocaine into the VP. For details on microinfusion and training procedures, see Floresco et al.[8] Three groups of rats received infusions of lidocaine and saline into the VP either: (1) prior to the training phase of the delayed SWSh task ($n = 7$), (2) prior to the test phase of the delayed SWSh task ($n = 9$), or (3) prior to a daily trial of the RF task ($n = 7$).

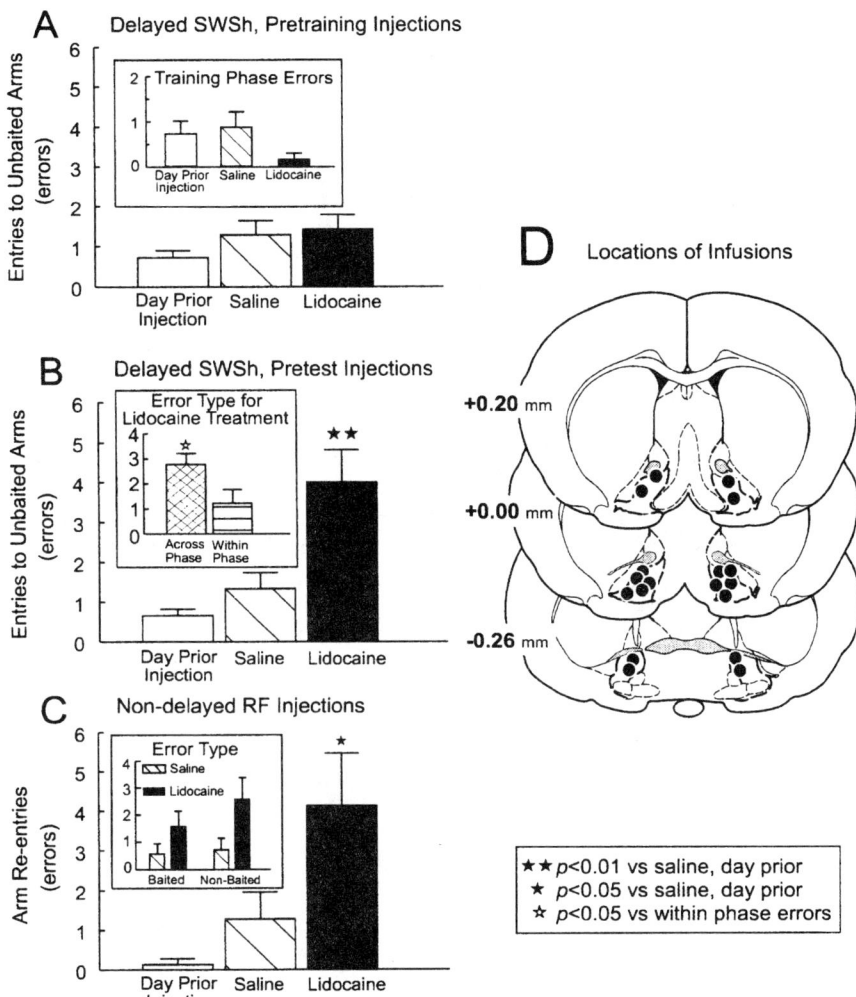

FIGURE 2. The effects of bilateral inactivation of the VP on performance of delayed and nondelayed radial-arm maze tasks. **A:** Number of errors (mean ±SEM) made by rats during the test phase or the training phase (2A, *inset*) on the day prior to the first injection and following pretraining phase infusions of saline or lidocaine into the VP prior to the training phase of the delayed SWSh task. **B:** Number of errors made by rats during the test phase following pretest infusions of saline or lidocaine into the VP. *Inset* shows number of across-phase errors and within-phase errors. **C:** Number of errors made by rats following infusions of saline and lidocaine into the VP prior to the RF task. *Inset* shows number of reentries to baited and nonbaited arms. **D:** Location of infusions (black circles) for all rats receiving infusions into the VP prior to the test phase of the delayed SWSh task. Numbers beside each slide correspond to mm from bregma.

RESULTS

Infusions of lidocaine into the VP prior to the training phase of the delayed SWSh task did not increase the number of errors made by rats on either the training phase ($F_{2,10} = 1.73$ ns.; see FIG. 2A inset) or the test phase ($F_{2,10} = 1.34$ ns.; see FIG. 2A). In addition, there were no significant differences in latencies to reach the first food cup or in the average time per subsequent choice of arms on both the training and test phases (all Fs < 1.3 ns). By contrast, infusions of lidocaine into the VP prior to the test phase of the delayed SWSh task significantly increased the number of errors made during the test phase, relative to saline infusions or the day prior to the first injection ($F_{2,14} = 11.86$, $p < 0.001$, and Tukey's, $p < 0.001$; see FIG. 2B). Rats made significantly more across-phase errors than within-phase errors ($F_{1,8} = 7.84$, $p < 0.05$; see FIG. 2B, inset). Lidocaine infusions also significantly enhanced the average time per subsequent choice (M = 21.3 s) relative to saline treatments (M = 12.8) ($F_{2,16} = 6.39$, $p < 0.01$).

Rats receiving infusions of lidocaine into the VP prior to the RF task made significantly more errors relative to saline infusions or the day prior to the first injection ($F_{2,10} = 5.631$, $p < 0.05$, and Tukey's, $p < 0.05$; see FIG. 2C). Rats made an equal number of reentries to both baited and nonbaited arms ($F_{1,6} = 1.64$ ns.; see FIG. 2C, inset). Lidocaine inactivations of the VP significantly increased the latencies to reach the first food cup (M = 48.7) relative to saline infusions (M = 6.8) ($F_{2,12} = 5.17$, $p < 0.05$).

The location of the infusions for all rats receiving inactivation of the VP prior to the test phase of the delayed SWSh task is shown in FIGURE 2D. The location of infusions for rats receiving infusions prior to the training phase, or prior to the RF task, was similar to those shown in FIGURE 2D. All acceptable placements were at the level of the anterior subcommisural VP. Rats whose infusions were not located in the VP or were asymmetrical in the rostral/caudal plane were not included in the analysis ($n = 6$). These rats were generally not impaired on any of the tasks.

DISCUSSION

The present study highlights the importance of the VP in spatially mediated search behavior on a radial-arm maze that is guided by two different forms of working memory. Reversible lesions of the VP administered prior to the training phase of the delayed SWSh task did not impair foraging during either the training phase or the test phase of this task. However, similar inactivations of the VP did disrupt performance of both the nondelayed RF task and the delayed SWSh task when inactivations were administered prior to the test phase. The failure to observe a disruption of foraging behavior in the training phase of the delayed SWSh task may reflect a minimal memory load (i.e., which of 4 arms had been entered previously on the trial) as compared to the greater memory load imposed by 8 open arms on the RF task. These data are consistent with other studies that report impairments in appetitively motivated tasks following lesions or pharmacological manipulations of the VP. These tasks include the acquisition of a conditioned place preference,[4] conditional visual discriminations,[9] and food-hoarding behavior.[10]

It is noteworthy that the pattern of deficits following transient lesions of the VP was strikingly similar to those observed following lidocaine-induced inactivations of the nucleus accumbens.[6] Lidocaine infusions into the nucleus accumbens increased the number of errors made by rats performing either the delayed SWSh or the RF tasks. Moreover, reversible lesions of the nucleus accumbens also resulted in enhanced latencies to initiate arm entries, as did inactivations of the VP. Given the similar behavioral impairments following inactivations of either the VP or the nucleus accumbens, and in light of the dense connectivity between these two regions, it is reasonable to conjecture that these two regions may participate in control of a similar behavioral function. Contemporary theory of nucleus accumbens function posits that this nucleus plays an essential role in integrating information from various limbic and cortical regions into goal-directed behaviors.[8,11,12] Thus it is plausible that the VP represents the next stage of limbic-motor integration, serving as a relay of cortico-limbic information processed by the ventral striatum/extended amygdala to motor effector sites that lead in to meaningful patterns of adaptive behaviors. With respect to the present study, the disruption in foraging behavior following VP inactivations may be attributed to an inability of hippocampal or prefrontal cortical inputs that interact with the ventral striatum to access motor effector sites that are downstream of the VP. Thus, the present results support the hypothesis that the VP is part of a larger, cortical-limbic-striatal neural circuit that governs search behavior that is guided by working memory.

ACKNOWLEDGMENT

This research was supported by a Grant from the Natural Sciences and Engineering Research Council of Canada to A.G.P.

REFERENCES

1. ALHEID, G.F. & L. HEIMER. 1988. New perspectives in basal forebrain organization of special relevance for neuropsychiatric disorders: the striatopallidal, amygdaloid, and corticopetal components of substantia innominata. Neuroscience 27: 1–39.
2. ZAHM, D.S. & L. HEIMER. 1990. Two transpallidal pathways originating in the rat nucleus accumbens. J. Comp. Neurol. 302: 437–446.
3. MOGENSON, G.J. et al. 1993. From motivation to action: a review of dopaminergic regulation of limbic→nucleus accumbens→ventral pallidum→pedunculopontine nucleus circuitries involved in limbic-motor integration. In Limbic Motor Circuits and Neuropsychiatry. P.W. Kalivas & C.D. Barnes, Eds.: 193–263. CRC Press, Boca Raton, FL.
4. MCALONAN, G.M., T.W. ROBBINS & B.J. EVERITT. 1993. Effects of medial dorsal thalamic and ventral pallidal lesions on the acquistion of a conditioned place preference: further evidence for the involvement of the ventral striatopallidal system in reward-related processes. Neuroscience 52: 605–620.
5. EVERITT, B.J. et al. 1991. The basolateral amygdala-ventral striatal systems and conditioned place preference: further evidence of limbic-striatal interactions underlying reward-related processes. Neuroscience 41: 1–18.
6. SEAMANS, J.K. & A.G. PHILLIPS. 1994. Selective memory impairments produced by transient lidocaine-induced lesions of the nucleus accumbens in rats. Behav. Neurosci. 108: 456–468.

7. SEAMANS, J.K., S.B. FLORESCO & A.G. PHILLIPS. 1995. Functional differences between the prelimbic and anterior cingulate regions of rat prefrontal cortex. Behav. Neurosci. **109:** 1063–1073.
8. FLORESCO, S.B., J.K. SEAMANS & A.G. PHILLIPS. 1997. Selective roles for hippocampal, prefrontal cortical and ventral striatal circuits in radial-arm maze tasks with or without a delay. J. Neurosci. **17:** 1880–1890.
9. EVERITT, B.J. et al. 1987. The effects of excitotoxic lesions of the substantia innominata, ventral and dorsal globus pallidus on the acquisition and retention of a conditional visual discrimination: implications for cholinergic hypothesis of learning and memory. Neuroscience **22:** 441–469.
10. MOGENSON, G.J. & M. WU. 1988. Disruption of food hoarding behavior by injections of procaine into the mediodorsal thalmus, GABA into subpallidal region and haloperidol into accumbens. Brain Res. Bull. **20:** 247–251.
11. PENNARTZ, C.M.A., H.J. GROENEWEGEN & F.H. LOPES DA SILVA. 1994. The nucleus accumbens as a complex of functionally distinct neuronal ensembles: an integration of behavioural, electrophysiological and anatomical data. Prog. Neurobiol. **42:** 719–761.
12. ROBBINS, T.W & B.J EVERITT. 1996. Neurobehavioural mechanisms of reward and motivation. Curr. Opin. Neurobiol. **6:** 228–236.

NMDA Glutamatergic Blockade of Nucleus Accumbens Disrupts Acquisition but Not Consolidation in a Passive Avoidance Task

P.A. GARGIULO,[a,b,c] G. MARTÍNEZ,[a,b] C. ROPERO,[a,b] A. FUNES,[a,b] AND A.I. LANDA[b]

[a]*Unidad de Farmacología del Comportamiento (UNIFCO-CONICET),*
Cátedra de Farmacología, Facultad de Ciencias Médicas,
Universidad Nacional de Cuyo, Casilla de Correo 33, Mendoza (5500), Argentina
[b]*Laboratorio de Neurociencias y Psicología Experimental, Cátedra de Neuropatología,*
Facultad de Humanidades y Ciencias de la Educación, Universidad Católica Argentina,
Perú 1160, Mendoza (5500), Argentina

The nucleus accumbens septi (Acc) of the basal forebrain is a major component of the ventral striatum of the rat.[8] It receives a dopaminergic projection from the ventral tegmental area and afferents from olfactory and limbic cortex.[6] A glutamatergic pathway from the limbic system reaches the Acc, as a part of the ventral striatum.[2] An Acc is also present in birds,[5] and evidence that it is involved in cognitive functions has been recently reported.[4]

The Acc appears to be involved in several behavioral processes: locomotion,[7,13] stereotypies,[3] motivation,[15] reward,[12,19] and some cognitive functions, such as learning,[17,18] memory,[9,16] and visual discrimination.[4] The aim of the present work was to examine the action of the blockade of N-methyl-D-aspartate (NMDA)–type glutamatergic receptors in the Acc during different phases of a learning process.

Male rats of a Holtzman-derived colony, aged 90 days and weighing 240–270 g were used ($n = 64$). They were maintained under controlled temperature conditions (22–24°C) and lighting (lights on 05.00–19.00 hours). Standard rat chow and water were freely available.

Animals were anesthetized with ether and stereotaxically implanted with bilateral stainless-steel cannulae into the Acc. The cannulae were double barreled, and the set was composed of an outer guiding cannula (stainless-steel tubing, 23 gauge, 15 mm in length), provided with a removable stylet (30 gauge, 15 mm in length) to avoid its obstruction. After surgery, rats were housed individually and maintained undisturbed for a week recovery period.

A passive avoidance task (step through paradigm) was used. The apparatus consisted of a brightly illuminated white chamber (30 × 30 × 30 cm) that communicated through a vertical slide door with a darkly illuminated black chamber (10 × 10 × 5 cm). The latter was fitted with an electric floor grid connected to an electric source.

For training, the animals were placed into the white chamber for one minute. After that, the door was elevated, and the animals stepped into the dark chamber. Im-

---

[c]Voice: 54.261.4238383; fax: 54.261.2487370; gargiulo@fmed2.uncu.edu.ar

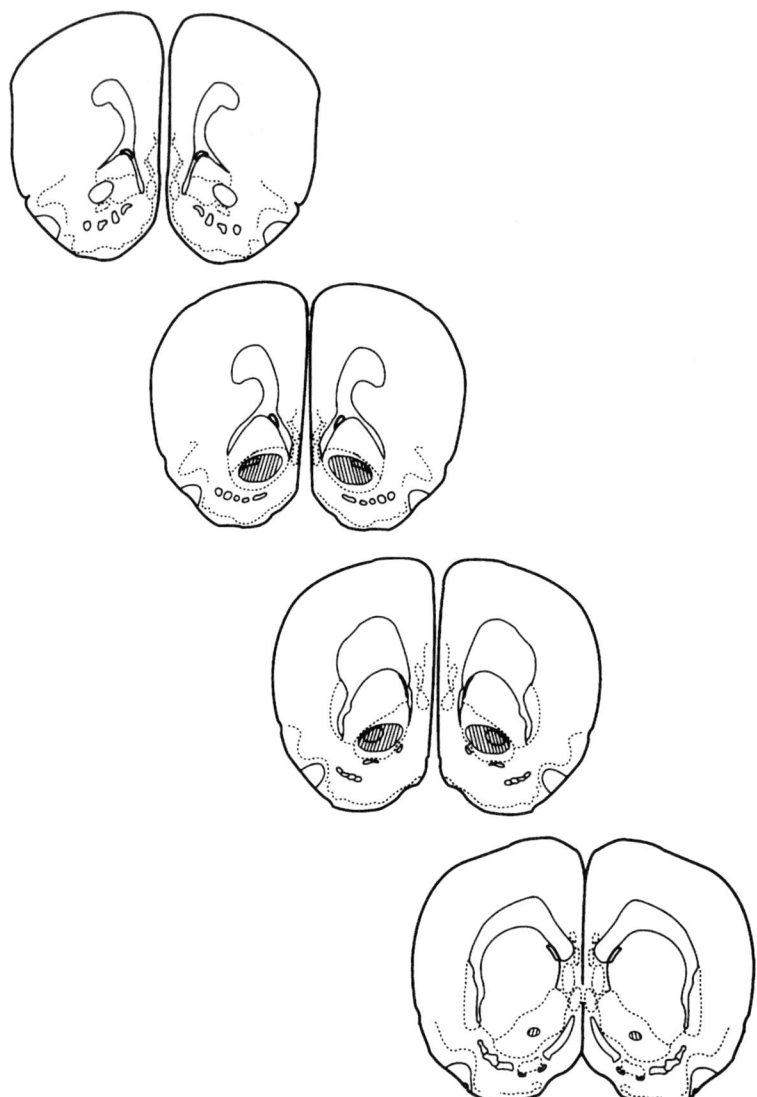

FIGURE 1. Frontal brain sections showing the location of the injection site. Schematic representation of histological findings.

mediately after that, the door was closed, and an electric shock was applied to the rats through the electric grid (1 mA, 3 s). The door was opened again; the rats returned to the white chamber and were removed.

A 30 gauge, 17 mm long stainless-steel injection cannula (designed to precisely reach the Acc) attached to a 10 µL microsyringe (Hamilton) was introduced into the guide cannula. Volumes of a 1 µL solution were gradually injected over a 2-min period into both the left and right Acc. The injection cannulae were left in place for an additional minute to allow for diffusion. The rats bilaterally received either saline or a 7-aminophosphonoheptanoic acid (AP-7, Research Biochemicals) solution (1 µg/ 1 µL) 10 minutes before training (pretraining schedule) or immediately after the shock (posttraining schedule). The injections in the latter schedule were completed within 6 minutes or less after the punishment.

For testing 24 hours later (under drug- and saline-free conditions), the animals were again placed in the white chamber for a 1-min period, and the door was removed. The elapsed times between the removal of the door to the introduction of the head into the dark chamber (latency 1) and the placement of the four paws on the grid (latency 2) were recorded.

At the end of testing, rats were killed by an overdose of ether. Brains were removed from the skull and fixed in a 10% formalin solution. The brains were then mounted and frozen in a cryotome and cut into 40 µm sections. The block face was examined with a 10 × magnifying lens, and the sections containing the injection sites were saved. Microscopic inspection of these sections served to ascertain the location of these sites. The locations were transferred to standard sections taken from a brain atlas.[10] We only report data for those rats with correct Acc placements (FIG. 1).

Nonparametric Mann-Whitney tests were used to evaluate significances. In all cases, a $p < 0.05$ was considered significant. The results reported are medians and interquartile intervals.

Regarding the pretraining injection schedule, the drug treatment did not modify latency 1 but significantly reduced latency 2 when compared with the saline control group ($p < 0.05$, $n = 17$ each group; FIG. 2A). The posttraining injection schedule drug treatment did not lead to any significant latency differences ($n = 15$ each group; FIG. 2B).

The results show that the postshock consolidation was not affected by AP-7 glutamatergic blockade of the Acc. However, the acquisition process was interfered with by previous AP-7 administration. The fact that, here, latency 2, but not latency 1, was affected shows that acquisition was disrupted without interference of exploratory motivation. This suggests that the glutamatergic transmission in the Acc is subject to a particular temporal pattern in the step-through one-trial learning.

We have previously found that intra-accumbens administration of AP-7 led to a disruption of discrimination of visual stimuli in the pigeon.[4] Like here, treatment did not interfere with the mere execution of the task, and we assumed that the blocking affected a more specific process than motivational drive or motor coordination. We considered that the effect that we obtained was due to an attentional impairment.[4] A similar explanation has been adduced for the deficits of Acc-lesioned rats performing a complex visual discrimination task.[14]

It has been reported that intra-accumbens administration of AP-7 produces impairments in a spatial water maze task both during initial training and when the task is well learned.[17] A maintained attentional level is probably required for the linkage of visual cues to the position of the platform. Generally these effects of glutamatergic blockade could be considered as due to alterations of working memory. In all these instances the solution of the relevant behavioral tasks can be considered to require a raised level of attention.

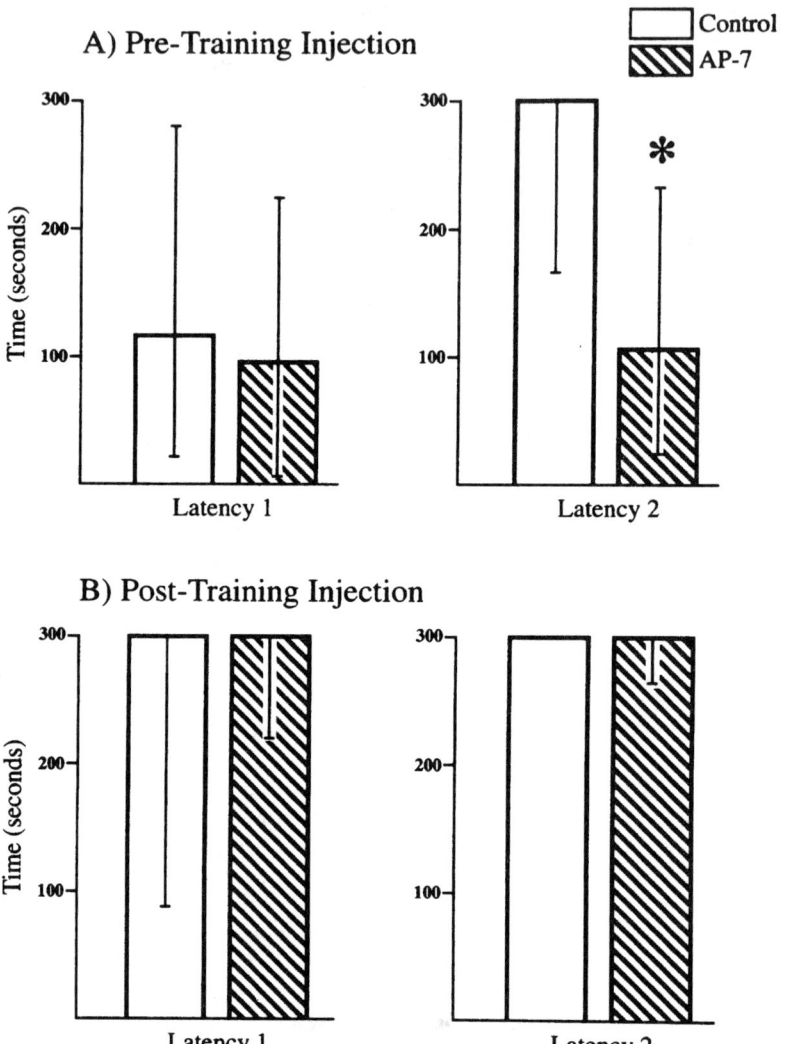

FIGURE 2. Effects of 7-aminophosphonoheptanoic acid injected into the Acc on latency 1 and latency 2 in the passive avoidance task (pretraining and posttraining injection schedules). Results are reported as medians and interquartile intervals ($n = 15$–17 rats).

Previously, unspecific blockades of striatum with lidocaine[11] or lesions[1] have been employed to interfere with cognitive functioning. Here we use a more specialized instrument to study the neural transmission involved in this function.

We conclude that a NMDA-glutamatergic blockade of the Acc appears to lead to cognitive disturbances and that these could be due to interference with working memory processes necessary for the acquisition, but not for the consolidation, of a learned task in rats.

ACKNOWLEDGMENTS

We thank Professor Dr. Juan D. Delius for comments and for editing of the manuscript. The work reported is part of the collaboration with the Allgemeine Psychologie, Universität Konstanz, Germany. We also thank G. Maravilla and C. Blotta for their assistance with the experiments, and Professors Drs. E. Rodriguez Echandia, E. O. Alvarez, D. Cardozo Biritos, and R. Furlan for their institutional support.

REFERENCES

1. ANNETT, L.M., A. MCGREGOR & T.W. ROBBINS. 1989. The effects of ibotenic acid lesions of the nucleus accumbens on spatial learning and extinction in the rat. Behav. Brain Res. **31:** 231–242.
2. CARLSSON, M. & A. CARLSSON. 1990. Schizophrenia: a subcortical neurotransimtter imbalance syndrome? Schizophr. Bull. **16** (3): 425–432.
3. GARGIULO, P.A. 1996. Thyrotropin releasing hormone injected into the nucleus accumbens septi selectively increases face grooming in rats. Braz. J. Med. Biol. Res. **29:** 805–810.
4. GARGIULO, P.A., M. SIEMANN & J. DELIUS. 1998. Visual discrimination in pigeons impaired by glutamatergic blockade of nucleus accumbens. Physiol. & Behav. **63** (4): 705–709.
5. KARTEN, H.J. & W. HOODS. 1967. A Stereotaxic Atlas of the Brain of the Pigeon. Johns Hopkins Press. Baltimore. MD.
6. KOOB, G.F. 1992. Neural mechanisms of drug reinforcement. In The Neurobiology of Drug and Alcohol Adiction. P.W. Kalivas & H.H. Samson, Eds.: **654:** 171–191. Annals of the New York Academy of Sciences. New York.
7. MOGENSON, G.J., M. WU & S.K. MANCHADA. 1979. Locomotor activity initiated by microinfusion of picrotoxin into the ventral tegmental area. Brain Res. **161:** 311–319.
8. MOGENSON, G.J., C.R. YANG & C.Y. YIM. 1988. Influence of dopamine on limbic inputs to the nucleus accumbens. In The Mesocorticolimbic Dopamine System. P.W. Kalivas & C.B. Nemeroff, Eds.: **537:** 86–100. Annals of the New York Academy of Sciences. New York.
9. PACKARD, M.G. & N.M. WHITE. 1990. Lesions of the caudate nucleus selectively impair "reference memory" acquisition in the radial arm maze. Behav. Neural Biol. **53:** 39–50.
10. PELLEGRINO, L.J., A.S. PELLEGRINO & A.J. CUSHMAN. 1979. A Stereotaxic Atlas of the Rat Brain. Plenum Press. New York.
11. PÉREZ RUIZ, C. & R.A. PRADO ALCALÁ. 1989. Retrograde amnesia induced by lidocaine injection into the striatum: protective effect of the negative reinforcer. Brain Res. Bull. **22:** 599–603.
12. PHILLIPS, A.G. & H.C. FIBIGER. 1978. The role of dopamine in maintaining intracranial self-stimulation in the ventral tegmentum, nucleus accumbens and medial prefrontal cortex. Can. J. Psychol. **32:** 58–66.
13. PIJNENBURG, A.J.J., W.M.M. HONIG, J.A.M. VAN DER HAYDEN & J.M. VAN ROSSUM. 1976. Effects of chemical stimulation of the mesolimbic dopamine system upon locomotor activity. Eur. J. Pharmacol. **35:** 45–58.
14. READING, P.J., S.B. DUNNETT & T.W. ROBBINS. 1991. Dissociable roles of the ventral, medium and lateral striatum on the acquisition and performance of a complex visual stimulus-response habit. Behav. Brain Res. **45:** 147–161.

15. SALAMONE, J.D. 1994. The involvement of nucleus accumbens dopamine in appetitive and aversive motivation. Behav. Brain Res. **61:** 117–133.
16. SCHACTER, G.B., C.R. YANG, N.K. INNIS & G.J. MOGENSON. 1989. The role of the hippocampal-nucleus accumbens pathway in radial-arm maze performance. Brain Res. **494:** 339–449.
17. SCHEELKRUGER, J. & P. WILLNER. 1991. The mesolimbic system: principles of operation. *In* The Mesolimbic Dopamine System: From Motivation to Action. P. Willner & J. Scheel-Kruger, Eds.: 559–597. Wiley. New York.
18. SEAMANS, J.K. & A.G. PHILLIPS. 1994. Selective memory impairments produced by transient lidocaine-induced lesions of the nucleus accumbens in rats. Behav. Neurosci. 108 (3): 456–468.
19. WISE, R.A. & M.A. BOZARTH. 1981. Brain substrates for reinforcement and drug self-administration. Prog. Neuropsychopharmacol. **5:** 467–474.

Disrupted and Undisruptable Latent Inhibition following Shell and Core Lesions

I. WEINER,[a,c] G. GAL, AND J. FELDON[b]

[a]*Department of Psychology, Tel Aviv University,
Ramat-Aviv, Tel Aviv, Israel 69978*
[b]*Behavioural Biology Laboratory, Swiss Federal Institute of Technology Zurich,
Schorenstrasse 16, CH-8603 Schwerzenbach, Switzerland*

In the latent inhibition (LI) paradigm, subjects are repeatedly presented in the first stage (preexposure) with a stimulus, which is paired with a reinforcement in the second stage (conditioning). LI consists of retarded conditioning to the preexposed stimulus; in other words, subjects are under the control of the previous stimulus–no event contingency rather than the changed, stimulus-reinforcement, contingency. LI is disrupted in amphetamine-treated rats and humans, normal humans with high schizotypy scores, and in some subsets of schizophrenic patients. Consequently, LI disruption has received an increasing interest as an animal model of cognitive deficits in schizophrenia. Furthermore, consistent with the central role of mesolimbic dopamine and temporal lobe pathology in schizophrenia, lesion and intracerebral injections studies in the rat have pointed to the involvement of the hippocampus/entorhinal cortex and the nucleus accumbens (NAC) in LI. Based on the latter, the switching model of LI proposed that (1) the mechanism responsible for LI disruption, that is, switching to respond according to the stimulus-reinforcement contingency, resides in the NAC; and (2) LI, that is, continuing to respond according to the stimulus–no event contingency, is mediated by signals from the hippocampal formation that inhibit the switching mechanism of the NAC (for reviews, see refs. 2, 3). Because the NAC is divided into shell and core subregions, which are cytoarchitecturally, physiologically, pharmacologically, and functionally distinct (e.g., ref. 5), we tested this hypothesis using lesions to these two subregions.[4] Our results showed that electrolytic lesions to the shell abolished LI, whereas core lesions left LI intact. Although this could be interpreted as showing that the core is not involved in LI, we interpreted these outcomes differently: rats with intact core (shell-lesioned) switched to respond according to the stimulus-reinforcement contingency (disrupted LI). Consequently, we proposed that the switching mechanism of the NAC resides in the core and that the switching mechanism is inhibited by the shell. This implies that it should be impossible to disrupt LI in rats with a core lesion and leads to the counterintuitive prediction that a lesion that destroyed both shell and core would leave LI intact. This prediction was tested here by comparing LI in rats sustaining an electrolytic shell lesion and a combined shell–core lesion.

[c]Voice: +972-3-6408993; fax: +972-3-640 7391; weiner@post.tau.ac.il

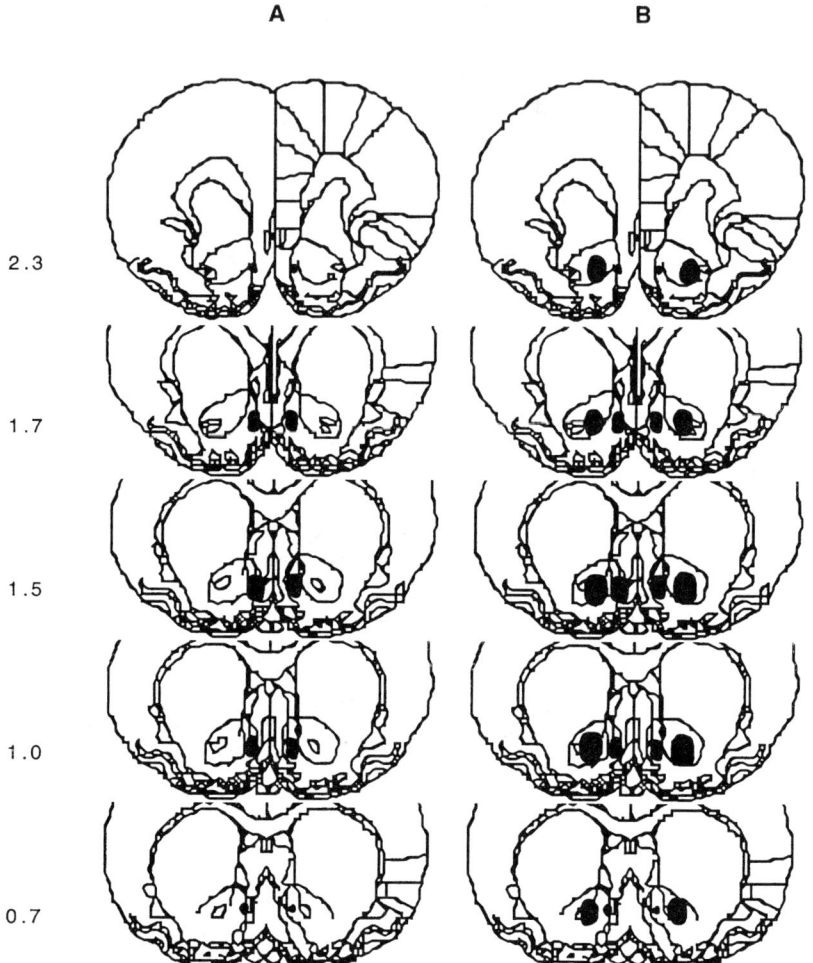

FIGURE 1. Schematic reconstructions of a representative shell (A) and a combined shell–core (B) lesion.

METHODS

Male Wistar rats approximately 4 months old sustained bilateral electrolytic lesions, using a 0.3 mm electrode insulated except for the tip, either in the shell (one anterior and one posterior lesion bilaterally using a 1 mA, 8-s current at coordinates: anterior: 1.7 mm anterior to bregma, 0.8 mm lateral to the midline, and 6.5 mm ventral to dura; posterior: 1.1 mm anterior to bregma, 0.8 mm lateral to the midline, and 6.5 mm ventral to dura) or in both shell and core (shell lesion as above in addition to an anterior and a posterior bilateral core lesion using a 1 mA, 15-s current at coordinates: anterior: 2.0 mm anterior to bregma, 1.8 mm lateral to the midline, and 6.5 mm ventral to dura; posterior: 1.4 mm anterior to bregma, 1.8 mm lateral to the midline, and 6.8 mm ventral to dura). Half of the sham-operated rats underwent a surgical procedure identical to shell and half identical to combined-lesion rats, but the electrodes were inserted 1 mm ventral to dura, and no current was passed.

LI was tested in standard Campden Instruments shuttle boxes.

Preexposure. The preexposed (PE) rats received 50 10-s, 2.8 kHz, 80 dB tones, whereas the nonpreexposed (NPE) rats were simply confined to the box.

Conditioning. Twenty-four hours later, all rats received 100 avoidance trials on a VI 60-s schedule. Each trial began with a 10-s tone followed by a 5-s 0.5 mA footshock, the stimulus remaining on with the shock. The number of avoidance responses (crossing to the opposite compartment during tone) were recorded in 10 trial blocks.

RESULTS

Schematic reconstructions of a representative shell (left) and a combined shell–core (right) lesion, based on assessment of sections stained with cresyl violet, are presented in FIGURE 1. FIGURE 2 presents the mean number of avoidance responses of the preexposed and nonpreexposed groups in sham, shell, and combined shell–core conditions. As can be seen, LI, that is, poorer avoidance performance of the preexposed as compared to the nonpreexposed rats, was evident in the sham condition from the 3rd to the 10th block, and in the combined shell–core condition from the 1st to the 8th block. By contrast, there was no LI in the shell-lesioned rats throughout the 10 blocks. A $2 \times 3 \times 10$ ANOVA yielded significant main effects of preexposure ($F_{(1,42)} = 5.24, p < 0.05$) and operation ($F_{(2,42)} = 3.60, p < 0.05$), as well as a significant preexposure $\times$ operation $\times$ blocks interaction ($F_{(18,378)} = 1.63, p = 0.05$), and the linear trend of this interaction ($F_{(2,42)} = 4.53, p < 0.05$).

CONCLUSION

As predicted, shell lesion abolished LI, but the addition of a core lesion prevented such disruption. In a subsequent series of experiments, we showed that rats with a combined lesion show LI under two conditions that disrupt it in normal rats, namely, a context change between preexposure and conditioning, and a high number of conditioning trials. Thus, in a two-way avoidance procedure as described above, sham rats showed LI when the same, but not when a different context, was used in preexposure and conditioning, whereas rats with a combined lesion showed LI in both conditions. Likewise, in a conditioned emotional response procedure, sham rats showed LI with 30 preexposures and 2 tone-shock pairings but not with 5 pairings; by contrast, rats with a combined lesion showed LI under both conditions. Finally, we found that excitotoxic (NMDA) lesions to the shell abolished LI, whereas core lesions led to LI with a high number of conditioning trials and with context shift.[1]

Taken together, these results demonstrate that shell and core lesions produce opposite effects on LI: Shell lesions disrupt LI, whereas core lesions produce an "un-

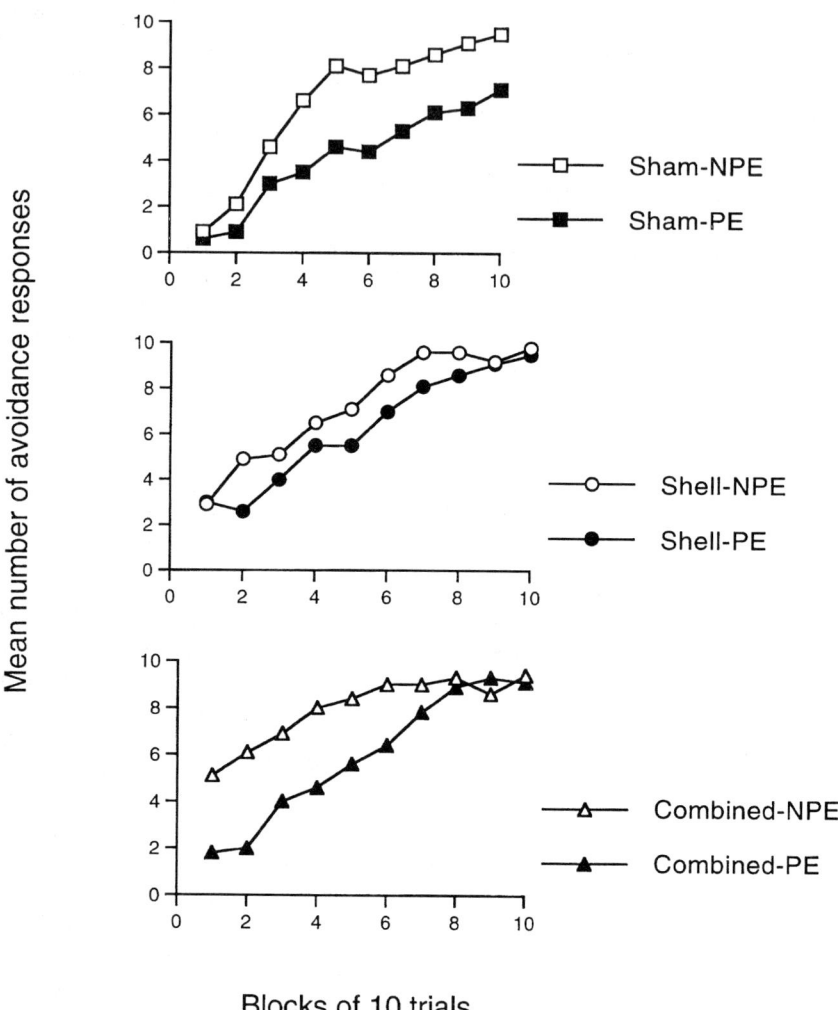

FIGURE 2. Mean number of avoidance responses, in 10 blocks of 10 trials, of the preexposed and nonpreexposed groups in sham (upper panel), shell (middle panel), and combined shell–core (lower panel) conditions.

disruptable LI," that is, LI that persists under conditions that disrupt it in normal rats. This supports our proposition that in the intact brain, the switching mechanism resides in the core, and the shell inhibits the switching mechanism of the core. We further propose that the function of the two subregions in LI is to determine which of the two contingencies, stimulus–no event (acquired in preexposure) or stimulus-reinforcement (acquired in conditioning) gains control over behavior. More specifically, the switching mechanism of the core is activated at the time of conditioning, when the previously nonreinforced stimulus is followed by reinforcement. Under conditions that lead to LI, the shell inhibits the switching mechanism of the core, so that the stimulus–no event contingency gains control over behavior; under conditions that do not lead to LI, the shell's inhibition is removed, allowing the expression of the stimulus-reinforcement contingency. Finally, we propose that whereas disrupted LI provides an animal model of disrupted LI found in some subsets of schizophrenic patients, undisruptable LI can provide an animal analogue to spared/reinstated LI found in other subsets of schizophrenic patients.

REFERENCES

1. GAL, G. 1998. The role of the shell and core in latent inhibition. PhD thesis, in preparation. Tel-Aviv University. Tel-Aviv.
2. WEINER, I. 1990. Neural substrates of latent inhibition: the switching model. Psychol. Bull. **108:** 442–461.
3. WEINER, I. & J. FELDON. 1997. The switching model of latent inhibition: an update of neural substrates. Behav. Brain Res. **88:** 11–25.
4. WEINER, I. et al. 1996. Differential involvement of the shell and core subterritories of the nucleus accumbens in latent inhibition and amphetamine induced activity. Behav. Brain Res. **81:** 123–133.
5. ZAHM, D.S. & J.S. BROG. 1992. On the significance of subterritories in the "accumbens" part of the rat ventral striatum. Neuroscience **50:** 751–767.

Freezing Behavior in BNST-lesioned Wistar Rats

DANIELA SCHULZ[a] AND RESIT CANBEYLI[b]

Department of Psychology, Bogazici University, Bebek 80815, Istanbul, Turkey

The bed nucleus of the stria terminalis (BNST) forms intricate anatomical links with the amygdala and is today viewed to function as part of the "extended amygdala."[1] Recent studies suggest an involvement of the BNST in anxiety or fear.[2,3] It appears that BNST lesions mediate hormonal reactions to fearful conditioned stimuli[2] and aspects of unconditioned fear, such as light-enhanced startle,[3] but not open-arm avoidance in the elevated plus-maze or suppression of shock-probe burying.[4] The present study examined the effects of BNST lesions on unconditioned contextual fear to uncontrollable and inescapable aversive tones. Previous work in our laboratory demonstrated that BNST lesions are sensitive to behavioral measures that involve uncontrollable stress. BNST compared to sham lesions resulted in increased learned despair or depression, as measured by forced swimming tests (FSTs).[5]

METHOD

Subjects were 9 BNST-lesioned and 8 sham-operated adult, male Wistar rats. They were maintained on a 12-h light/dark cycle (lights on at 7:00 a.m.) with food and water available ad libitum. Lesions were placed under ketamine anesthesia (155 mg/kg). Coordinates relative to bregma were +0.5 mm anteroposterior (AP), +1.1 mm mediolateral (ML), and −6.6 mm dorsoventral (DV) from dura for both BNST and sham-operated animals. For BNST lesions an anodal electric current was passed at 1.5 mAmp for 25 seconds. In sham operations the electrode was lowered into the brain for 25 seconds, but no current was applied.

Twenty days after surgery, freezing behavior was assessed in a sound attenuated, ventilated chamber (75 × 75 × 75) into which a Skinner box (30 × 30 × 30) was placed. The chamber was illuminated by a 60 W light bulb. Each animal was exposed to 5 tones (120 dB, 2000 Hz) of 5-s duration, with intertrial intervals of 25 seconds. Before the tones each animal was allowed to habituate to the chamber for 10 minutes. After the tones each animal remained in the box for another 10 minutes. Freezing behavior was coded during periods of immobility when all four paws touched the floor and the animal did not make any moves except those required for breathing. Total amounts of freezing and freezing latencies were coded both before and after the tones. Two types of freezing latencies were measured. Latency to become immobile was recorded when the animal became immobile for the first time for a period of at least five seconds. By contrast, latency to become mobile was recorded when

---

[a]Voice: +49-211-811-3491; fax: +49-211-811-2024; schulzd@uni-duesseldorf.de
[b]Voice: +90 212 263 1540, ext: 2129; fax: +90 212 287 2472; canbeyli@boun.edu.tr

TABLE 1. Means and SD of total immobility (seconds) and latency scores (seconds) as a function of group and time of test

Group/Time	Immobility	Latency-Mobility	Latency-Immobility
BNST ($n = 9$)			
Prior to tones			
Mean	95.80^d	7.10^d	177.80
SD	51.02	11.41	185.78
After tones			
Mean	405.60^a	166.80^b	6.00
SD	80.25	127.15	12.08
SHAM ($n = 8$)			
Prior to tones			
Mean	113.30^d	6.80^d	119.50^c
SD	74.95	11.91	114.79
After tones			
Mean	571.40	520.00	4.40
SD	30.30	116.26	12.37

NOTE: Significance levels for between-group comparisons: a, $p < .001$; b, $p < .0001$. Significance levels for within-group comparisons: c, $p < .05$; d, $p < .01$.

for the first time activity lasted for a period of at least five seconds. Mobility was defined as absence of immobility (i.e., any moves over and above those needed for breathing).

RESULTS

Histological examinations revealed that BNST lesions included bilateral damage to medial and lateral and mostly rostral portions of the BNST.

Results are presented in TABLE 1. Analyses of variance for a two-factor mixed design with repeated measures indicated that the main effects for the group were significant in the case of total immobility (freezing) [$F(1,14) = 17.52, p < 0.01$] and latency scores for mobility [$F(1,14) = 33.31, p < 0.0001$]. Comparisons for the repeated measures revealed main effects in all three cases, total immobility [$F(1,14) = 276.76, p < 0.0001$], latency scores for mobility [$F(1,14) = 116.26, p < 0.0001$], and latency scores for immobility [$F(1,14) = 11.64, p < 0.01$]. Interaction effects were significant for total immobility [$F(1,14) = 10.88, p < 0.01$] and latency scores for mobility [$F(1,14) = 33.27, p < 0.0001$]. Thus, the influence of time of the test (before versus after tones) on total amount of freezing as well as latency to become active depended upon the group. One-way analyses of variance revealed no significant differences between the groups, either in total freezing (immobility) durations [$F(1,15) = .32, p > 0.05$] or latencies to become mobile [$F(1,15) = 0.30, p > 0.05$] before the tones. By contrast, animals with BNST lesions froze significantly less after the tones [$F(1,14) = 29.87, p < 0.001$] and started to become active significantly earlier [$F(1,14) = 33.63, p < 0.0001$] than the control group. Both BNST-lesioned [$F(1,7) = 96.70, p < 0.0001$] and control [$F(1,7) = 183.94, p < 0.0001$] animals froze significantly more after tone stress compared to before. Both the lesion [$F(1,7) = 11.10, p < 0.05$] and the control

$[F(1,7) = 157.95, p < 0.0001]$ groups also started moving significantly earlier before than after the tones. Moreover, sham controls became immobile significantly earlier after than before the tones $[F(1,7) = 8.02, p < 0.05]$.

DISCUSSION

The present study showed that animals with BNST lesions were less fearful compared to controls, as assessed by total amounts of freezing and freezing latencies for mobility after the tone stress. BNST-lesioned rats were less immobile and became active earlier than controls after the tones. This suggests that BNST may mediate unconditioned fear in an uncontrollable aversive situation.

Previous work by Henke[6] suggested that BNST lesions result in increased perceived aversiveness in rats. Perceived aversiveness is thought to be greater during uncontrollable compared to controllable stress.[7] Perhaps because BNST-lesioned rats are most strongly affected by uncontrollable stress, no antifear effects were found in tests of open-arm avoidance in the elevated plus-maze and shock-probe burying.[4] In both tests, the animal had the choice to refrain from being exposed to the fear-inducing stimulus. By contrast, light-enhanced startle is a reflex[3] and, by definition, uncontrollable. In this paradigm, BNST lesions attenuated startle.

The BNST has also been implicated in coping behavior during stress.[6] Findings point to the possibility that BNST integrity carries protective functions.[8] Freezing behavior is protective; it is a natural and adaptive (coping) response exhibited by many species to avoid attack.[9] Thus, BNST lesions that lead to reduced freezing in the present study might have disrupted a coping response.

ACKNOWLEDGMENT

This work was supported by Bogazici University Research Grant 97B0703 to R.C.

REFERENCES

1. SUN, N. *et al.* 1991. Rat central amygdaloid nucleus projections to the bed nucleus of the stria terminalis. Brain Res. Bull. **27:** 175–191.
2. LEE, Y. *et al.* 1997. Role of the hippocampus, the bed nucleus of the stria terminalis. and the amygdala in the excitatory effect of corticotropin-releasing hormone on the acoustic startle reflex. J. Neurosci. **17:** 6434–6446.
3. WALKER, D.L. *et al.* 1997. Double dissociation between the involvement of the bed nucleus of the stria terminalis and the central nucleeus of the amygdala in the startle increases produced by conditioned versus unconditioned fear. J. Neurosci. **17:** 9375–9383.
4. TREIT, D. *et al.* 1998. Does the bed nucleus of the stria terminalis mediate fear behaviors? Behav. Neurosci. **112:** 379–386.
5. SCHULZ, D. *et al.* 1998. Effects of BNST lesions on learned despair as measured by forced swimming tests in male Wistar rats [abstract]. Soc. Neurosci. **24:** 1194.
6. HENKE, P.G. 1984. The bed nucleus of the stria terminalis and immobilization-stress: Unit activity, escape behavior, and gastric pathology in rats. Behav. Brain Res. **11:** 35–45.

7. OSBORNE, F.H. *et al.* 1975. Factors affecting the measurement of classicaly conditioned fear in rats following exposure to escapable versus inescapable signaled shock. J. Exp. Psychol. **1:** 364–373.
8. CASADA, J.H. *et al.* 1992. Evidence for two different pathways carrying stress-related information (noxious and amygdala stimulation) to the bed nucleus of the stria terminalis. Brain Res. **579:** 93–98.
9. KALIN, N.H. 1993. The neurobiology of fear. Sci. Am. **268:** 95–101.

A Functional Role for Dopamine Transmission in the Amygdala during Condtioned Fear

FAY A. GUARRACI,[a] RUSSELL J. FROHARDT, STACEY L. YOUNG, AND BRUCE S. KAPP

Department of Psychology, University of Vermont, Burlington, Vermont 05405, USA

INTRODUCTION

Recent research suggests that the mesencephalic dopaminergic system is activated by conditioned fear-arousing stimuli.[4,9] Research also strongly suggests that the amygdala is a critical component of the neural circuitry essential for conditioned fear, inasmuch as various manipulations of the amygdala disrupt both the acquisition and expression of conditioned fear.[3,6,8] Although, the amygdala has been identified as a site of dopamine release in response to fear-arousing stimuli,[2,5] surprisingly little effort has been devoted to investigating the specific contribution of the mesoamygdaloid dopamine system to fear conditioning. The present study was designed to investigate the effects of intra-amygdaloid infusions of a dopaminergic agonist and antagonist on the *acquisition* and *expression* of pavlovian fear, conditioned to acoustic and contextual stimuli in the rat.

EXPERIMENT 1

The purpose of experiment 1 was to assess the effects of infusions of the D_1 receptor antagonist, SCH 23390 (2.0 µg/0.5 µL; RBI, Natick, MA), into the amygdala on the acquisition and expression of conditioned fear using a 2×2 factorial design. Fear conditioned to both acoustic and contextual cues in Long Evans female rats was assessed by measuring freezing behavior, a well-established measure of conditioned fear in the rat.[1] Immediately prior to acquisition training, the animals received infusions of either SCH 23390 or saline vehicle, depending on group assignment. The animals were placed in conditioning chambers and received three tone-footshock pairings. Immediately prior to retention testing 24 hour later, the animals received infusions of either SCH 23390 or saline vehicle, depending on group assignment. The animals were again placed in the conditioning chambers and received three tone-alone presentations.

Thirty-one animals with microscopically verified guide cannulae tips located no more than 0.7 mm dorsal to the surface of the amygdaloid central nucleus (ACe) were included in the final analyses. Animals receiving pretraining SCH 23390 did not differ from animals receiving pretraining vehicle during acquisition training. The two groups demonstrated a similar increase in freezing behavior across trials to both acoustic and contextual conditioned stimuli. However, during the retention test, the

---

[a]Voice: 802-656-2670; fax: 802-656-8783; fguarrac@zoo.uvm.edu

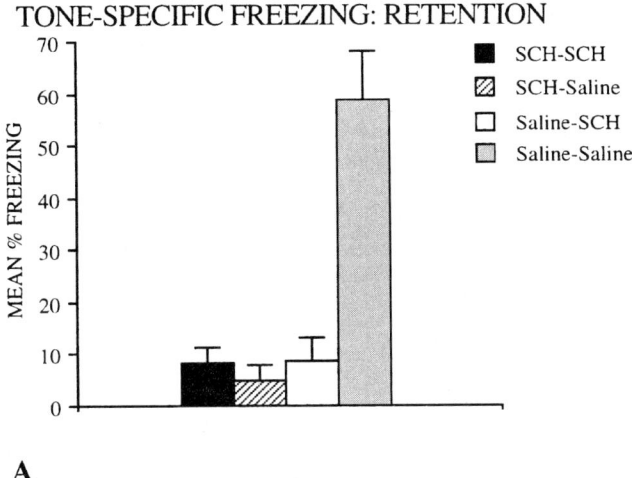

A

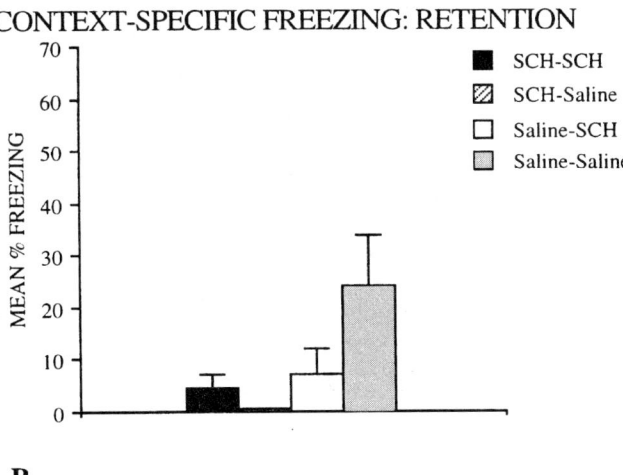

B

FIGURE 1. Freezing behavior during retention testing in experiment 1. **A:** Mean percent freezing behavior collapsed across trials during the retention test to the three tone presentations. The SCH-SCH group ($n = 6$) received pretraining and pretesting SCH 23390. The SCH-Saline group ($n = 9$) received only pretraining SCH 23390. The Saline-SCH group ($n = 7$) received only pretesting SCH 23390. The Saline-Saline group ($n = 9$) received pretraining and pretesting saline. The Saline-Saline group froze significantly more than all three drug groups. **B:** Mean percent freezing collapsed across the three 24 s pretone periods during the retention test. The Saline-Saline group froze more than all three drug groups. Error bars represent standard error of the mean.

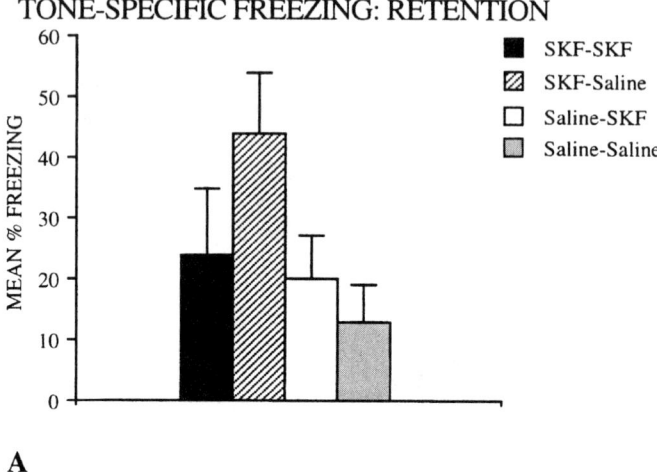

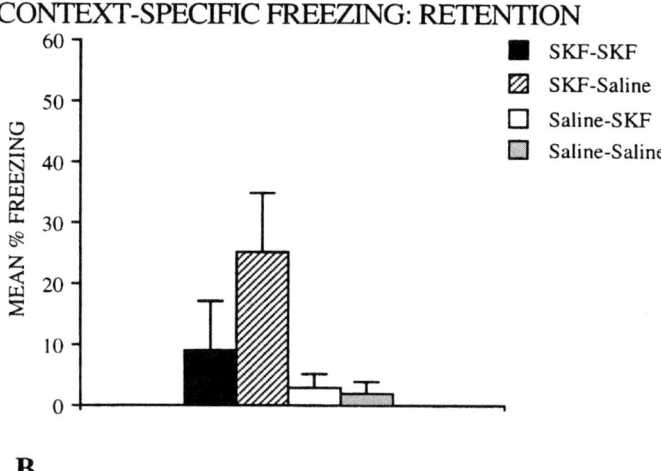

FIGURE 2. Freezing behavior during retention testing for experiment 2. **A:** Mean percent freezing behavior collapsed across trials during the retention test to the five tone presentations. The SKF-SKF group ($n = 8$) received pretraining and pretesting SKF 82958. The SKF-Saline group ($n = 8$) received only pretraining SKF 82958. The Saline-SKF group ($n = 10$) received only pretesting SKF 82958. The Saline-Saline group ($n = 10$) received pretraining and pretesting Saline. The SKF-Saline group froze significantly more than the Saline-Saline group. **B:** Mean percent freezing collapsed across the five 24 s pretone periods during the retention test. The SKF-Saline group froze significantly more than the Saline-Saline group. Error bars represent standard error of the mean.

animals that received SCH 23390 either prior to acquisition training, prior to retention testing, or prior to both demonstrated attenuated freezing behavior (FIG. 1).

EXPERIMENT 2

If the effects of SCH 23390 observed in experiment 1 were due to a selective effect on amygdaloid dopamine transmission, then one prediction would be that a D_1 receptor agonist would facilitate conditioned fear. Experiment 2 was designed to test the validity of this prediction by examining the effects of intra-amygdaloid administration of the D_1 receptor agonist, SKF 82958 (2.0 µg/0.5 µL; RBI, Natick, MA), on the acquisition and expression of conditioned fear. The methods and procedures of experiment 2 were similar to those of experiment 1. However, two procedural changes were made. The intensity of the footshock was reduced during acquisition training, and two additional acoustic-conditioned stimuli presentations were administered during retention testing. These changes were made in order to mitigate the possibility of a ceiling effect on freezing behavior for the SALINE-SALINE control animals, which could mask any drug-induced facilitation of conditioned fear.

Thirty-six animals with microscopically verified guide cannulae tips located no more than 0.7 mm dorsal to the surface of the ACe were included in the final analyses. Animals receiving pretraining SKF 82958 did not differ from animals receiving pretraining vehicle during acquisition training. The two groups demonstrated a similar increase in freezing behavior across trials to both acoustic and contextual- conditioned stimuli. However, during the retention test, the animals that received SKF 82958 prior to training demonstrated facilitated freezing behavior (FIG. 2).

DISCUSSION

The present experiments demonstrated that pretraining infusions of either SCH 23390 or SKF 82958 altered retention testing without effecting acquisition, suggesting that D_1 receptors within the amygdala may play a specific role in modulating of long- term memory consolidation following pavlovian fear conditioning. Dopamine may also be important for the normal expression of emotional motor responses, given that pretesting infusions of SCH 23390 attenuated freezing behavior during retention testing. This interpretation is consistent with the recently published results of Lamont and Kokkinidis[7] who found that intra-amygdaloid infusions of SCH 23390 immediately prior to testing blocked the expression of conditioned fear in the fear-potentiated startle paradigm in rats. Although the exact mechanism(s) by which dopamine exerts its effects on the amygdaloid circuits involved in the acquisition and expression of conditioned fear is presently unknown, the results clearly suggest a prominent role for the amygdaloid dopaminergic system in these phenomenon.

ACKNOWLEDGMENT

This research was supported by NIMH NRSA Fellowship MH11627-02 awarded to F.A.G.

REFERENCES

1. BOLLES, R.C. & A.C. COLLIER. 1976. Effect of predictive cues on freezing in rats. Anim. Learn. Behav. **4:** 6–8.
2. COCO, M.L., C.M. KUHN, T.D. ELY & C.D. KILTS. 1992. Selective activation of mesoamygdaloid dopamine neurons by conditioned stress: Attenuation by diazepam. Brain Res. **590:** 39–47.
3. DAVIS, M. 1992. The role of the amygdala in conditioned fear. *In* The Amygdala: Neurobiological Aspects of Emotion, Memory and Mental Dysfunction. J.P. Aggleton, Ed.: 255–306. Wiley-Liss, Inc. New York.
4. GUARRACI, F.A. & B.S. KAPP. 1999. Characterization of ventral tegmental dopamine neurons in the awake rabbit. Behav. Brain Res. **99:** 169–179.
5. INOUE, T., K. TSUCHIYA & T. KOYAMA. 1994. Regional changes in dopamine and serotonin activation with various intensity of physical and psychological stress in the rat brain. Pharmacol. Biochem. Behav. **49:** 911–920.
6. KAPP, B.S., A.J. SILVESTRI & F.A. GUARRACI. 1998. Vertebrate models of learning and memory. *In* Neurobiology of Learning and Memory. J.L. Martinez, Jr. & R.P. Kesner, Eds.: 289–332. Academic Press, Inc. San Diego.
7. LAMONT, E.W. & L. KOKKINIDIS. 1998. Infusion of the dopamine D_1 receptor antagonist SCH 23390 into the amygdala blocks fear expression in potentiated startle paradigm. Brain Res. **795:** 128–136.
8. LEDOUX, J.E. 1995. Emotion: Clues from the brain. Annu. Rev. Psychol. **46:** 209–235.
9. TRULSON, M.E. & D.W. PREUSSLER. 1984. Dopamine-containing ventral tegmental area neurons in freely moving cats: activity during sleep-waking cycle and effects of stress. Exp. Neurol. **83:** 367–377.

Effect of Amygdala Kindling on Emotional Behavior and Benzodiazepine Receptor Binding in Rats

LISA E. KALYNCHUK,[a,c] DEBRA M. PEARSON,[a] JOHN P.J. PINEL,[b] AND MICHAEL J. MEANEY[a]

[a]*Douglas Hospital Research Center, McGill University, 6875 LaSalle Boulevard, Verdun, Quebec, Canada H4H 1R3*
[b]*Department of Psychology, University of British Columbia, Vancouver, British Columbia, Canada V6T 1Z4*

Interictal (i.e., between seizure) emotional disturbances, such as fear, anxiety, and depression are often associated with temporal lobe epilepsy.[1] Although the presence of these interictal emotional disturbances has been repeatedly documented, considerable controversy still remains over their nature and cause. This controversy has proven troublesome to resolve because of difficulties inherent in the experimental study of epileptic patients.

We have found that long-term kindling (i.e., 100 stimulations) in rats produces substantial changes in emotional behavior that model those often observed in temporal lobe epileptics. For example, amygdala kindling in rats decreases open-field activity in an unfamiliar open field, increases thigmotaxia, increases resistance to capture, and increases escape behavior from an elevated plus maze.[4] Although we have determined that this emotionality depends on the number of stimulations the rats receive,[4] the site of stimulation,[3] and the time since the last stimulation,[5] the neural correlates that underlie it remain unknown. Because benzodiazepines (BZ) have been repeatedly implicated in the mediation of emotional behavior,[6] in the present experiment we investigated the effect of amygdala kindling on emotional behavior and on BZ receptor binding.

METHODS

A single bipolar electrode was implanted in the left basolateral amygdala of each of 44 adult male Long-Evans rats. After a postsurgical recovery period, the rats were divided into six groups: Three stimulation groups received 20 ($n = 11$), 60 ($n = 10$), or 100 ($n = 12$) amygdala stimulations; and three sham-stimulation groups received either 20 ($n = 4$), 60 ($n = 4$), or 100 ($n = 3$) sham stimulations. A sham stimulation entailed attaching the stimulation lead to a rat's electrode but not passing any current through it. The stimulations were delivered 3 times per day, 5 days per week, with a minimum of 2 h between consecutive stimulations. One day after the final kindling stimulation, each rat was placed by itself in a corner of a novel open field (i.e., 60 ×

[c]Voice: 514-762-3048; fax: 514-762-3034; mdk3@musica.mcgill.ca

60 × 60 cm wooden box with no top) for 5 minutes. After the 5 min, each rat was picked up from above by an experimenter who was wearing a leather glove that was unfamiliar to the rat. The rat's resistance to being captured was scored according to the following 7-point scale: 0, easy to pick up; 1, vocalizes or shies away from hand; 2, shies away from hand and vocalizes; 3, runs away from hand; 4, runs away and vocalizes; 5, bites or attempts to bite; 6, launches a jump attack.

Each rat was sacrificed approximately 72 h after the resistance to capture testing, and its brain was rapidly removed and frozen in isopentane and dry ice. Frozen 16 μm coronal sections were cut on a cryostat through the frontal cortex, septum, and hippocampus; thaw-mounted on poly-L-lysine-coated slides; dessicated under a vacuum at 4°C; and stored at −80°C until assay. For the BZ receptor assay, the slides were placed in preincubation buffer (i.e., 0.17 M Tris-HCl, pH 7.4) for 30 min at 4°C and then incubated for 60 min at 4°C in the same buffer plus a saturating 0.5 nM concentration of [^{3}H]flunitrazepam (84.5 Ci/nmol, New England Nuclear). Nonspecific binding was determined by incubation of adjacent brain sections in incubation buffer with the addition of 1 μM clonazepam. After incubation, the slides were rinsed in preincubation buffer twice for 30 s at 4°C, dipped in ice cold distilled water, and air dried under a fan. The next day, the slides were apposed to ^{3}Hyperfilm along with ^{3}H microscales for 14 days at 4°C. Autoradiograms were analyzed by obtaining optical densities determined by computer-assisted densitometry using an MCID image analysis system (Imaging Research, St. Catherine's, ON).

RESULTS AND DISCUSSION

FIGURE 1A illustrates the mean resistance to capture displayed by the rats in each group. The resistance to capture increased dramatically as the rats received more kindling stimulations. Statistical analyses of the differences in resistance to capture revealed a significant group effect [Kruskal-Wallis ANOVA: H (3, 44) = 22.66, $p < 0.0001$], and post hoc multiple comparisons revealed significant differences between the 100-stim and the sham-stim rats ($p < 0.01$), between the 100-stim and the 20-stim rats ($p < 0.05$), and between the 60-stim and the sham-stim rats ($p < 0.01$).

FIGURE 1B illustrates the mean density of [^{3}H]flunitrazepam binding to benzodiazepine receptors in various brain regions from the rats in each group. Only the differences in [^{3}H]flunitrazepam binding in the dentate gyrus [F (3, 40) = 9.77, $p < 0.0001$] and the CA1 subfield of the hippocampus [F (3, 40) = 5.765, $p < 0.002$] were statistically significant. In the dentate gyrus, [^{3}H]flunitrazepam binding was significantly increased in the 100-stim ($p < 0.05$), 60-stim ($p < 0.05$), and 20-stim rats ($p < 0.05$), compared to the sham-stim rats. By contrast, in the CA1 subfield of the hippocampus, [^{3}H]flunitrazepam binding was significantly decreased in the 100-stim rats ($p < 0.05$), compared to the sham-stim rats.

FIGURES 2A and 2B depict the correlation between resistance to capture and [^{3}H]flunitrazepam binding in the dentate gyrus and CA1 region of the hippocampus, respectively. In both cases, the correlations were statistically significant (dentate gyrus: $r = +0.518, p < 0.005$; CA1: $r = -0.367, p < 0.01$). This suggests that kindling-induced emotionality could be at least partly mediated by changes in BZ receptors in specific regions of the hippocampus. In fact, there is support for the idea that seizures produce regionally distinct changes in GABAergic neurotransmission: Gibbs

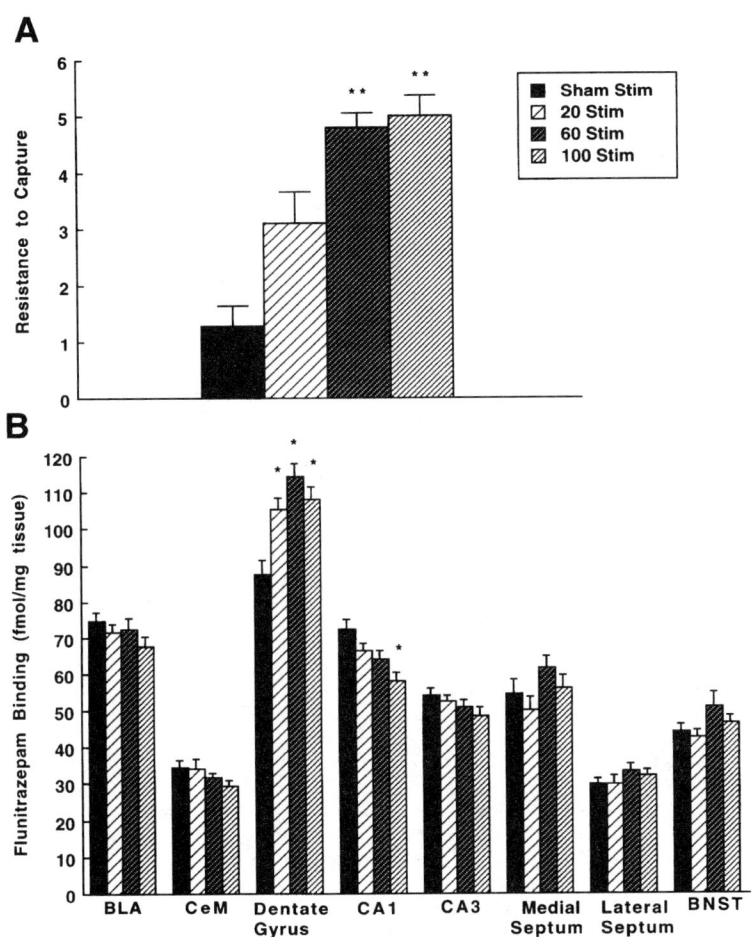

FIGURE 1. A: The mean (±SEM) resistance to capture displayed by the rats in each group. The three sham-stimulation groups were combined for the purposes of the statistical analyses. Resistance to capture increased dramatically as the rats received more kindling stimulations. The 100-stim rats were significantly more resistant to capture than both the 20-stim and the sham-stim rats; the 60-stim rats were significantly more resistant to capture than the sham-stim rats. **B:** The mean (±SEM) [^{3}H]flunitrazepam binding (in fmol/mg wet tissue) in various brain regions from the sham-stim, 20-stim, 60-stim, and 100-stim rats. Values represent specific binding (total binding minus nonspecific binding). Only the differences in binding in the dentate gyrus and CA1 were statistically significant. The 20-stim, 60-stim, and 100-stim rats all had significantly increased binding in the dentate gyrus compared to the sham-stim rats; the 100-stim rats had significantly decreased binding in the CA1 region compared to the sham-stim rats. BLA, basolateral nucleus of the amygdala; CeM, central nucleus of the amygdala; BNST, bed nucleus of the stria terminalis. * $p < 0.05$; ** $p < 0.01$.

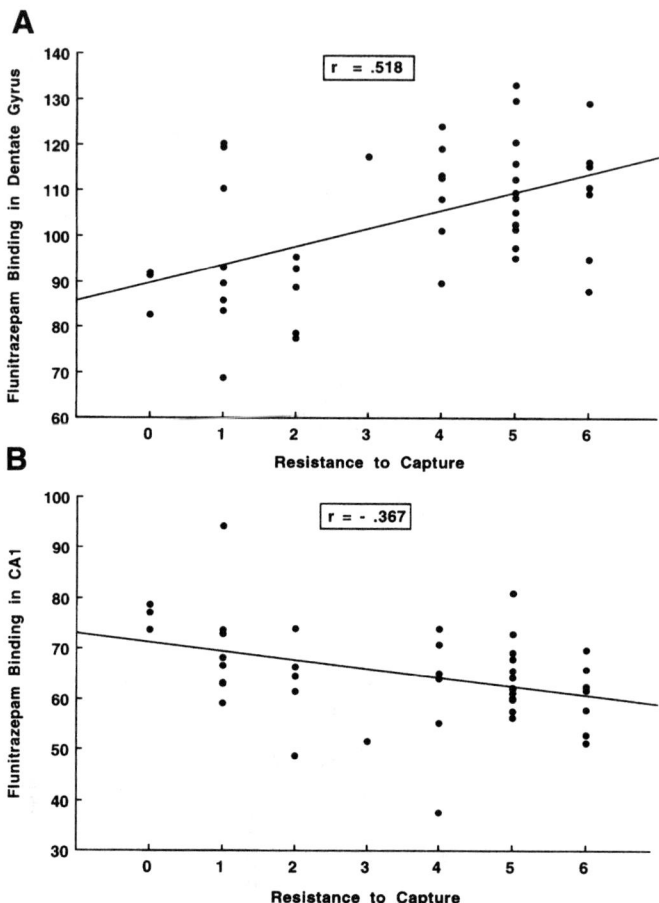

FIGURE 2. Scattergrams depicting the correlation between [^{3}H]flunitrazepam binding in the dentate gyrus (**A**) and CA1 region of the hippocampus (**B**), and the resistance to capture displayed by each rat. In both cases, the correlations were significant.

et al.[2] reported that the efficacy of GABA in activating $GABA_A$ receptors in epileptic tissue is increased by 78% in dentate granule neurons and decreased by 52% in CA1 neurons. Accordingly, it would be interesting to determine the effect of infusions of benzodiazepine agonists and antagonists into specific hippocampal regions on the development of interictal emotionality in kindled rats.

REFERENCES

1. DODRILL, C.B. & L.W. BATZEL. 1986. Interictal behavioral features of patients with epilepsy. Epilepsia **27** (suppl.2): S64–S76.

2. GIBBS, J.W. et al. 1997. Differential epilepsy-associated alterations in postsynaptic GABA(A) receptor function in dentate granule and CA1 neurons. J. Neurophysiol. **77:** 1924–38.
3. KALYNCHUK, L.E. et al. 1998. Long-term kindling and interictal emotionality in rats: Effect of stimulation site. Brain Res. **779**(1-2)**:** 149–157.
4. KALYNCHUK, L.E. et al. 1997. Changes in emotional behavior produced by long-term amygdala kindling in rats. Biol. Psychiatry **41:** 438–451.
5. KALYNCHUK, L.E. et al. 1998. Persistence of the interictal emotionality produced by long-term amygdala kindling in rats. Neuroscience **85**(4)**:** 1311–1319.
6. TALLMAN, J.F. et al. 1980. Receptors for the age of anxiety: Pharmacology of the benzodiazepines. Science **207:** 272–281.

Does Chronic Activity-Stress Produce Hippocampal Atrophy and Basal Forebrain Lesions?

A Preliminary Analysis

KELLY G. LAMBERT,[a,c] PRINCY QUADROS,[b] CATHERINE AURENTZ,[a] CATHERINE LOWRY,[a] AND CRAIG H. KINSLEY[b]

[a]*Randolph-Macon College, Department of Psychology, Ashland, Virginia 23005, USA*
[b]*University of Richmond, Richmond, Virginia 23173, USA*

INTRODUCTION

Although the stress response is adaptive for overcoming acute physical stressors, research suggests that the chronic stress response may be more damaging than the stressor itself, resulting in the emergence of many stress-related diseases. Much of the stress research has focused on the hippocampus because of the location of glucocorticoid receptors in this limbic structure.[1] Focusing on rats, exposure to chronic stress negatively affects the hippocampus by reducing the complexity and length of apical dendrites in the CA1 and CA3 pyramidal neurons.[2] Does stress threaten the hippocampus in other species? Uno *et al.*[3] reported a 30% reduction in the hippocampus of rhesus monkeys that received dexamethasone injections during prenatal development (which produced an increased baseline plasma cortisol level when the brains were quantified at 20 months of age). Early exposure to stress and accompanying elevated cortisol levels also seem to be a threat to human children. Mary Carlson's[4] work with children living in the harsh conditions of Romanian orphanages has indicated increased cortisol levels at certain times of the day; further, the high cortisol was correlated with diminished mental and motor development. Thus, it appears that stress influences the hypothalamic-pituitary axis and, at least in nonhuman animals, the resulting increases in glucocorticoids result in compromised hippocampal neurons. The effect of elevated cortisol on the developing human brain is an important question yet to be answered.

The effect of chronic stress was investigated in the present study by exposing rats to activity-stress (A-S), which consists of housing animals in activity wheels and feeding them one hour per day. Typically, within just one week, animals increase running to about seven miles per day and, upon autopsy, show evidence of significant weight loss, stress ulcers, atrophied thymus glands, and atrophied hippocampal CA1 and CA3 pyramidal neurons.[2] The brains in the present study were subjected to immunocytochemistry for an investigation of the involvement of glial cells in the chronic stress-induced hippocampal neuronal atrophy. During the histological process, however, it became apparent that the stressed and, to a lesser degree, the pair-fed

---

[c]Voice: 804-752-4717; fax: 804-752-7345; klambert@rmc.edu

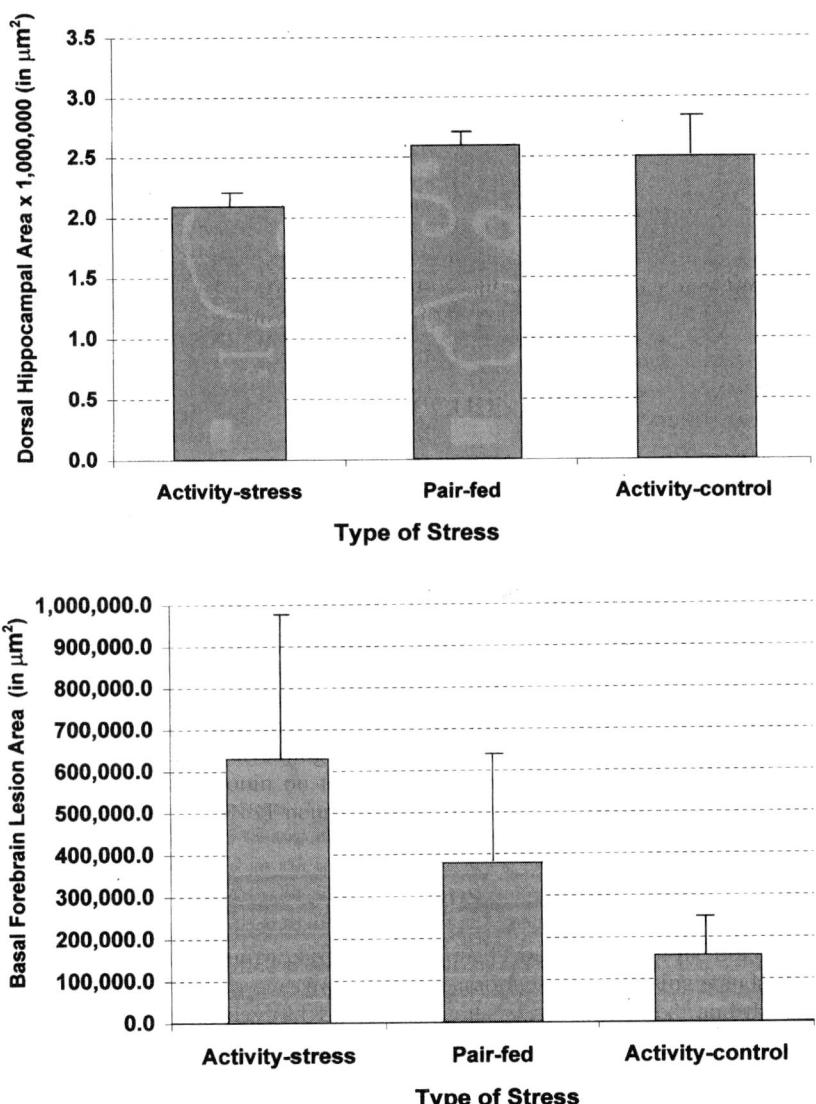

FIGURE 1. The effect of stress on dorsal hippocampal area (top) and basal forebrain lesion area (bottom).

brains had hippocampal atrophy and, in some animals, accompanying basal forebrain lesions in the amygdaloid area, when compared to nonactive, nonfood-restricted controls. Because this observation had not been made previously in our laboratory, we investigated possible differences between the current study and past studies. Interestingly, the animals in the current study were about 11 days younger than animals used

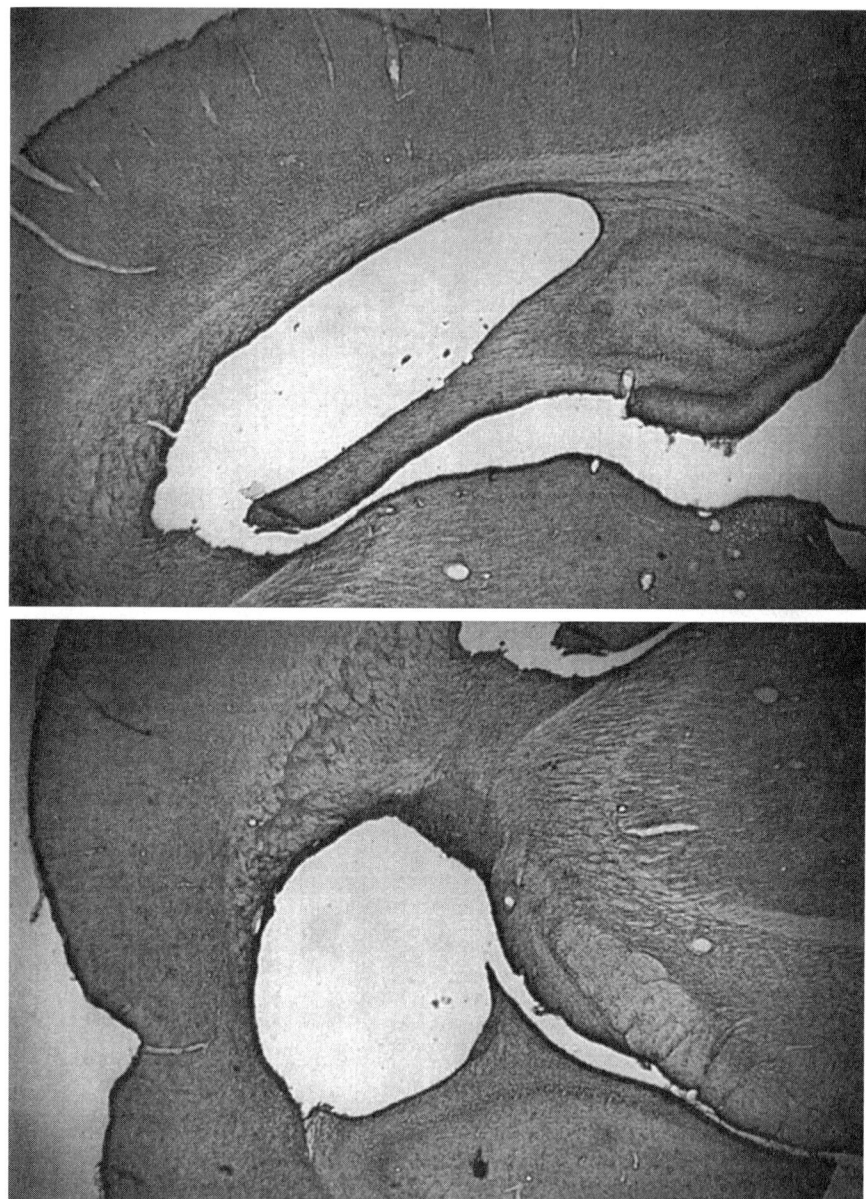

FIGURE 2. Photomicrographs of hippocampal area (top) and basal forebrain lesion area (bottom) in activity-stress rat.

in prior studies in our laboratory. These findings suggest that the brains of prepubescent animals may be especially vulnerable to exposure to chronic stress.

METHOD

Eighteen male Long-Evans rats (38 days of age) were randomly assigned to either an activity-stress (A-S) group, a pair-fed (P-F) group, or an activity-control (A-C) group ($n = 6$ in each group.) The activity animals were housed in activity wheels, which had adjoining cages; the P-F group was housed in standard suspended cages. After one week of habituation to the appropriate cages, the A-S paradigm commenced. Initially, the food was removed for the A-S animals and, on each of the next 4 days, the animals received one hour to eat ad libitum. The P-F animals were also food restricted for one day, and on subsequent days, each animal was given the same amount of food as the assigned food-yoked animal consumed the prior day. The A-C animals were not food restricted.

After the animals were exposed to the A-S paradigm for five days, they were sacrificed so their brains could be prepared for immunocytochemistry (gFAP) and Neutral Red staining. Ten sections (50 microns) were made through the dorsal hippocampus of each brain. Neurolucida software was used to trace (at 1.25×) and quantify the areas of both dorsal hippocampus and the basal forebrain lesions. In order to quantify the basal forebrain lesions, observers were instructed to go to the amygdalohippocampal area and trace any absence of tissue (which included portions of the lateral ventricles in some animals—hence the apparent appearance of lesions in the control animals).

RESULTS

A 3 × 1 ANOVA was used to determine the effect of type of stress (A-S, P-F, or A-C) on the mean hippocampal and basal forebrain lesion areas. The structural and lesion areas represent the area for each hemisphere. Results indicated a significant effect of stress on the dorsal hippocampal area [$F (2,14) = 4.64$; $p = 0.028$]; specifically, the A-S animals had a smaller hippocampal area than the P-F and A-C animals. Further, a nonsignificant trend was found in the basal forebrain lesion data. Although the A-S group had 300% and 65% larger lesion areas than the A-C and P-F groups, respectively, the variability was excessive. See FIGURE 1 for graphs of hippocampus and amygdaloid data and FIGURE 2 for photomicrographs of A-S hippocampal and amygdaloid areas.

CONCLUSIONS

Although these results are preliminary, it appears that A-S compromises the size of the dorsal hippocampus. Certainly more research needs to be conducted to more firmly establish the effect of this animal model of chronic stress on hippocampal and amygdaloid morphology. Most importantly, these results suggest that the stress response needs to be investigated across the life span to determine critical developmental periods in which the brain may be especially vulnerable to the negative effects of stress.

REFERENCES

1. MCEWEN, B.S., J.M. WEISS & L.S. SCHWARTZ. 1968. Selective retention of corticosterone by limbic structures in the brain. Nature **220**: 911–912.
2. LAMBERT, K.G., S.K. BUCKELEW, G. STAFFISO-SANDOZ, S. GAFFGA, W. CARPENTER, J. FISHER & C. H. KINSLEY. 1998. Activity-stress induces atrophy of apical dendrites of hippocampal pyramidal neurons in male rats. Physiol. Behav. **65**: 43–49.
3. UNO, H., R. TARARA, J.G. ELSE, M.A. SULEMAN & R.M. SAPOLSKY. 1989. Hippocampal damage associated with prolonged and fatal stress in primates. J. Neurosci. **9**: 1705–1711.
4. CARLSON, M. & F. EARLS. 1997. Psychological and neuroendocrinological sequelae of early social deprivation in institutionalized children in Romania. *In* The Integrative Neurobiology of Affiliation. C.S. Carter, I.I. Lederhendler & B. Kirkpatrick, Eds.: **807**: 419–428. Annals of the New York Academy of Sciences. New York.

Role of the Basolateral Amygdala in Panic Disorder

A. SHEKHAR,[a] T. S. SAJDYK, S. R. KEIM, K. K. YODER, AND S. K. SANDERS

Departments of Psychiatry, Pharmacology and Toxicology and Program in Medical Neurobiology, Institute of Psychiatric Research, Indiana University Medical Center, 791 Union Drive, Indianapolis, Indiana 46202, USA

INTRODUCTION

Anxiety disorders are the most prevalent of all psychiatric problems. The neurobiological mechanisms of severe anxiety states, such as panic disorder, are still poorly understood. A number of CNS areas have been implicated in the generation of panic responses, and it is likely that a "network" of interconnected nuclei may regulate this important survival reflex under normal circumstances. In pathological conditions, such as panic disorder, one or more critical regulatory sites may be dysfunctional, such that a panic response is elicited with minimal or inappropriate stimuli. One such regulatory area is the dorsomedial hypothalamus (DMH), where chronic GABA dysfunction results in a panic-like response.[1] Another area is the anterior basolateral amygdala (aBLA), where blocking a tonic GABAergic inhibition results in physiological and behavioral responses associated with panic attacks. The aBLA has pyramidal cells that are probably glutamatergic and nonpyramidal cells that contain GABA and presumably function as inhibitory neurons on the pyramidal cells.[2] Blockade of $GABA_A$ receptors in the aBLA with bicuculline methiodide (BMI) elicits increases in heart rate (HR), blood pressure (BP), respiratory rate, and anxiety, as measured by the social interaction (SI) test,[3] suggesting a panic-like response. In addition, injecting repeated subthreshold doses of BMI into the aBLA induces long-term synaptic plasticity (termed "priming") in the aBLA, such that the animals become chronically anxious and reactive to previously subthreshold stimuli.[4] Further, there appears to be a tonic GABAergic inhibition and EAA-mediated excitation within the aBLA,[5] and the panic-like responses following $GABA_A$ receptor blockade or the priming phenomenon seen with subthreshold GABA blockade is an *N*-methyl-D-aspartate (NMDA) receptor-dependent phenomenon.[6] Also, if priming of aBLA is similar to the development of pathological anxiety states, such as panic disorder, then the primed animals would be predicted to become responsive to sodium lactate (and yohimbine) infusions that provoke panic attacks clinically. This study reports some preliminary findings about the panic responses in rats primed with repeated subthreshold $GABA_A$ receptor blockade in the aBLA.

---

[a]Address correspondence to Dr. Anantha Shekhar, Institute of Psychiatric Research, 791 Union Drive, Indianapolis, IN 46202. Voice: 317-274-3685; fax: 317-274-1365; ashekhar@iupui.edu

TABLE 1. Effects on heart rate (HR, beats/min) and mean arterial blood pressure (BP, mm of hg) following iv infusions of either saline (10 ml/kg), sodium lactate (10 ml/kg of 0.5 N soln.), or yohimbine (0.4 mg/kg) in aBLA-primed and sham-primed rats

	aBLA-primed rats		Sham-primed rats	
Intravenous Infusion	HR	BP	HR	BP
Saline	18 ± 6	−4 ± 7	−23 ± 19	−14 ± 9
Sodium lactate	98 ± 17*	52 ± 12	−46 ± 22	−8 ± 11
Yohimbine	135 ± 8	45 ± 10	23 ± 27	10 ± 14

The sham-primed groups that received saline and lactate infusions were given repeated injections of saline into the aBLA, whereas the sham-primed group that received yohimbine was injected with BMI in areas adjacent to the aBLA. Data are represented as mean ± SEM. *Significantly different from saline by ANOVA, coupled with Newman-Keul's test; $p < 0.05$.

EXPERIMENTS AND RESULTS

Experiment 1: Primed Rats May Become Reactive to Peripheral Lactate and Yohimbine Infusions Similar to Patients with Panic Disorder

This was tested in two groups of rats ($n = 6$ each) that were fitted with arterial and venous catheters as well as bilateral injection cannulae in the aBLA. Both groups were tested with intravenous (iv) infusions of sodium lactate (10 mL/kg of 0.5 N solution) at baseline to confirm that they were not reactive to lactate. Then, one group ($n = 6$) was primed by daily injections of BMI (6 pmoles/100 nL/side) for the next 5 days, while the other group ($n = 6$) received daily injections of a-CSF (sham priming). Afterwards, separated by 48 hours, the two groups of rats were infused iv (in random order) with either saline (10 mL/kg) or lactate (10 mL/kg of 0.5 N), and their HR, BP, and SI responses were measured. Similarly, yohimbine infusions (0.4 mg/kg) were also tested in a preliminary study. Only the primed and not sham-primed animals elicited significant and dramatic increases in their HR and BP, as well as significant decreases (i.e., further increases in anxiety) in the SI test following lactate infusions (TABLE 1). Further, pretreatment with the antipanic agent alprazolam before lactate infusions blocked the panic responses.

Experiment 2: Third Ventricular Circumventricular Organs (CVOs) May Be the Relay Sites for the Lactate Response

In the case of chronic GABA dysfunction in the DMH, the CVOs (particularly the organum vasculosum lamina terminalis, OVLT) appear to be critical sensory sites that activate the DMH following peripheral lactate infusions and elicit a panic response.[1] Similarly, in a preliminary series of experiments, we tested the role of the third ventricular CVOs in the elicitation of lactate responses in the aBLA-primed rats. Two groups of animals were implanted with femoral arterial and venous catheters, as well as bilateral microinjection cannulae in the aBLA. In addition, one group ($n = 4$) had third microinjection cannulae implanted in the subfornical organs (SFO), while the other group ($n = 3$) had cannulae in the OVLTs. Both groups of rats underwent the

TABLE 2. Effects on heart rate (HR, beats/min) and mean arterial blood pressure (BP, mm of Hg) following iv infusions of either saline (10 mL/kg), sodium lactate (10 mL/kg of 0.5N soln), or sodium lactate after injections of tetrodotoxin (TTY, 1 pmole/100 nL) into the subfornical organ (SFO) in aBLA-primed rats

Intravenous Infusion	Changes in aBLA-primed Rats	
	HR	BP
Saline	-30 ± 12	-13 ± 8
Sodium lactate	100 ± 18*	61 ± 18*
Sodium lactate + TTX in SFO	$3 \pm 6^{\#}$	$-2 \pm 6^{\#}$

Data are represented as mean ± SEM. Significantly different from saline (*) and from lactate ($^{\#}$) infusions alone by ANOVA, coupled with Newman-Keul's test; $p < 0.05$.

priming procedure. They were then tested with iv lactate infusions (10 mL/kg) to ensure the development of the typical panic-like response. On two experimental days, separated by 48 hours, the rats were injected in random order with either a-CSF (vehicle) or the neurotransmission blocker, tetrodotoxin (TTX; 100 nL of 10 µM solution), into the CVO sites and then retested with iv lactate infusions. Injecting TTX and not a-CSF into the SFO completely blocked the iv lactate response, suggesting that the SFO is the primary sensor for the lactate response in the BLA priming model. Injection of TTX into the OVLT failed to block the lactate response in the second group of BLA-primed rats (TABLE 2).

Experiment 3: Efferent Pathways for the Panic Response Elicited in the aBLA

Finally, another study was conducted in order to begin elucidating the efferent pathways involved in the responses elicited by GABA$_A$ receptor blockade in the aBLA. One group of rats ($n = 4$) was implanted with specially constructed double-microinjection cannulae separated by 1.2 mm (Plastics One, Roanoke, VA), such that the lateral of the two cannulae was in the aBLA on either side, while the medial cannula was in the central nucleus (CE) on either side. Such bilateral double cannulae preparation permitted us to preinject the neuronal blocker TTX (100 nL of 10 µM solution) or a-CSF (vehicle) into the CE and then test the effects of BMI injected into the aBLA. The results of this study showed that blocking neurotransmission in the CE with TTX completely blocked the increases in HR and BP (data not shown) elicited by BMI injections into the aBLA, suggesting that the pathway for the autonomic components of the BLA response synapses at the CE. Another control group of rats ($n = 4$) was implanted similarly with a 1.2-mm double cannulae, such that one of the cannula was in the aBLA on either side, while the other cannula was 1.1 mm lateral to the BLA site in the lateral amygdala (LA). When TTX was injected in the LA, the HR and BP responses elicited by injecting BMI in the aBLA were not blocked. This suggests that the TTX was not simply diffusing back to the aBLA from the CE site and blocking the BMI responses, because passive diffusion of TTX back to the BLA would be expected to be similar in both groups.

CONCLUSIONS

Repeated activation of the aBLA by $GABA_A$ receptor blockade produces a long-term synaptic plasticity termed priming, resulting in chronic anxiety and reactivity to peripheral lactate infusions, similar to patients with panic disorder.

ACKNOWLEDGMENT

This study was supported by MH 52691.

REFERENCES

1. SHEKHAR, A. & S.R. KEIM. 1997. The circumventricular organs form a potential neural pathway for lactate sensitivity: implications for panic disorder. J. Neurosci. **17:** 9726–9735.
2. MCDONALD, A.J. 1985. Immunohistochemical identification of gamma-aminobutyric acid containing neurons in the rat basolateral amygdala. Neurosci. Lett. **53:** 203–207.
3. SANDERS, S. & A. SHEKHAR. 1995. $GABA_A$ receptors in the basolateral amygdala of rats regulate "anxiety." Pharmacol. Biochem. Behav. **52:** 701–706.
4. SANDERS, S.K., S.L. MORZORATI & A. SHEKHAR. 1995. Priming of physiological and anxiety responses by repeated subthreshold GABA blockade in the rat amygdala. Brain Res. **699:** 250–259.
5. RAINNIE, D.G., E.K. ASPRODINI & P. SHINNICK-GALLAGHER. 1991. Excitatory transmission in the basolateral amygdala. J. Neurophysiol. **66:** 986–998.
6. SAJDYK, T.J. & A. SHEKHAR. 1997a. Excitatory amino acid receptor antagonists block the cardiovascular and anxiety responses elicited by gamma-aminobutyric acid—a receptor blockade in the basolateral amygdala. J. Pharmcol. Exp. Ther. **283:** 969–977.

Changes in Nociceptive and Anxiolytic Responses following Herpes Virus-mediated Preproenkephalin Overexpression in Rat Amygdala Are Naloxone-reversible and Transient

WEN KANG, STEVEN P. WILSON, AND MARLENE A. WILSON[a]

Department of Pharmacology and Physiology, University of South Carolina School of Medicine, Columbia, South Carolina 29208, USA

To investigate the role of amygdalar opioid peptides in the control of anxiety, the anxiolytic effects of benzodiazepines, and nociception, a herpes virus vector (SHPE) expressing human preproenkephalin was stereotaxically delivered to the rat amygdala. Studies examined viral expression and behavioral responses at 3–4 days or 9–10 days postinjection, and the ability of systemic injections of the opioid antagonist naloxone to block the actions of enkephalin overexpression in rat amygdala.

VIRAL EXPRESSION

The recombinant SHPE virus was constructed by inserting the human preproenkephalin cDNA under control of the human cytomegalovirus promoter into the thymidine kinase locus. Control animals received a similar replication-defective SHZ.1 virus that contains lacZ.[1] Adult male rats (225–280 g) received SHZ.1 virus, SHPE virus (2×10^6 pfu, 1 µL), or vehicle (10% glycerol in culture medium) injected bilaterally into the amygdala (AP–2.4, LM ±4.6, DV–8.5 from bregma) under phenobarbital anesthesia. After behavioral analysis, rats were sacrificed for histological analysis of needle placement, β-galactosidase expression in SHZ.1-infected rats, and human preproenkephalin mRNA expression by nonradioactive *in situ* hybridization in SHPE-treated rats (ref. 1 and Kang *et al.*, submitted).

Compared with sham-injected animals, SHPE- and SHZ.1-infected animals showed no apparent behavioral or neurological abnormalities except for slight weight loss, and microscopic inspection suggested neural damage from the viral infection was minimal.[1] Viral infection in the amygdala resulted in strong, localized expression of the gene products in the first 2–3 days with little or no expression after one week (Kang *et al.*, submitted). Histochemical analysis confirmed that gene expression was predominantly in the central nucleus of the amygdala with some spread into the basolateral region (ref. 1 and Kang *et al.*, submitted). This was confirmed

---

[a]Corresponding author: Dr. Marlene A. Wilson. Voice: 803-733-3258; fax: 803-733-1523; marlene@med.sc.edu

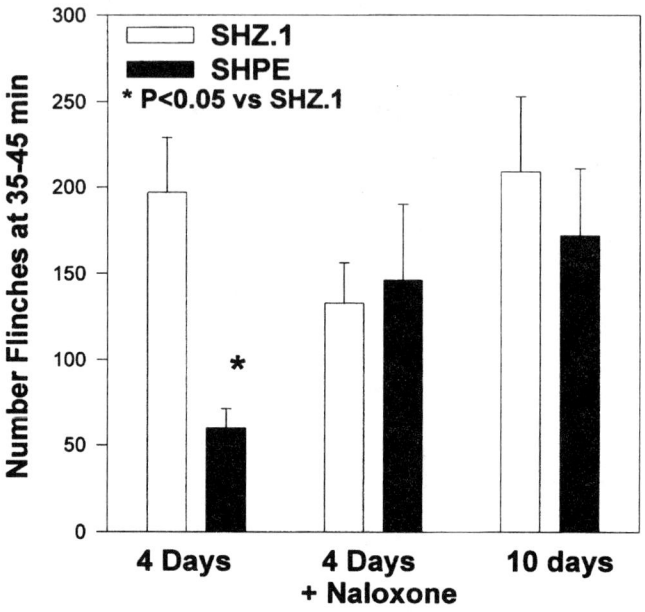

FIGURE 1. Four days after SHPE injection into the amygdala, rats show a reduced number of flinches in the second phase of the formalin test ($p < 0.05$), which is reversed by 5 mg/kg naloxone and dissipated at 10 days postinfection.

using a sensitive chemiluminescent assay for quantifying β-galactosidase,[2] which showed relatively little expression in brain areas outside the amygdalar region.

NOCICEPTIVE RESPONSES: FORMALIN TEST

To examine the effects of enkephalin overexpression in amygdala on supraspinal nociception, the formalin test was conducted in separate groups of animals either 4 or 10 days postinfection. Formalin (50 µL, 1%) was injected subcutaneously into the dorsal surface of the left hind paw, and the number of flinches was recorded during 5-min epochs for 60 minutes. Data were analyzed using analysis of variance (ANOVA) with repeated measures (time; $\alpha = 0.05$) and post-hoc Neuman-Keuls tests. A biphasic flinching response was seen, with an acute phase over 0–10 min and a tonic phase from 25–60 minutes. When compared to infection with SHZ.1, infection with SHPE caused a reduction of the flinching behavior in the second phase of the formalin test without affecting the first phase response.[1] As seen in FIGURE 1, the peak responses (flinches at 35–45 min) were reduced by enkephalin overexpression in the amygdala at 4 days postinfection. This reduction in tonic-phase flinching be-

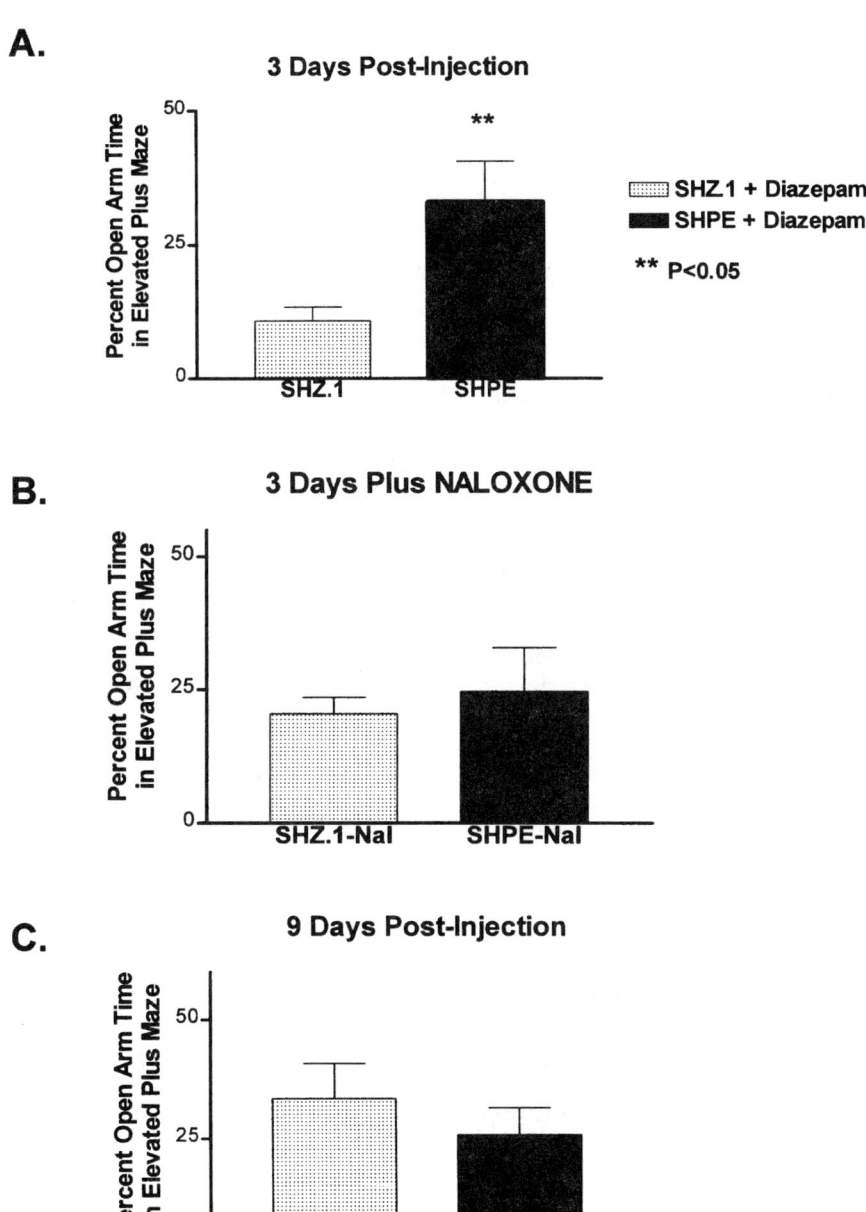

FIGURE 2. Three days after SHPE injection into the amygdala, rats show enhanced anxiolytic responses to diazepam, as shown by increased open arm time (panel **A**; $p < 0.05$) and open arm entries (data not shown) in the elevated plus maze. These enhanced responses to diazepam were reversed by 5 mg/kg naloxone (panel **B**) and not apparent at 9 days postinjection (panel **C**).

havior in SHPE-infected animals was reversed by the opioid antagonist naloxone hydrochloride (5 mg/kg, ip), given 10 min before formalin testing. No difference between SHZ.1 and SHPE-injected animals was seen at 10 days postinfection, suggesting that the antinociceptive effects of enkephalin overexpression had diminished by this time point.

ANXIOLYTIC EFFECTS OF BENZODIAZEPINES: ELEVATED PLUS MAZE

Anxiety levels and the effectiveness of the anxiolytic benzodiazepine agonist, diazepam, were examined at 3 days or 9 days after surgery using the elevated plus maze task.[3] Rats received either vehicle (10% ethanol, 40% propylene glycol, ip), or diazepam (1 mg/kg, ip) 30 min before testing, and naloxone hydrochloride (5mg/kg ip) was given simultaneously with diazepam in some rats. A reduced anxiety state was indicated by increased open arm activities, and the number of closed arm entries was used as a measure of locomotor activity. The behavioral measures were compared using t-tests (experiments with 2 groups) or ANOVA with post-hoc Bonferroni's multiple comparison tests.

Although SHPE infection alone did not reduce anxiety at 3 days postinjection, rats infected with SHPE exhibited a greater response to the anxiolytic effect of diazepam, when compared to rats infected with a control virus containing the lacZ gene (SHZ.1). FIGURE 2 shows the enhanced open arm time induced by SHPE injection in the amygdala compared with responses in SHZ.1-treated rats following diazepam administration, with no change in closed arm entries (data not shown). This enhancement of diazepam action was reversed by naloxone and correlated with preproenkephalin expression because the behavioral changes disappeared after gene expression dissipated at day 9 postinfection (FIG. 2).

SUMMARY

These results using herpes virus-mediated gene transfer to overexpress enkephalin in the amygdala support the role of amygdalar opioids in the anxiolytic actions of benzodiazepines and supraspinal nociception[4-7](see ref. 1). These studies also demonstrate the usefulness of recombinant herpes virus in evaluating the role of single gene products within specific brain sites in pharmacological responses and complex behaviors.

ACKNOWLEDGMENT

This work was supported by the USC Venture Fund, the SOM Research Development Fund, and the NIDA KO2 00249 to M.A.W.

REFERENCES

1. KANG, W., M.A. WILSON, M.A. BENDER, J.C. GLORIOSO & S.P. WILSON. 1998. Herpes virus-mediated preproenkephalin gene transfer to the amygdala is antinociceptive. Brain Res. **792:** 133–135.
2. JAIN, V.K. & I.T. MAGRATH. 1991. A chemiluminescent assay for quantitation of β-galactosidase in the femtogram range: application to quantitation of β-galactosidase in lacZ-transfected cells. Anal. Biochem. **199:** 119–124.
3. PELLOW, S., P. CHOPIN, S.E. FILE & M. BRILEY. 1985. Validation of open:closed arm entries in the elevated plus-maze as a measure of anxiety in the rat. J. Neurosci. Methods **14:** 149–167.
4. GOOD, A.J. & R.F. WESTBROOK. 1995. Effects of a microinjection of morphine into the amygdala on the acquisition and expression of conditioned fear and hypoalgesia in rats. Behav. Neurosci. **109:** 631-641.
5. DAVIS, M., D. RAINNIE & M. CASSELL. 1994. Neurotransmission in the rat amygdala related to fear and anxiety. Trends Neurosci. **17:** 208–214.
6. SCHEEL-KRUGER, J. & E.N. PETERSEN. 1982. Anticonflict effect of the benzodiazepines mediated by a GABAergic mechanism in the amygdala. Eur. J. Pharmacol. **82:** 115–116.
7. PESOLD, C. & D. TREIT. 1994. The septum and amygdala differentially mediate the anxiolytic effects of benzodiazepines. Brain Res. **638:** 295-301.

Enduring Neurochemical Effects of Early Maternal Separation on Limbic Structures

S.L. ANDERSEN,[a] P.J. LYSS, N.L. DUMONT, AND M.H. TEICHER

Department of Psychiatry, Harvard Medical School and McLean Hospital, Belmont, Massachusetts 02478, USA

Animal studies have shown us that exposure to a chronic stressor has enduring effects on brain development.[6,11] Subjects show a variety of responses, including increased anxiety in novel situations, dexamethasone resistance,[1] decreased growth hormone levels,[7] and increased corticosteroid levels.[9,11] Victims of early childhood abuse show an overall pattern of behavioral and biological dysregulation.[5,13] However, very little is known about the neurochemistry of these effects outside of the classic stress-related brain regions.

We have previously documented that maternal deprivation produces enduring behavioral changes that are apparent in adulthood. Chronic maternal deprivation subjects show activity patterns that are best characterized as restless with mild hyperactivity and reductions in serotonin (5-HT) and norepinephrine in key limbic targets.[2] The purpose of this study was to replicate and to better localize these effects with antibodies for 5-HT and tyrosine hydroxylase (TH).

Sprague-Dawley rats were bred in our colony, culled to 12 pup litters at P2, and weaned on P25. Rats were cross-fostered across three conditions, and randomly assigned to one of three conditions for 4 hr/day between P2 and P20. In the first condition (*colony control*), cross-fostered animals constituted litters that were unhandled except for weighing and marking on P2. Subjects in the second and third conditions were heterogeneously mixed into the other newly constituted litters. Subjects in the *stress condition* were removed from the litter, weighed, and marked with an indelible maker, and were then isolated in individual cups. Littermates in the *with mom condition* were similarly removed from the dam, weighed and marked, before being returned to the dam, during which time the stress group was isolated. After the four-hour deprivation period, the stressed pups were returned to the litters to rejoin the dam and with *mom* littermates.

At P60, all subjects were deeply anesthetized and transcardially perfused with 4% paraformaldehyde, and the brains were cryoprotected. Free-floating sections (40 μm thick) were washed in phosphate buffered saline (PBS) with 0.2% Tri-X, blocked in 10% serum (horse serum for the TH antibody and goat for the 5-HT antibody), and incubated overnight in primary antibody solution (5-HT: 1:10,000; Arnel; TH: 1:1,000; Chemicon). Sections, visualized with DAB, were quantified by an observer blind to the conditions with a BioQuant System for each ROI.

TH-stained varicosities in the accumbens shell, but not the core, were significantly reduced in the stress group and the group of subjects that were handled daily

---

[a]Corresponding author: S.L. Andersen, Ph.D., McLean Hosptial, 115 Mill Street, Belmont, MA 02478. Voice: 617-855-3211; fax: 617-855-3479; andersen@mclean.org

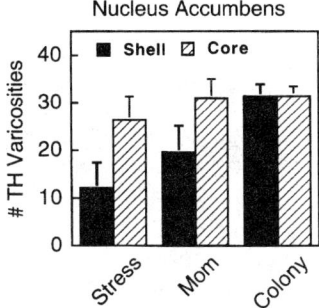

FIGURE 1. TH immunoreactivity is reduced significantly in the shell region of the nucleus accumbens ($F(2,9) = 4.32$, $p < 0.05$). No significant effects were observed in the core ($p = 0.6$).

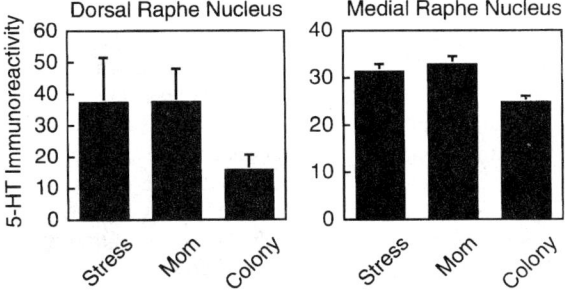

FIGURE 2. Serotonergic immunoreactive cell bodies in the dorsal and medial raphe nucleus were elevated in both the stress group and the mom group relative to the colony control.

(*mom*; see FIG. 1). 5-HT immunoreactivity was elevated in both the dorsal and medial raphe nucleus (FIG. 2). In addition, 5-HT innervation to the amygdala was reduced following maternal deprivation (data not shown).

The findings of reduced 5-HT and TH immunoreactivity in key limbic regions of the brain have implications for understanding behavioral underpinnings of the effects of early childhood abuse. Specifically, hyperactivity in the dorsal raphe system may manifest itself in terms of increased anxiety and avoidance behavior.[3] The restlessness characterized in our stress animals is consistent with this notion, but bears future testing. The detrimental effects of stress may have a greater impact on the accumbens and the amygdala, underscoring this region's importance in mediating fear responses, aggression, and its role in limbic kindling that is observed with repeated trauma.[14]

These data are also consistent with the notion of arrested development that may occur during the time of severe stress.[12] 5-HT typically serves as a trophic factor for the development of its projection systems.[8] A decline in 5-HT in the amygdala might limit branching and arborization of serotonin terminals entering the amygdala, and may increase dendritic arborization in the raphe.

Alterations in TH in the accumbens shell, but not the core, is a curious finding. TH immunoreactivity was not significantly different in the cell bodies of the ventral tegmental area, substantia nigra, nor the striatum (data not shown), nor did HPLC analysis in separate studies reveal any attenuation in dopamine levels.[2] However, we did find a 54% reduction in norepinephrine (NE) content in the accumbens of comparably stressed rats.[2] Hence, reduced TH immunoreactivity in accumbens shell may reflect diminished noradrenergic innervation.

It is important to note that both the *isolated* animals and their handled and marked littermate controls were different than nonhandled colony controls on the immunochemical measures. To some extent, the effects were more marked in the isolated animals (e.g., 50 vs 30% reduction in TH staining in accumbens shell), but are present in both groups. Additional controls are being run to determine if marked and handled animals raised in homogeneous litters without isolated littermates show comparable changes. Previous research has shown that control pups are seriously affected as a consequence of rearing in litters with manipulated pups.[10] It is conceivable that the repeated isolation paradigm exerted a highly disruptive effect on the dam that was translated to both groups of pups. Clinically, research has shown that it is the caregiver's response after a significant separation that is the critical variable in determining any enduring effects.[4,13] Nevertheless, the present study provides further support that early experience exerts enduring effects on monoamine innervation into ventral striatum, and also affects density of 5-HT cell bodies in the raphe nuclei. These enduring effects on 5-HT and NE systems may have implication for adult vulnerability to emergence of posttraumatic stress disorder, borderline personality disorder, substance abuse and depression found in individuals who have been seriously abused in childhood.

REFERENCES

1. ADER, R. & L.J. GROTON. 1969. Effects of early experience on adrenocortical reactivity. Physiol. Behav. **4:** 303–305.
2. ANDERSEN, S.L., P.J. LYSS, N.L. DUMONT & M.H. TEICHER. 1998. Early maternal separation produces enduring neurochemical and behavioral changes in the rat: Implications for child abuse. Int. Behav. Neurosci. Soc. [Abstract] Richmond, VA.
3. DEAKIN, J.F.K. 1990. Depression and 5-HT. Int. Clin. Psychopharmacol. **6(S3):** 24–29.
4. FIELD, T.M. & M. REITE. 1984. Children's response to separation from mother during the birth of another child. Child Dev. **55:** 1308–1316.
5. GLOD, C.A. & M.H. TEICHER. 1996. Relationship between early abuse, posttraumatic stress disorder, and activity levels in prepubertal children. J. Am. Acad. Child Adolesc. Psychiatry **35:** 1384–1393.
6. HOFER. M. 1975. Studies on how early maternal deprivation produces behavioral change in young rats. Psychosom. Med. **37:** 245–264.
7. KUHN, C.M., J. PAUK & S.M. SCHANBERG. 1990. Endocrine response to mother-infant separation in developing rats. Dev. Psychobiol. **23:** 395–410.
8. LAUDER, J.M. 1990. Ontogeny of the 5-HT system in the rat: 5-HT as a developmental signal. Ann. N.Y. Acad. Sci. **600:** 297–313.
9. LEVINE S., D.F. JOHNSON & C.A. GONZALEZ. 1985. Behavioral and hormonal responses to separation in infant rhesus monkeys and mothers. Behav. Neurosci. **99:** 399–410.
10. PEARSON, D.E., M.H. TEICHER, B.A. SHAYWITZ, D.J. COHEN, J.G .YOUNG & G.M. ANDERSON. 1980. Environmental influences on body weight and behavior in developing rats after 6-hydroxydopamine. Science **209:** 715–717.
11. PLOTSKY, P.M. & M.J. MEANEY. 1993. Effects of early environment on hypothalamic corticotropin-releasing factor mRNA, synthesis, and stress-induced release. Brain Res. Mol. Brain Res. **18:** 195–200.

12. TEICHER, M.H., Y. ITO, C.A. GLOD, F. SCHIFFER & H.A. GELBARD. 1996. Neurophysiological mechanisms of stress response in children. *In* Severe Stress and Mental Disturbance in Children. C. Pfeffer, Ed.: 59–84. American Psychiatric Association Press. Washington, DC.
13. VAN DER KOLK, B.A. & R.E. FISLER. 1994. Childhood abuse and neglect and loss of self-regulation. Bull. Menninger Clin. **58:** 145–168.
14. VAN DER KOLK, B. & M.S. GREENBERG. 1987. The psychobiology of the trauma response: hyperarousal, constriction, and addiction to traumatic reexposure. *In* Psychological Trauma. B. Van der Kolk, Ed.: 63–87. American Psychiatric Association Press. Washington, DC.

Prenatal Stress-induced Modifications of Neuronal Nitric Oxide Synthase in Amygdala and Medial Preoptic Area

STEPHEN D. MILLER, ERIC MUELLER, GORDON W. GIFFORD, AND CRAIG HOWARD KINSLEY[a]

Department of Psychology, University of Richmond, Richmond, Virginia 23173, USA

INTRODUCTION

Prenatal and early postnatal sexual differentiation of the brain determines the quality and quantity of subsequent behavior, physiology and anatomy.[5,10] Prenatal stress (PS) alters these developing neural systems, disrupting the normal sequence of sexual differentiation and reducing adult social behaviors, such as aggression and copulation.[3,4,6] Through what neurotransmitter pathways could PS elicit its effects? Recent evidence suggests that nitric oxide (NO) may be sensitive to PS effects. A gaseous neurotransmitter found throughout the central nervous system,[1,2,8,11] NO regulates many different social behaviors, including aggression and copulation.[1,2,8] The medial preoptic area (mPOA) and basolateral amygdala (bAM) regulate, respectively, sexual and aggressive behavior.[4,5,7,9,10] Given that PS affects both aggression and sexual behavior, the current work examines NO (through its rate-limiting enzyme neuronal NO synthase [nNOS]) in the mPOA and bAM of PS male rats.

METHODS

Prenatal Stress Procedure

Adult nulliparous female Sprague-Dawley rats were timed mated in our laboratory. Food and water were available *ad libitum*, and all animals were housed in light (on: 0500–1900 hr) and temperature (21–24°C)-controlled testing rooms. On gestation day 15 (+sperm = day 1), one group of pregnant animals (PS, $n = 6$) was exposed to a thrice-daily, 30-min regimen of heat and restraint stress. The second group of females (non-PS control, $n = 7$) was left undisturbed for the duration of their pregnancies. At birth litters were culled to 7–10 pups, with weaning at day 21.

Immunocytochemistry Protocol

Animals were sacrificed between 90–120 days of age by lethal injection of sodium pentobarbital, followed by perfusion with PBS and paraformaldehyde. Following postfixation and cryoprotection, brains were frozen-sectioned (30 µm for mPOA,

---

[a]Address for correspondence: Craig H. Kinsley, Ph.D., Dept. of Psychology, University of Richmond, Richmond, VA 23173. Voice: 804-289-8132; fax: 804-289-8943; ckinsley@richmond.edu

40 μm for bAM; a total of ten sections per brain region were taken, the first section for mPOA beginning approximately where the anterior commissure [AC] bridged the midline; for bAM, approximately 1.5 mm behind the posterior decussation of the AC). A standard ICC-protocol included primary and secondary antibodies (nNOS, 1:1,500, Incstar Biochemicals and Vector Labs, respectively). nNOS immunoreactivity (IR) was assessed from within a 250 μm by 235 μm grid superimposed on each serial section through the mPOA and bAM, and quantified in two different ways using Bioquant (R&M Biometrics, Inc.): (1) as defined by darkly stained perikarya with small stained processes in each section; and (2) total amount of nNOS-IR identified by image analysis and subsequent calculation of the ratio between stained:unstained material (what we are calling total nNOS immunoreactivity).

RESULTS

The data were analyzed using one-way analysis of variance. For the mPOA cell counts, there was a nonsignificant trend with control animals having more nNOS-IR

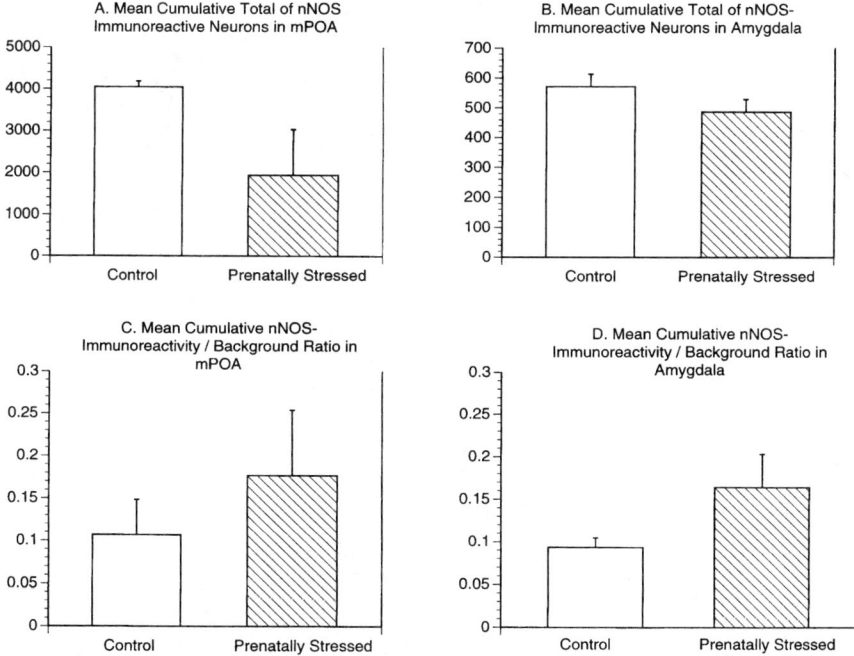

FIGURE 1. (**A**) Mean (+SEM) number of nNOS-IR neurons in mPOA of prenatally stressed and control male rats. (**B**) Mean (+SEM) number of nNOS-IR neurons in basolateral amygdala of prenatally stressed and control male rats. (**C**) Mean (+SEM) ratio of nNOS-IR stained:unstained tissue in mPOA of prenatally stressed and control male rats. (**D**) Mean (+SEM) ratio of nNOS-IR stained:unstained tissue in basolateral amygdala of prenatally stressed and control male rats.

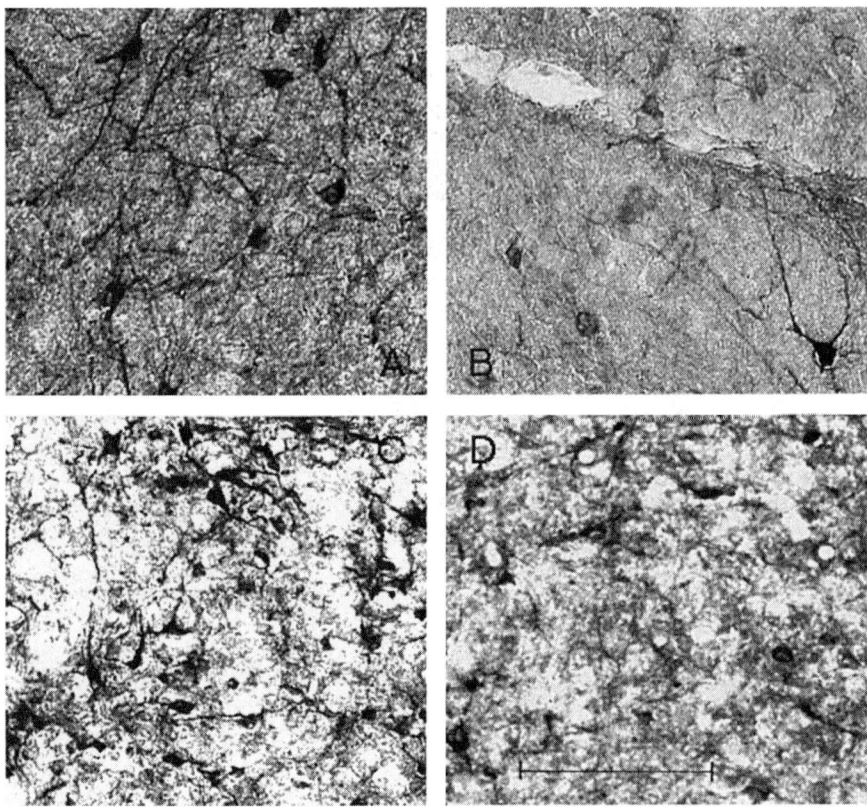

FIGURE 2. (**A**) nNOS-immunoreactive neurons in basolateral amygdala (bAM) of control male rats. Total magnification = 200× (bar = 100 μm). (**B**) nNOS-immunoreactive neurons in bAM of prenatally stressed male rats. Total magnification = 200× (bar = 100 μm). (**C**) nNOS-immunoreactive neurons in medial preoptic area (mPOA) of control male rats. Total magnification = 200× (bar = 100 μm). (**D**) nNOS-immunoreactive neurons in medial preoptic area (mPOA) of prenatally stressed male rats. Total magnification = 200× (bar = 100 μm).

neurons compared to PS animals ($M = 4048.00$ and $M = 1937.82$, respectively), $F(1,2) = 7.41$, $p > 0.05$. For the bAM, there was a significant difference in nNOS-IR neurons between control and PS animals, ($M = 571$ and $M = 487$, respectively), $F(1,2) = 12.6$, $p < 0.05$. Interestingly, with the mPOA ratio count, there was a nonsignificant trend with controls having a smaller stained:unstained ratio compared to PS animals ($M = 0.106$ and $M = 0.176$, respectively), $F(1,7) = 2.06$, $p > 0.05$. Lastly, when bAM sections were quantified by ratio count, again, the differences were opposite to what was observed when individual nNOS-IR neurons were counted. PS males had a significantly greater nNOS-IR stained:unstained ratio in the bAM ($M = 0.093$ and $M = 0.164$, respectively), $F(1,6) = 8.79$, $p < 0.05$.

CONCLUSIONS

PS, which demasculinizes male rats,[3,4,6] appears to alter nNOS in adult male rats in both mPOA and bAM. The number of neurons, as defined primarily by perikarya, expressing nNOS-IR is lower in PS animals in both mPOA and bAM. When we began this work we observed not just nNOS-IR cell bodies, but many processes also expressing nNOS. In order to determine overall levels of nNOS-IR (which would suggest other interpretations of the data), we then measured total amount of nNOS-IR that includes both cell bodies and processes. By using this more inclusive measure, however, nNOS-IR, as measured by the ratio of nNOS-IR to total area, is greater in PS males compared to control males in both mPOA and bAM. Such a paradox may reflect differential synthesis, storage and/or release of nNOS, and hence NO, in the brains of PS males. Though correlative at this time—and because the meaning of differences between cell body and process/fiber nNOS-IR is not clear—such alterations could affect both sexual and aggressive behaviors—behaviors identified as being modified by prenatal stress.[3,4,6] For example, too much nNOS or improper regulation of the enzyme may be associated with alterations of social behaviors such as sex and aggression.[11] The development of the regulation of nNOS, therefore, may include exposure to gonadal steroids with which PS effectively interferes.

REFERENCES

1. BENILLI, A., A. BERTOLINI, R. POGGIOLI, E. CAVAZZUTI, L. CALZA, L. GIARDINO & R. ARLETTI. 1995. Nitric oxide is involved in male sexual behavior of rats. Eur. J. Pharmacol. **294:** 505–510.
2. BIALY, M., J. BECK, P. ABRAMCZYK, A. TZEBSKI & J. PRZYBYLSKI. 1996. Sexual behavior in male rats after nitric oxide synthesis inhibition. Physiol. Behav. **60:** 139–143.
3. HARVEY, P.W. & P.F.D. CHEVINS. 1984. Crowding pregnant mice affects attack and threat behavior of male offspring. Horm. Behav. **18:** 101–110.
4. HUMM, J.L., K.G. LAMBERT & C.H. KINSLEY. 1995. Paucity of c-fos expression in the medial preoptic area of prenatally-stressed male rats following exposure to sexually receptive females. Brain Res. Bull. **37:** 363–363.
5. KELLEY, D. 1988. Sexually dimorphic behavors. Annu. Rev. Neurosci. **11:** 225–251.
6. KINSLEY, C.H. & B.B. SVARE. 1986. Prenatal stress reduces intermale aggression in mice. Physiol. Behav. **36:** 783–786.
7. MCGREGOR, A. & J. HERBERT. 1992. Differential effects of excitotoxic basolateral and corticomedial lesions of the amygdala on the behavioral and endocrine responses to either sexual or aggression-promoting stimuli in the male rat. Brain Res. **574:** 9–20.
8. NELSON, R.J., G.E. DEMAS, P.L. HUANG, M.C. FISHMAN, V.L. DAWSON, T.M. DAWSON & S.H. SNYDER. 1995. Behavioral abnormalities in male mice lacking neuronal nitric oxide synthase. Nature **378:** 383–386.
9. ROBERTSON, G., L. PFAUS, L. ATKINSON, A. PHILLIPS & H. FIBIGER. 1991. Sexual behavior increases c-fos expression in the forebrain of the male rat. Brain Res. **564:** 352–357.
10. SACHS, B.D. & R.L. MEISEL. 1988. The physiology of male sexual behavior. *In* The Physiology of Reproduction. E. Knobil & J.D. Neill, Eds.: 1393–1486. Raven Press. New York.
11. SNYDER, S.H. 1992. Nitric oxide: first in a new class of neurotransmitters? Science **257:** 494–496.

Amygdaloid and Hippocampal β-Adrenoceptors in the Olfactory Bulbectomy Syndrome: Effects of Desipramine

J. STEVEN RICHARDSON[a,b,c] AND ALEC H. K. TIONG[a]

Departments of [a]Pharmacology and of [b]Psychiatry, College of Medicine, University of Saskatchewan, Saskatoon, Saskatchewan S7N 5E5, Canada

Removing the olfactory bulbs (OBX) of rats induces behavioral deficits[1,2] that are improved only by interventions with therapeutic effects in people with major depressive disorder.[3,4] Due to this remarkable selectivity of the OBX deficits to reversal by antidepressants as reported by many authors over the past 20 years,[5,6] and to numerous behavioral and neurochemical similarities between people with major depression and rats with olfactory bulb lesions,[7,8] the OBX rat has become recognized not only as an effective screening system for identifying compounds with antidepressant actions, but also as the best available animal model of the patient with major depressive disorder.[9–11] In the intact organism, the olfactory bulbs appear to modulate the activity of limbic structures,[2] and the OBX syndrome reflects the consequences of disrupting the normal flow of neural traffic between the bulbs and the limbic system. In the present study, we monitored the time course effects of the antidepressant drug desipramine on OBX-induced changes in passive avoidance learning and in β-adrenergic receptors in the amygdala, hippocampus and cortex.

Under pentobarbital anesthesia, male Sprague-Dawley rats weighing 250–350 grams received OBX or a sham operation (SO) as described previously.[8] Starting 15 days post surgery, groups of OBX and SO rats received a daily intraperitoneal (i.p.) injection of desipramine at a dose of 10 mg/kg, or of a comparable volume of the saline vehicle. After 0, 3 or 15 days of injections, or 15 days after the last of 15 daily injections, the rats were trained on a step-down passive avoidance task to a criterion of remaining for 1 minute on a wooden platform located in the middle of an electrifiable metal grid. Trials to criterion were recorded. The rats were then sacrificed, the brains were removed, and the extent of the bulbectomy was determined visually for each rat. Only rats with complete bilateral destruction of the olfactory bulbs with no damage to frontal cortex or olfactory peduncle were accepted for data analyses. The amygdala, hippocampus and cortex from acceptable brains were dissected, frozen in liquid nitrogen and stored at −86°C. The β-adrenoceptors in these brain areas were characterized by standard ligand binding studies using [^{125}I]iodocyanopindolol plus 10 μM serotonin, and isoproterenol for displacement studies, and by measuring cyclic AMP formation following the stimulation of adenylyl cyclase by agents acting at various points in the signal transduction pathway. Isoproterenol was used as a direct β-adrenoceptor agonist, the G_S protein subunit was stimulated with sodium flu-

---

[c]Corresponding author: Dr J. S. Richardson, Department of Pharmacology, University of Saskatchewan, 107 Wiggins Road, Saskatoon, SK, S7N 5E5, Canada. Voice: 306-966-6301; fax: 306-966-6220; richardson@sask.usask.ca

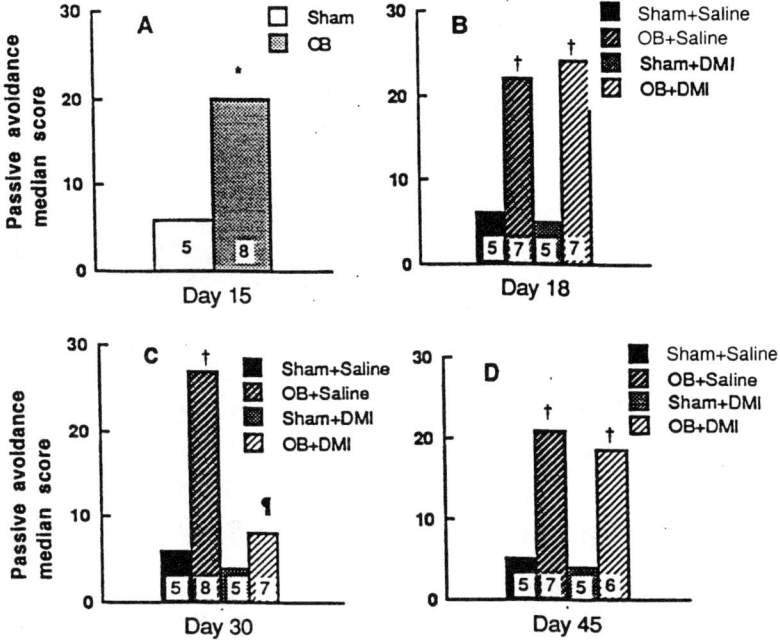

FIGURE 1. Effects of olfactory bulbectomy (OB) and daily desipramine treatment (10 mg/kg i.p.) on step-down passive avoidance learning by rats. **(A)** Rats were tested 15 days post lesion. **(B)** Rats were tested 18 days post lesion having received 3 days of desipramine. **(C)** Rats were tested on post lesion day 30 having received 15 days of desipramine. **(D)** Rats were tested on post lesion day 45, 15 days after the last of 15 daily injections of desipramine. Columns are median trials to learning criterion. Numbers in each column are the number of rats in that group. * = $p < 0.005$ versus OB rats. † = $p < 0.005$ versus sham saline rats. ¶ = $p < 0.005$ versus OB saline rats.

oride or guanylyl imidodiphosphate, and the catalytic unit of adenylyl cyclase was stimulated with forskolin. The behavioral data were analyzed statistically with the Mann-Whitney U test, and the binding and the cyclic AMP data were analyzed by 2-tailed unpaired Student's t-tests.

Passive avoidance learning was significantly impaired in OBX rats tested 15 days post lesion (FIG. 1). This deficit was not altered by 3 days of desipramine treatment (post lesion Day 18), was significantly attenuated after 15 days of desipramine administration (Day 30), and had returned 15 days after chronic desipramine had been discontinued (Day 45). The density of β-adrenoceptors, determined by competition binding assays, was significantly elevated (data not shown) in the amygdala and hippocampus but not in the cortex, 15 days after the OBX surgery and was still elevated after 3 days of desipramine, and in saline-treated OBX rats at all time points tested. In both OBX and SO rats, 15 days of desipramine treatment significantly reduced β-adrenoceptor density below that of SO-saline rats in all 3 brain areas. In preliminary studies, these changes in brain part β-adrenoceptor densities were seen in β-1 but not in β-2 adrenoceptors. The affinity of the β-adrenoceptors in the amygdala and in the

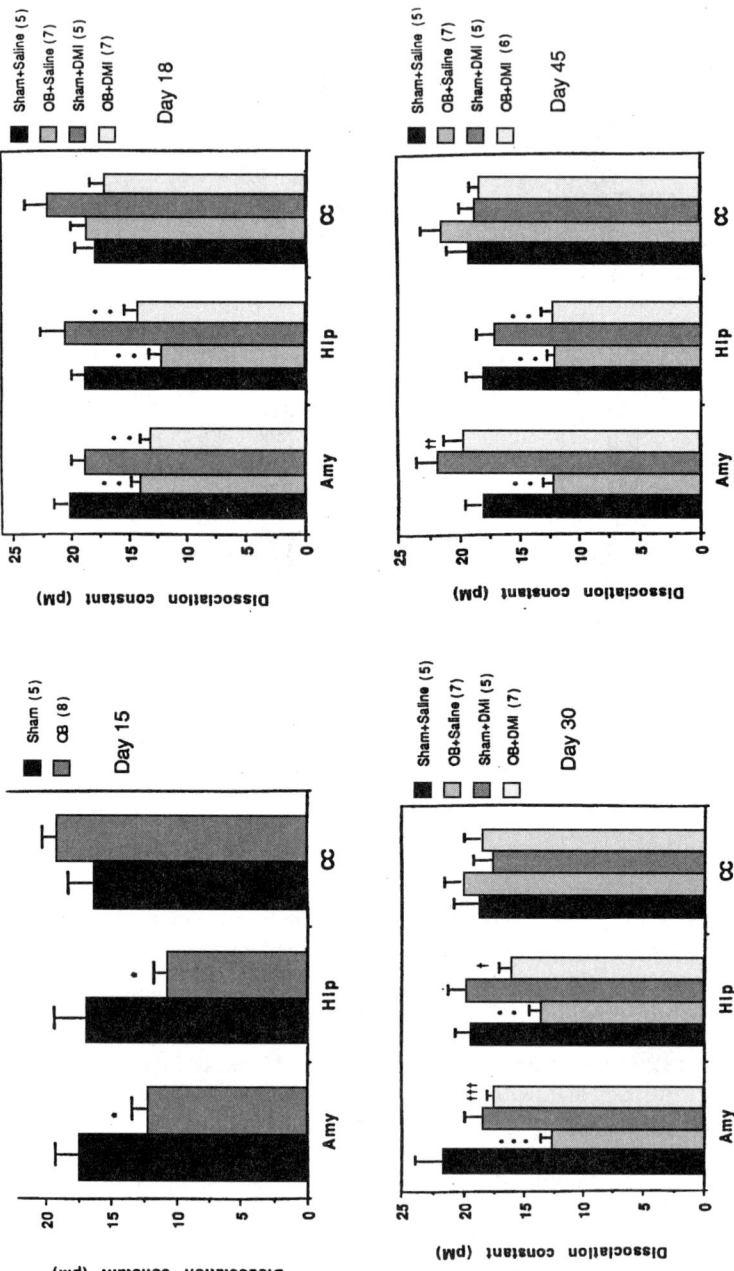

FIGURE 2. The affinity of β-adrenoceptors in the amygdala (Amy), hippocampus (Hip), and cerebral cortex (CC) following passive avoidance learning as described in FIGURE 1. Dissociation constants were determined in competition binding studies with isoproterenol and [^{125}I]iodocyanopindolol in the presence of 10 μM serotonin. The smaller the dissociation constant, the higher the affinity. The number of rats in each group is given in the parentheses in each key. ** = $p <0.01$, *** = $p <0.005$ versus sham saline rats. † = $p <0.05$, †† = $p <0.01$, ††† = $p <0.005$ versus OB saline rats.

hippocampus, but not in the cortex, was also elevated 15 days post OBX (FIG. 2). These receptor affinities were not altered by 3 days of desipramine treatment, but after 15 days of desipramine, the affinity of amygdaloid β-adrenoceptors had decreased to that of the SO rats, and the affinity of the hippocampal β-adrenoceptors was significantly reduced as well. Chronic desipramine did not change the affinity of the cortical β-adrenoceptors in either OBX or SO rats. Changes in stimulated cAMP formation comparable to receptor affinity were seen in each brain part in each group of rats (data not shown). Fifteen days after the discontinuation of 15 daily desipramine injections, the affinity of hippocampal β-adrenoceptors in OBX rats had increased to the level of the OBX-saline rats. However, the affinity of the amygdaloid β-adrenoceptors did not increase but remained the same as that of the SO rats.

Following OBX, rats show a deficit in passive avoidance learning that is alleviated by 15 days of desipramine treatment and that returns 15 days after desipramine is discontinued. Paralleling this learning deficit, the β-adrenoceptors in the amygdala and the hippocampus are upregulated by the OBX, downregulated by the chronic administration of desipramine, and at least in the hippocampus, upregulated again 15 days after the last desipramine dose. This suggests that upregulated hippocampal β-adrenoceptors impair step-down passive avoidance learning in the OBX rat. However, amygdaloid β-adrenoceptors have been shown to be involved in other forms of learning. In the first demonstration of β-adrenoceptors in the amygdala, the acquisition of DRL-20 responding by rats was facilitated by isoproterenol, and impaired by propranolol, injected into the basolateral amygdala.[12] And more recently, the formation of hippocampal long-term potentiation was also impaired by injections of propranolol into the basolateral amygdala.[13] The interaction of amygdaloid and hippocampal β-adrenoceptors in the modulation of behavioral output remains to be determined but may be profitably investigated in OBX rats.

REFERENCES

1. WATSON, J.B. 1906. Kinaesthetic and organic sensations: their role in the reactions of the white rat in the maze. Psychol. Bull. **8:** 1–100.
2. CAIN, D.P. 1974. The role of the olfactory bulb in limbic mechanisms. Psychol. Bull. **81:** 654–671.
3. LEONARD, B.E. 1984. The olfactory bulbectomized rat as a model of depression. Pol. J. Pharmacol. **36:** 561–569.
4. JESBERGER, J.A. & J.S. RICHARDSON. 1985. Animal models of depression: parallels and correlates to severe depression in humans. Biol. Psychiatry **20:** 764–784.
5. VAN RIEZEN, H. *et al.* 1977. Olfactory ablation in the rat: behavioural changes and their reversal by antidepressant drugs. Br. J. Pharmacol. **60:** 521–528.
6. MCGRATH, C. & T.R. NORMAN. 1998. The effect of venlafaxine treatment on the behavioural and neurochemical changes in the olfactory bulbectomized rat. Psychopharmacology **136:** 394–401.
7. JESBERGER, J.A. & J.S. RICHARDSON. 1988. Brain output dysregulation induced by olfactory bulbectomy: an approximation in the rat of major depressive disorder in humans? Int. J. Neurosci. **38:** 241–265.
8. RICHARDSON, J.S. 1991. The olfactory bulbectomized rat as a model of major depression. *In* Neuromethods: Animal Models in Psychiatry. II. M.T. Martin-Iverson, A.A. Boulton & G.B. Baker, Eds.: 61–79. Humana Press. Clifton, NJ.
9. RICHARDSON, J.S. 1991. Animal models of depression reflect changing views on the essence and etiology of depressive disorders in humans. Prog. Neuropsychopharmacol. Biol. Psychiatry **15:** 199–204.

10. GRECKSCH, G. *et al.* 1997. Influence of olfactory bulbectomy and subsequent imipramine treatment on 5-hydroxytryptaminergic presynapses in the rat frontal cortex: behavioural correlates. Br. J. Pharmacol. **122:** 1725–1731.
11. KELLY, J.P. *et al.* 1997. The olfactory bulbectomized rat as a model of depression: an update. Pharmacol. Ther. **74:** 299–316.
12. RICHARDSON, J.S. & R.E. MUSTY. 1974. Effects on the acquisition of DRL-20 performance of propranolol or isoproterenol injected into the basolateral amygdala of rats. Can. J. Physiol. Pharmacol. **52:** 1033–1035.
13. IKEGAYA, Y. *et al.* 1997. Amygdala β-noradrenergic influence on hippocampal long-term potentiation *in vivo*. Neuroreport **8:** 3143–3146.

Cholinergic, M_1 Receptors in the Nucleus Accumbens Mediate Behavioral Depression

A Possible Downstream Target for Fluoxetine

DAVID CHAU, PEDRO V. RADA, REBECCA A. KOSLOFF, AND BARTLEY G. HOEBEL[a]

Department of Psychology, Princeton University, Princeton, New Jersey 08544, USA

INTRODUCTION

Antidepressants alleviate behavioral depression via monoamines, notably serotonin,[1,2] but the next step in the mechanism is not established. A possible role of acetylcholine in mood disorders has been widely discussed,[3,4] although it is not clear which cholinergic system is involved nor where in the brain it might act. Brainstem serotonergic neurons innervate much of the brain, including the nucleus accumbens, a mesolimbic region important for reward, aversion and incentive motivation.[5] Local infusion into the posterior-medial nucleus accumbens (NAc) of serotonin, a serotonin 1-A receptor agonist (5-OH-DPAT) or a serotonin reuptake inhibitor (fluoxetine, Prozac) decreased extracellular acetylcholine (ACh).[6] This suggests that serotonin inhibits ACh interneurons in the NAc via $5-HT_{1A}$ receptors. Given that depression is associated with low serotonergic transmission in the brain,[2] it is possible that during depression ACh interneurons in the NAc are disinhibited. According to this theory, high synaptic ACh in NAc may be involved in depression. If so, extracellular ACh should rise as a correlate of behavioral depression. This was tested using microdialysis in the Porsolt swim test. The swim test is an animal model of depression that can effectively screen wide classes of antidepressants.[7] In this model, rodents placed in a swim tank vigorously try to escape for several minutes, then give up and just tread water displaying reduced motivation to escape. Antidepressants prolong the animal's escape behaviors. If antidepressants act in the nucleus accumbens (NAc), then serotonergic drugs such as 8-OH-DPAT might reduce depression (i.e., increase swimming time) when injected locally in the NAc. Further, if ACh plays a causal role in depression, then appropriate cholinergic receptor agonists injected in the NAc should increase immobility, and cholinergic antagonists should increase swimming. If successful, this series of results would suggest that fluoxetine alleviates some behavioral manifestations of depression via inhibition of ACh release in the NAc.

[a]Address for correspondence: Prof. Bart Hoebel, Department of Psychology, Princeton University, Princeton, NJ 08544. Voice: 609-258-4463; fax: 609-258-1113; hoebel@princeton.edu

MATERIALS AND METHODS

Surgery

Female, Sprague-Dawley rats ($n = 102$, 250–320 g) were housed individually on a 12:12-hr light-dark schedule with food and water *ad libitum*. Stainless steel cannulas (21 ga) to serve as guide shafts for microdialysis probes and drug injectors were implanted bilaterally (A: +1.2 mm, V: −4 mm, and L: 1.2 mm, relative to bregma, midsagittal sinus and level surface of the skull). Probes and injectors protruded another 4 mm to reach the posterior medial NAc.

Swim Tests

Rats were placed individually in a water tank for 10 min (tank diameter 27 cm; water depth 33 cm; 25–30°C). Subjects initially exhibit escape-directed behaviors such as diving, rigorous paddling with all four paws, clambering at the tank walls, propelling body out of water, circling around tank, and sometimes circling in place in the middle of tank to survey the outside. The rigor and duration of these behaviors gradually diminish until subjects exert just enough effort to stay afloat (i.e., all four paws immobile or slow, intermittent paddling with only one forepaw, and exhibiting piloerection and a hunched body posture). Escape-directed activity sometimes resumed intermittently. "Swimming" was defined by the escape behaviors, and "immobile" by floating behavior. At least two observers with stop watches and blind to experimental conditions independently recorded swimming time.

Locomotor Test

Motor activity was assessed in an enclosure with five equally spaced, infrared photocells on each of two adjacent walls, 2 mm above a 40 × 40 cm wire-grid floor. Subjects were adapted to this environment for 1 hr before tests. Activity tests began 30 min prior to vehicle or drug injection and continued for 70 min.

Drugs

The serotonergic drug used was 8-hydroxy-2-(di-*n*-propylamino)-tetralin hydrogen bromide (8-OH-DPAT, a specific 5-HT$_{1A}$ agonist; RBI Inc.). Cholinergic drugs used were: arecoline hydrobromide (a specific M$_1$ agonist; Sigma Chemical Co.), pirenzepine hydrochloride (a specific M$_1$ antagonist; Sigma), and scopolamine hydrobromide (a muscarinic M$_1$ and M$_2$ antagonist; Sigma).

Acute intracerebral drug administration was counterbalanced with vehicle Ringer as a control. Subjects received drug or vehicle on Day 2 or Day 3 of the swim test in counterbalanced order. The respective data were later combined. Injections into the NAc were administered 0.71 µl/min/side during 42 sec. To determine whether behavioral changes were due to drug reflux up the injector or probe track to other sites, pirenzepine was injected bilaterally, 2 mm more dorsal in the striatum of 10 control rats.

Microdialysis and Histology

ACh was analyzed in 5-min samples collected from rats 30 min before the swim test, during 10 min in the swim tank and for 30 min afterwards, using the techniques described previously.[6,8] Injection sites and microdialysis probe tracks were later identified in 40-μm brain sections.

RESULTS

Extracellular Acetylcholine in the Posterior-Medial Nucleus Accumbens Increases When Rats Become Behaviorally Depressed in the Forced Swim Test

On first exposure to water (Day 1), when rats persisted in escape behaviors (swam 465 ± 63 sec, $n = 8$), no significant changes in extracellular ACh occurred. However, subjects swam progressively less on subsequent exposures (Day 2, 444 ± 45 sec, $n = 7$; Day 3, 392 ± 61 sec, $n = 6$), and extracellular ACh increased significantly in the first 5 min (Day 2, $140 \pm 12\%$ of baseline, $F(0,13) = 7.39$, $p < 0.001$; Day 3, $130 \pm 12\%$ of baseline, $F(0,13) = 1.88$, $p < 0.05$). ACh levels were not significantly different from baseline during the second 5 min in the water or after the animals were removed from the water.

Muscarinic, M_1 Receptors in the Posterior-Medial Nucleus Accumbens Mediate Behavioral Depression

Muscarinic, M_1 agonists and antagonists acutely injected in the posterior medial NAc altered performance in swim tests. Arecholine, an M_1 agonist, at 40 and 80 μg/side decreased swimming dose-dependently to 59 and 34% of saline control days (40 μg/side, $n = 8$, $t = 3.53$ two-tailed, $p < 0.01$; 80 μg/side, $n = 6$, $t = 4.12$, $p < 0.01$). Conversely, pirenzepine, an M_1 antagonist, increased swimming 39% (17.5 μg/side, $n = 8$, $t = 3.63$, $p < 0.01$) and 40% (35 μg/side, $n = 9$, $t = 7.15$, $p < 0.001$). Scopolamine, an M_1 and M_2 antagonist, tended to decrease swimming time at 0.5 μg/side (−13%, $n = 10$, NS), but it increased swimming time 50% at 1.0 μg/side ($n = 10$, $t = 12.74$, $p < 0.001$). Behavioral changes were not due to fluid reflux up the injectors to other sites, because pirenzepine (17.5 μg/side) injected above NAc in the dorsal striatum did not increase swimming time ($n = 10$, NS).

The same drugs were tested in the photocell cage. Arecholine (40 μg/side) injected into NAc elicited a significant biphasic change in rats' locomotor activity ($n = 6$, $F(1,6) = 3.09$, $p < 0.01$). Activity was reduced 56% below control in the 10 min following the arecholine injections, but it rebounded above control in the next 20 min. Local pirenzepine or scopolamine did not elicit any significant changes in locomotor activity (pirenzepine, 35 μg/side, $n = 6$, NS; scopolamine, 1 μg/side, $n = 4$, NS).

Serotonergic, $5-HT_{1A}$ Receptors in the Posterior-Medial Nucleus Accumbens Reduce Behavioral Depression

8-OH-DPAT (2.5 μg/side), a highly specific $5-HT_{1A}$ agonist, dramatically increased swimming time 108% above control ($n = 8$, $t = 4.59$, $p < 0.005$).

DISCUSSION

The Porsolt swim test is an imperfect measure of depression; however, the swim test with rats is sensitive to some of the antidepressant properties of drugs used to treat humans successfully. Since we are only measuring behavior, this discussion is limited to "behavioral depression." It is conceivable that the neural mechanism discovered also plays a role in some of the learned despair, learned helplessness or mood characteristics of real depression.

The results of the present study suggest a mechanism and location for some of serotonin's antidepressant action. In a prior microdialysis study, serotonergic agonists injected systemically or into the accumbens caused a decrease in ACh release at that site.[6] Prior research on accumbens ACh suggests that it can inhibit the output of voluntary behavior. When ACh is in excess, it may create an aversive state. This view is based on findings that extracellular ACh increases during slowing of a meal, during the sexual refractory period after ejaculation, during conditioned taste aversion, and during opiate withdrawal.[5,9] Artificial elevation of synaptic ACh in the accumbens with an enzyme inhibitor (neostigmine) can substitute for nausea by generating a conditioned taste aversion.[5]

The present microdialysis results show that ACh is released when rats display behavioral depression in the Porsolt swim test. The further observation that local injection of a cholinergic receptor agonist (arecholine) caused behavioral depression (less escape swimming) suggests that endogenous ACh in the NAc plays a causal role. This interpretation is further supported by the antidepressant effect of a local cholinergic antagonist (pirenzepine) which presumably blocked endogenous ACh. Both arecholine and pirenzepine are relatively specific for M_1 receptors. This suggests that M_1 receptors in the NAc are partially responsible for behavioral depression when animals stop trying to escape and instead conserve energy.

It is difficult to know how much of the drugs' effects on escape behavior are due to changes in overall activity. The M_1 agonist arecholine reduced locomotion in the photocell cage. This result might be expected of cholinergic agents that produce symptoms of depression such as psychomotor retardation, anergia, and dysphoria.[4] For other drugs, the change did not reach statistical significance; perhaps because confinement in a cage is less stressful than confinement in a pool of water. The M_1 antagonist pirenzepine did not cause significant hyperactivity, even though it increased swimming. The drug is like classic antidepressants that increase escape swimming without hyperlocomotion, as originally described by Porsolt.[7] Similarly, scopolamine, a nonspecific M_1 and M_2 antagonist, increased swimming, but did not change activity in the photocell cage.

Muscarinic antagonists have long been suspected of antidepressant action and contributed to a cholinergic theory of depression.[3,4] Nonspecific muscarinic antagonists have many problems of interpretation when given systemically due to the variety of cholinergic systems in the nervous system and several different muscarinic receptor types. To obtain internally consistent results it was necessary to use relatively specific cholinergic drugs given locally and to measure ACh release as a function of behavioral depression. Then it becomes clear that ACh is released from the well-known cholinergic interneurons of the NAc when rats in the swim test stop trying to escape and begin to display immobility. ACh was released beginning on the second day, when the animals learned that attempts to escape were futile. The effect occurred in the first half of the swim test; thus showing a better correlation with swimming and stopping than with protracted immobility. This extracellular ACh presumably acts, in part, where local arecholine acts at M_1 receptors, thereby causing behavioral depression. The M_1 antagonist pirenzepine apparently blocks the endogenous ACh at the M_1 receptor and thus acts as an antidepressant as defined by more swimming and escape attempts.

This model may help explain part of the remarkable effectiveness of SSRIs in humans. By gradually increasing synaptic serotonin in the NAc, SSRIs may have the same effect as locally injected serotonin or 8-OH-DPAT, which is to inhibit ACh release. The effectiveness of this treatment at this site is shown in rats by the immediate antidepressant effect of locally administered 8-OH-DPAT.

In summary, microdialysis experiments and the swim tests suggest that behavioral depression involves the release of ACh in the NAc. Fluoxetine, by blocking serotonin reuptake in the NAc, raises the concentration of synaptic serotonin, which acts at 5-HT_{1A} receptors to inhibit ACh release. This reduces the concentration of ACh acting at accumbens M_1 receptors, thereby increasing instrumental behavior and increasing the possibility of positive reinforcement.

ACKNOWLEDGMENTS

This work was supported by USPHS Grants R01 DA 10608 and NS 30697.

REFERENCES

1. SKOLNICK, P., Ed. 1997. Antidepressants: New Pharmacological Strategies. Humana Press. Totowa, NJ.
2. MAES, M. & H.Y. MELTZER. 1995. The serotonin hypothesis of major depression, *In* Psychopharmacology: The Fourth Generation of Progress. F.E. Bloom & D.J. Kupfer, Eds.: 933–944. Raven Press, New York.
3. JANOWSKY, D.S. & D.H. OVERSTREET. 1995. The role of acetylcholine mechanisms in mood disorders. *In* Psychopharmacology: The Fourth Generation of Progress. F.E. Bloom & D.J. Kupfer. Eds.: 945-956. Raven Press. New York.
4. DILSAVER, S.C. 1986. Cholinergic mechanisms in depression. Brain Res. Rev. **11**: 285–316.
5. HOEBEL, B.G., P.V. RADA, G.P. MARK & E. POTHOS. Neural systems for reinforcement and inhibition of behavior: relevance to eating, addiction and depression. *In* Well-Being: Foundations of Hedonic Psychology. D. Kahneman, E. Diener & N. Schwarz, Eds. Russell Sage Foundation. New York. In press.
6. RADA, P.V., G.P. MARK & B.G. HOEBEL. 1993. *In vivo* modulation of acetylcholine in the nucleus accumbens of freely moving rats. I. Inhibition by serotonin. Brain Res. **619**: 98–104.
7. PORSOLT, R.D. 1990. Behavioral despair: present status and future perspectives. *In* Antidepressants: Thirty Years On. B.E. Leonard & P.J. Spencer, Eds.: 85–94. CNS Publishers. London.
8. MARK, G.P., D.H. SCHWARTZ, L. HERNANDEZ, H.L. WEST & B.G. HOEBEL. 1991. Application of microdialysis to the study of motivation and conditioning: measurements of dopamine and serotonin in freely-behaving rat. *In* Microdialysis in the Neurosciences. T.E. Robinson & J.B. Justice, Eds.: 359–385. Elsevier. Amsterdam.
9. LEIBOWITZ, S.F. & B.G. HOEBEL. 1998. Behavioral neuroscience of obesity. *In* Handbook of Obesity. G.A. Bray, C. Bouchard & W.P.T. James, Eds.: 313–358. Marcel Dekker. New York.

10. BLIER, P., R. BERGERON & C. DE MONTIGNY. 1997. Selective activation of postsynaptic 5-HT_{1A} receptors induces rapid antidepressant response. Neuropsychopharmacology **16:** 333–338.
11. DETKE, M.J., M. RICKELS & I. LUCKI. 1995. Active behaviors in the forced swimming test differentially produced by serotonergic and noradrenergic antidepressants. Psychopharmacology **121:** 66–72.

Pattern of Disturbance of Different Ventral Frontal Functions in Organic Depression

FRIEDEL M. REISCHIES[a]

Department of Psychiatry, Free University of Berlin, 14050 Berlin, Germany

INTRODUCTION

Neuropsychological data on deficits of frontal lobe functions in patients with depression syndromes (e.g., Ref. 7) together with subcortical vascular lesions (deep white matter lesions, DWML[3]) as probable neuropathological correlates support the idea that a dysfunction of the frontal lobe and frontal cortico-subcortical projection loops may be factors in the pathophysiology of depression. However, a major problem is that lesion studies have demonstrated (1) apathy without depressed mood (pseudodepression) after lesions of mediodorsal prefrontal cortex, and more specifically (2) euphoria with disinhibition[9] after ventral frontal lesions or their subcortical afferent and efferent connections.[5,7] The relation of frontal lobe dysfunction and depressed mood has to be clarified.

The orbitofrontal cortex (OFC) receives two divergent kinds of input. The first kind is visual object information from inferotemporal cortex and olfactory and gustatory information as well as reward information from ventral tegmental area (VTA).[11] Because of this and according to neurophysiological data (see, e.g., Ref. 10), it can be inferred that object-related reward information processing takes place in ventral frontal cortex. The second kind, a strong input from amygdala specifically to these cortex regions (see review, Ref. 2) and to the subcortical projection area, namely, n. accumbens, supports the view that object-related anxiety/behavioral control information processing takes place within the ventral and ventro-medial prefrontal cortex. Therefore, two antagonistic object-related types of information are processed in OFC.

In this study we asked whether depressed subjects are disturbed in an orbitofrontal test like the object reversal task,[9] and if so if there is a specific kind of disturbed behavior. The object reversal task was adapted for use in mildly impaired subjects. We constructed a probability variant of an object reversal task: the preferred choice has a clear advantage but there is some stochastic variation in reward value points, which additionally allow for testing reward-related behavior. The hypothesis was that performance of reward-related task demands should be disturbed in depression, and it had to be determined if performance in negative reinforcement-related task demands are normal.

---

[a]Address for correspondence: Friedel M. Reischies, MD, PhD, Department of Psychiatry, Free University of Berlin, Eschenallee 3, 14050 Berlin, Germany. Voice: +49-30-8445-8780; fax: +49-30-8445-8393; reischie@zedat.fu-berlin.de

SUBJECTS AND METHODS

Subjects with severe depressive episode (DSM-IV) were investigated in this pilot trial ($n = 8$, age 55.38, SD 16.37 yr, depression scale: Bech-Raffaelsen-MS 19.6, SD 2.9). Almost all had subcortical vascular type lesions in MRI. As control 8 education-matched subjects without psychiatric illness as well as without CNS disease or substance abuse were tested (age 47.50, SD 15.38 yr, statistical comparison: t-test, n.s.). For the probability object reversal test, subjects had to choose between 5 objects (1 through 5), which are randomly offered on a computer screen at 5 places for 3 sections of 30 decisions. One number was rewarded by 20 value points in 80%. Two others got 0 points in 70%, and two numbers got −10 points in 50%. After 30 trials the first preferred number changes to 0 point assignment and in the last part to −10 point assignment; each time a new preferred number has to be found.

RESULTS

Depressed subjects had less optimal choices per trial at the second half of the first 30 trials (20–60%, mean 35.0%, SD 17.7) compared with healthy control subjects (30–100%, mean 62.5%, SD 24.9, $t = -2.54$, $p < 0.05$), although they clearly experienced the optimal reward several times. Perservative choices after change of reinforcement schedule were found in both groups at approximately the same percentage (25.7, SD 7.9 vs 12.5, SD 14.9, n.s.). In the control tasks the depressed subjects had no deficit in psychomotor speed: Reitan Trail Making Test a (38.86, SD 9.82 vs 35.17, SD 24.85, n.s.). The digit span (working memory) was not disturbed (5.57, SD 0.79 vs 5.33, SD 1.03, n.s.).

DISCUSSION

Depressed subjects are disturbed in a task supposedly testing ventral frontal lobe functions, However, the impairment is not the kind expected in euphoria/disinhibition syndrome of ventral frontal lobe lesions.[9] The depressed subjects suffer from an impairment of reward-related behavior. Because the performance in the control tests was not impaired—especially the psychomotor speed was relatively high, which was tested after completion of the object reversal task—the data argue against a general demotivation or fatigue of these patients.

The neuropsychological data together with data of the literature (which cannot be mentioned in detail here) as well as earlier results of our group lead to the following neuropsychiatric hypothesis regarding the organic depression syndrome: Antagonistic functions of ventral frontal lobe seem to be disturbed in depression in a specific way (TABLES 1 and 2). (A) Object-related reward information processing of the ventral frontal cortex, which is associated to the function of the ventral tegmental area, is disturbed by disconnection because of, e.g., deep white matter lesions, disturbed subcortical centers of the orbitofrontal loops or cortical dysfunction. (A1) Ventral frontal neurons have influence on the VTA presumably partly via n. accumbens, and partly directly—where the temporal pattern of activation seems to be crucial.

TABLE 1. Two antagonistic functional systems of ventral frontal cortex in organic depression

Ventral frontal information processing	Object related reward	Object related anxiety/ behavioral control
Localization	*Distributed; predominantly ventral frontal efferents via n. accumbens (n. acc.) to ventral tegmental area (VTA) *Cognitive related motivational aspects: also dorsolateral pre-frontal cortex *Large overlap with anxiety/ behavioral control system in OFC	Specific area or specific afferent or efferent connections to or from ventral prefrontal cortex
Afferent information	Visual: inferotemporal object information; gustatory, olfactory etc.; reward information of VTA	Amygdala; object information about previous experience of fear/anxiety situations
Efferent information	Via n. acc. to (a) VTA (b) ventral pallidum (ventral striatal loops)	(a) Via n.acc. to extended amygdala; (b) to anterior cingulate
Lesion/ localization	Partial lesion of distributed system, cortex or afferent/efferent connections (by DWML/ stroke etc.)	Specific lesions of cortex or afferent/efferent connections; vulnerability: because of specific localization or critical threshold of large lesion
Activation	*Reward information processing (together with VTA) *Ventral striatum loop function: retrieval of behavioral programs *Presynaptic block of amygdala afferents in n.acc. by VTA neurons	*Inhibition of ventral striatal loop function *Interaction with extended amygdala partially via n. accumbens (see TABLE 2) * Behaviorally consequences of overactivation: depression symptoms (see TABLE 2)
Deactivation/ lesion	*Neuropsychology: deficits in reward related tasks and retrieval of memory *Behaviorally: depression symptoms (see TABLE 2)	*Neuropsychology: Perseveration (deficit of response to negative reinforcement). *Behaviorally: euphoria, disinhibition, utilization behavior, etc.
Interaction	Inhibition of object related anxiety/behavioral control information processing	Inhibition of object related reward information processing
Additional effects	Potential alternative pathophysiology: *metabolical disturbance affecting extended amygdala and VTA *Afferent aminergic systems to extended amygdala and frontal cortex disturbed	*Effects of subgenual cingulate cortex activation (possibly in perception of negative emotion and depressed mood)

TABLE 2. Relation of symptoms of the depression syndrome to disorder of function of ventral frontal cortex and related structures

Depression: Obligatory Symptoms DSM-IV	Pathophysiological factors	Commentary
Lack of positive emotion, loss of perception of joy	Disturbance: reward related neuronal information processing of OFC; disconnection: afferent and efferent connections (with VTA, see TABLE 1)	Disturbance of cortical representation of reward, of generally predominant positive emotional tone
Lack of interest	Disturbance: (a) motivation: reward related, see TABLE 1 (b) retrieval of behavioral programs via ventral striatal loops (c) goal directed drive: activation of inhibitory function of anterior cingulate cortex-relation to anterior cingulate attention and motor centers	
Increase of negative emotion	(a) activation of anxiety/behavioral control information processing and disinhibited amygdala input, see TABLE 1 (b) anterior cingulate activation	(b) Possible association to pain
Further symptoms		
Social withdrawal	Disturbance of extended amygdala - function (social vocalization, social behavior)	Related to lack of interest and initiative
Lack of emotional expression	Disturbance of extended amygdala as interface to emotional motor system	
Vegetative symptoms (nutrition, sexual behavior, sleep)	Interaction with extended amygdala (related to its conntecions to brain stem and hypothalamic centers)	
Loss of attentional effort	(a) Disorder of anterior cingulate and its influence on attentional/eye movement control (lateral OFC efferents to supracallosal anterior cingulate area) (b) n. accumbens/extended amygdala: influence on n. basalis Meynert (also directly from OFC)	
Depressive thought content and attentional / perceptual bias	(a) Extended amygdala (n.acc.) efferent connections with executive function loops; (b) anterior cingulate efferent connection with amygdala	Bias by deficit of representation and retrieval of reward related information

(A2) VTA neurons activate frontal cortex as well as frontal loop functions. They presynaptically inhibit amygdala afferents to the n. accumbens and control cortical afferents to this nucleus. (A3) Ventral frontal neurons are engaged in retrieval of behavior programs via ventral striatal reentering cortico-subcortical loops.

(B) There is some specificity in brain behavior relationship regarding ventral frontal lobe: euphoric and disinhibited behavior results if the presumed object-related anxiety/behavioral control information processing is disturbed,[5,7] which can obviously be considered as a kind of opposite to the depressive syndrome. (B1) In agreement with this, the data on ventral frontal hyperactivity (e.g., Ref. 6) may point to a hyperactivity of this system in depression.[4] (B2) The anterior cingulate area 24a[1,4] may be most parsimoniously related to perception of grief and depressed mood as in perception of pain and probably perception of effort for attention in more posterior parts of the cingulate cortex.

A reciprocal inhibition of the dorsal and ventral prefrontal cortex and related structures has been introduced in the revised model of Mayberg.[4] A reciprocal inhibition, however, between the two antagonistic functions of ventral frontal cortex, i.e., reward information processing and the anxiety/behavioral control information processing, may be implicated in OFC function itself. A further interaction may be effective via presynaptic inhibition of amygdala afferents to n. accumbens by the VTA dopamine neurons. This may add to an explanation why in depression the anxiety-behavioral control information processing is even overactive in case of an impairment of the reward-related system by neuronal damage or disconnection (see TABLE 1). Hitherto, it has not been determined whether there is to some extent a localizing segregation of the reward-related and anxiety/behavioral control related information processing in OFC. A more general or specific lesion will lead to a euphoric/disinhibition syndrome, whereas a partial lesion and in early stages of progressive diseases a depression syndrome will be elicited. These distinctions may help to model organic depression, which may in turn help to explain other but not all forms of depressive illnesses.

REFERENCES

1. DREVETS, W.C., J.L. PRICE, J.R. SIMPSON, JR., R.D. TODD, T. REICH, M. VANNIER & M.E. RAICHLE. 1997. Subgenual prefrontal cortex abnormalities in mood disorders. Nature **386:** 824–827.
2. GLOOR, P. 1997. The Temporal Lobe and Limbic System. Oxford University Press. New York.
3. KRISHNAN, K.R.R. 1993. Neuroanatomic substrates of depression in the elderly. J. Geriatr. Psychiatry Neurol. **1:** 39–58.
4. MAYBERG, H.S. 1997. Limbic-cortical dysregulation: a proposed model of depression. *In* The Neuropsychiatry of Limbic and Subcortical Disorders. S. Salloway, P. Malloy & J.L. Cummings, Eds.: 167–178. American Psychiatric Press. Washington.
5. REISCHIES, F.M., K. BAUM, H. BRÄU, J.P. HEDDE & G. SCHWINDT. 1988. Cerebral magnetic resonance imaging findings in multiple sclerosis: relation to disturbance of affect, drive, and cognition. Arch. Neurol. **45:** 1114–1116.
6. REISCHIES, F.M., J.P. HEDDE & R. DROCHNER. 1989. Clinical correlates of cerebral blood flow in depression. Psychiatry Res. **9:** 323–326.
7. REISCHIES, F.M., K. BAUM, C. NEHRIG & W. SCHÖRNER. 1993. Psychopathological symptoms and MRI-findings in multiple sclerosis. Biol. Psychiatry **33:** 676–678.
8. REISCHIES, F.M. 1993. Heterogeneity of the time course of cognitive performance of depressed patients. *In* Psychopharmacotherapy for the Elderly: Research and Clinical Implications. M. Bergener, R.H. Belmaker & M.S. Tropper, Eds.: 318–327. Springer-Verlag. New York.
9. ROLLS, E.T., J. HORNAK, D. WADE & J. MCGRATH. 1994. Emotion-related learning in patients with social and emotional changes associated with frontal lobe damage. J. Neurol. Neurosurg. Psychiatry **57:** 1518–1524.

10. ROLLS, E.T. 1996. The orbitofrontal cortex. Philos. Trans. R. Soc. Lond. B. Biol. Sci. **351:** 1433–1443.
11. SCHULTZ, W., P. DAYAN & R. MONTAGUE. 1997. A neural substrate of prediction and reward. Science **275:** 1593–1599.

Phasic Accumbal Firing May Contribute to the Regulation of Drug Taking during Intravenous Cocaine Self-administration Sessions

LAURA L. PEOPLES,[a] ANTHONY J. UZWIAK, FRED GEE,
ANTHONY T. FABBRICATORE, KATHRYN J. MUCCINO,
BINAIFER D. MOHTA, AND M.O. WEST

*Department of Psychology, Rutgers, The State University of New Jersey,
New Brunswick, New Jersey 08903, USA*

INTRODUCTION

Recent studies have applied chronic extracellular recording techniques to the intravenous cocaine self-administration paradigm to investigate the neurophysiological mechanisms that contribute to drug taking (e.g., Refs. 1–4). Data of one study suggest that a large percentage of nucleus accumbens (NAcc) neurons exhibit a change in firing during limited-access (fixed-ratio 1) self-administration sessions that is both synchronized to the self-infusion behavior and has a time course comparable to the interval that elapses between successive self-infusions. A firing pattern with such a time course may be involved in the regulation of the self-infusion behavior (cf. Ref. 4). The focus of the present study was to further characterize neurons that exhibit this firing pattern.

METHODS AND RESULTS

Male Long-Evans rats ($n = 32$)[5] were implanted with a catheter in the jugular vein and an array of microwires in the NAcc. Intravenous cocaine self-administration sessions were conducted daily (fixed-ratio 1 schedule of 0.7 mg/kg/0.2 ml cocaine infusion). Electrophysiological recording sessions were in most cases conducted on the fifteenth day of self-administration. The recording session consisted of 3 phases: 1) predrug period, 2) self-administration session, and 3) postdrug period.[4,5]

Animals exhibited typical self-administration behavior (FIG. 1: 1B,2B). Of 121 neurons, 84 exhibited a phasic change in firing rate during the mins before and after individual self-infusions. Consistent with our previous observations,[4] the most common (58/84, 69%) change consisted of an initial decrease in firing rate during the 1 min after self-infusion and a subsequent reversal of that decrease which occurred progressively during the remaining mins of the interinfusion interval (decrease + progressive reversal) (FIG. 1: 1D,2D).

---

[a]Corresponding author: Laura L. Peoples, Ph.D., Dept. of Psychology, Busch Science Campus, Rutgers, The State University of New Jersey, New Brunswick, NJ 08903. Voice: 732-445-4309, -5405; fax: 732-445-2263; llp@psych.rutgers.edu

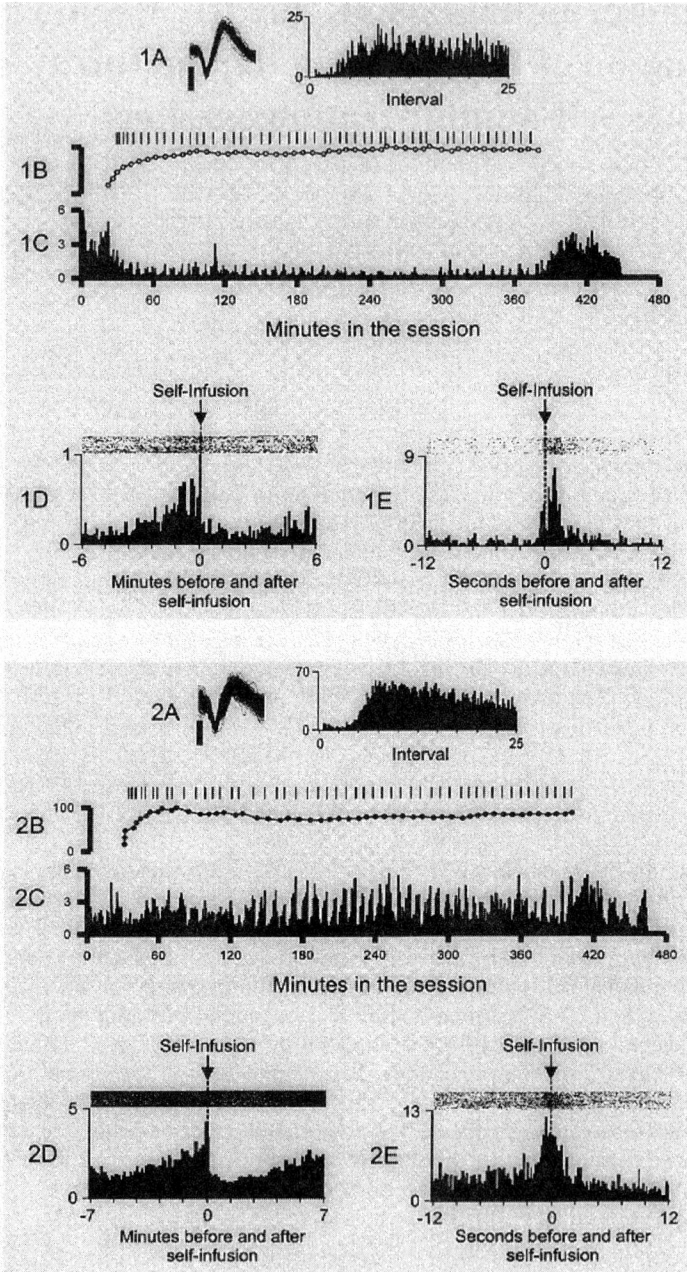

FIGURE 1. Neurons that showed the decrease + progressive reversal showed additional changes in firing. Part 1 and Part 2 each shows the behavior of a single animal and the tonic and phasic firing patterns of a single neuron recorded in that animal during one record-

Neurons that exhibited the decrease + progressive reversal firing pattern showed additional modulations in firing rate. First, almost all (51/58, 87.9%) the neurons showed either a decrease (33/58, 56.9%) (FIG. 1: 1C) or increase (18/58, 31.0%) (FIG. 1: 2C) in *tonic* firing rate during the self-administration session relative to the presession predrug recording period. Second, about half (27/58, 46.5%) of the neu-

---

ing session. Each Part consists of six Panels labeled A–E. *Panel A.* An interspike interval histogram shows the total number of interspike intervals in the recording session that were of durations ≥0.1 msec and ≤25.0 msec. The ordinate of the interspike interval histogram displays the number of counts (calculated as a function of 0.1 msec bins) and the abscissa displays the length (msec) of the interspike intervals. All neurons exhibited evidence of a minimum interspike interval consistent with the refractory period of a single neuron. To the left of the histogram are overlays of waveform traces (positive voltage is up). The vertical calibration bar on the left side of the waveform traces indicates 0.05 mV (i.e., amplitude of noiseband). Each waveform trace spans 0.64 msec. *Panel B.* Two functions are shown. At the top is a display of all lever presses made by the animal; underneath the display of lever presses is a graph of normalized calculated (cf. Ref. 12) drug level at the time of each reinforced lever press. Calculated drug level was normalized with respect to the maximum drug level attained in the session. The ordinate displays the percent (0–100%) of maximum drug level present at the time of the lever press (prior to the onset of the infusion). The display of lever presses and the graph of drug level are temporally aligned. Thus, the first and last point on the drug curve indicates the first and last self-infusion of cocaine, respectively. Although actual drug level (not shown) may have differed by some constant amount from that which was calculated, the drug accumulation curve demonstrates the degree to which the rate of self-infusion was likely to have maintained the level of drug in the body within stable limits. *Panel C.* A stripchart displays the tonic change in firing rate during the self-administration session relative to the presession predrug recording period. The ordinate displays firing rate (Hertz, Hz) and the abscissa displays time (min) during the recording session. The abscissa in Panel C is aligned temporally with the events shown in Panel B. Thus, in Panel C, firing during the self-administration session is shown directly below the drug curve, and firings during the predrug and postdrug recording periods are shown to the left and right of the drug curve, respectively. Panel 1C exemplifies a neuron that showed a decrease in tonic firing rate during the self-administration session, and Panel 2C exemplifies a neuron that showed an increase in tonic firing rate during the self-administration session. *Panel D.* A histogram shows the decrease + progressive reversal. Time "0" on the abscissa represents the occurrence of the reinforced lever press (i.e., self-infusion). Mins before and after the lever press are shown to the left and right of time "0", respectively. Average firing rate (i.e., average Hz per 0.1 min bin) is shown on the ordinate. Average firing was calculated across all lever-press trials, excluding both the first 8–10 presses and any lever presses bracketed by an interinfusion interval ≤6.0 min. Above the histogram is a raster display that shows firing of the neuron on a trial-by-trial basis. Lever-press trials are shown chronologically from the bottom row to the top row. As shown in the histogram, the firing rate decreased during the 1 min after self-infusion. Within 2 min after the infusion, the firing rate began to increase. The firing rate continued to progressively increase for the remainder of the interinfusion interval, until the firing rate approximated that present at the time of the previous self-infusion and the animal initiated the next self-infusion. *Panel E.* A histogram shows a phasic increase in firing during the secs before and after self-infusion. Time "0" on the abscissa represents the occurrence of the reinforced lever press. The secs before and after the lever press are shown to the left and right of time "0", respectively. The ordinate shows average firing rate (i.e., average Hz per 0.1 sec bin). Both 1E and 2E demonstrate common phasic changes in firing during the secs before and after self-infusion, i.e., an increase in the firing rate that began within the 3 secs before the cocaine reinforced lever press and ended within the 3 secs after self-infusion.[14] All tonic and phasic changes were statistically significant (Wilcoxon Matched Pairs test, $\alpha = 0.05$, unidirectional; cf. Refs. 4,5,9).

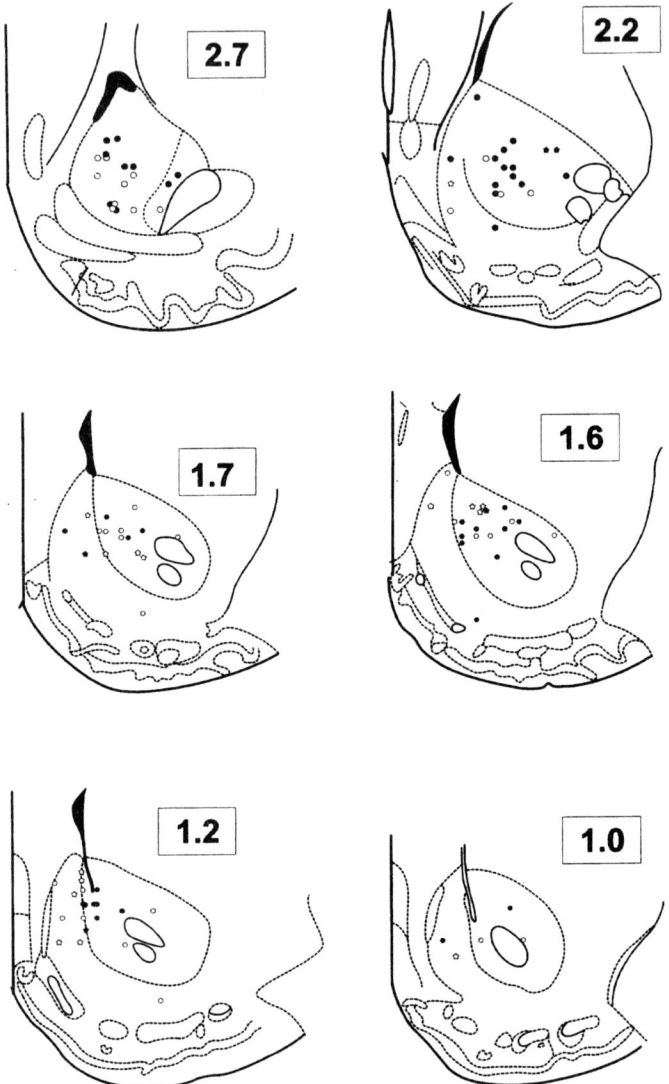

FIGURE 2. Histological localization of neurons. The nucleus accumbens is shown in each of six coronal plates (adapted from Paxinos and Watson[7]). The rostral-caudal position, relative to bregma is indicated by the number in the upper right of each plate. *Black symbols* indicate the locations of neurons that exhibited the decrease + progressive reversal; *gray symbols* indicate the locations of all other neurons. *Circles* indicate wire tips identified by a lesion mark. Histological procedures were described previously;[4] stars indicate neurons located by interpolation based on lesion marks corresponding to the adjacent rostral and caudal wires. When multiple neurons were recorded from the same location, symbols were slightly offset in order to show all neurons.

rons exhibited a third type of firing pattern which consisted of a *rapid* phasic change in firing during the few *secs* before and/or after self-infusion (e.g., FIG. 1: 1E,2E). Neurons that did not exhibit the decrease + progressive reversal firing pattern rarely exhibited the rapid phasic changes in firing (11/63, 17%). This latter finding is suggestive of a functional and perhaps necessary or limiting relationship between the decrease + progressive reversal pattern and most of the rapid phasic firing patterns.

Subterritorial Distribution

Neurons along the entire rostral-caudal extent of the NAcc[6,7] exhibited the decrease + progressive reversal firing pattern (FIG. 2). However, neurons of the shell[8] tended to be less likely to show decrease + progressive reversals (4/17, 23.5%) relative to neurons in either the rostral one-fourth of the NAcc (area defined as rostral pole[8]) (11/21, 52.4%) ($\chi^2 = 2.17$, $p > 0.05$), or the core (33/61, 54%) ($\chi^2 = 3.8$, $p < 0.05$). This trend was consistent with the significantly lower likelihood of shell neurons to exhibit any type of phasic change in firing during the mins and/or secs before and after self-infusion (9/17, 52.9%) than either the rostral pole (18/21, 85.7%) ($\chi^2 = 3.4$, $p < 0.05$) or the core (51/61, 83.6%) ($\chi^2 = 6.13$, $p < 0.05$).

DISCUSSION

The decrease + progressive reversal firing pattern is the most common phasic change in firing time locked to drug self-infusion and is exhibited by a relatively large number of neurons. The firing pattern is unique relative to other phasic changes in exhibiting not only a time-locked synchronicity with the self-infusion behavior but also a time course equal to the interval that separates successive self-infusions[4] (all other phasic changes show only the time-locked synchronicity). Furthermore, the present data suggest that the decrease + progressive reversal firing pattern may be necessary to, or permissive of, other phasic changes. These data suggest that the decrease + progressive reversal pattern may be a particularly important component of the neurophysiological mechanisms that mediate the contribution of the NAcc to self-administration behavior.

Self-infusion is importantly regulated by the pharmacokinetic time course of the self-administered drug (cf. Ref. 4). Certain data, some of which include the following (see also Refs. 4,9), indicate that the decrease + progressive reversal may be pharmacologically determined and may contribute to the mediation of the drug-induced regulation of self-administration behavior. First, the firing pattern closely mirrors changes in drug level as well as drug-induced changes in dopamine.[10] Second, a majority of neurons show a general inhibition of tonic firing rate during the self-administration session. Thus, the decrease + progressive reversal could reflect a repeating pharmacological cycle which consists of an initial inhibition of firing caused by the most recent drug infusion and a subsequent gradual recovery from that inhibition.

Other data are suggestive of a potential nonpharmacologic origin and function of the decrease + progressive reversal pattern. First, as noted above, about one third of the neurons show an overall increase in tonic firing during the self-administration session. Decrease + progressive reversal patterns exhibited by tonically *excited* neurons are unlikely to be due entirely to drug actions. Second, approximately half of all neurons that exhibit the decrease + progressive reversal pattern exhibit additional phasic increases in firing rate during the secs before and after self-infusion.[4,5] These rapid changes appear to be nonpharmacological and involved in the motivational (cf. Ref. 11) processing of the cocaine-related appetitive events.[1–3,12] Thus, at least half the decrease + progressive reversal neurons appear to be modulated by behaviorally related excitatory afferent input during the self-administration session. These data are consistent with the conclusion that there may be multiple, perhaps pharmacological and nonpharmacological, determinants of the decrease + progressive reversal firing pattern.

The subterritorial topographical distribution of phasic firing patterns observed in the present study (see also Ref. 13) should be viewed as preliminary, given the number of neurons currently included in the analysis. However, a differential distribution of phasic firing is consistent with what one might expect on the basis of other research. The shell shows a number of unique anatomical and neurochemical characteristics relative to the remainder of the NAcc[6,8,14,15] and plays a distinct role in drug reinforcement (e.g., Ref. 16).

ACKNOWLEDGMENTS

Ms. Linda King, Mr. Patrick Grace, and Dr. Donald McNeil contributed technical support. The research was supported by NIDA Grant DA 06886.

REFERENCES

1. BOWMAN, E.M., T.G. AIGNER & B.J. RICHMOND. 1996. Neural signals in the monkey ventral striatum related to motivation for juice and cocaine rewards. J. Neurophysiol. **75:** 1061–1973.
2. CARELLI, R.M. & S.A. DEADWYLER. 1997. Cellular mechanisms underlying reinforcement-related processing in the nucleus accumbens: electrophysiological studies in behaving animals. Pharmacol. Biochem. Behav. **57:** 495–504.
3. CHANG, J.-Y., S. F. SAWYER, R.-S. LEE & D.J. WOODWARD. 1994. Electrophysiological and pharmacological evidence for the role of the nucleus accumbens in cocaine self-administration in freely moving rats. J. Neurosci. **14:** 1224–1244.
4. PEOPLES, L.L. & M.O. WEST. 1996. Phasic firing of single neurons in the rat nucleus accumbens correlated with the timing of intravenous cocaine self-administration. J. Neurosci. **16(10):** 3459–3473.
5. PEOPLES, L.L., A.J. UZWIAK, F.X. GUYETTE & M.O. WEST. 1998. Tonic inhibition of single nucleus accumbens neurons in the rat: a predominant but not exclusive firing pattern induced by cocaine self-administration sessions. Neuroscience **86:** 13–22.
6. JONGEN-RÊLO, A.L., P. VOORN & H.J. GROENEWEGEN. 1994. Immunohistochemical characterization of the shell and core territories of the nucleus accumbens in the rat. Eur. J. Neurosci. **6:** 1255–1264.
7. PAXINOS, G. & C. WATSON. 1996. The Rat Brain in Stereotaxic Coordinates. Academic Press. New York.
8. ZAHM, D.S. & L. HEIMER. 1993. Specificity in the efferent projections of the nucleus accumbens in the rat: comparison of the rostral pole projection patterns with those of the core and shell. J. Comp. Neurol. **327:** 220–232.
9. PEOPLES, L.L., F. GEE, R. BIBI & M.O. WEST. 1998. Phasic firing time locked to cocaine self-infusion and locomotion: dissociable firing patterns of single nucleus accumbens neurons in the rat. J. Neurosci. **18(18):** 7588–7598.

10. WISE, R.A., P. NEWTON, K. LEEB, B. BRUNETTE, D. POCOCK & J.B. JUSTICE, JR. 1995. Fluctuations in nucleus accumbens dopamine concentration during intravenous cocaine self-administration in rats. Psychopharmacology **120:** 10–20.
11. DI CHIARA, G. 1995. The role of dopamine in drug abuse viewed from the perspective of its role in motivation. Drug Alcohol Depend. **38:** 95–137.
12. PEOPLES, L.L., A.J. UZWIAK, F. GEE & M.O. WEST. 1997. Operant behavior during sessions of intravenous cocaine infusion is necessary and sufficient for phasic firing of single nucleus accumbens neurons. Brain Res. **757:** 280–284.
13. UZWIAK, A.J., F.X. GUYETTE, M.O. WEST & L.L. PEOPLES. 1997. Neurons in accumbens subterritories of the rat: phasic firing time-locked within seconds of intravenous cocaine self-infusion. Brain Res. **767:** 363–369.
14. GROENEWEGEN, H.D., C.I. WRIGHT & A.V.J. BEIJER. 1996. The nucleus accumbens: gateway for limbic structures to reach the motor system? *In* Progress in Brain Research. Vol. 107. G. Holstege, B. Bandler & C.B. Saper, Eds.: 485–511. Elsevier Science. New York.
15. HEIMER, L., D.S. ZAHM, L. CHURCHILL, P.W. KALIVAS & C. WOHLTMANN. 1991. Specificity in the projection patterns of accumbal core and shell in the rat. Neuroscience **41**(1): 89–125.
16. CARLEZON, W.A. & R.A. WISE. 1996. Rewarding actions of phencyclidine and related drugs in nucleus accumbens shell and frontal cortex. J. Neurosci. **16:** 3112–3122.

Cocaine Is Self-administered into the Shell Region of the Nucleus Accumbens in Wistar Rats

D.L. McKINZIE, Z.A. RODD-HENRICKS, C.T. DAGON, J.M. MURPHY, AND W.J. McBRIDE[a]

Department of Psychiatry, Indiana University School of Medicine, and Department of Psychology, Purdue School of Science, IUPUI, Indianapolis, Indiana 46202, USA

INTRODUCTION

The mesolimbic dopamine (DA) system originating in the ventral tegmental area (VTA) and projecting to the nucleus accumbens (NAC) is thought to be a major neural substrate for mediating the reinforcing properties of abused drugs such as cocaine.[1,2] Evidence for the involvement of the mesolimbic DA system in mediating cocaine's reinforcing properties include studies showing that 6-hydroxydopamine (6-OHDA) lesions of the NAC dramatically reduce i.v. cocaine responding.[3] Additionally, conditioned place preference and drug discriminative properties of cocaine are attenuated by local administration of DA antagonists into the NAC.[4,5] However, most reports have indicated that rats will not self-administer cocaine directly into the NAC.[6]

Given increasing evidence that regional differences exist in the functioning of the NAC, it is possible that conflicting results concerning NAC-mediated intracranial self-administration (ICSA) for cocaine are related to anatomical placement of the injection site within the NAC. The core region receives substantial inputs from substantia nigra DA cell bodies, whereas the shell is largely innervated by DA projections from the VTA. It is this VTA-NAC pathway that is thought to be involved in incentive motivational aspects of drug reward.[7]

The objective of the present study was to determine whether regional heterogeneity exists in the NAC to the reinforcing properties of cocaine. Specifically, the efficacy of self-administration of cocaine into the NAC as a function of the location of injector tips in both the core and shell regions was examined. It was hypothesized that the shell, but not the core, region of the NAC would support ICSA behavior for cocaine.

METHODS

Subjects were adult female Wistar rats ($n = 5$–9 per group) weighing between 275–325 g prior to surgery. Rats were maintained on a reverse 12:12 dark:light cycle

---

[a]Corresponding author: Dr. W.J. McBride, Institute of Psychiatric Research, Indiana University School of Medicine, 791 Union Drive, Indianapolis, IN 46202-4887. Voice: 317-278-3820; fax: 317-274-1365; wmcbride@iupui.edu

TABLE 1. Infusions into the shell region of the NAC[a]

	Infusion Dose			
	aCSF	400 pmol	800 pmol	1200 pmol
Acquisition Day 4	5 ± 1.7	12 ± 3.2	28 ± 13*	45 ± 8.3*
Extinction Day 2	5 ± 1.8	12 ± 3.5	25 ± 10.4*	14 ± 2.3[#]
Reinstatement	5 ± 1.6	41 ± 11.7*[#]	27 ± 7.4*	58 ± 20.4*

[a]Mean number of self-infusions of rats administering aCSF, 400, 800, or 1200 pmol cocaine into the shell region of the nucleus accumbens (NAC). By the 4th day of acquisition, both the 800 and 1200 pmol cocaine groups received significantly more infusions than did aCSF and 400 pmol groups ($p < 0.05$). By the 2nd day of extinction training, total infusions decreased by almost 70% in the 1200 pmol group ($p < 0.05$). Reinstatement of cocaine-contingent infusions following extinction resulted in a return to Day 4 levels of infusions in the 1200 pmol group. Although the 400 pmol group did not differ from aCSF rats during acquisition, reinstatement of cocaine produced over a 3-fold increase in infusions over levels on Day 4 ($p < 0.05$). Data are means ±SEM. * $p < 0.05$ vs. aCSF group: [#] $p < 0.05$ vs. Day 4.

with food and water freely available except during operant sessions. Under halothane anesthesia, a unilateral guide cannula was stereotaxically implanted in the anterior NAC using the following coordinates: +1.7 AP, +2.4 L, −7.5 mm V (shell) or +1.7 AP, +2.6, −7.0 mm V (core).[8] All coordinates were calculated using a 10° angle. All rats received a 7–10 day recovery period before operant sessions were initiated.

Rats were then given the opportunity to respond in a 2-lever operant paradigm. One lever was designated the 'active' lever and each press resulted in a 5-sec, 100-nl infusion of 400, 800, or 1200 pmol cocaine or artificial cerebrospinal fluid (aCSF) vehicle. The other lever was inactive, with presses being recorded but producing no programmed consequence. Reinforcement availability was signaled by illumination of a single cue light over the active lever as well as an ambient houselight. A lever press on the active lever illuminated a second flashing cue light over the active lever for a 10-sec period. Additional lever presses during this period were recorded but produced no further infusions. Operant sessions were 4 hr in duration and conducted every other day for a total of seven sessions. In the first 4 operant sessions, rats responded for their designated dose of cocaine or vehicle. In sessions 5 and 6, extinction training was implemented in which all rats responded for aCSF. On session 7, the original infusate that was administered on the first 4 days was again reinstated. Following the last operant session, rats were euthanized and dye was injected through the cannula. Brains were then removed, sliced, and stained with cresyl violet. Anatomical placements were verified under a dissection microscope. Only animals with injection sites in the shell or core region of the NAC were analyzed.

RESULTS

NAC Shell

A Day (Days 4, 6, 7) × Drug (aCSF, 400, 800, 1200 pmol cocaine) mixed ANOVA was conducted on the total number of infusions received in the NAC shell. Main effects of both Day and Drug were found [$F(2,70) = 5.20$ and $F(3,31) = 4.43$, p values <0.01], as well as a Day × Drug interaction [$F(6,62) = 2.29$, $p < 0.05$]. Simple effects

TABLE 2. Infusions into the core region of the NAC[a]

	Infusion Dose		
	aCSF	800 pmol	1200 pmol
Acquisition Day 4	10 ± 3.6	9 ± 3.5	2 ± .6
Extinction Day 2	9 ± 3.8	5 ± 1.2	1 ± 0.3
Reinstatement	6 ± 1.7	8 ± 3.0	3 ± 1.8

[a]Mean number of self-infusions of rats administering aCSF, 800 or 1200 pmol cocaine into the core region of the nucleus accumbens (NAC). Cocaine was not reinforcing at either dose when infused into the NAC core as total infusions of cocaine groups on Day 4 and reinstatement remained at, or below, vehicle levels. Only a significant effect of Drug was found, indicating that the 1200 pmol group consistently responded less than either aCSF or 800 pmol groups ($p < 0.05$). Data are means ± SEM.

analysis revealed that by Day 4 of acquisition, both the 800 and 1200 pmol groups were receiving significantly more infusions than were vehicle controls. Operant behavior appeared to be contingent on cocaine reinforcement as the 1200 pmol cocaine group reduced the number of self-infusions by almost 70% on the second day of extinction (Day 6). When cocaine was reinstated on Day 7, the number of infusions returned to baseline levels in 800 and 1200 pmol cocaine groups. Moreover, 400 cocaine pmol rats increased ICSA behavior by greater than 3-fold over Day 4 infusion levels (TABLE 1).

To determine whether ICSA for cocaine in the shell NAC was response contingent and not due to nonspecific arousing properties of cocaine, lever discrimination was also analyzed over the first 4 days of acquisition. A Day (Days 1–4) × Drug (aCSF, 400, 800, 1200 pmol cocaine) × Lever (active vs inactive) mixed ANOVA was conducted. A significant Day × Drug × Lever interaction was found [$F(9,93) = 3.03$, $p < 0.003$]. Neither aCSF nor 400 pmol rats discriminated between active and inactive levers over the 4 days of acquisition. However, lever discrimination was observed in both the 800 and 1200 pmol cocaine groups as evidenced by significantly more lever presses on the active than inactive lever.

NAC Core

A Day (Days 4, 6, 7) × Drug (aCSF, 400, 800, 1200 pmol cocaine) mixed ANOVA on the total number of infusions revealed only a main effect of Drug [$F(2,14) = 4.88$, $p < 0.03$]. Analysis of this effect determined that the 1200 pmol group had generally lower numbers of infusions than did the aCSF and 800 pmol groups throughout training. Examination of lever pressing behavior again revealed that cocaine groups with core placements did not respond more than vehicle controls, nor did they exhibit lever discrimination [all F values <1.7] (TABLE 2).

DISCUSSION

These data indicate that regional differences exist in the ICSA of cocaine into the NAC. Doses of 800 and 1200 pmol cocaine resulted in robust operant responding in female Wistar rats as long as infusions were localized to the shell region of the NAC.

These same doses were not reinforcing when infused into the NAC core. The ICSA for cocaine was contingent upon operant conditioning, in that, (1) rats readily discriminated between active and inactive levers, (2) total responding and infusions significantly decreased following substitution of vehicle alone, and (3) cocaine reinstatement elevated active lever responding to levels observed prior to extinction.

Although anatomical placements were not shown in a previous failure to observe cocaine-mediated ICSA in the NAC, the results may have been due to preferential placements of the injection cannula into the core region.[6] Further support for this explanation comes from a recent paper examining the rewarding properties of nomifensine, which also noted that cocaine appeared to be reinforcing when injection sites were localized within the shell region of the NAC.[9] Taken together, the present study demonstrates that only the shell region of the NAC mediates ICSA of cocaine and that core-shell distinctions are potentially critical factors when determining behavioral aspects of NAC functioning.

ACKNOWLEDGMENTS

This study was supported by the National Institute on Alcohol Abuse and Alcoholism Grants AA07611, AA07462, AA10722 and AA11261. D.L.M. is a recipient of a Research Scientist Development Award (K01 AA00207).

REFERENCES

1. KOOB, G.F. 1992. Drugs of abuse: anatomy, pharmacology and function of reward pathways. TIPS **13:** 177–184.
2. TRUJILLO, K.A. *et al.* 1993. Drug reward and brain circuitry: recent advances and future directions. *In* Biological Basis of Substance Abuse. S.G. Korenman & J.D. Barchas, Eds.: 119–142. Oxford University Press. New York.
3. PETTIT, H.O. *et al.* 1984. Destruction of dopamine in the nucleus accumbens selectively attenuates cocaine but not heroin self-administration in rats. Psychopharmacology **84:** 167–173.
4. BAKER, D.A. *et al.* 1998. Effects of intraaccumbens administration of SCH-23390 on cocaine-induced locomotion and conditioned place preference. Synapse **30:** 181–193.
5. CALLAHAN, P.M. *et al.* 1997. Mediation of the discriminative stimulus properties of cocaine by mesocorticolimbic dopamine systems. Pharmacol. Biochem. Behav. **57:** 601–607.
6. GOEDERS, N.E. *et al.* 1983. Cortical dopaminergic involvement in cocaine reinforcement. Science **221:** 773–775.
7. ZAHM, D.S. *et al.* 1997. On the significance of subterritories in the "accumbens" part of the rat ventral striatum. Neuroscience **50:** 751–767.
8. PAXINOS, G. *et al.* 1986. The Rat Brain in Stereotaxic Coordinates. 2nd edit. Academic Press. Orlando, FL.
9. CARLEZON, W.A. *et al.* 1995. Habit-forming actions of nomifensine in nucleus accumbens. Psychopharmacology **122:** 194–197.

Involvement of Acetylcholine in the Nucleus Accumbens in Cocaine Reinforcement

GREGORY P. MARK,[a] ANTHONY E. KINNEY, MICHELE C. GRUBB, AND ALAN S. KEYS

Department of Behavioral Neuroscience, Oregon Health Sciences University, School of Medicine, Portland, Oregon 97201, USA

The nucleus accumbens (NAc) in the mesolimbic system has been identified as a key component of the neurobiological circuit that mediates the reinforcing properties of many drugs of abuse. The NAc consists primarily of GABAergic neurons but also contains a smaller population of acetylcholine (ACh)-containing interneurons.[1,2] These large aspiny interneurons may have an important integrative function, and their involvement in drug reward has not been systematically investigated. Our first studies using microdialysis found that cocaine self-administration increased ACh levels in the NAc to a greater extent than response-independent (i.e., yoked) cocaine.[3] These findings suggested that the context of drug experience may influence the neurochemical response to cocaine.

In the two experiments described here, we have examined the interaction between cocaine self-administration and the activity of cholinergic interneurons in the NAc using microdialysis for acetylcholine and intracerebral microinjections. In our first experiment, we sought to determine if the response of NAc ACh neurons to the glutamate agonist AMPA was different in animals that self-administered cocaine versus those that received passive cocaine exposure. In the second experiment, we measured cocaine self-administration on a progressive ratio schedule of reinforcement in rats that received intraaccumbens injections of cholinergic agonists.

EXPERIMENT 1: COCAINE EXPOSURE REDUCES AMPA-STIMULATED ACH RELEASE

Three groups of male Sprague-Dawley rats (300–340 g) were used for this experiment: drug naïve, cocaine self-administration (CSA) and cocaine yoked (CY). After preliminary food training, all animals were implanted with bilateral guide shafts (21 gauge) immediately above the NAc shell. Also at this time, CSA and CY animals were implanted with chronic, indwelling jugular vein catheters as described previously.[4] Following 5–7 days of postoperative recovery, subjects were run according to their respective treatment condition. CSA subjects were placed in individual test chambers and were trained to press a response lever for cocaine infusions (0.75 mg/kg/140 µl) on a FR1 schedule with a 20-sec time out. Upon stable responding, daily 3-hr sessions continued for 14 days. During this time, individual CY animals re-

[a]Corresponding author. Voice: 503-494-2680; fax: 503-494-6877; markg@ohsu.edu

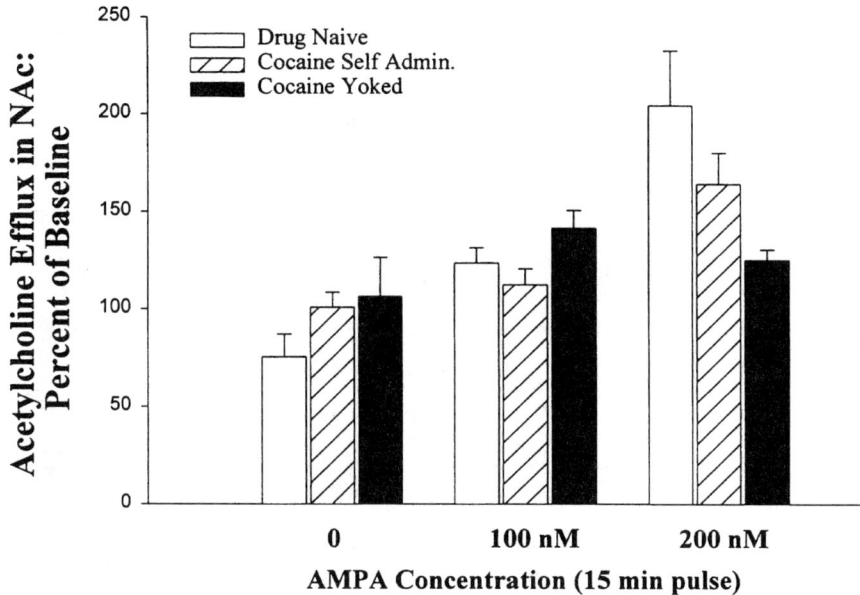

FIGURE 1. Acetylcholine release in the nucleus accumbens shell in response to a 15-min exposure to the non-NMDA agonist, AMPA (0, 100, and 200 nM) via reverse dialysis. Cocaine self-administration (*hatched bars*) and cocaine-yoked (*filled bars*) animals were tested 3 days after last cocaine access session. In drug-naïve animals (*open bars*), AMPA caused a dose-dependent increase in acetylcholine that reached a maximum of 205%. This increase was attenuated following cocaine self-administration and almost completely blocked in cocaine-yoked animals.

ceived response-independent cocaine infusions that were governed by the output from a corresponding CSA animal.

Three days following cocaine exposure, microdialysis sessions were conducted in both CSA and CY animals in the absence of cocaine (for microdialysis details, see Ref. 3). Baseline samples of ACh in the NAc were collected for at least 90 min prior to reverse dialysis perfusion of 15-min pulses of the non-NMDA agonist AMPA (100 and 200 nM) and perfusion ringer. Pulses were separated by 90-min recovery periods. An age-matched, drug-naïve control group underwent the same microdialysis procedure.

In drug-naïve animals, the ACh response to AMPA perfusion in the NAc followed a dose-dependent increase, thus supporting an excitatory glutamate-ACh connectivity within this region. The results in cocaine-exposed animals indicated that this response was attenuated at 3 days of withdrawal (FIG. 1). The 205% increase observed in naïve animals due to 200 nM AMPA was reduced in both cocaine exposure groups, with the CY animals exhibiting a near-complete blockade of this increase. The overall reduction of the glutamate-mediated facilitation of ACh efflux in this region provides evidence that glutamate mechanisms may play a role in withdrawal-dependent processes. Prior evidence has indicated that changes in glutamate mech-

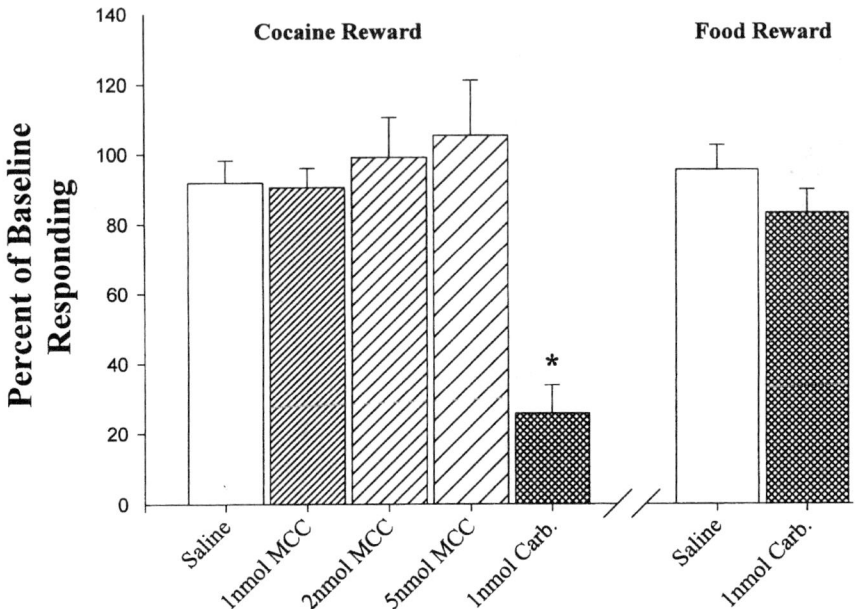

FIGURE 2. Percent change in baseline bar pressing for cocaine or food reward following bilateral microinfusions of saline, methylcarbamylcholine (MCC) or carbachol into the NAc shell. Carbachol dramatically reduced lever pressing for cocaine but not food reward. Conversely, MCC infusions caused a trend toward an increase in cocaine responding. *Asterisk* indicates $p < 0.05$ versus saline.

anisms accompany the well-documented phenomenon of withdrawal-dependent sensitization to cocaine. Furthermore, long-term depletions of presynaptic glutamate have been found following cocaine self-administration but not response-independent exposure.[4] The present results suggest that changes in the coupling of ACh and glutamate components within the NAc may play a role in the production of persisting, regimen-dependent neurochemical changes.

EXPERIMENT 2: EFFECTS OF CHOLINERGIC AGONISTS ON COCAINE SELF-ADMINISTRATION

Several lines of evidence suggest that both nicotinic and muscarinic drugs have effects on psychostimulant-induced locomotor activity and mesolimbic DA levels although perhaps in opposite directions.[5,6] In this experiment, we sought to determine the impact of intraaccumbens infusions of nicotinic and muscarinic agonists on cocaine seeking behavior.

Fifteen male Sprague-Dawley rats (300–340 g) were implanted with intravenous catheters and intracranial guide shafts aimed at the medial shell region of the NAc as described above. Animals were trained to lever press for cocaine or food reward on a progressive ratio schedule of reinforcement. The last successfully completed ratio before 1 hr of nonreinforcement was termed the break point. After a minimum of three days in which break points did not vary by more than 10%, rats received bilateral intra-NAc injections of saline, the nicotinic agonist methylcarbamylcholine (MCC) or the broad spectrum muscarinic agonist, carbachol and were then allowed to self-administer cocaine as before. A separate group of 6 rats received saline or carbachol injections before bar-pressing for 45 mg food pellets on the same progressive ratio schedule. Carbachol profoundly reduced break point measures of cocaine reinforcement but had little effect on food reward (FIG. 2). In contrast, injections of MCC caused a trend toward increasing the number of cocaine infusions relative to saline injections. These findings suggest that a general increase in cholinergic tone within the medial shell of the NAc can have different behavioral consequences depending on the type of cholinergic receptor activated. Evidence from previous reports using atropine or scopolamine have suggested that blockade of muscarinic receptors is associated with increases in psychostimulant reinforcement.[7] Our results suggest that activation of muscarinic receptors within the NAc is sufficient to generate the opposite effect.

REFERENCES

1. LEHMANN, J. & S.Z. LANGER. 1983. The striatal cholinergic interneuron: synaptic target of dopaminergic terminals? Neuroscience **10:** 1105–1120.
2. KAWAGUCHI, Y. *et al.* 1995. Striatal interneurons: chemical, physiological and morphological characterization. Trends Neurosci. **12:** 527–535.
3. MARK, G.P. *et al.* 1999. Self-Administration of cocaine increases the release of acetylcholine to a greater extent than response-independent cocaine in the nucleus accumbens of rats. Psychopharmacology **143:** 117–153.
4. KEYS, A.S. *et al.* 1998. Reduced glutamate immunolabeling in the nucleus accumbens following extended withdrawal from self-administered cocaine. Synapse **30:** 393–401.
5. BYMASTER, F.P. *et al.* 1993. Comparative behavioral and neurochemical activities of cholinergic antagonists in rats. J. Pharmacol. Exp. Ther. **267:** 16–24.
6. DI CHIARA, G. *et al.* 1994. Modulatory functions of neurotransmitters in the striatum: ACh/dopamine/NMDA interactions. Trends Neurosci. **17:** 228–233.
7. LYNCH, M.R. 1991. Scopolamine enhances expression of an amphetamine-conditioned place preference. Neuroreport **2:** 715–718.

Cocaine-seeking Behavior and Fos Expression in the Amygdala Produced by Cocaine or a Cocaine Self-administration Environment

DAVID A. BAKER,[a] RITA A. FUCHS,[a] LY T.L. TRAN-NGUYEN,[a] ART J. PALMER,[a] JOHN F. MARSHALL,[b] RON J. McPHERSON,[b] AND JANET L. NEISEWANDER[a,c]

[a]*Department of Psychology, Arizona State University, Tempe, Arizona 85287, USA*
[b]*Department of Psychobiology, University of California-Irvine, Irvine, California 92697, USA*

Incentive motivation elicited by cocaine or cocaine-associated stimuli is thought to contribute to craving and relapse in cocaine abusers, and cocaine-seeking behavior (nonreinforced operant responding) in rats. The aim of this study was to examine the involvement of the basolateral (BlA) and central (CeA) amygdala in incentive motivation produced by a cocaine primer and/or exposure to a cocaine self-administration (SA) environment by examining Fos expression as a general marker for neuronal activation.

Male Sprague-Dawley rats were trained to self-administer cocaine (0.5 mg/kg/ 0.1 ml, i.v.; $n = 25$) or received yoked-saline infusions ($n = 12$) for 15–21 days depending on performance. Cocaine-trained rats then received 21 daily 2-hr exposures to either the SA environment in the absence of cocaine reinforcement (i.e., extinction training) or an alternate environment (i.e., no extinction trainng). Extinction training was intended to decrease incentive motivation for cocaine elicited by the environment. The saline-yoked controls were treated identically; however, these groups were combined into a single control group, since extinction training did not alter any of the behavioral or neurochemical measures in these rats. Thus, the design yielded the following groups: Control, Extinction, and No Extinction.

Following extinction training, rats were tested for cocaine-seeking behavior for 90 min following exposure to the SA environment (extinction phase). The rats were then tested for reinstatement of cocaine-seeking behavior for 60 min following an i.p. saline injection, and 90 min following an i.p. cocaine injection (15 mg/kg). Rats from each group ($n = 5$–7) were sacrificed following either the extinction (i.e., exposure to the environment only) or the cocaine phase. Fos protein expression was then measured as described previously.[1]

Extinction training decreased cocaine-seeking behavior produced by exposure to the SA environment. There was a main effect of group ($F(2,34) = 38.4$, $p < 0.0001$), and post hoc comparisons indicated that the No Extinction group exhibited more cocaine-seeking behavior during the extinction phase relative to all other groups (Fisher LSD test, $p < 0.05$; FIG. 1) and there was no difference between the Extinction and

[c]Address for correspondence: Janet L. Neisewander, Ph.D., Dept. of Psychology, Arizona State University, Box 871104, Tempe, AZ 85287. Voice: 602-965-0635; fax: 602-965-8544; janet.neisewander@asu.edu

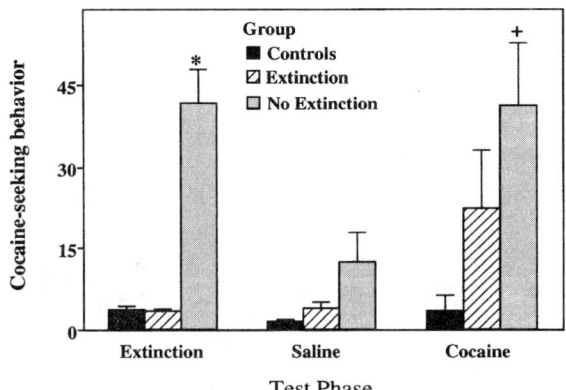

FIGURE 1. Effect of extinction training on cocaine-seeking behavior (nonreinforced responding) during extinction, saline reinstatement, and cocaine reinstatement test phases. Cocaine-seeking behavior is illustrated as the mean number of responses (±SEM) per 30-min interval during each phase. *Asterisk* represents a significant difference from all other groups, Fisher LSD, $p < 0.05$. *Plus sign* represents a significant difference from controls, Fisher LSD, $p < 0.05$.

Control groups. These findings suggest that extinction training effectively decreased incentive motivation elicited by the environment.

The saline injection did not reinstate cocaine-seeking behavior in any of the groups. Conversely, the cocaine-priming injection reinstated cocaine-seeking behavior regardless of group; however, this effect was more robust in the No Extinction group. There was a main effect of time between the last interval of the saline phase and the first interval of the cocaine phase ($F(1,15) = 7.6, p < 0.05$). There was also a main effect of group ($F(2,15) = 4.05, p <0.05$) with only the No Extinction group exhibiting enhanced cocaine-seeking behavior relative to Controls (Fisher LSD, $p < 0.05$), suggesting extinction training also attenuated cocaine-seeking behavior following a cocaine primer.

The cocaine priming injection produced an unconditioned increase in Fos expression in the CeA, but not the BlA. In contrast, the SA environment produced a conditioned increase in Fos expression in the BlA, but not the CeA. In the CeA, there was a main effect of stimulus exposure ($F(1,29) = 27.72, p < 0.001$), evident as an increase in Fos expression in rats receiving the cocaine primer relative to those exposed to the environment only, regardless of SA history or extinction training (FIG. 2A). In the BlA, there was a main effect of group ($F(2,29) = 5.58, p < 0.01$), and post hoc comparisons indicated that the SA environment elicited an increase in Fos expression in the No Extinction group relative to all other groups (Fisher LSD test, $p < 0.05$; FIG. 2B). There was only a trend toward an effect of the cocaine primer ($F(1,29) = 3.3, p = 0.08$) and no interaction with group. The increase in Fos expression in the BlA was not simply due to operant responding, since an additional No Extinction group was tested following exposure to the environment without levers present, and these rats exhibited similar Fos expression (mean ±SEM = 11.4 ± 1.4) as the No Extinction group allowed to engage in cocaine-seeking behavior.

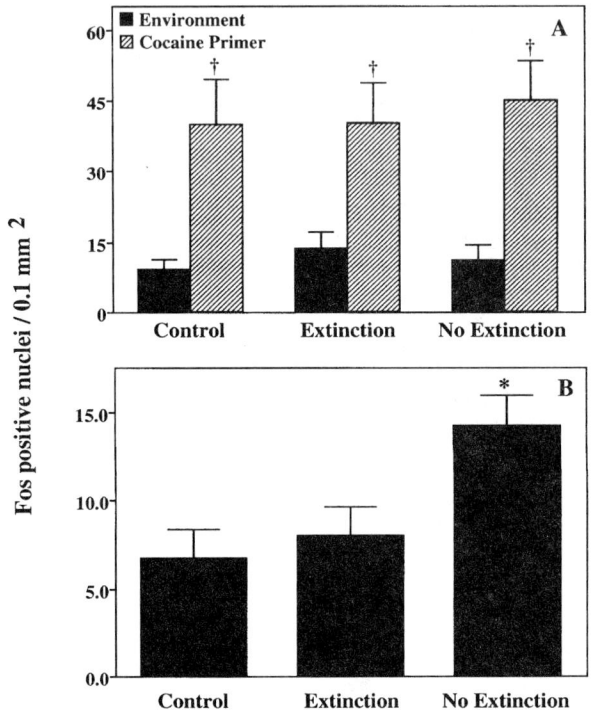

FIGURE 2. The mean number (±SEM) of Fos positive nuclei/0.1 mm^2 in the central (**A**) and basolateral (**B**) amygdala for each group. *Daggers* represent a significant difference from rats exposed only to the environment, ANOVA main effect, $p < 0.001$. *Asterisk* represents a significant difference from all other groups, Fisher LSD, $p < 0.05$.

Previous research has indicated that the amygdala is activated following either an acute cocaine injection in rats or exposure to cocaine-associated cues in humans and rats.[2,3] These studies, however, did not distinguish between the CeA and the BlA. In the present study, an unconditioned increase in Fos expression was observed in the CeA following the cocaine primer, which is consistent with previous research suggesting that the CeA is involved in initiating psychomotor stimulant reward.[4] In contrast, a conditioned increase in Fos expression was obtained in the BlA following exposure to a cocaine environment, which is consistent with previous research indicating that lesions of the BlA disrupt cocaine-seeking behavior elicited by cocaine-associated cues.[5,6] Furthermore, the findings suggest that different mechanisms are involved in incentive motivation produced by the environment versus a cocaine primer.

REFERENCES

1. RUSKIN, D.N. & J.F. MARSHALL. 1997. Differing influences of dopamine agonists and antagonists on Fos expression in identified populations of globus pallidus neurons. Neuroscience **81:** 79–92.

2. GRANT, S. *et al.* 1996. Activation of memory circuits during cue-elicited cocaine craving. Proc. Natl. Acad. Sci. **93:** 12040–12045.
3. BROWN, E. *et al.* 1992. Evidence for conditional neuronal activation following exposure to a cocaine-paired environment: role of forebrain limbic structures. J. Neurosci. **12:** 4112–4121.
4. O'DELL, L.E. *et al.* 1999. Behavioral effects of psychomotor stimulant infusions into amygdaloid nuclei. Neuropsychopharmacology **20:** 591–602.
5. MEIL, W.M. & R. E. SEE. 1997. Lesions of the basolateral amygdala abolish the ability of drug associated cues to reinstate responding during withdrawal from self-administered cocaine. Behav. Brain Res. **87:** 139–148.
6. WHITELAW, R.B. *et al.* 1996. Excitotoxic lesions of the basolateral amygdala impair the acquisition of cocaine-seeking behavior under a second-order schedule of reinforcement. Psychopharmacology **127:** 213–224.

Differences in Receptor System Participation between Nicotine- and Cocaine-induced Dopamine Overflow in Nucleus Accumbens

ISTVAN SZIRAKI,[a] HENRY SERSHEN, MYRON BENUCK, AUDREY HASHIM, AND ABEL LAJTHA[b]

Center for Neurochemistry, The Nathan S. Kline Institute, Orangeburg, New York 10962, USA

INTRODUCTION

The dopamine overflow in the nucleus accumbens represents a major neurochemical correlate of the reinforcing effects of drugs of abuse. A similar increase of dopamine induced by nicotine to that by cocaine has indicated similar mechanisms of action.[1] In addition to the reward system, nicotine has influence on several other systems that could alter behavior, including cognition, learning, memory, arousal, etc.[2,3] Our hypothesis is that some of the changes in various structures and in behavior are specific for nicotine, and that interaction of different receptor systems is involved in the various effects of nicotine. In the present study we investigated differences in receptor interactions involved in nicotine- and cocaine-induced changes of the levels of dopamine in the nucleus accumbens.

METHODS

Animals and Administration of Drugs

Male Sprague-Dawley rats (280–320 g) bred in our animal facility were used for the experiments. Nicotine, cocaine, and receptor subtype specific antagonists were administered through a cannula inserted under anesthesia into the right jugular vein.[4]

Brain Microdialysis and Determination of Dopamine

After the catheterization of the jugular vein, the rats were placed in a stereotaxic apparatus. A guide cannula was lowered to 2 mm above the selected site in the brain and fixed to the skull with dental cement. The coordinates (mm) for nucleus accumbens shell relative to the bregma were: AP: +2.0, ML: −1.2, DV: −6. A 2-mm probe was inserted into the guide cannula either in the morning of the day of an experiment or in the evening of the previous day. The dialysates of 15- to 30-min periods were

---

[a]On leave of absence from the Division of Biochemistry, Institute for Drug Research, Budapest, Hungary.
[b]Corresponding author: Abel Lajtha, Ph.D., The N.S. Kline Institute, 140 Old Orangeburg Rd., Orangeburg, NY 10962. Voice: 914-398-5530; fax: 914-398-5531; Lajtha@nki.rfmh.org

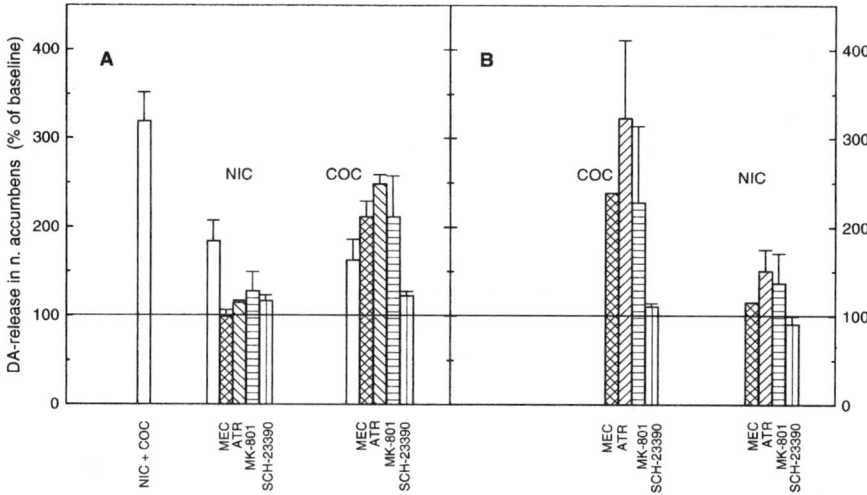

FIGURE 1. Effects of various antagonists on nicotine- and cocaine-induced accumbal dopamine release in rats. The *bars* represent peak heights (averages of three experiments ±SEM) after nicotine or cocaine injections in the presence or in the absence of antagonists. **(A)** The animals were treated through the jugular vein with nicotine (NIC; 50 µg/kg) in the presence of an antagonist as indicated and 2 hr later with cocaine (COC; 250 µg/kg). The antagonists were coadministered with nicotine or cocaine and then continously infused through the vena cannula until collecting the last sample after the cotreatment with cocaine. The doses (free base) of the antagonists were as follows: mecamylamine (MEC): bolus: 200 µg/kg, infusion: 120 µg/kg/hr; atropine (ATR): bolus: 50 µg/kg, infusion: 30 µg/kg/hr; dizocilpine (MK-801): bolus:500 µg/kg, infusion: 500 µg/kg/hr; SCH-23390: bolus: 30 µg/kg, infusion: 18 µg/kg/hr. In separate experiments (*empty bars*) the animals received nicotine (50 µg/kg) at zero time, the combination of nicotine and cocaine (50 µg/kg and 250 µg/kg, respectively) at 120 min, and then cocaine (250 µg/kg) alone at 240 min. **(B)** In the experiments represented in this panel, the animals received cocaine at zero time, and nicotine 2 hr later. Doses were the same as in the experiments represented in (A).

collected, and the dopamine levels in the samples were determined by a BAS 200 A HPLC system equipped with a BAS Unijet detector cell.

RESULTS AND DISCUSSION

HPLC analysis of the microdialysates from awake animals shows that intravenously administered 50 µg/kg of nicotine was equipotent with subsequently administered 250 µg/kg of cocaine in inducing dopamine overflow in the nucleus accumbens shell. When administered together, the effect of nicotine and cocaine was additive (FIG. 1A). Coadministration of the nicotinic antagonist mecamylamine, the muscarininc antagonist atropine, and the NMDA antagonist MK-801 each blocked nicotine-induced dopamine overflow but not the subsequent, cocaine-induced DA release (FIG. 1A). In fact, these compounds seem to potentiate the effect of cocaine. Coadministration of dopamine antagonist (D_1) SCH-23390, however, inhibited both the nicotine- and the cocaine-induced dopamine-release. Similar inhibition of the nicotine-induced accumbal dopamine overflow by mecamylamine, atropine, MK-801, and SCH-23390 was observed when the animals received first cocaine and then nicotine (FIG. 1B). Again, the cocaine-induced dopamine release was inhibited by SCH-23390, but not by mecamylamine, atropine, or MK-801.

Our results that coadministration of nicotine (50 µg/kg) and cocaine (250 µg/kg) induces a greater dopamine overflow in the nucleus accumbens shell than any of the two drugs alone are in agreement with recent finding of Zernig and co-workers,[5] and may provide neurochemical explanation for behavioral changes in subjects consuming both nicotine and cocaine.[6,7] It is of interest that nicotine did not trigger dopamine overflow when it was administered 2 hr after nicotine + cocaine treatment.[8]

The inhibition of nicotine-induced dopamine release by nicotinic, muscarinic, and NMDA antagonists shows the participation of several receptor systems in the nicotine-induced effect. Blocking of both nicotine- and cocaine-induced effects by a dopamine D_1 receptor antagonist, indicates the possible role of this receptor in nicotine-associated and also in cocaine-associated reward effects.

In conclusion, these results indicate several differences in receptor interactions that play a critical role in the induction of dopamine overflow in nucleus accumbens by nicotine and cocaine.

ACKNOWLEDGMENTS

The work was supported in part by a grant from Philip Morris, USA.

REFERENCES

1. PONTIERI, F.E. *et al.* 1996. Effects of nicotine on the nucleus accumbens and similarity to those of addictive drugs. Nature **382:** 255–257.
2. LEVIN, E.D. 1992. Nicotinic systems and cognitive function. Psychopharmacology **108:** 417–431.
3. BARDO, M.T. 1998. Neuropharmacological mechanisms of drug reward: beyond dopamine in the nucleus accumbens. Crit. Rev. Neurobiol. **12:** 37–67.
4. FLECKNELL, P.A. 1992. Catheterisation of the jugular vein. *In* Experimental and Surgical Technique in the Rat. H.B Waynforth & P.A. Flecknell, Eds.: 215–222. Academic Press. San Diego.
5. ZERNIG, G. *et al.* 1997. Nicotine and heroin augment cocaine-induced dopamine overflow in nucleus accumbens. Eur. J. Pharmacol. **337:** 1–10.
6. SCHORLING, J.B. *et al.* 1994. Tobacco, alcohol and other drug use among college students. J. Subst. Abuse **6:** 105–115.
7. BUDNEY, A. J. *et al.* 1993. Nicotine and caffeine use in cocaine-dependent individuals. J. Subst. Abuse **5:** 117–130.
8. SZIRAKI, I. *et al.* 1998. Receptor systems participating in nicotine-specific effects. Neurochem. Int. **33:** 445–457.

Modulation of Cocaine-induced Sensitization by κ-Opioid Receptor Agonists

Role of the Nucleus Accumbens and Medial Prefrontal Cortex

VLADIMIR CHEFER, ALEXIS C. THOMPSON, AND TONI S. SHIPPENBERG[a]

Integrative Neuroscience Unit, Behavioral Neuroscience Laboratory, NIDA Intramural Research Program, Baltimore, Maryland 21224, USA

INTRODUCTION

The behavioral effects of cocaine are enhanced in individuals with a prior history of intermittent cocaine use.[1] This phenomenon, referred to as behavioral sensitization, can persist for months following the cessation of drug use and has been implicated in the reinstatement of compulsive drug-seeking behavior.[2] Abstinence from cocaine also produces long-term alterations in mesocorticolimbic dopamine (DA) neurotransmission. Basal DA levels within the nucleus accumbens (NAC) are elevated during the early phase of abstinence from cocaine and there is a progressive increase in cocaine-evoked DA levels as abstinence proceeds.[1,3] These alterations in DA neurochemistry are thought to underlie the initiation and expression of behavioral sensitization.

The coadministration of κ-opioid receptor agonists with cocaine prevents the development of sensitization to cocaine.[4] Systemically administered κ-opioid agonists also prevent alterations in DA neurochemistry that occur within the NAC during abstinence from cocaine. The site of action of κ-opioid agonists in producing these effects is unknown. The present studies examined the role of κ-opioid receptors in the NAC and medial prefrontal cortex (mPFC) in mediating the interaction of κ-opioid agonists with cocaine.

METHODS

Male Sprague-Dawley rats were stereotaxically implanted with bilateral guide cannula aimed at the NAC or at the NAC and mPFC.[5] Drug treatments commenced one week later. Rats received once daily injections of cocaine (20.0 mg/kg, i.p.) or saline for five days. On days 3–5, they received intracranial infusions of the κ-opioid agonist, U69593 (1.0 µg/side), 5 min prior to i.p. injections. Microdialysis was conducted 3 and 21 days later. A 2.0-mm dialysis probe was perfused with artificial cerebrospinal fluid, and inserted into the NAC. Twelve hr later, 3 dialysis samples

---

[a]Address for correspondence: Toni S. Shippenberg, Integrative Neuroscience Unit, Behavioral Neuroscience Laboratory, NIDA Intramural Research Program, 5500 Nathan Shock Drive, Baltimore, MD 21224. Voice: 410-550-1451; fax: 410-550-1692; tshippen@intra.nida.nih.gov

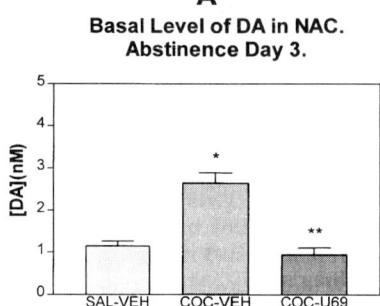
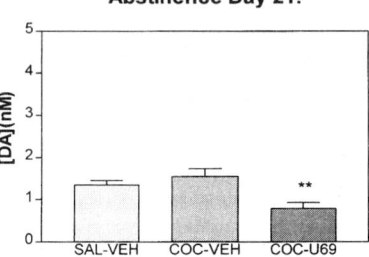

FIGURE 1. Influence of intra-NAC U69593 upon abstinence-induced alterations in basal DA levels in the NAC. **(A)** Abstinence day 3. **(B)** Abstinence day 21. * denotes significant difference from control (saline-treated) group; ** denotes significant difference from cocaine-treatment group, $p \leq 0.05$.

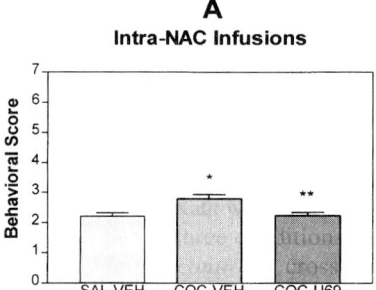
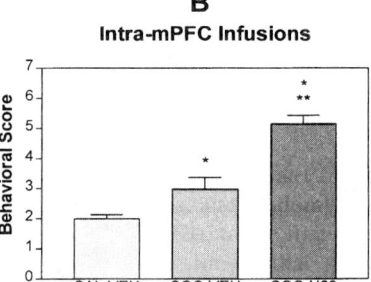

FIGURE 2. Influence of intra-NAC **(A)** and intra-mPFC **(B)** U69593 infusion upon sensitization to the psychomotor stimulant effects of cocaine. The data were obtained 3 days following the cessation of the cocaine- and U69593/cocaine-treatment regimens. * denotes significant difference from control (saline-treated) group; ** denotes significant difference from cocaine-treatment group, $p \leq 0.05$.

(perfusion rate: 1.1 μl/min) were collected at 25-min intervals for determination of basal DA levels. Animals were then injected with cocaine (20.0 mg/kg, i.p.) and samples were collected for 100 min. DA levels were quantified by HPLC/EC detection. Locomotor activity was rated during dialysis studies using a 9-point rating scale.[4] Data were analyzed using two factor analyses of variance and tests of contrast. Only data from animals with histologically correct cannula placements were used in statistical analyses.

RESULTS

DA levels in the NAC were elevated 3 days after the cessation of cocaine treatment. Although sensitization to the psychomotor stimulant effects of cocaine was evident at this time point, cocaine-evoked DA overflow was significantly less than that of control (saline-treated) animals. On abstinence day 21, basal DA levels had normalized (FIG. 1) and cocaine-evoked DA overflow was significantly enhanced relative to controls. In animals that had received intra-NAC infusions of U69593 with cocaine, the elevation of basal DA levels was prevented (FIG. 1) and no enhancement of cocaine-evoked DA overflow was seen. NAC infusions also attenuated sensitization to the psychomotor stimulant effects of cocaine (FIG. 2). In contrast, mPFC infusions of U69593 attenuated, but did not prevent, the elevation of basal DA levels that occurred on abstinence day 3. At this time point, the responsiveness of DA neurons to a challenge dose of cocaine was significantly enhanced, and the behavioral response to cocaine was significantly greater than that in cocaine-treated animals (FIG. 2).

DISCUSSION

Basal and cocaine-evoked DA levels in the NAC are increased following repeated cocaine administration. These neurochemical alterations are thought to result, in part, from cocaine-induced decreases in DA levels within the mPFC and disinhibition of pyramidal cells projecting to the ventral tegmental area and NAC.[7] Decreased DA in the mPFC and a reduction in D_2-receptor-mediated stimulation of GABA release in the mPFC have been implicated in the disinhibition process.[8] Increasing evidence suggests that these alterations in mesocorticolimbic neurotransmission underlie cocaine-induced behavioral sensitization.[7]

The activation of NAC κ-opioid receptors suppressed behavioral sensitization to cocaine and prevented cocaine-induced increases in basal and drug-evoked DA levels in the NAC. In contrast, the activation of mPFC κ-receptors exacerbated the development of behavioral sensitization and increased cocaine-evoked DA levels. The mechanisms mediating the opposing effects of κ-receptor activation in these two brain regions are unclear. κ-Agonists decrease DA release and downregulate D_2 receptors.[9] These actions may underlie the differing effects of U69593. Inhibition of DA release and D_2 receptor downregulation in the mPFC would disinhibit pyramidal cell firing and enhance the behavioral and neurochemical effects produced by the repeated administration of cocaine. In contrast, decreases in DA release within the NAC that occur following the activation of κ-opioid receptors in this brain region would oppose the increase in NAC DA levels that occur in response to the repeated administration of cocaine and attenuate behavioral sensitization. In conclusion, the activation of κ-opioid receptors in the NAC, but not the mPFC, prevents alterations in behavior and DA neurochemistry that occur during abstinence from cocaine. Similar effects are observed in response to systemically administered κ-opioid agonists. As such, an involvement of NAC κ-opioid receptors in mediating the interaction of systemically administered κ-opioid agonists with cocaine is indicated.

ACKNOWLEDGMENTS

This work was supported by the NIDA IRP and NIDA Grant DA 10084.

REFERENCES

1. KALIVAS, P.W. & J. STEWART. 1991. Dopamine transmission in the initiation and expression of drug- and stress- induced sensitization of motor activity. Brain Res. Rev. **16:** 223–244.
2. ROBINSON, T.E. & K.C. BERRIDGE. 1993. The neural basis of drug craving: an incentive-sensitization theory of addiction. Brain Res. Rev. **18:** 247–249.
3. HEIDBREDER, C. et al. 1996. Role of extracellular dopamine in the initiation and long-term expression of behavioral sensitization to cocaine. J. Pharmacol. Exp. Ther. **278:** 490–502.
4. HEIDBREDER, C. & T.S. SHIPPENBERG. 1994. U-69593 prevents cocaine sensitization by normalizing basal accumbens dopamine. Neuroreport **5:** 1797.
5. PAXINOS, G. & C. WATSON. 1982. The Rat Brain in Stereotaxic Coordinates. Academic Press. Sydney.
6. ELLINWOOD, E. & R. BALSTER. 1974. Rating the behavioral effects of amphetamine. Eur. J. Pharmacol. **38:** 35–41.
7. KALIVAS, P.W. 1995. Interactions between dopamine and excitatory amino acids in behavioral sensitization to psychostimulants. Drug Alcohol Depend. **37:** 95–100.
8. GROBIN, A.C. & A.Y. DEUTCH. 1988. Dopaminergic regulation of extracellular GABA levels in the prefrontal cortex of the rat. J. Pharmacol. Exp. Ther. **285:** 350–357.
9. IZENWASSER, S. et al. 1998. Repeated treatment with the selective κ-opioid agonist U69593 produces a marked depletion of dopamine D_2 receptors. Synapse **30:** 275–283.

SPECT following Intravenous Procaine in Cocaine Addiction

BRYON ADINOFF,[a,b,d] MICHAEL D. DEVOUS,[a] SUSAN BEST,[a,b]
MARK S. GEORGE,[c] DEANNA ALEXANDER,[a] AND KELLY PAYNE[a]

[a]*University of Texas Southwestern Medical Center, Dallas, Texas 75235, USA*
[b]*Veterans Affairs North Texas Health Care System, Dallas, Texas 75216, USA*
[c]*Medical University of South Carolina, Charleston, South Carolina 29425, USA*

INTRODUCTION

Cocaine has been shown to stimulate the limbic system in both preclinical and clinical studies, and the euphorigenic effects of cocaine have been correlated with limbic system activation. Previous investigators have suggested that a state of permanent limbic neuronal hyperexcitability may be present in cocaine addicts, such that spontaneous or cue-related episodes of limbic neuronal discharge may occur.[1] Limbic discharge may subsequently induce craving in cocaine-dependent patients, precipitating relapse.

Procaine has previously been shown to stimulate limbic regions in humans.[2] In order to explore the phenomena of sensitization in cocaine addicts, we administered procaine to cocaine-addicted patients and healthy controls. Subjective responses and regional cerebral blood flow (rCBF), by SPECT, were assessed following both placebo and procaine infusion. We hypothesized that, as a result of cocaine-induced limbic sensitization, patients with a history of cocaine dependence would demonstrate greater procaine-induced limbic activation compared to healthy controls.

METHODS

Ten male (37.1 ± 5.2 yr (mean ±SD)) cocaine-addicted patients were studied. Patients were 14–21 days abstinent and housed on a structured residential treatment unit. Patients' primary lifetime drug of choice was cocaine, they had experienced no other substance use disorder in the past year (except nicotine), there was no lifetime history of alcohol, sedative-hypnotic, or opiate withdrawal, and there was no lifetime history of non-substance-induced Axis I disorder.

Ten men (32.9 ± 7.1 yr) and ten women (32.7 ± 7.6 yr) were studied as controls. Controls had no lifetime history of Axis I disorders, were in good medical health, and had no family history of an Axis I disorder in a first degree relative.

Two study sessions (single blind) were 48 hours apart. Placebo was administered in the first session, and procaine 1.38 mg/kg was administered intravenously in the second session. Placebo and procaine administration was immediately followed by

---

[d]Address for correspondence: Bryon Adinoff, M.D., 116A, VA Medical Center, 4500 S. Lancaster Rd., Dallas, TX 75216. Voice: 214-857-0843; fax: 214-857-0902; bryadinoff@aol.com

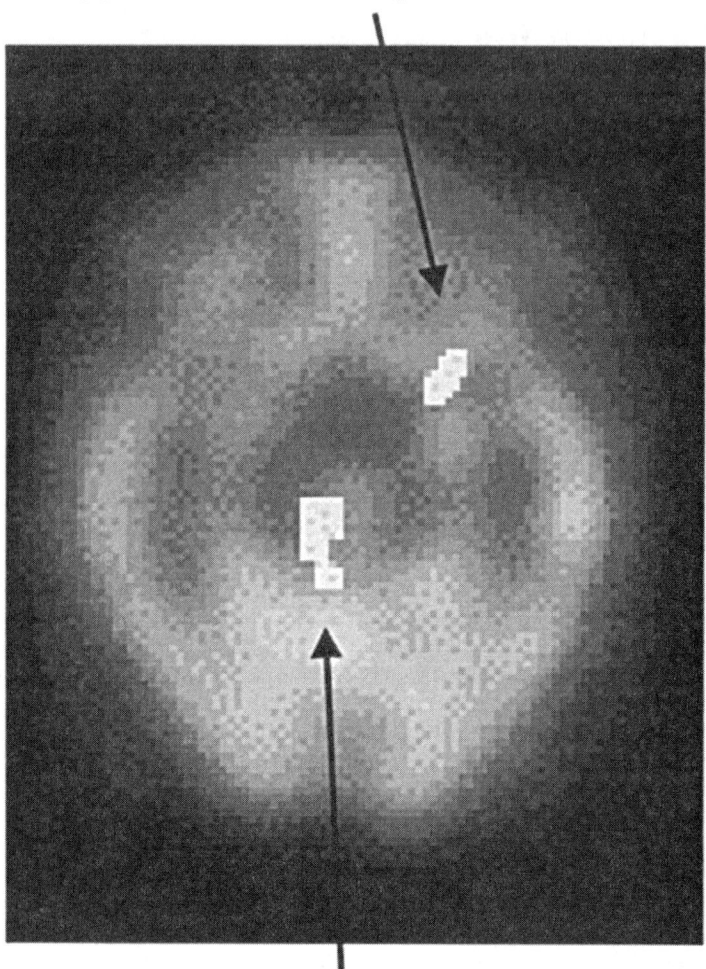

FIGURE 1. rCBF response to procaine in cocaine-addicted patients with a nonaversive response to procaine compared to patients with an aversive response. *White areas* show regions of increased rCBF ($p < 0.01$) in nonaversive patients compared to aversive patients. Left is to the reader's right. Transverse cut is at Talaraich coordinate $z = -10$.

^{99m}TcMH-PAO administration. Baseline measures included blood pressure, pulse, and the SCL 90-Revised. Post-drug measures included a Drug Effect Questionnaire and baseline measures. SPECT was obtained 90 min following drug administration on a PRISM (three-headed) scanner with 6 mm transverse plane resolution. Five 4-

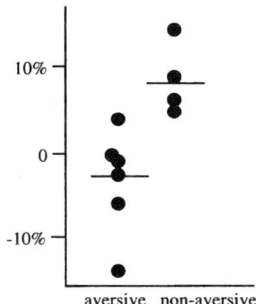

FIGURE 2. Amygdalar response to procaine in cocaine-addicted patients experiencing aversive vs. nonaversive subjective effects. The *y axis* is percent change between procaine and saline infusion in amygdalar fixed ROI (procaine-saline/saline*100).

min scans were summed and data normalized to whole brain counts. Image sets were coregistered within and between subjects, and each scan linearly registered to Talairach space and smoothed to 10 cm. Image analysis was performed by T-Image Analysis.

RESULTS

Drug Effects Questionnaire

The male and female healthy controls reported a significant drug effect, "bad" effect, and "dislike" of the procaine compared to placebo, whereas male patients reported only a significant drug and "bad" effect. Male controls reported significantly more drug effect and "bad" effect from procaine compared to patients. All but two controls (females) reported an "aversive" response (bad effect and dislike to procaine at least 5 (6 was maximum)), whereas four male patients reported a "nonaversive" response to procaine (bad effect or dislike 2 or less).

Changes ($p < 0.01$) in Regional Cerebral Blood Flow (rCBF)

There were significant baseline differences between male cocaine-addicted patients and male controls. Male patients had relative rCBF decreases in the bilateral mid and orbital frontal and right superior temporal areas, whereas male controls showed relative baseline decreases in the left posterior thalamic and brainstem regions.

Following procaine, female controls demonstrated rCBF increases in the bilateral orbital frontal and insular, bilateral amygdalar, hypothalamic, and cerebellar regions. Male controls demonstrated rCBF increases to procaine in the anterior cingulate, bilateral insular, right anterior/mesial temporal and hippocampal, and hypothalamic regions, whereas male patients showed rCBF increases in the right anterior temporal, bilateral orbital/posterior/inferior frontal, and right superior/posterior parietal areas.

The rCBF response to procaine in the nonaversive ($n = 4$) and aversive patients ($n = 6$) was also compared. Nonaversive patients showed significantly greater rCBF responses to procaine in the left inferior and superior frontal, left anterior temporal/amygdalar, and brainstem regions compared to the aversive patients (FIG. 1).

DISCUSSION

Cocaine addicted male patients show significantly lower rCBF in the bilateral mid/orbital frontal and right superior temporal regions compared to controls. This is similar to the reports of others.[3]

Following procaine administration, we observed that abstinent cocaine-addicted male patients show a qualitatively different response to the limbic stimulant procaine compared to healthy male controls. Preliminary data suggest that these differences may be related to differences in the subjective response in a subset of patients. These patients demonstrate a less aversive response and increased rCBF activation in the left anterior temporal/amygdalar brain regions in response to procaine compared to both patients and male controls with an aversive response to procaine. We suggest that the aversive patient group may show limbic hypersensitivity compared to the nonaversive patient group.

ACKNOWLEDGMENTS

This study was funded by NIDA Grant #1R21-DA10218-01 and the Sarah and Charles E. Seay Center for Research in Psychiatric Illness.

REFERENCES

1. POST, R.M. & S.R.B. WEISS. 1988. Psychomotor stimulant vs. local anesthetic effects of cocaine: role of behavioral sensitization and kindling. *In* Mechanisms of Cocaine Abuse and Toxicity. D. Clouet, K. Asghar & R. Brown, Eds.: 217–238. NIDA Research Monograph Series.
2. KETTER, T.A., P.J. ANDREASON, M.S. GEORGE *et al.* 1996. Anterior paralimbic mediation of procaine-induced emotional and psychosensory experiences. Arch. Gen. Psychiatry **53:** 59–69.
3. VOLKOW, N.D., R. HITZEMANN, G.J. WANG *et al.* 1992. Long-term frontal brain metabolic changes in cocaine abusers. Synapse **1:** 184–190.

A Multicomponent Learning Model of Drug Abuse

Drug Taking and Craving May Involve Separate Brain Circuits Underlying Instrumental and Classical Conditioning, Respectively

JOHN L. HARACZ,[a,c] DEBORAH C. MASH,[b] AND RATNA SIRCAR[a]

[a]*Department of Psychiatry, Albert Einstein College of Medicine, Bronx, New York 10461, USA*
[b]*Department of Neurology, University of Miami School of Medicine, Miami, Florida 33136, USA*

INTRODUCTION

Available treatments for cocaine abuse have achieved only modest success in facilitating abstinence.[1-4] Vulnerability to relapse persists even after sustained abstinence.[4] Clinical observations and laboratory experiments with cocaine abusers suggest that exposure to cocaine-associated environmental cues may trigger craving and relapse.[5-7] Thus, a major priority for developing new treatments is the identification of strategies to help the patient deal with continued exposure to drug-related cues.[8] Since classical conditioning enables these cues to elicit craving,[6] clinicians have started trials of cue-exposure treatment aimed at extinguishing cue-elicited craving in cocaine addicts.[5] However, these treatment sessions cannot encompass the wide variety of cues that addicts encounter in natural environments.[9] Furthermore, even after a successful extinction procedure, exposure to stress can reinstate craving in addicts[10] and drug self-administration in animals.[11,12] Therefore, the memory trace that survives behavioral extinction treatment may be more effectively reversed pharmacologically. Such drug treatment could counteract the neural plastic changes underlying classically conditioned cue-elicited craving[6] and instrumentally conditioned drug-taking habits.[13-16] Learning-based theories of drug addiction propose roles for both classical and instrumental conditioning, the latter of which is also called habit learning in this context.[13-18] These learning-based theories are supported by functional brain imaging studies, which show that the exposure of addicts to cocaine-related cues activates brain regions known to be involved in learning and memory.[19-25] Cue exposure also elicits what appears to be conditioned responses, which include craving and physiological signs of arousal.[5-7] The above evidence supports the conclusion that "drug-taking is learned behavior and is controlled by the normal principles of learning" (Ref. 26, p. 1). If learning is etiologically involved in

---

[c]Current address for correspondence: Dr. John L. Haracz, Dept. of Neurology, University of Miami School of Medicine, 1501 NW 9th Ave., Miami, FL 33136. Voice: 305-243-6219; fax: 305-243-3649; jharacz@hotmail.com

addiction, then a key research goal should be the identification of brain circuits and neural plastic changes mediating this learning. By bringing this goal within reach, the presently proposed model and associated studies can establish a research paradigm designed to facilitate the development of drugs that reverse the neural plasticity underlying learned drug taking. Such drug development may achieve a more sustained treatment for addiction than currently available drugs that mainly suppress symptoms of craving or withdrawal.[4,27] Recidivism associated with symptomatic treatments may reflect the failure of these drugs to reverse long-lasting neural plasticity underlying drug-seeking behavior.

METHODS

Animal Behavior Paradigm

Studies of the neural plasticity underlying learned drug taking must control for drug effects unrelated to mechanisms of drug-seeking behavior. This control is achieved by the triadic yoked cocaine self-administration paradigm (FIG. 1), which includes a self-administering (SA) rat group and yoked rats passively receiving cocaine (YC) or saline (YS) injections. This design enables neurobiological studies of learning-related neural plasticity underlying drug taking behavior. Brain changes reflecting this neural plasticity would be specific to SA rats. The YC rats control for diverse drug effects unrelated to the neural plasticity of learned self-administration (e.g., toxic and autonomic effects are controlled for). This group also controls for neurobiological changes reflecting neural plasticity underlying learning that is not specifically related to self-administration. For example, both SA and YC rats are

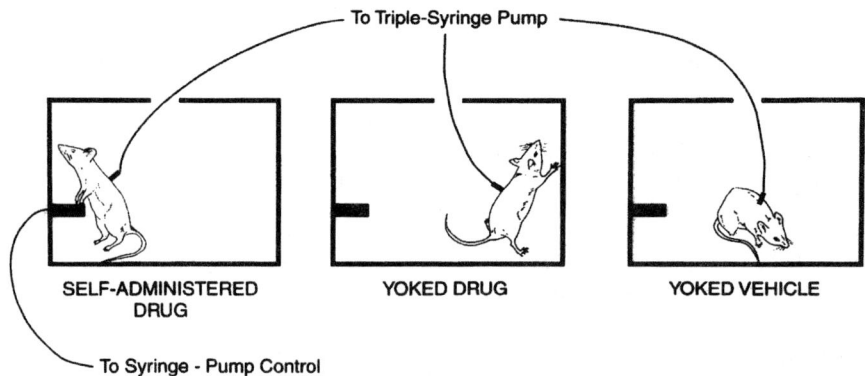

FIGURE 1. Triadic yoked cocaine self-administration paradigm. The self-administration (SA) rat (*left*) is trained to press a lever in an operant box in order to receive i.v. cocaine injections. The yoked-cocaine (YC) rat (*center*) passively receives the same number and pattern of i.v. cocaine injections as the SA rat. The yoked-saline (YS) rat (*right*) passively receives i.v. saline injections that are identical in number and pattern to the cocaine injections of the other two rats. A computer-controlled, three-chambered syringe pump enables the simultaneous delivery of these injections to SA, YC, and YS rats.

classically conditioned to associate cocaine administration with environmental cues. Neural plasticity underlying this classical conditioning probably differs from mechanisms of learned self-administration, which uniquely involves an instrumental response. By using YC rats to control for classical conditioning, this paradigm can focus on neural plasticity specifically relevant to the instrumental response of cocaine self-administration.

It is important to specifically link neurobiological findings to instrumental (i.e., habit) learning, because these brain changes may be a driving force for drug addiction. Recent reports emphasized the importance of identifying mechanisms involved in the switch that converts casual drug abuse into compulsive addiction.[28,29] Robbins[16] proposed that this switch may trigger a transition from classical conditioning, which occurs early upon drug exposure, to habit learning. Evidence of classical conditioning to drug-paired environmental stimuli is found in animals after a single exposure to cocaine.[30–32] On the other hand, habit learning develops after extended training,[33,34] which, in the case of drug self-administration in animals, involves repeated exposures to operant procedures that link drug delivery to instrumental responses. The multiple stages of drug experience leading to addiction prompted a call for stage-specific animal models.[13] The triadic yoked drug self-administration paradigm may be a useful model of classical and instrumental conditioning potentially involved in specific steps to addiction.

Neurobiological Research

Forms of neural plasticity are being revealed in basic research on animal learning and learning models such as long-term potentiation (LTP). TABLE 1 shows a partial list of neurobiological factors involved in this neural plasticity. The involvement of these or other factors in learned drug taking can be tested for in the triadic yoked self-administration paradigm. This research can provide a neurobiological target for the development of drugs that can reverse the neural plasticity underlying learned drug taking. Elucidation of this neural plasticity in animals will provide comparative data to guide future tests for similar neural plastic changes in postmortem brains from drug addicts. Such changes may reflect learning-related neural plasticity underlying drug addiction. If the changes in animals are confirmed in human postmortem studies, these neural adaptations would be candidate targets for drug development aimed at erasing memory traces that compel addicts toward drugs. In conclusion, this research program enables a new, etiology-based approach to developing pharmacotherapeutics. Such an approach may be significantly more successful than the current symptom-based approach to drug treatment (see Introduction). The very limited effectiveness of current pharmacotherapeutics led to the conclusion that a new paradigm is needed to develop treatments for cocaine addiction.[4] The present research program offers an initial step toward establishing a novel, etiology-based paradigm for anti-cocaine medication development.

MODEL

The Methods section noted that the triadic yoked cocaine self-administration paradigm can model classical and instrumental conditioning potentially involved in

TABLE 1. Neurobiological factors involved in neural plasticity of animal learning or learning models

Gene or Gene Product	Learning or Learning Model
Dopamine receptors	Learning (multiple types), LTP
NMDA receptors	Learning (multiple types), LTP
mGluR1	Learning (multiple types), LTP
I-Adenylate cyclase	Spatial learning, LTP
CREB	Learning (multiple types), LTP
Protein kinase A	Amphetamine CPP, LTP
Protein kinase C	Learning (multiple types), LTP
CaMKII	Spatial learning, LTP
fyn-tyrosine kinase	Spatial learning, LTP
β2 nACh receptor subunit	Passive avoidance learning
NCAM	Spatial learning
BDNF	LTP
NT-3	Long-term synaptic enhancement

Abbreviations and references: Dopamine receptors;[52,57,59] LTP, long-term potentiation; NMDA, *N*-methyl-D-aspartate;[60] mGluR, metabotropic glutamate receptor;[61] I-adenylate cyclase;[62] CREB, cAMP-responsive element-binding protein;[63] protein kinase A;[51,52,64] protein kinase C;[65,66] CaMK, calcium-calmodulin-dependent kinase;[67,68] fyn-tyrosine kinase;[69] nACh, nicotinic acetylcholine;[70] NCAM, neural-cell adhesion molecule;[71] BDNF, brain-derived neurotrophic factor;[72,73] NT, neurotrophin.[74]

drug addiction. In this paradigm, classical conditioning occurs in both SA and YC rats, whereas only SA rats learn the instrumental response of drug self-administration. While further delineating the multiple forms of learning in this paradigm, the present section presents a biobehavioral model in which the neural plasticity of specific brain circuits is linked to craving and drug taking.

Craving Arising from Amygdala-based Classical Conditioning

The multicomponent learning model (MLM) proposes that different brain circuits mediate multiple forms of learning underlying drug abuse.[14] In the triadic yoked cocaine self-administration paradigm, which models this learning, three forms of classical conditioning may be expected in both SA and YC rats, whereas only SA rats undergo habit learning and a fourth type of classical conditioning. The three common forms of classical conditioning are conditioned autonomic arousal, behavioral activation, and orientation to stimuli. These forms of conditioning are likely to involve different brain circuits. In rats and rabbits, conditioned autonomic responses to fear-provoking stimuli involve projections from the central nucleus of the amygdala to the lateral hypothalamus and cardioregulatory nuclei of the dorsal medulla.[35–37] Since the central nucleus is also involved in conditioning to attractive, appetitive stimuli,[38–40] these projections may mediate conditioned autonomic responses to cocaine-associated stimuli.[5,6] In contrast, lesions of the entire amygdaloid complex[41] or just the basolateral nucleus[42] did not affect locomotor activation conditioned to environments paired with stimulant drugs. This conditioned activation depends on dopaminergic and cholecystokinin$_A$-receptor function in nucleus accumbens.[43,44] Conditioned orienting responses to food-paired stimuli are impaired by lesioning a circuit from the central nucleus to dorsolateral striatum, via dopaminergic projections from substantia nigra.[38–40] This orienting response might also be conditioned to cocaine-linked stimuli in the self-administration paradigm. In addition to habit learning, SA rats are likely to undergo conditioned incentive learning, in which cocaine-induced behavioral and internal affective effects are classically conditioned to stimuli in an operant box.[13,15] Conditioned incentive learning promotes approach responses toward a drug-delivery apparatus, such as an operant lever, and may thereby facilitate the development of drug taking habit learning.[13,16] Therefore, any neurobiological changes specific to SA rats are potentially relevant to habit learning, either as a primary mechanism of such learning or as a mechanism of classical conditioning that supports habit learning. Conditioned incentive (or "stimulus-reward") learning, which is also elicited in the conditioned place preference paradigm, involves the basolateral and lateral nuclei of the amygdala, ventral tegmental area (VTA), nucleus accumbens, ventral pallidum, mediodorsal thalamic nucleus, and prefrontal cortex.[45–50]

The above results implicate the amygdala in 3 of the 4 forms of classical conditioning expected to occur in the drug self-administration paradigm. In human cocaine abusers, cue-elicited craving, which apparently is classically conditioned,[6] correlates with metabolic activation of the amygdala.[21] Thus, the drug self-administration paradigm may model amygdala-based classical conditioning relevant to drug craving.

Drug Taking Driven by Striatum-based Instrumental Conditioning (Habit Learning)

Corticostriatal projections are involved in habit learning.[33,34] Striatum-based habit learning was proposed to be involved in drug addiction.[13,15] Corticostriatal projections to nucleus accumbens may be involved in conditioned incentive learning,[51,52] which, as discussed above, supports habit learning.[13,16]

Potential Links between Classical and Instrumental Conditioning

Clinical studies indicate that, although craving may occasionally predispose to relapse, craving and drug use are not necessarily correlated.[53,54] Thus, the MLM proposes that craving, which may be classically conditioned,[6] can be a nonobligatory facilitator of drug taking, which involves instrumental conditioning.[13,15] As reviewed below, neuroanatomical studies of classical conditioning suggest pathways by which amygdala-based craving may facilitate drug taking driven by a striatum-based habit learning system. This facilitation may exemplify a common, general relationship between classical and instrumental conditioning. In both laboratory and natural conditions, learning commonly involves an initial phase of classical conditioning that facilitates a subsequent phase of instrumental conditioning.[55] This structure of learned behavior may be a necessary consequence of brain structure. The amygdala, particularly the basolateral nucleus, projects to medial areas of striatum, including the nucleus accumbens.[56] This projection is involved in conditioned incentive learning,[45,49] which, as noted above, is one of the types of classical conditioning that may model craving. The striatonigral projection from nucleus accumbens includes a significant input to medial substantia nigra, which, in turn, sends dopaminergic innervation to much of neostriatum.[56] Striatal dopamine may potentiate corticostriatal inputs involved in learning.[52,57,58] This circuitry could enable classically conditioned amygdala-based craving to facilitate striatum-based habit learning underlying drug taking. Studies of conditioned orientation suggest that this facilitation may also involve another circuit from amygdala to striatum. As noted above, conditioned orientation involves a circuit from the central amygdaloid nucleus to dorsolateral striatum, via dopaminergic projections from substantia nigra.[38–40]

CONCLUSIONS

Craving, which apparently is classically conditioned, can be a nonobligatory facilitator of drug taking, which may involve instrumental conditioning (i.e., habit learning). The triadic yoked drug self-administration paradigm may model amygdala-based classical conditioning relevant to drug craving. This paradigm may also model striatum-based instrumental conditioning relevant to drug taking habits. In this self-administration paradigm, neurobiological changes specific to self-administering (SA) rats may model the neural plasticity of habit learning involved in addiction. If these neurobiological changes in animals are confirmed in postmortem studies of human addicts, these neural adaptations would be candidate targets for drug development aimed at erasing memory traces that compel addicts toward drugs. This research program may lead to a new, etiology-based approach to developing antiaddiction pharmacotherapeutics.

REFERENCES

1. GAWIN, F.H. 1991. Cocaine addiction: psychology and neurophysiology. Science **251:** 1580–1586.
2. KOSTEN, T.R. 1993. Clinical and research perspectives on cocaine abuse: the pharmacotherapy of cocaine abuse. NIDA Res. Monogr. **135:** 48–56.
3. WITHERS, N.W. et al. 1995. Cocaine abuse and dependence. J. Clin. Psychopharmacol. **15:** 63–78.
4. NUNES, E. 1996. Search for anti-cocaine medications. Presented at the Symposium on Pharmacotherapy for the Addictions: Research and Clinical Issues. New York, NY, June 3, 1996.
5. O'BRIEN, C.P. et al. 1990. Integrating systematic cue exposure with standard treatment in recovering drug dependent patients. Addict. Behav. **15:** 355–365.
6. EHRMAN, R.N. et al. 1992. Conditioned responses to cocaine-related stimuli in cocaine abuse patients. Psychopharmacology **107:** 523–529.
7. BAUER, L.O. & H.R. KRANZLER. 1994. Electroencephalographic activity and mood in cocaine-dependent outpatients: effects of cocaine cue exposure. Biol. Psychiatry **36:** 189–197.
8. LESHNER, A.I. 1996. Drug abuse and addiction research: implications for the field of psychiatry. Mol. Psychiatry **1:** 168–169.
9. MARLATT, G.A. 1990. Cue exposure and relapse prevention in the treatment of addictive behaviors. Addict. Behav. **15:** 395–399.
10. MCLELLAN, A.T. et al. 1986. Extinguishing conditioned responses during treatment for opiate dependence: turning laboratory findings into clinical procedures. J. Subst. Abuse Treat. **3:** 33–40.

11. SHAHAM, Y. & J. STEWART. 1995. Stress reinstates heroin-seeking in drug-free animals: an effect mimicking heroin, not withdrawal. Psychopharmacology **119:** 334–341.
12. SHAHAM, Y. & J. STEWART. 1996. Effects of opioid and dopamine receptor antagonists on relapse induced by stress and re-exposure to heroin in rats. Psychopharmacology **125:** 385–391.
13. ALTMAN, J. et al. 1996. The biological, social and clinical bases of drug addiction: commentary and debate. Psychopharmacology **125:** 285–345.
14. HARACZ, J.L. & R. SIRCAR. 1996. A multi-component learning model of drug abuse: drug-taking, craving, and physiological changes may involve different brain circuits [abstract]. Soc. Neurosci. Abstr. **22:** 1930.
15. WHITE, N.M. 1996. Addictive drugs as reinforcers: multiple partial actions on memory systems. Addiction **91:** 921–949.
16. ROBBINS, T.W. 1997. Interaction of the dopaminergic system with mechanisms of associative learning and cognition: implications for drug abuse. Presented at the NIDA/APS Satellite Symposium, Cognitive Science Research: More Than Thinking About Drug Abuse. Washington, DC, May 23, 1997.
17. NEWLIN, D.B. 1992. A comparison of drug conditioning and craving for alcohol and cocaine. Recent Dev. Alcoholism **10:** 147–164.
18. O'BRIEN, C.P. et al. 1992. A learning model of addiction. In Addictive States. C.P. O'Brien & J.H. Jaffe, Eds.: 157–177. Raven Press. New York.
19. CHILDRESS, A.R. et al. 1996. Brain correlates of cue-induced cocaine and opiate craving [abstract]. Soc. Neurosci. Abstr. **22:** 933.
20. CHILDRESS, A.R. et al. 1998. Brain imaging during cue-induced opiate and cocaine craving [abstract]. NIDA Res. Monogr. **178:** 106.
21. GRANT, S. et al. 1996. Activation of memory circuits during cue-elicited cocaine craving. Proc. Natl. Acad. Sci. USA **93:** 12040–12045.
22. LONDON, E.D. 1996. Activation of memory circuits during cocaine craving: PET studies. Presented at the NIDA-sponsored symposium, Cognitive Neuroscience: What Can Cognitive Neuroscience Tell Us About Drug Abuse Disorders? Washington, DC, November 16, 1996.
23. SCHWEITZER, J. et al. 1996. The neuroanatomy of drug craving in crack cocaine addiction: a PET analysis [abstract]. Soc. Neurosci. Abstr. **22:** 933.
24. BONSON, K.R. et al. 1997. Regional cerebral glucose metabolism during induced craving for cocaine: a PET FDG study [abstract]. Soc. Neurosci. Abstr. **23:** 804.
25. MAAS, L.C. et al. 1997. Functional MRI studies of cue-induced cocaine craving [abstract]. Biol. Psychiatry **41:** 70S.
26. BIGELOW, G.E. 1995. President's comments: behavioral science is fundamental to drug abuse research and treatment. NIDA Res. Monogr. **152:** 1–5.
27. STIMMEL, B. 1996. Pharmacotherapies for opioid dependence. Presented at the Symposium on Pharmacotherapy for the Addictions: Research and Clinical Issues. New York, NY, June 3, 1996.
28. LESHNER, A.I. 1997. The need for cognitive science in understanding drug abuse and addiction. Presented at the NIDA/APS Satellite Symposium, Cognitive Science Research: More Than Thinking About Drug Abuse. Washington, DC, May 23, 1997.
29. AHMED, S.H. & G.F. KOOB. 1998. Transition from moderate to excessive drug intake: change in hedonic set point. Science **282:** 298–300.
30. WEISS, S.R.B. et al. 1989. Context-dependent cocaine sensitization: differential effect of haloperidol on development versus expression. Pharmacol. Biochem. Behav. **34:** 655–661.
31. PERT, A. et al. 1990. Conditioning as a critical determinant of sensitization induced by psychomotor stimulants. NIDA Res. Monogr. **97:** 208–241.
32. KALIVAS, P.W. & J.E. ALESDATTER. 1993. Involvement of N-methyl-D-aspartate receptor stimulation in the ventral tegmental area and amygdala in behavioral sensitization to cocaine. J. Pharmacol. Exp. Ther. **267:** 486–495.
33. MISHKIN, M. et al. 1984. Memories and habits: two neural systems. In Neurobiology of Learning and Memory. G. Lynch et al., Eds.: 65–77. Guilford Press. New York.

34. SALMON, D.P. & N. BUTTERS. 1995. Neurobiology of skill and habit learning. Curr. Opin. Neurobiol. **5:** 184–190.
35. LEDOUX, J.E. et al. 1988. Different projections of the central amygdaloid nucleus mediate autonomic and behavioral correlates of conditioned fear. J. Neurosci. **8:** 2517–2529.
36. DAVIS, M. 1992. The role of the amygdala in conditioned fear. In The Amygdala: Neurobiological Aspects of Emotion, Memory, and Mental Dysfunction. J.P. Aggleton, Ed.: 255–306. Wiley-Liss. New York.
37. KAPP, B.S. et al. 1992. Amygdaloid contributions to conditioned arousal and sensory information processing. In The Amygdala: Neurobiological Aspects of Emotion, Memory, and Mental Dysfunction. J.P. Aggleton, Ed.: 229–254. Wiley-Liss. New York.
38. GALLAGHER, M. & P. HOLLAND. 1992. Understanding the function of the central nucleus: is simple conditioning enough? In The Amygdala: Neurobiological Aspects of Emotion, Memory, and Mental Dysfunction. J.P. Aggleton, Ed.: 307–321. Wiley-Liss. New York.
39. GALLAGHER, M. & P. HOLLAND. 1994. The amygdala complex: multiple roles in associative learning and attention. Proc. Natl. Acad. Sci. USA **91:** 11771–11776.
40. IIAN, J.S. et al. 1997. The role of an amygdalo-nigrostriatal pathway in associative learning. J. Neurosci. **17:** 3913–3919.
41. BROWN, E.E. & H.C. FIBIGER. 1993. Differential effects of excitotoxic lesions of the amygdala on cocaine-induced conditioned locomotion and conditioned place preference. Psychopharmacology **113:** 123–130.
42. AHMED, S.H. et al. 1995. Amphetamine-induced conditioned activity in rats: comparison with novelty-induced activity and role of the basolateral amygdala. Behav. Neurosci. **109:** 723–733.
43. GOLD, L.H. et al. 1988. The role of mesolimbic dopamine in conditioned locomotion produced by amphetamine. Behav. Neurosci. **102:** 544–552.
44. JOSSELYN, S.A. et al. 1997. Evidence for CCK_A receptor involvement in the acquisition of conditioned activity produced by cocaine in rats. Brain Res. **763:** 93–102.
45. ROBBINS, T.W. et al. 1989. Limbic-striatal interactions in reward-related processes. Neurosci. Biobehav. Rev. **13:** 155–162.
46. GAFFAN, D. & E.A. MURRAY. 1990. Amygdalar interaction with the mediodorsal nucleus of the thalamus and the ventromedial prefrontal cortex in stimulus-reward associative learning in the monkey. J. Neurosci. **10:** 3479–3493.
47. HIROI, N. & N.M. WHITE. 1990. The reserpine-sensitive dopamine pool mediates (+)-amphetamine conditioned reward in the place preference paradigm. Brain Res. **510:** 33–42.
48. HIROI, N. & N.M. WHITE. 1991. The lateral nucleus of the amygdala mediates expression of the amphetamine-produced conditioned place preference. J. Neurosci. **11:** 2107–2116.
49. EVERITT, B.J. & T.W. ROBBINS. 1992. Amygdala-ventral striatal interactions and reward-related processes. In The Amygdala: Neurobiological Aspects of Emotion, Memory, and Mental Dysfunction. J.P. Aggleton, Ed.: 401–429. Wiley-Liss. New York.
50. GONG, W. et al. 1997. 6-Hydroxydopamine lesion of ventral pallidum blocks acquisition of place preference conditioning to cocaine. Brain Res. **754:** 103–112.
51. BENINGER, R.J. et al. 1996. Inhibition of protein kinase A in the nucleus accumbens blocks amphetamine-produced conditioned place preference in rats [abstract]. Soc. Neurosci. Abstr. **22:** 1127.
52. BENINGER, R.J. & R. MILLER. 1998. Dopamine D_1-like receptors and reward-related incentive learning. Neurosci. Biobehav. Rev. **22:** 335–345.
53. FISCHMAN, M.W. et al. 1990. Effects of desipramine on cocaine self-administration by humans. J. Pharmacol. Exp. Ther. **253:** 760–770.
54. MILLER, N.S. & M.S. GOLD. 1994. Dissociation of "conscious desire" (craving) from and relapse in alcohol and cocaine dependence. Ann. Clin. Psychiatry **6:** 99–106.
55. MACKINTOSH, N.J. 1983. Conditioning and Associative Learning. Oxford University Press. New York.

56. NAUTA, W.J. & V.B. DOMESICK. 1984. Afferent and efferent relationships of the basal ganglia. Ciba Found. Symp. **107:** 3–29.
57. WICKENS, J.R. 1990. Striatal dopamine in motor activation and reward-mediated learning: steps towards a unifying model. J. Neural Transm. **80:** 9–31.
58. HARACZ, J.L. et al. 1998. Amphetamine effects on striatal neurons: implications for models of dopamine function. Neurosci. Biobehav. Rev. **22:** 613–622.
59. FREY, U. et al. 1990. Dopaminergic antagonists prevent long-term maintenance of posttetanic LTP in the CA1 region of rat hippocampal slices. Brain Res. **522:** 69–75.
60. SAKIMURA, K. et al. 1995. Reduced hippocampal LTP and spatial learning in mice lacking NMDA receptor ε1 subunit. Nature **373:** 151–155.
61. RIEDEL, G. 1996. Function of metabotropic glutamate receptors in learning and memory. Trends Neurosci. **19:** 219–224.
62. WU, Z.-L. et al. 1995. Altered behavior and long-term potentiation in type I adenylyl cyclase mutant mice. Proc. Natl. Acad. Sci. USA **92:** 220–224.
63. BOURTCHULADZE, R. et al. 1994. Deficient long-term memory in mice with a targeted mutation of the cAMP-responsive element-binding protein. Cell **79:** 59–68.
64. ABEL, T. et al. 1997. Genetic demonstration of a role for PKA in the late phase of LTP and in hippocampus-based long-term memory. Cell **88:** 615–626.
65. ABELIOVICH, A. et al. 1993. Modified hippocampal long-term potentiation in PKCγ-mutant mice. Cell **75:** 1253–1262.
66. ABELIOVICH, A. et al. 1993. PKCγ mutant mice exhibit mild deficits in spatial and contextual learning. Cell **75:** 1263–1271.
67. SILVA, A.J. et al. 1992. Impaired spatial learning in α-calcium-calmodulin kinase II mutant mice. Science **257:** 206–211.
68. SILVA, A.J. et al. 1992. Deficient hippocampal long-term potentiation in α-calcium-calmodulin kinase II mutant mice. Science **257:** 201–206.
69. GRANT, S.G.N. et al. 1992. Impaired long-term potentiation, spatial learning, and hippocampal development in *fyn* mutant mice. Science **258:** 1903–1910.
70. PICCIOTTO, M.R. et al. 1995. Abnormal avoidance learning in mice lacking functional high-affinity nicotine receptor in the brain. Nature **374:** 65–67.
71. CREMER, H. et al. 1994. Inactivation of the N-CAM gene in mice results in size reduction of the olfactory bulb and deficits in spatial learning. Nature **367:** 455–459.
72. KORTE, M. et al. 1995. Hippocampal long-term potentiation is impaired in mice lacking brain-derived neurotrophic factor. Proc. Natl. Acad. Sci. USA **92:** 8856–8860.
73. PATTERSON, S.L. et al. 1996. Recombinant BDNF rescues deficits in basal synaptic transmission and hippocampal LTP in BDNF knockout mice. Neuron **16:** 1137–1145.
74. KANG, H. & E.M. SCHUMAN. 1996. A requirement for local protein synthesis in neurotrophin-induced hippocampal synaptic plasticity. Science **273:** 1402–1406.

Mesoaccumbens Dopamine and the Self-administration of Amphetamine

DANIEL S. LORRAIN, GRETCHEN M. ARNOLD, AND PAUL VEZINA[a]

Department of Psychiatry, The University of Chicago, Chicago, Illinois 60637, USA

Prior exposure to amphetamine leads to enhanced locomotor and nucleus accumbens (NAcc) dopamine (DA) responding to subsequent injections of the drug. Similarly, and more importantly, such preexposure also leads to long lasting enhancements in animals' incentive to self-administer the drug (for references, see ref. 2). Indeed, manipulations known to block induction of enhanced locomotor and NAcc DA responding to amphetamine (such as blocking D_1 DA receptors prior to each preexposure injection of amphetamine) also block the development of the facilitated responding for amphetamine in a drug self-administration paradigm.[4] This facilitation of amphetamine self-administration may thus represent an instance of amphetamine sensitization that is induced and expressed via potentially the same neuronal mechanisms leading to and underlying enhanced locomotor and DA responding to the drug.

Evidence that prior exposure to psychomotor stimulants enhances the subsequent self-administration of these drugs has been largely limited to that obtained in studies assessing rats' predisposition to self-administer relatively low doses of the drugs. The present study tested whether prior exposure to amphetamine would enhance rats' predisposition to self-administer a high dose of the drug under fixed (FR) and progressive (PR) ratios of reinforcement.[5]

Male Sprague-Dawley rats received either amphetamine (1.5 mg/kg) or saline once every three days for a total of five injections and were then fitted with intravenous catheters. Ten days following the final drug preexposure injection, rats were placed in the drug self-administration chambers and given the opportunity to self-administer amphetamine (200 mg/kg/infusion, iv). Animals were trained under an FR schedule and then tested under a PR schedule of drug reinforcement. During the training phase rats were allowed to self-administer 10 infusions of amphetamine. Once rats attained criterion (10 infusions within a 4-h session) under both FR1 and FR2 schedules, they were placed under a PR schedule for the remainder of the experiment. Break points, defined as the final ratio completed before a one-hour period expired without a drug infusion, were recorded per PR session.

Consistent with previous reports,[1,3,6] amphetamine- and saline-preexposed animals did not differ in their acquisition of the lever-press response for the high dose of drug (data not shown). Prior exposure to amphetamine did, however, promote subsequent self-administration of the drug when animals were tested under the PR schedule of reinforcement. Amphetamine-preexposed animals maintained higher

---

[a]Address for correspondence: Paul Vezina, Department of Psychiatry, The University of Chicago, 5841 S. Maryland Ave. MC3077, Chicago, IL 60637. Voice: 773-702-2890; fax: 773-702-0857; pvezina@yoda.bsd.uchicago.edu

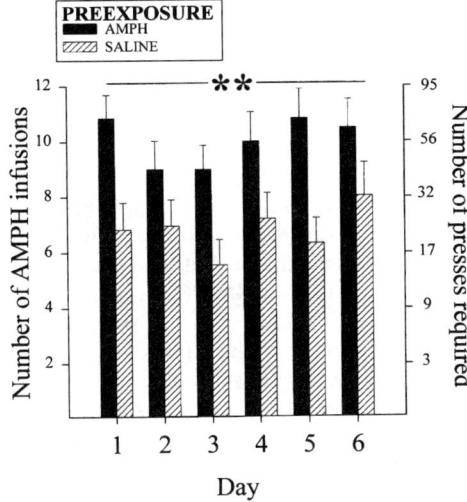

FIGURE 1. Preexposure to amphetamine (AMPH) enhanced the subsequent self-administration of the drug under a PR schedule of reinforcement in which the number of lever presses required increased following each drug infusion. Data are represented as the mean (±SEM) break point per self-administration session. Break point was defined as the final ratio completed before a one-hour period expired without a drug infusion. **$p < 0.01$ for overall ANOVA group effect; $n = 20$–23/group.

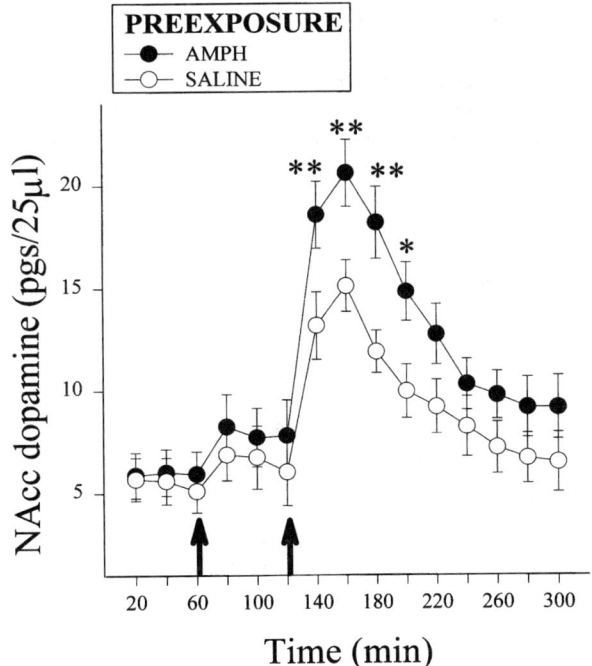

FIGURE 2. Prior exposure to amphetamine led to an enhanced NAcc DA response to the drug in comparison to that observed in saline preexposed animals. Rats remained in dialysis test chambers overnight, and the following day (after collection of baseline samples in this neutral environment) they were placed in a self-administration chamber (first arrow). After collection of additional baseline samples, they were given an ip priming injection of

break points compared to saline-preexposed animals across the six days of PR testing [$F(1,41) = 8.095, p <0.01$, FIG. 1].

Clearly, previous exposure to amphetamine leads to a persistent enhancement of behaviors directed at acquiring the drug. We next tested, using *in vivo* microdialysis, whether animals previously exposed to amphetamine and displaying enhanced self-administration behavior (as those reported here) would also display enhanced NAcc DA overflow when challenged with the drug.

Animals were preexposed to amphetamine, fitted with a jugular catheter and allowed to self-administer amphetamine in the same manner as outlined above. In addition, all animals were implanted with a guide cannula aimed at the NAcc. On the evening following the completion of either the 3rd or the 4th PR test session, rats were fitted with a microdialysis probe via the guide cannula. The following day they received an ip (priming) injection of amphetamine (1.0 mg/kg). Their NAcc DA response and lever pressing (without drug consequence) were subsequently measured.

In a manner paralleling the group differences in lever pressing described above, prior exposure to amphetamine led to an enhanced NAcc DA response to the drug in comparison to that observed in saline preexposed animals ($F(1,16) = 6.4, p <0.05$, FIG. 2). Because these latter results were obtained after animals received a systemic priming injection of amphetamine and exhibited lever pressing with no drug consequence, they clearly are not due to the presence of higher brain levels of self-administered drug.

The present findings establish that prior exposure to a sensitizing regimen of amphetamine injections leads to augmented self-administration of a high dose of the drug. Furthermore, this enhanced self-administration of amphetamine appears to be accompanied by enhanced mesoaccumbens DA neuron reactivity. Together these data suggest that changes in mesoaccumbens DA neurons produced by prior exposure to amphetamine and expressed as exaggerated responding to pharmacological and environmental challenges may contribute importantly to the persistent and excessive pursuit of the drug.

ACKNOWLEDGMENTS

This work was supported by Grant # DA-09397 to P.V. from the USPHS. D.S.L. was supported by USPHS Grant # T32-DA-07255.

REFERENCES

1. MENDREK, A., C.D. BLAHA & A.G PHILLIPS. 1998. Psychopharmacology **35:** 416–422.
2. PIERRE, P.J. & P. VEZINA. 1997. Psychopharmacology **129:** 277–284.
3. PIERRE, P.J. & P. VEZINA. 1997. NIDA Res. Monogr. **178:** 122.
4. PIERRE, P.J. & P. VEZINA. 1998. Psychopharmacology **138:** 159–166.
5. ROBERTS, D.C.S. & N.R. RICHARDSON. 1992. Neuromethods **24:** 233–269.
6. SCHENK, S. *et al.* 1993. Psychopharmacology **111:** 332–338.

---

amphetamine (1.0 mg/kg, second arrow). Data are represented as mean (±SEM) levels of DA in 25 µL of dialysate. *$p < 0.05$, **$p < 0.01$ vs saline animals revealed by post-hoc Sheffé comparisons following ANOVA; $n = 9$/group.

Amphetamine Microinfusion in the Dorso-Ventral Axis of the Prefrontal Cortex Differentially Modulates Dopamine Neurotransmission in the Shell-Core Subterritories of the Nucleus Accumbens

GAËL HEDOU, JUDITH HOMBERG, JORAM FELDON, AND CHRISTIAN A. HEIDBREDER[a]

Laboratory of Behavioral Biology, The Swiss Federal Institute of Technology Zürich (ETH), CH-8603 Schwerzenbach, Switzerland

The two main subdivisions of the nucleus accumbens (NAC), the dorsolateral core and the ventromedial shell, can be distinguished by a distinct connectivity pattern originating mainly from the prefrontal cortex (PFC).[1,2] More specifically, the core of the NAC receives major projections from the anterior cingulate and dorsocaudal prelimbic cortices, which are referred to as the dorsal PFC.[3,4] In contrast to the core, the shell of the NAC receives main afferents from the ventral prelimbic and rostral infralimbic cortices, which are termed the ventral PFC.[3,4] The present study sought to evaluate the contributions of the ventral prelimbic/infralimbic cortices and shell subterritory of the NAC as well as the dorsal prelimbic/anterior cingulate cortices and core subregion of the NAC to the microinfusion of amphetamine (AMPHE) on dialysate DA levels using a dual-probe microdialysis design. Male Wistar rats were anesthetized with sodium pentobarbital (60 mg/kg, i.p.) and mounted on a stereotaxic apparatus. The skull was exposed and two holes were drilled for unilateral placement of microdialysis probes into (1) the core of the NAC and the dorsal PFC, and (2) the shell of the NAC and the ventral PFC. One-hourly dose of chloral hydrate (100 mg/kg, i.p.) was administered to maintain a constant level of anesthesia throughout the experiment. Following the determination of basal DA levels, 5 increasing concentrations of AMPHE (1, 10, 100, 500, 1000 µM) were substituted for the dialysis perfusate in the PFC for 60 min each. Both microdialysis procedures and chromatographic analyses of brain microdialysates were the same as described previously.[5]

Basal DA levels were significantly higher in the ventral PFC compared with the dorsal PFC and higher concentrations of DA were also observed in the core of the NAC compared with its shell counterpart (FIG. 1A). Reverse microdialysis of AMPHE in the ventral PFC produced a significant dose-dependent decrease in dialysate DA levels. In contrast, no significant alterations in DA levels were observed following AMPHE microinfusion in the dorsal PFC (FIG. 2A). Furthermore, the

---

[a]Address for correspondence: Dr. Christian A. Heidbreder, Laboratory of Behavioral Biology, The Swiss Federal Institute of Technology Zürich (ETH), Schorenstrasse, 16, CH-8603 Schwerzenbach, Switzerland. Voice: +41-1-825-7371; fax: +41-1-825-7417; heidbreder@toxi.biol.ethz.ch

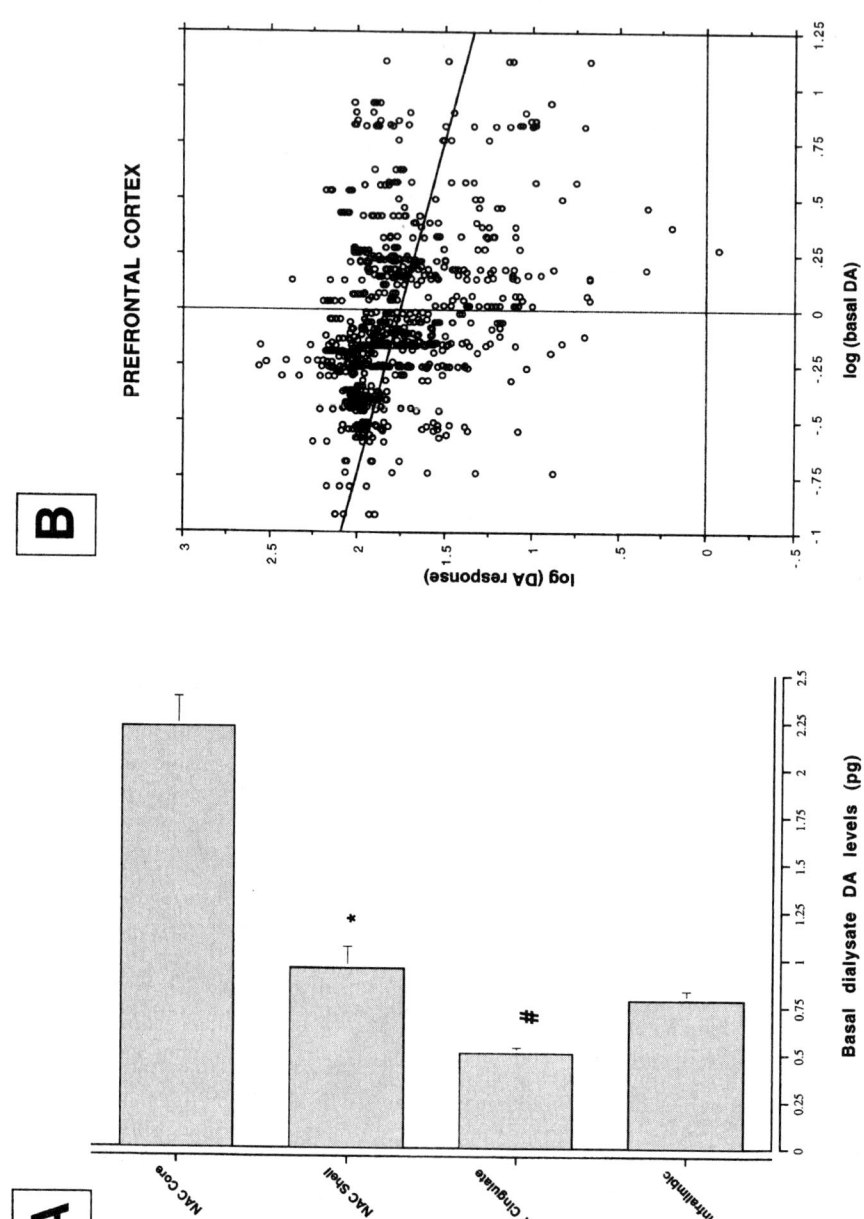

higher the basal DA concentrations, the lower the DA response to AMPHE in the PFC (FIG. 1B). Amphetamine-induced alterations of DA dynamics in subregions of the PFC also profoundly influenced DA function in subterritories of the NAC. Thus, dialysate DA levels were significantly reduced in both the shell and core subregions of the NAC. The magnitude of the effect was greater in the shell of the NAC compared with the core (FIG. 2B).

The observation that corticostriatal neurons from different laminae of the PFC terminate in different subregions of the striatum suggests that this pattern of innervation may provide a functional segregation for cortical control of striatal functions.[6] If this speculation has credence, it also suggests that neurons originating from deep layers of the prelimbic cortex control a very different aspect of striatal function compared with corticostriatal neurons from the superficial layers of the anterior cingulate cortex. This hypothesis is supported by the results of the present study showing a differentiation between the infralimbic and anterior cingulate cortices both in basal DA levels and DA response to AMPHE. Furthermore, our results revealed that the higher the basal DA concentrations, the lower the DA response to AMPHE in the PFC. The inverse relationship between basal and stimulated DA levels suggests that the responsiveness of DA terminals in the PFC to pharmacological challenge by AMPHE is proportionally reduced if the system is operating at a higher basal tone. These observations are consistent with the recent discovery that the DA transporter (DAT) is densely distributed in the dorsal anterior cingulate cortex and distributed only sparsely to the deep layers of the prelimbic cortex.[7] These findings together with the results of the present study demonstrate that both the ventral prelimbic and infralimbic cortices have a lower content of DAT and, hence, a reduced uptake capacity and a higher concentration gradient of extracellular DA. In contrast, the distribution of DAT-labeled axons is higher in the dorsal anterior cingulate cortex, which has an increased uptake capacity and a lower concentration gradient of extracellular DA. The question of whether DA release in subterritories of the PFC is *causally* related to DA activity in subregions of the NAC remains to be investigated. Despite the different subregions that characterize the medial PFC (medial precentral, medial orbital, anterior cingulate, prelimbic, and infralimbic cortices), most studies have considered the medial PFC as a whole entity. The results of the present study point to the importance of conducting a functional analysis of prefrontal subregions to understand further the role of the PFC in the regulation of subterritories of the ventral striatum.

FIGURE 1. (**A**) Basal dialysate DA levels in microdialysates from either the infralimbic cortex, the anterior cingulate cortex, the shell of the nucleus accumbens (NAC) or the core of the NAC. The *bars* represent the mean (±SEM) level of DA (pg) in each subterritory (Infralimbic, $n = 22$; Anterior Cingulate, $n = 19$; NAC Shell, $n = 19$; NAC Core, $n = 17$). Basal dialysate DA levels were significantly different between subregions of both the prefrontal cortex (PFC) (Fischer's LSD test, $^\#p < 0.01$) and NAC (Fischer's LSD test, $^*p < 0.0005$). (**B**) Double logarithmic plot of the dependence of the DA response to amphetamine (AMPHE) microinfusion (1, 10, 100, 500, and 1000 μM) into the PFC on basal DA concentrations in the PFC. The figure illustrates that the magnitude of the extracellular DA response becomes progressively smaller as basal DA levels increase. Regression analyses confirmed a significant relationship between DA response to AMPHE and basal DA levels in the PFC irrespective of AMPHE doses or PFC subterritories ($F(1,839) = 133.1$, $p < 0.0001$).

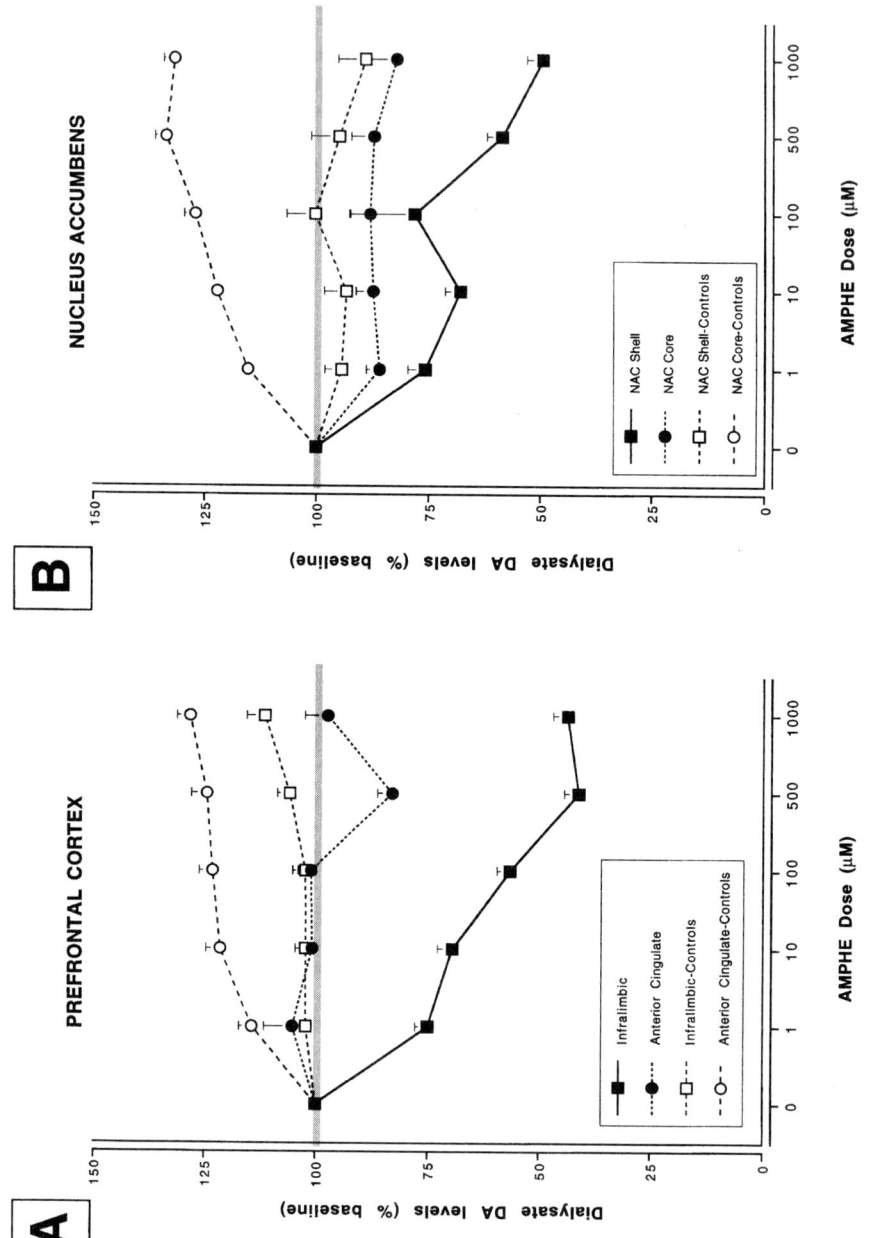

ACKNOWLEDGMENTS

This work was supported by the Swiss Federal Institute of Technology Zürich and the Swiss National Science Foundation (Grant No. 3100-051657).

REFERENCES

1. BERENDSE, H.W., Y. GALIS-DE GRAAF & H.J. GROENEWEGEN. 1992. Topographic organization and the relationship with ventral striatal compartments of prefrontal corticostriatal projections in the rat. J. Comp. Neurol. **316:** 314–347.
2. HEIMER, L., D.S. ZAHM, L. CHURCHILL, P.W. KALIVAS & C. WOHLTMANN. 1991. Specificity in the projection patterns of accumbal core and shell in the rat. Neuroscience **41:** 89–125.
3. GORELOVA, N. & C.R. YANG. 1997. The course of neural projection from the prefrontal cortex to the nucleus accumbens in the rat. Neuroscience **76:** 689–706.
4. ZAHM, D.S. & J.S. BROG. 1992. On the significance of subterritories in the "accumbens" part of the rat ventral striatum. Neuroscience **50:** 751–767.
5. HEIDBREDER, C. & J. FELDON. 1998. Amphetamine-induced neurochemical and locomotor responses are expressed differentially across the anteroposterior axis of the core and shell subterritories of the nucleus accumbens. Synapse **29:** 310–322.
6. GERFEN, C.R. 1989. The neostriatal mosaic: striatal patch-matrix organization is related to cortical lamination. Science **246:** 385–388.
7. SESACK, S.R., V.A. HAWRYLACK, C. MATUS, M.A. GUIDO & A.I. LEVEY. 1998. Dopamine axon varicosities in the prelimbic division of the rat prefrontal cortex exhibit sparse immunoreactivity for the DA transporter. J. Neurosci. **18:** 2697–2708.

FIGURE 2. Relationship between the dose of amphetamine (AMPHE) and the relative dopamine (DA) response in subregions of both the prefrontal cortex (**A**) and nucleus accumbens (**B**) following AMPHE microinfusion into either the infralimbic or anterior cingulate cortices. Control animals were perfused continuously with artificial cerebrospinal fluid. The data were analyzed by $2 \times 5 \times 6$ analyses of variance (ANOVAs) with main factors of subregion (infralimbic vs anterior cingulate, NAC shell vs NAC Core) and AMPHE dose (1, 10, 100, 500, 1000 µM) with a repeated measurements factor of 6 blocks of 10 min. In the prefrontal cortex, the ANOVA revealed significant main effects of subregion ($F(1,28) = 14.9$, $p < 0.0006$) and AMPHE dose ($F(4,112) = 9.5, p < 0.0001$) as well as significant time × subregion and time × AMPHE dose interactions ($F(5,140) = 5.9, p < 0.0001$ and $F(20,560) = 1.7, p < 0.02$, respectively). Direct comparisons with control animals showed a significant dose-dependent effect of AMPHE on dialysate DA levels in the infralimbic cortex but not the anterior cingulate cortex. In the NAC, no significant main effects or interactions were revealed by the ANOVA. However, direct comparison with control animals showed a significant main effect of AMPHE on dialysate DA levels both in the shell and core subterritories of the NAC.

Amphetamine Injections into the Nucleus Accumbens Enhance the Reward of Stimulation of the Subiculum

K. L. SWEET AND D. B. NEILL[a]

Department of Psychology and Graduate Program in Neuroscience, Emory University, Atlanta, Georgia 30322, USA

The mesolimbic dopamine (DA) pathway, originating from the ventral tegmental area (VTA) and projecting to the nucleus accumbens septi (NAS), has been the major focus of research on the neural basis of reward for the past 15 years. However, relatively little is known of what happens in rewarding circumstances beyond the dopamine synapse. Because most, if not all, DA terminal areas are abundantly supplied by glutamatergic afferents, it is probable that some sort of dopamine-glutamate interaction occurs. Mogenson and colleagues, in a landmark theoretical paper in 1980,[1] described the NAS as a "limbic-motor-interface." They presented anatomical, neurophysiological, and behavioral data suggesting that DA interacts in the NAS with glutamatergic inputs originating from forebrain cortical regions including the hippocampus.

Since the groundbreaking work of Mogenson and colleagues, much evidence has added to our knowledge of dopamine-glutamate interaction in NAS. For instance, Kalivas and Duffy[2] found intraaccumbens infusion of the dopamine agonist amphetamine decreased extracellular levels of glutamate. Kiyatkin and Rebec[3] presented electrophysiological data indicating that, while elevated DA transmission in NAS may suppress spontaneous activity of NAS neurons, it increases the neuronal response to glutamate relative to the baseline, i.e., enhances the signal-to-noise ratio. Robbins and Everitt[4] have argued that this dopamine-glutamate interaction is at the heart of the accumbal involvement in reward and motivation.

We have been developing a model system, using behavior as the dependent variable, to examine dopamine-glutamate interaction in the NAS. This model is based on the knowledge that the hippocampal complex, specifically the subiculum, sends a glutamatergic projection to the NAS[5] where it terminates on neurons which also receive a dopaminergic input.[6]

Our experiment was designed to determine if the subiculum supports ICSS and if so, whether a DA agonist injected into the NAS would affect the reward. Our experimental preparation is shown in FIG. 1. Sprague-Dawley rats were implanted with bipolar electrodes in the ventral subiculum of the hippocampus (AP 2.7, L 5.0, H 3.0) and bilateral cannulae in the medial core of the NAS (AP 10.2, L 1.5, H 3.5; atlas of Paxinos and Watson[7]). These rats were trained to self-stimulate in a test chamber where each depression of the lever elicited a stimulation (150 msec train; 0.5 msec

---

[a]Corresponding author: Dr. Darryl Neill, Dept. of Psychology, Emory University, Atlanta, GA 30322. Voice: 404-727-7445; fax: 404-727-0372; dneill@emory.edu

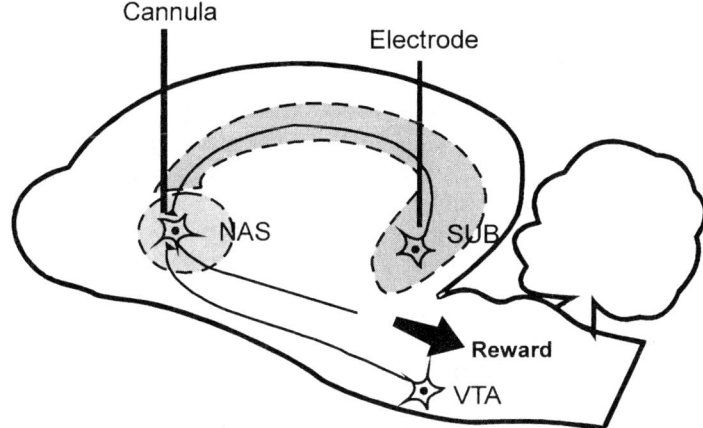

FIGURE 1. Proposed subicular stimulation reward circuit. Side view of a rat brain, showing the electrode and cannula placements used in the experiment described in this report. It is proposed that the reward signal, originating via self-stimulation of the subiculum, travels to the nucleus accumbens, where it is modulated by dopamine released from the terminals of ventral tegmental area neurons. NAS, nucleus accumbens septi; SUB, subiculum; VTA, ventral tegmental area.

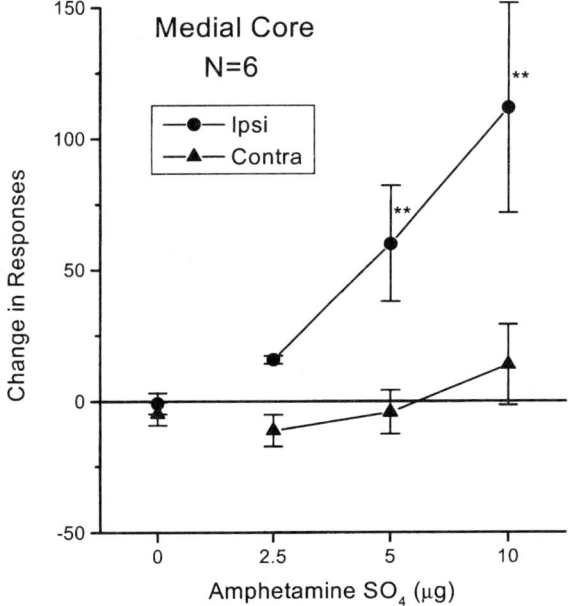

FIGURE 2. Injections of amphetamine sulfate into the nucleus accumbens ipsilateral to a subicular self-stimulation electrode increase responding in a 20-min test. Similar injections contralateral to the electrode are ineffective. **$p < 0.01$, compared to saline.

biphasic square waves; 100 pps). Approximately 3 weeks of daily 20-min sessions were required for maximal responding to develop (100–400 responses/session). Once responding was stable, unilateral injections of d-amphetamine sulfate (2.5, 5.0, 10.0 μg in 1 μl saline) were performed immediately before test sessions.

As shown in FIGURE 2, injections of amphetamine into the ipsilateral, but not the contralateral, medial core (L 1.5 mm) increased subicular ICSS in a dose-related fashion. We interpret this result as signifying enhancement of the subicular ICSS reward signal and not a generalized behavioral excitation, since the effect was only seen with the ipsilateral injection site. Ipsilateral injections of amphetamine into the shell subregion of NAS (L 0.8 mm) or lateral core (L 2.5 mm) were ineffective.

We believe that the results of this study show that the ventral subiculum of the hippocampus will support ICSS and that the reward of this ICSS can be enhanced by a dopamine agonist in a specific region of the NAS. Although these results agree with Mogenson's idea of the NAS as a region where dopamine modulates limbic inputs, it is also possible that the glutamate affects dopamine release.[8] We propose that the subicular ICSS preparation can be used as a neurobehavioral model system to gain insight into this glutamate-dopamine interaction, which occurs widely throughout the subcortical forebrain.

REFERENCES

1. MOGENSON, G.J., D.L. JONES & C.Y. YIM. 1980. From motivation to action: functional interface between the limbic system and the motor system. Prog. Neurobiol. **14:** 69–97.
2. KALIVAS, P.W. & P. DUFFY. 1997. Dopamine regulation of extracellular glutamate in the nucleus accumbens. Brain Res. **761:** 173–177.
3. KIYATKIN, E.A. & G.V. REBEC. 1996. Dopaminergic modulation of glutamate-induced excitations of neurons in the neostriatum and nucleus accumbens of awake, unrestrained rats. J. Neurophysiol. **75:** 142–153.
4. ROBBINS, T.W. & B.J. EVERITT. 1996. Neurobehavioural mechanisms of reward and motivation. Curr. Opin. Neurobiol. **6:** 228–236.
5. GROENEWEGEN, H.J., E. VERMEULEN-VAN DER ZEE, A. TE KORTSCHOT & M.P. WITTER. 1987. Organization of the projections from the subiculum to the ventral striatum in the rat. A study using anterograde transport of phaseolus vulgaris leucoagglutinin. Neuroscience **23:** 103–120.
6. SESACK, S.R. & V.M. PICKEL. 1990. In the rat medial nucleus accumbens, hippocampal and catecholaminergic terminals converge on spiny neurons and are in apposition to each other. Brain Res. **527:** 266–279.
7. PAXINOS, G. & C. WATSON. 1998. The Rat Brain in Stereotaxic Coordinates. Academic Press. San Diego.
8. BLAHA, C.D., C.R. YANG, S.B. FLORESCO, A.M. BARR & A.G. PHILLIPS. 1997. Stimulation of the ventral subiculum of the hippocampus evokes glutamate receptor-mediated changes in dopamine efflux in the rat nucleus accumbens. Eur. J. Neurosci. **9:** 902–911.

Asymmetrical Effects of Ethanol in Basal Ganglia Aldehyde Dehydrogenase Activity

V.I. SATANOVSKAYA[a] AND L.R. BARDINA

Institute of Biochemistry, National Academy of Sciences of Belarus, BLK 50, Grodno, 230017, Belarus

A factor governing the sensitivity of the CNS to the hypnotic effects of alcohol is the activity of the aldehyde-metabolizing systems—aldehyde dehydrogenase and reductase.[1] Earlier we showed a nonuniform distribution of these enzymes in brain regions.[2] Moreover, alcohol intoxication changed, to a variable extent, the activities of these enzymes in animals, initially differing in preference to ethanol or resistance to its hypnotic effects.[2,3] Little has been known about the asymmetry of aldehyde metabolism in paired structures of the brain, basal ganglia, and the response of aldehyde dehydrogenase to alcohol.

Male albino rats (the Rappolovo breeding colony, St. Petersburg, Russia) initially weighing 160–200 g received a morning intraperitoneal injection of ethanol (3.5 g/kg body weight, as a 20% w/v solution). According to the duration of ethanol-induced sleep, the animals were divided into a long sleep group (LS, sleep time > 66 min) and a short sleep group (sleep time < 10 min), and then four groups were formed: LS control and LS experimental, SS control and SS experimental. The experimental rats received ethanol singly at the above-mentioned dose and in the above way during a week. The control rats received equal volumes of an isotonic saline solution. The rats were decapitated following 30 min, 24 h, and 48 h after the last ethanol injection.

The brains were dried from the blood, and basal ganglia (right and left) were isolated at 0°C. The samples were stored in liquid nitrogen until required. Aldehyde dehydrogenase (ALDH) activity was measured in the supernatant (20,000 g × h) with 5 mM acetaldehyde as substrate.[4] The statistical analysis of the data was performed using Student's *t*-test. The results are expressed as mean ±SD.

By the end of the week, as a result of chronic ethanol administration, most of the animals from the SS and LS groups reduced their initial sleep time or did not fall asleep at all. This is indicative of the development of tolerance to the hypnotic effect of ethanol.

LS rats were found to have more left basal ganglia ALDH than SS (TABLE 1). This difference was retained in experimental rats 30 min after ethanol. Control LS rats had no difference between ALDH activities in right and left basal ganglia. However, at 30 min the experimental group of animals showed activated left basal ganglia ALDH, in comparison to right basal ganglia ALDH. SS rats had lower left basal ganglia ALDH activity in comparison to right basal ganglia ALDH as late as after 24 h following the ethanol injection. No such asymmetry in ethanol effects was found within the other periods studied.

[a]Fax: 0152-33-41-21; mag@biochem.belpak.grodno.by

TABLE 1. Aldehyde dehydrodenase activity (μmol NADH $\times$ h^{-1} $\times$ g^{-1} of protein) in basal ganglia (bg) of rats with long (LS) and short (SS) sleep time after chronic ethanol administration (3.5 g/kg BW, ip)

	SS		LS	
	left bg	right bg	left bg	right bg
Saline				
$n = 7$	84.8 ± 4.4	111.6 ± 12.3	117.0 ± 5.4^a	116.8 ± 13.5
Ethanol				
30 min, $n = 6$	78.3 ± 0.7	79.0 ± 17.6	171.6 ± 7.9^a	149.1 ± 7.6^a
24 h, $n = 6$	87.1 ± 4.4	116.5 ± 9.6^b	89.3 ± 6.5	107.2 ± 11.1
48 h, $n = 6$	68.0 ± 11.3	60.7 ± 16.4	118.3 ± 16.7^a	108.8 ± 21.0

^{a} $p < 0.001$, between the same brain regions of SS and LS rats.
^{b} $p < 0.001$, between left and right bg within each group.

Brain ALDH participates not only in the processes of acetaldehyde (exogeneous and endogeneous) detoxication but is also a neuronal component of the metabolism of neurotransmitters and fatty acid aldehydes. Therefore the results obtained allow us to suggest that brain adaptation to alcohol may be based on the asymmetrical functioning of the basal ganglia.

ACKNOWLEDGMENT

The authors would like to thank Mrs. L.G. Kiryukhina for help in preparing the English version of this manuscript.

REFERENCES

1. ERIKSSON, C.J.P. & R.A. DEITRICH. 1983. Metabolic mechanisms in tolerance and physical dependence on alcohol. *In* The Biology of Alcoholism, Vol.7. B. Kissin & H. Begleiter, Eds.: 253–283. Plenum Press. New York.
2. SATANOVSKAYA, V.I. 1992. System of aldehyde metabolism in brain of rats during development of tolerance to the hypnotic effect of ethanol. *In* The Neurobiology of Drug and Alcohol Addiction. P.W. Kalivas & H.H. Samson, Eds.: **654:** 517–518. Annals of the New York Academy of Sciences. New York.
3. SATANOVSKAYA, V.I., YU. M. OSTROVSKY & M.N. SADOVNIK. 1984. Brain aldehyde dehydrogenase and aldehyde reductase in rats with preference to water or ethanol after injection of calcium cyanamide. Alcoholism **8:** 330.
4. ERWIN, V. & R.A. DEITRICH. 1966. Brain aldehyde dehydrogenase. Localization, purification and properties. J. Biol. Chem. **241** (15): 3533–3539.

Index of Contributors

Acquas, E., 461–485
Adinoff, B., 807–810
Ahlenius, S., 292–308
Alexander, D., 807–810
Alheid, G.F., 645–654
Andersen, S.L., 756–759
Anstrom, K., 91–112
Arnold, G.M., 820–822
Arroyo, M., 412–438
Aston-Jones, G., 486–498
Augustinack, J.C., 575–594
Aurentz, C., 742–746
Azarov, A., 91–112

Baker, D.A., 796–799
Bardina, L.R., 831–832
Bassareo, V., 461–485
Beijer, A.V.J., 49–63
Beltramino, C.A., 645–654
Bengtson, C.P., 691–694
Benuck, M., 800–802
Best, S., 807–810
Braaksma, D.N., 711–716
Braff, D.L., 202–216
Breiter, H.C., 523–547
Bruno, J.P., 368–382

Cadoni, C., 461–485
Canbeyli, R., 728–731
Carboni, E., 461–485, 707–710
Carr, D.B., 676–678
Cassell, M.D., 217–241
Chang, J.-Y., 91–112
Chau, D., 769–774
Chefer, V., 803–806
Chiba, T., 667–670
Churchill, L., 64–70

Dagon, C.T., 788–791

Daunais, J.B., 700–702
Davis, M., 281–291, 309–338
de Olmos, J.S., 1–32, 258–280
Delfs, J.M., 486–498
Devous, M.D., 807–810
Di Chiara, G., 461–485, 707–710
Drevets, W.C., 614–637
Druhan, J., 486–498
Dumont, N.L., 756–759

Epstein, J., 562–574
Everitt, B.J., 412–438

Fabbricatore, A.T., 781–787
Feldon, J., 723–727, 823–827
Fenu, S., 461–485
Floresco, S.B., 711–716
Freedman, L.J., 217–241
Frohardt, R.J., 732–736
Fuchs, R.A., 796–799
Funes, A., 717–722

Gal, G., 723–727
Gallagher, M., 397–411
Gargiulo, P.A., 717–722
Gee, F., 781–787
George, M.S., 807–810
Geyer, M.A., 202–216
Gifford, G.W., 760–763
Grace, A.A., 157–175, 688–690
Gray, T.S., 439–444
Greene, J., 157–175
Groenewegen, H.J., 49–63
Grubb, M.C., 792–795
Guarraci, F.A., 732–736
Gurevich, E.V., 595–613

Haber, S.N., 33–48
Haracz, J.L., 811–819

Hashim, A., 800–802
Healy, D.J., 684–687
Hedou, G., 823–827
Heidbreder, C.A., 823–827
Heimer, L., 1–32
Hoebel, B.G., 769–774
Homberg, J., 823–827
Hurd, Y.L., 499–506

Janak, P., 91–112
Johnson, A.K., 258–280
Johnson, L.R., 661–666
Jonker, A.J., 671–675
Joyce, J.N., 595–613

Kalivas, P.W., 64–70
Kallo, I., 339–367
Kalynchuk, L.E., 737–741
Kang, W., 751–755
Kapp, B.S., 732–736
Kayahara, T., 667–670
Keim, S.R., 747–750
Kelley, A.E., 71–90
Keys, A.S., 792–795
Kinney, A.E., 792–795
Kinsley, C.H., 742–746, 760–763
Koob, G.F., 445–460
Kosloff, R.A., 769–774

Lajtha, A., 800–802
Lambert, K.G., 742–746
Landa, A.I., 717–722
Larsson, K., 292–308
Lewis, B.L., 157–175
Lorrain, D.S., 820–822
Lowry, C., 742–746
Lyss, P.J., 756–759

Mark, G.P., 792–795
Marshall, J.F., 796–799
Martínez, G., 717–722
Mash, D.C., 507–522, 811–819
McBride, W.J., 788–791
McDonald, A.J., 309–338
McFarland, N.R., 33–48

McGinty, J.F., xiii–xv, 129–139
McKinzie, D.L., 788–791
McPherson, R.J., 796–799
Meador-Woodruff, J.H., 684–687
Meaney, M.J., 737–741
Meredith, G.E., 140–156
Miller, S.D., 760–763
Mitrovic, I., 176–201
Mohta, B.D, 781–787
Morelli, M., 703–706
Muccino, K.J., 781–787
Mueller, E., 760–763
Murphy, J.M., 788–791

Nadasdy, Z., 339–367
Nader, M.A., 700–702
Nakano, K., 667–670
Napier, T.C., 176–201
Neill, D.B., 828–830
Neisewander, J.L., 796–799
Newman, S.W., 242–257

O'Donnell, P., 157–175
Olmstead, M.C., 412–438
Osborne, P.B., 691–694

Pabello, N., 157–175
Palmer, A.J., 796–799
Pang, K., 339–367
Parkinson, J.A., 412–438
Pastuskovas, C.V., 258–280
Payne, K., 807–810
Pearson, D.M., 737–741
Peoples, L.L., 781–787
Periasamy, S., 679–683
Phillips, A.G., 711–716
Pickel, V.M., 679–683
Pinel, J.P.J., 737–741
Pinna, A., 703–706
Pontén, M., 499–506
Pontieri, F., 461–485
Porrino, L.J., 700–702
Price, J.L., 383–396

Quadros, P., 742–746

INDEX OF CONTRIBUTORS

Rada, P.V., 769–774
Rainnie, D.G., 695–699
Redman, S.J., 575–594
Reischies, F.M., 775–780
Richardson, J.S., 764–768
Robbins, T.W., 412–438
Robledo, P., 412–438
Rodd-Henricks, Z.A., 788–791
Rolando, M.T.P., 707–710
Romanides, A., 64–70
Ropero, C., 717–722
Rosen, B.R., 523–547

Sajdyk, T.S., 747–750
Sanders, S.K., 747–750
Santiago, A.C., 655–660
Sarter, M., 368–382
Satanovskaya, V.I., 831–832
Schoenbaum, G., 397–411
Schulz, D., 728–731
Sershen, H., 800–802
Sesack, S.R., 676–678
Shammah-Lagnado, S.J., 309–338, 645–654, 655–660
Shekhar, A., 747–750
Shi, C., 217–241, 281–291, 309–338
Shippenberg, T.S., 803–806
Silbersweig, D., 562–574
Silvagni, A., 707–710
Sircar, R., 811–819
Smith, H.R., 700–702
Somogyi, J., 339–367
Staley, J.K., 507–522
Stern, E., 562–574
Stevens, J.R., 548–561
Svensson, P., 499–506
Svingos, A.L., 679–683
Sweet, K.L., 828–830
Swerdlow, N.R., 202–216

Sziraki, I., 800–802

Tanda, G., 461–485
Teicher, M.H., 756–759
Thompson, A.C., 803–806
Tiong, A.H.K., 764–768
Tjon, G., 671–675
Todd, C.L., 688–690
Tran-Nguyen, L.T.L., 796–799
Trimble, M.R., 638–644
Turchi, J., 368–382

Uzwiak, A.J., 781–787

Van de Witte, S., 671–675
Van Elst, L.T., 638–644
Van Hoesen, G.W., 575–594
Vezina, P., 820–822
Vivas, L., 258–280
Voorn, P., 49–63, 671–675

Weiner, I., 723–727
West, M.O., 781–787
Wilson, M.A., 751–755
Wilson, S.P., 751–755
Wood, R.I., 661–666
Woodward, D.J., 91–112
Wright, C.I., 49–63

Yoder, K.K., 747–750
Young, S.L., 732–736

Zaborszky, L., 339–367
Zahm, D.S., 113–128
Zardetto-Smith, A.M., 258–280
Zhu, Y., 486–498